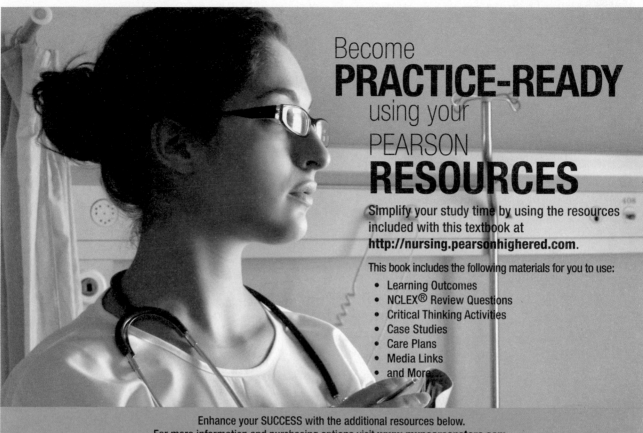

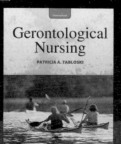
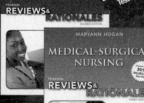

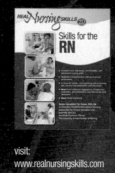

MyNursingLab®

www.mynursinglab.com

Learn more about and purchase
access to MyNursingLab.

MyNursingApp™

www.mynursingapp.com

MyNursingApp puts all the information
you need in the palm of your hand.

myPEARSONstore.com

Find your textbook and everything
that goes with it.

THIRD EDITION

Gerontological Nursing

PATRICIA A. TABLOSKI

PhD, RN-BC, GNP-BC, FGSA, FAAN
William F. Connell
School of Nursing at Boston College

PEARSON

Boston   Columbus   Indianapolis   New York   San Francisco   Upper Saddle River
Amsterdam   Cape Town   Dubai   London   Madrid   Milan   Munich   Paris   Montreal   Toronto
Delhi   Mexico City   São Paulo   Sydney   Hong Kong   Seoul   Singapore   Taipei   Tokyo

Publisher: Julie Levin Alexander
Publisher's Assistant: Regina Bruno
Executive Acquisitions Editor: Pam Fuller
Editorial Assistant: Cynthia Gates
Development Editor: Kim Wyatt
Managing Editor, Production: Patrick Walsh
Production Liaison: Yagnesh Jani
Director of Marketing: David Gesell
Senior Marketing Manager: Phoenix Harvey
Marketing Coordinator: Michael Sirinides
Manufacturing Buyer: Lisa McDowell
Senior Art Director: Christopher Weigand
Cover Designer: Wanda España
Media Project Manager: Leslie Brado/Michael Dobson
Composition and Production: S4Carlisle
Publishing Services
Production Editor: Amy Gehl
Printer/Binder: Courier Kendallville
Cover Printer: Lehigh-Phoenix Color/Hagerstown
Cover Images: © Blend Images/Alamy

Notice: Care has been taken to confirm the accuracy of information presented in this book. The authors, editors, and the publisher, however, cannot accept any responsibility for errors or omissions or for consequences from application of the information in this book and make no warranty, express or implied, with respect to its contents.

The authors and publisher have exerted every effort to ensure that drug selections and dosages set forth in this text are in accord with current recommendations and practice at time of publication. However, in view of ongoing research, changes in government regulations, and the constant flow of information relating to drug therapy and drug reactions, the reader is urged to check the package inserts of all drugs for any change in indications of dosage and for added warnings and precautions. This is particularly important when the recommended agent is a new and/or infrequently employed drug.

A note about Nursing Diagnoses: Nursing Diagnoses in this text are taken from *Nursing Diagnoses – Definitions and Classification 2012-2014.* Copyright © 2012, 1994-2012 by NANDA International. Used by arrangement with John Wiley & Sons Limited. In order to make safe and effective judgments using NANDA-I nursing diagnoses it is essential that nurses refer to the definitions and defining characteristics of the diagnoses listed in this work.

QSEN reprinted with permission. Cronenwett, L., Sherwood, G., Barnsteiner, J., Disch, J., Johnson, J., Mitchell, P., Sullivan, D., & Warren, J. (2007). *Quality and safety education for nurses. Nursing Outlook,* 55(3): 122–131.

Library of Congress Cataloging-in-Publication Data
Tabloski, Patricia A.
 Gerontological nursing / Patricia A. Tabloski. — 3rd ed.
  p.; cm.
 Includes bibliographical references and index.
 ISBN-13: 978-0-13-295631-4
 ISBN-10: 0-13-295631-4
  I. Title.
 [DNLM: 1. Geriatric Nursing. WY 152]
 LC Classification not assigned
 618.97'0231—dc23
                          2012026383

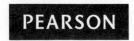

10 9 8 7 6 5 4 3 2 1
ISBN-10:   0-13-295631-4
ISBN-13: 978-0-13-295631-4

PATRICIA A. TABLOSKI, PhD, RN-BC, GNP-BC, FGSA, FAAN

Patricia Tabloski possesses three degrees in nursing. She received her BSN from Purdue University, her MSN from Seton Hall University, and her PhD from the University of Rochester. As a gerontological nurse practitioner, Dr. Tabloski has provided primary care to older patients in a variety of settings, including acute care facilities, geriatric outpatient clinics, long-term care facilities, and hospice programs. She has taught graduate and undergraduate students about gerontology since 1981 and presently is an Associate Professor at the William F. Connell School of Nursing at Boston College. In 2002, Dr. Tabloski was honored as a Fellow in the Gerontological Society of America and in 2010 was honored as a Fellow in the American Academy of Nursing. She has numerous publications and presentations relating to gerontological nursing and has lectured internationally in Hungary, China, Switzerland, and the United Kingdom. Dr. Tabloski has chaired the Test Development Committee for the Gerontological Nurse Practitioner examination by the American Nurses Credentialing Center and is a member of the American Nurses Association, the Gerontological Society of America, the American Geriatrics Society, the National Organization of Nurse Practitioner Faculties, Sigma Theta Tau, and the Eastern Nursing Research Society. Dr. Tabloski is a federally funded researcher and conducts clinically based outcome studies related to nonpharmacological interventions designed to improve sleep and ease agitation in older persons in community and institutional settings. Additionally, Dr. Tabloski has received federal funding to establish an Advanced Practice Nursing Program in Palliative Care.

DEDICATION

To the students with the clarity of vision to see beauty and strength in aging and to my family for their ever-present love and support.

THANK YOU

We extend a heartfelt thanks to the contributors who gave their time, effort, and expertise generously to the development and writing of chapters and resources.

TEXT CONTRIBUTORS

Susan K. Chase, EdD, RN, FNP-BC
Associate Dean for Graduate Affairs
 and Professor, University of Central
 Florida
Chapter 15

Laurel Eisenhauer, RN, EdD, FAAN
Professor Emeritus
William F. Connell School
 of Nursing at Boston College
Chestnut Hill, Massachusetts
Chapter 6

Terry Fulmer, PhD, RN, FAAN
Dean, Bouve College of Health
 Sciences, Northeastern University
Chapter 10

Gail A. Harkness, DrPH-RN, FAAN
Professor Emeritus
University of Connecticut
Storrs, Connecticut
Chapter 23

Rita J. Olivieri, PhD, RN
Associate Professor, Retired
William F. Connell School of Nursing
 at Boston College
Chestnut Hill, Massachusetts
Chapters 12 and 18

Rachel E. Spector, PhD, RN, FAAN
CultureCare Consultant
Needham, Massachusetts
Chapter 4

**Katherine Tardiff, RN, MSN,
 GNP-BC**
Manager of Clinical Operations,
 Senior Care Options
Tufts Health Plan
Chapters 9 and 11

Sheila Tucker, RD
Dietitian and Part-time Faculty Member
Boston College
Chestnut Hill, Massachusetts
Chapter 5

**Tamara Zurakowski, PhD, RN,
 GNP-BC**
Lecturer/Clinical Specialist
School of Nursing
University of Pennsylvania
Philadelphia, Pennsylvania
Chapter 17

REVIEWERS

We extend sincere thanks to our colleagues from schools of nursing across the country who gave their time generously to help create this new edition of *Gerontological Nursing*. These professionals helped us plan and shape our book and resources by reviewing chapters, art, design, and more.

**Melissa J. Benton, PhD, RN,
 GCNS-BC, FACSM**
Associate Professor, Valdosta
 State University
Valdosta, GA

Deborah Brabham, MSN, RN
Program Coordinator, Florida State
 College at Jacksonville
Jacksonville, FL

Patricia J. Bresser, PhD, RN
Associate Professor, St. Cloud
 State University
St. Cloud, MN

Annie Collins
Professor, Washburn University
Topeka, KS

**Charlotte S. Connerton, RN,
 MSN, FCN, CNE**
Lakeview College of Nursing
Charleston, IL

Maria Derylo
Professor, Northern Illinois University
DeKalb, IL

Sarah Doty, MSN, FNP, BC
Full-time Instructor, Southeast
 Missouri Hospital College of
 Nursing & Health Sciences
Cape Girardeau, MO

M. Kathleen Ebener, PhD, RN
Associate Dean of BSN Program,
 Florida State College at Jacksonville
Jacksonville, FL

Mary L. Edwards, RN, MSN
Full-time Instructor, Lakeview
 College of Nursing
Charleston, IL

**Rowena W. Elliott, PhD, RN, CNN,
 BC, CNE, FAAN**
Professor, University of Southern
 Mississippi
Hattiesburg, MS

Kathleen A. Ennen, PhD, RN, CNE
Professor, University of North
 Carolina Wilmington
Wilmington, NC

Amy L. Feaster, RN, MSN
Director of Nursing Programs,
 Johnston Community College
Smithfield, NC

**Sarah Gilbert, MSN, RN, G-CNS,
 BC, FNGNA**
Full-time Instructor, Radford University
Radford, VA

Sister Janet Goetz
Part-time/Adjunct Instructor,
 Gannon University
Erie, PA

**Joni C. Goldwasser, DNP, APRN,
 FNP-BC**
Part-time/Adjunct Instructor,
 Radford University
Radford, VA

Kathryn Harward
Professor, Florida State College
 at Jacksonville
Jacksonville, FL

**Angela Heckman, MSN, RN,
 PHCNS, CNE**
Associate Professor, Indiana
 University Kokomo
Kokomo, IN

**James D. Holland, MSN, PhDc, RN,
 RRT, RCP**
Assistant Professor, Valdosta State
 University
Valdosta, GA

Carolyn Hulsen, MSN, RN
Professor, Black Hawk College
Moline, IL

Brenda P. Johnson, PhD, RN
Professor, Southeast Missouri State
 University
Cape Girardeau, MO

Kelli Kusisto, MSN, RN
Full-time Instructor, Siena Heights
 University
Adrian, MI

**Susan J. Lamanna, RN, MA, MS,
 ANP, CNE**
Professor, Onondaga Community
 College
Syracuse, NY

**Cecilia Langford, EdD, MSN,
 ARNP-BC, PMHNP-BC**
Full-time Instructor, Florida
 State College
Jacksonville, FL

Linda Lott, RN, MSN
Full-time Instructor, Itawamba
 Community College
Fulton, MS

**Lisa Martin, PhD, MS,
 RN, PHN**
University of Minnesota
Minneapolis, MN

Melinda Martinson, RN, MSN
Full-time Instructor, Southeast
 Community College
Lincoln, NE

**Kristen L. Mauk, PhD, DNP, RN,
 CRRN, GCNS-BC, GNP-BC,
 FAAN**
Professor, Valparaiso University
Valparaiso, IN

Janet Minzenberger, MSN, RN
Full-time Instructor, Gannon
 University–Villa Marie School
 of Nursing
Erie, PA

Debra Murphy, RN, MS, WCC
Full-time Instructor, Methodist
 College of Nursing
Peoria, IL

Elizabeth Peterson
Professor, Bethel University
St. Paul, MN

Nancy L. Price, MSN, RN, CNE
Full-time Instructor, Delaware
 Technical and Community College
Newark, DE

**Christine Osborne Reardon,
 RN, MSN**
Assistant Professor, Samuel Merritt
 University
Oakland, CA

**Desma R. Reno, MSN, APRN,
 GCNS-BC**
Assistant Professor, Southeast
 Missouri State University
Cape Girardeau, MO

Tara C. Rich, RN, MSN
Department Chair, James Sprunt
 Community College
Kenansville, NC

**Theresa Schwindenhammer,
 PhD(c), MSN, RN**
Assistant Professor, Methodist
 College of Nursing
Peoria, IL

Sigrid Sexton, RN, MSN, FNP
Professor, Long Beach City College
Long Beach, CA

Joy A. Shepard, PhD(c), MSN, RN, CNE, BC
Professor, East Carolina University
  College of Nursing
Greenville, NC

Paula L. Sullivan, DHSc, MSN, RN, BC
Department Chair, Brunswick
  Community College
Supply, NC

Patricia A. Thielemann, PhD, RN
Professor, St. Petersburg College
St. Petersburg, FL

Rachel Thomas, PhD, MSN, ARNP-BC
Assistant Professor, Florida State
  College at Jacksonville
Jacksonville, FL

Beth Thompson, MSN, RN, CNE
Associate Professor, Sentara College
  of Health Sciences
Chesapeake, VA

Gladdi Tomlinson, RN, MSN
Professor, Harrisburg Area
  Community College
Harrisburg, PA

Brenda K. Trigg, DNP, GNP-BC, APRN, CNE
Professor, Henderson State
  University
Arkadelphia, AR

Paige Whitney
Full-time Instructor, Methodist
  College of Nursing
Peoria, IL

Donna Williams, DNP, RN
Full-time Instructor, Itawamba
  Community College
Fulton, MS

Rita K. Young, MSN, RN, CNS
Full-time Instructor, The University
  of Akron
Akron, OH

FOREWORD

Dramatic changes in American health care will dominate the 21st century. Advances in science, new theories of caring, and the application of knowledge into practice contribute to this changing environment and affect the education and delivery of nursing services. The challenges to nursing education for preparing tomorrow's practitioner are huge. Evidence-based practice generated from real-life situations will enhance patient care. The older patient will dominate nursing care, and stands to gain from this changing environment.

Additions to this edition further elaborate the care described in the original text. The inclusion of QSEN standards and healthy aging tips expands the nurse's repertoire of strategies in caring for the older person.

This text offers the nursing professional a valuable direction in caring for life, care that is research based, logical, and humane. The authors are experts in their fields and offer the reader a virtual tour on caring for the older person. Dr. Tabloski is an eminent researcher and practitioner and has been a lifelong advocate for responsible, considerate, and expert nursing care for the older person. She has been a champion for the aging population. Along with her colleagues, she presents challenges and solutions for caring for our aging population. She and her colleagues make it fun to care for those who are aging, and have influenced many nurses over the years toward this new attitude and vision. The users of this text will discover this vision and will come to know the pleasure of caring for the older person.

Jean E. Steel, PhD, FAAN
Professor Emerita
MGH Institute of Health Professions
Boston, Massachusetts

PREFACE

This book is intended to guide the reader in the care of older people. All patients, regardless of age, deserve expert and dignified nursing care, and the challenge is to encourage our patients to grow and evolve throughout the entire life span. The work of our hands and our hearts contributes much to the dialogue between nurses and patients and softens the sometimes harsh boundaries between humanity and technology.

The older population is the largest consumer of healthcare and nursing services. This population will present societal challenges to nurses and citizens as we plan to meet the healthcare needs of an increasingly diverse group with higher expectations regarding quality of life and health in old age. Nurses and other healthcare workers in a wide range of settings will find themselves caring for larger numbers of older persons with a variety of healthcare needs. Additionally, we are all aging and encountering issues of aging within our own families, so there is a tremendous need for increased knowledge and preparation in gerontological nursing.

The new focus of research and health care for older persons involves "adding life to years" rather than a singular focus on "adding years to life." This new focus acknowledges that merely extending life without attention to the quality of life may lead to a life that is neither active nor fulfilling. This new focus calls for health care delivery within the context of a multidisciplinary team with recognition that nurses play a key and vital role in the function of this team. Highly specialized and expert health care is needed when caring for older adults, including emergency treatment of life-threatening illness; management of chronic health problems; primary healthcare services with emphasis on disease prevention and health promotion; support for professional and family caregivers; provision of culturally appropriate care to an increasingly diverse older population; removal of barriers to emotional, educational, and financial resources; and providing expert palliative and hospice care to frail older adults and those at the end of life. There are expert nursing faculty and graduate and undergraduate curricula available to instruct students, research-based journals and websites with current information to assist clinicians, and a variety of specialized textbooks, such as this, designed to prepare the nurse to meet these crucial challenges.

New To This Edition

- QSEN Feature
- Healthy Aging Tips
- Application of New NANDA-I Diagnoses
- *Healthy People 2020* Goals for Older Adults
- More Evidence-Based Practice
- Current Demographics Using the 2010 Census

The third edition of *Gerontological Nursing* comes at a critical time in the continuing evolution of our healthcare system. Not only are the demographics of aging changing in our country, but also nurse educators have been encouraged to add content to the curriculum that relates to the care of older adults. *Gerontological Nursing* is a comprehensive, research-based text to guide nursing students in their care of older adults. This text presents information related to the normal and pathological changes of aging, healthy aging tips, commonly encountered diseases of aging, and the broad psychosocial, cultural, and public health knowledge required to provide expert nursing care to older persons. The emphasis is on providing the critical information needed to engage in the nursing process of assessment, diagnosis, planning, and evaluating outcomes of care.

The current emphasis on evidence-based practice and the appropriate delivery of scarce healthcare resources are factors that have guided the development of this textbook. Several chapters provide information on "Best Practices" in the nursing care of older adults and cutting-edge information on QSEN standards. The nursing student of today will need to possess as much knowledge as possible regarding the care of the older person. It is no longer sufficient to utilize basic medical-surgical knowledge and modify it for use with the older person. The knowledge needed by the nurse caring for the older patient must be grounded in gerontology with emphasis on holistic assessment, setting realistic goals, use of appropriate pain assessment and pain management, recognition of cognitive impairment and frailty, and provision of end-of-life care. This text provides the comprehensive information that the nurse will use to practice safely, effectively, and appropriately when caring for the older patient in the home, hospital, long-term care, and hospice settings. Whether the goal is to return the older patient to his or her previous levels of health and function, improve overall health status, provide supportive care, or prepare for death by instituting hospice care, the nurse assumes a pivotal role on the interdisciplinary healthcare team and this text will provide crucial information in preparation for that role.

Organization of the Text

The text is organized to facilitate student learning. Unit One is composed of three chapters that form the foundations of gerontological nursing practice. In these chapters the principles of gerontology, identification of key gerontological nursing issues, and the principles of geriatrics are covered. Unit Two describes the challenges of aging and the cornerstones of excellence in nursing care and includes information on cultural diversity, nutrition, pharmacology, psychological and cognitive function, sleep, pain

management, violence and elder mistreatment, and care of the dying. Unit Three describes the physiological basis for nursing practice in gerontology with information on body systems, including the integument, the mouth/oral cavity, sensation, circulatory, respiratory, genitourinary, musculoskeletal, endocrine, gastrointestinal, hematologic, nervous, immune, and multisystem problems relating to care of the frail older adult.

The chapters in Units Two and Three begin with an overview of the content, describing the normal changes of aging, and the common diseases of aging, and move toward the assessment, diagnosis, management, and evaluation of nursing care. This framework allows the student to integrate the basic knowledge presented in Units One and Two with the clinical issues presented in Unit Three.

Throughout the text, issues related to cultural diversity are integrated into the discussions of disease and care. Increasingly large numbers of older adults will be from ethnically diverse cultures, and threats to healthy aging can vary according to cultural heritage.

Key Components of the Text

The following features will help students integrate the theoretical and clinical information essential to the understanding and practice of gerontological nursing.

New to the Third Edition:

- **QSEN Feature**—This four-column table appears in clinical/systems chapters and addresses competencies in phase 1 of the Quality and Safety Education for Nurses (QSEN) project. These competencies included patient-centered care, teamwork and collaboration, evidence-based practice, quality improvement, and informatics as well as safety.

Meeting QSEN Standards: Frailty

	KNOWLEDGE	SKILLS	ATTITUDES
Patient-Centered Care	Involvement of patient and family in plan of care is crucial.	Family assessment and adult learning principles.	Appreciate uniqueness of each patient/family.
	Examine barriers that may keep patients from being active in formulating their plan of care.	Evaluation for depression, vision/hearing, tobacco use, and cognitive and functional status.	Provide patient-centered care to improve successful nursing outcomes.
Teamwork and Collaboration	Recognize scope of practice for interdisciplinary team members.	Use leadership skills to coordinate team and share knowledge.	Value the contribution of each member of the team to improve outcomes.
	Be aware of organizational problems that can inhibit effective team functioning.	System assessment skills. Plan for patient care at the appropriate level to maximize functioning and quality of life.	Be open to input from team members on effective means to improve communication and collaboration.
Evidence-Based Practice	Describe effective interventions to decrease iatrogenic risk factors and improve overall health and functioning.	Access current evidence-based protocols to guide interventions.	Possess confidence in necessary skills to evaluate and incorporate nursing interventions from the literature about caring for frail older adults.

HEALTHY AGING TIPS

Musculoskeletal Improvement

At home: walk on toes around the house, and stand on one foot at a time for as long as possible.

These activities will decrease risk for falling by improving balance.

Exercise routinely: find activities you like and find a partner to do them with.

Having a schedule with a friend improves your chances of keeping fit.

Implement healthy eating habits.

Weight loss decreases risk of osteoarthritis.

- **Healthy Aging Tips**—A new, boxed feature designed for health promotion in older adults.

NORMAL CHANGES OF AGING

Most of the changes of aging in the hematologic system are the result of the bone marrow's reduced capacity to produce RBCs quickly when disease or blood loss has occurred. However, without major blood loss or the diagnosis of a serious illness, the bone marrow changes of aging are not clinically significant. Figure 21-1 ▶▶▶ illustrates the normal changes of aging in the hematologic system.

At about age 70, the amount of bone marrow in the long bones (where most RBCs are formed) begins to decline steadily. Additional changes of aging in the hematologic

- **Common Diseases of Aging**—Each clinical chapter emphasizes the common diseases (acute and chronic) that afflict older people, nursing implications of these diseases, atypical presentation of disease in older persons, functional implications of these diseases, pharmacological treatment, and evaluation of care. Etiology, risk factors, function, and complications are included.

- **Normal Changes of Aging**—Each of the clinically based chapters covers the normal changes of aging as a basis for the nursing assessment and care to follow. Full-color illustrations and photographs complement the text, allowing for a more meaningful synthesis of information.

Common Diseases of Aging Related to the Mouth and Oral Cavity

Oral diseases and conditions are common to those older people who grew up without the benefit of community water fluoridation and other fluoride products. More than 25% of older adults have not seen a dental professional within the past 5 years (Centers for Disease Control and Prevention [CDC], 2011b). About 25% of adults ages 65 and older no longer have any natural teeth and are **edentulous** (without teeth). Rates of edentulism vary, from a high of 37.8% of older Americans in West Virginia, followed by Tennessee and Mississippi, compared to only 13% in Maryland (CDC, 2011b). Having missing teeth can affect nutrition because older adults with no teeth have difficulty chewing and swallowing foods with fiber and texture. Poor oral hygiene and ill-fitting dentures can exacerbate oral problems with an older person's self-esteem and speech, serve as a source of halitosis, increase the risk of aspiration pneumonia, and negatively alter facial appearance (Reuben et al., 2011). Even those with dentures and partial plates may choose softer foods and avoid fresh fruits and vegetables because artificial teeth are not as efficient as natural teeth in the chewing and biting process. **Periodontal disease** (gum disease) or dental **caries** (cavities) most often cause tooth loss. The severity of periodontal disease increases with age. About 20% of people from the ages of 65 to 74 have severe periodontal disease, measured by a 6-mm loss of attachment of the tooth to the adjacent gum (receding gum dis-

poor oral health. About 1/5 of older adults rep had tooth pain at least twice during the past 6 mo adults who belong to racial or ethnic minorities o a low level of education are more likely to re pain than older adults who are Caucasian or bette (CDC, 2011a).

Many Americans lose their dental insurance retire, and hence do not have access to regular c The situation may be even worse for older wo generally have lower incomes and may neve dental insurance. Medicare does not cover rou care or most dental procedures such as cleanin tooth extractions, or dentures. Additionally, Me not pay for dental plates or other dental devic for Medicare and Medicaid Services, 2012). Me jointly funded federal–state health insurance p low-income people, funds dental care in some reimbursement rates are so low that it is often locate a dentist who will accept Medicaid patien

Oral and pharyngeal cancers, diagnosed in 30 icans every year, result in about 8,000 deaths an proximately 3% of all malignancies occur in th neck. These cancers, primarily diagnosed in ol carry a poor prognosis. The 5-year survival rat Americans is 50% and for African Americans is (CDC, 2011b). Early detection is the key for inc survival rate.

Most older Americans take prescription an counter medications that can decrease salivary f sult in xerostomia or dry mouth. It is estimated t

- **Complementary and Alternative Therapies**—Learners are introduced to therapies used by patients to supplement mainstream medicine. Nurses need to understand the therapies themselves and how they interact with more traditional therapies.

- **Drug Alerts and Practice Pearls** supply students with crucial information and call attention to key issues.

COMPLEMENTARY AND ALTERNATIVE THERAPIES

Pain is among the most common reasons that adults use complementary and alternative therapies (National Center for Complementary and Alternative Medicine [NCCAM], 2011). Nontraditional methods to control pain can be effective as stand-alone treatments and adjuncts to traditional pharmacological interventions with the potential to reduce dosages of medications and thus reduce the risk of adverse drug reactions. Nurses can assess older patients' preferences and attitudes toward nontraditional methods of relieving pain and

Drug Alert! ▶▶▶ Instruct older patients to take blood pressure medication at the same time each day and as prescribed and to never abruptly stop taking a prescribed medication without consulting care provider first. It is important to kee drug levels for effective blood pressure c rapid discontinuation of medication can rebound hypertension.

Practice Pearl ▶▶▶ Oral medications should be given with a nutritious liquid (e.g., juice) rather than water if a patient is anorexic or is likely to refuse to take adequate amounts of liquid. This maximizes the nutritional values of liquids ingested. (Do not use liquids that are contraindicated due to drug–food interactions.)

- The **Best Practices** feature presents an assessment instrument, protocol, or nursing intervention that recommends the best practice for an older patient with the particular health problem under discussion.

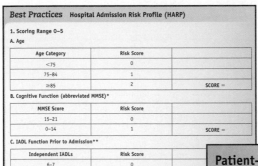

Best Practices   Hospital Admission Risk Profile (HARP)

1. Scoring Range 0–5

A. Age

Age Category	Risk Score	
<75	0	
75–84	1	
≥85	2	SCORE =

B. Cognitive Function (abbreviated MMSE)*

MMSE Score	Risk Score	
15–21	0	
0–14	1	SCORE =

C. IADL Function Prior to Admission**

Independent IADLs	Risk Score
6–7	0
0–5	2

2. Risk Categories

Total Score	Risk of Decline in ADL Function
4 or 5	High risk
2 or 3	Intermediate risk
0 or 1	Low risk

- **Patient–Family Teaching Guidelines** include sample questions and answers an older patient and his or her family may pose when receiving care for a particular problem. A rationale is given for each answer to assist the student in gaining valuable insights into how best to provide succinct, focused answers to patient and family questions within the context of a busy and sometimes hectic clinical setting. When educating patients and families about a life-altering chronic illness such as diabetes, teaching priorities are described.

Patient–Family Teaching Guidelines

The following are guidelines that the nurse may find useful when instructing older persons and their families about mental health.

MENTAL HEALTH AND THE OLDER ADULT

Many older people think it is normal to have a variety of physical and mental problems. However, mental health problems, including depression and anxiety, are not part of the normal aging process. If you, a family member, or friend experience a sudden change in mood, the way you think, or your memory, see your healthcare professional as soon as possible.

1 What causes mental health problems?

Some mild memory or mood problems can occur in healthy older adults, but serious problems can be a sign of underlying mental health disease.

RATIONALE:

Chronic unrelieved pain, some physical illnesses, problems with eyesight and hearing, certain medications, and use of alcohol can cause mental health problems. To further complicate things, serious physical illnesses can cause delirium or acute mental status changes that will usually resolve when the un—

hopeless, loss of interest in sex, or difficulty concentrating and making decisions, you may be depressed. Some older people say that they just do not feel like their old self. Others gain or lose weight because they change the way they eat. Others may avoid going out to social events and prefer to stay home alone. Everyone is different, so it is important to think broadly and look for a variety of symptoms.

RATIONALE:

Recognition of depression in the older person is a key skill for every clinician working with older patients. Depression is a treatable disease and may masquerade as a symptom of illness or be falsely attributed to normal aging.

4 Is suicide a problem with older people?

Yes, some groups of older people (especially older Caucasian men) have high suicide rates. If you have persistent thoughts of death

- **Nursing Care Plans** illustrate the nursing process. A case study is used to tie together content described in the chapter and provide an example of various nursing interventions and the planning and implementation of nursing care. Each case study presents an **ethical dilemma** in anticipation of the kinds of situations the student will encounter when delivering care to older persons. The case studies present the real-world experience of the author and contributors of this book and encourage the student to participate in the assessment and planning process.

CARE PLAN   A Patient With Alterations in Nutrition

Case Study

Mrs. McGillicuddy is a 78-year-old woman admitted 2 weeks ago to a nursing home following a complicated hospital stay for a cerebrovascular accident. While hospitalized, she lost 10 lbs in 1 month and developed a stage II decubitus ulcer. Her prior medical history was significant for hypertension managed with an ACE inhibitor and low-sodium diet.

On admission to the nursing home, she was found to weigh 115 lbs and reported a height of 5'5". Her albumin was 3.0 mg/dL and complete blood cell count was normal. Physical examination revealed residual right-sided weakness. Mrs. McGillicuddy reported that she had been feeding herself in the hospital and felt she could manage. A therapeutic 2-g low-sodium diet was ordered.

Now, 2 weeks later, it is discovered that she has lost another 4 lbs. Her urine is dark in color and a mouth examination reveals dry mucosa and long tongue furrows. Pocketed food was noted along the gum line as well.

Mrs. McGilliuddy's roommate has noticed that she "gravelly." Her decubitus ulcer is reportedly unch

Upon further discussion with Mrs. McGillicu comes apparent that she has been having diff self-feeding and managing the utensils. Freq spills food from the spoon or fork and feels e about this. She is experiencing particular troub liquids. It is difficult to hold the cup handle, seem to be spilling out of her mouth. This e her as well. Lately, she has just been moving around on her plate to make it look like she Her nursing care assistant has been recording cal chart reports that 75% to 90% of food wa most meals.

Mrs. McGillicuddy also reports that the food bland and she often has a bad taste in her reduces her appetite.

- **Critical Thinking Exercises** follow the case studies, encouraging the student to engage in additional learning activities that stimulate and support learning. The exercises may be done individually or within a group setting. The insights gained from the exercises will form the basis of individualized and empathetic nursing practice and widen the student's understanding of the older patient's situation. Answers to these exercises are found in Appendix B ⊂▭ of this book.

Critical Thinking and the Nursing Process

1. Why is cardiac rehabilitation indicated following angioplasty or revascularization with coronary artery bypass grafting?
2. How is knowing and following up with a cardiovascular patient over time important to the caring process?
3. How do you respond when a patient says, "I don't want to run a marathon. Why should I go to rehab?"
4. What supports are necessary to assist older adults who live alone to maintain their independence when they are diagnosed with heart failure?
5. Imagine you are designing an intergenerational program in an inner-city community center. What health issues would benefit both older and younger people?

■ Evaluate your responses in Appendix B. ⊂▭

Physical examination revealed residual right-sided weakness. Mrs. McGillicuddy reported that she had been feeding herself in the hospital and felt she could manage. A therapeutic 2-g low-sodium diet was ordered.

Now, 2 weeks later, it is discovered that she has lost another 4 lbs. Her urine is dark in color and a mouth examination reveals dry mucosa and long tongue furrows. Pocketed food was noted along the gum line as well.

around on her plate to make it look like she has eaten. Her nursing care assistant has been recording her intake due to the report of weight loss on admission. The medical chart reports that 75% to 90% of food was eaten at most meals.

Mrs. McGillicuddy also reports that the food tastes too bland and she often has a bad taste in her mouth that reduces her appetite.

Applying the Nursing Process

Assessment

The nurse should think broadly and assess a variety of factors, including the following:

- **Physical.** Assess for signs or symptoms of dehydration—tongue furrows, dry oral mucosa; dysphagia symptoms—drooling, food pocketing, voice alterations, coughing during swallowing or afterwards. Reassess decubitus ulcer stage.

- **Diet.** Assess appetite; observe self-feeding and dietary intake, especially of calories and protein; note food textures that are difficult to swallow.
- **Laboratory.** Assess plasma levels for blood urea nitrogen, creatine, and sodium, and urine for sedimentation rate.

Diagnosis

Appropriate nursing diagnoses for Mrs. McGillicuddy may include the following:

- *Nutrition, Imbalanced: Less Than Body Requirements* related to increased need for nutrition with hypermetabolic state (decubitus ulcer) and decreased intake

- *Fluid Volume: Deficient*
- *Aspiration, Risk for*
- *Swallowing, Impaired*

NANDA-I © 2012.

- **NANDA-I Nursing Diagnoses** are suggested for many of the common diseases presented to help students categorize the nursing problems that accompany the medical diagnoses.

Acknowledgments

I wish to thank the many older patients and families I have worked with and cared for through the years. They have been wise teachers and provided the impetus for me to pursue my education, undertake my research, and write this text. I also wish to thank my students who have an insatiable desire to provide the highest quality nursing care possible and improve the quality of their patients' lives. The reviewers of this text have provided suggestions that have strengthened and improved the content, and I am most appreciative of their thoughtful suggestions. I also wish to express my appreciation to the expert contributors who generously agreed to share their knowledge and expertise even though they lead busy and overcommitted lives.

Additional thanks go to my family who has provided support, encouragement, and advice when needed. I especially want to thank the editorial and production staff of Pearson Health Science, including Pamela Fuller, Kim Wyatt, Cynthia Gates, Yagnesh Jani, Pat Walsh, and Amy Gehl at S4Carlisle Publishing Services.

CONTENTS

LIST OF SPECIAL FEATURES

MEETING QSEN STANDARDS

Foundations of Nursing Practice

Principles of Gerontology

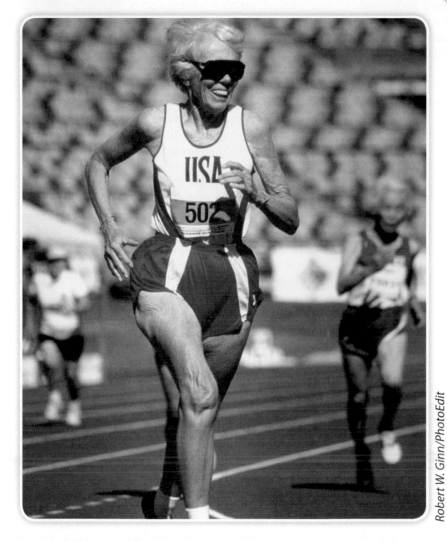

KEY TERMS

epidemiology *9*
geriatrics *4*
gerontologists *4*
gerontology *4*
homeostasis *17*
homeostenosis *17*
life expectancy *4*
life span *11*
risk factors *8*
senescence *16*

LEARNING OUTCOMES

On completion of this chapter, the reader will be able to:

1. Interpret demographic data according to race, gender, and age.
2. Relate leading causes of morbidity and mortality among older adults.
3. Identify common myths of aging and their contribution to ageism.
4. Describe the effects of chronic disease.
5. Contrast several major theories of aging.
6. Evaluate the natural history of disease using principles of epidemiology.

The aging of America will trigger a huge demand for increased healthcare services. Nurses with skills in caring for older people, or gerontological nurses, will be especially in demand because of their understanding of the normal changes of aging and the ways that symptoms of illness and disease present differently in the older adult. Gerontological nurses recognize that the presentation of disease is often more subtle and less typical when compared to the younger adult and response to treatment differs in the older adult when compared to other groups of patients. The care of the frail older person, defined as the older person with multiple chronic conditions or comorbidities, presents a unique challenge. This book addresses the key issues involved in caring for the older person, with an emphasis on health problems encountered by nurses caring for older persons in clinical settings.

The diverse health needs of an older person mandate that care be holistic and delivered by professionals with varying but complementary viewpoints; the study of aging combines or integrates information from several separate areas of study including biology, psychology, and sociology but also considering public policy, economics, and the arts.

Gerontology is the holistic study of the aging processes and individuals as they mature throughout the adult life span and includes the following: *mind, body, spirit*

- Study of the physical, mental, and social changes of aging
- Analysis of the changes in society as a result of an aging population
- Application of this knowledge to policies and program development *PT, OT, dietary*

As a result of the multidisciplinary focus of gerontology, professionals from diverse fields, including nurses, call themselves **gerontologists.**

Geriatrics is the field more closely aligned with medicine and involves:

- Study of health and disease in later life
- Comprehensive health care of older persons and the well-being of their caregivers

The fields of gerontology and geriatrics are of interest to nurses, and some nurses providing care to older people call themselves *geriatric nurses* while others prefer the term *gerontological nurses* (Association for Gerontology in Higher Education, 2012).

Older people receive nursing care in skilled nursing facilities, retirement communities, adult day care, residential care facilities, transitional care units, rehabilitation hospitals, community-based home care, and a variety of other settings. The underlying core values and principles of gerontological nursing include health promotion, health protection, disease prevention, and treatment of disease, with emphasis on evidence-based best practices and current clinical practice guidelines. A well-educated and confident gerontological nurse is a vital member of the healthcare team and brings improved health outcomes to older patients and their families by providing appropriate skilled nursing care, preventing adverse outcomes, and improving quality of life.

Aging is an inevitable and steadily progressive process that begins at the moment of conception and continues throughout the remainder of life. The life or aging process is artificially divided into stages and usually includes antepartum, neonate, toddler, child, adolescent, young adult, middle age, and older adult. The final stage of life, called *old age* (this term usually applies to those over the age of 65), can be the best or worst time of life and requires work and planning throughout all of the previous stages to be a successful and enjoyable period. Old age can be further subdivided to reflect the longer **life expectancy,** defined as number of years from birth that an individual can expect to live, in the United States and other developed countries and includes the young-old (ages 65–74), middle-old (ages 75–84), and old-old (ages 85+). This designation reflects the philosophy that a 65-year-old will be as developmen-[tally] a 20-year-old is dif-fe[rent]

[handwritten note over text:] *old-old is the fastest growing segment of the population*

[handwritten note over text:] *centenary population: growing # of people living beyond 100 years old.*

du[...] ssues related to aging
to[...] ess they have reason
le[...] r instance, some ado-
m[...] age of 16 so that they
tic[...] rhaps others will an-
ev[...] in the military. How-
a[...] in to dread our own
a[...] isease, disability, and
[...] of the aging process.

[...] r people can be con-
s[...] e stereotypes of aging.
[...] e facts that prove them

[...] teach an old dog new
[...] hange negative health
[...] may think that every-
[...] for sex and label older
[...] st in another person a
[...] gh comments such as
[these can be hurtful and reflect] poorly on the speaker, they do further damage by perpetuating stereotypes. Negative stereotypes of aging make it more difficult to recruit the best and the brightest nurses to work with older patients, limit the opportunities for rehabilitation and health promotion services offered to older people, and segregate older

---

BOX 1-1 ▸ Myths of Aging

- Myth: Being old means being sick.
  - Fact: Fewer than 5% of people over the age of 65 are frail enough to require care in a skilled nursing facility.
  - Fact: Many older adults have chronic diseases but still function quite well.
- Myth: Most older people are set in their ways and cannot learn new things or take up new activities.
  - Fact: Older people can learn new things and should be challenged to stay mentally active.
  - Fact: Healthy older adults find hobbies that they can enjoy to give life meaning and pleasure.
- Myth: Health promotion is wasted on older people.
  - Fact: It is never too late to begin good lifestyle habits such as eating a healthy diet and engaging in exercise.
  - Fact: Although it may not be possible to reverse all of the damage caused by bad habits, it is never too late to stop smoking cigarettes or drinking too much alcohol. Even people who quit smoking at older ages enjoy better health outcomes than those who continue to smoke.

- Myth: Older adults do not pull their own weight and are a drain on societal resources.
  - Fact: Older people contribute greatly to society by supporting the arts, doing volunteer work, and helping with grandchildren.
  - Fact: Paid employment is not the only measure of value and productivity and older people continue to make contributions to society into advanced old age and many continue working, volunteering, and mentoring others long after formal retirement.
- Myth: Older people are isolated and lonely.
  - Fact: Many older people join clubs and do volunteer work to stay active and connected.
  - Fact: There are many ways to maintain contact with people and healthy older adults have a variety of great options for staying connected with others.
- Myth: Older people have no interest in sex.
  - Fact: Although sexual activity does decrease in some older people, there are tremendous differences. Most often, the human need for affection and physical contact continues throughout life.

Source: Adapted from Saison, Smith, Segal, & White, 2010.

---

people from mainstream society. Gerontological nurses can help by educating others when they hear these negative attitudes about aging from their colleagues and peers.

The study of gerontology is a relatively new science. Congress created the National Institute on Aging (NIA) in 1974 as part of the National Institutes of Health. In the 1950s and 1960s, little was known about aging. Much of the knowledge resulted from the study of diseases associated with aging. This practice resulted in the widespread idea that decline and illness were inevitable in old age (Hamerman & Butler, 2007). The focus of gerontology and gerontological nursing at this time was to study, diagnose, and treat disease. However, in recent years, the study of gerontology has moved beyond the disease focus to the improvement of health holistically, including physical, mental, emotional, and spiritual well-being. Health promotion and "Tips for Healthy Aging" are a key component of the practice of gerontological nursing and many of the chapters in this book include this feature. The addition of a health promotion focus in the nursing care plan is appropriate for essentially well older persons in order to maintain and improve their state of good health; for those with chronic illness, so they can prevent or delay the progression of their disease; and even for those in hospice, so they can retain function in order to enjoy every minute of their limited life span.

Nurses should test their knowledge about aging to find out if they have the needed knowledge to provide the best gerontological nursing care to their patients. Nurses can take the aging IQ quiz developed by the NIA (2011). The NIA conducts and supports research on aging and educates the public about the findings.

The study of aging and health is imperative for older people to enjoy quality of life in their final years. The new reality of aging reflects our understanding that there has been a dramatic reduction in the prevalence of the precursors to chronic disease including hypertension, high cholesterol, and smoking. The enlightened nurse now knows that having a healthy and productive old age is possible for growing numbers of aging Americans. Those persons who suffer from inherited illnesses such as cancers and blood dyscrasias that present in youth and middle age, weak immune systems, and the inevitable damage from devastating poverty and substance abuse do not usually live to be old. Often, they carry the burden of chronic disease and poor health developed in younger years into old age, resulting in disability at the end of life. For those older persons who are fortunate enough to enter old age in relatively good health, growing older is a reward and a time to be treasured and enjoyed. Some of the benefits of healthy aging are listed in Box 1-2.

> ### BOX 1-2
>
> ### Benefits of Healthy Aging
>
> - Creativity and confidence are enhanced.
> - Coping ability increases.
> - Gratitude and appreciation deepen.
> - Confidence increases with less reliance on the approval of others.
> - Self-understanding and acceptance increase.

The goal for nurses who provide health care to older people is not only to improve the length of life, but also to improve the quality of life. The healthcare needs of older patients are unique because of their stage of life, just as the health needs of children are different from those of adults. Most healthcare professionals do not receive the education and training necessary to respond to the unique and complex health needs of older adults; however, it is now recognized that content and learning opportunities related to the care of older adults should be incorporated throughout the education of all nurses to ensure that the nurse of the future will be able to provide high-quality nursing care to the nation's aging population (Hartford Institute for Geriatric Nursing, 2011). As a result, many older people who in the past received inappropriate health care that was unnecessary, harmful, or even dangerous will now have access to more appropriate health care with the desired outcome of improving their quality of life.

Demographics and Aging

Countries all over the world are facing demographic aging. In the United States, we often speak of "the graying of America," but all nations are—or soon will be—faced with important issues regarding the provision of health care to older persons. As illustrated in Figure 1-1 ▶▶▶, the proportion of persons over the age of 60 is projected to double worldwide during the next 50 years (United Nations, 2012). The greatest increases will be seen in developing countries, many of which do not have healthcare systems geared to the health needs of older people. During the first half of the current century, the global population age 60 or over is projected to expand by more than three times to reach nearly 2 billion in 2050. Declining fertility and improved health care have increased the number of older persons worldwide at a dramatic rate. By 2050, the United Nations estimated that the proportion of the world's population ages 65 and older will more than double from 7.6% today to 16.2%. Countries in the world with the largest numbers of older people today include China (129 million older persons), India (77 million), the United States (40 million), and the Russian Federation (27 million) (United Nations, 2012).

Industrialized countries made great progress in extending life expectancy at birth. Japan has the highest life expectancy of the world's major nations, with the average Japanese born today expecting to live 82.9 years, while the

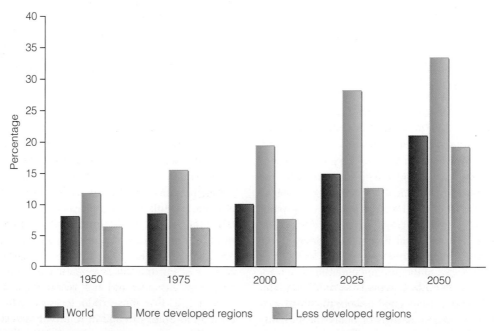

Figure 1-1 ▶▶▶ Population over the age of 60, worldwide and developing regions.

Source: United Nations, Population Division. (2012). *World population aging 1950–2050.* Retrieved from http://www.un.org/esa/population/publications/worldageing19502050/pdf/80chapterii.pdf.

Central African Republic has the lowest average life expectancy at 47 years (World Bank, 2011).

The United States is projected to experience rapid growth in its older population as well. In 1930, America's older population numbered less than 7 million—about 5.4% of the population. According to the 2010 census, the population of the United States was 308.7 million. Those age 65 and over numbered 40.3 million persons, about 13% of the population (U.S. Census Bureau, 2010). By 2050, the number of Americans ages 65 and older is projected to be 88.5 million—more than twice today's population of older adults. The "baby boomers" (those born between 1946 and 1964) are mostly responsible for the growth of older persons because they began crossing into the age 65+ category on January 1, 2011. By 2030, about one in five U.S. residents will be age 65 or older. The United States will also become more racially and ethnically diverse and in 2042, the aggregate minority population is projected to become the majority (Vincent & Velkoff, 2010).

Aging trends occurring now and into the future will affect each of the three subgroups of older people in different ways:

- **The young-old (ages 65–74):** During the next 20 years, 74 million baby boomers will retire. Medicare and Social Security will add 10,000 new retirees *per day*.
- **The middle-old (ages 75–84):** During the next decade, increased life expectancy will add to the numbers of aging baby boomers and increase the total numbers in this category.
- **The old-old (ages 85+):** The old-old are the fastest growing segment of the population, growing at twice the rate of those ages 65 and over and four times faster than the total U.S. population. This group will triple from the current 5.7 million to over 19 million by 2050 (U.S. Census Bureau, 2010).

Past fertility trends exerted the strongest influence on the U.S. age structure in the 20th century. Relatively high fertility at the start of the century, lower fertility in the late 1920s and 1930s, and higher fertility after World War II during the baby boom all affected the U.S. age composition. In 1950 there were 3.01 children born to each woman in the United States; in 2000 the average was one child lower at 2.01 (U.S. Census Bureau, 2010). At the beginning of the 20th century, half of the U.S. population was younger than 22.9 years. At the century's end, half of the population was younger than 35.3 years, the country's highest median age ever (U.S. Census Bureau, 2010). The baby boomers ("boomers") have had—and will continue to have—a profound impact on American culture and demographics. Figure 1-2 ▶▶▶ illustrates the "bulge" in the U.S. population pyramid and the changes by age and sex as the baby boomers have aged between 2000 and 2010.

Longevity and the Gender Differential

Prior to 1950, the male population outnumbered the female population. In 1950, this trend reversed. Women now comprise the majority of the older population (55%) in all nations, and the majority of these women (58%) live in developing countries. In the United States, women outnumber men and the ratio of men to women over the age of 65 is 49 men to every 100 women (U.S. Census Bureau, 2010). In the United States in 2010, the average life expectancy was 78.3 years, with the life expectancy of men at 75.7 years and of women at 80.8 years (U.S. Census Bureau, 2010). Disparities in life expectancy remain according to the race/gender of the population, although all populations have enjoyed increases in life expectancy during the past decade. For instance, at the age of 65 a Caucasian male has a life expectancy of 17.3 remaining years, whereas an African American male is projected to have 15.5 remaining years. A Caucasian female has 19.9 remaining years, whereas an African American female has 18.9 projected years (U.S. Census Bureau, 2010). In recognition of this fact, *Healthy People 2020* was recently released with one of its four major goals being to "achieve health equity, eliminate disparities, and improve the health of all groups" including the growing number of racially and ethnically diverse older persons (U.S. Department of Health and Human Services [USDHHS], 2010).

> **Practice Pearl ▶▶▶** Older women greatly outnumber older men in most nations. Therefore, the study of gerontology is closely linked to the study of women's health.

Older women face different socioeconomic circumstances than men as they age. They are more likely to be widowed, to live alone, to be less educated, and to have fewer years of labor experience, making older women (especially those over the age of 75) more likely to live in poverty (Health Resources and Services Administration, 2010). By 2025, nearly three quarters of the world's older women are expected to reside in what is known today as the developing world. The term *feminization of later life* describes how women predominate at older ages and how the proportions increase with advancing age (Transgenerational Design Matters, 2011). In most countries, including the United States, the relative female advantage due to increased life expectancy increases with advancing age and the number of males relative to females decreases as age increases (U.S. Census Bureau, 2010) (Figure 1-3 ▶▶▶).

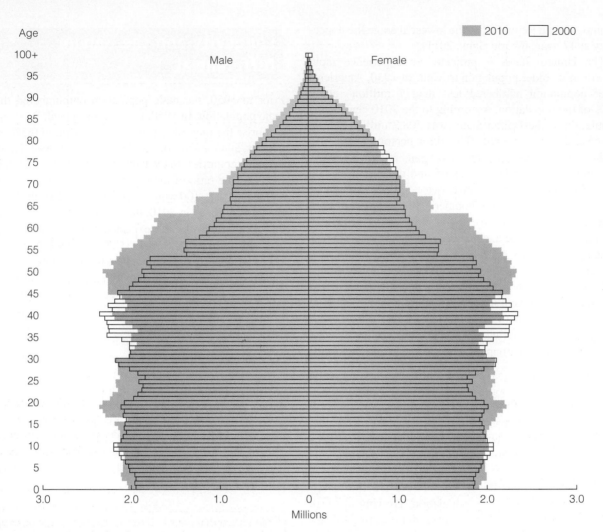

Figure 1-2 ▶▶▶ Population by age and sex: 2000 and 2010.
Source: U.S. Census Bureau, 2010.

The gender differences in life expectancy may be explained by the complex interaction among biological, social, and behavioral factors. Greater male exposure to **risk factors** (factors whose presence are associated with an increased probability that disease will develop at a later time) such as tobacco, alcohol, and occupational hazards might negatively affect male life expectancy. If women begin to approach the rates of tobacco and alcohol use and face the same environmental hazards as men, the gender gap may narrow (U.S. Census Bureau, 2010).

In the 2010 U.S. census, more than 40 million people were over the age of 65. The most rapid growth of the older population occurred in the oldest age groups. People ages 65+ represented 13.1% of the population in the year 2010, but are expected to grow to be 19.3% of the population by 2030. The 85+ population is projected to increase from 5.5 million in 2010 to 6.6 million in 2020 (19%) (U.S.

Census Bureau, 2010). The implication of the rapid growth of the population over age 85 (old-old) is that there will be larger numbers of older people with normal changes of aging, diagnosed chronic illness, and a greater demand for preventive health services. Gerontological nurses will find greater demand for their services in home, community-based, and institutional settings.

Life After Age 65

This increase in life expectancy has been attributed to improved health care, increased use of preventive services, and healthier lifestyles. Experts disagree as to whether this trend in life expectancy can continue without major treatment advances or even cures in heart disease and cancer, which account for nearly half (48.5%) of all deaths in older persons (Centers for Disease Control and Prevention [CDC], 2009).

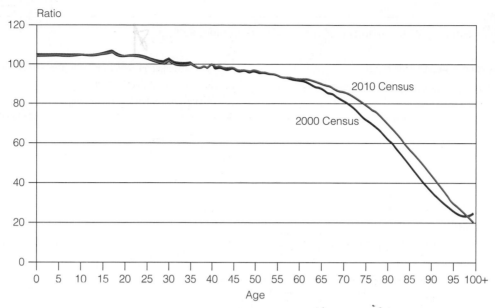

Figure 1-3 ▶▶▶ Number of males per 100 females by age, 2010. *healthy aging*
Source: U.S. Census Bureau, 2010.

However, nurses should be aggressive in health promotion efforts and rehabilitation after surgery or illness, because the 65-year-old man or woman has the potential for many additional years of life. Health promotion efforts can assist the older person to enjoy these years and enhance quality of life and functional ability rather than living out their final years with significant disability. Most older people would prefer to live out their final years independently and reside in their own homes, rather than living in extended care facilities and relying on others for care, making health promotion and rehabilitation efforts essential.

Chronic conditions usually develop over long periods and thus offer ample opportunity for nurses and other healthcare professionals to screen, detect, educate, and intervene. Using the principles of **epidemiology,** which is the study of health and disease determinants and patterns among populations, the stages of chronic disease have been documented to start at about age 20. The disease process may be altered or change course with a resultant increase or decrease in symptoms. The actions that older persons, families, and healthcare professionals take can alter and change the course of a chronic illness.

The aging of America is triggering a higher demand for healthcare and social services. Chronic conditions can cause years of disability, pain, and loss of function. Three million older adults indicate that they cannot perform basic activities of daily living such as bathing, shopping, dressing, and eating. Their quality of life suffers as a result, and demands on family and caregivers can be challenging.

In general, older people in the United States are healthier than in the past, with lower rates of disability. Still, a significant proportion of the older population suffers from health problems and chronic disease, and causes of death have not changed dramatically:

■ About 80% of seniors have at least one chronic health condition, which often leads to disability. Arthritis, hypertension, heart disease, diabetes, and respiratory disorders are some of the leading causes of activity limitations among older people.
■ The rates of disability and functional limitation among the older population have declined substantially since the 1980s; about one in five older Americans reports having a chronic disability.
■ Data comparing people from the ages of 65 to 74 in 1988–1994 and 1999–2000 show a startling rise in the percentage of people considered obese—in men, the proportion grew from about 24% to 33% and in women from about 27% to 39% (CDC, 2010b).

During the many years it takes most chronic diseases to develop, nurses have the opportunity to intervene using the three levels of prevention designated as primary, secondary, and tertiary. Box 1-3 illustrates nursing interventions to promote health in older people.

The best strategy for the control of diagnosed chronic disease in the older adult is to employ tertiary prevention and attempt to slow the progression of the illness and prevent or reverse disabling loss of function. However, the nurse will

---

BOX 1-3   ## Nursing Interventions to Promote Health in Older People

Primary Prevention—Health Promotion

- Education about a healthy lifestyle
- Injury prevention
- Nutritional assessment and guidance
- Exercise prescriptions as appropriate
- Avoidance of tobacco
- Moderation of alcohol
- Limiting exposure or avoiding known carcinogens

Secondary Prevention—Early Diagnosis and Prompt Treatment

- Screening questions and health assessment (use of standardized assessment instruments appropriate for older adults, including

function, cognition, mood, mobility, pain, skin integrity, quality of life, nutrition, neglect, and abuse)
- Referral for examination and testing
- Disease cure and aggressive treatment to limit disability and stop disease progression

Tertiary Prevention—Restoration and Rehabilitation

- Multidisciplinary rehabilitation (physical, occupational, speech, and recreational therapy)
- Short-term placement in rehabilitation facilities or aggressive in-home rehabilitation
- Appropriate services and aids to increase independence (walkers, canes, homemaker/home health aid, visiting nurse)

Source: U. S. Department of Health and Human Services. (2010). *Healthy people, 2020. What are its goals?* Rockville, MD: Author.

---

have the opportunity to use primary and secondary prevention techniques in other areas of the older person's risk profile. For instance, when caring for an older patient after a surgical intervention to repair a broken wrist suffered in a fall, the nurse may avert a future stroke or myocardial infarction by carefully noting and reporting a consistently elevated blood pressure. Remembering that the person at age 65 has another 16 to 19 years of life expectancy, the nurse may employ all three levels of health prevention simultaneously even in the older person diagnosed with chronic illness.

In recent years, Medicare, the national health insurance for older Americans, has expanded coverage of preventive services to encourage older people to stay healthy. Changes in coverage occur on an ongoing basis, and the gerontological nurse should keep track of these changes by visiting the Medicare website at www.medicare.gov or calling 1-800-MEDICARE (1-800-633-4227). At the present time, Medicare will pay for a yearly wellness visit and routine physical examination. It also covers a "Welcome to Medicare" physical exam so that risk factors and/or health problems can be identified and treated in order to promote health and prevent disability. This one-time Welcome to Medicare preventive physical exam is given within the first 12 months that the older person is enrolled in Part B of Medicare. The examination covers a medical and social health history with attention to modifiable risk factors for disease, education and counseling about preventive services, and referrals for care if needed. Services covered during this examination include measurement of height and weight and blood pressure, vision screening, an electrocardiogram (EKG), routine immunizations as needed, education and counseling on how to stay well, and a list of recommended screening tests and a

timetable for when they should be obtained. The following screening tests and timetable are recommended by Medicare:

- Screenings for breast, cervical, vaginal, colorectal, and prostate cancer
- Fecal occult blood testing (once yearly)
- Flexible sigmoidoscopy (once every 4 years)
- Colonoscopy (every 10 years for those with normal risk levels and once every 2 years for those at high risk)
- Lipids, triglycerides, and cholesterol levels (every 5 years)
- Barium enema (once every 4 years for those with normal risk levels or every 2 years for those at high risk)
- Mammograms (routine screenings once yearly)
- Pap smears and pelvic examination (once yearly)
- Prostate-specific antigen (PSA) test (once yearly)
- Digital rectal exam (once yearly)
- Bone mass screening—once every 2 years for those at risk
- Fasting blood glucose screening (every 6 months for those at high risk)
- Diabetes monitoring—glucose monitors, test strips, lancets, and self-management training for those with diabetes
- Flu, pneumonia, and hepatitis B vaccinations—annual flu vaccine, pneumonia vaccine at the physician's discretion, and hepatitis B vaccine for those at medium to high risk for hepatitis
- Nutrition assessment and counseling for those with diabetes or renal disease
- Glaucoma screening (yearly for those with high risk of glaucoma)
- Smoking cessation counseling (eight face-to-face visits during a 12-month period for those with smoking-related illness or those taking medicine that may be affected by tobacco)

Medicare Covered Test/Screening/Service	Date You Got This Test/ Screening/Service	Next Test/Screening Service Due
Abdominal aortic aneurysm screening		
Bone mass measurement		
Cardiovascular screening		
Colorectal cancer screening		
Fecal occult blood test		
Flexible sigmoidoscopy		
Colonoscopy		
Barium enema		
Diabetes screening		
Diabetes self-management training		
Flu shot		
Pneumococcal shot		
Hepatitis B shot		
Glaucoma test		
HIV screening		
Mammogram		
Medical nutrition therapy services		
Pap test and pelvic exam (includes breast exam)		
"Welcome to Medicare" preventive visit*		
Yearly wellness visit		
Prostate cancer screening		
Smoking cessation counseling		

*__Important:__ Make your appointment for this exam within the first 12 months of enrolling in Medicare Part B.

Figure 1-4 ▶▶▶ Preventive services checklist.

Source: Centers for Medicare and Medicaid Services, 2012.

Figure 1-4 ▶▶▶ may be useful to nurses when helping older patients prepare for their initial Medicare examination. In addition to helping patients prepare for this examination, this checklist can also serve as an important patient education tool and help the patient to plan for and schedule future preventive services.

As nurses and other healthcare professionals continue to work on closing the gap between **life span** (defined as the biologic limit to the length of life varying by species) and healthy life span, the older adult should be urged to assume more responsibility for healthy aging. About 70% of physical decline that occurs with aging is related to modifiable factors such as smoking, poor nutrition, lack of physical activity, injuries from falls, and failure to use Medicare-covered preventive services (CDC, 2010a). Older people should be educated regarding the need to start exercise programs, stop smoking, and engage in other healthy behaviors (USDHHS, 2010). Nurses often interact with older patients when they are suffering an acute health problem or traumatic injury. This interaction is considered to be a "teachable moment" when an older person who may take his or her health for granted is interested in hearing about health promotion and the nurse can seize this opportunity to achieve broader goals and improve the long-term health status of older people by reducing health risk behaviors.

> **Practice Pearl** ▶▶▶ The three major misconceptions about aging and health are that most older people are sick, older adults have no future and therefore health promotion efforts are wasted, and physical aging is primarily determined by genetics (Family Education, 2011). The gerontological nurse can help dispel these misconceptions and serve as a role model by making health promotion activities a major focus of nursing care.

Living Longer or Living Better?

From 2009 to 2010, the death rates for older persons declined significantly for 7 of the 10 leading causes of death. The death rate for the leading cause of death, heart disease, decreased by 2.4%. The death rate for malignant neoplasms decreased by 0.6%. Deaths from these two diseases combined accounted for 47% of deaths in the United States in 2010. Although heart disease mortality has exhibited a fairly steady decline since 1980, cancer mortality began to decline only in the early 1990s. Of the 10 leading causes of death, the death rate also decreased significantly for chronic lower respiratory diseases (1.4%), stroke (1.5%), accidents (unintentional injuries) (1.1%), and influenza and pneumonia (8.5%). The death rate increased significantly from 2009 to 2010 for Alzheimer's disease (3.3%) and nephritis, nephrotic syndrome, and nephrosis (1.3%). The observed changes in the age-adjusted death rates from 2009 to 2010 were not significant for diabetes mellitus, intentional self-harm (suicide), or renal disease (Murphy, Xu, & Kochanek, 2012). Figure 1-5 ▶▶▶ illustrates the leading causes of death in people over 65 years of age.

Five chronic diseases—heart disease, cancer, stroke, chronic obstructive pulmonary disease, and diabetes—cause more than two thirds of all deaths each year. The number of deaths alone, however, fails to convey the toll of chronic disease. More than 130 million Americans live with these diseases, and millions of new cases are diagnosed each year. Although treatable, these diseases are not curable. The disability and diminished quality of life that result from these diseases is a great burden. Chronic, disabling conditions cause major limitations in activity for 1 of every 10 Americans, or 30 million people. Costs of caring for chronic illness are staggering both to older persons and their family members and to society. The cost of medical care for Americans with chronic illness was $470 billion in 1995, and these costs are projected to be as high as $864 billion in 2040 as the baby boomers continue to age (CDC, 2010a). Box 1-4 lists the most common causes of disability in the United States.

Because the population will be older and greater in number in the coming years, overall U.S. healthcare costs are projected to increase 25% by 2030 (Partnership to Fight Chronic Disease, 2009). Preventing health problems is one of the few known

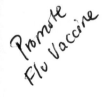

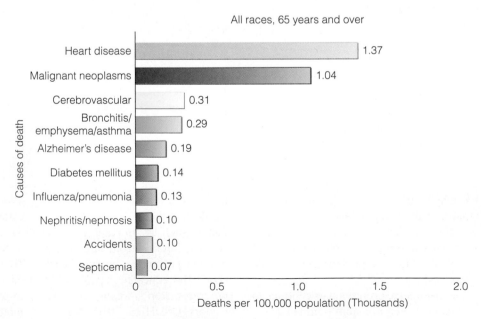

Figure 1-5 ▶▶▶ Leading causes of death for men and women 65 years and older.

Source: Centers for Disease Control and Prevention (2011); National Center for Health Statistics, data from the National Vital Statistics System (2006).

KATZ Independence in Activities of Daily Living Website

BOX 1-4 ▷ **Most Common Causes of Disability in the United States**

- Degenerative joint disease
- Chronic back pain
- Atherosclerosis
- Lung or respiratory problems
- Deafness or hearing problems
- Mental or emotional problems
- Diabetes mellitus
- Blindness or vision problems
- Stroke

Source: Centers for Disease Control and Prevention (2011).

ways to stem rising healthcare costs. By preserving function and preventing injury, we also can help older adults remain independent for as long as possible, which can improve their quality of life and delay the need for costly long-term care.

Many people who have chronic conditions and disabilities lead active, productive lives, but some require assistance with activities of daily living (ADLs). About 41 million Americans with chronic conditions require assistance daily. In general, older people with lower incomes are more likely to have conditions that are difficult or costly to treat. African Americans are more likely than Caucasians to have limitations in ADLs when chronically ill. Older African American men and women with arthritis are more likely to have activity limitations than other older people (National Center for Health Statistics [NCHS], 2010). Nearly 60% of older African Americans report high blood pressure, and a growing number of older African Americans and Hispanics are reporting diabetes, probably related to the increasing rates of obesity in these populations (CDC, 2010b). The Hartford Institute of Geriatric Nursing recommends the Katz Independence in Activities of Daily Living (ADL) scale as a Best Practices in Nursing Care to older adults (see page 14). This scale has been used in many clinical settings for over 30 years. The scores can be recorded in the older patient's medical record so that progress toward independence can be measured over time.

The number of Americans with chronic conditions is expected to increase significantly during the next several years. This will pose a challenge for nurses and other healthcare providers. The hospitalization rates are higher for those with arthritis and hypertension, two common chronic conditions of older people. In general, women of all ages require more help with ADLs than do men and the need for assistance tends to increase with age. Figure 1-6 ▶▶▶ illustrates this relationship.

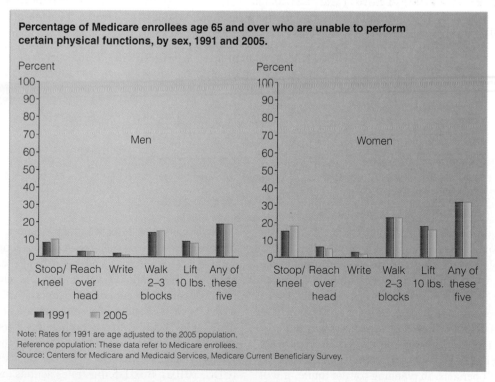

Percentage of Medicare enrollees age 65 and over who are unable to perform certain physical functions, by sex, 1991 and 2005.

Note: Rates for 1991 are age adjusted to the 2005 population.
Reference population: These data refer to Medicare enrollees.
Source: Centers for Medicare and Medicaid Services, Medicare Current Beneficiary Survey.

Figure 1-6 ▶▶▶ Older Americans, key indicators of well-being, 2008.

Source: Federal Interagency Forum on Aging-Related Statistics. (2008, March). *Older Americans 2008: Key indicators of well-being.* Washington, DC: U.S. Government Printing Office.

Best Practices Katz Index of Independence in Activities of Daily Living

ACTIVITIES	INDEPENDENCE	DEPENDENCE
POINTS (1 OR 0)	(1 POINT) **NO** supervision, direction, or personal assistance	(0 POINTS) **WITH** supervision, direction, personal assistance, or total care
BATHING POINTS:_____	**(1 POINT)** Bathes self completely or needs help in bathing only a single part of the body such as the back, genital area, or disabled extremity.	**(0 POINTS)** Needs help with bathing more than one part of the body, getting in or out of the tub or shower. Requires total bathing.
DRESSING POINTS:_____	**(1 POINT)** Gets clothes from closets and drawers and puts on clothes and outer garments complete with fasteners. May have help tying shoes.	**(0 POINTS)** Needs help with dressing self or needs to be completely dressed.
TOILETING POINTS:_____	**(1 POINT)** Goes to toilet, gets on and off, arranges clothes, cleans genital area without help.	**(0 POINTS)** Needs help transferring to the toilet, cleaning self, or using bed-pan or commode.
TRANSFERRING POINTS:_____	**(1 POINT)** Moves in and out of bed or chair unassisted. Mechanical transferring aids are acceptable.	**(0 POINTS)** Needs help in moving from bed to chair or requires a complete transfer.
CONTINENCE POINTS:_____	**(1 POINT)** Exercises complete self-control over urination and defecation.	**(0 POINTS)** Is partially or totally incontinent of bowel or bladder.
FEEDING POINTS:_____	**(1 POINT)** Gets food from plate into mouth without help. Preparation of food may be done by another person.	**(0 POINTS)** Needs partial or total help with feeding or requires parenteral feeding.
TOTAL POINTS = _____ 6 = High (*patient independent*) 0 = Low (*patient very dependent*)		

Source: Sidney Katz, et al., Progress in Development of the Index of AD. *The Gerontologist,* Vol. 10(Part 1), 1970: 20-30. Copyright © The Gerontological Society of America. Reproduced by permission of Oxford University Press.

Chronic conditions also affect emotional health. Women with chronic conditions are more likely to rate their health as poor, and older African American women provide the least positive assessment of their emotional well-being (NCHS, 2010). The combined effects of poor health status with the negative impact of age and racial discrimination may be responsible for these assessments. With the cost of health care rising each year, the United States already faces the challenge of providing appropriate and accessible health care to all persons. In planning for the future, it will also be important to recognize that different groups of older and chronically ill persons have different healthcare needs.

Americans can improve their chances for a healthy old age by simply taking advantage of recommended preventive health services and by making healthy lifestyle changes. The challenge for nurses and other healthcare professionals is to encourage people at all stages of life to reduce their chances of disability and chronic illness by undertaking healthy lifestyle changes. This strategy will improve quality of life, delay disability, and increase the number of healthy years an older person is expected to live (CDC, 2010a). Box 1-5 illustrates actions nurses and other healthcare professionals can take to improve older Americans' health and quality of life.

BOX 1-5 | **Opportunities to Improve Older Americans' Health and Quality of Life**

Poor health and loss of independence are *not* inevitable consequences of aging. The following strategies have proven effective in promoting the health of older adults:

- **Healthy lifestyles.** Research has shown that healthy lifestyles are more influential than genetic factors in helping older people avoid the deterioration traditionally associated with aging. People who are physically active, eat a healthy diet, do not use tobacco, and practice other healthy behaviors reduce their risk for chronic diseases and have half the rate of disability of those who do not lead healthy lifestyles.
- **Early detection of diseases.** Screening to detect chronic diseases early in their course, when they are most treatable, can save many lives; however, many older adults have not had recommended screenings. For example, 60% of Americans over age 65 have not had a sigmoidoscopy or colonoscopy in the previous 5 years to screen for colorectal cancer, even though Medicare covers the cost.
- **Immunizations.** More than 40,000 people age 65 or older die each year of influenza and invasive pneumococcal disease. Immunizations

reduce a person's risk for hospitalization and death from these diseases. Yet in 2010, 34% of Americans age 65 or older had not had a recent flu shot, and 37% had never received a pneumonia vaccine.

- **Injury prevention.** Falls are the most common cause of injuries to older adults. More than one third of adults age 65 or older fall each year. Of those who fall, 20% to 30% suffer moderate to severe injuries that decrease mobility and independence. Removing tripping hazards in the home and installing grab bars are simple measures that can greatly reduce older Americans' risk for falls and fractures.
- **Self-management techniques.** Programs to teach older Americans self-management techniques can reduce the pain and costs of chronic disease. For example, the Arthritis Self-Help Course, disseminated by the Arthritis Foundation, has been shown to reduce arthritis pain by 20% and visits to physicians by 40%. Unfortunately, less than 1% of Americans with arthritis participate in such programs, and courses are not available in many areas.

Source: Centers for Disease Control and Prevention. (2011b). *Chronic disease prevention. Healthy aging: Helping people to live long and productive lives and enjoy a good quality of life.* Retrieved from http://www.cdc.gov/chronicdisease/resources/publications/AAG/aging.htm

---

Healthy People 2020

Healthy People 2020 is the prevention agenda for the United States. It is a statement of national health objectives designed to identify the most significant preventable threats to health and to establish national goals to reduce these threats. The U.S. Department of Health and Human Services (2010) recently published this document with specific areas for health improvement. The four basic goals of this document are:

1. Attain high-quality, longer lives free of preventable disease, disability, injury, and premature death.
2. Achieve health equity, eliminate disparities, and improve the health of all groups.
3. Create social and physical environments that promote good health for all.
4. Promote quality of life, healthy development, and healthy behaviors across all life stages.

The first goal signals the importance of quality of life as well as length of life. By placing emphasis on these two vital concepts in one goal, the link between the two is reaffirmed. The second goal, eliminating health disparities, addresses the growing problems related to access to quality health care and differences in treatment based on age, race,

gender, and insurance coverage. The goals of *Healthy People 2020* serve as a guide for healthcare research, practice, and policy, and set the agenda for healthcare reform during the next 10 years. The focus areas pertinent to older people are listed in Box 1-6. It is apparent when reviewing this list that nurses can intervene in most of these focus areas to promote health and wellness in older people. Many of the focus areas are linked to one another, and intervening in one area may stimulate a positive outcome in several other areas. For instance, by educating an older person about the benefits of a healthy nutritious diet, the nurse may decrease the chance of cancer, obesity, diabetes, heart disease, and stroke, and improve mobility to prevent falls. Further, the older person who eats a nutritious diet will probably have more energy to engage in social and recreational activities, thereby decreasing the chance of depression and social isolation.

Additionally, *Healthy People 2020* highlights emerging issues for improving the health of older adults including the need to coordinate care; helping older adults manage their own healthcare needs; establishing quality measures; identifying minimum levels of training for people who care for older adults; and supporting research and analysis and appropriate training to equip providers with the tools they need to meet the needs of older adults. Further noted

Healthy People 2020 Website

> **BOX 1-6** **Focus Areas in *Healthy People 2020* Applicable to Older Persons**
>
> - Access to quality health services
> - Arthritis, osteoporosis, and chronic back conditions
> - Cancer
> - Chronic kidney disease
> - Dementia
> - Diabetes
> - Disability and secondary conditions
> - Educational and community-based programs
> - Environmental health
> - Food safety
> - Health communication
> - Heart disease and stroke
> - Human immunodeficiency virus
> - Immunization and infectious diseases
>
> - Injury and violence prevention
> - Medical product safety
> - Mental health and mental conditions
> - Nutrition and obesity
> - Occupational safety and health
> - Oral health
> - Physical activity and fitness
> - Public health infrastructure
> - Respiratory diseases
> - Sexually transmitted diseases
> - Substance abuse
> - Tobacco use
> - Vision and hearing

Source: U.S. Department of Health and Human Services. (2010). *Healthy people, 2020: Older adults.* Rockville, MD: Author.

is the need to gather more data relating to the healthcare needs of aging lesbian, gay, bisexual, and transgender populations.

View the entire *Healthy People 2020* report online, where detailed information is provided regarding each focus area, and specific objectives are suggested for each age group.

Theories of Aging

The study of aging continues to grow and evolve, and scientists uncover new insights daily. The quest to understand aging, which began as the pursuit of one all-encompassing theory, has evolved to the knowledge that multiple processes can affect how humans age. These processes combine and interact on many levels, and individual cells, proteins, tissues, and organ systems are all involved. Some of the changes of aging are benign and superficial such as graying of the hair and wrinkling of the skin. Others, however, increase the risk of disease and disability, such as arteriosclerosis. Gerontologists prefer to use the term **senescence** when characterizing the aging process. Senescence is defined as the progressive deterioration of body systems that can increase the risk of mortality as the individual gets older.

The rate and progression of aging varies greatly from one individual to the next. Even identical twins who possess the same genetic makeup will age differently.

If everyone aged at the same rate and in the same way, we would become more alike as we get older. However, just the opposite is true. When a group of older people gathers, there is a great variety in the way they look, express their attitudes, engage in recreational and social activities, and relate health problems. Notice the variety and differences in the older persons depicted in Figure 1-7 ▶▶▶.

Generally, each body system is affected by aging. Some of the changes can begin in the 20s and 30s. "Plastic" or modifiable changes can be slowed by exercise, good nutrition, and other elements of a healthy lifestyle. For example, most people can avoid lung disease by not smoking and avoiding secondhand smoke exposure. There is a growing understanding of what is considered to be a disease or common problem of aging and what is considered to be part of the "normal" aging process. Normal aging consists of those universal changes that occur in all older people. It is generally accepted that the level of organ reserve declines as we grow older. Longitudinal studies such as the Baltimore Longitudinal Study of Aging have supplied valuable information that can help to define normal aging. However, even within one person's organs and organ systems there are different rates of decline. Understanding these changes can help to distinguish chronological age (number of years from birth) from physiological age (degree of senescence experienced by each body system). Figure 1-8 ▶▶▶ illustrates normal changes of aging.

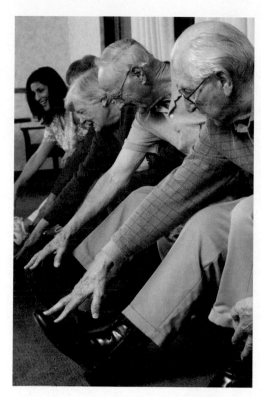

Figure 1-7 ▶▶▶ Good health can last long into old age.

Source: gwimages/Fotolia

Normal aging includes but is not limited to the following changes:

1. **Heart.** Heart muscles thicken with age. The heart's maximum pumping rate and the body's ability to extract oxygen from blood diminish with age.

2. **Arteries.** Arteries tend to stiffen with age. The older heart has to beat harder to supply the energy needed to propel the blood forward through less elastic arteries.

3. **Lungs.** Maximum breathing capacity may decline by about 40% between the ages of 40 and 70.

4. **Brain.** With age, the brain loses some of the axons and neurons that connect with each other. Recent studies indicate that the older brain can be stimulated to produce new neurons, but the exact conditions that stimulate this growth are unknown.

5. **Kidneys.** Kidneys gradually become less efficient at removing waste from blood.

6. **Bladder.** Bladder capacity declines.

7. **Body fat.** Body fat typically increases until about middle age and then stabilizes until late life when weight tends to decline. When weight declines, older people lose both muscle and fat. With age, fat is redistributed to the deeper organs from the skin. Fat that is redistributed to the abdomen rather than the hips (being apple shaped rather than pear shaped) makes older men and women more vulnerable to heart disease.

8. **Muscles.** Without exercise, muscle mass declines 22% for women and 23% for men between the ages of 30 and 70. Exercise can slow this rate of loss.

9. **Bones.** Bone mineral is lost and replaced throughout life, but the loss outpaces the replacement for women at about age 35. This loss is accelerated at menopause. Regular weight-bearing exercise and high calcium intake can slow bone loss.

10. **Sight.** Difficulty focusing close up may begin in the 40s. After age 50, there is increased sensitivity to glare, greater difficulty in seeing at low levels of light, and more difficulty in detecting moving objects. Adapting to light changes and nighttime driving become more difficult. At age 70, ability to distinguish fine details begins to decline.

11. **Hearing.** It becomes more difficult to hear higher frequencies with aging and this loss begins to accelerate in middle age. Even older adults with good hearing may have difficulty distinguishing vowels and understanding speech, especially in situations with high levels of background noise. Hearing declines more quickly in men than women.

12. **Personality.** Personality is remarkably stable throughout adult life, and rarely do healthy older people show signs of personality change during their final years. Personality usually does not change radically even as a result of major lifestyle changes such as retirement or death of a loved one. Older people who experience health problems, chronic illness, and pain are at risk for depression and social isolation (Schaie & Willis, 2010).

The final result of all the normal changes of aging is the loss of organ reserve, or the ability of a given organ to react quickly and efficiently to physiological stress. When an individual is very young, the heart can increase its output during exercise sixfold, the kidneys can excrete efficiently if 80% of the nephrons are damaged or destroyed, and surgeons can remove a lung or three fourths of the liver without loss of life or function. The organ systems of the body combine their efforts and orchestrate a complicated set of responses designed to maintain equilibrium. This equilibrium consists of temperature, acid–base balance, body chemicals, and other vital life components. This tendency of the body toward maintaining equilibrium is defined as **homeostasis.** The loss of organ reserve that can occur with aging can lead to **homeostenosis,** or inability of the body to restore homeostasis after even minor environmental challenges such as trauma or infection. Therefore, an older person may die from pneumonia or influenza, which may have been only a minor illness to a younger person (CDC, 2010a).

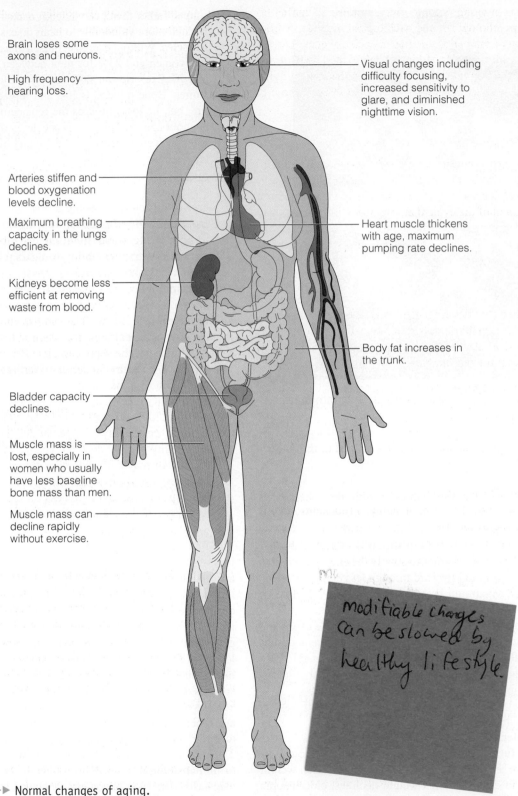

Brain loses some axons and neurons.

High frequency hearing loss.

Visual changes including difficulty focusing, increased sensitivity to glare, and diminished nighttime vision.

Arteries stiffen and blood oxygenation levels decline.

Maximum breathing capacity in the lungs declines.

Heart muscle thickens with age, maximum pumping rate declines.

Kidneys become less efficient at removing waste from blood.

Body fat increases in the trunk.

Bladder capacity declines.

Muscle mass is lost, especially in women who usually have less baseline bone mass than men.

Muscle mass can decline rapidly without exercise.

modifiable changes can be slowed by healthy lifestyle.

Figure 1-8 ►►► Normal changes of aging.

Theories of aging fall into several groups, including biological, psychological, and sociological theories. A brief description of the major theories in each category follows; however, with the tools of biotechnology and new knowledge regarding aging, all-encompassing theories of aging are giving way to a more diverse perspective (Schaie & Willis, 2010).

Biological Aging Theories

Biological aging theories fall into two groups: programmed theories and error theories. Programmed theories assert that aging follows a biological timetable and may represent a continuation of the cycle that regulates childhood growth and development. The error theories emphasize environmental assaults to the human system that gradually cause things to go wrong.

Programmed Theories

Programmed theories hypothesize that the body's genetic codes contain instructions for the regulation of cellular reproduction and death. The following are some of the most popular programmed theories.

Programmed Longevity Aging is the result of the sequential switching on and off of certain genes, with senescence defined as the point in time when age-associated functional deficits are manifested. Persons who endorse this theory are interested in studying the human genome and genetic theories of aging.

Endocrine Theory Biological clocks act through hormones to control the pace of aging. Proponents of this theory ascribe to the use of various natural and synthetic hormones, such as testosterone, estrogen, and human growth hormone, to slow the aging process.

Immunological Theory A programmed decline in immune system functions leads to an increased vulnerability to infectious disease, aging, and eventual death. Declines in immune system function can affect the outcomes of many illnesses such as postoperative infections, diabetes, urinary tract infections, and pneumonia. It is generally accepted that a healthy diet and lifestyle coupled with preventive health measures, such as a yearly flu shot and limiting exposure to pathogens, can support immune function in the older person.

Error Theories

The most popular error theories are listed below and hypothesize that environmental assaults and the body's constant need to manufacture energy and fuel metabolic activities cause toxic by-products to accumulate. These toxic by-products may eventually impair normal body function and cellular repair.

Wear-and-Tear Theory Cells and organs have vital parts that wear out after years of use. Proponents of this theory see the human body as a machine. They believe that a "master clock" controls all organs and that cellular function slows down with time and becomes less efficient at repairing body malfunctions that are caused by environmental assaults. Abusing or neglecting one organ or body system can stimulate premature aging and disease (e.g., a person who drinks excessive amounts of alcohol may develop liver disease).

Cross-Link Theory In this theory, an accumulation of cross-linked proteins resulting from the binding of glucose (simple sugars) to protein (a process that occurs under the presence of oxygen) causes various problems. Once the binding occurs, the protein cannot perform normally, which may result in visual problems such as cataracts or wrinkling and skin aging. The modern diet is often high in sugar and carbohydrates, and some nutritionists believe that low-carbohydrate diets can slow the development of cross-links (American Federation for Aging Research, 2011).

Free Radical Theory Accumulated damage caused by oxygen radicals causes cells, and eventually organs, to lose function and organ reserve. The use of antioxidants and vitamins is believed to slow this damage.

Somatic DNA Damage Theory Genetic mutations occur and accumulate with increasing age, causing cells to deteriorate and malfunction. Proponents believe that genetic manipulation and alteration may slow the aging process.

Emerging Biological Theories Study and mapping of the human genome have led to the belief that many genes may be responsible for human aging. These genes may be activated by certain enzymes and/or environmental conditions and may account for the influence of toxins, stress, and lifestyle choices. As these studies progress during the next decade, much more will be known about the aging process, and scientists may be able to explain why individuals age differently.

Psychological Aging Theories

Most psychological theories maintain that various coping or adaptive strategies must occur for a person to age successfully. The triggers might be the physical changes of aging, issues of retirement, dealing with the death of a spouse or friends, and perhaps declining health. Major psychological aging theories include Jung's theory of individualism and Erikson's developmental theory.

Jung's Theory of Individualism

This theory hypothesizes that as a person ages, the shift of focus is away from the external world (extroversion) toward the inner experience (introversion). At this stage of life, the older person will search for answers to many of life's riddles and try to find the essence of the "true self." To age successfully, the older person must accept past accomplishments and failures (Jung, 1960). Older persons subscribing to Jung's theory may spend a lot of time in contemplation and introspection.

Erikson's Developmental Theory

According to Erikson (1950), there are eight stages of life with developmental tasks to be accomplished at each stage. The task of the older adult includes ego integrity versus despair. Erikson advanced that during this stage, the older adult will become preoccupied with acceptance of eventual death without becoming morbid or obsessed with these thoughts. If major failures or disappointments have occurred in the older person's life, this final stage may be difficult to accomplish because the older person may be despairing rather than accepting of death. Older persons who have not achieved ego integrity may look back on their lives with dissatisfaction and feel unhappy, depressed, or angry over what they have done or failed to do. Psychological counseling can help to resolve some of these issues.

Sociological Aging Theories

Sociological theories of aging differ from biological theories because they tend to focus on roles and relationships that occur in later life. Each of the theories must be judged within the context of time that they were formulated. Major sociological theories of aging include disengagement theory, activity theory, and continuity theory.

Disengagement Theory

Introduced by Cummings and Henry in 1961, this controversial theory asserts that the appropriate pattern of behavior in later life is for the older person and society at large to engage in a mutual and reciprocal withdrawal. Thus, when death occurs, neither the older individual nor society is disadvantaged and social equilibrium is maintained. Mandatory retirement forces some older people to withdraw from work-related roles, accelerating the process of disengagement. In some cultures, older people remain engaged, active, and busy throughout their lives.

Activity Theory

This theory contradicts the disengagement theory by proposing that older adults should stay active and engaged if they are to age successfully (Havighurst, Neugarten, & Tobin, 1963). By staying active and extending the activities enjoyed in middle age, the older person has a better chance of enjoying old age. Happiness and satisfaction with life are assumed to result from a high level of involvement with the world and continued social involvement. According to this theory, when retirement occurs, replacement activities must be found.

Continuity Theory

This theory advances that successful aging involves maintaining or continuing previous values, habits, preferences, family ties, and all other linkages that have formed the basic underlying structure of adult life. Older age is not viewed as a time that should trigger major life readjustment, but rather just a time to continue being the same person (Havighurst et al., 1963). According to this theory, the pace of activities may be slowed. Activities pursued in earlier life that did not bring satisfaction and genuine happiness may be dropped at the discretion of the older person. For some, gaining relief from constant time pressures and deadlines is one of the bounties of old age.

Patient and Family Teaching

Gerontological nurses require skills and knowledge related to teaching patients and families about the key concepts of gerontology and the role of gerontological nurses. The patient–family teaching guidelines in the following feature will assist the nurse to assume the role of teacher and coach. Educating patients and families is critical so that older patients can assume a larger role in health promotion activities.

Patient–Family Teaching Guidelines

The following are guidelines that the nurse may find useful when instructing older persons and their families about gerontology in health care.

LEARNING ABOUT GERONTOLOGY

1 What is gerontology?

Gerontology is the study of aging. It involves all aspects of an older person's life, including physical, social, psychological, and spiritual function.

RATIONALE:

Many people, including some healthcare professionals, are unaware that gerontology is holistic, encompasses more than the medical model, and involves all aspects of an older person's life.

2 Why is this important to an older person like me?

With aging, an older person's health status can be affected by many factors. Gerontologists and geriatricians have extra training to become experts in the factors that can affect health status and function, including management of chronic illness, proper medication use, lifestyle changes to improve health, disease prevention and health promotion techniques, and early detection of diseases.

RATIONALE:

Nurses can educate older patients and their families regarding the many factors that contribute to maintaining and improving health status and function throughout the entire life span with emphasis on staying healthy in old age.

3 Is it too late for me to do anything to make myself healthier?

It is never too late to address behaviors and lifestyle choices that can contribute to premature death or disability. The top killers in the United States are heart disease, cancer, and stroke. Smoking, poor nutrition, and physical inactivity all can contribute to the formation and progression of these diseases.

RATIONALE:

The nurse should educate older persons and their families regarding the link between lifestyle choices and unfavorable health outcomes in an attempt to provide motivation and incentive for improving health behaviors.

4 Where should I go to get further information?

Many hospitals, community health agencies, and healthcare professionals can guide you to choose an appropriate source of information. Look for a specialty clinic with a geriatrician, advanced practice gerontological nurse, gerontological nurse, social worker, nutritionist, physical therapist, occupational therapist, and geropsychiatrist as part of a team to specialize in caring for older adults. These experts can address many common health problems of older people, including falls, medication side effects, pain, sleep disorders, memory problems, and urinary incontinence.

RATIONALE:

Many older persons and their adult children are interested in learning more about staying healthy and seeking resources specific to aging and geriatrics. The nurse can make a referral to a geriatric specialty clinic or specially trained healthcare professional in order to make the search easier.

5 Should all older people be cared for by a team of geriatric experts?

Many older people receive their health care from generalists and primary care providers. Others with special problems related to aging would benefit from seeing specialists in aging. If you take many medications, have been diagnosed with multiple chronic illnesses, or think you may be having problems with your memory, you may benefit from seeing an aging specialist such as a geriatrician or an advanced practice gerontological nurse.

RATIONALE:

There is great diversity in health needs of people over the age of 65. While it is generally agreed that all older people would benefit from receiving their health care from geriatric specialists, many older people are well cared for by primary care physicians, advanced practice nurses, and family physicians; geriatricians are sought to provide care for frail older persons with complicated medical problems. Regardless of a person's age or healthcare status, a geriatric specialist should be consulted when placement in a long-term care facility is being considered for an older person, family members are feeling stressed or burdened, or the older person is not coping well with illness or disability.

CARE PLAN   A Patient Who Experiences a Fall

Case Study

Mrs. Kane is a 78-year-old retired teacher. She was brought to the emergency department by ambulance after she fell and injured her right wrist. An X-ray reveals an acute problem of a fractured right wrist and notes the presence of significant osteoarthritis and osteoporosis (degenerative joint changes and thinning of the bones).

Mrs. Kane lives independently and manages adequately since the death of her husband about 8 years ago, although she gave up driving because she has difficulty seeing oncoming cars in intense sunlight or when headlights are on at night. She has a daughter who visits her often and helps with heavy cleaning and grocery shopping.

The patient reports she was bending over to feed some neighborhood stray cats when she lost her balance and reached out to break her fall. It was dark and she did not notice the loose rug on the back porch that may have contributed to her fall. On further questioning, she remembers that she may have fallen one or two times before, both in the house and on the back porch, during the past several months.

Applying the Nursing Process

Assessment

When an older person falls and experiences injury, the nurse should identify the factors of normal aging, disease, and environment that may have contributed to the fall. Just noting that an older person has fallen is an incomplete assessment. Further information is needed.

> The nurse must recognize that a fall may be the result of an unfortunate accident (anyone can trip and fall, especially in a dark environment), but certainly Mrs. Kane's report of previous falls and visual impairment are red flags. Further, the X-ray reveals the presence of osteoarthritis and osteoporosis, both of which can contribute to mobility problems and risk of serious injury. Because the patient is 78 years old, she is experiencing many normal changes of aging, including declines in neurologic, cardiovascular, and musculoskeletal reserve that ultimately result in

> homeostenosis, or an inability of her body to maintain regular function under adverse conditions. Whereas a younger person might not have fallen at all or might have fallen without becoming injured, Mrs. Kane was unable to correct her balance and broke her wrist as a result of the fall. The nurse must think broadly and consider the fall the result of normal changes of aging, chronic disease processes, and environmental circumstances. A careful past medical history should include any diagnosed illnesses, significant health problems, surgeries or trauma, medications taken, health maintenance activities, name and address of her primary care provider, assessment of mood and mental status, environmental hazards, and baseline ADLs. This information is needed to gain a baseline understanding of Mrs. Kane and her health status.

Diagnosis

Some appropriate nursing diagnoses for Mrs. Kane include the following:

- *Ineffective Health Maintenance* demonstrated by lack of adaptive behaviors to internal and external environmental changes (bending over in the dark with a loose scatter rug)

- *Impaired Physical Mobility* (due to osteoporosis and degenerative joint disease)
- *Risk for Falls, Acute Injury,* and *Pain*

NANDA-I © 2012.

Expected Outcomes

Expected outcomes for the plan of care specify that Mrs. Kane will:

- Become aware of the dangers of injury resulting from falling and institute appropriate safety measures in her home.

- Use appropriate visual aids and reduce safety hazards such as loose rugs and inadequate lighting to increase safety in the home.

CARE PLAN   A Patient Who Experiences a Fall *(continued)*

- Develop a therapeutic relationship with the nurse and develop a mutually agreed-on plan for health and safety.
- Agree to a pharmacological and nonpharmacological pain management plan with assistance or temporary placement in a rehabilitation facility while her wrist is healing.

Planning and Implementation

The following nursing actions may be appropriate for Mrs. Kane:

- Mrs. Kane requires pain management secondary to her wrist fracture with appropriate pharmacological and nonpharmacological techniques.
- Because her wrist is to be set in a cast, Mrs. Kane will require assistance from a home health aide or short-term placement in a rehabilitation center until she can safely cook, clean, and manage her own personal hygiene and ADLs.
- She requires further assessment of her health status and treatment and monitoring of her osteoporosis.
- She should be referred to an ophthalmologist and a low-vision clinic for further assessment of her vision and assessment of appropriate visual aids.

Evaluation

The nurse hopes to work with Mrs. Kane over time and realizes the chronic nature of falls in older people. The nurse will consider the plan a success based on the following criteria:

- Mrs. Kane will not experience any more falls during the next 6 months.
- She will accept temporary placement in a rehabilitation facility or assistance from a home health aide while her wrist heals.

- Schedule medical appointments for health promotion activities and ongoing treatment and assessment of her osteoporosis.

- Question Mrs. Kane regarding the establishment of advance directives such as naming a durable power of attorney or establishing a living will (depending on the laws of the state where she resides). If no advance directives have been established, urge Mrs. Kane and her daughter to discuss this with her primary care provider at her next visit.
- Both Mrs. Kane and her daughter would benefit from counseling and education regarding appropriate levels of social involvement, balance training, reduction of environmental safety hazards, and health maintenance activities.

- She will use appropriate visual aids and home safety interventions to promote safety.
- She will establish advance directives and communicate her desires for health care should she be unable to speak for herself.
- Finally, Mrs. Kane will follow up and receive ongoing treatment for her chronic medical conditions and visit her primary healthcare provider within 1 month of discharge from the rehabilitation facility.

Ethical Dilemma

The nurse finds that Mrs. Kane's blood pressure is highly elevated, and an electrocardiogram reveals significant cardiac ischemia with evidence of recent myocardial infarction. When questioned about the presence of cardiac symptoms, Mrs. Kane states, "Yes, I've had chest pain on and off but I didn't mention it to anyone. Honestly, I don't want to have cardiac surgery like my friend Louise. They cut her open and now she can't even walk across the room, because she is so weak. I just decided I'm not going to say a thing to anyone. Besides I don't want to bother my daughter. She is so busy with her own family. The last thing she needs to worry about is me." What is the best course of action for the nurse to follow?

(continued)

A Patient Who Experiences a Fall *(continued)*

Mrs. Kane has the right to autonomy and to refuse medical interventions assuming that she is cognitively intact and competent. However, she would benefit from education regarding pharmacological and behavioral techniques that can control blood pressure, prevent stroke, relieve the symptoms of chest pain, and improve the quality of life. As medical technology extends the options for older people, healthcare providers must function as patient educators and advocates so that appropriate care is provided to those who will benefit from these procedures. Because the patient is generally healthy, she may be a good candidate for angiography and stent placement; both are minimally invasive techniques that have the potential to improve and maintain the quality of her life. The geriatric social worker should be consulted to talk with Mrs. Kane and her family (if she is willing). The conversation should be recorded in the confidential medical record.

Critical Thinking and the Nursing Process

1. Imagine yourself at age 80. What will you be like? What will you like best about being older? What are your fears regarding your own aging?
2. Examine your lifestyle. Are you engaging in behaviors that will support and encourage healthy aging? Are you engaging in risky behaviors that might promote the development of chronic illnesses?
3. Think of older people you know who have aged successfully. What are some characteristics they possess that might have contributed to a healthy older age?
4. Examine the website that describes your school of nursing. Is care of the older person mentioned? If not, do you think it should be?

■ Evaluate your responses in Appendix B.

Chapter Highlights

■ The population of the world is aging. This trend is seen in all developed and most developing countries.

■ Women comprise the majority of older people and outlive men by about 6 years. Older people are more likely to suffer from chronic illnesses that have the potential to cause disability and limitations in ADLs.

■ Nurses and other healthcare professionals have the opportunity to engage in health promotion activities at all stages of life, including old age. *Healthy People 2020* specifies goals for older Americans.

■ With normal aging, there is loss of organ reserve that contributes to homeostenosis or narrowing of the zone of adaptation. Older persons with decreased organ reserve are unable to respond to physiological or psychological stress and need a more supportive environment to maintain function.

References

American Federation for Aging Research. (2011). *Biology of aging: Theories of Aging.* Retrieved from http://www.afar.org/infoaging/biology-of-aging/theories-of-aging/

Association for Gerontology in Higher Education. (2012). *Careers in aging: Consider the possibilities.* Retrieved from http://www.careersinaging.com/careersinaging/what.html

Centers for Disease Control and Prevention (CDC). (2009). *National vital statistics report.* Retrieved from http://www.cdc.gov/media/pressrel/1009/r/090819.htm

Centers for Disease Control and Prevention (CDC). (2010a). *Chronic disease prevention and health promotion.* Retrieved from http://www.cdc.gov/chronicdisease/overview/index.htm

Centers for Disease Control and Prevention (CDC). (2010b). *Prevalence of overweight and obesity.* Retrieved from http://www.cdc.gov/NCHS/data/hestat/obesity_adult_07_08/obesity_adult_07_08.pdf

Centers for Disease Control and Prevention (CDC) (2011a). *47.5 million U.S. adults report a disability: Arthritis remains most common cause.* Retrieved from http://www.cdc.gov/Features/dsAdultDisabilityCauses/

Centers for Disease Control and Prevention (CDC). (2011b). *Healthy aging: Helping people to live long and productive lives and enjoy a good quality of life.* Retrieved from http://www.cdc.gov/chronicdisease/resources/publications/AAG/aging.htm

Centers for Medicare & Medicaid Services. (2012). *Welcome to Medicare preventive visit.* Retrieved from http://www.medicare.gov/navigation/manage-your-health/preventive-services/medicare-physical-exam.aspx

Cummings, E., & Henry, W. (1961). *Growing old: The process of disengagement.* New York, NY: Basic Books.

Erikson, E. (1950). *Childhood and society.* New York, NY: W.W. Norton.

Family Education. (2011). *Misconceptions about aging.* Retrieved from http://life.familyeducation.com/health/social-emotional/47269.html

Hamerman, D., & Butler, R. (2007). *Geriatric bioscience : The link between aging and disease.* Baltimore, MD: Johns Hopkins University Press.

Hartford Institute for Geriatric Nursing. (2011). *Recommended baccalaureate competencies and curricular guidelines for the nursing care of older adults.* Retrieved from http://www.hartfordign.org/Education/Baccalaureate

Havighurst, R., Neugarten, B., & Tobin, S. (1963). Disengagement, personality and life satisfaction in the later years. In P. Hanse (Ed.), *Age with a future.* Copenhagen, Denmark: Munksgoard.

Health Resources and Services Administration, U.S. Department of Health and Human Services. (2010). *Women's health USA 2010.* Retrieved from http://mchb.hrsa.gov/whusa10/popchar/pages/102usfp.html

Jung, C. (1960). *The stage of life in collected works: Vol. 8. The structure and dynamics of the psyche.* New York, NY: Pantheon Books.

Katz, S., Down, T. D., Cash, H. R., & Grotz, R. C. (1970). Progress in the development of the index of ADL. *The Gerontologist, 10*(1), 20–30.

Miniño, A. (2011). *Death in the United States, 2009.* National Center for Health Statistics (NCHS) data brief, no 64. Hyattsville, MD: National Center for Health Statistics.

Murphy, S. L., Xu, J. Q., & Kochanek, K. D. (2012). Deaths: Preliminary data for 2010. *National Vital Statistics Reports, 60*(4), 7–9.

NANDA International. (2012). *NANDA International nursing diagnoses: Definitions and classification, 2012–2014.* Philadelphia, PA: Wiley-Blackwell.

National Center for Health Statistics (NCHS). (2010). *Depression in the United States household population.* Retrieved from http://www.cdc.gov/nchs/data/databriefs/db07.htm

National Center for Health Statistics (NCHS). (2011). Death in the United States 2009. Retrieved from http://www.cdc.gov/nchs/data/databriefs/db64.pdf

National Institute on Aging (NIA). (2011). *What's your aging IQ?* Retrieved from http://www.niapublications.org/quiz/index.php

Partnership to Fight Chronic Disease. (2009). *Almanac of chronic disease.* Retrieved from http://www.fightchronicdisease.org/sites/default/files/docs/PFCDAlmanac_ExecSum_updated81009.pdf

Saison, J., Smith, M., Segal, J., & White, M. (2010). *Healthy aging tips.* Retrieved from http://www.helpguide.org/life/healthy_aging_seniors_aging_well.htm

Schaie, K., & Willis, S. (2010). *Handbook of the psychology of aging.* Burlington, MA: Academic Press.

Transgenerational Design Matters. (2011). *The demographics of aging.* Retrieved from http://transgenerational.org/aging/demographics.htm

United Nations, Population Division. (2012). *World population aging 1950–2050.* Retrieved from http://www.un.org/esa/population/publications/worldageing19502050/pdf/80chapterii.pdf

U.S. Census Bureau. (2010). *Current population survey. Population 65 and over in the US.* Retrieved from http://www.census.gov/population

U.S. Department of Health and Human Services (USDHHS). (2010). *Healthy people 2020.* Retrieved from http://www.healthypeople.gov/2020/default.aspx

Vincent, G., & Velkoff, V. (2010). *The next four decades. The older population in the United States: 2010–2050.* Retrieved from http://www.census.gov/prod/2010pubs/p25-1138.pdf

Wan, H., Sengupta, M., Velkoff, V. A., & DeBarros, K. A. (2005). *Current population reports, P 23-209, 65+ in the United States, 2005.* Washington, DC: U.S. Government Printing Office.

World Bank. (2011). *Life expectancy at birth.* Retrieved from http://data.worldbank.org/indicator/SP.DYN.LE00.IN

Contemporary Gerontological Nursing

KEY TERMS

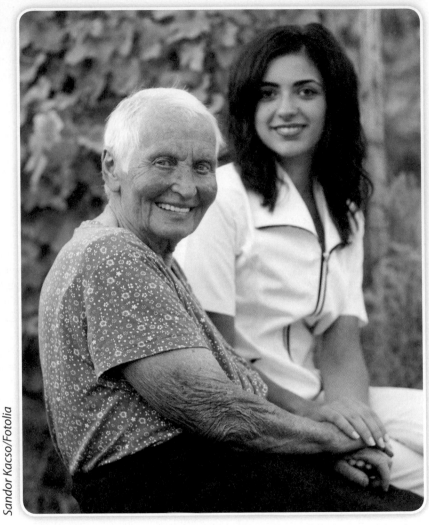

Sandor Kacso/Fotolia

LEARNING OUTCOMES

On completion of this chapter, the reader will be able to:

1. Discuss the nurse's role in caring for older adults.
2. List appropriate educational preparation and certification requirements of the gerontological nurse generalist and specialist.
3. Identify components of the long-term care system.
4. Describe the ANA standards and scope of practice for gerontological nursing.

5. Apply the use of functional health patterns in the formulation of a nursing diagnosis.
6. Recognize the basis and use of QSEN standards to support and improve quality nursing care.
7. Relate the uses and need for gerontological nursing research as support for evidence-based practice.
8. Summarize effective communication techniques appropriate for use with the older adult.

Working with older people is one of the most rewarding and challenging opportunities in the nurse's professional career. Sometimes seen as a difficult or depressing specialization, gerontological nursing offers unique joys and rewards. Many nurses enjoy working with older people because they enjoyed a special relationship with a positive role model of aging such as a grandparent. Those of us lucky enough to have laughed with and loved an older person know the joy of caring and the wisdom that can be gained in these relationships.

We owe a debt of gratitude to the pioneer gerontological nurses who paved the way for us. In the 1920s, a few visionary nurses began to identify the need for a specialization in caring for older people. This need was based on observations and evidence that older people responded differently to illness, disease, and treatments based on their age and general state of health. These nurses also recognized that institutional settings such as old age homes or boarding houses were appropriate settings for gerontological nurses to deliver health care outside of the traditional acute care hospital. In 1925, geriatrics, the medical specialty focusing on diagnosing and treating disease of older people, began to emerge. Nursing soon followed and nursing leaders began to call for nurses to consider gerontological nursing a specialty. This was based on the need for nursing services for larger numbers of older people and the trend toward increasing life expectancy.

Scope of Practice

The American Nurses Association (ANA) is responsible for defining the **scope of practice** and **standards** of nursing practice. The scope of practice is defined as a range of nursing functions that are differentiated according to the level of practice, the role of the nurse, and the work setting. The parameters of nursing practice are determined by each state's nurse practice act, professional code of ethics, and nursing practice standards and include each nurse's competency to perform particular nursing activities or functions. The standards are defined as authoritative statements enunciated and promulgated by the profession by which the quality of practice, service, or education can be judged.

The three elements of the scope of practice consist of quality, evidence, and safety. These three elements combined with professional standards, code of ethics, certification, practice rules and regulations, and institutional policies and procedures enable and empower the nurse to achieve self-determination in practice (American Nurses Association, 2010c). The scope of practice encourages gerontological nurses to be creative and individualize care in order to improve the older adult's health care status and quality of life.

In 1966, the ANA established the Division of Geriatric Nursing Practice with the mission of creating standards for quality nursing care for aging persons in all settings. In 1976, the division's name was changed to the Division on Gerontological Nursing Practice to reflect the idea that nursing care of the older adult is holistic and emphasizes health as well as common diseases of old age. In 1970, the ANA published *A Statement on the Scope of Gerontological Nursing Practice*, which established the foundation for the nature and scope of current gerontological nursing practice and addressed the concepts of health promotion, health maintenance, disease prevention, and self-care. This document was revised and updated periodically and the latest revision of this ANA publication involves collaboration between the ANA and selected members from several national nursing organizations. It is intended to be a guide to current practice in conjunction with other documents that articulate the values of professional nursing. While the *Scope and Standards of Gerontological Nursing Practice* (ANA, 2010c) apply to all professional nurses, the gerontological standards contain specific criteria for defining expectations and competent care associated with basic and advanced clinical practice of gerontological nursing. As in the past, the primary goal of **gerontological nursing** is defined as the provision of high-quality care to older adults. Gerontological nurses additionally employ a shared body of skills and knowledge to address the full range of needs related to aging. These specialists lead interprofessional teams and collaborate with older adults and their significant others to promote autonomy, wellness, optimal functioning, and comfort and quality of life from healthy aging to end of life (ANA, 2010c).

These standards apply in all clinical practice settings, including acute care institutions, ambulatory treatment centers and clinics, home care, long-term care facilities, and adult day care centers. The ongoing revision and refinement of these standards reflect the rapid growth of the practice of gerontological nursing and the challenges that result from the evolving healthcare needs of older adults. The ANA envisions the standards of practice, the *Code of Ethics for Nurses*, and specialty certification as the basis for high-quality, safe, and evidence-based nursing practice.

Gerontological Specialty Certification

In 1973, the first gerontological nurses were certified by the ANA to provide tangible recognition of professional achievement in a defined functional or clinical area of nursing. **Certification** is defined as the formal process by which clinical competence is validated in a specialty area of practice (ANCC, 2012). The certification process consists of a written examination developed and reviewed by nursing experts. Certification as a gerontological nurse assures the public, nursing colleagues, and the employer that the nurse possesses specialized skills and knowledge in providing care to older people. Certified nurses may be eligible for additional monetary compensation and promotion or advancement.

Nurses can become certified as gerontological nurses or as **advanced practice registered nurses (APRNs)** based on their education and knowledge, skills, and experience. Nurses with associate, diploma, or baccalaureate degrees in nursing can seek certification as gerontological nurses if they are currently registered as a nurse in the United States or one of its territories, have practiced the equivalent of 2 years full time as a registered nurse (RN), and have a minimum of 2,000 hours of clinical practice within the past 3 years (see the American Nurses Credentialing Center website for complete eligibility requirements). Specialist nurses function in a variety of settings and may coordinate services and manage care for older people. They may serve as direct care providers, case managers, and nurse leaders and administrators within many settings of the healthcare system. Once certified, nurses may indicate their certification by signing their name and the initials RN-BC (Registered Nurse, Board Certified).

APRNs with master's degrees (clinical nurse specialists and nurse practitioners) may seek certification as adult-gerontology specialists. Once certified, they may use the credentials AGNP-BC (Adult-Gerontological Nurse Practitioner, Board Certified) or CNS-BC (Clinical Nurse Specialist, Board Certified). The different credentials distinguish among levels of certification within the nursing profession, to other healthcare professionals, and to patients and their families. Advanced practice adult-gerontological nurses serve as primary care providers and focus on health promotion, disease prevention, and long-term management of chronic conditions and their exacerbations that require prompt and intensive nursing interventions. AGNPs deliver primary care to older patients and have considerable autonomy addressing healthcare problems, often with prescriptive authority. CNSs provide direct and indirect care to patients and their families and serve as consultants to staff on complex issues of patient care. In some instances, the roles of the CNS and AGNP are interchangeable, but often the AGNP focuses more attention on the direct provision and evaluation of care, whereas the CNS focuses more attention on the educator and consultative role. Advanced practice nurses play an important role in caring for older patients by preventing, recognizing, and treating common problems and illnesses that are major causes of morbidity and mortality in the older adult. Timely care in the nursing home setting has been shown to decrease inappropriate hospital admissions and transfers.

On October 25, 2004, the members of the American Association of Colleges of Nursing (AACN) endorsed the *Position Statement on the Practice Doctorate in Nursing* (DNP). The AACN members voted to move the current level of preparation necessary for advanced nursing practice from the master's degree to the doctorate level (DNP) by 2015. Although master's education will continue, it is envisioned that the master's degree will be reconceptualized to be a generalist degree as a clinical nurse leader (CNL) and specialty education will occur at the doctoral level. The DNP will not replace the PhD, the research doctorate, but is designed for those in direct clinical practice who will be able to apply the principles of evidence-based practice. The transition date of 2015 for the DNP was set far enough in the future to give programs enough time to make a smooth transition and address the role of master's education (AACN, 2011). Table 2-1 summarizes the pathways to certification in gerontological nursing.

The American Nurses Credentialing Center (ANCC) supports the development and administration of the certification examinations based on the ANA's scope and standards of practice. ANCC defines practice for the gerontological nurse as follows:

> Nurses who work primarily with older adults incorporate gerontological competencies in order to assess, manage and implement health care to meet the specialized needs of older adults and evaluate the effectiveness of such care. The nurse's primary challenge is to identify and use the strengths of older adults and assist them to maximize their independence, minimize disability, and where appropriate,

TABLE 2-1	Pathways to Certification in Gerontological Nursing		
Academic Degree	**Required License**	**Certification Eligibility**	**Credential**
Associate degree (ADN) Baccalaureate degree (BSN)	Registered nurse with 2 years of practice, 2,000 hours of clinical practice, and 30 continuing education hours in the past 3 years	Gerontological nurse	RN-BC (Registered Nurse, Board Certified)
Master's degree with APRN specialization (MSN) Doctor of nursing practice (DNP) with APRN specialization	RN licensure and completion of a minimum of 500 supervised clinical hours; completion of advanced pathophysiology, pharmacology, and health assessment courses	Adult-gerontological nurse practitioner or clinical nurse specialist	AGNP-BC (Adult-Gerontological Nurse Practitioner, Board Certified) or AGCNS-BC (Adult-Gerontological Clinical Nurse Specialist, Board Certified)

BOX 2-1 — Example of Nursing Actions Based on Knowledge and Skills for Gerontological Nurses (ANA, 2010)

1. Inform and assist patients with clinical capacity to make health care decisions. Avoid jargon and provide adequate time and information.
2. Implement nursing interventions based upon current evidence and guidelines.
3. Collaborate with inter-professional team members to improve the care and quality of life of older adults.
4. Provide expert nursing care across the spectrum of health care settings including acute care, rehabilitation, institutional and community-based long-term care, and palliative and hospice care when appropriate.
5. Advocate for older patients and their families when indicated to assist them to maximize services within a complex health care system.
6. Promote ethical practice by recognizing ethical dilemmas and referring these dilemmas to colleagues and/or ethical committees for discussion and resolution.
7. Ensure a complete and holistic patient assessment has been performed in order to identify, plan, deliver and evaluate the nursing care plan.
8. Become expert in the recognition and differences between normal changes of aging versus disease-related signs and symptoms in order to identify atypical and subtle signs and symptoms of disease in the older adult.
9. Utilize evidence-based communication techniques appropriate for older adults to establish a therapeutic relationship.
10. Recognize and respect the provisions of advance directives if already in place or assist the older adult to establish advance directives if not previously specified.
11. Engage in lifelong learning and continued professional development in order to provide high quality and safe nursing care.
12. Provide ongoing support to caregivers, spouse, significant others and family members.
13. Educate the older adult and family about healthy behaviors, care and monitoring of chronic illness, and ways to prevent acute illness.
14. Serve as a role model for other caregivers by advocating for the autonomy of the older adult and providing holistic, dignified care.

achieve a peaceful death. Nurses actively involve older adults and family members, where possible, in decision making which impacts the quality of the older adult's everyday life (ANCC, 2008).

The responsibilities of the gerontological nurse include direct care, management and development of the professional and other nursing personnel, and evaluation of care and services for the older adult. All professional nurses practicing gerontological nursing need the basic knowledge and skills to perform the highest level of care. Box 2-1 lists the ANA-required knowledge and skills for gerontological nurses.

Standards and Practice of Gerontological Nursing

The *Standards of Clinical Gerontological Nursing Care* describe the necessary competencies of care for each step of the nursing process, including assessment, diagnosis, outcome identification, planning, implementation, and evaluation (Box 2-2). These competencies are the essential foundation of the actions taken by gerontological nurses when caring for their patients.

These standards enable the nursing profession to identify and meet the professional responsibility to deliver quality patient care to older persons. For further information about the *Scope and Standards of Gerontological Nursing Practice,* go to the ANA website. Performance standards are defined and each includes measurement criteria.

Nurses can be proud of a long history as leaders in public health and home care nursing, because these systems address many needs of older people. Nurses provide valuable primary care to older people, seek out needed referrals, eliminate costly duplication of services, and provide continuity of care within a chaotic healthcare system. Nurses comprise the greatest number of healthcare providers to older people in hospitals, long-term care facilities, and community-based settings including home care.

There are approximately 3 million registered nurses in the United States, with 85% actively practicing nursing. Ninety percent of these nurses are female, 16.8% come from minority backgrounds, 62% work in hospitals, 34% have baccalaureate degrees, 4% have master's degrees, and 0.03% hold doctorates. Most nurses have associate degrees (45%) and the majority of new graduates come from associate degree programs (5.4%) (Health Resources and Services Administration [HRSA], 2010).

Workforce and Quality of Care

Teachers with master's-level preparation have a mean age of 49, and doctorally prepared teachers have a mean age of 53.5, indicating that within the next 10 to 20 years, large numbers of nursing faculty members will be leaving teaching and retiring. Faculty shortages limit the number of students that can be admitted to nursing programs and many schools are unable to accept qualified applicants because of inadequate faculty size. The recent slowdown in

---

BOX 2-2   **Examples and Application of the ANA Standards of Clinical Gerontological Nursing Care**

Standard I: Assessment

A systematic and complete assessment that is culturally appropriate is the basis for development of the nursing care plan. Many common problems affecting the older adult begin with vague signs and symptoms. In order to adequately treat the problem, a careful assessment is needed.

Standard II: Diagnosis

Organizing the assessment information independently or with other members of the interprofessional team into medical and nursing diagnoses helps form the basis for care interventions.

Standard III: Outcome Identification

Identifying and setting mutually agreed upon goals or outcomes with the older person's and family's input can help with resource allocation and indicate which members of the interprofessional team are needed to improve health and functional status.

Standard IV: Planning

The plan establishes the interventions needed to achieve the stated outcomes.

Standard V: Implementation

The gerontological nurse along with others on the interprofessional team implements the plan and notes the response to the various interventions. Evidence-based nursing interventions might be direct (direct provision of nursing care) or indirect (e.g., advocacy, sharing information with others on the team, referral to ethics committees). Input from the older person and family is crucial during the implementation process.

Standard VI: Evaluation

The older adult's response to the plan is noted and used to evaluate the effectiveness of nursing care. Progress towards the identified outcomes may be satisfactory or it may be necessary to modify the plan and begin the process again by collecting new data, revising the nursing diagnoses and modifying the plan of care.

economic growth has resulted in many nurses delaying retirement or moving from part-time to full-time positions in order to increase earnings. Despite these factors, new job advertisements were up 46% from last year, indicating that nurses continue to be sought after in the job market (Raphael, 2011).

Despite the current easing of the nursing shortage due to the recession, the U.S. nursing shortage is projected to grow to 260,000 registered nurses by 2025 (Buerhaus, Auerbach, & Staiger, 2009). A shortage of this magnitude would be twice as large as any nursing shortage experienced in this country since the mid-1960s. There is a growing demand for nurses with skills to treat patients with complex health needs, and the shortage is expected to worsen as the aging population increases. More than 19,400 RN vacancies exist in long-term care facilities and 116,000 open positions exist in acute care hospitals, translating into a national RN vacancy rate of 8.1% (American Healthcare Association, 2010).

A nursing shortage has serious implications for the quality of patient care. Registered nurses play an important role in all sites where older people receive care including acute care hospitals. A recent study examined the relationship between RN staffing levels and patient mortality and found that below-target nurse staffing and high patient turnover are independently associated with the risk of death among patients. These findings suggest that hospitals, payers, and those concerned with the quality of care should pay increased attention to assessing the frequency with which actual RN staffing levels match patients' needs for expert nursing care (Needleman et al., 2011).

Another recent study found that inadequate RN staffing at mealtime is a barrier to adequate nutritional intake in nursing homes. Serious consequences related to poor nutrition include dehydration and aspiration leading to pneumonia (Smith, Greenwood, Payette, et al., 2007). A more recent analysis found a direct relationship between nurse staffing levels in nursing homes and the quality of resident care. It was noted that approximately 30% of nursing homes surveyed reported that they were not staffed at the minimum RN staffing level. By hiring more nursing staff, nursing home providers can lower deficiency scores and improve quality. In doing so, they can improve their ability to attract consumers who are exploring long-term care options (Hyer et al., 2011). Consumers can visit the Nursing Home Compare website to find nursing homes in their area, compare quality, and choose a home that meets their needs.

Hospitals remain the major employer of nurses, although the number of nurses employed in other sectors has increased. During 2010–2011 about 60% of RNs worked in hospitals (down from 66% in 1980). Public and community health settings, ambulatory care, and other noninstitutional health settings increased RN employment by 155% during the same 20-year period. Hospital lengths of stay have decreased, and many older patients are now recuperating in long-term care facilities or at home (U.S. Bureau of Labor Statistics, 2010). Consequently, nursing homes and home care nurses are caring for patients with a greater range of clinical needs.

While the job opportunities for RNs will continue to grow, opportunities will vary at different employment sites. For instance, hospital openings will grow at a rate of 17%, nursing facility openings at 25%, and positions in physicians' offices at 48%. The increasing diversity of the U.S. population, the growing number of vulnerable individuals, and the challenges of caring for increasing numbers of people with complex chronic illnesses call for revised thinking about the delivery of health care and the education of health professionals (Genworth, 2011). Nurse educators and policymakers are addressing the crucial issues of student recruitment and strengthening the infrastructures within the healthcare system to support health care and education of health professionals (HRSA, 2011).

Long-Term Care

In the United States, there are approximately 16,000 nursing homes and 1.7 million nursing home beds. The current nursing home occupancy rate is about 86%, and the number of beds and nursing home residents began to decline in 1999 (Centers for Disease Control and Prevention [CDC], 2011). This decline has been attributed to the rise of assisted living facilities and community-based services that can delay or prevent nursing home placement in older persons requiring assistance with activities of daily living. Also interesting to note is that the number of discharges has increased each year. This indicates that many long-term care facility residents are short-stay rehabilitation patients who receive skilled nursing services and then are discharged to home, while the number of patients requiring ongoing custodial care for chronic illnesses such as Alzheimer's disease has remained relatively stable.

Currently, about 3.2 million Americans will spend at least some time in a long-term care facility, but this percentage is declining based on better health status of many older persons and more choices for care including assisted living facilities and community-based home care (Comarow, 2011). About 7.1% of Americans ages 75 and older lived in nursing homes in 2010, compared with 8.1% in 2000 and 10.2% in 1990 (CDC, 2011). The average nursing home resident is an older woman, age 83.2 years, with at least one disability that necessitates the need for placement in a long-term care facility (U.S. Census Bureau, 2010). Given that nurses assist nursing home residents with bathing, dressing, eating, toileting, walking, and medications, staffing is a serious concern (Harrington, 2010). The National Consumer Voice for Quality Long-Term Care has called for safe staffing standards mandating that long-term care facility residents receive at least 4.13 hours of direct nursing care each day. These requirements should be in place for all residents, regardless of payment source and no waivers of these standards should be allowed. Staffing must be adjusted upward for residents with higher nursing care needs (Harrington, 2010). Surveys indicate that nurse staffing time averaged just 3.5 hours per resident per day (little more than 1 hour per shift) and has decreased 14% since 2000 (American Society on Aging, 2007). There is cause for concern given the dangerously low RN staffing levels in nursing homes, the larger numbers of nursing home residents recuperating from acute illness, and the need for professional nursing judgment to monitor these residents for unpredictable healthcare events. Lower nurse staffing levels are associated with higher rates of urinary catheter use, increased pressure ulcer rates, and lower resident participation in activities. Higher RN staffing levels were found to reduce the likelihood of death (American Association of Retired Persons, 2011).

> **Practice Pearl** ▶▶▶ Safe RN staffing levels save lives!

The Role of the Gerontological Nurse

As the consistent caregivers in most healthcare settings, nurses assume responsibility for providing care and coordinating services throughout a 24-hour period. In addition to focusing on the physical health and function of their patients, gerontological nurses also address issues of access to healthcare services, quality and affordability of health care, and coordination of services by the interdisciplinary team. As health care continues to evolve, new roles will emerge for gerontological nurses. Strong linkages between nurse educators and practicing nurses will be vital to ensure appropriate education and inclusion of relevant clinical experiences in gerontology. This support for emerging clinicians will prepare them to play an important role in providing high-quality nursing care to patients and shaping the healthcare system throughout the remainder of the 21st century. In addition to the traditional role of clinical practitioner, the gerontological nurse may also serve in the role of patient advocate, nurse educator, nurse manager, nurse

consultant, and nurse researcher. Key aspects of each role are as follows:

- **Advocate.** Advances the rights of older persons and educates others regarding negative stereotypes of aging.
- **Educator.** Organizes and provides instructions regarding healthy aging, disease detection, treatment of disease, and rehabilitation to older patients and their families. Also participates in in-service education, continuing education, and training of ancillary personnel as appropriate.
- **Manager.** Maintains current relevant information regarding federal and state regulations, and provides nursing leadership in a variety of healthcare settings.
- **Consultant.** Consults with and advises others who are providing nursing care to older patients with complex healthcare problems. Participates in the development of clinical pathways and quality assurance standards and the implementation of evidence-based practices.
- **Researcher.** Collaborates with established researchers in the development of clinically based studies, assists with data collection and the identification of appropriate research sites, communicates relevant research findings to others, and participates in the presentation of findings at gerontological conferences and publications.

Because they view patients holistically, nurses are in an ideal position to serve in these roles. The primary goal of the gerontological nurse is to help patients achieve their optimal level of physical, mental, and psychosocial well-being.

Quality and Safety Education for Nurses (QSEN)

The overall goal for the Quality and Safety Education for Nurses (QSEN) project is to meet the challenge of preparing future nurses who will have the knowledge, skills, and attitudes (KSAs) necessary to continuously improve the quality and safety of the healthcare systems within which they work (Ironside, 2007).

Funded by the Robert Wood Johnson Foundation, the QSEN project has developed KSAs that nursing students should master during their pre-licensure education. The purpose of these KSAs is to improve patient care and serve as the basis for quality standards and improvement both now and well into the future. The KSAs address the importance of delivering patient-centered nursing care that respects the values, beliefs, and unique needs of each individual patient. This care should be delivered within the context of a well-functioning interprofessional team. Well-functioning teams are characterized by their ability to engage in transparent and respectful methods of communication, collaborate with other team members in decision-making, and reach agreement on overall goals of care with realistic time-frames for achievement.

This care should be based upon current research evidence in order to ensure that the individual goals developed for each patient will be successfully achieved. The appropriate use of informatics and health care technology has the potential to greatly assist health care providers as they function within these interprofessional teams. This technology will provide enhanced methods for effective communication, access to evidence-based protocols, reduce the probability of error by accessing current and relevant patient information, and document progress towards mutually developed goals.

Improvement of patient safety is a prime area of concern in order to minimize risk and harm to patients in the health care system. Areas of focus related to patient safety include analysis of both health care system-related issues and evaluation of outcomes of care delivered by individual healthcare providers. In order to document that these efforts improve the quality of care delivered to patients, the KSAs suggest collection of data on patient outcomes and processes. This data collected over time will provide crucial information needed to evaluate the effectiveness of these efforts to improve overall patient safety and quality (QSEN, 2011).

The Future of Nursing

In 2010, the Institute of Medicine (IOM) published *The Future of Nursing: Leading Change, Advancing Health.* The report notes that the number of nurses has doubled since 1980 and the nursing workforce represents the largest segment of the healthcare workforce. The report advances that nursing must address the increasing demand for safe, high quality, and effective health care and identifies aging and the need to provide complex care to a more diverse population with chronic conditions as one of five national health challenges for the 21st century. This seminal report also notes the need for nurses to take the lead in coordination of the long-term and palliative care provided to chronically ill older persons. The report recommends that the nursing profession double the number of nurses with doctorates by 2020, ensure that nurses engage in lifelong learning, and prepare all nurses to lead change to advance health (IOM, 2010).

Functional Health Pattern Assessment and Nursing Diagnosis

A systematic nursing assessment is necessary to provide holistic care to the older person (ANA, 2010b). This nursing assessment, called **functional health patterns,** is defined as an interrelated group of behavioral areas that provides a view of the whole person and his or her relationship with the environment. This assessment goes beyond physical

function and the diagnosis of disease (the medical model) by also focusing on the interaction of the older person with the environment. Gordon (1994) developed a set of health-related behaviors that form an assessment framework for nurses. This framework consists of 11 functional health patterns that can interact and form the basis for an older person's lifestyle. Although these functional health patterns were not specifically developed for older patients, they are ideally suited for use by gerontological nurses. An older person's functional status is a primary concern because it addresses key issues, including how the patient sees his or her present level of health, usual and preferred lifestyle and activities, demands of daily life and existing support systems, and functional ability. Each of the 11 functional areas guides the nurse to seek information about the older patient and forms a crucial foundation to the care planning process and diagnosis of the patient's nursing needs. The 11 functional health patterns are listed in Table 2-2.

Each of these patterns represents an expression of function within a whole individual and indicates the underlying physical, social, psychological, and spiritual foundations of the individual and his or her relationship with the environment (Gordon, 1994). By concentrating on these 11 crucial areas, the nurse can identify actual or potential health problems and each individual's health and life goals. When this information has been systematically gathered through a nursing assessment, the nurse can make a **nursing diagnosis,** defined as the naming of an individual's response to actual or potential health problems or life processes (Gordon, 1994; NANDA International, 2012).

Nursing Diagnosis

Nursing diagnoses provide the basis for selection of interventions to achieve outcomes for which the nurse is accountable. NANDA International has developed standardized descriptions of human responses frequently encountered by nurses while providing health care to patients. Health problems are defined as dysfunctional patterns, and nursing's major contribution to health care is in preventing and treating these patterns (Gordon, 1994). A pattern is dysfunctional when it deviates from established norms or from an individual's previous condition or goals. These dysfunctional patterns may generate concern on the part of the older person, family members or significant others, healthcare professionals, or others knowledgeable of health promotion and health maintenance activities. Problems or dysfunctional patterns may be identified as actual or potential threats to health, allowing the nurse an opportunity to intervene.

For example, suppose an older man with type 1 diabetes mellitus has a long-established pattern of good control by careful and frequent blood glucose monitoring and

TABLE 2-2	Gordon's Functional Health Patterns
Functional Health Pattern	**Behavioral Area**
Health perception– health management	The older individual's perceived health and well-being along with self-management strategies
Nutritional–metabolic	Patterns of food and fluid consumption relative to metabolic need and nutrient supply
Elimination	Patterns of excretory function and elimination of waste (e.g., bowel, bladder)
Activity–exercise	Patterns of exercise and daily activity. Includes leisure and recreation
Sleep–rest	Patterns of sleep, rest, and relaxation
Cognitive–perceptual	Patterns of thinking and ways of perceiving the world and current events
Self-perception–self-concept	Patterns of viewing and valuing self (body image and psychological state, self-image, etc.)
Roles–relationships	Patterns of engagement with others, ability to form and maintain meaningful relationships, assumed roles
Sexuality–reproductive	Patterns of sexuality and satisfaction with present level of interaction with sexual partners
Coping–stress tolerance	Patterns of coping with stressful events and level of effectiveness of coping strategies
Values–beliefs	Patterns of beliefs, values, and perception of the meaning of life that guide choices or decisions

Source: Adapted from Gordon, 1994. *Nursing diagnosis: Process and application.* St. Louis, MO: Mosby.

appropriate administration of insulin. However, his wife notes that within the past 2 months he has tested his blood glucose less frequently, has failed to administer his pre-meal insulin bolus, and as a result has frequently recorded very high glucose levels. No actual harm has resulted as yet, but the nurse realizes that this behavior increases the patient's risk for complications of diabetes such as damage to the eyes and kidneys and decreased immune function. Further, this behavior is a deviation from previously well-established patterns and indicates a potential health problem. Therefore, the nurse may suspect that something has changed in the patient's underlying physical, social, psychological, and spiritual foundation, and in his relationship to the environment. After systematic assessment in each of the 11 functional health patterns, the nurse may make the diagnosis of *Health Maintenance, Ineffective.* The ability to formulate an accurate nursing diagnosis will depend on the nurse's adherence to a systematic approach, the application of relevant clinical skills, the nurse's experience, and the nurse's knowledge of the norms and presentation of disease in the older person.

Care Planning and Setting Realistic Goals

After completing an assessment and reaching appropriate nursing diagnoses, the nurse formulates a plan of care. The goals of the care planning process should be individualized

> **Practice Pearl** ▶▶▶ A common omission made by gerontological nurses is to implement a nursing care plan without first obtaining an accurate diagnosis of the patient's problem. For instance, an older person may be placed on a liquid nutritional supplement to reverse weight loss without an understanding of why the person is losing weight. The patient may be depressed, have a developing cancer, or be unable to chew because of ill-fitting dentures. Appropriate nursing interventions would vary in each of these circumstances.

to reflect the older adult's values. The overall goals of nursing care are to influence health outcomes, to improve or maintain the older person's health status, or to provide comfort care at the end of life. Gerontological nurses will often focus on improvement of the patient's quality of life, improvement of functional status, and promotion of well-being.

The clarity and achievability of the goals are critical to the development of an effective plan of care. Goals of nursing care should:

- Be linked to the nursing diagnoses.
- Be mutually formulated with the older adult, family, and interdisciplinary team whenever possible.
- Be culturally appropriate.

- Be attainable in relationship to available resources and the care setting.
- Include a time frame for attainment.
- Adequately reflect associated benefits and costs.
- Provide direction for continuity of care.
- Be measurable.

ANA, 2010c.

Beginning gerontological nurses are sometimes overwhelmed with the many problems identified by the older adult and the numerous nursing diagnoses generated from the assessment. One of the first steps is to assign priority to the problems diagnosed. Problems with high priority include those that have a potential for immediately impacting negatively on health status, those of concern to the older person and the family, and those that negatively affect function and quality of life. Other problems can be deferred and addressed at a later time. Patients can become overwhelmed when well-meaning healthcare providers attempt to do too much at one time.

For instance, imagine the situation in which Mr. Jones, 84 years old, visits a blood pressure screening clinic in a senior citizen center and is found to have an extremely elevated blood pressure reading of 158/92. During the encounter with the nurse, the patient relates that although he has a primary care physician, he has not seen his physician for several years. He further reports that his wife was very ill and recently passed away, but during her illness, he focused all his time and attention on the provision of her care. In her role as *clinician*, the nurse is alarmed that Mr. Jones has an elevated blood pressure, has not had his cholesterol checked in several years, has not had a screening colonoscopy, and has never received the pneumococcal vaccine. Further, the nurse notes that Mr. Jones is actively grieving his wife's recent death. However, the nurse realizes that the most immediate need Mr. Jones has at this time is to visit his physician for further evaluation and treatment of his elevated blood pressure. In her *advocate* role, the nurse advises Mr. Jones to phone his physician to request a problem-focused evaluation at this time and to follow up with an appointment for a full physical examination and screening at a later date. The nurse offers to assist Mr. Jones should he have trouble arranging an appointment within the next few days. Further, in her *educator* role, the nurse discusses the health risks associated with hypertension so that Mr. Jones understands the need for the appointment with his physician. Additionally, the nurse questions Mr. Jones about his grief and assesses his depression utilizing the Geriatric Depression Scale.

The nurse hopes to develop a trusting relationship with the patient, encouraging him to express his values and concerns, and to work with him over time on issues relating to his health. To increase the chance of success, the nurse will address one problem at a time (Blissmer et al., 2010).

Mr. Jones's nursing diagnoses include *Health Maintenance, Ineffective* and *Grieving, Risk for Complicated.* Desired goals for Mr. Jones include the following:

1. Identifies positive beliefs regarding the benefits of taking action to seek medical attention to promote health and prevent illness.
2. Achieves a therapeutic relationship with a nurse at the senior center in order to develop a long-range plan to reduce risk of future illness or disease.
3. Identifies resources that will assist him to engage in appropriate action.

Nursing interventions appropriate to these goals might include the following:

1. Urge Mr. Jones to phone his physician or healthcare provider within the next 3 days to schedule a blood pressure evaluation. Provide him with a written copy of his blood pressure reading to take to the physician.
2. Educate Mr. Jones regarding the immediate health risks associated with an elevated blood pressure.
3. Assess insurance status and availability of the patient's healthcare provider.
4. Assess need for transportation to and from the provider's office and identify community resources available to assist if needed.
5. Identify family members or significant others who may accompany the patient and provide comfort and support, if he so desires.
6. Schedule a follow-up appointment with Mr. Jones to return to the screening clinic next week.

> ***Practice Pearl*** ▶▶▶ Use measurable verbs when establishing goals of care. The nurse should use the words *states, performs, identifies, has an increase/decrease in, specifies,* and *administers*. The words *accepts, knows, appreciates,* and *understands* should be avoided because they are not measurable (Carpenito-Moyet, 2011).

Assigning priority to problems is usually done with input from the patient and family as well as the interdisciplinary team. Some problems needing immediate attention can be resolved by nursing interventions, and some require referral to others, including family members, nursing colleagues, or interdisciplinary members of the healthcare team. A well-functioning interdisciplinary team demands that the participants take into account the contributions of other team members and communicate effectively in all phases of the care planning process (American Chronic Pain Association, 2011).

> **Practice Pearl** ▶▶▶ It is generally accepted that an interdisciplinary team can deliver the best health care to the older person. The complexity of problems and concerns common to the older person often requires a team approach to practice. The gerontological nurse is a key member and often serves as leader of the interdisciplinary healthcare team.

Another critical issue in goal formulation is the ability of the gerontological nurse to set realistic and achievable goals. When the nurse sets goals that are unattainable, the nurse positions the patient for failure. Once older patients feel they have failed to meet the goals established by their healthcare providers, they may not keep follow-up appointments, they may become depressed and blame themselves for being weak or lazy, or they may manufacture excuses to protect themselves from criticism. For instance, a 74-year-old obese woman was informed by her healthcare provider that she must lose weight to ease her back pain and increase her mobility. The unrealistic goal set by the provider was to lose 10 lbs within the next month. This was extremely difficult for the patient, because she was unable to exercise or move freely because of her back pain. At the end of the month she felt as if she had failed because she had only lost 5 lbs. She failed to return for her follow-up appointment, fearing she had disappointed her healthcare provider. If the provider had gained input from the patient and set a more realistic goal, the patient's weight loss could have been seen as a valuable first step in a long process toward achieving an ideal body weight.

> **Practice Pearl** ▶▶▶ When older people have made poor lifestyle choices for many years, the result is often progressive chronic illness. It is unreasonable to think that these chronic health problems can be resolved within a short period of time. The nurse should work with older patients over time as they begin the journey toward lifestyle modification and activities aimed at reducing risk and promoting health.

Implementation of the Nursing Care Plan

After the goals of care have been carefully selected, the gerontological nurse will choose appropriate direct and indirect interventions in collaboration with the older adult, the family (if appropriate), and the interdisciplinary care team. The nursing profession must identify its unique focus

and demonstrate accountability in terms of that focus. The nursing interventions identified on the nursing care plan demonstrate that accountability and communicate to the nursing staff the particular problems of the older patient and the prescribed interventions for directing and evaluating the care given (Carpenito-Moyet, 2011). The interventions are selected on the basis of the needs, desires, and resources of the older adult and accepted nursing practice (ANA, 2010a). Appropriate nursing interventions may include the following:

- Assisting the older patient to a higher level of function or self-care
- Identifying health promotion activities
- Identifying disease prevention and screening activities
- Health teaching
- Counseling
- Seeking consultation
- Collecting data on an ongoing basis and refining the initial nursing assessment
- Exploring treatment choices, including pharmacological and nonpharmacological options
- Implementing palliative care and holistic care of the dying or seriously ill patient
- Referring the patient to community resources
- Managing the patient's case
- Evaluating and educating ancillary caregivers and family

ANA, 2010a.

Nursing interventions will be selected based on the following:

1. Linkage to the desired outcome
2. Characteristics of the nursing diagnosis
3. Strength of the research associated with the intervention
4. Probability of successfully implementing the intervention
5. Acceptability of the intervention to the older person and others involved in the plan of care
6. Assurance that the intervention is safe, ethical, culturally competent, and appropriate
7. Documentation of the intervention
8. Knowledge, skills, experience, and creativity of the nurse

ANA, 2010c.

The *Nursing Outcomes Classification (NOC)* is a comprehensive, standardized classification of patient/client outcomes developed to evaluate the effects of nursing interventions (Iowa Intervention Project, 2008). These standardized outcomes are useful for ensuring quality documenting in electronic records, providing standardized outcomes for nursing research, and guiding nursing education. The outcomes have been tested in hospitals, community settings, long-term care facilities, and other clinical sites. Further, the NOC outcomes assist in tracking patient outcomes over long periods of time and across various settings. NOC is one of the standardized languages recognized by the ANA (Iowa Intervention Project, 2008).

The *Nursing Interventions Classification (NIC)* provides examples of nursing interventions based on theoretical or clinical perspectives (Iowa Intervention Project, 2008). NIC is a comprehensive, research-based, standardized classification of interventions that nurses perform. It is useful for clinical documentation, communication of care across settings, integration of data across systems and settings, effectiveness research, productivity measurement, competency evaluation, reimbursement, and curricular design. The classification includes the interventions that nurses do on behalf of patients, both independent and collaborative interventions, both direct and indirect care. NIC can be used in all settings (from acute care intensive care units, to home care, to hospice, to primary care) and all specialties (from critical care to ambulatory care and long-term care).

Nursing interventions based on clinical guidelines are sometimes published with a coding system that indicates the strength of the research associated with a particular recommendation. The gold standard for achieving the highest ranking is an intervention that has been tested in a randomized controlled clinical trial. Randomized controlled clinical trials are thought to have the strongest design and thus have the best chance of establishing a cause-and-effect relationship between a nursing intervention and the desired outcome of care. When the Agency for Healthcare Research and Quality (formerly known as the Agency for Health Care Policy and Research) first published its clinical practice guidelines in 1993, the expert panel charged with developing the guidelines developed a coding system to indicate the strength of the available evidence on the recommended interventions. This system includes criteria for classification and level of evidence as illustrated in Table 2-3.

For example, the gerontological nurse wishing to engage in evidence-based practice regarding cardiovascular disease prevention in women can visit the National Guideline Clearinghouse website to find the recommendation that women should engage in 30 minutes of moderate intensity exercise on most or all days of the week in order to prevent cardiovascular disease (National Guideline Clearinghouse, 2007). This recommendation is graded Class I Level B indicating that the recommendation is useful and effective based on limited evidence; however, it is rated as useful

TABLE 2-3	Classification and Level of Evidence
Classification	**Relative Utility in Clinical Practice**
Class I	Intervention is useful and effective
Class IIa	Weight of evidence/opinion is in favor of usefulness/efficacy
Class IIb	Usefulness/efficacy is less well established by evidence/opinion
Class III	Intervention is not useful/effective and may be harmful
Level of Evidence	**Recommendation Based On**
A	Sufficient evidence from multiple randomized trials
B	Limited evidence from single randomized trial or other nonrandomized studies
C	Based on expert opinion, case studies, or standard of care

Source: U.S. Department of Health and Human Services. Agency for Healthcare Research and Quality (AHRQ). (2002).

and effective in practice. This classification system guides nursing interventions and identifies interventions that may not be useful or may even be harmful. These guidelines are periodically updated as new evidence becomes available.

Gerontological nurses choose appropriate nursing interventions based on their knowledge of practice and the supports available in the practice environment. In the dependent role, the nurse will implement physician orders according to safe and acceptable standards of practice. Administration of treatments, medications, therapeutic diets, and preparation for diagnostic testing will usually be specified in writing for implementation by the nursing staff. In the independent role, the nurse will establish and implement nursing actions to carry out the nursing care plan. The goal of the nursing action is to direct individualized care of the older patient and prescribe care to prevent, reduce, or eliminate the actual or potential problem identified in the nursing diagnosis.

The nursing care plan also identifies nursing interventions that have proven successful based on trial and error. These interventions when recorded can be helpful to nurses working other shifts, nurses "floating" to the unit who may not know the patient well, or agency or temporary nurses

Weblink: National Guideline Clearinghouse

who do not know the patient at all. For instance, when nurses are attempting to increase fluid intake to an older patient who is at risk for a fluid volume deficit, a nursing intervention may be as follows:

Goal: Increase Fluid Intake
1. Increase fluids to 2,500 mL/24 hours:
   a. 1,500 mL on day shift
   b. 700 mL on evening shift
   c. 300 mL on night shift
2. Prefers apple juice or cool water.
3. Offer fluids between meals with patient in sitting position.
4. Record fluid intake on the intake/output sheet at patient's bedside.
5. Assess and note patient's satisfaction with the fluid intake plan and modify schedule/routine as needed.

Carpenito-Moyet, 2011.

During implementation of the nursing intervention, the gerontological nurse will carefully monitor the patient's response, the response of others involved in the care delivery, achievement of the outcome, alternative interventions that may supplement or replace the specified interventions, the accuracy and safety of the intervention, the competency of others in delivering the care, and validation of the appropriateness of the intervention (Carpenito-Moyet, 2011). Nursing interventions can be added, deleted, or modified as part of the ongoing process of providing individualized care.

Evaluation

Evaluation is the final component of the nursing process. To obtain the data needed for the evaluation, the gerontological nurse systematically gathers and records actual patient outcomes and compares these outcomes to the patient outcomes set as goals in the nursing care plan. The nurse will seek input from the patient, family, and others involved in the care as appropriate and as necessary. It is important to consider information from the physical, social, and psychological assessment of the patient; information from diagnostic testing; level of satisfaction with care; and documentation of the costs and benefits associated with the treatment. The initial assessment and nursing diagnosis may be revised with new goals and nursing interventions specified if appropriate: the problem has been resolved and the plan should be continued as specified, the problem has been resolved and the nursing interventions can be revised or discontinued, or the problem still exists. If the problem still exists despite implementation of the nursing care plan, that may indicate the interventions were not carried out as specified, the interventions

were not effective in alleviating the problem, or there was an error or omission in the initial nursing assessment and diagnosis. At this point, the nurse has the opportunity to modify and revise the nursing care plan.

Some healthcare institutions routinely gather evaluation data as part of an ongoing quality assurance project. By gathering outcome data on large numbers of older patients, nurse managers and clinicians can identify opportunities for improvement. Quality assurance data will often focus on negative outcomes such as falls with injury, medication errors, unintentional weight loss, development of decubitus ulcers, and incidence of urinary tract infections. Should problems in these areas be identified, the gerontological nurse may become involved in the development of policies, procedures, and practice guidelines to improve quality of care and quality of life for the older adult (ANA, 2010c).

Research Agenda

Per ANA Standard VII, gerontological nurses interpret, apply, and evaluate research findings to inform and improve gerontological nursing practice (ANA, 2010c). The gerontological nurse participates by identifying clinical problems appropriate for study, gathering data, and interpreting findings to improve the nursing care provided to older adults. Additionally, gerontological nurses use research findings to provide evidence-based nursing interventions to their patients. The use of evidence-based practice is considered the best method for delivery of skilled and compassionate care to older adults.

Many gerontological nurses work as part of research teams and collaborate with nursing colleagues with advanced education and research training. Further, the gerontological nurse may serve on an institutional review board in order to give input on the protection of rights for research subjects involved in clinical research activities.

Nurses have long been recognized as direct healthcare providers, but the role of nurse as scientist is less recognized. In the United States, federal funding for nursing research began in the 1950s. It was not until 1986 that the National Center for Nursing Research, later to become the National Institute of Nursing Research (NINR), was established within the National Institutes of Health (NIH). NINR's mission is to support the science that advances the knowledge of nurses in order to:

- Build the scientific foundation for clinical practice.
- Prevent disease and disability.
- Manage and eliminate symptoms caused by illness.
- Enhance end-of-life and palliative care.

National Institute of Nursing Research [NINR], 2011.

Several private foundations (Robert Wood Johnson, Soros, Hartford Foundation, Research Retirement Foundation, American Association of Retired Persons) as well as federal agencies (National Cancer Institute, National Institute of Mental Health, National Institute on Aging) have lobbied for greater funding for gerontological nursing research. Nursing research efforts are needed to improve the delivery of health care to older adults. The demographics of an aging population make this imperative.

During the past 10 years, knowledge regarding the aging process and the heterogeneity of older adults, as well as their special needs and strengths, has made gerontology a viable area of study and clinical practice. Many of the issues affecting older people have been traditionally managed by nurses. It is not surprising that much of the research in these areas has been done by nurse researchers and that findings from many nursing studies have been used by practicing nurses. The NINR Strategic Plan for 2006–2010 identifies four current areas to advance nursing science: promoting health and preventing disease; improving quality of life through self-management, symptom management, and caregiving; eliminating health disparities; and taking the lead in end-of-life research. Often, nursing research focuses on the development of noninvasive, cost-efficient behavioral techniques as alternatives or supplements to the usual care provided to older patients.

Nursing research can lead to broad policy and practice changes. For instance, studies by nurse researchers identified the problems that can result from the use of physical restraints in the clinical setting. Increases in agitation, falls, decubitus ulcers, and urinary and fecal incontinence were documented as harm that can result from physical restraints (Strumpf & Evans, 2008). As a result, the standard of practice and federal law now mandate that physical restraints be used only on an emergency basis when all other methods have been tried without success. This has improved the quality of life for many older patients.

The NINR is the lead institute at NIH in advancing the science of end-of-life care. A nurse researcher and her colleagues have studied quality-of-life issues and have moved beyond the focus of relieving suffering to identify and build on positive psychological strengths and traits in seriously ill people. This radical shift in thinking has led to the establishment of a NINR/NIH funded Center of Excellence in the Francis Payne Bolton School of Nursing with Barbara Daly, PhD, RN, FAAN, as the director and principal investigator (Daly, 2011).

The development of doctoral programs in nursing has played a major role in the production of gerontological research. Nursing research can address basic science and clinical questions. Gerontological nurse researchers have participated in and chaired many review panels across various institutes at NIH. Doctorally prepared nurse researchers now are urged to seek postdoctoral positions and funding.

Only a small percentage of NINR-funded research can be called basic or bench research (NINR, 2011). Most nurse investigators have a clinical background, and the problems they choose to study arise from their interactions with older patients. Nurse researchers are now being urged to collaborate with people from other disciplines, such as engineers and pharmacists, in order to extend the reach of their work beyond nursing alone and make the work easily applicable to real-world settings.

Many nurse researchers present their findings at specialized nursing meetings and interdisciplinary conferences, and publish in nursing and interdisciplinary journals. The relationship between gerontological nursing practice issues and nursing research should be a dynamic one, with each informing the other. However, there is sometimes a lag between the dissemination of a research finding and the use of that finding in clinical practice. This may be the result of four factors:

1. Some nurses may have a natural reluctance to change the way things are done.
2. Some nurses lack training or education in the use and interpretation of research and are hesitant to endorse the findings of research studies.
3. Many practicing nurses do not read research-based journals and therefore are unaware of the findings.
4. Many nurses may doubt the validity or generalizability of the findings and be unwilling to try new techniques in their clinical setting.

NINR, 2011.

Nurse researchers continue to search for effective ways to inform and educate practicing nurses, older patients, and families about important research findings. Websites for specific diseases and problems are useful for those who have access to the Internet; however, some Internet sites are not entirely reputable and older patients may need help and guidance judging the reliability of information found on various websites. Additionally, nurse researchers should publish important clinical findings in practice-based journals and popular magazines read by the general public. Making the research more accessible to the public will better serve patients and their families. In addition, increased media coverage would serve to further the status and credibility of nursing research while showing that nurses' professional knowledge can, and does, make a difference in the health of people (NINR, 2011).

Role by Setting

Gerontological nurses are employed in most healthcare settings. In the United States, the term *long-term health-care delivery system* is now used to designate several types of non–acute care settings in which gerontological nurses have opportunities for practice. Patients requiring long-term care have varying degrees of difficulty in performing activities of daily living. They may have a mental impairment such as Alzheimer's disease, be physically frail, or both. Approximately 8.6 million older adults needed assistance in 2007, with 38% of older adults reporting at least one disability requiring them to seek help with activities of daily living (U.S. Census Bureau, 2010).

> **Practice Pearl** ▶▶▶ Long-term care is different from acute health care. It encompasses services related to maintaining quality of life, preserving individual dignity, and satisfying preferences in lifestyle for someone with a disability severe enough to require the assistance of others in everyday activities (U.S. Department of Health and Human Services, 2011).

About 64% of older people requiring assistance for a disability rely on unpaid care from family or other informal caregivers. Others rely on formal assistance from the long-term healthcare system. These sites of care include the following:

- **Skilled nursing facilities.** Skilled care is delivered by nurses and others to residents. Care may be subacute (Medicare reimbursed, short stay) or chronic (private pay or Medicaid) for older adults requiring custodial care and assistance with activities of daily living.
- **Retirement communities.** Senior citizen retirement communities range in size and scope of services. Some are life care communities and offer coordinated independent living in apartments, assisted living apartments, and nursing home care. Residents can move from one level of care to another as their situation demands. Some retirement communities offer a narrower range of services such as independent apartments only. Others have a clubhouse with activities; some have indoor or outdoor pools, dining rooms with optional meal services, healthcare facilities, and a range of housekeeping services. Usually the resident pays an admission fee and then a monthly fee for rent and services. Some communities have 24-hour supervision and concierge services.
- **Adult day care.** Adult day care is an option for older adults with multiple comorbidities or people who require daytime supervision and activities. Sometimes an older person lives with an adult child who may have to work during the day or otherwise be absent from the home. Some day care centers offer transportation and others do not. Usually the older person and family are offered options for attendance ranging from 1 or 2 days per week to daily attendance. Day care is usually paid for privately and not covered by insurance. Usually meals are served, planned activities are provided, and some health services (e.g., podiatry, immunizations, monitoring of blood pressure, blood glucose testing) may be offered on a private pay basis.
- **Residential care facilities.** Previously called rest homes, these facilities are sometimes large private homes that have been converted to provide rooms for residents who can provide most of their own personal care, but may need help with laundry, meals, and housekeeping. Supervision and health monitoring are usually provided.
- **Transitional care units.** Many acute care hospitals have established transitional care units to provide subacute care, rehabilitation, and palliative care health services to patients who no longer require acute care. Most of these patients are recuperating from major illness or surgery, have complex health monitoring needs, or require palliative care with pain and symptom control. Diagnostic and support services of the acute care facility support the care given on transitional care units as needed.
- **Rehabilitation hospitals or facilities.** Special facilities exist to provide subacute care to patients with complex health needs. These patients may have head injuries or be on ventilators, require aggressive rehabilitation after injury or surgery, or require services and intensive treatments from specialists such as physical therapists, occupational therapists, dietitians, and physiatrists. Usually rehabilitation in these facilities is covered by the patient's private insurance or Medicare.
- **Community nursing care.** Visiting nurse services are an option for many older patients requiring skilled care in the home. The nurse may visit the patient on a regular basis to monitor vital signs, provide education or counseling, administer intramuscular injections, change a dressing and deliver wound care, and provide supervision to home health aides or homemakers. Usually home care is covered by Medicare for the time period when the need for skilled nursing services exists under the direction of a physician.

Many of the long-term care options previously listed are considered private pay and are not covered by insurance. Nationally, spending from all public and private sources for long-term care totaled about $203 billion in 2009, accounting for nearly 10% of all healthcare expenditures (The George Washington University National Health Policy

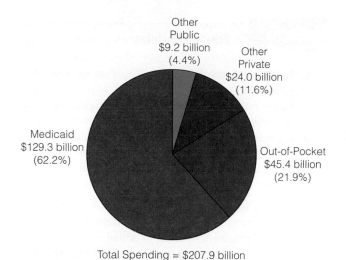

Other
Public
$9.2 billion
(4.4%)

Other
Private
$24.0 billion
(11.6%)

Medicaid
$129.3 billion
(62.2%)

Out-of-Pocket
$45.4 billion
(21.9%)

Total Spending = $207.9 billion

Figure 2-1 ▶▶▶ National spending for long-term care.

Source: National Health Policy Forum. (2011). *The basics: National spending for long-term care and supports.* Washington, DC.

Forum, 2012). Over 66% of expenditures for long-term care services are paid by public programs, primarily Medicaid and Medicare. About 22.6% is paid by patients and their families. Figure 2-1 ▶▶▶ shows the major sources financing long-term care expenditures.

Medicaid, the joint federal and state program for low-income individuals, is the largest funding source for long-term care. To qualify for Medicaid, older persons must "spend down" their assets to cover the costs of long-term care. In 2011, the national median yearly rate for a semiprivate room in a nursing home was $68,708 (Genworth, 2011). Medicaid covers about 55% of long-term care spending.

Medicare is a federal program for older people and younger people with disabilities and certain chronic conditions. Medicare offers prescription drug coverage to everyone with Medicare. To get Medicare prescription drug coverage, the older person must join a plan run by an insurance company or other private company approved by Medicare. Each plan can vary in cost and drugs covered. In 2011, after paying a yearly deductible, a copayment is required on covered drugs until the total spent on drugs reaches $2,840. At this point, the older person falls into the "donut hole" or coverage gap where all drugs are paid out-of-pocket up to a yearly limit ($4,550 in 2011). Many legislators are trying to close the gap by offering rebates directly to older persons and discounts on brand-name drugs. Medicare recipients can purchase drug discount cards to help defray some of the cost of their prescription medications. Some older people are forced to choose between buying medicine or buying food. In the Northeast area of the United States, some seniors charter buses to go to Canada where drug prices are much lower. Medicare spending

accounted for only a small percentage of long-term care, covering only up to 100 days of skilled nursing care and rehabilitation after a 3-day hospital stay. Private insurance covers only about 1% of long-term care expenses.

Trends in Financing Health Care for Older Persons

The United States faces unprecedented demographic challenges with the aging of the baby-boom generation. As the share of the population ages 65 and over climbs, federal spending on older people will absorb a larger and ultimately unsustainable share of the federal budget. Federal spending for Medicare, Medicaid, and Social Security are expected to surge, nearly doubling by 2035, as people live longer and spend more time in retirement. Further, advances in medical technology and prescription drugs will likely keep pushing up the costs of health care (Kimbuende, Ranji, Lundy, et al., 2010). A rational approach to these problems with input from gerontological nurses is needed.

It is impossible to predict what will happen in the future, but it is clear that larger numbers of nurses and other healthcare providers with specialized knowledge and training regarding caring for older persons will be needed. Gerontological nurse clinicians, researchers, and educators are needed to prepare the quantity and quality of nurses needed to meet the needs of the older person. Additional needs include more opportunities for ongoing continuing education regarding new nursing interventions and health promotion techniques appropriate for older persons.

Nurses should assume a leadership position in all debates and discussions regarding healthcare reform and financing relating to older people. Gerontological nurses recognize the benefits, burdens, and costs of informal caregiving and the need for respite services. Society has a responsibility to maintain a safety net for older people without resources, but the costs of this safety net may mean that choices and options are limited. Debate must ensue around the fundamental question of how much of the financing of long-term care should depend on the individual's own resources and how much is a societal responsibility. Everyone should be educated and urged to become personally prepared. One of the factors contributing to lack of preparation for long-term care is a widespread misunderstanding about what services Medicare will cover. Gerontological nurses can play a key role in this education process.

A number of barriers prevent gerontological nurses and others from being able to respond effectively to rapidly changing healthcare settings and an evolving healthcare system. These barriers need to be overcome to ensure that nurses are well positioned to lead change and advance health.

In 2008, the Robert Wood Johnson Foundation and the IOM launched a 2-year initiative to respond to the need to assess and transform the nursing profession. Through its deliberations, the committee developed four key messages:

- Nurses should practice to the full extent of their education and training.
- Nurses should be full partners, with physicians and other healthcare professionals, in redesigning health care in the United States.
- Nurses should achieve higher levels of education and training through an improved education system that promotes seamless academic progression.
- Effective workforce planning and policy making require better data collection and information infrastructure.

This seminal report has generated an action plan that has generated much needed discussions among nurses and other healthcare professionals. Demonstration projects have been and will be funded in all parts of the United States in order to gather data and generate evidence to implement these goals (IOM, 2010).

Ethics

Gerontological nurses are required to provide nursing services and health care that are responsive to the public's trust and the older person's rights. This ethical practice is guided by the *Code for Nurses with Interpretive Statements* (ANA, 2001).

The gerontological nurse is concerned with the following ethical issues:

- Obtaining informed consent for research and clinical treatment
- Obtaining, clarifying, and carrying out advance directives
- Appropriateness of emergency treatment
- Provision of palliative care, including pain and symptom control, need for self-determination, quality of life, and treatment termination
- Elimination of the use of chemical and physical restraints
- Patient confidentiality including electronic records
- Surrogate decision making
- Access to complementary treatments
- Fair distribution of resources
- Economic decision making

ANA, 2001.

The gerontological nurse follows all ethical principles in the roles of clinician, advocate, case manager, researcher, and administrator. See Box 2-3.

BOX 2-3   **Ethical Principles**

- **Beneficence/nonmaleficence.** To do good and not harm patients.
- **Justice.** To be fair and distribute scarce resources equally to all in need.
- **Autonomy.** To respect patients' needs for self-determination, freedom, and patient rights.

In addition, the nurse is required to follow federal, state, and local law governing aspects of gerontological nursing practice. For instance, suspected or actual abuse or neglect of elders must be reported as required by law. Additionally, the nurse's own value system will influence all clinical and ethical decision making. Each nurse has a unique set of values, morals, and life experiences. In a society with many divergent opinions regarding what can and should be done, the gerontological nurse may engage in ethical inquiry to determine the appropriate course of action. This decision-making process involves examination by the nurse facing a moral dilemma and consideration of conflicting opinions about the applicability of specific ethical rules in an attempt to discover what the best outcome might be in a specific situation. Advances in healthcare technology, changes in social and family systems, the advent of managed care, and an unlimited variety of healthcare choices have added to the complexity of caring for the older adult. Although decisional authority may ultimately be the older patient's responsibility, the decision evolves within the therapeutic relationship with the nurse. The goal is to assist patients to identify and articulate genuine preferences and to make authentic choices.

Ethical decision-making competency involves the acquisition of knowledge and skills, knowledge application, and the creation of an environment that minimizes barriers to ethical practice (Federal Emergency Management Agency, 2010):

- **Knowledge and skills.** Ethical theories, professional codes, professional standards, identification of issues, state and federal regulations
- **Application.** Decision-making theory, mediation, facilitation of strategies to address ethical problems
- **Ethical environment.** Support from nursing administration, role models, mentors, and a system to address and rectify barriers

Our society is comprised of individuals from diverse cultural and ethnic backgrounds. Cultural norms and practice are critical parts of any assessment of patients and families.

Different subgroups respond to various situations in ways that do not always reflect the views of the dominant culture (ANA, 2001). A conflict commonly encountered when caring for older people centers around the issue of disclosure. The family may request that the older patient not be told the diagnosis because of legitimate fears or anxiety about the patient's coping abilities. The healthcare providers may feel that the patient has a right to know. In many cultures (e.g., Asian and Native American), nondisclosure may be the norm. (Refer to Chapter 4 ⬤▭.)

Important aspects of ethical decision making include the following:

- **Assessment.** The older patient's condition, including medical problems, nursing diagnosis, prognosis, treatment goals, and treatment recommendations
- **Relevant contextual factors.** Age, education, life situation, family relationships, setting of care, language, culture, religion, and socioeconomic factors
- **Capability of the patient to make decisions.** Legally competent, clearly incapacitated, diminished capacity, fluctuating mental status, presence of drugs or illness to cloud capacity
- **Patient preferences.** Understanding of condition, views on quality of life, values regarding treatment, and advance directives
- **Needs of the patient as a person.** Psychic suffering, interpersonal dynamics, resources and coping strategies, adequacy of the environment for care
- **Preferences of the family.** Competence as surrogate decision maker, judgment and evidence of knowledge of patient preferences, opinions on quality of life
- **Competing interests.** Interests of family, healthcare providers, healthcare organization, and futile utilization of scarce resources
- **Issues of power or conflict.** Between clinicians and family/patient, among family, among healthcare workers
- **Opportunity for all involved to speak and be heard.** Includes respect for opinions

Perlman, 2006.

After completing the ethical assessment, the nurse should consider ethical standards and guidelines, analyze similar cases in the literature or practice environment, and identify morally acceptable options for resolving the dilemma. The nurse may consult with an ethics team if one is in place, a nursing mentor, or a trusted ethics advisor. All healthcare institutions should have access to an ethics committee. The purpose of the committee is to provide a forum for ethical reflection and discussion of values, to build a moral community, and to attempt to meet the needs

of the patient and other affected individuals through group process and consensus. Ethics committees often validate or provide options regarding ethical dilemmas and support the care team in relation to already planned options (ANA, 2010b).

The interdisciplinary care team can also be convened to address the issue and assist in the process toward consensus. Often, the team can negotiate an acceptable plan of action. If satisfactory resolution cannot be achieved, the team may have to consider judicial review (Perlman, 2006). If a satisfactory resolution is achieved and the plan of action is implemented, evaluation of the plan should be ongoing.

It is the gerontological nurse's responsibility to ensure that the patient and family fully understand treatment options in order to make informed decisions. The nurse also clarifies their wishes to others involved in the care. Gerontological nurses often engage in the process of ethical discernment, discourse, and decision making. Application of ethical principles can assist in the search for the best solutions to complex treatment problems of the older person. Gerontological nurses need to work closely with other disciplines to address ethical issues surrounding care of older adult patients.

> **Practice Pearl ▶▶▶** When an ethical dilemma arises in a clinical practice, nurses should begin an ethical analysis and communicate with colleagues to seek a solution. The process is a way to seek balance, address issues, and understand the needs of all involved.

Communication

Communication is especially important to gerontological nurses. The lines of communication must be clear to develop an appropriate nursing care plan. Gerontological nurses need to communicate effectively with older patients with a variety of physical and cognitive impairments in order to develop a therapeutic relationship with each patient.

Communication is an ongoing, continuous dynamic process including verbal and nonverbal signals. Nonverbal communication is thought to comprise 80% of the communication process and includes body language such as position, eye contact, touch, tone of voice, and facial expression. Nurses should follow these guidelines for verbal communication:

- Do not yell or speak too loudly to patients. Not all older people are hard of hearing. If they are wearing a hearing

aid, yelling can be disturbing. Lowering the tone of your voice is helpful for older persons with presbycusis or loss of hearing for high-frequency tones.

- Try to be at eye level with the patient. Sit down if the patient is sitting or lying down.
- Try to minimize background noise, because it can make it difficult for the patient to hear.
- Monitor the patient's reaction. A puzzled look may mean the patient cannot hear but is ashamed to interrupt.
- Touch the patient if appropriate and acceptable. Many older patients report that they are hardly touched by their caregivers and they appreciate the human contact.
- Supplement verbal instructions with written instructions as needed.
- Do not give long-winded speeches or complicated instructions to persons with cognitive impairment, anxiety, or pain.
- Ask how the patient would like to be addressed. Avoid demeaning terms like *sweetie, honey,* or *dearie.*

Practice Pearl ▶▶▶ An older nursing home patient wears a button stating "Touch me. Wrinkles aren't catching!"

An important part of communication involves attentive listening. Many healthcare providers try to anticipate what may be said and interrupt silent pauses. A careful listener will be rewarded with additional information. Open-ended statements will encourage the patient to talk. It is helpful to practice saying "Tell me more about that . . . " or "How does this affect you?" The nurse should avoid misunderstandings by saying "I'm not sure what you mean" or "On one hand you say. . . , but yet. . . ."

Nurses should not be afraid to acknowledge their feelings. At times, a nurse may feel very sad when a patient is suffering and may even feel like crying. The older patient will probably not expect the nurse to have all the answers or know exactly what to do in all circumstances. The nurse may say, "I don't know how I can help you with this problem" or "I wish there was something I could do to make it better for you." Many times just the caring response and careful listening of the nurse will be a comfort to the patient.

Encouraging reminiscing is usually fruitful when communicating with older patients. Reminiscence involves the

---

BOX 2-4 ▶ **Barriers That Can Disrupt the Communication Process**

1. Fear of one's own aging
2. Fear of showing emotion or being around emotional patients
3. Fear of missing something and feeling the need to write down every detail of the encounter
4. Fear of being called on to rectify every problem verbalized by the patient
5. Lack of knowledge of the patient's culture, goals, and values
6. Unresolved issues with aging relatives in the nurse's own family that can lead to insensitivity
7. Feeling that professional distance must be maintained at all cost
8. Being overworked, or overscheduled, and lacking proper time to communicate with older patients

---

recall of pleasant memories or circumstances. It often gives comfort and reassurance to patients that they can talk about a time in their life when circumstances were better. It also allows the nurse to see the patient as an entire person with a life history and survival skills. If a patient cries, the nurse should offer a tissue, hold the patient's hand if appropriate, and wait a few minutes. Crying can be therapeutic to the older patient and offer release from persistent feelings of sadness. Box 2-4 identifies barriers that can disrupt the communication process.

Many schools of nursing offer students the opportunity to role-play various patient encounters while being videotaped. This is a valuable learning experience. The student may say, "I can't believe I actually said that!" or "Why did I wrinkle my nose and look away when the patient brought that topic up?" Remember, practice makes perfect.

Patient and Family Teaching

Gerontological nurses require skills and knowledge related to teaching patients and families about the key concepts of gerontology and gerontological nursing. The guidelines in the following feature will assist the nurse to assume the role of teacher and coach.

Patient–Family Teaching Guidelines

The following are guidelines that the nurse may find useful when instructing older persons and their families about gerontological nursing in health care.

LEARNING ABOUT GERONTOLOGICAL NURSING

1 What is gerontological nursing?

Gerontological nurses specialize in the nursing care and the health needs of older adults. They plan, manage, and implement health care to meet those needs, and evaluate the effectiveness of such care. They try to maximize independence and function by recognizing the strengths each older person has. Also, gerontological nurses actively involve older adults and family members as much as possible in the decision-making process, which has an impact on the quality of everyday life.

RATIONALE:

Educating the older person and his or her family regarding the goals of gerontological nursing helps to establish credibility and can form the foundation of a trusting and therapeutic relationship.

2 Why is this important to an older person like me?

With aging, an older person's health status can be affected by many factors. Gerontological nurses have extra training to become experts in the factors that can affect health status and function, including management of chronic illness, proper medication use, lifestyle changes to improve health, disease prevention and health promotion techniques, and early detection of diseases.

RATIONALE:

When older persons and their families begin to think of health in old age in a holistic manner, they can move beyond the medical model and begin to understand the importance of making appropriate lifestyle choices in order to stay healthy.

3 What factors do gerontological nurses consider important?

Gerontological nurses consider functional health patterns important. These are the key factors they consider when caring for older patients. These patterns include health management, nutrition, elimination, activity and sleep, cognition and self-perception, role, sexuality, coping and stress, and values and beliefs.

RATIONALE:

The health of older people depends on all of these patterns and as nurses, we consider them all.

4 Where should I go to get further information?

Many hospitals, community health agencies, and clinics have hired and support nurses with special knowledge and expertise in caring for the older person. Ask your healthcare provider for a referral if you would like a visit or consultation with a gerontological nurse. Many gerontological nurse practitioners and clinical specialists work along with physicians and provide care to older people who want to stay healthy or recover after an illness.

RATIONALE:

Seeking information from geriatric specialists and specialty clinics can facilitate the search for resources and help ensure appropriate and accurate sources of information.

5 Should all older people be cared for by gerontological nurses?

The health needs of people over the age of 65 vary greatly. While all nurses caring for adults possess knowledge and skills in caring for older persons, sometimes a specialist is required. Regardless of a person's age or healthcare status, a gerontological nurse is helpful when placement in a long-term care facility is being considered for an older person, family members are feeling stressed or burdened, and the older person is not coping well with illness or disability.

RATIONALE:

Older persons with complicated health problems, frailty, families experiencing stress, or those who are at risk for entering a nursing home should receive care from a gerontological nurse. These elders at risk are the most likely to benefit from specialty care.

CARE PLAN   A Patient With a Cognitive Impairment

Case Study

Mrs. Kepler is an 85-year-old woman recovering from hip surgery. She smiles, nods her head, and looks away whenever any of the nursing staff tries to speak to her. Some staff members think the patient suffers from dementia and lacks the ability to stay focused long enough to carry on a conversation.

Applying the Nursing Process

Assessment

The nurse cannot assume the patient has a cognitive impairment based on this information alone. Further assessment is clearly needed. Perhaps the woman is depressed, is in pain, or suffers from severe hearing loss. Many older patients will look away for fear that the nurse will ask a question that they cannot answer because they have not heard the question.

Diagnosis

Possible nursing diagnoses for Mrs. Kepler include the following:

- *Communication: Verbal, Impaired*
- *Social Interaction, Impaired*

The nurse's goal would be to begin a systematic assessment of all 11 functional health patterns in order to set realistic goals and devise a nursing care plan.

NANDA-I © 2012.

Expected Outcomes

Expected outcomes for the plan of care specify that Mrs. Kepler will:

- Begin to make eye contact and appropriately respond to questions from the nurse.
- Make some effort to communicate level of comfort or presence of pain using verbal or nonverbal techniques.
- Begin to form a therapeutic relationship with the nursing staff and respond appropriately to nursing interventions designed to increase her security and comfort.

Planning and Implementation

The following nursing interventions may be appropriate for Mrs. Kepler:

- Establish a therapeutic relationship.
- Avoid being frustrated or angry when she fails to respond to communication attempts.
- Encourage a family meeting to talk about health issues in general with Mrs. Kepler's permission.

- Examine Mrs. Kepler's ears with an otoscope to check for impacted cerumen.
- Begin a functional health pattern assessment to establish the underlying cause of the patient's communication problems.
- Observe the patient carefully for signs of pain, depression, or discomfort.

Evaluation

The nurse realizes that it may take time to establish a trusting therapeutic relationship with Mrs. Kepler. The nurse will consider the plan a success based on the following criteria:

- Mrs. Kepler will progress through recuperation from her hip surgery with improving function and communication skills.
- A family meeting will be held to discuss the patient's overall health.

CARE PLAN | A Patient With a Cognitive Impairment *(continued)*

■ Mrs. Kepler will use appropriate assistive devices such as hearing aids and eyeglasses to improve communication.

■ Mrs. Kepler will communicate pain or discomfort to the nurses so that appropriate pharmacological and nonpharmacological pain control methods can be administered.

Ethical Dilemma

Other nurses on the floor state, "I never even try to talk to her anymore, because she just gives you that same silly smile in response. It's just more efficient to give her care without even trying to talk with her." How should the nurse respond?

By providing care without explanation, the principle of autonomy is being violated. Although the care is being delivered carefully and competently, the patient may feel anxiety and may not be prepared for what is about to happen to her. The patient may come to dread and fear nursing care and even become defensive or resistive to the care. It may be helpful to role-model appropriate verbal communication with the patient and the careful use of touch and nonverbal communication, consult with the patient's family if appropriate, and seek advice and consultation from others on the healthcare team.

Critical Thinking and the Nursing Process

1. Spend a day or two getting to know older people in your family, community, or church. Ask about their lives, struggles, successes, and regrets.
2. Try to discuss aging with colleagues from other professions such as social work, law, or premedicine. What is their view of gerontological nursing? Do they have accurate information and a good understanding of the nursing role?
3. Do you sometimes feel that nurses are underappreciated? Do your colleagues think of nurses as "pill pushers" and "bandage appliers"? Try to educate them about the importance and autonomy of the nurse's role.
4. How does nursing diagnosis complement medical diagnosis? How does medical diagnosis complement nursing diagnosis?
5. What are the greatest assets the gerontological nurse can contribute to the multidisciplinary team?

■ Evaluate your responses in Appendix B.

Chapter Highlights

■ Gerontological nurses work in a variety of settings and assume a variety of roles in order to improve the quality of life for older people and their families.

■ Nurses are in an ideal position to encourage and support this new focus because of the variety of settings in which they encounter older people. All nurses will encounter older adults in their practice setting.

■ With the percentage of older Americans increasing and the percentage of old-old people growing the fastest, even nurses in pediatrics will be addressing the needs of caregiving grandparents, as well as giving advice to family and friends regarding issues of aging.

■ Because aging is a progressive and universal process, it will happen to everyone. The nurse who is adequately prepared and educated to work with older people can face a long and enjoyable career.

Pearson Nursing Student Resources
Find additional review materials at
nursing.pearsonhighered.com

Prepare for success with additional NCLEX®-style practice
questions, interactive assignments and activities, web links,
animations and videos, and more!

References

American Association of Colleges of Nursing (AACN). (2004). *AACN position statement on the practice doctorate in nursing.* Retrieved from http://www.aacn.nche.edu/DNP/DNPPositionStatement.htm

American Association of Colleges of Nursing (AACN). (2011). *Nursing faculty shortage.* Retrieved from http://www.aacn.nche.edu/media-relations/fact-sheets/nursing-faculty-shortage

American Association of Retired Persons. (2011). *Improving the quality of care.* Retrieved from http://www.theconsumervoice.org/sites/default/files/advocate/policy-resources/Quality-Care-and-Increased-Nursing-Staffing-Minimum-Hours-in-Kansas-Nursing-Facilities.pdf

American Chronic Pain Association. (2011). *Pain management programs.* Retrieved from http://www.theacpa.org/26/PainManagementPrograms.aspx

American Healthcare Association. (2010). *Report of findings: 2008 nursing facility staff vacancy, retention, and turnover survey.* Retrieved from http://www.ahcancal.org/research_data/staffing/Documents/Retention_Vacancy_Turnover_Survey2008.pdf

American Nurses Association (ANA). (2001). *Code for nurses with interpretive statements.* Washington, DC: Author.

American Nurses Association (ANA). (2010a). *ANCC certification.* Washington, DC: Author.

American Nurses Association (ANA). (2010b). *Position statement: Registered nurses' roles and responsibilities in providing expert care at the end of life.* Retrieved from http://www.nursingworld.org/MainMenuCategories/EthicsStandards/Ethics-Position-Statements/etpain14426.aspx

American Nurses Association (ANA). (2010c). *Scope and standards of gerontological nursing practice.* Washington, DC: Author.

American Nurses Credentialing Center (ANCC). (2008). *Gerontological nurse certification.* Retrieved from http://www.nursecredentialing.org

American Nurses Credentialing Center (ANCC). (2012). *ANCC certification center.* Retrieved from http://www.nursecredentialing.org/Certification.aspx

American Society on Aging. (2007). How to improve nursing homes: One expert's 30 year view. *Aging Today, XXVII*(5). Retrieved from http://allhealth.org/BriefingMaterials/AgingToday-Harrington-985.pdf

Blissmer, B., Prochaska, J., Velicer, W., Redding, C., Rossi, J., Greene, G., ... Robbins, M. (2010). Common factors predicting long-term changes in multiple health behaviors. *Journal of Health Psychology, 15*(2), 205–214.

Buerhaus, P., Auerbach, D., & Staiger, D. (2009). *The recent surge in nurse employment: Cause and implications.* Retrieved from http://content.healthaffairs.org/content/28/4/w657.abstract

Carpenito-Moyet, L. J. (2011). *Nursing care plans and documentation package.* Philadelphia, PA: Lippincott Williams & Wilkins.

Centers for Disease Control and Prevention (CDC). (2011). *Nursing home care.* Retrieved from http://www.cdc.gov/nchs/fastats/nursingh.htm

Comarow, A. (2011). *Best nursing homes: Behind the rankings.* Retrieved from http://health.usnews.com/health-news/best-nursing-homes/articles/2011/02/07/best-nursing-homes-behind-the-rankings-2011

Daly, B. (2011). *Francis Payne Bolton Sixth Center of Excellence.* Retrieved from http://fpb.case.edu/Centers/BEST/index.shtm

Federal Emergency Management Agency. (2010). *Decision making and problem solving.* Retrieved from http://training.fema.gov/EMIWeb/IS/IS241A.pdf

Genworth. (2011). *Cost of care survey.* Retrieved from http://www.genworth.com

Gordon, M. (1994). *Nursing diagnosis: Process and application.* St. Louis, MO: Mosby.

Harrington, C. (2010). *Nursing home staffing standards in state statutes and regulations.*

The National Consumer Voice for Quality Long Term Care. Retrieved from http://www.theconsumervoice.org/sites/default/files/advocate/action-center/Harrington-state-staffing-table-2010.pdf

Health Resources and Services Administration (HRSA). (2010). *The registered nurse population: Findings from the national sample survey of registered nurses.* Retrieved from http://bhpr.hrsa.gov/healthworkforce/rnsurveys/rnsurveyfinal.pdf

Health Resources and Services Administration (HRSA). (2011). Nursing—Mission. Retrieved from http://bhpr.hrsa.gov/nursing/index.html

Hyer, K., Thomas, L., Branch L., Harmon, J., Johnson, C., & Weech-Malconada, R. (2011). The influence of nurse staffing levels on quality of care in nursing homes. *The Gerontologist.* Retrieved from http://www.commonwealthfund.org/Publications/In-the-Literature/2011/Jul/Influence-of-Staffing-on-Quality-of-Care-in-Nursing-Homes.aspx

Institute of Medicine (IOM). (2010). *The future of nursing: Leading change, advancing health.* Retrieved from http://www.iom.edu/Reports/2010/The-Future-of-Nursing-Leading-Change-Advancing-Health.aspx

Iowa Intervention Project. (2008). J. C. McCloskey & G. M. Bulechek (Eds.), *Nursing interventions classification (NIC).* Retrieved from http://www.nursing.uiowa.edu/excellence/nursing_knowledge/clinical_effectiveness/nicoverview.htm

Ironside, P. M. (2007). *Exploring the complexity of advocacy: Balancing patient-centered care and safety.* Retrieved from http://www.qsen.org/teachingstrategy.php?id=58

Kimbuende, E., Ranji, U., Lundy J., & Salganicoff, A. (2010). *U.S. health care costs.* Kaiser Family Foundation. Retrieved from http://www.kaiseredu.org/Issue-Modules/US-Health-Care-Costs/Background-Brief.aspx

NANDA International. (2012). *NANDA International nursing diagnoses: Definitions and classification, 2012–2014.* Philadelphia, PA: Wiley-Blackwell.

National Guideline Clearinghouse. (2007). *Evidence-based guidelines for prevention of cardiovascular disease in women: 2011 update.* Retrieved from http://www.guideline.gov/content.aspx?id=10948&search=exercise

National Institute of Nursing Research (NINR). (2011). *Mission.* Retrieved from http://www.nih.gov/about/almanac/organization/NINR.htm

Needleman, J., Buerhaus, P., Pankratz, S., Leibson, C., Stevens, S., & Harris, M. (2011). Nurse staffing and inpatient hospital mortality. *New England Journal of Medicine, 364*, 1037–1045.

Perlman, D. (2006). Putting the "ethics" back into research ethics: A process for ethical reflections for human research protection. *Journal of Research Administration, 36*(1), 13–22.

Quality and Safety Education for Nurses (QSEN). (2011). *Competency KSAs (prelicensure).* Retrieved from http://www.qsen.org/ksas_prelicensure.php

Raphael, T. (2011). Nurse turnover in hospitals. *ERE.net.* Retrieved from http://www.ere.net/2011/06/08/nurse-turnover-in-hospitals

Smith, K., Greenwood, C., Payette, H., & Alibhai, S. (2007). *An approach to the nonpharmacologic and pharmacologic management of unintentional weight loss among older adults.* Retrieved from http://www.medscape.com/viewarticle/555217

Strumpf, L., & Evans, L. (2008). *Individualized restraint free care.* University of Pennsylvania, Hartford Center for Geriatric Nursing Excellence. Retrieved from http://www.nursing.upenn.edu/centers/hcgne/restraints.htm

The George Washington University, National Health Policy Forum. (2012). National Spending for Long-Term Services and Supports (LTSS). Washington, DC: The George Washington University.

U.S. Bureau of Labor Statistics. (2010). *Occupational outlook handbook, 2010–11 edition, registered nurses.* Retrieved from http://www.bls.gov/oco/ocos083.htm

U.S. Census Bureau. (2010). *Profile America: Facts for features.* Retrieved from http://www.census.gov/newsroom/releases/archives/facts_for_features_special_editions/cb10-ff13.html

U.S. Department of Health and Human Services. Agency for Healthcare Research and Quality (AHRQ). (2002). Systems to rate the strength of scientific evidence. (AHRQ Publication No. 02-E015).

U.S. Department of Health and Human Services. (2011). *Glossary of terms—Long term care.* Retrieved from http://aspe.hhs.gov/daltcp/diction.shtml#L

Principles of Geriatrics

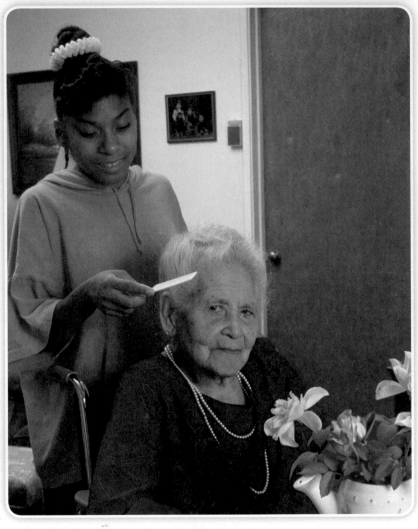

Michael Newman/PhotoEdit

LEARNING OUTCOMES

On completion of this chapter, the reader will be able to:

1. Define interdisciplinary geriatric assessment and terminology.
2. Apply appropriate guidelines for health promotion and disease prevention.
3. Identify the nurse's role in the geriatric assessment process.

4. Recognize the importance of identifying the presence of advance directives and communicating the information contained in those directives to others when caring for the older adult.
5. Identify ethical, legal, and public policy issues affecting care of the older patient.

The medical care of the older patient is known as *geriatric medicine.* **Comprehensive geriatric evaluation,** defined as an interdisciplinary process to assess older people using a biopsychosocial functional model to systematically collect data, is essential to fully understand the health needs of an older person. A key part of the geriatric evaluation is the **functional assessment** or systematic evaluation of the older person's level of function and self-care. The comprehensive evaluation is usually interdisciplinary and multidimensional and will address function in the physical, social, and psychological domains. The **gerontological nurse** is a nurse who works primarily with older adults by incorporating gerontological competencies in order to assess, manage, and implement health care to meet the specialized needs of older adults and evaluate the effectiveness of such care. The nurse's primary challenge is to identify and use the strengths of older adults and assist them to maximize their independence, minimize disability, and, where appropriate, achieve a peaceful death (American Nurses Credentialing Center, 2012). Key members of the interdisciplinary team are the gerontological nurse, the social worker, and the geriatric physician. Other healthcare professionals can be included in the evaluation or consulted depending on the needs and problems exhibited by the older patient. Sometimes advanced practice nurses, physical therapists, occupational therapists, clinical pharmacists, psychologists, psychiatrists, podiatrists, dentists, and other professionals are called in to consult and evaluate an older patient with complex needs.

A comprehensive geriatric evaluation should be carried out on a regular basis, including at these times:

1. After hospitalization for an acute illness
2. When nursing home placement or a change in living status is being considered
3. After any abrupt change in physical, social, or psychological function
4. Yearly for the older person with complex health needs during the annual visit for routine health maintenance with the primary healthcare provider
5. When the older patient or family would like a second opinion regarding an intervention or treatment protocol recommended by the primary care provider

Not all older people will have need for, or access to, trained interdisciplinary teams; however, the careful clinician can incorporate holistic assessment techniques and standardized instruments into routine evaluations. Gerontological nurses are in an ideal position to advocate for older patients who would benefit from holistic assessment and to urge them to seek the services of specialized geriatric assessment teams.

Comprehensive geriatric evaluation should be the standard of practice for older adults. Research evaluating the clinical outcomes of comprehensive geriatric evaluation with older patients reveals reduced hospital use, reduced mortality rates, improved mental status, lower health costs, improved functional ability, and lower hospital readmission rates (Stuck & Iliffe, 2011). The vision for the future is that every older person will have access to appropriate interdisciplinary health care and that every healthcare organization and setting providing care to older adults will have financial support for an interdisciplinary geriatric service or program (Capezuti, Siegler, & Mezey, 2008). The demand for RNs who can care for older persons is expected to increase dramatically in the next 20 years. Not every older person would require care from an interdisciplinary team, but the team would be available for those older patients whose complex health needs require holistic evaluation.

The gerontological nurse utilizes a different perspective during the geriatric evaluation process, and special instruments are needed to gather appropriate data (see Best Practices: Instruments for Use With Older Adults). The members of the team must not only be knowledgeable in the content area of gerontology and geriatrics, but also be educated regarding the issues of team dynamics. Essential skills in team dynamics include awareness of the roles and contributions of all team members, excellent communication skills in order to share information, conflict resolution skills, and the ability to see beyond their unique professional perspective that assumes only one's own discipline is enough to solve the problems of the older patient. Many schools of nursing and medicine offer interdisciplinary courses and educate students to work together and share knowledge to solve complex patient problems.

Collaboration implies the process of shared planning, decision making, accountability, and responsibility in the care of the patient (Hartford Institute for Geriatric Nursing, 2011b). Reasons for collaborative care for older adults include those depicted in Box 3-1. The Veterans Administration (VA) system has provided funding to research and evaluate the geriatric evaluation process. In 1979, the Interdisciplinary Team Training in Geriatrics program was established to provide leadership in **interdisciplinary education** (education encouraging the integration of different professional perspectives) and training using a team approach to service delivery throughout the VA system. Approximately 50 clinical teams have been formed, and over 5,000 VA personnel have been trained in the principles of teamwork. Geriatric research, education, and clinical centers have been formed to evaluate and meet the health needs of older veterans. The Health Resources and Services Administration has funded over 30 projects in underserved rural areas to educate health professionals in the principles of interdisciplinary

Best Practices **Instruments for Use With Older Adults**

The Hartford Institute recommends the following instruments for use when assessing the function of older adults. These instruments have been used clinically for many years, are commonly referred to in practice, and have been validated on large patient groups. Additional assessment tools that focus on specific problems will be included in the appropriate chapters in this text. Recommended functional assessment tools include:

1. Katz Index of Independence in Activities of Daily Living (Katz, Down, Cash, et al., 1970).
2. PULSES Profile. Measures general functional performance in mobility and self-care, medical status, and psychosocial factors.
   P = physical condition
   U = upper limb function
   L = lower limb function
   S = sensory components
   E = excretory functions
   S = support factors (Granger, Albrecht, & Hamilton, 1979)

3. SPICES. An overall assessment tool used to plan, promote, and maintain optimal function in older adults.
   S = sleep disorders
   P = problems with eating and feeding
   I = incontinence
   C = confusion
   E = evidence of falls
   S = skin breakdown

Source: Hartford Institute for Geriatric Nursing, 2011a.

BOX 3-1 > **Reasons for Interdisciplinary Collaboration to Improve Care**

- Older adults may face a multitude of complex problems requiring assessment and intervention from various healthcare professionals.
- Assembling a group of knowledgeable providers can enhance problem solving and the delivery of health care.
- Coordination of services can be enhanced by various professionals working together.
- The patient will have access to a comprehensive and integrated care plan.
- Care can be safer for patients, more cost effective, and efficient.
- Healthcare professionals can feel supported and encouraged by the input and collaboration from other professionals. Interdisciplinary care has the potential to decrease feelings of "burnout" when caring for older patients with complex health needs.

Source: Hartford Institute for Geriatric Nursing, 2011b.

education and patient care. In 1994, the Joint Commission on Accreditation of Healthcare Organizations (now called The Joint Commission) established standards that emphasize the importance of an interdisciplinary approach to providing patient care. Healthcare personnel working in Joint Commission–approved healthcare facilities must possess the knowledge and skills to participate in **interdisciplinary teams** (groups of people from differing professions who collaborate in the assessment and care of the older person) in order to mobilize internal and external resources to meet patients' needs and assume responsibility for care coordination (Joint Commission, 2011).

Geriatric evaluation can be conducted by teams within the acute care hospital setting, on an outpatient basis at an ambulatory clinic, or even in the home setting. Results of the assessment and recommendations can be implemented by the team or conveyed to the primary healthcare provider for implementation or follow-up as appropriate. Leadership of the team is based on expertise rather than discipline or authority. Gerontological nurses assume team leadership when the older patient's problems reside within the primary domain of nursing. Social workers assume leadership for social problems, and physicians assume leadership for the assessment and diagnosis of illness and disease.

Components of Comprehensive Geriatric Assessment

Despite variations in instruments, structure of the interdisciplinary team, and methods employed, several strategies have been proven to make the evaluation process more effective. These include the development of a close-knit interdisciplinary team with minimal redundancy in the assessments performed, the use of carefully designed questionnaires that reliable older patients or their caregivers can complete beforehand, and the effective use of assessment forms that are utilized by all team members and are easily incorporated into the electronic medical record (Kane, Ouslander, Abrass et al., 2009).

There are three underlying principles of comprehensive geriatric assessment:

1. Physical, psychological, and socioeconomic factors interact in complex ways to influence the health and functional status of the older person.
2. Comprehensive evaluation of an older person's health status requires an assessment in each of these domains. The coordinated efforts of various healthcare professionals are needed to carry out the assessment.
3. Functional abilities should be a central focus of the comprehensive evaluation. Other more traditional measures of health such as medical diagnosis, nursing diagnosis, physical examination results, and laboratory findings form the basic foundation of the assessment in order to determine overall health, well-being, and the need for and intensity of social services.

Kane et al., 2009.

Contextual Variables Affecting Holistic Geriatric Assessment

The interrelationships between the physical, social, and psychological aspects of aging and perhaps illness present a challenge to the gerontological nurse when beginning the geriatric evaluation. The gerontological nurse is often charged with the responsibility of obtaining the patient's past health history and history of the present illness. The following contextual variables should be considered.

Evaluation of the Environment

To make the older patient and family comfortable, environmental modifications should be made, if possible. Environmental modifications may include adequate lighting, decreased background noise, comfortable seating for the older patient and family, easily accessible restrooms, examination tables that can be raised or lowered to assist patients with disabilities, and availability of water or juice for patient use. Patient comfort will ease communication and improve the data-gathering process.

Accuracy of the Health History

Clear instructions should be provided to the patient and family beforehand regarding the parking arrangements and registration process. Many assessment clinics mail an information packet in advance so that the older patient can come prepared. This packet might include:

1. A past medical history form. This form can be completed at home and is helpful for patients with

complicated medical histories. The dates of hospitalizations, operations, serious injuries or accidents, procedures, and so on can be ascertained beforehand to save time during the assessment appointment. The form would also include history of adverse drug effects or allergies.
2. Instructions to bring in all prescription, over-the-counter, and herbal medications for review by the gerontological nurse.
3. Instructions to bring any medical records, laboratory or X-ray reports, electrocardiograms, reports of vaccination, and other pertinent health records that the patient or family may possess.
4. Instructions to write down and bring the names of all healthcare providers involved with the patient's health care, including primary care providers, specialists, and alternative medicine practitioners (e.g., acupuncturists, massage therapists, chiropractors).

The more information that the patient and family can organize ahead of time, the better and more efficient the assessment will be. Patience is a virtue when obtaining a history because many times the thought and verbal processes are slower in the older person. Patients should be allowed adequate time to answer questions and report information

Kane et al., 2009.

> **Practice Pearl ▶▶▶** When the older patient is asked to bring all medications to the geriatric evaluation session and he or she arrives carrying a large bag of medication bottles, the gerontological nurse knows that the first problem identified on the problem list is likely to be "at risk for adverse drug reaction related to polypharmacy."

The history should include emphasis on the following:

- Review of acute and chronic medical problems (sometimes called "the presenting complaint")
- Medications (prescription, over the counter, herbals, and dietary supplements)
- Disease prevention and health maintenance review: vaccinations, PPD (tuberculosis), cancer screenings
- Functional status (activities of daily living)
- Social supports (family, caregiver stress, safety of living environment)
- Finances
- Driving status and safety record
- Geriatric review of symptoms (patient/family perception of memory, dentition, taste, smell, nutrition, hearing, vision, falls, fractures, bowel and bladder function)

Ward & Reuben, 2011.

Often, a standardized form is used to guide and direct the process of obtaining the health history. The gerontological nurse should be aware of potential difficulties that may arise when obtaining health histories from older persons, including those identified in Box 3-2.

Social History

Holistic evaluation is not complete without an assessment of the social support system. Many frail older persons receive support and supervision from family members and significant others to compensate for functional disabilities.

Key elements of the social history include the following:

- Past occupation and retirement status
- Family history (helpful to construct a family genogram)
- Present and former marital status, including quality of the relationship(s)
- Identification of family members, with designation of level of involvement and place of residence
- Living arrangements
- Family dynamics
- Family and caregiver expectations
- Economic status, adequacy of health insurance
- Social activities and hobbies
- Mode of transportation
- Community involvement and support
- Religious involvement and spirituality

Older persons who exhibit symptoms of sadness, social isolation, questioning their existence, feeling they are being punished by God, or asking about availability of religious or spiritual counseling should be asked if they would like help with their spiritual concerns. Religion and spirituality can be a great source of hope and strength in times of need and crisis. Many healthcare facilities and community agencies have access to religious and spiritual counselors who can meet with older persons and their families if the need arises and the older person does not have an ongoing relationship with a priest, minister, rabbi, or spiritual counselor.

If there is a social worker on the assessment team, the gerontological nurse may collaborate with the social worker closely to identify and address social problems. Older patients with inadequate health insurance can often be helped by accessing community services, free hospital care, hardship funds established for indigent patients by major drug companies, and referrals to community-based free clinics. This information is helpful to nurses working with older persons in many settings but is absolutely necessary for those being admitted to long-term care facilities and those expressing feelings of loneliness or absence of significant persons in their lives.

Psychological History

Another key component of the holistic geriatric assessment is evaluation of psychological and cognitive function. A significant proportion of older patients with mental illness remain unrecognized and untreated; when treated, the use of healthcare services decreases (National Alliance on Mental Illness, 2009). The reported range of adults over the age of 65 with mental disorders, both in institutions and in the community, is estimated to be between 20% and 30%.

The older person is more likely to use general healthcare services than to seek specialized services with mental health professionals. Many older people are fearful of seeing a psychiatrist, psychiatric social worker, or psychiatric–mental health advanced practice nurse because they fear being labeled as "crazy." All healthcare workers working with older patients should be aware of the mental health problems common in the older adult, diagnostic instruments appropriate for screening and diagnosing mental health problems, and the resources for treatment and referral within their practice site. Mental and emotional problems are not a normal part of aging. When mental health problems manifest themselves in the older adult, they should be evaluated, diagnosed, and treated. By forming a trusting therapeutic relationship, the gerontological nurse can demonstrate caring, warmth, respect, and support for the older person who may be hesitant to verbalize feelings of low self-esteem, depression, bizarre thought patterns, or phobias and anxieties.

Key elements of the psychological history include:

- Any history of past mental illness
- Any hospitalizations or outpatient treatments for psychological problems
- Current and past stress levels and coping mechanisms

BOX 3-2 ▸ **Potential Difficulties in Obtaining Health Histories**

- **Communication difficulties.** Decreased hearing or vision, slow speech, and use of English as a second language have an effect on communication.
- **Underreporting of symptoms.** Fear of being labeled as a complainer, fear of institutionalization, and fear of serious illness can influence symptom reporting.
- **Vague or nonspecific complaints.** These may be associated with cognitive impairment, drug or alcohol use or abuse, or atypical presentation of disease.
- **Multiple complaints.** Associated "masked" depression, presence of multiple chronic illnesses, and social isolation are often an older person's cry for help.
- **Lack of time.** New patients scheduled for geriatric assessment should have the minimum of a 1-hour appointment with the gerontological nurse. Shorter appointments will result in a hurried interview with missed information.

Source: Kane et al., 2009.

- Current and past levels of alcohol or recreational drug use
- Medications taken for anxiety, insomnia, or depression
- Identification of any problems with memory, judgment, or thought processing
- Any changes in personality, values, personal habits, or life satisfaction
- Identification of feelings regarding self-worth and hopes for the future
- Feelings of appropriate emotions related to present life and health situation (feelings of sadness regarding losses, etc.)
- Presence of someone to love, support, and encourage the older patient
- Feelings of hopelessness or suicidal ideation

The accuracy of the health history and identification of problems depend on adequate mental and affective functioning. The higher the level of cognitive impairment, the more likely the older patient is to report inaccurate information. Problems with short-term memory can cause older people to forget to report adverse events such as falls, safety issues in the home, or other relevant problems that could influence the plan of care. Further, depressed older patients may score poorly on instruments used to assess psychological function because they do not have the energy or motivation to concentrate or answer questions. These older persons continuously appear sad and state, "I don't know" or "I couldn't tell you" when responding to questions. The nurse should refer these patients for further psychological evaluation because they may be exhibiting signs and symptoms of depression.

There is benefit from interviewing the older person with and without the family or significant others present. Some older patients will confide difficulties to the gerontological nurse in private that they may be hesitant to report in the presence of family. These issues may encompass family dynamics, sexuality, matters relating to bowel and bladder function, or other personal issues. Many older patients are hesitant to complain when family members are present because they are afraid to be seen as being critical or labeled as a complainer. When the older person has memory impairments, however, the family presence may assist in obtaining an accurate health history. A good strategy is to seek permission from the older patient to include the family to verify or gather additional information. An older patient with depression may feel demoralized and be unable to take part in rehabilitation or health promotion activities based on lack of energy and motivation. Family members and involved caregivers are often in a position to report subtle changes in personality and function that may go undetected by others.

Instruments commonly used in clinical practice to assess psychological function include the following:

- **Geriatric Depression Scale (Kurlowicz & Greenberg, 2007).** The short form includes 15 questions and measures depression in the older adult. The answers in **bold** indicate depression. Score 1 point for each bolded answer. A score of greater than 5 is suggestive of depression and indicates the need for further screening. Refer to Chapter 7 ⊂⊃ for further discussion of depression.
- **The Mini-Cog.** The Mini-Cog consists of three item recalls and a clock drawing test (CDT). The Mini-Cog takes about 3 minutes to administer and is not affected by language, education, or culture. The tool can differentiate older persons with dementia from those without dementia (see Best Practices: The Mini-Cog) (Borson, Scanlan, Chen et al., 2003).

Home Environment / usually only can ask

Some geriatric assessment teams have the time and resources to visit the older patient's home and conduct an assessment of the environment. While this direct observation is the best way to gather accurate and reliable data, it is time consuming and can be expensive. Therefore, many geriatric assessment teams question the older person and the family regarding the adequacy of the home environment and the available resources to maintain adequate levels of function.

Factors to be considered when assessing the home environment are included in Table 3-1.

Culture and Education

The increasing need for healthcare providers to care for older adults from diverse backgrounds means that gerontological nurses must consider how assessment and development of a treatment plan are modified to avoid misunderstanding or ineffective care. Caution is urged when users of assessment instruments draw conclusions from test scores that are derived from patients of different cultures and various educational backgrounds (American Psychological Association, 2011). Some instruments such as the Mini-Mental Status Examination (MMSE) have developed and validated scoring norms based on level of education. The examination has a component that is dependent on reading a sentence and following instructions, writing a sentence, performing complex mathematical calculations, and spelling a word backwards. Older patients may be reticent to tell a healthcare provider that they are unable to read or write and may score poorly as a result. Low scores could falsely be attributed to cognitive impairment rather than low reading literacy. The gerontological nurse should always consider and assess educational level, language barriers, reading levels, and cultural background before using standardized instruments.

Best Practices The Mini-Cog

Administration

The test is administered as follows:

1. Instruct the patient to listen carefully to and remember three unrelated words and then to repeat the words.
2. Instruct the patient to draw the face of a clock, either on a blank sheet of paper or on a sheet with the clock circle already drawn on the page. After the patient puts the numbers on the clock face, ask him or her to draw the hands of the clock to read a specific time.
3. Ask the patient to repeat the three previously stated words.

Scoring

Give 1 point for each recalled word after the clock drawing test (CDT) distractor.
Patients recalling none of the three words are classified as demented (Score = 0).
Patients recalling all three words are classified as nondemented (Score = 3)
Patients with intermediate word recall of one or two words are classified based on the CDT
(Abnormal = demented; Normal = nondemented)

Note: The CDT is considered normal if all numbers are present in the correct sequence and position, and the hands readably display the requested time.
Source: Borson, S., Scanlan, J., Brush, M., Vitaliano, P., & Dokmak, A. (2000). The mini-cog: A cognitive "vital signs" measure for dementia screening in multilingual elderly. *International Journal of Geriatric Psychiatry, 15*(11), p. 1024. Copyright John Wiley & Sons Limited. Reproduced with permission.

It is important to understand and elicit the beliefs, attitudes, values, and goals of older people relating to their lives, illness, and health states in order to provide culturally appropriate care. Cultural competence in health care consists of at least four components:

1. Knowing the prevalence, incidence, and risk factors (epidemiology) for diseases in different ethnic groups
2. Understanding how the response to medications and other treatments varies with ethnicity
3. Focusing on relational ethics and identifying the culturally held beliefs and attitudes toward illness, treatment, and the healthcare system
4. Keeping an open mind and approaching each older person as a unique individual.

Adapted from Bearskin, 2011.

To avoid stereotypical thinking, the nurse must recognize that there is heterogeneity within various ethnic groups, and the provision of culturally sensitive care dictates that each person be approached as a unique individual. Patient age, place of birth, where childhood was spent, and how the older person was socialized to American culture can all affect performance on standardized assessment instruments. Many of the instruments used by clinicians to assess older patients have not been validated for use with cultural minorities (Bearskin, 2011). The members of some ethnic groups are less willing to report difficulty

taking care of themselves and may fear admitting their dependence on others. Refer to Chapter 4 ⬚⬚ for a thorough discussion of culture.

Minimum Data Set

Assessment of an older person for appropriate placement within the nursing home or within the long-term care system is done using the Minimum Data Set (MDS). The MDS is a comprehensive multidisciplinary assessment that is used throughout the United States. It was devised and passed into law because of the belief that a better, more holistic patient assessment will facilitate improved patient care. The Omnibus Budget Reconciliation Act of 1987 (OBRA 87) contained a provision mandating that all residents of facilities that collect funds from Medicare or Medicaid be assessed using the MDS. The Minimum Data Set is a standardized, primary screening and assessment tool of health status that forms the foundation for the comprehensive assessment of all residents of long-term care facilities certified to participate in Medicare or Medicaid. The MDS is used for validating the need for long-term care, reimbursement, ongoing assessment of clinical problems, and assessment of and need to alter the current plan of care.

Categories of data gathered for the MDS 3.0 include items that measure physical, psychological, and psychosocial functioning. The items in the MDS give a multidimensional view of the patient's functional capacities, and can be used to present a nursing home's profile. The MDS now plays a key role in the Medicare and Medicaid reimbursement system and in monitoring the quality of care provided to nursing facility residents (Research Data Assistance Center, 2011).

Certain patient information gathered for the MDS such as unanticipated functional decline or a poorly managed chronic disease may trigger the need for further assessment. The MDS process begins with the care area assessment (CAA), care plan development, care plan implementation, and evaluation. See Table 3-2 for care area assessments as defined by the MDS process, which is illustrated in Figure 3-1 ►►►. The CAA process identifies areas that the interdisciplinary team will address further to develop the interdisciplinary care plan. The team, in collaboration with the long-term care facility resident and/or the resident's representative will identify issues that:

- Warrant intervention.
- Impact the resident's functioning in order to assist with development of interventions for improvement, or maintenance of the present level of functioning or to prevent decline based on the resident's condition and choices and preferences for interventions.

TABLE 3-1	Factors to Consider When Assessing the Home
Item Assessed	**Assessment Parameters**
Stairs	Narrow stairs with poor lighting, inadequate railings, and uneven steps are fall risks. Does the older person have the strength and balance to climb stairs? If a wheelchair or walker is used, are ramps present or is there space for them to be added?
Bathing and Toileting	Can the older person safely transfer on and off the toilet? Is a raised toilet seat needed? Are grab bars present? Is there an adequate bath mat in the tub? Is a shower seat needed? Is lighting adequate?
Medications	Where are medications stored? Are there grandchildren in the home who are at risk because of open storage or nonreplacement of caps? Are old and outdated medications disposed of to prevent accidents? Are medications refilled on time to prevent on–off dosing patterns? Is there a list of medications available for use in emergencies?
Advance Directives	Has the older person named a health proxy or established a living will? (See Chapter 11 ⬤▭.) If so, do the family and primary care provider have a copy? Is the healthcare proxy knowledgeable regarding the patient's preferences? Is the proxy's number posted in an easily visible position (e.g., on the refrigerator)? Is the value quality of life or length of life specified?
Nutrition and Cooking	Is there adequate food in the home? Is there a stove or microwave to cook? Are any safety problems reported with the stove or microwave? If a gas stove, is it safe? Is the pilot functioning properly? Are there gas leak detectors? Is food storage adequate? Is spoiled food present? Is the food preparation environment clean? Who does the grocery shopping? How are trash and garbage disposed?
Falls	Are the floors free of cords, debris, and scatter rugs? Is there adequate lighting? Are there night-lights? Are there pets that dart around quickly? If there is a history of falls, would the older person consider wearing an emergency alert system around the neck?
Smoke Detectors	Are there functioning smoke detectors? Are batteries changed yearly?
Emergency Numbers	Are emergency phone numbers posted or preprogrammed into the phone?
Temperature of Home	Is there adequate heat in the winter and cooling in the summer?
Temperature of Water	Is the hot water set below 120°F?
Safety of the Neighborhood	Can the older person venture outside without fear of becoming a crime victim? Are there adequate door locks and latches? How close is the nearest neighbor? Is there help nearby if it is needed?
Financial	Are there stacks of unpaid bills? Are services such as phone and electricity in good working order? Are there large amounts of cash hidden or stored around the house? Is there adequate money to purchase nutritious food?

TABLE 3-2	Care Area Assessments in the Resident Assessment Instrument, Version 3.0
Delirium	Cognitive Loss/Dementia
Visual function	Communication
Activity of daily living (ADL) functional/rehabilitation potential	Pain
Urinary incontinence and indwelling catheter	Return to community referral
Psychosocial well-being	Mood state
Behavioral symptoms	Activities
Falls	Nutritional status
Feeding tubes	Dehydration/fluid maintenance
Dental care	Pressure ulcer
Psychotropic medication use	Physical restraints

Source: Centers for Medicare and Medicaid Services [CMS], 2010.

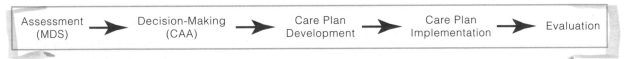

Figure 3-1 ▶▶▶ The MDS process.
Source: Centers for Medicare and Medicaid Services.

- Minimize decline for those at risk in order to avoid functional complications, to the extent possible, including pain or the development of contractures.
- Address symptom relief or pain management and/or the provision of palliative care.

MDS version 3.0 was introduced in 2010 and builds on lessons used in testing and using the earlier versions. Like earlier versions, it focuses on clinical assessment of nursing home residents and screens for common unrecognized or undertreated conditions and problems but, based on feedback from families and resident advocates, new goals were added including these:

- **Obtaining information directly from the residents— "Giving Residents Voice."** Residents and their families appreciate the opportunity to answer direct and specific questions regarding their preferences for care and the adequacy of that care to improve the quality of their lives. Often, the most accurate way to collect data is to directly ask the resident. Even residents with cognitive impairments can provide data on how they feel, what they like about their care, and how they think things might be improved. The interview items have been tested to find the best way to measure the topic in question and have been shown to work well with frail nursing home residents.
- **Inclusion of assessment items used in other healthcare settings.** Items that are used to measure potential risk of skin breakdown, delirium, and activities of daily living in the acute care environment are now included in the MDS to improve communications across settings and providers.
- **Begin movement toward the electronic health record format.**

The changes described above make the MDS more efficient: the new version takes 45% less time to complete and provides higher quality information than the older version. Items that did not supply accurate information were eliminated and the form was redesigned for ease of use with larger fonts, logical page breaks, fewer items per page, and more critical instructions on the form. The MDS is still used as a basis for payment and provides data to assess quality of care for each individual long-term care facility.

The gerontological nurse will provide valuable input into the formation of the care plan and may serve as leader of the interdisciplinary team. New provisions in the MDS mandate that the care plan must be oriented toward:

1. Preventing avoidable declines in functioning or functional levels
2. Managing risk factors
3. Addressing resident's strengths
4. Using current standards of practice in the care planning process

5. Evaluating treatment objectives and outcomes of care
6. Respecting the resident's right to refuse treatment
7. Offering alternative treatments
8. Using an interdisciplinary approach to care plan development to improve the resident's functional abilities
9. Involving family and other resident representatives
10. Assessing and planning for care sufficient to meet the care needs of new admissions
11. Involving the direct care staff with the care planning process relating to the resident's expected outcomes
12. Addressing additional care planning areas that could be considered in the long-term care setting

CMS, 2010.

The MDS can be viewed as a start in acquiring the broad base of clinical information necessary to provide quality long-term care. The gerontological nurse with excellent clinical skills will often be called on to individualize the predetermined structured assessment and the interventions. For example, a nursing home resident with severe Alzheimer's disease may be losing weight. The probable cause of the weight loss is probably not a gastrointestinal problem, but rather the result of the older person's cognitive impairment and loss of appetite and food recognition. Clinical experts in geriatrics and gerontology are working with federal regulators to develop a risk stratification system that would be better able to measure quality and trigger the need for further assessments based on the risks associated with severe cognitive impairment.

Health Promotion and Disease Screening
[handwritten: ∅ quality ∅]

Health for older adults is a complex interaction of physical, functional, and psychosocial factors. Clearly, it is not just the absence of disease, because many people diagnosed with a chronic disease consider themselves to be healthy. Health may be considered a state of physical, mental, and social functioning that realizes the potential of which a person is capable. Margaret Newman (2010) has developed a theory of health as expanding consciousness that was stimulated by concern for those for whom health as the absence of disease or disability was not realistic or possible. The World Health Organization (1946) has defined health as "the state of complete physical, mental, and social well-being and not merely the absence of disease and infirmity."

Others speak of health and illness as opposite ends of a continuum with the midpoint forming the demarcation between illness and health (Figure 3-2 ▶▶▶). The person is envisioned to move back and forth on the continuum in response to a variety of factors such as ability to function adequately, feelings of control of chronic illness, clinical markers, environmental supports, and rate and degree of disease progression. Nursing goals for improving health in older persons with altered health maintenance are listed in Box 3-3. These interventions are intended to move the older person along the continuum toward health and away from illness. The gerontological nurse formulates indicators of movement on the health continuum by specifying markers, targets, and time intervals that are appropriate for assessing the older patient's progress.

The older person's health beliefs will indicate the motivational support and perceived benefits of action. Indicators of health beliefs and examples of how these beliefs relate to an older patient's decisions include the following: *[handwritten: what is important to them?]*

- Perceived importance of taking action—*I know if I exercise regularly, I am less likely to have a heart attack.*
- Perceived threat of inaction—*If I don't eat more healthy foods, I will not be able to control my blood sugar and may need to take more medicine.*
- Perceived benefits of action—*I should schedule my mammogram because the earlier a mass is found, the better the chance of cure.*
- Perceived internal control of action—*I know the choices I make will affect my present and future health.*
- Perceived control of health outcome—*I should schedule an appointment with my primary care provider so that I can stay healthy.*
- Perceived improvement in lifestyle from action—*If I lose weight, it will be easier for me to tend to my garden.*

BOX 3-3 **Nursing Interventions for Altered Health Maintenance Goals**

1. Lifestyle changes
2. Acquisition of new health-promoting thought patterns and behaviors
3. Self-care in managing chronic health conditions or risks

Source: Scherb et al., 2011.

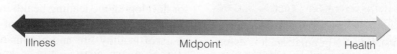

Illness   Midpoint   Health

Figure 3-2 ▶▶▶ The health continuum.

- Perceived resources to perform action—*My health insurance covers immunizations, so I think I will get a flu shot this year.*
- Perceived absence of barriers to action—*My health insurance pays for part of a membership in a health club and my physician has urged me to exercise. I think I'll enroll this week!*
- Perceived reduction of threat from action—*I know if I quit smoking, I will reduce my risk of getting lung disease or cancer.*

Scherb et al., 2011.

The older person who indicates strong health beliefs in these indicators will have a higher probability of being able to take positive action to move toward health on the continuum.

According to Pender, Murdaugh, and Parsons (2010), health promotion is a "multidimensional pattern of self-initiated actions and perceptions that serve to maintain or enhance the level of wellness, self-actualization and fulfillment of the individual" (p. 9).

Such behaviors often include:

- Engaging in regular physical activity
- Engaging in challenging mental activity
- Eating a healthy, balanced diet
- Getting 8 hours of sleep a night
- Having at least one friend to trust and confide in
- Having some relaxing and pleasant activities to look forward to
- Having the self-discipline to enjoy pleasant things in moderation
- Trying to view things positively and have hopes for the future

Health promotion for the older adult is not focused on disease or disability, but rather on the individual's strengths, abilities, and values. It is important to recognize the "cohort effect" or the impact of history on the older person and others in his or her generation. For instance, older men who have fought in the Vietnam War may have experienced a lifelong struggle with post-traumatic stress disorder (PTSD). Recognition of these cohort effects can be important foundational information useful in the formulation of the nursing care plan. By maximizing strengths, identifying resources, and identifying values that guide behaviors, the gerontological nurse has the opportunity to greatly influence positive health behaviors in the older adult.

Health Status

To understand the health status of a population, it is essential to monitor and evaluate the determinants of health and their consequences. The health status of the United States is a description of the health of the total population, using information representative of most people living in this country. The goal of eliminating health disparities will necessitate improved collection and use of standardized data to correctly identify disparities among select population groups (U.S. Department of Health and Human Services [USDHHS], 2011b).

Health status can be measured by birth and death rates, life expectancy, quality of life, morbidity from specific diseases, risk factors, use of ambulatory care and inpatient care, accessibility of health personnel and facilities, healthcare financing, health insurance coverage, and many other factors. The information used to report health status comes from a variety of sources, including birth and death records, hospital discharge data, and health information collected from healthcare records, personal interviews, physical examinations, and telephone surveys (USDHHS, 2011b).

The leading causes of death are used frequently to describe the health status of the nation. During the past 100 years, the United States has seen a great deal of change in the leading causes of death. Currently, most older people die from chronic illness such as cardiovascular disease and malignant neoplasms. At the beginning of the 1900s, infectious diseases were common in the United States and worldwide and topped the leading causes of death. A century later, with the control of many infectious agents and the increasing age of the population, chronic diseases top the list (USDHHS, 2011b).

A very different picture emerges when the leading causes of death are viewed for various population groups. Unintentional injuries, mainly motor vehicle crashes, are the fifth leading cause of death for the total population, but they are the leading cause of death for people ages 1 to 44 years. Similarly, HIV/AIDS is the 14th leading cause of death for the total population but the leading cause of death for African American men ages 25 to 44 years (USDHHS, 2011b).

The leading causes of death in the United States generally result from a mix of behaviors: injury, violence, and other factors in the environment, as well as the unavailability or inaccessibility of quality health services. Understanding and monitoring behaviors, environmental factors, and community health systems may prove more useful to monitoring and improving the nation's *true* health than the death rates that reflect the cumulative impact of these factors. This more complex approach has served as the basis for developing the leading health indicators.

From the overarching goals of increasing quality and years of healthy life and eliminating disparities, specific *Healthy People 2020* goals have been developed that focus

Weblink: *Healthy People 2020*

on increasing health promotion activities and decreasing morbidity and mortality in persons of all ages. To view the complete report, go to the *Healthy People 2020* website. The goals included in *Healthy People 2020* form the foundation of professional activities, influence the allocation of health resources, and will direct clinical research activities during the next several years. Some of the goals that pertain to older adults are listed in Box 3-4.

Many older adults are willing and eager to engage in health promotion activities. They may have seen their friends and relatives become ill, go to nursing homes, or die. As a result, they have come to realize how important it is to protect and maintain good health. Additionally, many older people fear they will become a

---

BOX 3-4	**Selected *Healthy People 2020* Health Promotion Goals Applicable to Older People**

- Increase the proportion of older adults who use the Welcome to Medicare benefit.
- Increase the proportion of older adults who are up to date on a core set of clinical preventive services.
- Increase the proportion of older adults with one or more chronic health conditions who report confidence in managing their conditions.
- Increase the proportion of older adults who receive diabetes self-management benefits.
- Reduce the proportion of older adults who have moderate to severe functional limitations.
- Increase the proportion of older adults with reduced physical or cognitive function who engage in light, moderate, or vigorous leisure-time physical activities.
- Increase the proportion of the healthcare workforce with geriatric certification.
- Reduce the proportion of noninstitutionalized older adults with disabilities who have an unmet need for long-term services and supports.
- Reduce the proportion of unpaid caregivers of older adults who report an unmet need for caregiver support services.
- Reduce the rate of pressure ulcer–related hospitalizations among older adults.
- Reduce the rate of emergency department visits due to falls among older adults.
- Increase the number of states, the District of Columbia, and tribes that collect and make publicly available information on the characteristics of victims, perpetrators, and cases of elder abuse, neglect, and exploitation.

Source: U.S. Department of Health and Human Services. (2011b). *Healthy people 2020: What are its goals?* Rockville, MD: Author. Retrieved from http://healthypeople.gov/2020/topicsobjectives2020/objectiveslist.aspx?topicId=31.

---

burden on their children and therefore do everything they can to remain active, healthy, and independent. Health maintenance practices should also include regular visits to a primary care provider and appropriate diagnostic and screening tests as recommended. Table 3-3 lists recommended health screenings for older persons.

Legal Issues

Legal issues affecting older adults are increasingly common based on the number of people living longer, fuller lives. The gerontological nurse should be aware of all the rules, regulations, and standards that govern professional practice. When patients suffer injury or receive inappropriate care, patients or families may file a lawsuit seeking damages for personal injury. If a suit is filed, the care and treatment offered the patient will be compared with standards of care. Usually an expert witness will review the medical records and offer an opinion regarding whether the standard of care was met. Sources for establishing the nursing standard of care include the American Nurses Association, state nurse practice acts, nursing home regulation and standards, Joint Commission standards, nursing journals, nursing textbooks, specialty websites, and expert opinions.

OBRA 87 requires all states to operate long-term care ombudsmen programs and to notify patients about their rights. These programs provide trained people to investigate complaints made by residents and families about poor care or violation of patients' rights within the nursing home. If a violation is found, the ombudsman may seek administrative or legal action.

Older patients have the right to:

- Receive individualized care.
- Be free from abuse, neglect, and discrimination.
- Be free from chemical and physical restraints.
- Have privacy.
- Control their funds.
- Be involved in decision making.
- Raise grievances and make complaints.
- Vote.
- File lawsuits.
- Practice religion.
- Marry.
- Participate in facility and family activities.
- Have freedom to leave the facility.
- Make a will and dispose of property.
- Enter into contracts.

The healthcare facility is required to post the bill of rights in a conspicuous place and list the name and telephone

TABLE 3-3 Recommended Health Screenings and Interventions for Older Persons

Screening/Intervention	Recommended Interval
For Primary Prevention	
Bone mineral density (women)	At least once after the age of 65
Blood pressure	Yearly
Diabetes screening	Every 3 years in people with BP > 135/80
Herpes zoster immunization	Once after the age of 60
Influenza immunization	Yearly
Lipid disorder screening	Every 5 years, more often in older people with coronary artery disease, diabetes, peripheral artery disease or history of prior stroke
Obesity (height and weight)	Yearly
Pneumonia immunization	Usually once. Revaccination for healthy persons is not recommended. However, if a patient received the first dose prior to age 65, give a single revaccination at age 65 (or older) if at least 5 years have elapsed since the previous dose.
Smoking cessation	Every health encounter
Tetanus booster	Every 10 years. Verify that the primary series was received.
For Secondary Prevention	
Abdominal aortic aneurysm	Once between ages 65–75 in men who are smokers or have a history of smoking
Alcohol abuse	Periodically
Depression screening	Yearly
Sigmoidoscopy/colonoscopy	Every 10 years from ages 50–75
Fecal occult blood	Yearly
Mammography/clinical breast exam	Every 2 years in women ages 50–74
Hearing/vision screening	Yearly
Pap smears	Limited benefit in women over the age of 65 or those without a cervix after hysterectomy.

Sources: Centers for Disease Control and Prevention (2011); U.S. Preventive Services Task Force (2011).

number of the ombudsman so patients know who to contact if they feel that their rights have been violated.

All nurses should adequately prepare themselves for safe practice, question any action or physician's order that seems inappropriate or unsafe, and seek advice or guidance from their superior whenever they are unsure of the safety of an action. Additionally, all nurses are urged to purchase individual professional liability insurance to pay financial damages should they be the target of a lawsuit. Even if the healthcare facility where the nurse is employed offers liability coverage, the nurse should consider purchasing individual coverage to ensure that the individual nurse's professional interests will be defended as well as the nurse's interests as an employee of the institution.

Nursing care that violates the standards of practice can be considered malpractice. The legal definition of standard of care is to consider what a reasonable nurse would do if placed in a similar situation according to professional standards. When the nurse's performance does not meet that standard of care, malpractice can be charged. Situations that can lead to malpractice include the following:

- Not adequately assessing or monitoring patients as to change in condition
- Not safeguarding the environment of a cognitively impaired patient
- Not informing the physician that a patient is in need of medical care
- Medication errors (wrong dose, wrong patient, wrong time, wrong route of administration)
- Incorrectly performing a nursing intervention that results in patient injury (placing a feeding tube in the lung, etc.)
- Failing to carry out positioning or treatment orders (e.g., not offering fluids, changing dressing, repositioning the patient), resulting in patient injury

Careful documentation of nursing care is the best way to defend oneself should a legal suit be filed. Charting should be legible, accurate, timely, and specific enough to describe

---

BOX 3-5 ▷ **Documentation Guidelines**

- Write clearly and legibly so others can read the record without struggling or ambiguity.
- Record all significant nursing interventions and patient responses.
- Record all significant nursing interventions withheld or deferred (e.g., "laxative not given as patient has diarrhea").
- Record any unusual event or circumstances (falls, patient or family comments, concerns).
- Record routine and ongoing nursing care.
- Record conversations and phone calls to physicians, advanced practice nurses, families, diagnostic facilities, and so on.
- Record recommended actions or inactions ("no new orders received") in response to phone calls and inquiries.
- When taking verbal medication orders by phone, request the physician repeat doses at least twice to verify accuracy. For example, "Dr. Jones, I would like to confirm that you ordered Compazine, 25 milligrams, be given orally every 6 hours for complaint of nausea. Is that correct?"
- Ask the physician or advanced practice nurse to fax the information conveyed in the telephone order if possible, as an additional safeguard.
- Record thoughts when any actions are taken or not taken as the result of nursing judgments. For example, "Oral fluids withheld as patient lacks gag reflex and is at risk for aspiration. Dr. Jones notified by phone and IV fluid rate increased by 50 mL/hr to prevent dehydration."
- Do not scratch out, white out, enter notes later, or obliterate any part of the patient record. If an error is made, draw a single line through the entry and write "mistaken entry" (or, e.g., "incorrect patient") and sign your name.

BOX 3-6 ▷ **Recommended Documentation After a Fall**

- Time of day
- Outcomes of the fall (e.g., injury, changes in vital signs, pain, deformity)
- What the patient said ("I forgot my glasses!")
- Whether mechanical devices were involved (e.g., walkers, bed alarms, wheelchairs)
- Whether the nursing staff was aware of the fall risk
- What fall-reducing measures (if any) were in place (e.g., placing the bed in the position closest to the floor, presence of bed alarm, use of protective floor mat, scheduling of frequent observations, patient placed close to nurses' station, use of protective hip pads)

---

the care given. Nurses should follow the guidelines listed in Box 3-5 when documenting care.

When documenting an adverse event occurring in the clinical environment, the standard of practice is to record all circumstances surrounding the event. For instance, if a patient falls, the nurse should carefully document the circumstances of the fall, as indicated in Box 3-6.

Not all falls can be prevented, even with the highest quality nursing care. When frail older adults move about on their own, falls will occur. The nurse can take steps to minimize the risks for fall and injury. See Chapter 18 for further information on patient falls.

At one time, physical restraints were routinely used in nursing homes and hospitals to prevent falls. Waist restraints, bed rails, vests, and lap belts were used to limit movement and keep patients confined to their bed or chair. However, since the passage of OBRA 87, restraints are now limited to short-term use (2 hours or less) and only with a

physician's order in emergency situations. This is because nursing research illustrated the relationship between the use of physical restraints and many problems of immobility, including decubitus ulcers, fecal and urinary incontinence, increased agitation, and physical deconditioning. Now gerontological nurses are urged to develop alternatives to physical restraints such as addressing patient and environmental factors. Patient factors include making sure the resident is wearing eyeglasses and safe footwear, has discontinued all unnecessary medication, has supervision if it is required, has appropriate assistive devices such as canes and walkers, has frequently scheduled opportunities to use the toilet, and has the benefit of frequent nursing observation. Environmental factors include placing the bed in a low position, not using side rails to limit movement, having adequate environmental lighting, and reducing fall hazards such as dangling electrical cords, scatter rugs, and wet surfaces.

OBRA 87 also limits the use of chemical restraints, or the use of sedating psychotropic drugs to control behavior. It is now mandated that psychotropic drugs should be used only in circumstances where they will clearly benefit the older patient and improve the patient's quality of life. They are not to be used in circumstances where behavior such as calling out is annoying to the nurses. See Chapter 6 for further information regarding OBRA 87 and medication regulation.

Practice Pearl ▶▶▶ Try to limit the use of wheelchairs to the smallest number of older patients possible. Older people who learn to rely on wheelchairs are likely to suffer from muscle atrophy, making them less able to move about on their own. Also, many older patients get their feet tangled in the foot rests or sit down into unlocked wheelchairs, increasing the chance of falls with injury.

Patient Confidentiality

The healthcare record and information regarding the care and treatment of the patient must be kept confidential. Patients have the right to view their medical record if they choose and to ask questions regarding information contained in the record. Patients can ask for copies of their medical records, and their request must be granted in a timely manner. Healthcare facilities must maintain medical records for at least 7 years. Each healthcare facility is required to develop policies and procedures to maintain the medical record and ensure confidentiality.

Healthcare providers should not discuss patients in elevators, cafeterias, or other public areas where they can be overheard. Even if patient names are not used, it is sometimes possible to determine who is being discussed by the clinical information provided in the conversation.

Use of Technology in Assessment

The use of technology in many healthcare facilities leads to additional problems with patient confidentiality and privacy. Computers should have passwords that limit access to authorized providers only. Healthcare providers must be reminded to log off after using a computer to access a patient's medical record so that an unauthorized person cannot come along and gain access to medical records. Electronic health records (EHRs) have the potential to improve patient care through efficient access to complete patient health information. Benefits of the EHR include less reliance on paper charts, improved billing, easier and quicker access to patient information, improved visit coding, and reduced transcription costs. Additional potential benefits may include population management and proactive patient reminders; improved reimbursement from payers due to EHR usage; and participation in pay-for-performance programs. There is a need to harmonize this information across different EHR systems so that data are easily accessible between healthcare providers from differing healthcare systems (Estabrooks et al., 2012).

E-mails and fax machines can also transmit confidential patient information that unauthorized persons may have access to. Fax machines should be used only when it is understood that the authorized provider is the only receiver or that the authorized receiver will "stand by" a shared fax machine to receive confidential information. When e-mail is used to transmit confidential information, only secure networks should be used. Larger healthcare facilities address this issue by offering private entry codes to authorized users. These codes are changed routinely, and caregivers are urged never to share them with others. Smaller facilities and individual providers should work with computer security consultants to ensure that their e-mail systems and networks are secure and that patients' records and communications cannot be read, deleted, or altered by unauthorized persons.

Patients must sign a permission form to authorize release of information before medical records can be copied, faxed, electronically transmitted, or released to others. Technology has the tremendous potential to enhance access to healthcare services for older patients, but extra efforts are needed to ensure privacy. The gerontological nurse should be informed of all regulations and restrictions governing emerging technologies and access to patient records.

Health Insurance Portability and Accountability Act

In 1996, the Health Insurance Portability and Accountability Act (HIPAA) was signed into law (Public Law 104-191) with the broad goal of improving the efficiency and effectiveness of the healthcare system. It is the first national legislation that protects every patient's health information through the establishment of standards and requirements for the electronic transmission of certain health information (eligibility, referrals, and claims). Healthcare providers were required to comply with privacy rules as of April 1, 2003.

HIPAA standards include:

- Confidentiality—Only the right people can see protected information.
- Integrity—The information is supposed to be without alteration or destruction.
- Availability—The right people can see it when needed.
- The information is protected against reasonably anticipated threats and hazards to its security or integrity.
- The information is protected against reasonably anticipated uses and disclosures not permitted by privacy rules.
- The provider will ensure compliance by the agency workforce.

USDHHS, 2011a.

Most larger healthcare institutions have developed HIPAA training and certification to educate their employees regarding the new requirements for the protection of patient privacy. The cornerstone of the training is that privacy and confidentiality are basic rights in our society and it is now the legal and ethical obligation of all healthcare providers to protect that right.

The following healthcare information is considered confidential:

- Patient-identifying information (name, medical record number)
- Health information relating to past, present, or future health status or condition
- Documentation regarding the provision of health care
- Past, present, or future payment for the provision of health care

During their initial visit to a healthcare provider, it is mandated that all patients will receive a privacy notice. The privacy notice is a written statement of how their healthcare information will be used and disclosed. The patient is asked to sign a form acknowledging receipt of the privacy notice.

If HIPAA standards are not followed and breaches in privacy occur, healthcare institutions can be held accountable for wrongful disclosures. Severe civil and criminal penalties will be brought forward, including fines and sanctions against business associates and workforce members in violation.

Examples of breaches or seemingly innocent activities that can lead to breaches include the following:

- Throwing test results or patient reports into the regular trash
- Failing to log off after checking a patient record on the computer
- Leaving a medical record open at the nurses' station, in the hallway, or in a conference room
- Sending a patient report to be printed and forgetting to take it off the printer
- Discussing patient information with a family member without the patient's permission
- Failing to check the ID badge or reason for needing the chart when a coworker in scrubs or a lab coat asks for a patient chart

Various policies have been developed to assist healthcare workers to practice safely and meet the new confidentiality legislations. Policies vary from institution to institution; however, Box 3-7 lists guidelines typical of the kinds of safeguards that can be instituted. For more complete information on HIPAA and to follow the development and implementation of new regulations, visit the U.S. Department of Health and Human Services website.

Informed Consent and Competence

The Patient Self-Determination Act requires providers to seek informed consent from all patients before they receive health care or engage in a research protocol. Older patients are entitled to be told the full implications of their treatment or nontreatment and then have the freedom to make an independent decision, without coercion, whether or not to receive the care. Older persons have the

---

BOX 3-7 ▶ Guidelines for Computer Security

- Do not share passwords.
- Always log off after reviewing a patient record.
- Do not let others glance over your shoulder when you are reviewing a patient record at a computer workstation.
- Limit your viewing of patient records to only those patients for whom you are providing care or who are participating in a valid research study and have given informed consent.

Faxing

- Use caution with fax machines, because they are the least secure of all technologies.
- When faxing information, always use a cover sheet with a confidentiality statement.
- Never leave fax machines sitting unattended.
- Always verify the fax number before faxing patient information, verify the receiver is available to immediately receive the fax, and verify patient permission to release the information before faxing.

E-Mail

- When sending e-mail, never use a patient's name or medical record number in the subject line.
- Attach a confidentiality statement as part of your automatic signature. For example, "The information contained in this e-mail is intended only for the person to whom it is addressed and may contain confidential and/or privileged information. If you received this e-mail in error, please contact the sender and delete the material from your computer."
- An e-mail with confidential patient information should not be sent over the Internet (public access), because security cannot be guaranteed. Use only Intranet secure systems (limited to use by authorized providers) to ensure privacy.

right to make informed decisions about all care and treatment unless they have been determined to be incompetent (unable to make decisions) by a court of law. Failure to receive consent before a medical or surgical procedure is carried out can be considered assault and battery, a criminal offense.

Often, upon admission to a healthcare facility, the older person will sign a consent for routine care, which gives permission to others to provide care with bathing, dressing, feeding, and medication administration. However, these general consent forms do not cover specialized procedures such as blood transfusions, electroshock therapy, experimental procedures, and invasive procedures.

For consent to be truly informed, the nurse must explain to the older patient in language that he or she can understand the benefits and burdens of the procedure being proposed. Benefits are considered to be outcomes of treatment that would improve the care or comfort of the patient. Burdens are considered to be any potential pain and suffering the patient may have to endure as a result of treatment. Ideally, treatments should offer benefits to the patient without overwhelming burdens. However, when burden is high and chance of benefit is low, the intervention may be considered medically futile. For instance, an older patient with widespread metastatic cancer may be offered one more surgery or one more round of chemotherapy, even though there is little chance of cure, remission, or improvement in quality of life. If the older patient and the family make an informed decision to receive this care after the risks and benefits have been explained, the care may be considered legal but probably not ethical.

To feel comfortable gaining consent from older patients, the gerontological nurse will want to assess capacity for consent. To be considered capable of providing consent, older patients should have the ability to:

- Comprehend information (understand).
- Contemplate options (reason).
- Evaluate risks and consequences (problem solve).
- Communicate that decision (make their decision known).

While *competence* is a legal term, *capacity* is a clinical term. Gerontological nurses are called on to assist in the determination of decisional capacity of older patients. When a patient lacks decisional capacity because of severe illness, sedating drugs, or cognitive impairment, there are mechanisms and laws that dictate who may make a decision for the patient. If the patient has a living will, a healthcare proxy or surrogate decision maker, durable power of attorney, or involved family member, these persons or documents will be used to decide whether to proceed with the treatment or procedure in question (see Chapter 11). If an older person lacks decisional capacity and has no predetermined wishes, family, or healthcare proxy, the care facility may seek a court-appointed guardian. A guardian is appointed by a judge to act on behalf of a *ward* when the judge has determined that the ward is incapacitated and in need of a decision maker. Guardians may be relatives, friends, or strangers. Usually wards are people with advanced dementia, untreated mental illness, developmental disabilities, head injuries, strokes, or long-standing drug addictions (Seniors for Living, 2011).

Assessment of decisional capacity is an ongoing dynamic process. Patients have the right to make decisions that do not follow the recommendations of healthcare providers and to change their mind at any time. Even if patients have dementia or cognitive impairments, it does not mean that they should not be consulted regarding treatment decisions. Often, while true consent cannot be obtained from an older person, *assent* should be sought. If the older person does not assent to the care to be given, it ethically cannot be offered. For instance, if the healthcare proxy consents to a blood transfusion for an older patient with dementia, the patient may not agree to having the needle inserted into the arm and may violently resist the procedure. To avoid conflict and the risk of potential harm to the patient, assent for all procedures should be obtained from the older patient before beginning any treatment or procedure. Patients with dementia are assumed to be unable to participate in decision making, but current research indicates that this is an inaccurate assumption (Alzheimer's Association, 2011).

End-of-Life Issues

When the end of life is approaching, a variety of legal as well as ethical issues may emerge. (Chapter 11 provides a complete discussion of these issues.) An older patient who is approaching death may not be able to make ongoing treatment decisions. Confusion as to how to provide appropriate care may arise. If the person has named a healthcare proxy to make a decision or has an advance directive such as a living will, then healthcare professionals will have guidance through the decision-making process at the end of life. However, most older patients have not

Weblink: Five Wishes Form Website

completed an advance directive or named a proxy. Barriers to the completion of an advance directive include the following:

- Inability to speak English
- Religious or ethnic beliefs
- Poor eyesight, cognitive impairment, and/or hearing
- Standardized forms that are too technical or print that is too small to read
- Procrastination
- Dependence on family for all decisions
- Lack of knowledge about advance directives
- Belief a lawyer is necessary
- Fear of being written off or signing life away
- Acceptance of the will of God

Fried et al., 2010.

Do-not-resuscitate (DNR) or the newer term *allow-natural-death* orders may appear on the charts of many frail older patients. They are written and signed by the physician or advanced practice nurse and are legally valid orders. *Allow natural death* (AND) is a formal designation that can replace the DNR order in some hospitals and other healthcare facilities. AND is also a model of care that acknowledges aging and death as a natural part of life—one that foregoes aggressive technologies that treat aging as if it were a disease requiring curative interventions. While DNR orders describe patient wishes for intubation or chest compressions or the administration of intravenous medications, AND orders additionally describe the patient's instructions for the use of feeding tubes, administration of antibiotics, use of catheters and intravenous fluids, and other methods of prolonging life. Without exception, AND orders emphasize provisions for comfort measures as needed (Taft & Daniels, 2010). A useful form available

online or print called *Five Wishes* assists an older person to express how he or she would want to be treated in the event of serious illness and inability to speak for himself or herself. This form addresses the older person's needs including medical, personal, emotional, and spiritual needs.

Some healthcare facilities mandate that if these orders are not in place, then the older person should be a candidate for cardiopulmonary resuscitation (CPR) and other heroic measures. Unfortunately, CPR is not very successful in older people who experience cardiac arrest in the nursing home or community setting. Monitoring equipment, intravenous access, and equipment to reverse cardiac arrhythmias are usually not readily available and delays in treatment often occur. Older patients who survive the cardiac arrest may suffer brain damage or broken ribs and have an even poorer quality of life than they experienced before the cardiac arrest.

The gerontological nurse should consult the patient, the family, and advance directives when a patient's code status is being considered. All discussions with the patient and the family should be documented in the patient chart. If there are problems or disagreements within the family, the nurse should involve the patient, family, physician, social worker, clergy, or the ethics team.

Patient and Family Teaching

Gerontological nurses require skills and knowledge related to teaching patients and families about the key concepts of gerontology and gerontological nursing. The guidelines in the following feature will assist the nurse to assume the role of teacher and coach.

Patient–Family Teaching Guidelines

The following are guidelines that the nurse may find useful when instructing older persons and their families about gerontological nursing in health care.

PRINCIPLES OF GERIATRICS

1 What should I look for when choosing a physician?

Look for a physician who is well trained, competent, and conveniently located. Additional things to consider include:

- *Board certification.* Choose a physician who is a specialist in geriatrics, internal medicine, or other area such as cardiology to treat your specific problem.
- *Type of insurance.* Choose a physician who accepts Medicare or is in your managed care network.
- *Hospital affiliation.* Choose a physician who admits patients to a hospital you have faith in and is convenient to you and your family.
- *Interdisciplinary team.* Choose a physician who works with others who can help you to stay healthy, including gerontological nurses, social workers, nutritionists, physical therapists, and so on.

RATIONALE:

Choosing a physician wisely is key to good health care. Older patients should benefit from having a physician who is convenient to see and who accepts their insurance. The website Physician Compare helps older people find a physician in their geographic area and provides maps, directions, and details about the practice.

2 What type of physician is best for me?

It is always good to choose a geriatrician, family practitioner, or internist for your primary care physician. Some things to consider include the following:

- Family practitioners can treat a wide range of problems and do not specialize in any one area.
- Internists are physicians for adults. Some take extra training and specialize in a certain area like cardiology.
- Geriatricians focus specifically on problems of aging and are trained in family practice and internal medicine. Geriatricians usually work with a team of healthcare professionals.

RATIONALE:

Talk to your family, friends, healthcare professionals, and neighbors when choosing a physician. Ask how they chose their physician and what they like and dislike about him or her. When a physician is described consistently as "great," "approachable," "caring," "takes time to get to know you," you can feel confident in choosing this physician. When you need a specialist, get advice from a healthcare professional and be sure to pick someone who is knowledgeable and competent.

3 How can I increase my chances of making an informed choice?

Here are some questions to ask the nurse or receptionist in the office of a physician you are considering:

- What age patients do you treat?
- Do you specialize in any areas such as cardiology, dermatology, or orthopedics? (Choose areas to ask about that are of interest to you.)
- How long do I have to wait for an appointment?
- How long does the physician spend with each patient?
- May I bring a family member with me?
- Is the physician comfortable in including patients in healthcare decisions?
- Where are the laboratory tests and X-rays performed?

RATIONALE:

After asking these questions, the older person should meet with the physician and decide whether to proceed with the relationship.

4 What should I do to prepare for the first appointment?

During your first visit, your physician and nurse will probably take a health history and ask you about your health. You can help by bringing a list of medications, medical diagnoses, tests and operations you have had, and any significant events like hospitalizations, accidents, and injuries. Make a list of any drug allergies or serious drug reactions you have had. Be prepared to describe what a typical day is like for you. During this visit, take time to ask questions and get comfortable with your new physician. Leave time to discuss how you wish to be treated should you become unable to make your own healthcare decisions. For example, do you want to have CPR if your heart stops beating? Would you want to have aggressive care like intravenous fluids if you had dementia or Alzheimer's

Patient–Family Teaching Guidelines *(continued)*

disease? Discuss these issues with your new physician and nurse and name a person whom you trust to make decisions if you are unable to make them yourself.

RATIONALE:

Finding a good physician is just the first part of the caring process. The older patient should enter into an active *partnership with the physician and nurse to solve health problems and improve function. Good communication is the key. Stay involved and advocate for your health and well-being!*

CARE PLAN   A Patient With Multiple Diagnoses

Case Study

Mrs. Cooper is an 83-year-old woman who is admitted to the hospital for observation following a fall in her home. She lives alone with support from her daughter who visits once or twice a week to bring food and check up on her mom. Mrs. Cooper has several diagnoses including hypertension, nervous anxiety, macular degeneration, and arthritis. Neither Mrs. Cooper nor her daughter can name all of the physicians and healthcare specialists she has seen in the past few years because she has received many referrals, has been evaluated by a variety of consultations, and does not have a stable primary care provider.

The patient reports she takes many medicines, most of which she cannot name. The daughter reports Mrs. Cooper does not eat very well and has lost weight recently. She worries that her mom has had other falls that she has not reported to anyone, because she is fearful of having to go to a nursing home.

Applying the Nursing Process

Assessment

The nurse should obtain further information. Mrs. Cooper may have many physical, social, and psychological issues that could be influencing her health status. She needs a complete geriatric assessment with input from a variety of team members.

Diagnosis

Several nursing diagnoses could be considered. The hospitalization and immediate problem is related to a fall. Therefore, *Risk for Falls* might be the most immediate problem. If Mrs. Cooper is released from the hospital without adequate assessment of her fall risks, she may suffer another fall with significant injury or even premature death. The immediate need is to complete a fall history and subsequent interdisciplinary review to determine why falls are occurring. Additional diagnoses to be considered might include the following:

- *Failure to Thrive, Adult*
- *Injury, Risk for*
- *Coping, Ineffective*
- *Health Maintenance, Impaired*
- *Knowledge, Deficient* related to medications and therapeutic regimen management
- *Nutrition, Imbalanced*: Less than Body Requirements

NANDA-I © 2012.

(continued)

CARE PLAN   **A Patient With Multiple Diagnoses** *(continued)*

Expected Outcomes

Expected outcomes for the plan of care specify that Mrs. Cooper will:

- Become aware of the harmful effects of poor nutrition on health status and function.
- Accept family or paid help with grocery shopping and/or meal preparation to improve her nutritional status.
- Use appropriate safety measures in the home to decrease falling including elimination of clutter, placing handrails if needed, and use of mats and grab bars in the bathroom.
- Develop a stable, caring relationship with a primary healthcare provider to oversee and coordinate visits to specialists as evidenced by visiting the healthcare provider every 6 months or more often if needed.
- Agree to establish a therapeutic relationship with the nurse and develop a mutually acceptable plan to work toward these outcomes.

Planning and Implementation

The following nursing interventions may be appropriate for Mrs. Cooper:

- Establish a therapeutic relationship.
- Consult with nutritionist, social worker, and other members of the healthcare team.
- Encourage a family meeting with the daughter present to talk about health issues in general, with Mrs. Cooper's permission.
- Carefully assess all functional health patterns, noting strengths in order to maximize function.
- Begin a values clarification to establish long-term goals and facilitate end-of-life planning.

Evaluation

Mrs. Cooper has several strengths, including a stable home environment, an involved daughter living close by, a history of adequate and appropriate self-care, and motivation to continue to live independently.

The nurse will consider the plan a success based on the following criteria:

- Improvement in functional ability and health status
- Reduction in risk for injury
- Identification of a stable primary care provider
- Improvement of trust in the healthcare system
- Reduction of possible feelings of strain and burden as verbalized by Mrs. Cooper's caregiver daughter

Ethical Dilemma

A second daughter from California pages the nurse at the hospital. She introduces herself and requests information regarding her mom's condition. The nurse asks why she has not spoken with her mom or her sister directly. She states she had a disagreement with them several years ago and is not on good terms, but wants to stay informed of her mom's condition. Because information cannot be shared with the daughter without the consent of the patient, the nurse can suggest she leave her phone number and have Mrs. Cooper give her a call if she is willing. The nurse could validate the daughter's concern and offer to share with Mrs. Cooper the fact that she phoned and is requesting information. HIPAA guidelines do not allow the sharing of confidential patient information with others (even families) without the consent of the patient. Violation of the regulations could result in fines and censure.

CARE PLAN A Patient With Multiple Diagnoses *(continued)*

Critical Thinking and the Nursing Process

1. Imagine that you are caring for Mr. Turner, a hospice patient. He is dying of esophageal cancer and is cognitively intact. He asks you to make sure no one puts a tube down his throat when he is near death. His family is worried that when the end is near and he becomes short of breath, he may change his mind and will be unable to communicate his wishes. What strategies would you use to communicate and reassure this patient?

2. Imagine you are caring for Mrs. Lee. She lives alone and can no longer care for herself due to severe cognitive impairment. She has no family and refuses to discuss leaving her home. What is the best course of action to pursue?

3. You have a colleague who consistently forgets to log off from the computer when checking patient records. Once, you found a confidential psychiatric record clearly displayed on the computer terminal at the nurses' station. What action is appropriate?

■ Evaluate your responses in Appendix B. ⫸

Chapter Highlights

■ Providing holistic care to the older patient is a joy and a challenge. An interdisciplinary team can provide a comprehensive evaluation to fully understand the health needs of an older person and to form the basis for the plan of care.

■ Standardized instruments are available to assist in the evaluation process and monitor patient progress over time.

■ The gerontological nurse is a key member of the interdisciplinary team, often taking the lead and coordinating care.

■ A comprehensive geriatric assessment includes emphasis on physical, psychological, and socioeconomic factors, and input from various health professionals. Functional ability is the central focus of the examination.

■ Contextual variables such as the older person's culture and level of education can affect the assessment process and should be addressed to facilitate the gathering of accurate and complete patient information.

■ Health for older adults is a complex interaction of physical, functional, and psychosocial factors. The gerontological nurse can play a key role in the implementation of the goals of *Healthy People 2020*. The overarching goals for health promotion and disease prevention include increasing quality and years of healthy life and eliminating health disparities. Recommended health screenings and interventions for older persons can assist in meeting these goals.

■ Legal issues and the protection of patient privacy present challenges to gerontological nurses and other healthcare providers who often must seek or ask to share confidential patient information with others, obtain informed consent, and assist patients and families with end-of-life decision making. Guidelines for documentation, safeguarding confidentiality, and assessing decisional capacity are suggested.

Pearson Nursing Student Resources
Find additional review materials at
nursing.pearsonhighered.com

Prepare for success with additional NCLEX®-style practice questions, interactive assignments and activities, web links, animations and videos, and more!

References

Alzheimer's Association. (2011). *The national Alzheimer's project act (NAPA)*. Retrieved from http://napa.alz.org/wp-content/uploads/2011/11/2011-NAPA-Factsheet-Post-Report.pdf

American Nurses Credentialing Center. (2012). *Gerontological nurse*. Retrieved from http://consultgerirn.org/uploads/File/ANCC_Gerontologica_Nursing_Cert_Brochure.pdf

American Psychological Association. (2011). *What practitioners should know about working with older adults*. Retrieved from http://www.apa.org/pi/aging/resources/guides/practitioners-should-know.aspx

Bearskin, R. (2011). A critical lens on culture in nursing practice. *Nursing Ethics, 15*(4), 548–559.

Borson, S., Scanlan, J., Chen, P., & Ganguli, M. (2003). The Mini-Cog as a screen for dementia: Validation in a population-based sample. *Journal of the American Geriatrics Society, 51*(10), 1451–1454.

Capezuti, L., Siegler, E., & Mezey, M. (2008). *Encyclopedia of elder care* (2nd ed.). New York, NY: Springer.

Centers for Disease Control and Prevention. (2011). *MMWR—Recommended adult immunization schedule—US 2011*. Retrieved from http://www.cdc.gov/vaccines/recs/schedules/downloads/adult/mmwr-adult-schedule.pdf

Centers for Medicare and Medicaid Services (2010). *RAI version 3.0 manual*. Retrieved from http://www.polaris-group.com/Press%20Releases/Chapter%204%20-%20CAA_Process%20and%20Care%20Planning.pdf

Estabrooks, P., Boyle, M., Emmons, K., Glasgow, R., Hesse, B., Kaplan, R., Krist, A., Moser, R., & Taylor, M. (2012). Harmonized patient-reported data elements in the electronic health record: Supporting meaningful use by primary care action on health behaviors and key psychosocial factors. *Journal of the American Medical Informatics Association*. Retrieved from http://jamia.bmj.com/content/early/2012/04/16/amiajnl-2011-000576.abstract

Fried, T., Redding, C., Robbins, M., Paiva, A., O'Leary, J., & Iannone, L. (2010). States of change for the component behaviors of advance care planning. *Journal of the American Geriatrics Society, 58*, 2329–2336.

Granger, C., Albrecht, G., & Hamilton, B. (1979). Outcomes of comprehensive medical rehabilitation: Measures of PULSES profile and the Barthel index. *Archives of Physical Medicine and Rehabilitation, 60*, 145–154.

Hartford Institute for Geriatric Nursing. (2011a). *Assessment tools: Try this*. Retrieved from http://hartfordign.org/Practice/Try_This

Hartford Institute for Geriatric Nursing. (2011b). *GITT—Dynamic team building guidance to enhance care*. Retrieved from http://hartfordign.org/Education/GITT

Joint Commission. (2011). *Joint Commission primary care medical home (PCMH) model*. Retrieved from http://www.jointcommission.org/assets/1/18/Joint_Commission_PCMH_model.pdf

Kane, R., Ouslander, J., Abrass, I., & Resnick, B. (2009). *Essentials of clinical geriatrics* (6th ed.). New York, NY: McGraw-Hill.

Katz, S., Down, T. D., Cash, H. R., & Grotz, R. C. (1970). Progress in the development of the index of ADL. *The Gerontologist, 10*(1), 20–30.

Kurlowicz, L. M., & Greenberg, S. (2007). The Geriatric Depression Scale (GDS). *Try this: Best practices in nursing care for older adults*. Hartford Institute of Geriatric Nursing. Retrieved from http://www.hartfordign.org/publications/trythis/issue04.pdf

National Alliance on Mental Illness. (2009). *Mental illnesses*. Retrieved from http://www.nami.org/Template.cfm?Section=By_Illness&template=/ContentManagement/ContentDisplay.cfm&ContentID=7515

Newman, M. (2010). *Health as expanding consciousness*. Retrieved from http://www.healthasexpandingconsciousness.org/home

Omnibus Budget Reconciliation Act (OBRA). (1987). Washington, DC: U.S. Department of Health and Human Affairs.

Pender, N., Murdaugh, C., & Parsons, M. (2010). *Health promotion in nursing practice* (6th ed.). Upper Saddle River, NJ: Prentice Hall Health.

Research Data Assistance Center. (2011). Resident level assessment data. Retrieved from http://www.resdac.org/mds/data_available.asp

Scherb, C., Head, B., Maas, M., Swanson, E., Moorhead, S., Reed, D., Conley, D., & Kozel, M. (2011). Most frequent nursing diagnoses, nursing interventions, and nursing-sensitive patient outcomes of hospitalized older adults with heart failure: Part 1. *International Journal of Nursing Knowledge*. Retrieved from http://onlinelibrary.wiley.com/doi/10.1111/j.1744-618X.2010.01164.x/full

Seniors for Living. (2011). *Guardianship and patient advocacy protects elders, prevents abuse*. Retrieved from http://www.seniorsforliving.com/blog/2011/09/26/guardianship-patient-advocacy-for-older-adults

Stuck, A., & Iliffe, S. (2011). Comprehensive geriatric assessment for older adults. *British Medical Journal, 343*, d6799.

Taft, R., & Daniels, S. (2010). Allow natural death. *Dorland Health*. Retrieved from http://www.dorlandhealth.com/adult_and_senior/cip_magazine/Allow-Natural-Death_804.html.

U.S. Department of Health and Human Services [USDHHS]. (2011a). *Health information privacy*. Retrieved from http://www.hhs.gov/ocr/privacy/hipaa/understanding/coveredentities/index.html

U.S. Department of Health and Human Services [USDHHS]. (2011b). *Healthy people 2020: What are its goals?* Rockville, MD: Author. Retrieved from http://www.healthypeople.gov

U.S. Preventive Services Task Force. (2011). *The guide to clinical preventive services*. Retrieved from http://www.uspreventiveservicestaskforce.org/index.html

Ward, K., & Reuben, D. (2011). *Comprehensive geriatric assessment*. Retrieved from http://www.uptodate.com/contents/comprehensive-geriatric-assessment

World Health Organization. (1946). *Preamble to the constitution of the World Health Organization*. Retrieved from http://www.who.int/about/definition/en

Challenges of Aging and the Cornerstones of Excellence in Nursing Care

Cultural Diversity

Rachel E. Spector, PhD, RN, CTN-A, FAAN

VISITING DISTINGUISHED SCHOLAR, INSTITUTE FOR PATIENT CARE, MASSACHUSETTS GENERAL HOSPITAL, BOSTON, MA

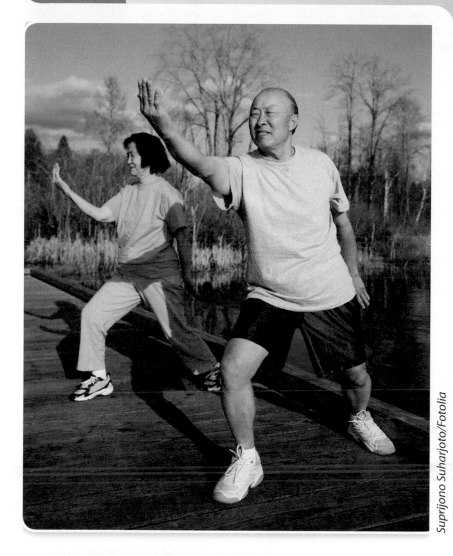

Suprijono Suharjoto/Fotolia

KEY TERMS

CLAS standards 77
communication 77
CULTURALCARE 76
culturally appropriate services 76
culturally competent care 76
culturally sensitive 78
culture 81
demographic disparity 79
demographic parity 78
ethnicity 81
heritage consistency 81
heritage inconsistency 81
life trajectory 78
religion 81
respectful care 77
socialization 81
Transcultural Nursing Society
    Standards 76

LEARNING OUTCOMES

On completion of this chapter, the reader will be able to:

1. Discuss the importance of the Transcultural Nursing Society's care standards and the culturally and linguistically appropriate services (CLAS) in health care.
2. Apply the CULTURALCARE triad to the complex interrelationships of the nurse, caregiver, and patient within community and institutional (home or residential) settings.
3. Identify potential areas of conflict derived from the demographic, ethnocultural, and life trajectory variables of the people within the triad.
4. Describe the value and process of heritage and life trajectory assessments of nurses, caregivers, and patients.
5. Create a plan of care for the older adult integrating CULTURALCARE.

Not only does cultural diversity have significant implications for healthcare delivery and policy making throughout the United States, it also has profound implications in the delivery of safe nursing care to older adult patients from diverse cultural backgrounds. People from the world's 251 sovereign states, dependent areas, or disputed territories are well represented in the United States, and their cultures are continually being blended and merged, in part because mobility is an ingrained feature of our society. Cultural diversity has been expanding into all regions of the country—not just inner city and coastal areas, but throughout the Midwest, suburbs, and small towns of America (Office of Minority Health, 2001).

In all clinical practice areas—nurse practitioner and doctor's offices, clinics, acute care settings, and long-term care settings—one sees this diversity every day. The need to provide culturally and linguistically competent healthcare services to diverse populations is attracting increased attention from health providers and those who judge their quality and efficiency. Although certain providers, such as nurses, have struggled to deliver **culturally appropriate services**—those in which providers have an underlying knowledge of specific cultural needs—to diverse populations for many years, this has not been the case in many mainstream settings. Now, as the mainstream begins to treat a more diverse patient population as a result of demographic changes and participation in insurance programs, the interest in designing culturally and linguistically appropriate services that lead to improved nursing care outcomes, efficiency, and patient satisfaction has increased.

Cultural background and language have a considerable impact both on how patients access and respond to healthcare services and on how the caregivers work within the system. The two main goals relating to the delivery of **culturally competent care,** in which the provider understands the total context of the patient's situation and attends to individualized needs, are:

1. To develop cultural and linguistic competence by nurses and other healthcare providers
2. For healthcare organizations to understand and respond effectively to the cultural and linguistic needs brought by both patients and caregivers to the healthcare experience

This two-pronged phenomenon recognizes the diversity that exists among the patients, nurses, and caregivers. It is not limited to the changes in the patient population. It also embraces the members of the workforce—both the nurses who may be from other countries and the caregivers. Many of the people in the workforce are new immigrants or are from ethnocultural backgrounds that are different from those of their patients.

This chapter presents an overview of the salient content and complex processes necessary to enable professional nurses to develop knowledge and skills related to the development of culturally competent care, or CULTURALCARE, and to integrate CULTURALCARE into their gerontological nursing practice and into the practice environment. CULTURALCARE is the term coined by Spector (2009) to describe nursing care that is culturally competent, culturally appropriate, and culturally sensitive.

Transcultural Nursing Care Standards

The Transcultural Nursing Society (n.d.), a professional nursing organization whose mission is to "enhance the quality of culturally congruent, competent, and equitable care that results in improved health and well being for people worldwide," has developed 12 standards for cultural competence in nursing practice (Box 4-1).

BOX 4-1   **Twelve Standards for Cultural Competence**

Standard 1. Social Justice—Promote social justice for all

Standard 2. Critical Reflection—Understand one's own values, beliefs, and cultural heritage to have awareness of how these attributes affect culturally congruent care

Standard 3. Knowledge of Cultures—Develop understanding of the perspectives, traditions, and so forth of the communities of the populations they care for

Standard 4. Culturally Competent Practice—Use cross-cultural knowledge and culturally sensitive skills in implementing care

Standard 5. Cultural Competence in Healthcare Systems and Organizations—Provide the structure and resources necessary to meet the cultural and language needs of patients

Standard 6. Patient Advocacy and Empowerment—Advocate for the inclusion of patient's cultural beliefs and practices in all facets of health care

Standard 7. Multicultural Workforce—Engage in efforts to ensure a multicultural workforce

Standard 8. Education and Training in Culturally Competent Care—Educational preparation to provide culturally competent care

Standard 9. Cross-Cultural Communication—Knowledge of verbal and nonverbal communication skills

Standard 10. Cross-Cultural Leadership—Development of knowledge and skills to influence others to achieve culturally competent care

Standard 11. Policy Development—Development of knowledge and skills to establish comprehensive policies in both the public and private sectors

Standard 12. Evidence-Based Practice and Research—Research-based practice that will be effective in multi-cultural populations

Source: Douglas, M. K., Pierce, J. U., Rosenkoetter, M., et al. (2011). Standards of practice for culturally competent care. *Journal of Transcultural Nursing, 22*(4), 318.

National Standards

In 1997, the Office of Minority Health undertook the development of national standards to provide a much-needed alternative to the patchwork that had been available in the field of cultural diversity. They developed the *National Standards for Culturally and Linguistically Appropriate Services in Health Care* (**CLAS standards**). These 14 standards (Box 4-2) must be met by most healthcare-related agencies. The standards are based on an analytical review of key laws, regulations, contracts, and standards currently in use by federal and state agencies and other national organizations. They were developed with input from a national advisory committee of policy makers, healthcare providers, and researchers. (Revised standards of care were expected to be published sometime in 2012.) Once published, they can be accessed from the Office of Minority Health Information. Accreditation and credentialing agencies can assess and compare providers of culturally competent services and ensure quality care for diverse populations. These agencies include The Joint Commission (TJC), the National Committee on Quality Assurance, professional organizations such as the American Medical Association and the American Nurses Association, and quality review organizations such as peer review organizations. It is a given that comprehensive nursing care depends on effective **communication** (the exchange of information, thoughts, or feelings) between patients and all nursing care providers. Ineffective communication can lead to improper nursing diagnoses and delayed or improper nursing care. Effective communication with persons who have limited English proficiency (LEP)—as

---

BOX 4-2 ▶ **National Standards for Culturally and Linguistically Appropriate Services (CLAS) in Health Care**

1. Healthcare organizations should ensure that patients/consumers receive from all staff members effective, understandable, and **respectful care** (care reflecting consideration of the values, preferences, and needs of the patient/family) that is provided in a manner compatible with their cultural health beliefs and practices and preferred language.

2. Healthcare organizations should implement strategies to recruit, retain, and promote at all levels of the organization a diverse staff and leadership that are representative of the demographic characteristics of the service area.

3. Healthcare organizations should ensure that staff at all levels and across all disciplines receive ongoing education and training in culturally and linguistically appropriate service delivery.

4. Healthcare organizations must offer and provide language assistance services, including bilingual staff and interpreter services, at no cost to each patient/consumer with limited English proficiency at all points of contact, in a timely manner during all hours of operation.

5. Healthcare organizations must provide to patients/consumers in their preferred language both verbal offers and written notices informing them of their right to receive language assistance services.

6. Healthcare organizations must assure the competence of language assistance provided to limited English proficient patients/consumers by interpreters and bilingual staff. Family and friends should not be used to provide interpretation services (except on request by the patient/consumer).

7. Healthcare organizations must make available easily understood patient-related materials and post signage in the languages of the commonly encountered groups and/or groups represented in the service area.

8. Healthcare organizations should develop, implement, and promote a written strategic plan that outlines clear goals, policies, operational plans, and management accountability/oversight mechanisms to provide culturally and linguistically appropriate services.

9. Healthcare organizations should conduct initial and ongoing organizational self-assessments of CLAS-related activities and are encouraged to integrate cultural and linguistic competence–related measures into their internal audits, performance improvement programs, patient satisfaction assessments, and outcomes-based evaluations.

10. Healthcare organizations should ensure that data on the individual patient's/consumer's race, ethnicity, and spoken and written language are collected in health records, integrated into the organization's management information systems, and periodically updated.

11. Healthcare organizations should maintain a current demographic, cultural, and epidemiological profile of the community as well as a needs assessment to accurately plan for and implement services that respond to the cultural and linguistic characteristics of the service area.

12. Healthcare organizations should develop participatory, collaborative partnerships with communities and utilize a variety of formal and informal mechanisms to facilitate community and patient/consumer involvement in designing and implementing CLAS-related activities.

13. Healthcare organizations should ensure that conflict and grievance resolution processes are culturally and linguistically sensitive and capable of identifying, preventing, and resolving cross-cultural conflicts or complaints by patients/consumers.

14. Healthcare organizations are encouraged to regularly make available to the public information about their progress and successful innovations in implementing the CLAS standards and to provide public notice in their communities about the availability of this information.

Source: U.S. Department of Health and Human Services. (2001). *National standards for culturally and linguistically appropriate services in health care: Final report.* Washington, DC: Author.

well as persons who are deaf or hard-of-hearing—often requires interpreters. Title VI of the Civil Rights Act of 1964 prohibits discrimination on the basis of race, color, and national origin. Under these laws, nursing personnel must communicate effectively with patients, family members, and visitors who are deaf or hard of hearing. They must take reasonable steps to provide meaningful access to their nursing care plans for persons who have limited English proficiency. Complementing these obligations are the new accreditation provisions promulgated by TJC, including the recently adopted requirement that nurses and other care providers collect information about the language and communications needs of patients.

To ensure both equal access to quality health care by diverse populations and a secure work environment, nurses should "promote and support the attitudes, behaviors, knowledge, and skills necessary for staff to work respectfully and effectively with patients and each other in a culturally diverse work environment" (Office of Minority Health, 2001, p. 7). This is the first of the 14 CLAS standards in health care.

CULTURALCARE Nursing

CULTURALCARE is professional nursing care that is culturally competent, culturally appropriate, and culturally sensitive. CULTURALCARE nursing is critical to meet the complex nursing care needs of a given person, family, and community. It is the provision of nursing care across cultural boundaries and takes into account the context in which the patient lives as well as the situations in which the patient's health problems arise.

■ **Culturally competent.** The nurse understands and attends to the total context of the patient's situation. It is a complex combination of knowledge, skills, and attitudes.

Example: If the patient has dietary practices such as not mixing meat and dairy foods, food and beverage combinations that the patient prefers can be readily supplied. An exploration of dietary beliefs and practices will be inherent in the orientation of all nurses and assistive personnel.

■ **Culturally appropriate.** The nurse applies the underlying background knowledge that must be possessed to provide a given patient with the best possible health care.

Example: If the patient values modesty, the nurse will strive to have care provided by a person of the same sex and to protect the patient's personal privacy at all times. If the staff member is reluctant to provide care

to a person of the opposite sex because of cultural or religious beliefs, the nurse will respect the beliefs and interpret them to the staff.

■ **Culturally sensitive.** The nurse possesses some basic knowledge of, and constructive attitudes toward, the health traditions observed among the diverse cultural groups found in the practice setting.

Example: If a given patient does not desire adult immunizations, blood transfusions, or invasive procedures of any sort, the patient's, family's, or healthcare proxy's wishes will be granted and respected.

CULTURALCARE expresses all that is inherent in the development of nursing practice to meet the mandates of the Transcultural Nursing Society's standards and the CLAS standards. Countless conflicts in the healthcare delivery arena have been predicated on cultural misunderstandings. Many of these misunderstandings are related to universal situations such as verbal and nonverbal language misunderstandings, the conventions of courtesy, sequencing of interactions, phasing of interactions, and objectivity. However, many cultural misunderstandings are unique to the delivery of nursing care. The necessity to provide CULTURALCARE demands that nurses be able to assess and interpret a given patient's health beliefs and practices and cultural needs. CULTURALCARE alters the perspective of nursing care delivery as it enables the nurse to understand the manifestations of the patient's cultural, ethnic, and religious heritage and **life trajectory,** or passage and experiences of a given person as his or her life unfolds from birth to death. The nurse must serve as a bridge in the community and long-term care settings between the patient and the direct caregivers who are from different cultural backgrounds. This is accomplished by serving as a role model.

CULTURALCARE Triad

The delivery of CULTURALCARE to the entire population, especially the older population, is extremely complex. It grows from an understanding of the ethnocultural religious heritages and life trajectories of the people involved in the CULTURALCARE triad. The triad is set within the demographic change that has swept the United States during the past 35 years. It is composed of three distinct populations: the nurse, the direct caregiver, and the patient. Each of the populations enters into the patient care arena with different backgrounds that are predicated on their ethnocultural religious heritage and life trajectory; hence, the relationship between the parties is complex. In addition, no **demographic parity** (an equal distribution of a given entity) exists between the three populations; hence, the

demographic disparity (a variation below given percentages of the total population with a specific entity) is striking.

Demographic Change

As of the 2010 U.S. census, the population of the United States included a White, non-Hispanic majority at 63.7%. For comparison, it was 83.2% in 1980, 75.6% in 1990, and 69.1% in 2000. People of color were over 36.3% of the population, and the numbers are growing. More than half of the growth in the total U.S. population between 2000 and 2010 resulted from an increase in the Hispanic population. Between 2000 and 2010, the Hispanic population grew by 43% and, by 2010, Hispanics comprised 16% of the total U.S. population (U.S. Census Bureau, 2010).

By the year 2020, it is predicted that people of color will be the majority population, and the major source of people for population growth will be immigrants. In addition, millions of immigrants were admitted to the United States during the 1990s and 2010s. In 2010 alone, a total of 1,042,625 people became legal permanent residents (LPRs) of the United States. The majority, 54%, already resided here. Among the LPRs, Mexico at 13%, China at 7%, and India at 7% were the leading countries of birth (Monger & Yankay, 2011, p. 1). In the years between the official decennial censuses, it is possible to gather demographic information from the American Community Survey (www.uscensus.gov). The survey presents estimates of the population, gathered through random sampling, immigration records, births, and deaths. Table 4-1 and Figure 4-1 ▶▶▶ review the results of Census 2010.

The Nurse

Of the 2,843,000 employed registered nurses in 2010, 78.6% were White, 12% were Black, 7.5% were Asian, and 4.9% were Hispanic (Figure 4-1A) (U.S. Department of Labor, 2011). The registered nurse (RN), in general, is a White, non-Hispanic woman between the ages of 40 and 59 years, with a median age of 46 years. Just over 41% of RNs are 50 years of age or older and only 8% of RNs are under the age of 30, compared with 25% in 1980. The majority of nurses (74%) are married, and more than three-fourths of all nurses (77%) have children (U.S. Department of Health and Human Services [USDHHS], 2010). The demographic profile of professional nurses represents a demographic disparity from the overall demographic profile of the United States. In 2008, most working RNs spoke only English fluently. Just 5.1% of RNs spoke Spanish, and 3.6% spoke Tagalog or another Filipino language. About 1.1% spoke French, while less than 1% of RNs spoke any Chinese dialect, German, American Sign Language, or other language.

In 2010 there were 573,000 licensed practical nurses (LPNs); 69.3% were White, 24.4%, Black, 3.8% Asian, and 6.2% Hispanic (U.S. Department of Labor, 2011, p. 19). Indeed, LPNs are also highly represented by Whites, but there is a larger percentage of Blacks and Hispanics involved in this discipline (Figure 4-1B).

White, non-hispanic, married, English speaking women

TABLE 4-1 Population by Race for the United States: 2000 and 2010

	2000	2010
Total Population	281,421,906	308,745,538
	Percentage of Total Population	Percentage of Total Population
Hispanic or Latino	12.5	16.3
Not Hispanic or Latino	87.5	83.7
White Alone	69.1	63.7
Race		
One race	97.6	97.1
White	75.1	72.4
Black or African American	12.3	12.6
American Indian and Alaska Native	0.9	0.9
Asian	3.6	4.8
Native Hawaiian and other Pacific Islander	0.1	0.2
Some other race	5.5	6.2
Two or more races	2.4	2.9

Source: Humes, K. R., Nicholas, A. J., & Ramirez, R. (2011). Overview of race and Hispanic origin: 2010. *Census Briefs*, p. 4. Retrieved from http://2010.census.gov/2010census/data

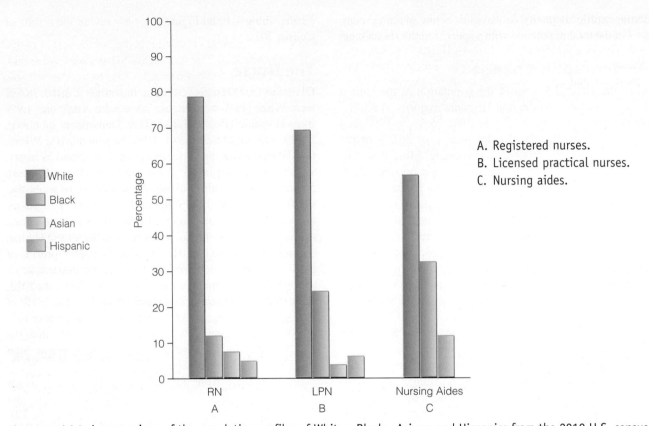

A. Registered nurses.
B. Licensed practical nurses.
C. Nursing aides.

Figure 4-1 ▶▶▶ A comparison of the population profiles of Whites, Blacks, Asians, and Hispanics from the 2010 U.S. census.

Sources: Humes, K. R., Nicholas, A. J., & Ramirez, R. (2011). Overview of race and Hispanic origin: 2010. *Census Briefs,* p. 4. Retrieved from http://2010.census.gov/2010census/data; U.S. Census Bureau, *Census 2000 Redistricting Data (Public Law 94-171) Summary File,* Tables PL1 and PL2; and *2010 Census Redistricting Data (Public Law 94-171) Summary File,* Tables P1 and P2. Retrieved from http://www.census.gov/prod/cen2010/briefs/c2010br-02.pdf.

The Caregiver

In 2010, there were 3,332,000 people employed in healthcare support occupations, including 1,928,000 as nursing, psychiatric, and home health aides. Of this population, 58.6% were White, 34.6% Black, 4.0% Asian, and 14.7% Hispanic (U.S. Department of Labor, 2011, p. 20). The proportions found in this demographic breakdown again illustrate a demographic disparity and are not consistent with the overall demographic proportions of the United States, because 43.1% of the low-paid workers represent minority populations. A greater percentage of Blacks are represented in these positions than are in the general population. Hispanics represent 16.3% of the general population and are slightly less in this workforce population. In many long-term care facilities, the setting may be one in which the nurses are White and the staff, especially the certified nurses' aides who provide hands-on care, is composed of many people of color. Figure 4-1C illustrates the

percentages of nursing aides. A high school diploma is required in most settings; however, many of the caregivers are new immigrants and may have difficulty speaking and understanding English. Both the native workers and immigrants may well have limited understanding of the ethnocultural religious heritages and life trajectories of the patients and nurses, who in turn have a limited understanding of the natives' and immigrants' backgrounds.

The Patient

The third party in the triad is the patient. The 2010 census required respondents to report their age and date of birth. The population of people 65 years and over has grown significantly since the 2000 census. The older population of today was born many years after the beginning of the 20th century. In 1910, the life expectancy at birth was 47.3 years; and in 1930 it was 59.7 years. Currently, on average adults in the U.S. reaching the age of 65 can expect nearly 20 more years of additional life. The number of people 100 years and over (53,364) is the highest it has ever been (Howden & Meyer, 2011, p. 4). Scottsdale, Arizona; Clearwater, Florida; and Cape Coral, Florida; have the highest median ages. The generation of women born in 1910 was the first generation in which the majority (58%) of women lived to see their children become adults. In 2009, more than 1.4 million people 65 years and over lived in nursing homes (National Center for Health Statistics, 2011, p. 359). This population grew up without gadgets—without the cell phones, computers, remote controls for televisions, microwave ovens, and countless other things taken for granted by younger generations.

Ethnocultural Heritage

A person's ethnocultural heritage is predicated on the concept of **heritage consistency,** which was developed by Estes and Zitzow (1980) to describe the degree to which a person's lifestyle reflects his or her respective tribal culture. The theory has been expanded in an attempt to study the degree to which a person's lifestyle reflects his or her traditional culture, whether European, Asian, African, or Hispanic. The values indicating heritage consistency exist on a continuum, and a person can possess value characteristics that are both heritage consistent (traditional) and heritage inconsistent (acculturated or modern). The concept of **heritage inconsistency,** observance of the beliefs and practices of one's acculturated belief system, includes a determination of one's cultural, ethnic, and religious background (Spector, 2009, p. 8).

Culture

There is no single definition of culture, and all too often definitions tend to omit salient aspects of culture or to be too general to have any real meaning. One definition of **culture** is that it is "the language, thoughts, communications, actions, beliefs, values, and institutions of racial, ethnic, religious, or social groups" (USDHHS, 2001, p. 4).

Culture is a complex whole in which each part is related to every other part. The capacity to learn culture is genetic, but the subject matter is not genetic and must be learned by each person in the family and social community. Furthermore, culture determines how healthcare information is received, how rights and protections are exercised, what is considered to be a health problem, and how symptoms and concerns about the problem are expressed (USDHHS, 2011).

Ethnicity

Cultural background is a fundamental component of one's ethnic background. The term **ethnicity** pertains to a social group within the social system that claims to possess variable traits such as a common religion or language. The term *ethnic* has for some time aroused strongly negative feelings and often is rejected by the general population. The upsurge in the use of the term may stem from the recent interest of people in discovering their personal backgrounds, a fact used by some politicians who overtly court "the ethnics." Paradoxically, in a nation as large as the United States and comprising as many different peoples as it does—with American Indians being the only true native population—many people are still reluctant to speak of ethnicity and ethnic differences. Most foreign groups that came to this land often shed the ways of the "old country" and quickly attempted to assimilate themselves into the mainstream, or the so-called melting pot (Novak, 1973).

Religion

The third major component of a person's heritage is **religion.** Religion is "the belief in a divine or superhuman power or powers to be obeyed and worshipped as the creator(s) and ruler(s) of the universe; and a system of beliefs, practices, and ethical values," and is a major reason for the development of ethnicity (Abramson, 1980, pp. 869–875). The practice of religion is revealed in numerous cults, sects, denominations, and churches. Ethnicity and religion are clearly related, and religion quite often is the determinant of a person's ethnic group. Religion gives a person a frame of reference and a perspective with which to organize information. Religious teachings about health help to present a meaningful philosophy and system of practices within a system of social controls having specific values, norms, and ethics. Adherence to a religious code is conducive to spiritual harmony and health. Evidence shows a correlation between this and decreased morbidity and mortality in older adults as well as increased reported quality of life. Illness is sometimes seen as punishment for the violation of religious codes and morals.

It is not possible to isolate the aspects of culture, religion, and ethnicity that shape a person's worldview. Each is part of the others, and all three are united within the person. When writing of religion, one cannot eliminate culture or ethnicity, but descriptions and comparisons can be made (Spector, 2009, p. 17).

Socialization

Socialization is the process of being raised within a culture and acquiring the characteristics of that group.

Education—be it elementary school, high school, college, or nursing—is a form of socialization. For many people who have been socialized within the boundaries of a "traditional culture" or a nonmodern culture (usually associated with emerging nations), modern "American," or Western, culture becomes a second cultural identity. Those who immigrate here from non-Western or emerging countries may find socialization into the American culture to be a difficult and painful process. As time passes, many people experience biculturalism, which is a dual pattern of identification that often involves divided loyalty (LaFrombose, Coleman, & Gerton, 1993). Many people who have been socialized in cultures that use traditional healthcare resources may prefer this type of care even when residing in a modern cultural setting with modern healthcare resources.

> **Practice Pearl** ▶▶▶ Do not make assumptions about the way older patients have been socialized to their racial identities. For example, some older African Americans identify themselves as Black, persons of color, colored persons, or African Americans. Racial identity can vary by generation, geographical region of the country, and other subgroups.

Examples of Heritage Consistency

The following are the factors indicative of heritage consistency. These factors may determine the depth to which members of the CULTURALCARE triad identify with their traditional heritage:

1. Childhood development occurred in the person's country of origin or in an immigrant neighborhood in the United States of like ethnic group. For example, the person was raised in a specific ethnic neighborhood, such as an Italian, Black, Hispanic, or Jewish one, in a given part of a city and was exposed only to the culture, language, foods, and customs of that particular group.
2. Extended family members encouraged participation in traditional religious and cultural activities. For example, the parents sent the person to religious (parochial) school, and most social activities were church related.
3. The individual engages in frequent visits to the country of origin or returns to the "old neighborhood" in the United States. The desire to return to the old country or to the old neighborhood is common; however, many people cannot return for various reasons. Those who came here to escape religious persecution or

whose families were killed during World War II, during the Holocaust, in the killing fields of Cambodia, or in other recent massacres, may not want to return to their homelands. Other reasons people may not return to their native country include political conditions or lack of relatives or friends in the homeland.
4. The individual's family home is within the ethnic community of which he or he is a member. For example, as an adult the person has elected to live in the ethnic neighborhood where the people are from a similar heritage.
5. The individual participates in ethnic cultural events, such as religious festivals or national holidays, sometimes with singing, dancing, and costumes. For example, the person is active in social and cultural groups and participates in festivities with family members.
6. The individual was raised in an extended family setting. For example, when the person was growing up, grandparents or aunts and uncles may have been living in the same household or close by. The person's social frame of reference was the family.
7. The individual maintains regular contact with the extended family. For example, the person maintains close ties with family members of the same generation, the surviving members of the older generation, and members of the younger generation.
8. The individual's name has not been Americanized. For example, the person has restored the family name to its original European, or other national, name if it had been changed at the time the family immigrated or if the family changed the name at a later time in an attempt to assimilate to the dominant culture.
9. The individual was educated in a parochial (nonpublic) school with a religious or ethnic philosophy similar to the family's background. For example, the person's education plays an enormous role in socialization, and the major purpose of education is to socialize a given person into the dominant culture. Children learn English and the customs and norms of American life in the schools. In the parochial or private schools, they not only learn English but also are socialized in the culture and norms of the religious or ethnic group that is sponsoring the school.
10. The individual engages in social activities primarily with others of the same religious or ethnic background. For example, the major portion of the individual's personal time is spent with primary structural groups—family and close friends.
11. The individual has knowledge of the culture and language of origin. For example, the person has been socialized in the traditional ways of the family and expresses this as a central theme of life.

12. The individual expresses pride in his or her heritage. For example, the person may identify himself or herself as ethnic American and be supportive of ethnic activities to a great extent (Spector, 2009, pp. 13–14).

Ethnocultural Life Trajectories

Generational differences have been described as deep and gut-level ways of experiencing and looking at the cultural events that surround us. "The differences between generations—and the determination of who we are—are more than distinct ways of looking at problems and developing solutions for problems" (Hicks & Hicks, 1999, p. 4). Changes in the past several decades have created cultural barriers that openly or more subtly create misunderstandings, tensions, and often conflicts between family members, coworkers, and individuals—and between patients and caregivers in the practice of gerontology. The cycle of life is an ethnocultural journey, and many aspects of this journey are derived from the social, religious, and cultural context in which a person is raised. Factors that imprint our lives are the characters and events that we interacted with at 10 years of age, more or less (Hicks & Hicks, 1999, p. 25).

People who reside in either the community or in institutional settings may be cared for not only by people who are much younger but also by people who are immigrants and have limited knowledge as to the life trajectory of each patient. Figure 4-2 ▶▶▶ illustrates one ethnocultural heritage life trajectory model. The patient may also be an immigrant who experienced a much different life trajectory from his or her caregivers and even other neighbors or residents of the same age living in the community or nursing home. Table 4-2 lists events during the past century that have had a profound impact on the lives of older patients as a cumulative experience. The early events set the background for later events and the later events have affected the nurses and caregivers. Depending on the heritage of the individuals, the experiences differ. Several

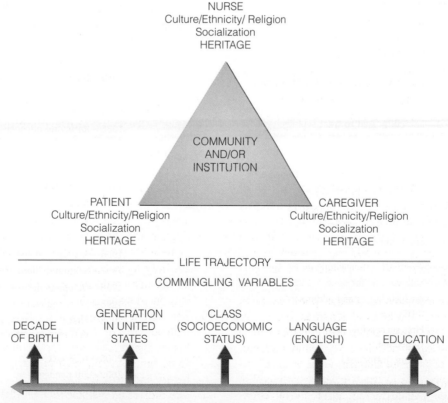

Figure 4-2 ▶▶▶ Ethnocultural heritage/life trajectory model. The complex relationship of nurse, caregiver, and patient in community and/or institutional settings and commingling variables.

Source: Spector, R. E. (2009). CULTURALCARE consultant. Needham, MA. © 2009. Reprinted with permission.

TABLE 4-2   **Selected Healthcare-Related Events From 1920 to 2012 That Profoundly Impacted the Lives of Patients, Nurses, and Caregivers in the United States and World**

Date	Healthcare-Related Events	Date	Healthcare-Related Events
1920–1929	1923—Dick test to determine susceptibility to scarlet fever 1923—Ethylene introduced as an anesthetic 1923—Mitral valve surgery introduced 1923—Peritoneal dialysis introduced 1924—BCG tuberculin test introduced 1924—Scratch test to determine susceptibility to diphtheria introduced 1925—Exchange transfusions introduced 1929—Blue Cross begun		1963—Measles vaccine 1963—Trivalent oral polio vaccine 1964—Surgeon General's report on smoking 1965—War on Poverty; Medicare/Medicaid passed 1969—Rubella vaccine developed 1967—First human heart transplant
1930–1939	1931-39—Pertussis immunization introduced 1932—Tuskegee syphilis experiment begun 1933—Tetanus toxoid immunization introduced 1933—Diphtheria immunization introduced 1933—Divinylether used 1934—Mumps virus isolated 1935—Sulfa drugs 1935—Insulin developed to treat diabetes 1936—Poliomyelitis virus isolated; cortisone developed 1937—First blood banks and blood transfusions; TB patch test developed 1938—Typhoid antiserum prepared	1970–1979	1970—Earth Day; EPA founded 1970s—Biotechnical explosion 1970s—Clotbusters introduced; interferon 1971—CT scans developed 1971—Measles, mumps, rubella vaccine 1972—Tuskegee experiment ends; PSROs established; Clean Water Act 1973—Emerging infections identified 1973—*Roe v. Wade* decision legalized abortion 1978—First test-tube baby 1978—Love Canal; hepatitis B (HBV) vaccine developed 1979—Three Mile Island
1940–1949	1943—Penicillin used to treat syphilis 1944—DDT insecticide introduced 1944—Hearing tests introduced Mid-1940s—Tetanus antitoxin developed 1944—Artificial kidney introduced 1945—Streptomycin used to treat TB 1947—Kolff-Brigham artificial kidney 1949—Cortisone discovered	1980–1989	1982—Hepatitis B vaccine 1984—Bhopal, India, chemical leak 1984—Monoclonal antibodies 1985—Emergence of crack cocaine 1985—Retroviral oncogenes
1950–1959	1952-53—Heart-lung machine perfected 1954—Salk vaccine for polio 1954—Antipsychotics and neuroleptics introduced 1954—First successful organ (kidney) transplant 1957—Valium introduced	1990–1999	1992—Human Genome Project 1993—Family and Medical Leave Act 1993—Hantavirus pulmonary syndrome 1993-94—Failure of Health Reform 1995—Varicella vaccine 1995—Hepatitis A vaccine 1996—Assisted suicide—Dr. J. Kevorkian 1997—Sextuplets born and survive 1998—Octuplets born—7 survive 1998—Stem cell cloning medical events 1998—First drug to treat erectile dysfunction introduced
1960–1969	1961—External cardiac pacing 1961—Thalidomide disaster 1962—Rachel Carson, *Silent Spring* 1963—Liver transplant method developed 1963—Mumps live virus vaccine developed	2000–2012	2006—HPV vaccine 2009—Flu pandemic 2010—Affordable Care Act passed 2012—Individual mandate provision of the Affordable Care Act challenged and upheld as constitutional by the U.S. Supreme Court

variables relate to this overall situation, and they may serve as potential sources of conflict. These include:

1. **Decade of birth.** One's life experiences will vary greatly depending on the events of the decade in which they were born and the cultural values and norms of the times. People who tend to be heritage consistent (i.e., have a high level of identification and association with a traditional heritage) tend to be less caught up in the secular fads of the time and popular sociocultural events.

2. **Generation in United States.** Worldviews differ greatly between the immigrant generation, subsequent generations, and people who score high as heritage consistent.

3. **Class.** Social class or socioeconomic status is an important factor among older persons. It includes analysis of one's education, economics, and background. There are countless differences among people based on social class or socioeconomic status. In 2009, 16.4% of the foreign-born Americans were 100% below the poverty level as compared to 13.0% of the native-born Americans (U.S. Census Bureau, 2010).

4. **Language.** When people who are hard of hearing attempt to understand others with limited English speaking skills, many cultural and social misunderstandings can develop. Frequent misunderstandings also occur when people who do not understand English must care for or receive care from English speakers. Younger immigrants often possess greater confidence in their English-speaking abilities than older immigrants. When surveyed about their ability to speak English, recent data document that younger immigrants were three times more likely than older immigrants over the age of 65 to choose the response "very well" when asked "How do you rate your ability to speak and understand English?" (U.S. Census Bureau, 2010).

5. **Education.** In 2009, the percentage of the foreign-born population with less than a high school education was 32.2% as compared to 12.3% of native-born Americans. This means that only 67.8% of foreign-born people have a high school diploma (U.S. Census Bureau, 2010). Many of the elders have experienced college and place an extremely high value on education (Spector, 2009, p. 23). Given that many low-paying positions require only a high school diploma, this educational situation can present cultural bias and even conflict.

Heritage Assessment Tool

A tool, or interview guide, has been developed to determine how deeply a given person identifies with a traditional heritage or is acculturated into the modern, dominant culture (Spector,

2009, pp. 321–323). Once a conversation begins and the person describes aspects of his or her cultural heritage, it becomes possible to develop an understanding of the person's unique health and illness beliefs and practices and cultural needs.

Figure 4-3 ▶▶▶ depicts the questions to ask in the heritage assessment interview. The tool was developed to create a way of interviewing a given person about sociocultural background. It facilitates communication with patients and their families, staff members, and colleagues. The tool is designed to enhance the interviewing process to determine if a given person is identifying with a traditional cultural heritage (heritage consistent) or if the person has acculturated into the dominant culture of the modern society (heritage inconsistent). The tool may be used in any setting and can facilitate conversation and help in the planning of CULTURAL-CARE. Many questions must be added regarding the person's life trajectory to integrate the cultural and historical events in the lives of each party into the work environment.

Providing CULTURALCARE

There are several ways to develop and implement the knowledge and skills necessary to incorporate CULTURALCARE into nursing care. Professional nurses are the leaders and bridges in this sensitive endeavor. Gerontological nurses can develop appropriate knowledge and skills needed to establish a CULTURALCARE practice environment. This includes the following:

1. Developing cultural sensitivity   *what*
2. Determining what care is culturally appropriate for a given patient   *How*
3. Developing cultural competency   *why*

Cultural Sensitivity

Sensitivity indicates a high level of awareness as to what is meaningful to the person. The assessment of heritage and ethnocultural life trajectory is important. How and when questions are asked requires both clinical judgment and sensitivity. The timing and phrasing of questions needs to be adapted to the individual. Sensitivity is needed when phrasing questions and determining what questions are appropriate at a given time. Trust must be established before patients and caregivers can be expected to share sensitive information. The nurse needs to spend time with patients, their families, and the caregivers; introduce some social conversation; and convey a genuine desire to understand their values, beliefs, ethnocultural background, and life trajectories. (See the Best Practices feature on page 88.)

Before a cultural assessment begins, the nurse must determine what language the person speaks and the degree

1. Where was your mother born? _____

2. Where was your father born? _____

3. Where were your grandparents born?
   a. Your mother's mother? _____
   b. Your mother's father? _____
   c. Your father's mother? _____
   d. Your father's father? _____

4. How many brothers _____ and sisters _____ do you have?

5. What setting did you grow up in?
   Urban _____ Rural _____

6. What country did your parents grow up in?
   Father _____   Mother _____

7. How old were you when you came to the United States? _____

8. How old were your parents when they came to the United States?
   Father _____   Mother _____

9. When you were growing up, did you live in an extended family?
   (1) Yes _____   (2) No _____

10. Have you maintained contact with
    a. Aunts, uncles, cousins?   (1) Yes _____   (2) No _____
    b. Brothers and sisters?   (1) Yes _____   (2) No _____
    c. Parents?   (1) Yes _____   (2) No _____
    d. Your own children?   (1) Yes _____   (2) No _____

11. Did most of your aunts, uncles, cousins live near your home?
    (1) Yes _____   (2) No _____

12. Approximately how often did you visit family members who lived outside of your home?
    (1) Daily _____   (4) Once a year or less _____
    (2) Weekly _____   (5) Never _____
    (3) Monthly _____

13. Was your original family name changed?
    (1) Yes _____   (2) No _____

14. What is your religious preference?
    (1) Catholic _____   (4) Other _____
    (2) Jewish _____   (5) None _____
    (3) Protestant _____
        Denomination _____

15. Is your spouse the same religion as you?
    (1) Yes _____   (2) No _____

16. Is your spouse the same ethnic background as you?
    (1) Yes _____   (2) No _____

Figure 4-3 ▶▶▶ The heritage assessment tool.   *(continued)*

Source: Spector, R. E. © 2009. *Cultural diversity in health and illness* (7th ed., pp. 321–323). Reprinted and electronically reproduced by permission of Pearson Education, Inc. Upper Saddle River, NJ.

17. What kind of school did you go to?
    (1) Public _____   (3) Parochial _____
    (2) Private _____

18. As an adult, do you live in a neighborhood where the neighbors are the same religion and ethnic background as you?
    (1) Yes _____   (2) No _____

19. Do you belong to a religious institution?
    (1) Yes _____   (2) No _____

20. Would you describe yourself as an active member?
    (1) Yes _____   (2) No _____

21. How often do you attend your religious institution?
    (1) More than once a week _____   (4) Special holidays only _____
    (2) Weekly _____   (5) Never _____
    (3) Monthly _____

22. Do you practice your religion in your home?
    (1) Yes _____ (if yes, please specify)
    (2) No _____
    (3) Praying _____
    (4) Bible reading _____
    (5) Diet _____
    (6) Celebrating religious holidays _____

23. Do you prepare foods special to your ethnic background?
    (1) Yes _____   (2) No _____

24. Do you participate in ethnic activities?
    (1) Yes _____ (if yes, please specify)   (5) Dancing _____
    (2) No _____   (6) Festivals _____
    (3) Singing _____   (7) Costumes _____
    (4) Holiday celebrations _____   (8) Other _____

25. Are your friends from the same religious background as you?
    (1) Yes _____   (2) No _____

26. Are your friends from the same ethnic background as you?
    (1) Yes _____   (2) No _____

27. What is your native language? (other than English)

28. Do you speak this language?
    (1) Prefer _____   (3) Rarely _____
    (2) Occasionally _____

29. Do you read your native language?
    (1) Yes _____   (2) No _____

Directions: Score one point for each positive answer except if a person has NOT changed his or her family name. That gets a point if negative. The greater the number of points, the greater the likelihood that the person identifies with a traditional culture and is not assimilated into the mainstream culture.

Figure 4-3 ▶▶▶ (*continued*)

Best Practices   Ethnogeriatrics and Cultural Competence for Nursing Practice

The Hartford Institute for Geriatric Nursing (2012) has recommended recognition of cultural and religious beliefs, practices and life experiences of ethnic groups, and the influence of these on attitudes toward aging and health care. It is important for nurses to understand the following categories of belief from the perspective of their older patients:

- **Respect.** What does this person from another culture believe about the roles and responsibilities of older persons, children, doctors, nurses, and others? Does the person desire that personal care be gender specific?
- **Death and dying.** What are the cultural and religious perspectives regarding death, life-sustaining treatments, care of the person when death is imminent, and treatment of the body after death and funeral rituals?
- **Pain.** What is the cultural perspective toward pain? Is there a view that it is punishment for past behaviors? What are the socially accepted behaviors of a person in pain (e.g., crying, wailing, moaning, stoicism)?
- **Medicines and nutrition.** What is the role of folk and home remedies and caregiving practices? Does the person have specific dietary practices? What foods or food combinations are taboo?
- **Independence.** How does the culture value independence in old age? Are older people expected or encouraged to stay active in their health care and living arrangements?
- **Manners.** How does the patient prefer to be addressed: by his or her last name, or Mr. or Mrs.? Or, does the patient prefer to be addressed by the first name? Is it appropriate to shake hands with an introduction? Is it appropriate to touch the person?

How is the care provider dressed? Older adults often expect a professional, clean, and neat appearance.
- **Gender-Specific Care.** Is the patient from an ethnoreligious heritage where it is forbidden for men to care for women or women to care for men?
- **Modesty.** Is the patient from an ethnoreligious heritage that teaches strict adherence to rules regarding body coverings?
- **Touch.** Is the patient from an ethnoreligious heritage that teaches that men cannot be touched by women or touch women?
- **Space.** Does the person need a place for privacy for prayer or other personal activities?

The nurse is urged to discuss these key issues with the older patient and the family. It would be wrong to make assumptions based on stereotypes, so each person should be approached as a unique individual. When the heritage assessment is complete, the nurse will have a clear understanding of the unique anticipated needs of the given patient.

There are many ways that a given person's life trajectory can be discussed. The nurse can inquire about historical events that occurred during the person's lifetime. Did the person serve in the military? What was that experience like? What was school like when the person was young? What was it like without television? What was it like without a computer or a cell phone? Once people begin to recall life experiences, they generally feel free to discuss them. For many people, sharing experiences can also be painful. Talk of World War II, for example, can be difficult for people who are Holocaust survivors or who lost family in the military. People born before 1935 may not have had childhood immunizations except smallpox. Vaccines for pertussis did not become available until 1931 to 1939, and other vaccines came later.

of fluency in the English language. It is also important to learn about the person's communications patterns and space orientation. When the person does not speak and/or understand English, a competent interpreter must be available. This is accomplished by observing both verbal and nonverbal communication:

1. For example, does the person do the speaking or defer to another?

2. What nonverbal communication behaviors are exhibited (e.g., touching, eye contact)?
3. What significance do these behaviors have for the interaction between the nurse and the patient or caregiver?
4. What is the person's proximity to other people and objects within the environment?
5. How does the person react to the nurse's movement toward him or her?

> ## BOX 4-3   Steps to Attaining Cultural Sensitivity
>
> 1. Always address patients, support people, and other healthcare personnel by their last names (e.g., Mrs. Cohen, Dr. Foley) until they give you permission to use other names. In some cultures, the more formal style of address is a sign of respect, whereas the informal use of first names may be considered disrespectful. It is important to ask people how they wish to be addressed. It is critical to not address people by "hey" and use the term "guys" for women.
> 2. When meeting a person for the first time, introduce yourself by your full name, and then explain your role (e.g., "Hello, Mrs. Cohen, my name is Lillian Cook and I am the registered nurse on this unit"). This helps establish a relationship and provides an opportunity for patients, others, and nurses to learn the pronunciation of one another's names and their roles.
> 3. Be authentic with people, and be honest about the knowledge you lack about their ethnocultural heritage and life trajectory. When you do not understand a person's actions, politely and respectfully seek information.
> 4. Do not make any assumptions about the patient and your coworkers; always tactfully ask about anything you do not understand.
> 5. Respect the ethnocultural values, beliefs, and practices of others, even if they differ from your own or from those of the dominant culture.
> 6. Show respect for the patient's support people. In some cultures, males in the family make decisions affecting the patient, whereas in other cultures, females make the decisions.
> 7. Make a concerted effort to obtain the trust of patients and coworkers, but do not be surprised if it develops slowly or not at all.

TABLE 4-3   Common Cultural Conflicts

Situation	Consequence	Patient Outcome
Linguistic barriers	Inadequate assessments (e.g., pain, needs, preferences)	Decreased quality of life
Dietary blunders	Refusal to eat specific foods, such as pork; and food combinations, such as milk and meat	Decreased oral intake Weight loss Dehydration
Missed cues	Inappropriate interventions Power struggles between nurses and family and patient	Withdrawal, depression, anger Loss of communication
Misunderstanding of religious or cultural beliefs and/or practices such as modesty and the need for gender-specific care	Avoid encounters Resist care Female refuses male caregiver or male refuses female caregiver	Fear Withdrawal Increased anxiety
Avoid scheduling elective procedures on religious holidays	Patient and family may refuse procedures	Delays in gathering necessary medical data
Family dynamics	Controversies Confusion	Hostility Withdrawal
Violation of manners	Avoid encounters Resist touch	Withdrawal

It is vital to be culturally sensitive (possessing basic knowledge of and constructive attitudes toward health traditions observed by diverse groups) and to convey this sensitivity to patients, support people, and other healthcare personnel. Box 4-3 lists some steps for conveying cultural sensitivity.

The heritage assessment and life trajectory interview takes time and usually extends over several time periods. Table 4-3 illustrates several examples of common cultural blunders, the potential consequences, and possible patient outcomes.

Cultural Appropriateness

The determination of culturally appropriate care is necessary so that the comfort levels of both the patient and the caregivers are met and respected. The case study that appears later in this chapter describes a culturally appropriate response. *How are we going to do this?*

The provision of the recommended interventions demonstrates the level of sensitivity and responses necessary to meet the patient's needs. The skills necessary to incorporate CULTURALCARE into standard nursing require a broad base of knowledge about the different ethnocultural heritages and life trajectories from which a given patient, colleague, or caregiver comes. It is an ongoing process, and both the skills and knowledge bases grow over time. As one's knowledge base grows, the ability to convey cultural sensitivity also grows.

Steps to Cultural Competency

The following are examples of the necessary steps toward cultural competency:

1. Become aware of your own ethnocultural heritage:
   - Where were your parents and grandparents born?
   - What are examples of their ethnocultural life trajectories?
   - Do they value stoic behavior? What kinds of behavior do they value?
   - Are the rights of the individual valued over and above the rights of the family?
   - What did they experience either as new immigrants or as children growing up in the United States?
   - What do they see as seminal cultural events of their lifetime?
   - Only by knowing one's own culture (values, practices, and beliefs) can a person be ready to learn about another's. Providers can conduct the heritage assessment on themselves.
2. Become aware of the ethnocultural heritage and life trajectory described by both the patient and the caregivers. It is important to avoid assuming that all people of the same ethnic, religious, or national background have the same cultural beliefs and values. Questions similar to those previously listed may be asked in conversation. When there is knowledge of the patient's and caregiver's ethnocultural heritage and life trajectories, mutual respect between patient, caregiver, and nurse is more likely to develop. The triad can become more unified.

3. Become aware of adaptations the patient and caregivers made to live in the North American culture. During this part of the process, a nurse can also identify the patient's and caregivers' preferences in health practices, diet, hygiene, and so on.
4. Form a CULTURALCARE nursing plan with the patient and caregivers that incorporates their cultural beliefs regarding care. In this way, cultural values, practices, and beliefs can be incorporated with the necessary nursing care.

Implementing CULTURALCARE Nursing

CULTURALCARE nursing involves the presentation of culturally related customs and values into a given setting, such as the common patient areas in a long-term care facility. Recognizing the patient's and caregiver's viewpoints and finding mutually agreeable solutions requires expert communication skills. An attempt must be made to bridge the gaps between the perspectives of the people in the CULTURALCARE triad. During this process, the views of each party must be explored, acknowledged, and valued. If there are views that could lead to harmful outcomes or behaviors, attempts are made to shift the perspectives to an acceptable view. Every action must be taken to recognize potential conflict before the situation becomes irreversible. This may be all that is realistically possible to achieve. If a crisis develops, it may be possible to return to original care approaches.

CULTURALCARE nursing is challenging. It requires discovery of the meaning of the patient's or staff member's ethnocultural heritage and life trajectory, flexibility, creativity, and knowledge to adapt interventions. There must be a cumulative effort to learn from each experience. This knowledge and experience will improve the delivery of CULTURALCARE to future patients and staff members.

Patient and Family Teaching

Gerontological nurses require skills and knowledge related to teaching patients and families about the key concepts of gerontology and gerontological nursing. The patient–family teaching guidelines in the following feature will assist the nurse to assume the role of teacher and coach. Educating patients and families is critical so that nurses can interpret scientific data and individualize the nursing care plan.

Patient–Family Teaching Guidelines

The following are guidelines that the nurse may find useful when instructing older persons and their families about cultural competence in health care.

CULTURAL COMPETENCE

1 **As a person from a different culture, what can I expect of my healthcare provider?**

You can expect to receive culturally competent care. This means that you will be provided the highest quality of care, regardless of your race, ethnicity, cultural background, English proficiency, or literacy. Some common services provided may include:

- Interpreter services
- Attempts to recruit persons from your culture (if possible) to work in health facilities in your area
- Coordination with traditional healers
- Respect for your values, beliefs, and traditions
- Printed health information in your language and appropriate to your reading level

Source: Georgetown University Center for Research and Policy, 2004.

RATIONALE:

Many older persons and their families are not aware of the services that healthcare facilities are urged to develop in order to provide culturally competent care. Informing patients will empower them to be more proactive with their healthcare providers.

2 **Why is culturally competent care important?**

A culturally competent healthcare system can help improve health outcomes and quality of care, and can contribute to the elimination of racial and ethnic health disparities. It is both to your advantage and to the advantage of your healthcare providers to eliminate any barriers that stand in the way of improving your health and caring for you when you are ill.

RATIONALE:

Persons of color and ethnic minorities experience a disproportionate amount of chronic illness and disability with aging. Because the treatment of chronic illness is a long-term process requiring many lifestyle changes and adaptations, any barriers to effective communication should be removed to increase the odds of successful disease management.

3 **What can I do to increase my chances of obtaining culturally competent health care?**

Try to find a healthcare provider you can relate to. People who do not have a regular doctor or healthcare provider are less likely to obtain preventive services or diagnosis, treatment, and management of chronic conditions. Health insurance coverage is also an important determinant of access to health care. People without healthcare insurance often wait longer to seek health care, delay treatment once diagnosed with an illness, and as a result suffer more serious health problems. Social workers and community clinics often have services for persons without health insurance and can direct you to receive free or low-cost care. Once you have located a healthcare provider, inform him or her about yourself and your culture. If your provider recommends an intervention that is not consistent with your beliefs, discuss this right away. Let your provider know if you cannot understand written material given to you, if verbal instructions contain too much medical jargon that you cannot understand, or if you are given forms to fill out that are inconsistent with your level of reading in English. Providing culturally competent health care is an ongoing learning process. Your healthcare provider will be grateful to hear your constructive comments and receive your support.

RATIONALE:

It is almost impossible to know everything about every culture. Training approaches that focus only on facts are best combined with the ongoing feedback from patients, families, and other healthcare providers. Curiosity, empathy, respect, and humility are some basic attitudes that can help the clinical relationship and yield useful information about the patient's beliefs and preferences. An approach that focuses on inquiry, reflection, and analysis throughout the care process is most useful for the healthcare provider who is attempting to provide culturally competent care.

CARE PLAN A Patient Requiring CULTURALCARE

Case Study

Mr. Hernandez, a 73-year-old man of Mexican heritage, was admitted to a long-term care facility and presented the following challenges for nurses, other healthcare staff, caregivers, and the institution:

- He and his family could not read, speak, nor understand English.

- His strong Catholic faith and Hispanic cultural traditions required modesty during physical examinations and when personal care was delivered.
- His family had both religious and cultural reasons for not discussing end-of-life concerns or his impending death.

Applying the Nursing Process

Assessment

Mr. Hernandez will require a complete health assessment in order to provide him with culturally appropriate nursing care. The nurse should admit the patient to his room, make him comfortable, and begin to assess basic necessities such as dietary preferences, level of pain, safety, current medications taken, and strength and availability of the family support system. If the nurse does not speak Spanish, every attempt must be made to obtain an interpreter. If a bilingual family member (not a child) is present, the nurse could rely on that person to establish immediate communication, but it is now mandatory to use a professional interpreter for ongoing communication with the patient.

Diagnosis

Appropriate nursing diagnoses for Mr. Hernandez might include the following:

- *Nutrition, Imbalanced: Less Than Body Requirements* (if culturally appropriate foods cannot be provided)
- *Injury, Risk for* (if safety precautions cannot be communicated)
- *Communication: Verbal, Impaired* because patient does not understand English

- *Loneliness, Risk for* (if social interactions are precluded by language difficulties)
- *Spiritual Distress* (if appropriate religious traditions are not heeded)
- *Decisional Conflict*, relating to end of life care (if the care providers request the family and patient to discuss his impending death)
- *Pain* (if levels cannot be communicated)

NANDA-I © 2012.

Expected Outcomes

Expected outcomes for the plan of care specify that Mr. Hernandez will:

- Accept nursing care and pain relief.
- Communicate his needs through a competent interpreter.
- Maintain adequate weight and levels of hydration.

- Carry out cultural and religious rituals as appropriate to Mexican culture.
- Have access to family, religious clergy, and healers as appropriate to his culture.
- Experience a peaceful death without suffering.

Planning and Implementation

The nurse should develop a plan of care to include culturally and linguistically appropriate responses such as:

- Locate interpreter staff to not only translate but also explain the cultural meanings of beliefs and practices.
- Provide translated and understandable written materials at the reading level of the family.

- Provide sensitive and comprehensive explanations and discussions about treatment, informed consent, and advance directive forms.
- Locate clinical nurses and caregivers who know how and what to ask about perceived needs and recognized cultural issues.

CARE PLAN

A Patient Requiring CULTURALCARE *(continued)*

- Obtain appropriate food choices.
- Limit caregivers to male care providers to the maximum extent possible.

- Obtain input from appropriate family members and patient regarding plan of care for pain, nutrition, safety, etc.

Evaluation

The nurse hopes to work with the patient and his family over time to provide culturally appropriate care. The nurse will consider the plan a success based on the following criteria:

- Mr. Hernandez will accept nursing care and pain control interventions.
- The patient and family will be in agreement with the plan of care.

- Mr. Hernandez will suffer no adverse events (falls, decubitus ulcers, adverse drug events) while receiving care in the long-term care facility.
- He will experience a peaceful death with adequate pain control, family and religious support, and attention to cultural rituals.

Ethical Dilemma

One of the nurse's colleagues feels strongly that Mr. Hernandez should be told of his impending death. This colleague feels that truth telling is important and that patients should have access to all information regarding their condition. When this colleague attempts to tell Mr. Hernandez of his condition, the patient and family become very upset and ask the nurse to intervene. The nurse takes the colleague aside and urges the colleague to examine any personal beliefs or cultural bias that may be present and influencing this behavior. The colleague should be urged to attempt to meet the needs of Mr. Hernandez and his family rather than his or her own needs. The patient's right to know (or in this case, not to know) is overridden by the mandate to "do no harm." Blunt and inappropriate truth telling in this case is culturally insensitive and likely to cause harm to Mr. Hernandez and his family.

Critical Thinking and the Nursing Process

1. At your next clinical session, evaluate care plans you and others have created for older patients as evidence of consideration of cross-cultural influences.
2. Interview a nurse who practices in your clinical setting. Ask him or her whether the age of the patient influences cultural aspects reflected in the planning or delivery of nursing care.
3. Pick a topic such as "truth telling," and research the customs of different cultures related to that topic. Enlist the help of your fellow students.

4. Write a reflective narrative about how your ethnic and cultural background influences your values and beliefs regarding life, death, health, and aging.
5. Interview an older patient regarding his or her traditional cultural/native health practices and medicine.
6. How do family and community support systems vary by culture?

- Evaluate your responses in Appendix B.

Chapter Highlights

- The people residing in North America come from a variety of ethnic and cultural backgrounds, and each person has a unique ethnocultural heritage and life trajectory.

- Culturally and linguistically appropriate services in health care are now mandated by the federal government and regulating bodies.

- The CULTURALCARE triad represents the complex interrelationships of the nurse, patient, and caregivers within community and institutional (home or residential) settings.

- Many groups in North America may be living within their traditional heritage, or they may embrace their original ethnocultural traditional heritage and a North American, modern culture.

- Potential areas of conflict derive from the demographic, ethnocultural, and life trajectory variables of the people within the CULTURALCARE triad.

- When assessing a patient, self, or caregiver, the nurse considers the patient's cultural values, beliefs, practices, and life trajectory.

- The integration of CULTURALCARE into the plan of care and workplace environment requires both thought and action.

Pearson Nursing Student Resources
Find additional review materials at
nursing.pearsonhighered.com

Prepare for success with additional NCLEX®-style practice questions, interactive assignments and activities, web links, animations and videos, and more!

References

Abramson, H. J. (1980). Religion. In S. Thernstrom (Ed.), *Harvard encyclopedia of American ethnic groups.* Cambridge, MA: Harvard University Press.

Douglas, M. K., Pierce, J. U., Rosenkoetter, M., Pacquiao, D., Callister, L. C., Hattar-Pollara, M., Lauderdale, J., Milstead, J., Nardi, D., & Purnell, L. (2011). Standards of practice for culturally competent care. *Journal of Transcultural Nursing, 22*(4), 317–333.

Estes, G., & Zitzow, D. (1980). *Heritage consistency as a consideration in counseling Native Americans.* Paper presented at the National Indian Education Association Convention, Dallas, TX, November 1980.

Georgetown University Center for Research and Policy. (2004). *Cultural competence in health care: Is it important for people with chronic conditions?* (Issue Brief 5). Washington, DC: Institute for Health Care Research and Policy.

Hartford Institute for Geriatric Nursing. (2012). *Ethnogeriatrics and cultural competence for nursing practice..* Retrieved from http://consultgerirn.org/topics/ethnogeriatrics_and_cultural_competence_for_nursing_practice/want_to_know_more

Hicks, R., & Hicks, K. (1999). *Boomers, Xers, and other strangers.* Wheaton, IL: Tyndale House.

Howden, L. M., & Meyer, J. A. (2011). *Age and sex composition: 2010.* Washington, DC: U.S. Census Bureau.

Humes, K. R., Nicholas, A. J., & Ramirez, R. (2011). Overview of race and Hispanic

origin: 2010. *Census Briefs*, p. 4. Retrieved from http://2010.census.gov/2010census/data

LaFrombose, T., Coleman, L. K., & Gerton, J. (1993). Psychological impact of biculturalism: Evidence and theory. *Psychological Bulletin, 114*(3), 395.

Monger, R., & Yankay, J. (2011). *U.S. legal permanent residents: 2010* (p. 3). Washington, DC: U.S. Department of Homeland Security. Retrieved from http://www.dhs.gov/ximgtn/statistics/publications/index.shtm

National Center for Health Statistics. (2011). *Health, United States 2010.* Washington, DC: U.S. Department of Health and Human Services.

Novak, M. (1973). How American are you if your grandparents came from Serbia in 1888? In S. TeSelle (Ed.), *The rediscovery of ethnicity: Its implications for culture and politics in America.* New York, NY: Harper & Row.

Office of Minority Health. (2001). *National standards for culturally and linguistically appropriate services in health care.* Washington, DC: U.S. Department of Health and Human Services.

Spector, R. E. (2009). *Cultural diversity in health and illness* (7th ed.). Upper Saddle River, NJ: Prentice Hall.

U.S. Census Bureau. (2010). *American community survey: Selected characteristics of the native and foreign-born population, 2010.* Retrieved from http://factfinder2.census.gov/faces/tableservices/jsf/pages/productview.xhtml?pid=DEC_10_SF1_QTP3&prodType=table

U.S. Department of Health and Human Services. (2001). *National standards for culturally and linguistically appropriate services in health care: Final report.* Washington, DC: Author.

U.S. Department of Health and Human Services. (2010). *The registered nurse population: Findings from the 2008 national sample survey or registered nurses.* Retrieved from http://bhpr.hrsa.gov/healthworkforce/rnsurveys/rnsurveyinitial2008.pdf

U.S. Department of Labor, Bureau of Labor Statistics. (2011). *Occupational outlook handbook, 2010–2011 edition.* Retrieved from http://www.bls.gov/oco/ocos166.htm

Selected Texts Related to CULTURALCARE Nursing Authored by Nurses

The following texts have been authored by nurses and may be helpful in developing CULTURALCARE knowledge:

Andrews, M. M., & Boyle, J. S. (2007). *Transcultural concepts in nursing care* (5th ed.). Philadelphia, PA: Lippincott.

Douglas, M., & Pacquiao, D. (2010). *The core curriculum for transcultural nursing and health care.* Los Angeles, CA: Sage.

Galanti, G. (2009). *Caring for patients from different cultures* (4th ed.). Philadelphia, PA: University of Pennsylvania Press.

Jeffreys, M. (2009). *Teaching cultural competence in nursing and health care* (2nd ed.). New York, NY: Springer.

Leininger, M., & McFarland, M. R. (Eds.). (2010). *Cultural care diversity and universality: A worldwide nursing theory* (2nd ed.). New York, NY: McGraw-Hill.

Lincoln, B. (2010). *Reflections from common ground . . . Cultural awareness in healthcare.* Eau Claire, WI: PESI Healthcare.

Purnell, L. D., & Paulanka, B. J. (2008). *Transcultural health care* (3rd ed.). Philadelphia, PA: F. A. Davis.

Ray, M. (2010). *Transcultural caring dynamics in nursing and health care.* Philadelphia, PA: F. A. Davis.

Spector, R. E. (2009). *CULTURALCARE: Guides to heritage assessment and health traditions.* Upper Saddle River, NJ: Prentice Hall Health. Available at www.prenhall.com/spector on companion web page with each chapter.

Spector, R. E. (2013). *Cultural diversity in health and illness* (8th ed.). Upper Saddle River, NJ: Pearson.

Transcultural Nursing Society. (n.d.). *Standards of practice for culturally competent nursing care.* Retrieved from http://www.tcns .org/TCNStandardsofPractice.html

U.S. Department of Health and Human Services. (2001). *National standards for culturally and linguistically appropriate services in health care: Final report.* Washington, DC: Author.

U.S. Department of Health and Human Services. (2011). *What is cultural competency?* Retrieved from http:// minorityhealth.hhs.gov/templates/browse .aspx?lvl=2&lvlid=11

Nutrition and Aging

Sheila Buckley Tucker, MA, RD, CSSD, LDN

PART-TIME FACULTY, CONNELL SCHOOL OF NURSING AND EXECUTIVE DIETITIAN, BOSTON COLLEGE

KEY TERMS

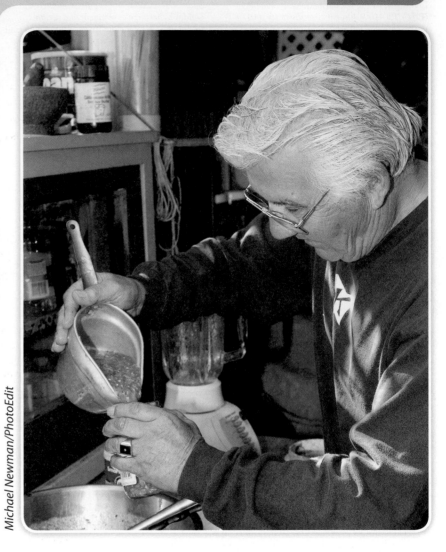

Michael Newman/PhotoEdit

LEARNING OUTCOMES

On completion of this chapter, the reader will be able to:

1. Classify the normal changes of aging in body composition and digestion, absorption, and metabolism of nutrients.
2. Differentiate between normal and disease-related changes in risk factors for undernutrition in older persons.
3. Identify normal nutrition requirements of the older person.
4. Analyze the causes and consequences of undernutrition in the older person.
5. Evaluate tools and parameters used to assess nutrition status.
6. Develop appropriate nursing interventions and treatment for nutrition-related problems of the older person.
7. Compare current dietary approaches to chronic disease in the older person.

The biological process of aging proceeds at an individualized pace, yet predictable changes can place older persons at a disproportionate risk of **undernutrition,** or **malnutrition,** compared to younger adults. Both undernutrition and diseases associated with overnutrition, such as obesity, degenerative joint disease, hypertension, and type 2 diabetes, can adversely affect vitality and quality of life. Lifelong eating habits can help promote health maintenance into older personhood. Independent older persons may only require regular nutritional screening during routine health checks, whereas others may require intervention for unintentional weight loss or drug–nutrient interactions. Hospitalized or frail older persons in long-term care deserve additional nutritional consideration because they are at highest risk for malnutrition. The wide spectrum of well-being in the older person presents nutritional challenges along a continuum.

dev life long eating habits early in life

Normal Changes in Aging

The normal aging process can result in biological changes that may place the older person at risk for malnutrition. The effects of these normal changes should be considered even in a healthy individual.

Changes in Body Composition *↑ in body fat*

Lean muscle mass diminishes with aging. The term **sarcopenia** refers to these age-related phenomena. Muscle loss occurs for a variety of reasons, including lessened physical activity, whether from disability or disease or related to a sedentary lifestyle; decreased anabolic hormone production (testosterone, growth hormone, dehydroepiandrosterone); increased cytokine activity; and decreased nutrition (Rolland, Dupuy, van Kan et al., 2011). Regardless of the etiology, loss of muscle mass can lead to a spiral of negative physical and functional changes. Resting energy expenditure, or metabolic rate, is largely driven by lean body mass and will decrease with loss of muscle. A coincidental increase in body fat occurs because of changes in hormonal status and reduced activity, among other reasons (Ahmed & Haboubi, 2010). This shift in body composition is not always apparent and cannot be discerned by measuring body weight alone.

Loss of muscle can lead to a functional decline because both strength and endurance are affected by specific loss of type II muscle fibers (von Haehling, Morley, & Anker, 2010). Fatigue, increased weakness, and slow walking speed often ensue, furthering the downward spiral in physical activity and increasing the risk of falls (Rolland et al., 2011; von Haehling et al., 2010). Fat-free mass, comprised of bone and muscle, is approximately 73% water content. The loss of muscle leads to lower total body water in the older person.

> **Practice Pearl** ▶▶▶ Unintentional weight loss of 5% of body weight in 1 month or 10% in 6 months should not be considered a normal part of aging and requires intervention.

Bone mineral density commonly is lost with age in both men and women. Suboptimal bone growth in younger years, medications, and disease can cause preexisting compromised bone density to which age-related bone losses are added. Bone loss puts women at risk for osteoporosis following menopause; men are at risk later in life.

Oral and Gastrointestinal Changes With Aging

Multiple changes may occur with age in the regulation of both appetite and fluid status. Additionally, gastrointestinal changes that may occur with aging can lead to altered dietary intake and eventually diminished nutritional status.

Dentition

By the age of 65 years, over 20% of Americans suffer from **edentulism,** or lack of teeth (Centers for Disease Control and Prevention, 2009). Poor dental health, missing or loose teeth, and ill-fitting dentures can affect the type and amount of food eaten and interfere with proper nutrition. Several studies have found an association between an edentulous state and poor intake of protein, vitamins, and minerals. Additionally, having fewer pairs of posterior teeth may result in less variety in the diet and is associated with compromised nutritional health (American Dietetic Association [ADA], 2007). Mandibular bone loss related to osteoporosis or periodontal disease can cause changes in structural tissue that affects chewing.

poor fitting dentures

Xerostomia

Saliva production declines with age and can be further exacerbated by excessive loss of fluid from the body (**dehydration**), medications, or disease. Lack of sufficient saliva production is termed **xerostomia.** Dry mouth can affect taste perception, hinder swallowing, and cause insufficient retention of poorly fitting dentures.

head + neck radiation dries mouth out

psych meds (side effect of dry mouth)

Atrophic Gastritis

In the stomach, decreases in the size and number of glands and mucous membranes can lead to **atrophic gastritis.** Lack of hydrochloric acid production, or **achlorhydria,** is common in the aging process. Iron and vitamin B_{12} require an acid medium in the stomach to begin absorption; lack of adequate hydrochloric acid production can limit absorption of both nutrients.

Chronic h.pylori   *Stomach pain*

Gastric production of intrinsic factor, which is necessary for vitamin B_{12} absorption in the ileum, may also decrease.

Drug Alert ▶▶▶ Medications that alter gastric pH such as antacids, proton pump inhibitors, H_2 receptor blockers, and potassium salts may also alter iron, calcium, and B_{12} absorption because of the alkalinizing effects of these medications.

Appetite Dysregulation

Cholecystokinin production increases with age and can cause early satiety and low hunger as a result. Early satiation also occurs due to changes in gastric emptying and central neurotransmitters responsible for the feeding drive. These physiological changes have been called the **anorexia of aging** (Chapman, MacIntosh, Morley et al., 2002).

Constipation

Slowed intestinal peristalsis, inadequate intake of fluid and fiber, illness, medications, and a sedentary lifestyle are contributing factors to the prevalence of constipation in the older person.

Thirst Dysregulation

Aging blunts the thirst mechanism. Additionally, the ability of the kidney to concentrate urine and the functional status of the renin–aldosterone system are all diminished. Together, this increases the risk of uncompensated dehydration in a population that already experiences lower total body water than do younger adults. Symptoms of dehydration such as confusion or lethargy can go unrecognized while hydration status continues to worsen without a strong thirst response. Dehydration risk can be worsened by voluntary fluid restriction in the older person trying to cope with incontinence, nocturia, or the need for assistance with toileting. Individuals with cognitive or physical limitations may have inadequate access to free fluids in addition to thirst dysregulation. Refer to Box 5-1 for dehydration risk factors and symptoms.

Sensory Changes

Age-related changes in vision, hearing, taste, and smell (see Chapter 14 ⬯) can have a negative impact on nutrition.

Vision

Cataracts, macular degeneration, and general poor vision can make shopping, food preparation, and even eating a burden. Fine-print food labels and cooking directions are difficult to read; handling hot foods or using a stove can be hazardous. Dim or harsh lighting in the dining area can

---

BOX 5-1   **Dehydration Risk Factors and Symptoms in the Older Adult**

Dehydration Risk Factors

Physical changes of aging

- ↓ Lean body mass ⟶ ↓ total body water
- ↓ Thirst from aging, medication, or disease
- Impaired angiotensin production

Lack of free access to fluids:

- Dependency on others
- Cognitive impairment
- Physical impairment

Voluntary fluid restriction to manage:

- Incontinence
- Nocturia
- Diuretic side effect
- Limited physical movement due to mobility or pain issues

Increased insensible fluid losses:

- Sweating from fever or climate
- ↑ Respiratory rate
- Vomiting
- Diarrhea
- Polyuria
- Exudative wound or fistula

Symptoms of Dehydration

Darkened urine
↓ Urine output
Confusion
Lethargy
Headache
Light-headedness
Sunken eyes
Dry mucous membranes
Dry axillae
Long tongue furrows
Postural changes in pulse and blood pressure

---

make it difficult to see a meal and reduce enjoyment associated with eating.

Practice Pearl ▶▶▶ Individuals with poor vision can benefit from mealtime assistance using the clock analogy with their dinner plate: "Your carrots are at two o'clock and the chicken is at six o'clock."

Hearing

Hearing losses that occur with age can make social dining a difficult experience. Some older persons may choose to dine alone rather than be embarrassed by not hearing well or frustrated trying to interact with others. Social isolation is considered a risk factor for undernutrition in the older person (ADA, 2010a).

Taste and Smell

Olfactory and taste perceptions are intertwined. Both senses diminish with age. Over 25% of adults older than age 60 years have olfactory impairment, a statistic that increases further with each subsequent decade of life (Karpa et al., 2010). Reduced sense of taste and smell contributes to decreased enjoyment of food, has a negative influence on the variety of foods consumed, and is associated with overall diminished intake (Ahmed & Haboubi, 2010). Medications are responsible for some taste alterations. ACE inhibitors, anticholinergics, antidepressants, and antihistamines can cause xerostomia and diminished taste perception. Dentures, zinc deficiency, smoking, and cognitive and neurodegenerative disease, such as Alzheimer's and Parkinson disease, are also associated with loss of taste. Some older persons experience **dysgeusia,** or altered taste perception, and complain of metallic and chalky taste transmissions. Others report needing markedly increased salt and sweet levels to perceive taste.

Social and Economic Changes Affecting Nutrition

Retirement from the workforce can lead to a more sedentary lifestyle for some older persons. The effects of decreased activity on body composition may involve muscle loss and fat gain. Social isolation, loneliness, loss of a spouse, or bereavement can introduce additional influences that can alter adequacy of diet. Changes in socioeconomic status may occur. Food insecurity, or the lack of sufficient funds or access to food, can force an individual to decide between paying bills, buying medications, or buying groceries. Over 8% of older adults in the United States live in a household suffering from food insecurity (ADA, 2010b). African American and Hispanic households are at disproportionate risk [*higher*] of food insecurity compared with other households. Living alone is associated with food insecurity for both older men and women. Food insecurity places the older adult at increased risk of nutrient deficiencies and functional limitations (ADA, 2010a). Box 5-2 outlines age-related nutritional changes in the body.

The benefits of healthy eating for older persons include increased functional capacity, more energy, quicker recovery from injury and/or surgery, and better immune system function. Sharing tips for healthy eating is an important part of health promotion and disease prevention.

HEALTHY EATING TIPS

▸ **Reduce sodium (salt).** This helps prevent water retention and high blood pressure.

> ### BOX 5-2 ▸ Nutrition-Related Changes Associated With Aging
>
> - ↓ Lean body mass
> - ↓ Metabolic rate
> - ↓ Bone mineral density
> - ↑ Cholecystokinin and early satiety
> - ↓ Saliva production
> - ↓ Thirst perception
> - ↓ Taste and smell
> - ↓ Production of gastric acid and fluids

▸ **Enjoy good fats.** Reap the rewards of olive oil, avocados, salmon, walnuts, flaxseed, and other monounsaturated fats.

▸ **Increase fiber.** To avoid constipation enjoy raw fruits and veggies, whole-grains, and beans.

▸ **Eat whole grains whenever possible.** Processed grains digest quickly and cause spikes in blood sugar levels and short-lived energy. For long-lasting energy and stable insulin levels, choose "good" or complex carbs such as whole grains, beans, fruits, and vegetables.

▸ **Look for hidden sugar.** Added sugar can be hidden in foods such as bread, canned soups and vegetables, pasta sauce, instant mashed potatoes, frozen dinners, fast food, and ketchup. Check food labels for alternate terms for sugar such as corn syrup, molasses, brown rice syrup, cane juice, fructose, sucrose, dextrose, or maltose. Opt for fresh or frozen vegetables instead of canned goods, and choose low-carb or sugar-free versions of products such as tortillas, bread, pasta, and ice cream.

▸ **Eat a variety of foods.** Variety is the spice of life. Enjoy fruits and veggies rich in taste and color to keep your meals interesting.

▸ **Slow down at mealtime.** Don't rush through your meals. Take the time to savor each bite and enjoy the mealtime experience.

Adapted from Segal & Kemp, 2012.

not knowing when you get your next meal.
- don't know when they go to store - can't drive

Nutritional and Disease-Related Health Changes

Many chronic diseases that affect older persons have nutritional implications on the disease and its treatment. Altered nutritional needs, therapeutic diets, and changes in nutrient utilization impact an individual's nutritional status. One example of this is cognitive impairment and mental illness, such as dementia, depression, or anxiety. Both the disease process itself and the medications used to treat these diagnoses can negatively impact appetite, taste, nutrient absorption, and metabolism; diminish saliva production; and cause gastrointestinal side effects. Numerous other diseases and medications have nutritional implications. Table 5-1 outlines some common medications with nutritional implications.

Nutritional Requirements and Aging

The older person has some unique nutritional requirements due to the physical and functional changes that occur with aging. Although many older persons experience a decline in physical activity level and have lower calorie needs,

there is not a decreased need for most vitamins and minerals with age. In fact, the dietary requirement for some nutrients increases with age. Obtaining a well-balanced diet while consuming fewer calories overall can present a challenge to many older persons.

There are several dietary standards that outline nutritional recommendations for older persons. The focus here is on recommendations that are unique to healthy older persons. The dietary reference intakes (DRIs) and the U.S. Dietary Guidelines are two distinctly different approaches to providing nutritional recommendations that work well together as assessment and educational tools. These two standards are not intended to be guidelines for use when making recommendations for older persons at risk for undernutrition or those with illness. The DRIs provide specific nutrient recommendations and are the larger umbrella under which exist the recommended dietary allowances

TABLE 5-1	Medications With Nutritional Implications	
Drug	**Side Effect**	**Explanation**
ACE inhibitors	Altered taste, dry mouth	Causes metallic taste/reduced taste perception
Alcohol	↓ Absorption and metabolism	Thiamin, folic acid, B_{12}, magnesium, B_6 affected
Antacids	↓ Absorption, constipation	Iron, calcium, B_{12}, need acid pH
Antianxiety agents	Dry mouth	Affects taste and swallowing
Antidepressants and antipsychotics	↓ Intake and dry mouth	Affects taste, smell, swallowing
Antiparkinson agents	↓ Intake and dry mouth	Nausea, vomiting, taste changes
Colchicine	↓ Absorption	Vitamin B_{12}, calcium, and iron affected
Corticosteroids	↓ Intake, ↓ nutrition	Nausea, vomiting; affects calcium, vitamin D, B_6, folate
Digoxin	↓ Intake	Anorexia and nausea
Diuretics, thiazide	↑ Losses	Urinary loss of potassium, magnesium, thiamin
Isoniazid	Altered metabolism	Vitamin B_6 affected
KCl (potassium chloride)	↓ Intake, ↓ absorption	Nausea; B_{12} and iron affected
Metformin	↓ Intake, ↓ absorption	Anorexia; B_{12} affected
Methotrexate	↓ Intake, ↓ absorption	Nausea; folate, B_{12}, calcium affected
Narcotics and sedatives	↓ Intake, constipation	Nausea, vomiting, sedation
Penicillamine	↓ Intake, ↓ nutrition	Anorexia, B_6 affected
Phenytoin	↓ Intake, ↓ nutrition	Altered taste and smell; folate, B_6, vitamin D affected. Drug interaction with enteral nutrition formula
Sulfasalazine	↓ Absorption	Folate and iron affected
Theophylline	↓ Intake, ↓ nutrition	Nausea, vomiting, anorexia; B_6 affected

(RDAs) and the newer adequate intakes (AIs) and tolerable upper limits (TULs). The RDAs are researched to meet the needs of 97% to 98% of healthy people within specific age and gender groups. Recommendations for older persons are categorized in two age groups: 51 to 70 years and over 70 years. When insufficient data exist to establish an RDA for a nutrient, an AI recommendation is made instead. The newest vitamin D recommendation is an example of an AI and not an RDA. The TUL guidelines have been included in the DRI umbrella to provide guidelines for a safe upper limit of intake for a nutrient. The saying "if some is good, more must be better" does not hold for all nutrients, as some have pharmacological action at high intakes. While a nurse can always refer to references for specific needs of random nutrients, knowledge of the unique nutritional needs and risk factors for the older person can be important to everyday practice. Knowledge of the TULs of commonly supplemented nutrients better allows a nurse to give crucial advice on supplement safety.

The U.S. Department of Agriculture (USDA) Dietary Guidelines translate the scientific recommendations of the DRIs into recommendations for daily eating. The focus is on variety, balance, and moderation in all food groups while providing adequate nutrient intake. The Tufts University MyPlate for Older Adults is a modification of the former USDA Food Guide Pyramid and is a useful complement to the DRIs when evaluating the nutritional history of an older person (Figure 5-1 ▶▶▶).

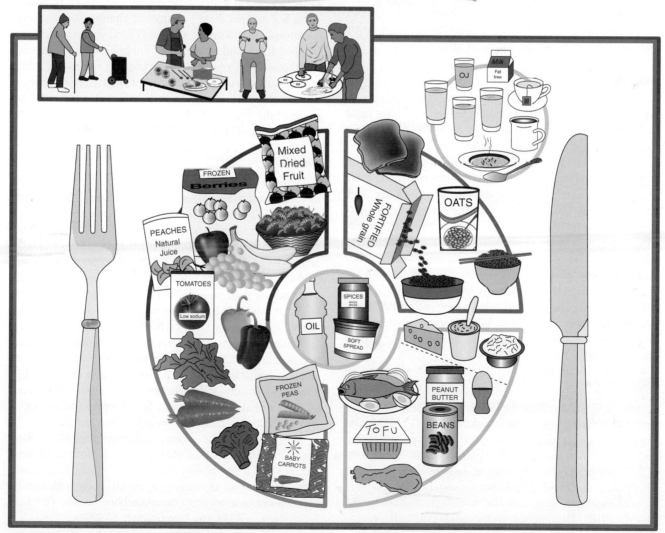

Figure 5-1 ▶▶▶ MyPlate for older adults.

Source: Copyright 2011 Tufts University. For details about the MyPlate for Older Adults, please see http://nutrition.tufts.edu/research/myplate-older-adults. Reprinted with permission.

Unique Nutrient Recommendations

The DRIs for the general adult population and the older adult population are the same with the exception of vitamin D, calcium, vitamin B_{12}, vitamin B_6, and energy. There is some dispute about whether the older person should have an altered protein requirement due to the prevalence of sarcopenia, yet the current RDA for protein remains unchanged at 0.8 g/kg body weight with no unique recommendation for the older person (Institute of Medicine [IOM], 2002). It is known that protein breakdown exceeds protein synthesis in the body with aging, but insufficient research exists to draw a definitive conclusion about a change in protein needs for this population (Rolland et al., 2011). Insufficient calorie intake is responsible for excessive protein breakdown regardless of the adequacy of dietary protein intake because the body's priority is for calories first. The MyPlate for Older Adults icon serves as a reminder that one-quarter of a meal should be comprised of protein-containing foods such as dairy, eggs, beans, meat, poultry, and fish.

Energy

The DRIs for energy, or estimated energy requirements (EERs), for all adults are based on gender, age, body mass index (BMI), and activity level. The EER is adjusted for age to account for both losses in lean muscle mass and diminished physical activity level. However, individuals with higher lean body mass or higher activity levels require more energy than those at lower levels for any given age. The reduced physical activity level seen in many older adults is largely felt to be the main contributor to decreased energy needs with aging (Frisard et al., 2007). The modified MyPlate makes overall recommendations for individual food groups to provide sufficient energy and nutrients together. Following the lowest daily recommended values for all the food groups will result in approximately 1,600 cal of energy. Use of this tool to guide energy recommendations is often more practical to the nurse and the patient than calculating EER.

Vitamin D

Vitamin D is required for its role in maintaining bone mineralization and proper serum calcium levels. Inadequate vitamin D levels can lead to poor bone mineralization, rickets, and osteomalacia. Adequate vitamin D intake is a component of reducing risk of falls in the older adult (Kalyani et al., 2010). The AI for vitamin D is 600 IU up to age 70 years and then increases to 800 IU for those older (IOM, 2010). Diminished endogenous synthesis of vitamin D with age, limited sun exposure, and potentially reduced absorption of vitamin D have guided these increased

recommendations aimed at reducing bone loss, fracture risk, and risk of some chronic diseases.

Food sources of vitamin D include liver, fortified milk, and fish liver oils. Note that it would require approximately six cups of milk consumption per day to meet the daily recommendation for vitamin D. Cheeses and yogurt are not mandated to be fortified with vitamin D and should not be considered good sources. Intake of dietary sources of vitamin D is insufficient in many population groups. Adults most at risk for poor vitamin D status include those who do not consume milk, have limited sun exposure, or take anticonvulsant medication or corticosteroids. The Modified MyPlate recommends a supplement of vitamin D in addition to the three dairy servings per day recommended. The authors acknowledge the limited intake of good sources of vitamin D and limited endogenous vitamin D synthesis with aging (Lichtenstein, Rasmussen, Yu et al., 2008). Table 5-2 outlines dietary sources of vitamin D. A thorough nutritional assessment of vitamin D food sources, including fortified foods and existing vitamin habits, should precede the recommendation of a supplement. Excessive intake of fortified foods or doubling up of multivitamin doses to achieve adequate vitamin D intake is not recommended because of the risk of unsafe levels of vitamin A intake. The TUL of vitamin D is 4,000 IU or 100 mcg (IOM, 2010).

Calcium

Calcium in the diet is required for the maintenance of bone mineral density and plasma calcium levels. The majority of the body's calcium reserves are in bone and teeth with only 1% of total body calcium in plasma. The AI for calcium in adults over 50 years of age is increased to 1,200 mg compared to 1,000 mg for adults 19 to 50 years of age (IOM, 2010). Despite higher calcium supplement use by older adults than younger counterparts, total calcium intake in this population is reportedly insufficient (Mangano, Walsh, Insogna et al., 2011). Inadequate intake of calcium and vitamin D may contribute to the prevalence of osteoporosis among the older population. Low dietary intake of calcium is also indicative of periodontal disease risk, while adequate calcium intake has been associated with reduced incidence of alveolar bone loss in older men (ADA, 2007). Box 5-3 lists risk factors for poor calcium nutrition.

See Table 5-3 for serving recommendations to meet the calcium needs of an older person. Recommendations are also given for lactose-intolerant or vegan individuals. Adequate vitamin D status is essential along with recommended calcium intake to maintain bone health. The TUL for calcium is 2,000 mg (see Chapter 18 ⬭).

The Dietary Approaches to Stopping Hypertension (DASH) initiative also recommends adequate dietary

TABLE 5-2	Vitamin D Amounts of Common Food Sources*	
Food	**Serving Size**	**Vitamin D Amount (International Units)**
Milk, vitamin D fortified	1 cup	127
Margarine, vitamin D fortified	1 tbsp	60
Egg yolk, large	1 ea	18
Beef liver, cooked	3.5 oz	30
Sardines with bones, canned, drained	3.5 oz	280
Salmon, cooked	3.5 oz	360
Cod liver oil	1 tbsp	1,360
Cereal, vitamin D fortified only	1/2 cup to 1 cup	~20–50 but varies—check label
Juice, vitamin D fortified only	1 cup	~20–50 but varies—check label
Soy milk or soy yogurt, vitamin D fortified only	1 cup	~100–150 but varies—check label

Note: Dairy sources such as cheese, yogurt, and ice cream contain calcium but are not good sources of vitamin D unless specifically fortified.

Sources: Adapted from U.S. Department of Agriculture, http://www.nal.usda.gov/fnic/foodcomp; National Institutes of Health Clinical Center, http://www.cc.nih.gov/ccc/supplements/vitd.html#food; and product labels.

Drug Alert ▶▶▶ Fat-soluble vitamins A, D, E, and K are stored in the body in larger amounts than are water-soluble vitamins (vitamin C and all the B vitamins). Taking large amounts of some fat-soluble vitamins could lead to toxicity due to continued storage in adipose and other tissue. In many clinic or office settings, the nurse may be the only clinician who has the opportunity to assess supplement use. The nurse should pay particular attention to the TUL for vitamins A, D, and E (vitamin K has no TUL due to lack of data on toxicity). When assessing nutritional status, the nurse should ask about all dietary supplements and fortified foods, like breakfast cereals and meal replacement drinks and bars.

High vitamin E intake can interact with anticoagulant therapy as well as potentiate the antiplatelet effects of other supplements such as ginkgo biloba, ginger, ginseng, and garlic. The TUL of vitamin E is 1,000 mg/day (IOM, 2000).

| BOX 5-3 | **Risk Factors for Poor Calcium Nutrition** |

- Low or absent intake of dairy products, especially milk and yogurt
- Lack of fortified calcium products in diet (fortified juices, soy products, and cereals)
- Excessive protein or caffeine intake (causes urinary calcium losses)
- Medications that alter calcium absorption or metabolism: corticosteroids, colchicine, phenobarbital, methotrexate, cholestyramine
- Poor vitamin D status (need adequate vitamin D to absorb calcium)

Vitamin B_{12}

Vitamin B_{12} (cyanocobalamin) is required in cell division and to maintain the myelin sheaths of the central nervous system. The RDA for vitamin B_{12} is 2.4 mcg. Exclusive to adults over the age of 50 years, the DRI, the Modified MyPlate, and the U.S. Dietary Guidelines recommend B_{12} fortified foods or a vitamin B_{12} supplement because of decreased absorption of the vitamin associated with atrophic gastritis and altered gastric pH (Lichtenstein et al., 2008). It is reported that up to 30% of adults over the age of 50 years have atrophic gastritis and decreased excretion of stomach acid (Stover, 2010).

calcium intake in the form of three dairy servings daily because of the association between adequate calcium, potassium, and magnesium intake from foods and lowered blood pressure (National Institutes of Health [NIH], 2006).

TABLE 5-3	Calcium Amounts of Common Food Sources	
Food	Serving Size	Calcium Amount (mg)
Milk, 1% low fat	1 cup	300
Cheese, American	1 oz	174
Cottage cheese, low fat	1/2 cup	78
Yogurt, low fat	1 cup	345
Ice cream, hard	1 cup	176
Juice, calcium-fortified	1 cup	200–300
Soy milk, calcium-fortified	1 cup	300
Custard or pudding, avg	1 cup	297
Chowder or cream soup, avg	1 cup	180
Sardines, with bones	3 oz	371
Figs, dried	5 ea	134
Almonds, slivered	1/4 cup	90
Spinach, cooked	1/2 cup	127

Source: Adapted from U.S. Department of Agriculture, http://www.nal.usda.gov/fnic/foodcomp.

> ***Practice Pearl*** ▶▶▶ Vitamins D and B_{12} and calcium are the only nutrients with routine consideration given to supplementation in the older person. The nurse should give careful consideration if an older person reports routine use of other supplements without medical need.

Supplemental B_{12} is not bound to protein, as it is in food sources, and hence does not require an acid medium to cleave the bond between the two nutrients. Vitamin B_{12} in fortified foods like breakfast cereals also is not bound to protein and therefore is more bioavailable than in natural food sources. Food sources include animal products like meats, fish, poultry, dairy, and eggs. Vegans must use nutritional yeast or consume fortified versions of foods like cereals and soy products to obtain B_{12} in the diet. Supplemental

forms of vitamin B_{12} generally are synthetic and acceptable to vegetarians and vegans. There is no TUL published for B_{12}. Symptoms of vitamin B_{12} deficiency include macrocytic anemia and neurologic problems such as peripheral neuropathy, irritability, depression, and poor memory. In addition to those with atrophic gastritis, older persons at risk for poor B_{12} status include individuals who use antacids and other gastric pH–altering medications and have malabsorptive disease or gastric resection (B_{12} is absorbed in the ileum bound to intrinsic factor made in the stomach). Gastric bypass surgery for obesity is associated with malabsorption of food-bound vitamin B_{12}, a risk that may increase the prevalence of deficiency found in the population as these individuals age (Frank & Crookes, 2010).

> ***Practice Pearl*** ▶▶▶ Folic acid supplementation can mask a B_{12} deficiency by treating the macrocytic anemia indices. However, neurologic symptoms will continue to progress without adequate B_{12}. It is important not to dismiss memory loss, depression, or irritability as age associated. A B_{12} assessment should be part of any workup for these neurologic symptoms.

Vitamin B_6

Vitamin B_6 (pyridoxine) is required as a coenzyme in metabolism of protein, fat, and other biochemical reactions. The DRI for B_6 in adults over 50 years of age is 1.5 mg per day for women and 1.7 mg per day for men. Younger adults require only 1.3 mg daily (IOM, 1998). Neither the DRIs nor the Modified MyPlate recommend a supplement of B_6 as it is widely available in the diet from meat, fish, poultry, legumes, and whole grains. A B_6 deficiency is unlikely to occur as a single event due to diet, but is more often found in combination with deficiencies of other B vitamins in chronic alcoholics. Medications that alter B_6 metabolism include isoniazid, theophylline, and penicillamine. Supplemental B_6 is routinely prescribed with isoniazid therapy. Symptoms of deficiency include an inflamed tongue and oral mucosa, called **glossitis and cheilosis,** depression, and confusion.

> ***Drug Alert*** ▶▶▶ The TUL for B_6 is 100 mg. This dose is easily available over the counter. Toxicity can cause sensory neuropathy, which occurs with as little as 200 mcg daily but diminishes when supplementation stops.

Fluid

Adequate fluid intake is important throughout the life cycle to ensure sufficient water is available to regulate body temperature, to provide a medium for biochemical reactions, and to eliminate the waste products of metabolism and digestion. Blunted thirst perception, altered hormone response, and decreased total body water can predispose the older person to dehydration, especially when additional hydration stressors like fever or exudative wounds occur. The RDAs estimate general water requirements at 1.0 to 1.5 mL/cal of energy intake. Specific daily total water recommendations for adults older than 51 years, including water from all foods and beverages, are 3.7 and 2.7 L for men and women, respectively (IOM, 2004). This includes a recommendation that daily total water from beverages alone reach 13 cups for men and 9 cups for women.

Critics have faulted the water requirement being linked to energy intake by some recommendations as this could underestimate fluid needs for poor eaters. The RDA is targeted at healthy individuals only. Older adults at risk for dehydration because of poor intake deserve close attention and intervention to assure adequate intake, but do not warrant a separate recommendation for higher than normal fluid intake. Likewise, those with excessive water losses because of wounds, fever, or intestinal loss require adjustment in fluid intake to compensate for these losses, which are not covered by the recommendations made for healthy persons.

The MyPlate for Older Adults emphasizes hydration by placing 8 servings of various fluids next to the plate icon. Individuals may require increased fluid intake during increased activity or higher ambient temperature or when taking medications such as diuretics. Other insensible fluid losses occur with fever, increased respiration, exudative wounds, and gastrointestinal losses. Increases in insensible losses over baseline should be accounted for when determining fluid needs. Alcohol and caffeine-containing beverages each have a temporary diuretic effect, but are included in the fluid total (IOM, 2004). Older persons with poor renal function need their fluid requirements individually prescribed based on clinical parameters and urine output. A minimum of 1,000 mL is needed to compensate for insensible losses even with anuria.

The older person can benefit from drinking to a schedule rather than waiting until thirsty. A drinking schedule can be adjusted for individuals requiring assistance with toileting or hesitant about nocturia or incontinence. Cognitive adults with these symptoms may be voluntarily restricting fluid intake to manage symptoms and may already be at risk for dehydration. Adults with cognitive impairment should be offered fluids throughout the day, as altered thirst perception and ability to communicate thirst are not reliable. Box 5-1 on page 98 outlines risks and symptoms of dehydration.

> **Practice Pearl ▶▶▶** Checking hydration by looking for "tenting" on the forearm or sternum is not a valid measure in the older person due to loss of skin elasticity. Instead, symptoms felt to be better indicators of dehydration include darkened urine, confusion, lethargy, long tongue furrows, sunken eyes, and dry mucous membranes. Postural changes in pulse and blood pressure may exist with larger volume deficits.

Supplement Savvy: Beyond the RDAs

Instead of taking dietary supplements to correct a nutritional problem, many consumers are swayed by early medical reports, the media, or their next-door neighbor to take a supplement for its purported disease-fighting or age-delaying properties. Gone are the days when supplements meant only vitamins, and minerals were just for preventing or correcting deficiencies. Current estimates report 70% of older adults take any type of dietary supplement, with one third taking a multivitamin/multimineral supplement (Bailey et al., 2011). Botanical dietary supplement use is more prevalent among older adults that other age groups (Bailey et al., 2011). There is substantial use of concomitant medications and dietary supplements among this population, increasing the risk of drug interactions especially with anticoagulants (Nahin et al., 2009; Qato et al., 2008).

Many adults believe that because nutritional supplements are natural, they are nontoxic and well tested before being placed on the market. The Dietary Supplements and Health Education Act, which covers vitamins, minerals, herbals, weight loss products, and other dietary supplements, does not require manufacturers to seek premarket approval from the Food and Drug Administration (FDA) for safety, purity, or product efficacy of any of these products. It is important to inquire about all dietary supplements in a nonjudgmental fashion as part of a patient history to help guide individuals about safe choices regarding supplements. This area of nutrition has little peer-reviewed research to guide the clinician and requires constant vigilance to remain up to date.

Here are some common supplements that older persons may be taking for reasons other than prevention of deficiencies:

■ **Vitamins E or B_{12} or ginkgo biloba and Alzheimer's disease:** Early research on high-dose vitamin E reported a delay in the progression of existing Alzheimer's disease, but more recent studies have failed to support any beneficial use of vitamin E in this population (Winslow, Onysko, Stob et al., 2011).

The herb ginkgo biloba had been associated with slight cognitive improvements in some patients with existing Alzheimer's disease. However, a consistent clinically recognizable benefit has not been demonstrated (Snitz et al., 2009; Winslow et al., 2011). Despite this, the findings have been captured by the popular press and consumers fearful of developing Alzheimer's disease. Combining vitamin E with ginkgo or any other supplement or medication with antiplatelet or anticoagulant effects could result in increased bleeding.

> **Practice Pearl** ▶▶▶ Supplements with antiplatelet effects include fish oils, garlic, ginseng, ginkgo biloba, evening primrose oil, and vitamin E. Thoughtful analysis of supplement intake by the nurse should yield whether an older person is at risk for this form of **polypharmacy** (use of multiple medications) and altered blood clotting. An assessment should also consider whether such supplements are being used with medications that alter clotting, such as warfarin and aspirin.

- **Antioxidants and age-related macular degeneration:** Age-related macular degeneration (AMD) is the most common cause of blindness in Americans over the age of 60 years. Initial nutrition-related research on AMD focused on antioxidant and zinc supplementation with recommendations for vitamins C and E, B-carotene, and zinc intake. More recently, it has been postulated that B-carotene and vitamin E may negatively affect disease progression in its later stage and plant pigments lutein and zeaxanthin may play a positive role along with omega-3 fatty acids (Olson, Erie, & Bakri, 2011). No recommendations can be made for nutritional supplementation used in treating this disease until further research findings have been completed.

The use of supplements continues as a widespread health behavior. These examples are indicative of the more common choices of supplementation but are not exhaustive. The wide variance in nutrient intake, unpredictable use of dietary supplements, and unique nutritional needs of older persons reinforce the necessity of good nutritional assessment tools and sharp clinical judgment.

Alcohol and Vitamins

Chronic alcohol intake affects nutritional status in many ways. More than 20% of older adults qualify as heavy drinkers, having more than eight drinks per week (Aalto, Alho, Halme et al., 2011). Older persons who ingest alcohol are at risk for deficiencies of thiamin, riboflavin, folate, vitamin B_6, and magnesium because of the direct negative effects of alcohol on gastric mucosa, nutrient absorption, metabolism, and excretion. When alcohol replaces food intake, additional effects of undernutrition occur.

Nutritional Assessment

Both undernutrition and overnutrition in the older person can affect quality of life, morbidity, and mortality. Malnutrition is associated with adverse outcomes such as poor wound healing, skeletal muscle loss, functional decline, altered immune response, altered pharmacokinetics, and increased risk of institutionalization (Chapman, 2011). Overnutrition can also affect quality of life in the older person when it is manifested as obesity, degenerative joint disease, diabetes, hypertension, and cardiovascular disease. Excess weight and elevated cholesterol have less clinical significance in those over 70 years of age, but remain important individual psychosocial and functional considerations (Houston, Nicklas, & Zizza, 2009; Witham & Avenell, 2010).

There is no gold standard to define malnutrition nor is there a consensus on one tool or a set of tools to be used to assess nutritional status in the older person. Several validated screening tools exist and many more have been proposed. Although the parameters evaluated in each are different, assessment of nutritional risk factors for undernutrition should be routinely incorporated into the routine health screening of the older person.

Nutritional Assessment Parameters

A comprehensive nutritional assessment reviews anthropometric measurements, laboratory values, and clinical findings from the physical examination and patient history.

Anthropometrics

Anthropometric measurements include any scientific measurement of the body. Height, weight and weight history, muscle mass, and fat mass measurements are included. Alternative techniques for obtaining anthropometric measurements may be necessary in the frail older person.

Weight Current measured body weight and weight history are an important component of a good nutritional assessment. If an older person is unable to stand to be weighed, use of a chair scale or bed scale is indicated (Figure 5-2 ▶▶▶). The nurse should not use verbal recall of current weight as a documented weight for anyone. Recorded weights on admission and at regular intervals are essential for hospitalized and long-term care patients. Individuals should be weighed with a minimum of clothing and after voiding. The nurse should note any presence of edema. A weight history that reveals unintentional weight loss of 5% body weight over a month or 10% over 6 months is clinically significant and should trigger further investigation.

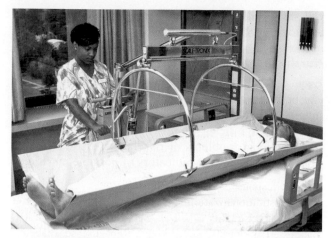

Figure 5-2 ▶▶▶ Nurse weighing patient on a bed scale.
Source: Michal Heron/Pearson Education/PH College.

Height Height can be measured using a standing measure or in a recumbent position. Recumbent measurements can be made with an individual lying flat and straight in bed with light pencil marks made on bed linens at head and heel. The distance between marks is then measured with a cloth tape. In most patients, the recumbent measurement is greater than standing height because of the relaxation of the spine in this position. Indirect height measurement can be done measuring knee height and arm span estimations. Arm span or demi–arm span does not require any special calculations but does require some mobility on the part of the older person, because either one or both arms and hands must be extended fully. Measurement is made from left-hand fingertip to right-hand fingertip; demi–arm span is made from fingertip to sternal notch and the value is doubled or entered into an equation (Hirani, Tabassum, Aresu et al., 2010). A knee height measurement is done with a sliding caliper that keeps the foot at a 90-degree angle to the leg during the measurement. A formula calculates height from the results (Chumlea, Roche, & Mukherjee, 1984). Impaired leg and foot flexibility can impede knee height measurements.

Body Mass Index Body mass index is derived using measured height and weight with the following formula: BMI = weight (kg)/height^2 (m). Parameters have been established to delineate underweight, normal weight, and overweight in the general population, but these generally are not applicable to the older person. Decreased BMI below 22 in the older person is predictive of undernutrition and associated with mortality (Chapman, 2011). While a BMI of 25 to 30 is considered overweight and carries an increased mortality risk for the general population, the relative risk of death associated with being overweight decreases after age 65, with little or no association between BMI and mortality after age 75 years (Chapman, 2011).

Body Fat Measurement The tricep skinfold measurement measures the subcutaneous fat over the triceps muscle at the back of the upper arm using a caliper. Fat mass measurements are derived from a formula using tricep measurements. Reliable use of the calipers takes practice and should be done by an experienced person. Skinfold measurements can be done on other sites on the body such as subscapular, ileac crest, and thigh, but the tricep is most easily accessed.

Indirect measurement of body fat can be done with technology such as bioelectrical impedance or near-infrared devices. Such equipment requires proper hydration of the person to avoid inaccurate measurements. Their use in the older population is largely for research purposes.

Muscle Mass Measurements Loss of lean body mass, or muscle, occurs with aging and is more pronounced in the inactive person. This loss may be visible to the eye or when measuring body weight, but may also be masked due to increased fat mass or edema. Midarm circumference is a measurement used to derive lean body mass. Arm circumference is measured at the midarm using a cloth tape. The measurement and the tricep skinfold measurement are together incorporated into a formula to derive midarm muscle circumference and an estimate of lean muscle mass. Measurement of midarm circumference alone is of no clinical value.

Laboratory Values

Several laboratory parameters are used to assess nutritional status. No one parameter is unique in its sensitivity to malnutrition; each has confounding reasons for abnormal values. Laboratory measurements should be part of an overall nutritional assessment and not relied on as a sole measurement of undernutrition. Recommendation of laboratory assessment should be in accordance with any advance directives for an individual. Box 5-4 outlines common laboratory measurements used in nutritional assessment.

Plasma Proteins Albumin, prealbumin, and transferrin are all used to assess visceral protein status. Albumin levels < or

---

BOX 5-4 **Laboratory Values Used in a Routine Nutritional Assessment**

- Albumin
- Retinol-binding prealbumin
- Transferrin
- Complete blood count (CBC) for:
  - Mean cell volume (MCV)
  - Hemoglobin
  - Hematocrit
- Serum folate and B$_{12}$ assays

equal to 3.5 mg/dL are considered indicative of mild malnutrition. Albumin values can be affected by disease. Nephrotic syndrome causes increased urinary loss of albumin. Liver disease can lead to decreased albumin synthesis. Dehydration or overhydration will cause false albumin values. Additionally, albumin is an acute-phase reactant protein, and levels will diminish during inflammation or infection. Relying on serum albumin alone as a nutritional indicator may lead to discordance with clinical assessment when this occurs. Using albumin in a nutritional assessment does not give the most current picture since the half-life of albumin is approximately 21 days.

Prealbumin and transferrin have shorter half-lives than albumin (2 to 3 days and 8 days, respectively), so they give more current information on protein status. They are not generally part of routine blood work and thus are less often a component of an assessment. Prealbumin is an acute-phase reactant protein as well. Transferrin measurements are often derived from total iron-binding capacity and therefore would be affected by anemia states.

Folate and Vitamin B₁₂ Assessment Evaluation of vitamin B_{12} and folic acid status is particularly pertinent due to the effects of aging, disease, and medications on absorption and metabolism of both vitamins. A high red blood cell mean cell volume (MCV) should be followed up by assessments of plasma folic acid and vitamin B_{12}.

Nursing Assessment

Even with limited resources, a nutritional assessment can be performed using sharp clinical observation and judgment. Examining the older person from head to toe can reveal significant findings that may indicate existing nutritional problems or risk factors for undernutrition. See Table 5-4 for indicators of possible nutritional problems.

The nursing assessment should focus on skin condition, including turgor, lesions, nonhealing ulcers, color variations, and excessive dryness or cracking. Additionally, the nurse should inspect the condition and distribution of the hair. The oral cavity is inspected for tooth or denture condition, oral lesions, hyperplasia of the gums, fissures around the lips, oral hygiene, and any coatings on the tongue. The abdomen should be palpated for firmness or tenderness. The bowel record should be checked for date of the last bowel movement, because constipation and fecal impaction will inhibit appetite. The nurse should observe the patient eating and drinking, note any swallowing difficulties or positioning problems, and consult with occupational

TABLE 5-4	Physical Findings on Examination Related to the Nutritional Status of Older Adults	
System	**Area of Focus**	**Potential Physical Findings**
Head	Mouth	Taste perception changes, swollen tongue, saliva production, angular lesions at lips, swollen gums, mouth sores
	Teeth	Loose or missing teeth, caries, dentures
	Chewing and swallowing	Pocketing food, drooling, note any complaints
	Hearing	Note alteration
	Vision	Note alteration
	Overall appearance	Note any temporal wasting
Trunk	Overall appearance	Note wasting of muscle or subcutaneous fat
	Skin turgor	Note presence of wounds, pressure ulcer
Extremities	Overall appearance	Note presence of edema, wasting of muscle or subcutaneous fat
Gastrointestinal Tract		Note complaints of nausea, vomiting, diarrhea
Genitourinary Tract		Note complaints of incontinence or nocturia with regard to voluntary fluid restriction
Neurologic		Note tremors, neuropathy, depressive symptoms, impaired cognition
Functional Capacity		Note ability to perform activities of daily living relative to eating

therapy should adaptive tableware be needed to encourage independence and maximum nutritional intake.

It is important to assess pain levels and administer PRN (as needed) medications 1 hour before mealtime if unrelieved pain appears to be a factor. The nurse should consult with the older patient and family regarding food preferences and timing, food dislikes, religious preferences, and cultural or ethnic traditions that could be negatively affecting nutritional intake.

Finally, the medication list should be reviewed for any medications (long-standing or newly prescribed) that could be causing loss of appetite or depression. Many medications have the side effects of early satiety, alterations of taste, lethargy, and appetite suppression. Common offenders are digoxin, diuretics, chemotherapy agents, some antibiotics, and some antidepressants. The older patient should be questioned regarding any feelings of depression, because changes in appetite are often associated with depression in the older person. Nurses should ask, "Do you feel sad or blue?" as a screening question that, if answered positively, could set in motion a complete depression assessment (Hartford Institute for Geriatric Nursing, 2008a). (See Chapter 7 ⬛▭ for further information on depression.)

It is also important to evaluate the eating environment. Some nursing home residents are assisted to the dining room over an hour before the meal is served. They may become restless, agitated, or bored and leave the dining room without eating. Many persons with dementia do better by eating smaller, more frequent meals. It helps to remove all unappetizing smells and provide a pleasant environment with music, small bouquets of flowers, and colorful tablecloths. Extra light should be supplied for older persons with visual limitations. The nurse should assist the older person with preparation for eating including opening straws and milk cartons, cutting meat, and so on. The food served to the residents should be warm (not too hot) and tasty. The family should be encouraged to dine with the resident if they are visiting. The same assessment parameters should be stressed for older patients living at home and being cared for by a family member or paid caregiver.

> **Practice Pearl** ▶▶▶ When serving food to an older person with dementia, it is best to serve one course at a time with the appropriate utensil. For instance, the nurse should serve the soup first with a spoon and then remove the soup and spoon before presenting the main meal. Supplying the appropriate utensil for the food will decrease frustration and encourage food intake.

Nutritional History

A careful nutritional history is part of a comprehensive assessment and can be accomplished in a variety of ways.

Like other screening tools, reliance on just one method will yield less valuable information than a combination of methods.

Diet Recall A 24-hour dietary recall can be done during an office visit or as part of an admission interview. It is important to ask open-ended questions that make no assumptions. For example, if the nurse asks, "What did you have for lunch?" some older persons may be too embarrassed to divulge that they had nothing and may fabricate the answer they think the nurse is seeking. It is better to ask, "What was the first thing you had to eat today?" and then "When was the next time you ate something?" Asking questions about weekend eating, which may be different than weekday habits, improves the value of the recall information. The nurse should ask questions about intake of dietary supplements, all fluids including alcohol, therapeutic diet, food intolerances, grocery shopping, food preparation frequency and ability, and any religious or cultural influences on diet. The nurse can ask, "Do you follow any special food guidelines or traditions? Are there any foods that you avoid or include in your diet?" The nurse should also ask how food is prepared. Diversity exists among and within religious and cultural groups; it is important to obtain a personal history without assumptions. The 24-hour recall is only a snapshot in time and is not always indicative of normal habits.

Food Frequency A food frequency assessment is an excellent tool to use with a 24-hour recall to fill in the gaps of missing information that occur with a 1-day snapshot. Simple questions about each food group can be asked to determine daily, weekly, or less often consumption of foods. For example, while a 24-hour recall may list only one glass of milk and no other dairy intake, a food frequency may show that cheese and milk are consumed more regularly. The nurse should ask about all food groups including fluids and supplements. Table 5-5 is an example of a food frequency questionnaire.

Food Record Asking a cognitively intact older person to record food intake for up to 3 days can provide a view of variable eating patterns. The recording of 2 weekdays and 1 weekend day works best. Food records beyond 3 days in length become cumbersome and may be filled out retrospectively right before being delivered.

Screening Tools

Nutritional screening and assessment tools exist to streamline the incorporation of nutritional status into routine healthcare processes. It is essential that any tool be used in the context for which it was developed and validated.

TABLE 5-5	Sample Food Frequency Quick Questionnaire				
Food	**Variety**	**Type**	**Per Day**	**Per Week**	**Or Less**
Fruit	Juice	Orange	4 oz		
	Fresh	None			
	Canned/frozen	Canned pears		1 cup	
Vegetables	Green	Varied		1–2×	
	Other	Carrots		1×	
Dairy	Milk	Low fat	2 cups		
	Cheese				1× month
	Yogurt	Never			
Protein	Animal	Poultry or fish	Each night		
	Plant	Hummus beans		1–2×	
Fats	Saturated	Butter	1–2 pats		
	Unsaturated				
Fluids	General	Water	4 oz 4 × with meds		
	Caffeine	Tea	Each a.m.		
	Alcohol	Wine			1–2× month
Sweets and Sugars		Cake or pie	After dinner		
Supplements		Multivitamin	One		

Nutrition Screening Initiative

The Nutrition Screening Initiative (NSI) was developed as a public health strategy. It consists of screening tools for use by individuals and healthcare providers to identify potential nutritional risk factors in community-dwelling older persons (Phillips, Foley, Barnard et al., 2010). The DETERMINE checklist is a mnemonic outlining nine warning signs that are predictive of poor nutrition. The tool is scored and stratified according to nutritional risk. Suggestions are given for professional intervention if needed. See Figure 5-3 ▶▶▶ for the NSI DETERMINE checklist. The checklist is used by some as a clinical screening tool, but it has not been validated for this use.

Mini Nutritional Assessment

The Mini Nutritional Assessment Short Form (MNA®-SF) is recommended for use by the Hartford Institute of Geriatric Nursing and has been validated as a clinical tool for use in screening nutritional status in the older person (Hartford Institute for Geriatric Nursing, 2008b; Kaiser, Bauer, Ramsch et al., 2009). The MNA®-SF can be used at the bedside or in the ambulatory care setting and takes less than five minutes to complete as part of a routine physical examination. The MNA®-SF (2009) has extensive research published on its use in the older person. When the older person's height

or weight cannot be determined, the MNA®-SF also allows for the substitution of the calf circumference in place of the body mass index (BMI). Please refer to the MNA website for further information and updates on the use of this instrument (www.mna-elderly.com). See Figure 5-4 ▶▶▶ for the Mini Nutritional Assessment.

Minimum Data Set

The Minimum Data Set (MDS) is a government-mandated component to the Resident Assessment Instrument used by all Medicare- or Medicaid-certified healthcare facilities. Assessments are done on admission, updated quarterly, and reassessed annually or whenever a significant change in resident status occurs. The MDS includes nutritional components such as weight status, swallowing difficulties, and intake of calories and fluid that must be assessed for all residents (Centers for Medicare and Medicaid Services, 2012). See Box 5-5 on page 113 for MDS nutrition-related criteria.

Other investigators have proposed different screening tools or edited versions of existing tools. Until a consensus is reached on a gold standard for use in nutritional assessment, new screening tools will continue to be developed. Formal, validated, and quick screening tools are helpful reminders of the importance of including a nutritional assessment when caring for the older person.

Read the statements below. Circle the number in the "yes" column for those that apply to you or someone you know. For each "yes" answer, score the number in the box. Total your nutritional score.

DETERMINE YOUR NUTRITIONAL HEALTH

	YES
I have an illness or condition that made me change the kind and/or amount of food I eat.	2
I eat fewer than 2 meals per day.	3
I eat few fruits or vegetables or milk products.	2
I have 3 or more drinks of beer, liquor or wine almost every day.	2
I have tooth or mouth problems that make it hard for me to eat.	2
I don't always have enough money to buy the food I need.	4
I eat alone most of the time.	1
I take 3 or more different prescribed or over-the-counter drugs a day.	1
Without wanting to, I have lost or gained 10 pounds in the last 6 months.	2
I am not always physically able to shop, cook and/or feed myself.	2
TOTAL	

Total Your Nutritional Score. If it's-

0-2 Good! Recheck your nutritional score in 6 months.

Remember that Warning Signs suggest risk, but do not represent a diagnosis of any condition.

3-5 You are at moderate nutritional risk. See what can be done to improve your eating habits and lifestyle. Your office on aging, senior nutrition program, senior citizens center or health department can help. Recheck your nutritional score in 3 months.

6 or more You are at high nutritional risk. Bring this Checklist the next time you see your doctor, dietitian or other qualified health or social service professional. Talk with them about any problems you may have. Ask for help to improve your nutritional health.

These materials are developed and distributed by the Nutrition Screening Initiative, a project of:

AMERICAN ACADEMY OF FAMILY PHYSICIANS

THE AMERICAN DIETETIC ASSOCIATION

THE NATIONAL COUNCIL ON THE AGING, INC.

The Nutrition Checklist is based on the Warning Signs described below. Use the word DETERMINE to remind you of the Warning Signs.

Disease   Any disease, illness or chronic condition which causes you to change the way you eat, or makes it hard for you to eat, puts your nutritional health at risk. Four out of five adults have chronic diseases that are affected by diet. Confusion or memory loss that keeps getting worse is estimated to affect one out of five or more of older adults. This can make it hard to remember what, when or if you've eaten. Feeling sad or depressed, which happens to about one in eight older adults, can cause big changes in appetite, digestion, energy level, weight and well-being.

Eating poorly   Eating too little and eating too much both lead to poor health. Eating the same foods day after day or not eating fruit, vegetables, and milk products daily will also cause poor nutritional health. One in five adults skip meals daily. Only 13% of adults eat the minimum amount of fruit and vegetables needed. One in four older adults drink too much alcohol. Many health problems become worse if you drink more than one or two alcoholic beverages per day.

Tooth loss/mouth pain   A healthy mouth, teeth and gums are needed to eat. Missing, loose or rotten teeth or dentures which don't fit well, or cause mouth sores, make it hard to eat.

Economic hardship   As many as 40% of older Americans have incomes of less than $6,000 per year. Having less— or choosing to spend less—than $25-30 per week for food makes it very hard to get the foods you need to stay healthy.

Reduced social contact   One-third of all older people live alone. Being with people daily has a positive effect on morale, well-being and eating.

Multiple medicines   Many older Americans must take medicines for health problems. Almost half of older Americans take multiple medicines daily. Growing old may change the way we respond to drugs. The more medicines you take, the greater the chance for side effects such as increased or decreased appetite, change in taste, constipation, weakness, drowsiness, diarrhea, nausea, and others. Vitamins or minerals, when taken in large doses, act like drugs and can cause harm. Alert your doctor to everything you take.

Involuntary weight loss/gain   Losing or gaining a lot of weight when you are not trying to do so is an important warning sign that must not be ignored. Being overweight or underweight also increases your chance of poor health.

Needs assistance in self care   Although most older people are able to eat, one of every five have trouble walking, shopping, buying and cooking food, especially as they get older.

Elder years above age 80   Most older people lead full and productive lives. But as age increases, risk of frailty and health problems increase. Checking your nutritional health regularly makes good sense.

The Nutrition Screening Initiative • 1010 Wisconsin Avenue, NW • Suite 800 • Washington, DC 20007
The Nutrition Screening Initiative is funded in part by a grant from Ross Products Division of Abbott Laboratories, Inc.

Figure 5-3 ▶▶▶ Nutrition Screening Initiative DETERMINE checklist. The warning signs of poor nutritional health are often overlooked. Use this checklist to find out if you or someone you know is at nutritional risk.

Source: Reproduced from the Nutrition Screening Initiative: Determine your nutritional health checklist. 2013 Reprinted with permission from Abbott.

Mini Nutritional Assessment
MNA®

Nestlé
NutritionInstitute

Last name: _____   First name: _____

Sex: _____   Age: _____   Weight, kg: _____   Height, cm: _____   Date: _____

Complete the screen by filling in the boxes with the appropriate numbers. Total the numbers for the final screening score.

Screening

A Has food intake declined over the past 3 months due to loss of appetite, digestive problems, chewing or swallowing difficulties?
0 = severe decrease in food intake
1 = moderate decrease in food intake
2 = no decrease in food intake ☐

B Weight loss during the last 3 months
0 = weight loss greater than 3 kg (6.6 lbs)
1 = does not know
2 = weight loss between 1 and 3 kg (2.2 and 6.6 lbs)
3 = no weight loss ☐

C Mobility
0 = bed or chair bound
1 = able to get out of bed / chair but does not go out
2 = goes out ☐

D Has suffered psychological stress or acute disease in the past 3 months?
0 = yes   2 = no ☐

E Neuropsychological problems
0 = severe dementia or depression
1 = mild dementia
2 = no psychological problems ☐

F1 Body Mass Index (BMI) (weight in kg) / (height in m^2)
0 = BMI less than 19
1 = BMI 19 to less than 21
2 = BMI 21 to less than 23
3 = BMI 23 or greater ☐

IF BMI IS NOT AVAILABLE, REPLACE QUESTION F1 WITH QUESTION F2.
DO NOT ANSWER QUESTION F2 IF QUESTION F1 IS ALREADY COMPLETED.

F2 Calf circumference (CC) in cm
0 = CC less than 31
3 = CC 31 or greater ☐

Screening score (max. 14 points)

12 - 14 points: Normal nutritional status
8 - 11 points: At risk of malnutrition
0 - 7 points: Malnourished ☐☐

References
1. Vellas B, Villars H, Abellan G, et al. Overview of the MNA® - Its History and Challenges. *J Nutr Health Aging*. 2006;**10**:456-465.
2. Rubenstein LZ, Harker JO, Salva A, Guigoz Y, Vellas B. Screening for Undernutrition in Geriatric Practice: Developing the Short-Form Mini Nutritional Assessment (MNA-SF). *J. Geront*. 2001; **56A**: M366-377
3. Guigoz Y. The Mini-Nutritional Assessment (MNA®) Review of the Literature - What does it tell us? *J Nutr Health Aging*. 2006; **10**:466-487.
4. Kaiser MJ, Bauer JM, Ramsch C, et al. Validation of the Mini Nutritional Assessment Short-Form (MNA®-SF): A practical tool for identification of nutritional status. *J Nutr Health Aging*. 2009; **13**:782-788.
® Société des Produits Nestlé, S.A., Vevey, Switzerland, Trademark Owners © Nestlé, 1994, Revision 2009. N67200 12/99 10M
For more information: www.mna-elderly.com

Figure 5-4 ▶▶▶ Mini Nutritional Assessment®.

Sources: Vellas B, Villars H, Abellan G, et al. Overview of the MNA®—Its History and Challenges. *J Nutr Health Aging 2006; 10*:456–465. Rubenstein L. Z., Harker J. O., Salva A, Guigoz Y, Vellas B. Screening for Undernutrition in Geriatric Practice: Developing the Short-Form Mini Nutritional Assessment (MNA-SF). *J Geront 2001; 56A:* M366–377. Guigoz Y. The Mini-Nutritional Assessment (MNA®) Review of the Literature—What does it tell us? *J Nutr Health Aging 2006; 10*:466–487. Kaiser M. J., Bauer J. M., Ramsch C, et al. Validation of the Mini Nutritional Assessment Short-Form (MNA®-SF): A practical tool for identification of nutritional status. *J Nutr Health Aging 2009; 13*:782–788. (for the MNA®-SF). © Nestle, 1994, Revision 2009. N67200 12/99 10M. www.mna-elderly.com. Reprinted with permission.

Common Nutritional Concerns in the Older Person

Both undernutrition and overnutrition can affect morbidity and mortality in the older person. Undernutrition, such as that which occurs with unplanned weight loss, is an important concern and deserves attention.

Unintentional Weight Loss

Adequate nutrition is an essential component for remaining autonomous into older personhood. Unfortunately, the prevalence of malnutrition in the older population is significant, especially among those who are institutionalized or hospitalized (ADA, 2010c; Chapman, 2011; Kaiser et al., 2010). Weight loss and undernutrition in nursing home residents is

---

BOX 5-5 Pertinent Risk Factors for Malnutrition From MDS Criteria

- Inability to feed oneself
- Chewing problems
- Swallowing problems
- Mouth pain
- Process: check mouth for food pocketing and abnormalities
- Weight loss
    ≥5% in 1 month
    ≥10% in 6 months
- Altered taste
- Hunger complaints
- Receives less than 25% of prescribed parenteral nutrition or tube feeding
- Nutrition approaches: Note parenteral/IV, tube feeding, mechanically altered diet, syringe feeding, therapeutic diet, supplement use, adaptive feeding equipment, or presence of weight gain program

Source: Adapted from Centers for Medicare and Medicaid Services Version 3.0 Manual, Chapter 3, MDS, https://www.cms.gov/NursingHomeQualityInits/45_ NHQIMDS30TrainingMaterials.asp#TopOfPage.

BOX 5-6 Causes of Unintentional Weight Loss

Insufficient Intake

- Depression or bereavement/loneliness
- Medication side effects
- Social isolation
- Dependency on others
- Improper feeding assistance
- Pain
- Xerostomia
- Dehydration
- Food insecurity
- Sensory changes in smell, taste, vision, hearing
- Chewing or swallowing difficulty
- Cognitive impairment
- Therapeutic diet
- Lack of personal, cultural, or religious food preferences
- Iatrogenic

Nutrient Losses

- Malabsorptive disease
- Medications
- Diarrhea/vomiting
- Alcoholism

Hypermetabolism

- Fever
- Infection or sepsis
- Wounds or pressure ulcers
- Bone fracture
- Tremors
- Disease, such as advanced chronic obstructive pulmonary disease

---

associated with an increased mortality compared with those residents with stable weight (ADA, 2010c). Independent older persons have a lower prevalence of undernutrition but should not be overlooked, especially those who experience food insecurity because they lack adequate funds for food or access to food. Food insecurity in older adults is associated with decreased intake of micronutrients (ADA, 2010a).

Etiology of Unintentional Weight Loss

The aging process alone is not the cause of unintentional weight loss. A complex assortment of contributing factors adds to the existing issues of the "anorexia of aging" and sarcopenia. Untreated malnutrition is followed by a sequela of negative consequences and poor outcomes that is difficult to stop. The known causes of unintentional weight loss fall into three general categories: insufficient intake of food and fluid, iatrogenic practices, increased losses of nutrients, and hypermetabolism. Box 5-6 outlines possible causes of unintentional weight loss.

Insufficient Intake Lack of adequate food and fluid intake occurs for multiple physical and psychosocial reasons.

Dehydration can be responsible for loss of weight. Lack of adequate fluid over time can cause a subtle and steady slip into hypovolemia. Dependence on others with lack of free access to fluids, altered thirst, and voluntary fluid restrictions for fear of incontinence or reliance on others

for toileting can precipitate inadequate intake. Exudative wounds, fever, or gastrointestinal losses can lead to negative fluid balance if not compensated. Hydration risks and symptoms are outlined in Box 5-1 on page 98.

Sadness and clinical depression are common causes of unintentional weight loss in both community-dwelling and long-term care older persons (Chapman, 2011). Social isolation, loneliness, and bereavement are associated with dietary inadequacy and weight loss (Ahmed & Haboubi, 2010). Medications used to treat depression can diminish appetite and cause xerostomia, leading to poor taste perception and difficulty swallowing. **Anorexia,** or lack of appetite, can be multifactorial. Polypharmacy is associated with undernutrition in part because many medications can cause a lack of appetite directly or from additional side effects, such as sedation (Stajkovic, Aitken, & Holroyd-Leduc, 2011). See Table 5-1 for specific medications contributing to anorexia.

Pain from arthritis or chronic disease can dull the appetite or cause nausea. Pain medications may have sedative or gastrointestinal side effects, which further curb intake. (See Chapter 9 ⟐ for a complete discussion of pain.)

Chronic diseases such as chronic obstructive pulmonary disease and congestive heart failure can contribute to anorexia. Shortness of breath can cause **aerophagia** while eating, a condition that results in bloating and early satiety from swallowing air. The physical effort of labored breathing can result in extreme fatigue with little energy left for the eating process. (See Chapter 24 ⟐.)

> *Practice Pearl* ▶▶▶ The nurse should discourage consumption of carbonated beverages, chewing gum, or use of straws in patients who complain of bloating, as these contribute to aerophagia.

Other chronic diseases or symptoms such as cancer, constipation or fecal impaction, and alcoholism can cause direct loss of appetite.

Difficulty swallowing, known as **dysphagia,** can result from difficulty chewing or swallowing or both. Chewing difficulties contribute to declining intake and risk of aspiration. Poor oral health, loose or missing teeth, ill-fitting dentures, and xerostomia can make the eating process uncomfortable, time consuming, and difficult. Generic texture-modified diets, often offered to those with chewing difficulties, are sometimes visually unattractive and can reduce interest in eating. (See Chapter 20 ⟐ for more information on the gastrointestinal system.)

> *Practice Pearl* ▶▶▶ Modification in diet texture runs along a continuum. For example, some older persons may be able to enjoy an apple if it is peeled and cut versus the usual applesauce. Texture-modified diets should be individualized. Collaborating with the registered dietitian (and speech pathologist if dysphagia is an issue) can often yield a more acceptable version of these diets.

Swallowing difficulties pose an immediate risk of aspiration and contribute to overall altered intake of both fluid and food. Pneumonia can result, especially if silent aspiration is occurring in those with insufficient coughing or cognitive impairment (Wieseke, Bantz, Siktberg et al., 2008). Dysphagia can occur as a result of neurologic disease or events such as Parkinson disease, multiple sclerosis, stroke, gastroesophageal reflux, cognitive impairment, esophageal motility disorders, cancer, and medications. Box 5-7 outlines symptoms to monitor for dysphagia. Presence or absence of a gag reflex is not a definitive screening tool for aspiration

> **BOX 5-7** ⟩ **Symptoms of Dysphagia**
>
> - Noticeable difficulty swallowing
> - Coughing or throat-clearing while eating or during swallowing process
> - Complaint of food sticking or chest pain with swallow
> - Multiple attempts to swallow single mouthful
> - Pocketing food along gum line
> - Inability to retain liquid bolus in mouth
> - Drooling
> - Voice changes
> - History of pneumonia or upper respiratory infections
> - Unexplained weight loss or dehydration

risk or dysphagia. Close observation for symptomatology and subsequent referral for clinical evaluation by a speech-language pathologist and a videofluoroscopic swallowing study or barium study are the recommended actions. Several bedside screening tools exist for nurses and other clinicians to assist with assessing symptoms (Wieseke et al., 2008).

Dependency on others for feeding or eating-related activities is associated with a risk of undernutrition. Much attention is being given to reports outlining poor feeding practices in long-term care. Inadequate length of time spent feeding patients, poor positioning, lack of social interaction with the feeding assistant, and inadequate supervision have been faulted. Although it has been shown that older persons consume meals more slowly than younger adults, study findings have reported as little as 5 minutes per meal is spent feeding residents while closer to 40 minutes is needed to provide feeding assistance (Simmons et al., 2008). Lack of free access to fluid and food between meals adds to the risk of those who are dependent on others.

Cognitive impairment is associated with unintentional weight loss. In addition to issues surrounding feeding dependency, cognitive impairment can impede the eating process. Cognitively impaired elders exhibit diminished ability to recognize food, failure to respond to hunger cues, difficulty with chewing and swallowing, and behavioral issues such as agitation contributing to declining intake. Feeding people with cognitive impairments can present unique challenges to caregivers, because it is often difficult to interpret aversive behaviors like clamping shut the mouth, expelling food, or turning the head. This can be interpreted as a desire to stop eating, but can also be dislike of the food, its temperature, or texture, or failure to recognize the eating process. A distracting environment, including too many foods on the plate, can also contribute to aversive behaviors during eating. Caregivers are faced with the dilemma of interpreting these behaviors and may feel burdened with feeding (Chang & Roberts, 2008). Poor eating manners such as drooling and expulsion of food can make the social dining experience unpleasant for others and lead to further social isolation of this population (Aselage, 2010). (See Chapter 22 ⬭.)

Sensory changes can make eating less pleasurable and lead to poor intake. Poorly lighted dining areas and busy patterns on dishes make seeing the meal harder for those with poor vision. Hearing problems can remove the pleasure from social dining. Taste and smell changes occur with age, medications, and chronic disease. Full dentures obscure the soft palate, affecting taste perception. Xerostomia, regardless of cause, contributes to reduced taste perception. Medications such as ACE inhibitors leave a metallic taste in the mouth. Olfactory changes further contribute to taste changes as the two senses are intertwined.

Improper diets can lead to diminished intake. Older persons in long-term care may be served unfamiliar foods after a lifetime of eating culturally familiar foods. Lack of food preferences and unpalatable textures can lead to lack of interest in eating.

Overzealous use of therapeutic diets may serve no clinical benefit if they are not eaten. Nursing home patients with evidence of malnutrition should have the risks and benefits of any proposed therapeutic diet assessed. Long-term care residents should be on liberalized diets unless deemed medically contraindicated following an individual assessment (ADA, 2010c).

Poverty and food insecurity can lead to poor nutritional health because of diminished intake. Lack of sufficient funds can result in both poor-quality food intake as well as limited quantity. Food insecurity issues arise from lack of financial resources, but also from lack of access to adequate food because of mobility or transportation issues. All of these factors can cause a decline in dietary intake.

Iatrogenic Practices Iatrogenic practices can put an individual at risk for undernutrition. Polypharmacy and improper feeding practices are considered iatrogenic in nature. Other contributors include prolonged nothing-by-mouth (NPO) status, reliance on clear liquid diet or routine intravenous fluids for nutrition, and improper recording of consumption.

Poor documentation of diminished intake has been observed in long-term care. Studies have noted that caregivers regularly overestimate documented consumption, with larger errors occurring with delayed reporting (Simmons, 2007). Subjective judgment as to what constitutes adequate intake and the perception that the amount a resident eats is indicative of caregiver job performance are theorized as reasons for the overestimation. Nutritional risk can be wrongly underestimated because of such errors.

Nutrient Losses Nutrient losses during absorption or metabolism can lead to undernutrition even with adequate dietary intake. Malabsorption from disease or its treatment can alter nutrient absorption. Inflammatory bowel disease, high-output ostomies, and radiation treatment to the abdominal area are such examples. Drugs, including alcohol, can alter nutrient status (see Table 5-1 on page 100 for drug and nutrient interactions).

Hypermetabolism Hypermetabolism warrants intake of increased energy and nutrients. When these increased needs are not met, undernutrition results. An older person with borderline nutritional status can easily be toppled into negative fuel balance by a hypermetabolic illness. Wounds, fever, infection, and fractures put difficult caloric and nutrient demands on an individual who may already be feeling and eating poorly. Cardiopulmonary disease can cause hypermetabolism due to the great physical effort of breathing when shortness of breath and diminished lung function occur. Tremors from neurologic disease such as Parkinson disease can increase metabolic rate due to increased physical movement.

Consequences of Unintentional Weight Loss and Undernutrition

Undernutrition is associated with poor clinical outcomes, including mortality. Hospitalized older persons or those in nursing homes with involuntary weight loss are at increased risk of mortality (Chapman, 2011). Malnutrition is associated with adverse outcomes such as poor wound healing, development of decubitus ulcers, skeletal muscle loss, functional decline, altered immune response, altered pharmacokinetics, longer length of hospital stay, and increased risk of institutionalization (Chapman, 2011; Stajkovic et al., 2011). Delayed wound healing in general occurs due to lack of nutritional substrates needed for each stage of tissue repair. Energy and protein deficits are often cited as limiting factors. Vitamins A and C and zinc have also been cited as necessary for wound closure (Kavalukas & Barbul, 2011). Altered immune response with increased susceptibility to infection puts the older person with malnutrition at further risk.

Low levels of plasma proteins that occur in malnutrition can alter drug metabolism. Low serum albumin can lead to decreased binding of certain drugs and resultant increased circulating free fraction of those medications. Polypharmacy can lead to multiple drugs competing for diminished protein binding sites and increase the likelihood of adverse drug reactions. Altered drug binding can go on to upset the balance of drugs at the cellular enzyme level. Over-the-counter and herbal medications are to be included in this effect.

Treatment of Unintentional Weight Loss and Undernutrition

It is intuitive to treat undernutrition and weight loss by targeting the cause. However, because almost 25% of all cases of weight loss in older persons occur for unknown reasons, targeting the symptoms is inherent in the overall treatment. This nonspecific and sometimes slowly occurring weight loss in the older person is often called "the dwindles."

Developing a nutritional care plan for an older person with undernutrition first requires a conversation with the individual or a proxy to determine the extent of personal wishes, quality-of-life issues, and advance directives before any aggressive interventions are begun.

Altering the quality of feeding assistance, the physical environment, and the food itself can encourage sufficient intake of fluid and food. Restrictive diets should be liberalized in long-term care unless an individual clinical assessment finds it contraindicated. Collaborating with the registered dietitian will help to optimize and individualize the nutritional care plan. Offending medications should be evaluated for alternatives and overall efficacy. Nutritional assessment laboratory values should be assessed, including folic acid and vitamin B_{12}. Appropriate referrals should be made for adaptive feeding equipment, financial assistance, swallowing evaluation, or psychosocial issues. See Box 5-8 for more specific treatment recommendations targeting causes and symptoms of undernutrition. Figure 5-5 ▶▶▶ is an important clinical algorithm for use in long-term care.

It is essential that caregivers in long-term care receive proper training on feeding assistance and documentation. See Box 5-8 for guidelines on proper positioning and assistance while feeding. Documentation of mealtime consumption will have improved accuracy if performed while actively observing what was eaten versus delayed documentation of intake. Training on interpretation of the MDS criteria for meal percentages is crucial.

Verbal prompting throughout the day has been shown to increase fluid intake by 78% in long-term care patients. Improvements in food and fluid intake have been demonstrated when fluid preferences were offered and verbal cueing and encouragement were provided (Chang & Roberts, 2008; Simmons, 2007). Increasing the volume of fluid given with each medication pass and snack is also beneficial.

> **Practice Pearl** ▶▶▶ Flagging the meal tray or door of long-term care patients at risk for dehydration can remind caregivers to provide extra prompting, and food service workers to leave unfinished beverages at the bedside, if safe to do so. Drinks can be provided in spillproof containers that can be left at the bedside. Cups should be of a size and weight that can be easily managed.

Social dining has been associated with an increase in dietary intake over dining alone (ADA, 2010a). Congregate meals in the community and family-style dining in long-term care provide older persons with opportunities for social interaction during a meal. Buffet-style dining offered to underweight nursing home residents was found to increase energy and protein intake when residents could self-select types and amounts of food (Desai, Winter, Young et al., 2007).

Alterations in the physical environment can benefit the older person with dementia. Music has been reported as the most common intervention used to reduce agitated behavior and increase dietary intake (Watson & Green, 2006). Limiting the amount of food presented at one time and the use of finger foods are suggested. An optimized breakfast, lunch, and early snacks should be offered to the older person with dementia who experiences sundowning and may eat poorly later in the day.

> **Practice Pearl** ▶▶▶ Some older persons with cognitive impairment may not recognize mealtime or the eating process and can benefit from cueing throughout the meal. Statements such as "Here is your soup and the spoon to eat it with" can help.

More aggressive intervention is indicated when other methods of improving nutritional status do not result in improvements. Such interventions should be in keeping with healthcare wishes and advance directives. Use of medications to promote weight gain is one consideration. Some medications used to treat depression may also lead to weight gain. Orexigenic medications, such as megestrol acetate, are sometimes considered, but negative side effects exist and scientific evidence of the efficacy in older adults is limited (Stajkovic et al., 2011).

Commercial oral supplements have been prescribed to boost intake with mixed results. Some studies have found that between-meal supplementation helps to increase overall intake while others have found that supplements simply replace food intake. Appropriate use of oral supplements as between-meal snacks has been demonstrated to improve nutrition status in underweight older adults (Hanson, Ersek, Gilliam et al., 2011; Silver, 2008).

> **Practice Pearl** ▶▶▶ Supplements should be liquid and not solid and should be given more than an hour before meals to minimize satiety. Providing a 4-oz serving of liquid supplement instead of other fluids with four medication passes each day can provide almost 500 kcal.

Nutritional supplementation and strength training are each recommended as components of treating unintentional weight loss in the older adult (Stajkovic et al., 2011). Progressive resistance training is specifically associated with slowing or reversing the loss of muscle mass and improved strength (Rolland et al., 2011).

BOX 5-8 **Nutritional Interventions for Undernutrition**

Enhanced Eating Environment

- Improve lighting
- Use plain dishes for those with poor vision
- Play familiar music from older adults' youth
- Encourage social dining
- Use attractive place settings
- Minimize distractions, medical trappings

Improved Taste Perception

- Avoid smoking
- Evaluate medication
- Add flavor enhancers to food
- Make changes in texture to increase appeal
- Optimize pleasant aromas

Increase Nutrient-Dense Intake

- Liberalize restrictive diets if indicated
- Offer juices, milk, shakes vs. water as fluid
- Add nonfat milk powder to soup, pudding, scrambled eggs, recipes for extra protein, nutrients
- Offer liquid supplements > 1 hour from meals
- Add sauces, butter, gravy to foods
- Serve desserts made with eggs/milk

ensure between meals

Saliva Stimulation for Xerostomia

- Medication assessment for contributors
- Use sugar-free candy and gum
- Encourage use of artificial saliva substitute
- Serve fluids with meals
- Add sauces, butter, gravy to foods
- Avoid overly hot or dry foods
- Maintain adequate hydration
- Optimize pleasant aromas

noalcohol-based mouthwash

Hydration

- Offer fluids frequently
- Provide regular prompting to drink
- Assess fluid preferences and provide preferred beverage choices
- Do not wait for report of thirst to offer fluid

- Calculate a daily fluid intake goal
- Provide cups that are easily handled

Alterations for Chewing Difficulty

- Dental consult if indicated
- Texture modification—individualize
- Find alternatives within food groups that are better tolerated (meat is hard to chew but tuna, eggs, hummus, beans, fish are easier to chew)
- Improve visual appeal of puree diet
- Do not mix puree diets into mush on plate when assisting with feeding
- Use attractive sauces, garnishes, molds

Improved Feeding Assistance

- Adequate unhurried time essential; include social interaction
- Proper posture: head and torso at 90-degree angle to lap
- Avoid head position tipped forward or back
- Avoid mixing foods together
- Encourage and assist with self-feeding where able
- Offer finger foods where appropriate
- Avoid straws if aspiration risk
- For cognitively impaired:
  - Minimize amount of foods on plate at once
  - Remind to swallow/brush cheek gently
  - Play music to ease agitation

Dysphagia Safety

- Clinical evaluation
- Gentle cough after each swallow
- Compensatory movements if prescribed
- Appropriately thinned or thickened foods
- Thin liquids or hard/dry/sticky foods only if prescribed since high aspiration risk
- Remain upright after meals

Alterations for Chewing Difficulty

- Cue throughout meal
- Match appropriate utensil with each food introduced

osteoporsis - to prevent do reg exercise

Alternative feeding routes can be considered when oral intake and supplementation fail following an earnest attempt at improving nutritional status via those routes. A nasogastric tube may be used for short-term feeding. A more permanent tube, such as a gastrostomy or jejunostomy tube, may be used for long-term feeding. Commercial enteral formulas provide between 1 cal and 2 kcal per milliliter. Most formulas that are 1 cal/mL are isotonic in nature, minimizing the osmotic draw of fluid into the gastrointestinal tract during feeding. Formulas with more than 1 cal/mL are generally hypertonic and need to be initiated at a dilute strength to minimize diarrhea. Full-strength delivery of these hypertonic

FOR NURSING STAFF AND DIETARY STAFF AND DIETITIANS (EVALUATE, DOCUMENT AND TREAT)

*The American Dietetic Association supports the Clinical Guide to Prevent and Manage Malnutrition in Long-Term Care.
Representatives from the American Dietetic Association were instrumental in its development.*

*These Guidelines were developed by the Council for Nutrition convened by Programs in Medicine under a grant
from Bristol-Myers Squibb. A special committee of The Gerontological Society of America (GSA) served as critical
reviewers and provided input and modification of the final Guidelines. While GSA does not endorse specific clinical
measures, we support the principles underlying these Guidelines and their potential to improve nutrition in the nursing home.*

Council for Nutrition

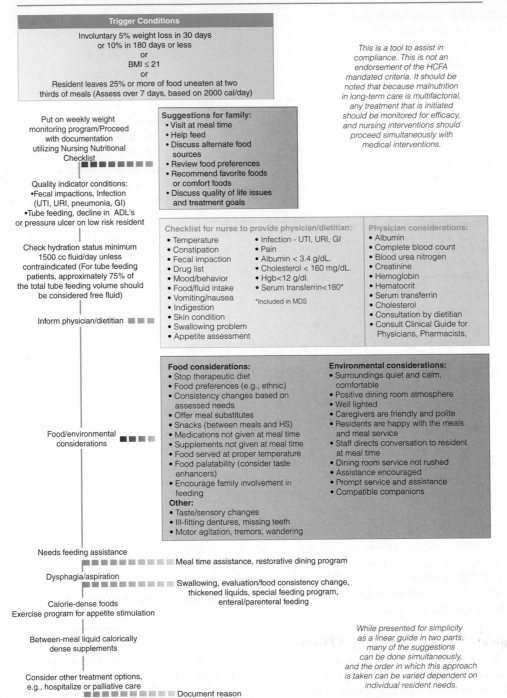

Trigger Conditions

Involuntary 5% weight loss in 30 days
or 10% in 180 days or less
or
BMI ≤ 21
or
Resident leaves 25% or more of food uneaten at two
thirds of meals (Assess over 7 days, based on 2000 cal/day)

*This is a tool to assist in
compliance. This is not an
endorsement of the HCFA
mandated criteria. It should be
noted that because malnutrition
in long-term care is multifactorial,
any treatment that is initiated
should be monitored for efficacy,
and nursing interventions should
proceed simultaneously with
medical interventions.*

Put on weekly weight
monitoring program/Proceed
with documentation
utilizing Nursing Nutritional
Checklist

Suggestions for family:
• Visit at meal time
• Help feed
• Discuss alternate food
  sources
• Review food preferences
• Recommend favorite foods
  or comfort foods
• Discuss quality of life issues
  and treatment goals

Quality indicator conditions:
•Fecal impactions, Infection
(UTI, URI, pneumonia, GI)
•Tube feeding, decline in ADL's
or pressure ulcer on low risk resident

Check hydration status minimum
1500 cc fluid/day unless
contraindicated (For tube feeding
patients, approximately 75% of
the total tube feeding volume should
be considered free fluid)

Checklist for nurse to provide physician/dietitian:
• Temperature
• Constipation
• Fecal impaction
• Drug list
• Mood/behavior
• Food/fluid intake
• Vomiting/nausea
• Indigestion
• Skin condition
• Swallowing problem
• Appetite assessment

• Infection - UTI, URI, GI
• Pain
• Albumin < 3.4 g/dL.
• Cholesterol < 160 mg/dL.
• Hgb<12 g/dl.
• Serum transferrin<180*

*Included in MDS

Physician considerations:
• Albumin
• Complete blood count
• Blood urea nitrogen
• Creatinine
• Hemoglobin
• Hematocrit
• Serum transferrin
• Cholesterol
• Consultation by dietitian
• Consult Clinical Guide for
  Physicians, Pharmacists,

Inform physician/dietitian

Food considerations:
• Stop therapeutic diet
• Food preferences (e.g., ethnic)
• Consistency changes based on
  assessed needs
• Offer meal substitutes
• Snacks (between meals and HS)
• Medications not given at meal time
• Supplements not given at meal time
• Food served at proper temperature
• Food palatability (consider taste
  enhancers)
• Encourage family involvement in
  feeding
Other:
• Taste/sensory changes
• Ill-fitting dentures, missing teeth
• Motor agitation, tremors, wandering

Environmental considerations:
• Surroundings quiet and calm,
  comfortable
• Positive dining room atmosphere
• Well lighted
• Caregivers are friendly and polite
• Residents are happy with the meals
  and meal service
• Staff directs conversation to resident
  at meal time
• Dining room service not rushed
• Assistance encouraged
• Prompt service and assistance
• Compatible companions

Food/environmental
considerations

Needs feeding assistance

Meal time assistance, restorative dining program

Dysphagia/aspiration

Swallowing, evaluation/food consistency change,
thickened liquids, special feeding program,
enteral/parenteral feeding

Calorie-dense foods
Exercise program for appetite stimulation

*While presented for simplicity
as a linear guide in two parts,
many of the suggestions
can be done simultaneously,
and the order in which this approach
is taken can be varied dependent on
individual resident needs.*

Between-meal liquid calorically
dense supplements

Consider other treatment options,
e.g., hospitalize or palliative care

Document reason

Figure 5-5 ▶▶▶ Clinical guide to prevent and manage malnutrition in long-term care.

Source: Thomas, D. R., et al. (2000). Nutrition management in long-term care: Development of a clinical strategy. *Journal of Gerontology: Medical Sciences, 55*(A), M725–M735,
by permission of Oxford University Press.

formulas is reached gradually. Hypertonic formulas contain less free water than do isotonic formulas, warranting close monitoring of hydration status. A registered dietitian will generally make an assessment and recommendation for appropriate formula type and volume. Cognitively intact older persons who are not at risk for aspiration can receive several small bolus feedings while sitting upright, amounting to prescribed volume over the day. Bolus feedings are contraindicated in others. Continuous drip-feeding with the head of the bed or chair upright at least at a 30- to 45-degree angle is necessary when there is risk of aspiration. These guidelines are for all types of feeding tubes because aspiration risk is not eliminated with temporary or permanent feeding tubes (Volkert et al., 2006). Feeding tubes should be flushed both before and after giving medications to avoid clogging the tube with precipitate. Smaller bore tubes, such as a jejunostomy tube, will become easily clogged from lack of flushing. Pharmacists can give guidance on suitability of medications for delivery through a feeding tube and recommendations for liquid versions when available. While flushing may take extra time, it will save time and patient comfort when tube replacement is avoided. Table 5-6 outlines nursing interventions for common problems with tube feedings.

The decision as to whether continued nutritional support will improve clinical outcome and quality of life in a terminally ill older person needs to include an assessment of all risks and benefits as well as the emotional, religious, cultural, and ethical considerations of the patient (Barrocas et al., 2010; Volkert et al., 2006). While use of tube feedings is beneficial in certain clinical situations, evidence in patients with advanced dementia suggests that tube feedings do not improve survival (Palecek et al., 2010). Increased risk of aspiration, gastrointestinal symptoms, discomfort, and other complaints are cited.

Medical Nutritional Therapy for Chronic Diseases

While liberalization of therapeutic diets is warranted for most older residents in long-term care, for some older persons a therapeutic diet is beneficial. Obesity in older persons can have functional and psychosocial consequences due to impaired mobility and the presence of comorbid conditions requiring intervention. The prevalence of weight concerns among older adults is increasing, with more than two thirds of those over age 60 years meeting criteria for overweight or obesity (Houston et al., 2009). While little evidence exists to recommend weight loss in the older adult based on weight alone, supervised weight loss can be beneficial for some older persons who are obese, though prognostic value is not equivalent to that seen in younger adults (Chapman, 2011). Those who may benefit from improved functional capacity with weight loss should have that benefit weighed against the risk of loss of muscle or bone that can accompany weight loss in this population already at risk for sarcopenia and osteoporosis (Houston et al., 2009). A registered dietitian should be consulted to provide nutritional education and to ensure preservation of nutritional status. Acceptable levels of appropriate physical activity should be incorporated to help preserve lean muscle mass and increase metabolic rate. Quick weight loss and dietary supplements for weight loss are contraindicated.

Nursing Diagnoses

The following nursing diagnoses are appropriate for use in patient care plans when problems relating to nutrition are encountered by the gerontological nurse. *Nurtrition, Imbalanced: Less Than Body Requirements* is appropriate when older persons do not consume enough calories to maintain their weight and are experiencing unintentional weight loss; are diagnosed with a malabsorption syndrome; are experiencing dysphagia or lower intestinal motility problems; or are lethargic or have a decreased level of consciousness. *Nurtrition, Imbalanced: More Than Body Requirements* is appropriate when older persons ingest more calories per day than needed or are unable to exercise and therefore experience weight gain. Older persons may also be diagnosed with *Knowledge, Deficient* related to diet when they make poor nutritional choices based on lack of education, cognitive impairment, or following fad diets or using dangerous weight loss products. *Noncompliance* to diet may be used when the older person is prescribed a therapeutic diet (e.g., low fat, 2 g sodium) and chooses not to follow recommendations

QSEN Recommendations Related to Nutrition

The Quality and Safety Education for Nurses (QSEN) project addresses the challenge of preparing future nurses with the knowledge, skills, and attitudes (KSAs) to continuously improve the quality and safety of the healthcare systems in which they work (Cronenwett et al., 2007). See the QSEN table on pages 121–122 for tips on meeting QSEN standards.

Patient and Family Teaching

Gerontological nurses require skills and knowledge related to teaching patients and families about the key concepts of gerontology and gerontological nursing. The guidelines in the following feature will assist the nurse to assume the role of teacher and coach.

TABLE 5-6	Nursing Interventions With Enteral Nutritional Support
Problem List	**Intervention**
Potential for Foodborne Illness	• Wash hands before handling formula and equipment. • Wipe off top of formula container before opening. • Label, cover, and store open formula in refrigerator for no more than 24 hours.
Aspiration	• Check for gastric residuals q4h. Hold for residual greater than ~100–150 mL and notify physician. • Ensure head of bed is elevated at least 30 degrees. • Avoid bolus feedings. • Consider smaller bore tube if nasally intubated. • Consider longer tube to reach duodenum or jejunum, if indicated. • Consider permanent feeding tube if on long-term feeding.

Clogged Tube	• Administer feeding with pump vs. gravity drip.
	• Administer room-temperature feeding. High-temperature storage or heating of formula will cause protein content to coagulate.
	• Follow guidelines for medication administration.
	  1. Flush tube with 20–30 mL water before, between, and after each single medication.
	  2. Consult pharmacist re: suitability of crushing medication with a small amount of water and availability of liquid versions of medications.
	  3. *Note: If using longer feeding tubes, ensure medication absorption site is not bypassed by tube.*

Diarrhea	• Administer feeding at room temperature. Cold feeding may cause increased gut peristalsis. • Consider lactose-free formula. • Consider medications that can cause diarrhea: antibiotics, magnesium, potassium, and digoxin, among others. • Administer continuous drip vs. bolus. • Consider temporarily altering formula concentration or rate of delivery: consult registered dietitian. • Consider medical causes.
Constipation	• Consider formula with added fiber. • Monitor hydration. Ensure adequate intake. • Encourage ambulation as indicated. • Assess for contributing medications, such as narcotics and some antacids among others. • Consider obstruction/medical causes.
Dehydration	• Monitor hydration. • Ensure adequate free water intake. • Need 1,500 mL minimum with 1 kcal/mL. • Most formulas are 50%–75% free water (high calorie/protein formulas have less free water than 1 cal/mL formula).

Meeting QSEN Standards: Nutrition

	KNOWLEDGE	SKILLS	ATTITUDES
Patient-Centered Care	Involvement of patient and family in the nutritional regimen is crucial.	Provide individual and cultural assessment of food preferences.	Appreciate uniqueness of each patient/family.
	Examine barriers to achieving nutritional goals.	Evaluate for depression, swallowing, dentition, vision/hearing, cognitive status.	Provide patient-centered care to improve successful nursing outcomes.
Teamwork and Collaboration	Recognize need for input from interdisciplinary team members including dietitian, pharmacist, physician, advanced practice nurses, and others on the team to reduce risk of adverse effects related to impaired nutrition and identify nutritional risks related to medication side effects.	Use leadership skills to coordinate team and share knowledge.	Value the contribution of each member of the team to improve outcomes.
	Be aware of organizational problems that can inhibit effective team functioning and establish plan for communication.	System assessment skills	Be open to input from team members on effective means to improve communication and collaboration.
Evidence-Based Practice	Describe effective interventions to decrease risk factors and improve overall health and function. Implement national nutritional guidelines and recommendations.	Access current evidence-based protocols to guide interventions.	Possess confidence in necessary skills to evaluate and incorporate nursing interventions from the literature.
Quality Improvement	Recognize the need for patient–family education regarding early recognition of impaired nutritional intake.	Skills in data management, technology, and U.S. government and ADA sites describing current dietary recommendations	Value the use of data and outcomes as a key component of QI efforts.

(continued)

Meeting QSEN Standards: Nutrition   *(continued)*

	KNOWLEDGE	SKILLS	ATTITUDES
Safety	Describe common problems that increase the likelihood of aspiration, protein calorie malnutrition, and excessive weight loss/gain.	Use appropriate strategies to provide written information to compensate for cognitive and sensory impairments (if any).	Appreciate the impact of cognitive and sensory impairments on the occurrence of nutritional problems.
Informatics	Provide input into the formation and maintenance of patient databases needed for gathering QSEN data and providing patient care.	Utilize the electronic health record.	Protect patient confidentiality according to HIPAA standards.

Patient–Family Teaching Guidelines

The following are guidelines that the nurse may find useful when instructing older persons and their families about dietary supplements (adapted from NIH, 2006).

CULTURAL COMPETENCE

1 Do I need a dietary supplement?

Dietary supplements can consist of vitamins, minerals, fiber, herbs, hormones, or a variety of other substances. While it is generally accepted that taking a multivitamin daily is a good idea, great controversy exists surrounding the use of other supplements. Many supplement manufacturers promise that their product will keep you young, make you feel better, and help you live longer. Because the FDA does not test or regulate these supplements, there is little evidence to back up these claims. In fact, some of these supplements can hurt you. Your best bet is to talk to your doctor, your nurse, or a dietitian about supplements if you are considering taking one.

RATIONALE:

Some older people think that supplements sold over the counter are safe and effective; however, many supplements can be dangerous and interact with prescription medications. It is always a good idea to consult with the physician, pharmacist, or dietitian about supplements. At best, they are harmless and a waste of money. At worst, they can be harmful and cause problems.

2 What about vitamins and minerals?

Vitamins and minerals are nutrients found naturally in food. The best way to get vitamins and minerals is by eating a balanced diet, not by taking supplements. Try to eat a variety of foods including meats, fruits, whole grains, and vegetables daily. Avoid foods that are low in fiber and high in fat and added sugar. If you occasionally skip meals or do not always eat right, taking a multivitamin may be a good choice for you. Remember:

- A regular multivitamin will do. It does not have to be a "senior" formula.
- Do not "megadose" (take large quantities of) any vitamin or mineral supplement.
- Generally, store or generic brands are fine and equivalent to more expensive preparations.

RATIONALE:

Some older people think if a little is good, then a lot is better. The nurse should urge older patients to eat well

(continued)

Patient–Family Teaching Guidelines *(continued)*

and enjoy the nutritious foods they consume daily. Taking large doses can be harmful depending on the patient's age, health, and dose. Some vitamins are stored and can reach toxic levels. Others are excreted in the urine and are a waste of money.

3 **What vitamins does my body need now that I am older?**

Depending on your age and level of health, you should take the following amounts of vitamins from food and supplements if needed:

- Vitamin B_{12}—2.4 mcg. Some foods, like cereal, are fortified with B_{12}, but many older people cannot absorb the B vitamins from food.

- Calcium—1,200 mg. As you age, you need more calcium to keep your bones strong. Vitamin D helps calcium to be absorbed, so look for a calcium preparation with this vitamin.

- Vitamin D—600 IU daily up to age 70 and 800 IU daily after age 70.

- Iron—up to 8 mg daily. Normally older people do not lose blood (as do menstruating women) but if you are recovering from surgery or you are a blood donor, be sure to eat foods high in iron or take a supplement. Be careful; it can be constipating.

- Vitamin B_6—1.7 mg for men and 1.5 mg for women. Found in some whole-grain products and fortified cereals.

RATIONALE:

Some older people may not eat well for a variety of reasons. They may have problems chewing whole-grain foods or fresh fruits and vegetables; they may buy prepackaged foods that have little nutritional value; they may have financial problems that limit their choices. The nurse should urge a balanced healthy diet that is acceptable to the older patient and the family. Older persons should use supplements as needed.

4 **How about herbal supplements?**

You may have heard of ginkgo biloba, ginseng, echinacea, ephedra, St. John's wort, and black cohosh. These are herbal supplements that are harvested from certain foods and plants.

Their ingredients will have some effect on your body, and they may interfere with medications you have been prescribed. Some herbal supplements can also cause serious side effects such as high blood pressure, nausea, diarrhea, constipation, fainting, headaches, seizures, heart attack, or even stroke. Play it safe. Check it out with your healthcare provider before you take any herbal supplement.

RATIONALE:

The safety and effectiveness of most herbals has not been documented by the FDA. Some herbals may be effective and others are not. The nurse should urge patients to consult with clinicians knowledgeable about herbal supplements to avoid problems.

5 **What is best for me if I am considering taking a dietary supplement?**

If you are thinking of taking an herbal supplement for any reason, consider this advice:

- Talk to your doctor, nurse, pharmacist, or dietitian. Do not believe the manufacturer's claims. Be cautious and careful.

- Use only the supplement recommended by your healthcare professional. Treat it as you would a prescription medication with careful dosing and monitoring for effect and side effects.

- If you decide to stop taking a supplement your doctor has recommended, make sure to let him or her know.

- Learn as much as you can about the supplement before taking it. Buy only from a reputable buyer. Avoid products sold over the Internet.

- If you are not sure, ask questions. Be an informed consumer.

RATIONALE:

Urging older patients to treat herbal supplements as they would prescription medications will underscore the seriousness and importance of safety and caution. Consult the Office of Dietary Supplements, National Institutes of Health, website for information and stay informed.

CARE PLAN   A Patient With Alterations in Nutrition

Case Study

Mrs. McGillicuddy is a 78-year-old woman admitted 2 weeks ago to a nursing home following a complicated hospital stay for a cerebrovascular accident. While hospitalized, she lost 10 lbs in 1 month and developed a stage II decubitus ulcer. Her prior medical history was significant for hypertension managed with an ACE inhibitor and low-sodium diet.

On admission to the nursing home, she was found to weigh 115 lbs and reported a height of 5'5". Her albumin was 3.0 mg/dL and complete blood cell count was normal. Physical examination revealed residual right-sided weakness. Mrs. McGillicuddy reported that she had been feeding herself in the hospital and felt she could manage. A therapeutic 2-g low-sodium diet was ordered.

Now, 2 weeks later, it is discovered that she has lost another 4 lbs. Her urine is dark in color and a mouth examination reveals dry mucosa and long tongue furrows. Pocketed food was noted along the gum line as well.

Mrs. McGillicuddy's roommate has noticed that she now sounds "gravelly." Her decubitus ulcer is reportedly unchanged.

Upon further discussion with Mrs. McGillicuddy, it becomes apparent that she has been having difficulty with self-feeding and managing the utensils. Frequently, she spills food from the spoon or fork and feels embarrassed about this. She is experiencing particular trouble drinking liquids. It is difficult to hold the cup handle, and liquids seem to be spilling out of her mouth. This embarrasses her as well. Lately, she has just been moving the foods around on her plate to make it look like she has eaten. Her nursing care assistant has been recording her intake due to the report of weight loss on admission. The medical chart reports that 75% to 90% of food was eaten at most meals.

Mrs. McGillicuddy also reports that the food tastes too bland and she often has a bad taste in her mouth that reduces her appetite.

Applying the Nursing Process

Assessment

The nurse should think broadly and assess a variety of factors, including the following:

- **Physical.** Assess for signs or symptoms of dehydration—tongue furrows, dry oral mucosa; dysphagia symptoms—drooling, food pocketing, voice alterations, coughing during swallowing or afterwards. Reassess decubitus ulcer stage.

- **Diet.** Assess appetite; observe self-feeding and dietary intake, especially of calories and protein; note food textures that are difficult to swallow.
- **Laboratory.** Assess plasma levels for blood urea nitrogen, creatine, and sodium, and urine for sedimentation rate.

Diagnosis

Appropriate nursing diagnoses for Mrs. McGillicuddy may include the following:

- *Nutrition, Imbalanced: Less Than Body Requirements* related to increased need for nutrition with hypermetabolic state (decubitus ulcer) and decreased intake

- *Fluid Volume: Deficient*
- *Aspiration, Risk for*
- *Swallowing, Impaired*

NANDA-I © 2012.

CARE PLAN **A Patient With Alterations in Nutrition** (continued)

Expected Outcomes

Expected outcomes for Mrs. McGillicuddy may include the following:

- Resident should safely consume adequate nutrients and fluid (consumes more than 75% of meal served at most meals) without aspiration.
- Decubitus ulcer should not increase in size and preferably reduce to stage I.

- Resident should report feeling improved self-feeding confidence.
- Resident's weight, hydration, and swallowing function should improve gradually without occurrence of adverse events.

Planning and Implementation

The following nursing interventions may be appropriate for Mrs. McGillicuddy:

- Consult to speech language pathologist for possible dysphagia as evidenced by symptoms of hoarse voice, inability to maintain a fluid bolus in the mouth, and food pocketing.
- Consult to occupational therapy for adaptive feeding equipment if indicated.
- Nutritional consult to coordinate swallowing recommendations and ensure nutritional needs are met by inclusion of appropriate foods. Resident food preferences as allowed.
- Consideration of an oral nutritional supplement if deemed safe for swallowing—may need texture alteration of supplement. Supplement must be given more than 60 minutes before meal.

- Consideration of a feeding tube if unable to consume adequate nutrition by mouth.
- Multivitamin and mineral supplement for adequate vitamins and minerals for wound healing.
- Adequate hydration—once swallowing consult indicates safety, put resident on fluid prompting program. Use adaptive cup to facilitate intake.
- Liberalization of low-sodium diet to improve intake.
- Medical and pharmacy evaluation of use of ACE inhibitor, which may be contributing to dry mouth, metallic taste residue and lack of taste perception of food, and difficulty swallowing.
- Reinforce nursing assistant training on recording accurate dietary intake.

Evaluation

The nurse hopes to work with Mrs. McGillicuddy over time and involve the interdisciplinary team in the plan of care. The nurse will consider the plan a success based on the following criteria:

- Mrs. McGillicuddy will stop losing weight and eventually begin to gain weight.

- Her decubitus ulcer will begin to heal.
- She will report increased satisfaction with the taste and quality of the food served.
- She will have improved oral hygiene and hydration.

Ethical Dilemma

After several days, Mrs. McGillicuddy tells the nurse in confidence that there are several reasons why she thinks she is losing weight:

- She is feeling sad and has no desire to eat.
- The food tastes awful and is very unappealing to her.

- She does not want to "bother" the nurses by asking for additional help with her meals.

The nurse informs Mrs. McGillicuddy that these feelings are commonly reported, and many can be addressed or remedied. Mrs. McGillicuddy asks that the nurse not tell

(continued)

CARE PLAN   **A Patient With Alterations in Nutrition** *(continued)*

anyone of their conversation. The nurse weighs the patient's request for privacy with the professional responsibility to assist the patient in her recovery. The nurse decides to consult with the physician and dietitian to see if Mrs. McGillicuddy can be placed on a regular, no-salt-added diet. This may make the food more appealing to her. Additionally, the nurse makes a note on the nursing care plan that the patient may not ask for assistance with meals but should be frequently observed to see if she needs assistance. Alerting others may alleviate some

of Mrs. McGillicuddy's feelings of dependency as she will not have to ask for help cutting her meat, opening milk containers, and so on. Finally, the nurse urges the patient to talk with a social work colleague so that she can discuss her recovery in general. Since Mrs. McGillicuddy is not suicidal, there is no need for immediate referral with violation of her right to privacy. A skilled social worker will determine the cause of her sadness and begin counseling her with referral to a geropsychiatrist or a psychiatric-mental health nurse practitioner if necessary.

Critical Thinking and the Nursing Process

1. Identify five or more risk factors for undernutrition in the older person. Pick three risk factors and outline appropriate nursing interventions for each factor. Which intervention would be a priority if all three factors were present in one person?
2. An older person is homebound with severe arthritis. What nutritional and hydration concerns should the nurse have?
3. An older person with cognitive impairment is admitted to a nursing home from the hospital with reports of inadequate dietary intake. The physician is contemplating insertion of a feeding tube. You note that there

is no documentation in the hospital record on self- or hand-feeding. What nursing interventions might you consider before consideration of a feeding tube?
4. What are some possible nursing interventions for the long-term care resident at risk for dehydration?
5. An older person recently had multiple teeth extracted and now is wearing dentures. On a subsequent clinic visit you note weight loss. What other physical and nutritional findings should you assess that are related to the specific issue of the changes in dentition?

■ Evaluate your responses in Appendix B. ▭▭

Chapter Highlights

■ Physiological changes associated with aging can have negative effects on the nutritional status of the older person.

■ Older persons are at disproportionate risk for unintentional weight loss and malnutrition, especially those in the hospital and long-term care.

■ Nutritional screening and assessment should be an essential component of routine health care for the older person.

■ Prevention and treatment of malnutrition should focus on the common etiologies: insufficient intake, increased nutrient losses, and hypermetabolism.

■ Aggressive nutrition support in advanced disease states should be in accordance with the advance directives of the older patient and include a thorough evaluation of the risks, benefits, and ethical considerations.

■ Most long-term care residents do not need a strict therapeutic diet, but rather can be prescribed a liberalized version.

Pearson Nursing Student Resources
Find additional review materials at
nursing.pearsonhighered.com

Prepare for success with additional NCLEX®-style practice
questions, interactive assignments and activities, web links,
animations and videos, and more!

References

Aalto, M., Alho, H., Halme, J. T., & Seppa, K. (2011). The Alcohol Use Disorders Identification Test (AUDIT) and its derivatives in screening for heavy drinking among the elderly. *International Journal of Geriatric Psychiatry, 26,* 881–885.

Ahmed, T., & Haboubi, N. (2010). Assessment and management of nutrition in older people and its importance to health. *Clinical Interventions in Aging, 5,* 207–216.

American Dietetic Association (ADA). (2007). Position of the American Dietetic Association: Oral health and nutrition. *Journal of the American Dietetic Association, 107,* 1418–1428.

American Dietetic Association (ADA). (2010a). Position of the American Dietetic Association, American Society for Nutrition, and Society for Nutrition Education: Food and nutrition programs for community residing older adults. *Journal of the American Dietetic Association, 110,* 463–472.

American Dietetic Association (ADA). (2010b). Position of the American Dietetic Association: Food insecurity in the United States. *Journal of the American Dietetic Association, 110,* 1368–1377.

American Dietetic Association (ADA) (2010c). Position of the American Dietetic Association: Individualized approaches for older adults in health care communities. *Journal of the American Dietetic Association, 110,* 1549–1553.

Aselage, M. B. (2010). Measuring mealtime difficulties: Eating, feeding, and meal behaviours in older adults with dementia. *Journal of Clinical Nursing, 19,* 621–631.

Bailey, R. L., Gahche, J. J., Lentino, C. V., Dwyer, J. T., Engel, J. S., Thomas, P. R., Betz, J M., Sempos, C. T., & Picciano, M.F. (2011). Dietary supplement use in the United States, 2003–2006. *Journal of Nutrition, 141,* 261–266.

Barrocas, A.,Geppert, C., Durfee, S., Maillet, J., Monturo, C., Mueller, C., Stratton, K., & Valentine, C. A.S.P.E.N. Board of Directors (2010). A.S.P.E.N. ethics position paper. *Nutrition in Clinical Practice, 25,* 672–679.

Centers for Disease Control and Prevention. (2009). *Summary health statistics for U.S. adults: National Health Interview Survey,*

2009. Retrieved from http://www.cdc.gov/nchs/data/series/sr_10/sr10_249.pdf

Centers for Medicare and Medicaid Services. (2012). *Minimum data set manual, version 3.0.* Retrieved from https://www.cms.gov/Medicare/Quality-Initiatives-Patient-Assessment-Instruments/NursingHomeQualityInits/MDS30RAIManual.html

Chang, C. C., & Roberts, B. L. (2008). Feeding difficulty in older adults with dementia. *Journal of Clinical Nursing, 17,* 2266–2274.

Chapman, I. M. (2011). Weight loss in older persons. *Medical Clinics of North America, 95,* 579–593.

Chapman, I. M., MacIntosh, C. G., Morley, J. E., & Horowitz, M. (2002). The anorexia of aging. *Biogerontology, 3,* 67–71.

Chumlea, W. C., Roche, A. F., & Mukherjee, D. (1984). *Nutritional assessment of the elderly through anthropometry.* Columbus, OH: Ross Laboratories.

Cronenwett, L., Sherwood, G., Barnsteiner, J., Disch, J., Johnson, J., Mitchell, P., Sullivan, D., & Warren, J. (2007). Quality and safety education for nurses, *Nursing Outlook,* 55(3) 122–131

Desai, J., Winter, A., Young, K. W., & Greenwood, C. E. (2007). Changes in type of foodservice and dining room environment preferentially benefit institutionalized seniors with low body mass index. *Journal of the American Dietetic Association, 107,* 808–814.

Frank, P., & Crookes, P. F. (2010). Short- and long-term follow-up of the postbariatric surgery patient. *Gastroenterology Clinics of North America, 39,* 135–146.

Frisard, M. I., Fabre, J. M., Russell, R. D., King, C. M., Delaney, J. P., & Wood, R. H. (2007). Physical activity level and physical functionality in nonagenarians compared with individuals aged 60–74 years. *Journals of Gerontology Series A: Biological Sciences and Medical Sciences, 62,* 783–788.

Guigoz, Y. (2006). The Mini-Nutritional Assessment (MNA®) Review of the literature—what does it tell us? *The Journal of Nutrition Health and Aging, 10,* 466–487.

Hanson, L. C., Ersek, M., Gilliam, R., & Carey, T. S. (2011). Oral feeding options for people with dementia: A systematic review. *Journal of American Geriatric Society, 59,* 463–472.

Hartford Institute for Geriatric Nursing. (2008a). Depression: Nursing standard of practice protocol. Retrieved from http://consultgerirn.org/topics/depression/want_to_know_more

Hartford Institute for Geriatric Nursing. (2008b). Nutrition in the elderly: Nursing standard of practice protocol. Retrieved from http://consultgerirn.org/topics/nutrition_in_the_elderly/want_to_know_more

Hirani, V., Tabassum, F., Aresu, M., & Mindell, J. (2010). Development of new demi-span equations from a nationally representative sample of adults to estimate maximal adult height. *Journal of Nutrition, 140,* 1475–1480.

Houston, D. K., Nicklas, B. J., & Zizza, C. A. (2009). Weighty concerns: The growing prevalence of obesity among older adults. *Journal of the American Dietetic Association, 109,* 1886–1895.

Institute of Medicine, Food and Nutrition Board [IOM]. (1998). *Dietary reference intakes for thiamine, riboflavin, niacin, vitamin B-6, folate, vitamin B-12, pantothenic acid, biotin and choline.* Washington, DC: National Academy Press.

Institute of Medicine, Food and Nutrition Board [IOM]. (2000). *Dietary reference intakes for vitamin C, vitamin E, selenium and carotenoids.* Washington, DC: National Academy Press.

Institute of Medicine, Food and Nutrition Board [IOM]. (2002). *Dietary reference intakes for energy, carbohydrates, fiber, fat, protein and amino acids (macronutrients).* Washington, DC: National Academy Press.

Institute of Medicine, Food and Nutrition Board [IOM]. (2004). *Dietary reference intakes for water, potassium, sodium, chloride, and sulfate.* Washington, DC: National Academy Press.

Institute of Medicine, Food and Nutrition Board [IOM]. (2010). *Dietary reference intakes for calcium, phosphorus, magnesium, vitamin D and fluoride.* Washington, DC: National Academy Press.

Kaiser, M. J., Bauer, J. M., Ramsch, C., et al. (2009).*Validation of the mini nutritional assessment Short-Form (MNA®-SF): A practical tool for identification of nutritional status. The Journal of Nutrition Health and Aging, 13,* 782–788.

Kaiser, M. J., Bauer, J. M., Ramsch, C., Uter, W., Guigoz, Y., Cederholm, T.,Thomas, D., Anthony, P., Charlton, K., Maggio, M., Tsai, A., Ellis, B., & Sieber, C. C. (2010). Frequency of malnutrition in older adults: A multinational perspective using the mini nutritional assessment. *Journal of the American Geriatric Society, 58,* 1734–1738.

Kalyani, R. R., Stein, B., Valivil, R., Manno, R., Maynard, J. W., & Crews, D. C. (2010). Vitamin D treatment for the prevention of falls in older adults: Systematic review and meta-analysis. *Journal of the American Geriatric Society, 58,* 1299–1310.

Karpa, M. J., Gopinath, B., Rochtchina, E., Wang, J., Cumming, R. G., Sue, C. M., & Mitchell, P. (2010). Prevalence and neurodegenerative or other associations with olfactory impairment in an older community. (2010). *Journal of Aging and Health, 22,* 154–168.

Kavalukas, S. L., & Barbul, A. (2011). Nutrition and wound healing: An update. *Plastic and Reconstructive Surgery, 127,* 38S–43S.

Lichtenstein, A. H., Rasmussen, H., Yu, W. W., Epstein, S. R., & Russell, R. M. (2008). Modified MyPyramid for older adults. *Journal of Nutrition, 138,* 5–11.

Mangano, K. M., Walsh, S. J., Insogna, K. L., Kenny, A. M., & Kerstetter, J. E. (2011). Calcium intake in the United States from dietary and supplemental sources across adult age groups: New estimates from the National Health and Nutritional Examination Survey 2003–2006. *Journal of the American Dietetic Association, 111,* 687–695.

Mini Nutritional Assessment. (2009). *Tool and information on usage.* Retrieved from http://www.mna-elderly.com

Nahin, R. L., Pecha, M., Welmerink, D. B., Sink, K., DeKosky, S. T., & Fitzpatrick, A. L. (2009). Concomitant use of prescription drugs and dietary supplements in ambulatory elderly

people. *Journal of American Geriatric Society, 57,* 1197–1205.

National Institutes of Health, National Heart, Lung, and Blood Institute. (2006). *Your guide to lowering your blood pressure with DASH.* Retrieved from http://www.nhlbi.nih.gov/health/public/heart/hbp/dash/new_dash.pdf

Olson, J. H., Erie, J. C., & Bakri, S. J. (2011). Nutritional supplementation and age-related macular degeneration. *Seminars in Ophthalmology, 26,* 131–136.

Palecek, E. J., Teno, J. M., Casarett, D. J., Hanson, L. C., Rhodes, R. L., & Mitchell, S. L. (2010). Comfort feeding only: A proposal to bring clarity to decision-making regarding difficulty with eating for persons with advanced dementia. *Journal of the American Geriatric Society, 58,* 580–584.

Phillips, M. B., Foley, A. L., Barnard, R., Isenring, E. A., & Miller, M. D. (2010). Nutritional screening in community-dwelling older adults: A systematic literature review. *Asia Pacific Journal of Clinical Nutrition, 19,* 440–449.

Qato, D. M., Alexander, G. C., Conti, R. M., Johnson, M., Schumm, P., & Lindau, S. T. (2008). Use of prescription and over-the-counter medications and dietary supplements among older adults in the United States. *Journal of the American Medical Association, 24,* 2867–2878.

Rolland, Y., Dupuy, C., van Kan, G., Gillette, S., & Vellas, B. (2011). Treatment strategies for sarcopenia and frailty. *Medical Clinics of North America, 95,* 427–438.

Rubenstein L. Z., Harker, J. O., Salva, A., Guigoz, Y., Vellas, B. (2001). Screening for Undernutrition in Geriatric Practice: developing the short-form mini nutritional assessment (MNA-SF). *The Journals of Gerontology, 56A,* M366–377.

Segal, J., & Kemp, G. (2012). *Senior nutrition and diet tips.* Retrieved from http://helpguide.org/life/senior_nutrition.htm

Silver, H. J. (2008). Oral strategies to supplement older adults' dietary intakes: Comparing the evidence. *Nutrition Reviews, 67,* 21–31.

Simmons, S. F. (2007). Quality improvement for feeding assistance care in nursing homes.

Journal of the American Medical Directors Association, 8, S12–S18.

Simmons, S. F., Keeler, E., Zhuo, X., Hickey, K. A., Sato, H. W., & Schnelle, J. F. (2008). Prevention of unintentional weight loss in nursing home residents: A controlled trial of feeding assistance. *Journal of the American Geriatric Society, 56,* 1466–1473.

Snitz, B. E., O'Meara, E. S., Carlson, M. C., Arnold, A. M., Ives, D. G., Rapp, S. R., . . . DeKosky, S. T. (2009). *Ginkgo biloba* for preventing cognitive decline in older adults: A randomized trial. *Journal of the American Medical Association, 302,* 2663–2670.

Stajkovic, S., Aitken, E. M., & Holroyd-Leduc, J. (2011). Unintentional weight loss in older adults. *Canadian Medical Association Journal, 183,* 443–449.

Stover, P. J. (2010). Vitamin B-12 and older adults. *Current Opinion in Clinical Nutrition and Metabolic Care, 13,* 24–27.

Vellas, B., Villars, H., Abellan, G., et al. (2006). Overview of the MNA®—Its history and challenges. *The Journal of Nutrition Health and Aging, 10,* 456–465.

Volkert, D., Berner, Y. N., Berry, E., Cederholm, T., Bertrand, P. C., Milne, A., . . . Lochs, H. (2006). ESPEN guidelines on enteral nutrition: Geriatrics. *Clinical Nutrition, 25,* 330–360.

Von Haehling, S., Morley, J. E., & Anker, S. D. (2010). An overview of sarcopenia: Facts and numbers on prevalence and clinical impact. *Journal of Cachexia, Sarcopenia, Muscle, 1,* 129–133.

Watson, R., & Green, S. M. (2006). Feeding and dementia: A systematic literature review. *Journal of Advanced Nursing, 54,* 86–93.

Wieseke, A., Bantz, D., Siktberg, L., & Dillard, N. (2008). Assessment and early diagnosis of dysphagia. *Geriatric Nursing, 29,* 376–383.

Winslow, B. T., Onysko, M. K., Stob, C. M., & Hazlewood, K. A. (2011). Treatment of Alzheimer Disease. *American Family Physician, 83,* 1403–1412.

Witham, M. D., & Avenell, A. (2010). Interventions to achieve long-term weight loss in older people. *Age and Ageing, 39,* 176–184.

Pharmacology and Older Adults

Laurel A. Eisenhauer, RN, PhD, FAAN
PROFESSOR EMERITUS WILLIAM F. CONNELL SCHOOL OF NURSING AT BOSTON COLLEGE

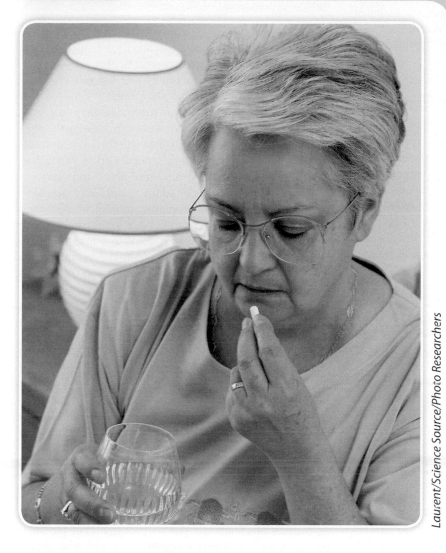

Laurent/Science Source/Photo Researchers

KEY TERMS

adverse drug events (ADEs) *132*
adverse drug experience *134*
adverse drug reactions (ADRs) *132*
chemical restraints *145*
first-pass effect drugs *131*
gradual dose reduction
    (GDR) *140*
iatrogenesis *132*
medication regimen
    review (MRR) *146*
over-the-counter (OTC)
    medication *134*
pharmacodynamics *131*
pharmacogenetics *130*
pharmacokinetics *131*
polypharmacy *140*

LEARNING OUTCOMES

On completion of this chapter, the reader will be able to:

1. Explain the interaction between normal aging and responses to drug therapy in older people.
2. Identify principles of safe medication management with older persons in a variety of patient care settings.
3. Discuss measures to prevent and reduce polypharmacy in older patients.
4. Describe assessments to monitor older patients for adverse drug effects and polypharmacy.

5. Apply principles of teaching and learning to promote compliance and adherence to the medication regimen.
6. List nonpharmacological therapies that may be useful as alternatives to medications.
7. Discuss issues related to ensuring the safe use of drug therapy by the older person.

The many advances in drug therapy and medical care have contributed to increased longevity and the promotion of greater health and well-being of adults. Reported estimates of the number of medications taken by older persons range from 8 to 13 (Farrell, Szeto, & Shamji, 2011). More than 40% of men and women older than age 65 take 5 or more medications per week; about 12% take 10 or more medications per week (Woodruff, 2010).

Drug therapy in the older person presents many challenges in ensuring the appropriate use of medications. Older persons have characteristics that affect the body's use of drugs; therefore, they are at greater risk for adverse drug events than are younger persons. Aging impacts the body's ability to handle and respond to medications. Chronic diseases and the multiple drugs used to treat them affect the physiological and adaptive responses of the older person. Psychosocial variables and cognitive changes may also affect the ability of older persons to manage their medications safely.

Adverse effects can be prevented to a great extent. The nurse is in a pivotal position to use nursing assessments and nursing interventions to promote the appropriate use of medications, to prevent or detect adverse drug events, and to prevent or reduce the need for drug therapy by the use of nursing interventions.

Even though many medications are used by older persons, their effects on older persons have not been studied extensively. Some drugs approved prior to 1989 were not studied in the older adult populations. Since 1989 the U.S. Food and Drug Administration (FDA) has required that applications for the approval of new drugs show that they have been studied in the populations in which they will be used. A section called *Geriatric Considerations* is now included in the packet inserts for new drugs. Although larger numbers of older people have been included in clinical trials, there is concern that those included have tended to be young-old persons (less than 75 years) and those with fewer medical problems who would be less likely to confound the study of a new drug. The young-old person, however, may not represent the old-old (85+ years of age) with multiple conditions and multiple drug therapies who are likely to receive the new drug after it has been approved by the FDA. However, chronological age alone is a poor indicator of how an older person will react to a medication. More appropriate predictors of medication response include the individual's general state of health, the number and types of other medications taken, liver and renal function, and presence of comorbidities or other diagnosed diseases.

Cultural Diversity and Medication Use

Cultural diversity and ethnic background can affect the older person's beliefs about health, illness, medications, and physiological response to medications.

Individuals from some cultures may use folk remedies and herbal preparations before they initiate treatment with prescription medications. Some may continue to use both types of treatments, sometimes without informing the physician. Delays in obtaining appropriate therapy can result in the older person beginning treatment later in the disease process, resulting in a more advanced illness trajectory.

In a study of urban older adults, Blacks were found to use complementary and alternative medicines more than whites. Hispanics were found to be more likely to choose herbal medications to self-treat colds and insomnia than whites or blacks. More Hispanics chose herbal treatments for insomnia rather than over-the-counter (nonprescription) or prescription medications (Cherniack et al., 2008).

Ethnic beliefs can also affect adherence to instructions to take medications as prescribed. For example, women from Islamic and African cultures who have vaginal yeast infections may prefer oral drugs rather than vaginally inserted medications due to cultural taboos restricting insertion of foreign bodies into the vagina. Asian patients tend to expect quick relief from symptoms yet are cautious about using American medicine; they may decrease dosages to avoid even minimal side effects (Grissinger, 2007). Some African Americans are distrustful of medicine and the healthcare system because of past history, for example, the Tuskegee Experiment in which African American men were not given treatment for syphilis as part of a research study.

Physiological response to medications may also depend on the race or ethnic and genetic background of the older person. A goal of **pharmacogenetics** research (how genetics affect the body's response to drugs) is to develop tests for genetic alterations in drug metabolism that can lead to prescribing of "personalized" medications. Such medications, with doses and targeted drugs unique to the individual's genetic makeup, may offer the opportunity for better initial therapeutic responses and decreases in many adverse effects. There are several drugs for which a person may be tested to determine if that person's genetic makeup would indicate the drug would be effective or ineffective or if it would cause an adverse effect. However, testing is quite expensive so it is not currently done on a routine basis. Some examples of drugs that may provide a genetics-based response are warfarin, clopidogrel, statins, tamoxifen, and vemurafenib.

Foods, herbal preparations, medications, alcohol, and tobacco can affect enzymes related to the metabolism of drugs. As immigrants change their lifestyle, their metabolic profile may change and could result in altered drug metabolism (Reyes, Van de Putte, Falcón et al., 2004). Religious practices related to fasting could interfere with drug absorption and schedules for taking medications (Grissinger, 2007).

See Chapter 4 ⊂⊃ for further information on the role of culture on illness, medications, and healing.

Pharmacokinetic Alterations in the Older Person

As people age, they become increasingly complex and develop their own patterns of physiological and psychosocial responses. Each older person's response to medications is unique.

Alterations in physiological function resulting from normal processes of aging must be carefully considered in prescribing, administering, and monitoring medications. Older persons tend to have acute and chronic conditions that may alter **pharmacokinetics** (what the body does to the drug) and **pharmacodynamics** (what the drug does to the body). The impact of the concurrent drug therapy to treat these conditions can also affect a person's response to other medications.

Aging affects the body's ability to handle drugs. This means that the recommended adult dose of many medications may need to be lowered for older adults. As individuals age, a variety of physiological changes affect pharmacokinetics and pharmacodynamics. Many of these changes do not result in clinically significant changes in fit older persons because they have sufficient renal and hepatic adaptability to respond. However, frail older persons with multiple pathological alterations in function are less able to respond effectively.

With aging, there is a decrease in body water (as much as 15%) and an increase in body fat. This could result in increased concentration of water-soluble drugs (e.g., alcohol) and more prolonged effects of fat-soluble drugs.

Hepatic blood flow may be decreased by as much as 50% in individuals over 65 years old. This could result in increased toxicity when they take usual doses of "first-pass effect" drugs because less of these drugs would be detoxified immediately by the liver. **First-pass effect drugs** are significantly metabolized when they first flow through the liver (first pass into the liver). Liver mass and overall metabolic activity decrease with aging but they are not usually clinically significant in relation to drug metabolism. The effect of aging on microsomal enzymes that regulate the rate of metabolism of drugs in the liver is believed to be minimal. Routine liver function tests, with the exception of a slight decrease in serum albumin, do not change significantly with age.

> **Practice Pearl** ▶▶▶ If a patient is receiving two or more drugs that are highly protein bound, the nurse should observe for drug interactions and variations in responses to each drug.

Decreases in serum albumin levels or binding capacity may result in increased serum levels of the "free" or unbound proportion of protein-bound drugs. This may result in toxic levels of highly bound drugs because more unbound drug is available to produce its effects. This is especially problematic in older patients with decreased liver or renal function.

> **Practice Pearl** ▶▶▶ Oral medications should be given with a nutritious liquid (e.g., juice) rather than water if a patient is anorexic or is likely to refuse to take adequate amounts of liquid. This maximizes the nutritional values of liquids ingested. (Do not use liquids that are contraindicated due to drug–food interactions.)

The kidneys excrete most drugs. Renal function generally decreases with age and thus should always be considered in the choice of a drug, in judging the appropriateness of a dose, and in evaluating adverse drug reactions. Estimates of decline in renal function based on aging vary. After age 30, creatinine clearance declines an average of 8 mL/min./1.73 m² each decade in about two thirds of people (Glassock & Winearls, 2009). However, individuals vary considerably in the degree of decline of renal function due to aging. Blood urea nitrogen (BUN) levels are poor indicators of renal function in the older person because of the decrease in muscle mass and other variables affecting BUN levels. Serum creatinine levels can be used to estimate creatinine clearance but are less reliable in older persons than in younger persons because older persons have less muscle mass, and creatinine is a product of muscle breakdown. A normal glomerular filtration rate (GFR) is considered to be equal to or greater than 90 mL/min/1.73 m². The FDA now requires that manufacturers provide dosing guidelines for patients with decreased creatinine clearance.

The formula usually used to calculate the GFR is that of Cockcroft and Gault (1976), which includes variables of age and lean weight and is adjusted for gender for women because of their having relatively less lean weight:

$$\text{creatinine clearance} = \frac{(140 - \text{age}) \times \text{lean wt (kg)}}{72 \times \text{serum creatinine}} \times 0.85 \text{ for women}$$

> **Practice Pearl ▶▶▶** Do not rely on BUN levels as an indicator of renal function in the older person. BUN is affected by muscle mass, level of hydration, diagnosis of anemia, and dietary intake of protein. Calculating the creatinine clearance using the formula above provides a more accurate assessment of how the drug will be metabolized and cleared by the kidneys.

Pharmacodynamic Alterations

Pharmacodynamic changes, which affect how the drug affects the body, can also occur because of the aging process. However, it is not always clear if changes in therapeutic responses are due to the pharmacodynamics or to the altered pharmacokinetics. Changes in pharmacodynamics in the older person may be due to decreases in the number of receptors, decreases in receptor binding, or altered cellular response to the drug–receptor interaction. An increased drug–receptor response can occur with benzodiazepines, opiates, and warfarin, resulting in increased sedation, increased analgesic effects and respiratory depression, and increased anticoagulation, respectively. The central nervous system, bladder, and heart tend to be more sensitive to medications with anticholinergic effects. (See later discussion of anticholinergic effects of medications.) In general, older adults have a decreased response to adrenergic agonists such as isoproterenol and an increased response to adrenergic blockers such as metoprolol (Hutchison & O'Brien, 2007).

> **Practice Pearl ▶▶▶** The general rule for drug prescription in the older person is "start low; go slow." For example, the drug should be prescribed at about one half the recommended adult dose, and the prescribing clinician should wait twice as long as recommended in the literature before increasing the dose. This tip will help to prevent toxic side effects and adverse drug reactions.

Concurrent Conditions and Drug Therapy

In addition to the alterations due to normal aging processes, older persons are more likely to have chronic pathological conditions that may affect responses to drugs. The older person is also more likely to be taking other drugs that may influence pharmacokinetics and pharmacodynamics. The increased emphasis on the use of drugs for prevention has also increased the use of medications in the absence of a pathological condition. Table 6-1 illustrates some of the alterations caused by the aging process, by pathological conditions, and by other concurrent drug therapy that may affect drug response in the older person.

> **Drug Alert ▶▶▶** Drugs that should be used with caution in older adults:
> - Drugs that are new to the market
> - Drugs with CNS effects
> - Drugs that are highly protein bound
> - Drugs that are eliminated by the kidneys
> - Drugs with a high first-pass effect
> - Drugs with a low therapeutic-to-toxicity ratio

Adverse Drug Reactions and Iatrogenesis

Adverse drug reactions (ADRs) are a particular problem in the older person. Almost 11% of hospital admissions of older adults are associated with adverse drug reactions (Kongkaew et al., 2008). Budnitz, Lovegrove, Shehab, and Richards (2011) found that four medications (warfarin, insulins, antiplatelet agents, and oral hypoglycemic agents) accounted for 67% of older adults' emergency hospitalizations for adverse drug events.

Older persons are more likely to have ADRs because of an inappropriate drug or dosing regimen, drug–drug interactions, **polypharmacy** (the prescription, administration, or use of more medications than are clinically indicated in a given patient), and nonadherence. **Adverse drug events (ADEs)** are injuries resulting from the use of a drug. **Iatrogenesis** refers to harm from a therapeutic regimen. Iatrogenic risks and ADRs from drug therapy are related to age, the number of drugs taken, and the complexity of pathophysiological alterations.

Research has found that approximately 16% of older persons in ambulatory care settings have experienced adverse drug events (Tache, Sonnichsen, & Ashcroft, 2011). Older people in nursing homes experience as many as 10.8 ADEs per 100 patient-months (or 135 events each year in an average size nursing home). Adverse drug events in nursing homes are estimated to cost as much as $4 billion in healthcare expenditures and are associated with 93,000 deaths each year (Handler & Hanlon, 2010).

Adverse drug event and adverse drug reaction are terms that usually refer to drug side effects that are serious.

TABLE 6-1	Normal Changes of Aging, Concurrent Conditions, and Other Drug Effects on Drug Therapy	
Physiological Changes of Aging	**Effects on Drug Therapy**	**Examples of Pathological Conditions or Drugs Also Affecting Drug Therapy**
Decreased gastrointestinal (GI) motility, decreased gastric acidity	Possible decreased or delayed absorption of acidic drugs; decrease in peak effect	Achlorhydria, malabsorption, diarrhea, gastric ulcers, pyloric obstruction or stenosis, pancreatitis, hypothyroidism, diabetic gastroparesis; antacids, H_2 blockers, proton pump inhibitors, anticholinergic drugs
Decrease in GI absorption surface of up to 20%	Effect on drug absorption believed to be minimal but possibly could decrease extent of absorption.	Surgery in the stomach or the small or large intestine
Dry mouth and secretions (xerostomia)	Difficulty in swallowing drugs	Dehydration, anticholinergic medications
Decreased liver blood flow; decreased liver mass; decrease in microsomal enzymes	Delayed and decreased metabolism of certain drugs	Liver disease, fever, malignancy, heart failure, severe anemia
Decreased lipid content in skin	Possible decrease in absorption of transdermal medications	Cachexia
Increase in body fat (from 18% to 36% in men and 33% to 45% in women); decrease in body water	Possible increased toxicity of water-soluble drugs; more prolonged and possible increased effects of fat-soluble drugs	Obesity, dehydration, diuretic drugs
Decrease in serum proteins	Possible increased effect/toxicity of highly protein-bound drug; increased possibility of interactions of two or more highly protein-bound drugs	Malnutrition, burns, liver disease
Decrease in renal mass, blood flow, and glomerular filtration rate (decline of 50% between ages 20 and 90, average of 35%)	Possible increased serum levels/toxicity of drugs excreted renally; NSAIDs may decrease renal blood flow and renal function	Renal insufficiency, heart failure, hypovolemia, NSAIDs, use of drugs excreted by kidneys
Changes in sensitivity of certain drug receptors	Increase in drug effects; e.g., anticholinergics, antihistamines, barbiturates (paradoxical excitation), benzodiazepines, digitalis, warfarin	Competition between drugs for receptor binding
	Decrease in drug effects; e.g., amphetamines, beta-blockers, quinidine	Cachexia, dehydration
Visual and hearing changes	Interference with learning and/or safe administration of medications	Anticholinergic drugs (vision changes); loop diuretics, certain antibiotics (e.g., aminoglycosides) (hearing)
Changes in brain/brain function	Changes in number and sensitivity of receptors and metabolism of neurotransmitters can cause imbalance in neurotransmitter functions and increased risk of anticholinergic effects; increased permeability of blood–brain barrier can result in increased central nervous system (CNS) adverse effects of drugs.	Anticholinergic drugs and drugs with anticholinergic side effects; sedative hypnotics, benzodiazepines; Alzheimer's and other dementias

---

> **BOX 6-1**   **Definitions of Adverse Drug Reactions and Adverse Drug Events**

- **Adverse drug reactions (ADRs):** Response to a medicine that is noxious and unintended, and that occurs at normal doses during normal use (World Health Organization, 2008). An undesirable response associated with use of a drug that either compromises therapeutic efficacy, enhances toxicity, or both (Joint Commission, 2007).
- **Adverse drug events (ADEs):** Any incident in which the use of a medication (drug or biologic) at any dose, a medical device, or a special nutritional product (for example, a dietary supplement, infant formula, medical food) may have resulted in injury or adverse outcome in a patient (Joint Commission, 2007).

- **Adverse drug experience**: Any adverse event associated with the use of a drug in humans, whether or not considered drug related, including the following: an adverse event occurring in the course of the use of a drug product in professional practice; an adverse event occurring from drug overdose whether accidental or intentional; an adverse event occurring from drug abuse; an adverse event occurring from drug withdrawal; and any failure of expected pharmacological action (FDA, 2011).

Definitions of an adverse drug reaction and an adverse drug event vary. Box 6-1 presents definitions of various terms. A *side effect* is any effect other than the intended therapeutic effect; the intended therapeutic effect depends on the particular condition for which the drug is prescribed and the expected therapeutic outcome. Differences in the terminology used to describe side effects may reflect degrees of alteration produced. In some references, side effects are considered to be expected effects that need to be tolerated and treated only if they are bothersome to the patient or cause noncompliance. However, inability to tolerate the side effects of some drugs can result in the patient deciding not to continue to take the medication. The nurse often can assist the patient in reducing the impact of some side effects of drugs, therefore enhancing compliance. For example, promoting the adequate intake of bulk in the diet and an adequate fluid intake can help to offset drug-induced constipation. The administration of diuretics can be scheduled so that the peak diuretic effect does not interrupt activities important to the patient. Frequent intake of liquids or the use of lozenges can help with dry mouth caused by medications.

Drug therapy for older persons requires a careful assessment of each patient's physiological and psychosocial status, the need for the drug, and the risk of an adverse drug reaction. Symptoms of many adverse drug effects may be similar to those of other conditions affecting the older person and therefore may be overlooked or not attributed to the drug therapy. Difficulties in the activities of daily living may provide clues to the presence of ADRs in an older person.

> **Practice Pearl** ▶▶▶ Suspect an adverse drug effect if a patient experiences cognitive changes, falls, anorexia, nausea, or weight loss that cannot be explained by any medical diagnoses.

Adverse Drug Events of Concern in Older Persons

Adverse drug events may manifest themselves differently in the older person. For example, digoxin side effects including amnesia, depression, nausea, vomiting, lethargy, confusion, and visual disturbances occur more often in older people than in younger people. Adverse drug events may be mistaken for common syndromes in the older person. Falls and fractures have been associated with the use of psychotropic and other medications. One study showed that the risk for falls in nursing home residents increased more than twofold within 1 day after patients received a new prescription for a diuretic or an increase in their diuretic dose (Berry, 2011).

Cognitive Effects

Cognitive impairment (e.g., delirium, dementia, depression) can be caused by a variety of medications. Delirium may be caused by drugs (including psychotropic medications) with anticholinergic effects. Changes in mood such as anxiety and depression can result from many types of drug therapy, such as antihypertensives (e.g., beta-blockers), antiparkinsonian agents, steroids, NSAIDs, narcotic analgesics, antineoplastic agents, CNS depressants, and psychotropics (e.g., alcohol, benzodiazepines, and other antianxiety agents).

Drugs with anticholinergic effects have been associated with cognitive decline (Fox et al., 2011; Low, Anstey, & Sachdev, 2009). In a study of older adults with memory problems, 10.3% were using one or more **over-the-counter (OTC) medication** or prescription medication with anticholinergic side effects that could contribute to memory problems and confusion (Kemper, Steiner, Hicks et al., 2007).

Metamucil - Psyllium seed
- can expand or swell in the esophagus without adaquate water
- take adaquate H2O

Chapter 6 Pharmacology and Older Adults   **135**

Diphenhydramine, which has anticholinergic effects, is an ingredient in commonly marketed sleep aids, often combined with acetaminophen and/or NSAIDS. Patients may not be aware of this and may experience decreased cognitive function, especially if used repeatedly and if used with other drugs with anticholinergic effects.

Cognitive changes from medications can lead clinicians to misinterpret these signs and possibly prescribe unnecessary medication to counteract them. Cognitive changes also may interfere with the clinician's ability to accurately assess the patient. This might occur if patients are unable to describe symptoms such as the location or degree of any pain they may be experiencing, to request PRN (*pro re nata* or as necessary) medications, or to describe side effects or changes in their well-being. Alterations in cognitive function can interfere with the patient's ability to manage the medication regimen and can pose additional dangers to level of functioning and quality of life.

Anticholinergic Effects

The use of drugs with anticholinergic effects presents a particular problem with the older person. This includes drugs classified as anticholinergics (e.g., atropine) as well as drugs in many pharmacological classifications that have anticholinergic side effects.

Many of the drug-related anticholinergic effects—both central and peripheral—can aggravate other conditions being experienced by the older person. Central anticholinergic effects include agitation, confusion, disorientation, poor attention, hallucinations, and psychosis. Peripheral effects include constipation, urinary retention, inhibition of sweating, decreased salivary and bronchial secretions, tachycardia, and mydriasis. Individuals with benign prostatic hypertrophy or other strictures of the urinary urethra may experience increased difficulty in initiating urine flow. Dryness of the mouth can slow the absorption of sublingual medications and may affect the ability to swallow oral preparations. Drugs with anticholinergic effects may also affect vision (blurred vision, dryness of the eyes). Anticholinergic effects on cardiac function may alter cardiovascular drug effects or lead to the possibly unnecessary prescription of cardiovascular drug therapy.

Anticholinergic effects are similar to the effects of atropine, a drug that can be used preoperatively to dry secretions and prevent aspiration during anesthesia. Anticholinergic or atropine-like side effects include bradycardia, dry mouth, decreased sweating, tachycardia, dilated pupils, blurred near vision, decreased intestinal peristalsis, dysphasia, dysphagia, urinary retention, hyperthermia and flushing, ataxia, hallucinations, delirium, and coma. The risk of these side effects increases directly in response to increasing doses of the drug. The nurse should carefully

BOX 6-2	Heuristic for Remembering Anticholinergic Effects
Dry as a bone	Inhibition of secretions
Red as a beet	Flushing related to absence of sweating
Hot as a hare	Temperature elevation from absence of sweating
Blind as a bat	Paralysis of the ciliary muscles and dilated pupils
Mad as a hatter	Cognitive status changes, delirium

observe older patients receiving large doses of these medications for extended periods of time and report any ADEs to the physician. A useful heuristic for remembering anticholinergic effects is given in Box 6-2.

Drugs with anticholinergic effects are also found in commonly prescribed medications (including antidepressants, antihistamines, antiparkinsonian agents, antipsychotics, and quinidine). The nurse should check each drug for its anticholinergic profile. The drugs within a certain pharmacological classification may differ in the severity of their anticholinergic effects; therefore, a drug from a different class of medications or a different drug from the same class might be chosen for its less severe anticholinergic effects. Table 6-2 provides examples of drugs that have anticholinergic effects.

Gastric and Esophageal Effects

Oral drugs that are swallowed but do not reach the stomach can result in esophageal obstruction or irritation of the esophageal lining. For example, it is important that enough water be taken with psyllium seed preparation (used to provide bulk to prevent constipation) to ensure that the medication reaches the stomach and does not swell in the esophagus and cause an obstruction. Box 6-3 provides strategies to prevent esophageal irritation from orally administered medications.

Loss of appetite, nausea, and weight loss may be the result of drug therapy. Drugs that decrease peristalsis can cause decreased appetite. Furthermore, nausea and loss of appetite may indicate toxic levels of drugs.

Gastric irritation can be caused by a variety of medications. This can lead to not only discomfort ("heartburn") but also gastric bleeding, which can be life threatening. Some drugs that have this effect are produced with an enteric coating that prevents the drug from dissolving until it reaches the alkaline environment in the duodenum. The coating of enteric-coated drugs (e.g., enteric-coated aspirin, erythromycin, oral bisacodyl tablets) may break down prematurely in the stomach if given with other drugs or foods that make the stomach alkaline; therefore, calcium,

TABLE 6-2	Examples of Medications With Anticholinergic Properties	
Antihistamines (H₁-Blockers)	**Antidepressants**	**Cardiovascular Medications**
Chlorpheniramine diphenhydramine, hydroxyzine	Amoxapine, amitriptyline, clomipramine, desipramine, doxepin, imipramine, nortriptyline, protriptyline, paroxetine	Furosemide, digoxin, nifedipine, disopyramide
Gastrointestinal Medications	**Antiparkinson Medications**	**Antipsychotic Medications**
Antidiarrheal, medications: diphenoxylate, atropine Antispasmodic medications: belladonna, clidinium, chlordiazepoxide, dicyclomine, hyoscyamine, propantheline Antiulcer medications: cimetidine, ranitidine	Amantadine, benztropine, biperiden, trihexyphenidyl	Chlorpromazine, clozapine, olanzapine, thioridazine
Muscle Relaxants	**Urinary Incontinence**	**Antivertigo Medications**
Cyclobenzaprine, dantrolene, orphenadrine	Oxybutynin, propantheline, solifenacin, tolterodine, trospium	Meclizine, scopolamine

Source: Centers for Medicare and Medicaid Services (CMS). (2011). *State operations manual appendix PP: Guidance to surveyors for long term care facilities.* Retrieved from http://www.cms.hhs.gov/manuals/Downloads/som107ap_pp_guidelines_ltcf.pdf

BOX 6-3 ▶ **Interventions to Prevent Esophageal Irritation From Drug Therapy**

- Patient should take medication while in an upright position and should remain upright for at least 30 minutes.
- Patient should swallow several sips of water to lubricate the throat and esophagus before taking the medication.
- Patient should not divide or break up tablets or capsules without consulting the pharmacist since some drugs may be enteric coated or compounded as a sustained-release preparation; chewing or breaking them apart could result in toxicity as more of the drug becomes immediately available for absorption.
- Patient should swallow medications with at least 8 oz of liquid, and one at a time.
- A dull aching pain in chest or shoulder after taking medication should be reported to the physician.
- A patient who has gastroesophageal reflux disorder should avoid use of medications that relax the lower esophageal sphincter and therefore would increase the reflux of stomach contents into the esophagus.

BOX 6-4 ▶ **Warning Signs of NSAID-Induced Gastric Irritation**

- "Heartburn" or burning sensation in stomach or back
- Blood in stool or positive test for occult blood
- Bloody vomit (including coffee-ground emesis), which may occur in older people without prior other symptoms
- Diarrhea

synthesis, which decreases resistance of the stomach lining to acid and other stomach contents. Additional effects of prostaglandin inhibition include slowing of blood clotting, therefore increasing the danger of gastric bleeding from these drugs. Box 6-4 lists warning signs of NSAID-induced gastric irritation. However, gastric bleeding in an older person may occur with little or no prior symptoms.

Medication-Related Falls

Medications have been associated with the occurrence of falls and related injuries. Falls may be due to the older person's alterations in vision and balance, decreases in reaction time, orthostatic hypotension, and decreased muscle strength. These alterations can be exacerbated by medications. The most common drugs with a significant association with falls in the older person are sedatives and hypnotics, antidepressants, and benzodiazepines (Woolcott et al., 2009).

dairy products, and antacids should not be given with enteric-coated preparations or within 2 hours.

Commonly used medications of concern are aspirin and nonsteroidal anti-inflammatory drugs (NSAIDs). These drugs not only cause irritation, but also block prostaglandin

Diuretics, alpha-adrenergic blockers, antihypertensives (e.g., nitrates, ACE inhibitors), antiparkinsonian agents, opioids, skeletal muscle relaxants, beta-blockers, anticholinergics, and phosphodiesterase type 5 inhibitors (used to treat erectile dysfunction) can cause or increase hypotension and lead to falls.

Exercise Effects

Nurses, older persons, and caregivers should be aware of the potential effects of exercise on a person's response to medications. Exercise can affect blood flow to skeletal muscles, skin, and internal organs and also affect the pH and motility of the gastrointestinal tract, drug metabolism, and renal excretion. Effects include the following: Drug absorption from the GI tract could be decreased; exercise decreases blood glucose, which could decrease the need for insulin or oral agents taken for diabetes; exercise decreases renal blood flow and glomerular filtration rate, which could decrease the renal excretion of drugs (Lenz, 2010). Statins can produce muscle aching, weakness, and cramps with excessive exercise. Hyperthermia can occur in patients taking diuretics or antipsychotics.

HEALTHY MEDICATION TIPS

▶ Take your medication exactly as prescribed.

▶ Ask about generic options.

▶ Keep a list of all your medications so you can share it with everyone involved in your care.

▶ Clean out your medicine cabinet at least once a year.

▶ Know the side effects of your medications and let your healthcare provider know immediately if you experience any of them.

▶ Consider lifestyle changes whenever possible to reduce medication use and minimize risk of side effects.

▶ Let your care providers know about all over-the-counter medications, vitamins, herbals, and dietary supplements you take.

▶ Have all your prescriptions filled at the same pharmacy.

▶ Store your medications in a safe place where they will be out of the reach of children.

Adverse Effects From Interactions

The potential for ADRs increases with increasing numbers of medications taken; this includes some complementary and alternative therapies as well. When multiple medications are used, there is a greater chance of drug–drug interactions, ADEs, and ADRs.

Over-the-Counter Medications

Increasingly, more medications are being approved by the FDA for nonprescription or over-the-counter (OTC) use, allowing patients access to these drugs without a prescription. Although this provides easier access, it also increases the possibility of inappropriate medication use by the patient. Patients increasingly are self-prescribing, using nonprescription medications, nutritional supplements, and herbal preparations. A study of community dwelling individuals ages 57 to 86 showed that 46% used OTC and prescription drugs concurrently (Qato et al., 2008).

The risk of drug interactions or an overdose is increased when OTC drugs are used that are identical or similar to a prescribed drug or another OTC medication. For example, acetaminophen is a common ingredient in OTC preparations for pain, sleep, colds, and arthritis. A person could inadvertently experience an overdose when taking multiple medications with acetaminophen in them.

The use of an OTC drug can also result in increased out-of-pocket costs to patients since health insurance usually does not pay for OTC medications. An additional concern is that self-medication with OTC drugs may delay the timely medical diagnosis and prescription of more appropriate and effective therapy.

Alcohol, which is a drug, can interact with medications, causing adverse effects. A 50% decrease in blood flow to the liver and kidneys may occur in older adults, resulting in decreased metabolism of other medications. Alcohol absorption is increased among older adults. Combining alcohol with other medications can cause CNS depression, falls, and other toxic effects. Concurrent use of alcohol and acetaminophen can result in serious liver damage.

Patients' use of alcohol should be carefully assessed since alcohol is a CNS depressant, may cause gastric irritation, and interferes with the metabolism of certain medications such as acetaminophen. Patients should be cautioned to use nonprescription drugs cautiously; some patients may think that these drugs are completely safe and that they can take as much as they want.

The use of psychoactive medications has been found to be associated with an increased risk of motor vehicle accidents requiring hospitalization in older individuals (Meuleners et al., 2011). In a study of 630 community-dwelling drivers ages 55 and older, only about 28% had awareness of potential driving-impairing medications. Few had received any warning about this from a healthcare professional (McClennon, Owlsey, Rue et al., 2009).

Table 6-3 provides examples of some common OTC drugs that can be associated with adverse drug effects if used inappropriately.

TABLE 6-3	Examples of Interaction of OTC Drugs With Prescribed Medications
OTC Drug	**Interactions**
Acetaminophen	Inhibits liver metabolism of warfarin leading to an increase in the International Normalized Ratio (INR). Limit to six or fewer regular-strength tablets per week unless INR is carefully monitored or if stable dose of acetaminophen is taken and warfarin dose is regulated while taking steady doses of warfarin. Alert patient to other OTC or prescription medications (e.g., Percocet) that may contain acetaminophen as an ingredient. Alcohol can cause increased production of toxic acetaminophen metabolites, which can result in irreversible liver damage. FDA-mandated labeling cautions against use of acetaminophen if a person takes three or more alcoholic drinks per day.
Alcohol	Blood pressure may be increased if a person drinks heavily or engages in binge drinking. The risk of gastric irritation and bleeding is increased when alcohol is consumed with NSAIDs; use of antacids may increase this risk even more. Bioavailability of alcohol is increased by the use of aspirin and H_2 antagonists within 2 hours due to inhibition of gastric alcohol dehydrogenase and more rapid gastric emptying.
Antacids and calcium supplements	Can cause premature dissolution of enteric-coated preparations (e.g., enteric-coated aspirin, erythromycin), resulting in premature dissolution of drug in the stomach and increased risk of gastric irritation. Should be taken 2 hours before or after these medications. The absorption of ciprofloxacin, digoxin, levothyroxine, phenytoin, tetracyclines, thiamine, vitamin B_{12}, and zinc may be disrupted.
Cimetidine	Inhibits microsomal enzymes, which could result in higher than usual levels of other drugs whose metabolism is regulated by the microsomal enzymes.
Decongestants	Have pressor effects and may increase blood pressure and/or counteract effect of antihypertensives. Alert patient to decongestants to avoid in cough or cold remedies (e.g., pseudoephedrine, phenylpropanolamine).
NSAIDs (e.g., aspirin, ibuprofen)	May cause renal toxicity and failure, especially in individuals with decreased glomerular flow and pressure (e.g., age-related renal failure, heart failure, volume depletion from diuretics)
Vitamin A	May interfere with absorption of calcium.
Vitamin E	May inhibit vitamin K synthesis and increase anticoagulant effects of coumarin.
Vitamin C	High doses acidify the urine and can affect the excretion of other medications.

Herbal Preparations

Increasingly, people of all ages are using alternative or complementary medicines such as homeopathic preparations and herbal medicines in addition to their routine medications. Homeopathic medications are well diluted and are not believed to interact with medications (National Center for Complementary and Alternative Medicine, 2010). Certain prescription medications (e.g., NSAIDs, antiulcer, and some pain medications), however, are considered by homeopathic practitioners to counteract the effectiveness of some homeopathic medicines. Because the FDA does not regulate herbal medicines, there is no assurance of standardization of their ingredients, purity, dosage, or potency. For most, there have not been sufficient clinical trials to demonstrate their effectiveness or appropriate dosage. Adverse effects may result from the herb itself as well as from contaminants in the preparation.

Herbs can interact with medications. Therefore, it is important to elicit from patients any herbs, home remedies, or dietary supplements that they take. If patients are to have anesthesia, it is important that they notify the anesthetist of what herbal remedies they have been using. Some herbs such as ginseng and ginkgo can inhibit platelet aggregation and increase bleeding time. Therefore, these drugs should be discontinued for several days before the anesthesia is given or surgery is scheduled. Table 6-4 highlights the uses and known drug interaction concerns of some commonly used herbs. Note, however, that other drug and herb interactions may occur that have not been reported to physicians or to an agency.

> **Practice Pearl** ▶▶▶ Discuss with prescribing clinician the possibility of discontinuing one drug when another is added to a drug regimen.

Reporting Adverse Drug Events

Once the FDA approves a new drug there is no requirement that clinicians report side effects. However, both manufacturers and the FDA have initiated measures to encourage the reporting of suspected adverse events of medications

TABLE 6-4	**Examples of Herbal Preparations and Interactions With Drugs**	
Herbal Preparation	**Use**	**Interactions/Precautions**
Echinacea	Stimulation of immunity	Counteracts effects of immunosuppressive drugs (e.g., cyclosporine). Avoid use with drugs toxic to liver.
Ephedra (ma huang) (no longer available in United States)	Promotion of weight loss, increasing energy, treatment of respiratory condition	Sympathomimetic effects can cause elevated blood pressure, stroke, and death.
Garlic	Reduction in risk of atherosclerosis by decreasing blood pressure, thrombin formation, and lipid and cholesterol levels	Inhibits platelet aggregation and potentiates effects of platelet inhibitor drugs (e.g., indomethacin, dipyridamole); increases INR if used with warfarin; hypoglycemia with chlorpropamide.
Ginseng	Protection against effects of stress, helps to restore homeostasis	Can cause bleeding problems and hypoglycemia; decrease in INR when used with warfarin; insomnia, headache, tremulousness, mania with phenelzine.
Ginkgo	Enhancement of cognitive performance, treatment of peripheral vascular disease, age-related macular degeneration, vertigo, tinnitus, erectile dysfunction, altitude sickness	Inhibits platelet-activating factor and can cause bleeding; bleeding with aspirin or warfarin; increased blood pressure with thiazide diuretic; increased sedation with trazodone.
Kava	Anxiolytic and sedative	Causes excessive sedation when used with other CNS depressants; sedation with alprazolam.
St. John's wort	Treatment of mild to moderate depression	May cause excess levels of serotonin if taken with selective serotonin reuptake inhibitors (SSRIs). Can increase the metabolism of many drugs, resulting in reduced effectiveness; reduced plasma concentrations of amitriptyline, cyclosporine, digoxin, indinavir, phenprocoumon, and theophylline. Decrease in INR with warfarin; symptoms of central serotonin excess with nefazodone, paroxetine, and sertraline. Altered menstrual bleeding with oral contraceptives.
Valerian	Sedative, hypnotic	Withdrawal from valerian mimics acute benzodiazepine withdrawal syndrome. Potentiates sedative effects of barbiturates and anesthetics and anesthetic adjuvants.

Sources: Ang-Lee, Moss, & Yuan (2001); Bent & Ko (2004); and Shiel (2009).

(drugs or biologicals), medical devices, special nutritional products, and other products regulated by the FDA. The FDA's MedWatch program provides a mechanism for the voluntary reporting of suspected problems; it is not necessary to have definitively established that the drug has caused the event. The patient's name is held in strict confidence; the name of the person reporting the problem may be provided to the product's manufacturer unless requested otherwise.

Adverse events that should be reported to MedWatch include serious events such as death, life-threatening events (real risk of dying), hospitalization (initial or prolonged), disability (significant, prolonged, or permanent), congenital anomaly, or required intervention to prevent permanent impairment of damage. A copy of the MedWatch reporting form can be obtained at the FDA website.

Most patient care institutions have a system for reporting adverse drug events. Clinicians need to be aware of policies and procedures within their practice settings related to adverse drug events as well as medication errors.

Weblink: Medwatch Reporting Form

Promoting Medication Effectiveness and Safety

The nurse has pivotal roles in ensuring that a person's drug therapy is effective for the person's condition and in preventing, detecting, or intervening as early as possible if the person develops adverse drug effects. This includes the "five rights" of medication administration (right patient, right drug, right dose, right route, and right time) but also goes beyond these rules; monitoring for and documenting a drug's therapeutic and adverse effects on the patient are essential. Nurses' clinical judgment and professional vigilance has been found to be an integral role of nurses in the medication management process (Eisenhauer, Hurley, & Dolan, 2007). In caring for older adults, this involves integration of knowledge about the aging process, drug therapy, and the unique physiological and psychosocial characteristics of each older person.

The prescribing of appropriate medications is a key step in ensuring appropriate medication effects and preventing adverse drug effects. The nurse may need to suggest to the prescribing clinician the possible need for reduced dosages of some medications, especially for a patient whose weight is less than average, who has decreased liver or renal function, or who is experiencing exaggerated responses to drugs that may reflect toxic levels. Box 6-5 summarizes the overall goals of medication regimens; although these are part of the Medicare regulations for long-term care facilities (from the Centers for Medicare and Medicaid Service's *State Operations Manual*), they are applicable in any setting.

The nurse has a major role in reducing the need for medications and in suggesting alternatives to their use. Many nursing interventions can prevent the need for some medications and/or reduce the dose or length of drug therapy. The nurse also should consider patient problems as having a possible basis in their drug therapy. Alternatives to the use of medications are featured in Table 6-5. These nursing interventions also can be used to reduce the dose or duration of a medication.

Drug therapy should be used only if there is a specific diagnosis or clearly documented symptom or condition to be treated. The use of a drug to treat the side effects of another drug should be avoided. It is usually much better to change the offending drug or decrease the dose to decrease the side effects and avoid the need for another medication. Box 6-6 lists Medicare's definition of an unnecessary drug.

Gradual dose reduction (GDR) of medications, especially psychotropic agents, is recommended, and is required by Medicare regulations for long-term care facilities. Gradual dose reduction is "the stepwise tapering of a dose to determine if symptoms, conditions, or risks can be managed by a lower dose or if the dose or medication can be discontinued. The

---

BOX 6-5 **Goals of Medication Regimens**

Each [person's] entire drug/medication regimen should be managed and monitored to achieve the following goals:

- The medication regimen helps promote or maintain the [person's] highest practicable mental, physical, and psychosocial well-being, as identified by the resident and/or representative(s) in collaboration with the attending physician and facility staff;
- Each [person] receives only those medications, in doses and for the duration clinically indicated to treat the [person's] assessed condition(s);
- Non-pharmacological interventions (such as behavioral interventions) are considered and used when indicated, instead of, or in addition to, medication;
- Clinically significant adverse consequences are minimized; and
- The potential contribution of the medication regimen to an unanticipated decline or newly emerging or worsening symptom is recognized and evaluated, and the regimen is modified when appropriate.

Source: Centers for Medicare and Medicaid Services (CMS). (2011). *State operations manual appendix PP: Guidance to surveyors for long-term care facilities.* Retrieved from http://www.cms.hhs.gov/manuals/Downloads/som107ap_pp_guidelines_ltcf.pdf.

---

goal of gradual dose reduction is to find an optimal dose for a particular patient or to evaluate if the continued use of the medication is benefiting the resident" (Centers for Medicare and Medicaid Services [CMS], 2011) (Box 6-7).

Polypharmacy is defined as the prescription, administration, or use of more medications than are clinically indicated in a given patient. This can include the use of a medication that has no apparent indication, continuing use of a medication after a condition has been resolved, use of a medication to treat the side effects of another medication, use of an inappropriate dose, and use of duplicate medications because the same drug has been prescribed by more than one prescriber. Patients may not be aware of the different names (e.g., generic and one or more brand names) used for the same medication. Polypharmacy may also occur when a patient self-medicates with OTC medications or herbal remedies to treat the same condition or to manage symptoms of an adverse drug effect. Some aspects of polypharmacy can be prevented by using the same pharmacy to fill all prescriptions so that the pharmacist can check for duplication or drug interactions. Patients should be encouraged to notify all prescribing clinicians about what other drugs they are taking.

Because more than one prescriber may treat a patient, the nurse should obtain a complete history of all drugs prescribed. Information about other drugs and remedies should also be elicited from the patient since they may be the basis for significant interactions with drug therapy. These include the use of

TABLE 6-5	Alternatives to Medications for Patient Problems	
Medication	**Patient Problem**	**Alternatives**
Laxatives, cathartics	Constipation	Increase bulk in diet (e.g., apple, bran muffin), avoid cheese and excessive use of other calcium products (including calcium in antacids); encourage exercise, ensure adequate fluid intake.
Hypnotics	Insomnia	Suggest warm milk (contains natural tryptophan); adapt environment to promote sleep (e.g., decrease noise and light, use of music if soothing to patient). Encourage patient to keep awake and active during the day. Review medications for those producing altered sleep patterns (e.g., sedative-hypnotics, benzodiazepines, psychotropics, anxiolytics, diuretics). Avoid caffeine drinks in the afternoon/evening.
Antacids	"Heartburn," sour stomach	Help patient to identify foods that precipitate symptoms and avoid them; use of small frequent meals; keep in upright position for at least 30 minutes after taking oral medication.
Antianxiety agents	Anxiety	Suggest counseling, biofeedback, and other stress reduction techniques; tai chi; yoga.
Analgesics	Pain	Suggest use of distraction, guided imagery, positioning (e.g., elevation of swollen limb), ice or heat, tai chi, or yoga.

BOX 6-6 Unnecessary Drugs

An *unnecessary drug* is any drug when used:

(i) In excessive dose (including duplicate therapy); or
(ii) For excessive duration; or
(iii) Without adequate monitoring; or
(iv) Without adequate indications for its use; or
(v) In the presence of adverse consequences which indicate the dose should be reduced or discontinued; or
(vi) Any combinations of the reasons above.

Source: Centers for Medicare and Medicaid Services (CMS). (2011). *State operations manual appendix PP: Guidance to surveyors for long-term care facilities.* Retrieved from http://www.cms.hhs.gov/manuals/Downloads/som107ap_pp_guidelines_ltcf.pdf.

BOX 6-7 Gradual Dose Reduction (GDR)

Tapering may be indicated when:

- the [patient's] clinical condition has improved or stabilized
- the underlying causes of the original target symptoms have resolved, and/or
- nonpharmacological interventions, including behavioral interventions, have been effective in reducing the symptoms.

Source: Centers for Medicare and Medicaid Services (CMS). (2011). *State operations manual appendix PP: Guidance to surveyors for long-term care facilities.* Retrieved from http://www.cms.hhs.gov/manuals/Downloads/som107ap_pp_guidelines_ltcf.pdf.

vitamins, OTC medications, dietary supplements, and herbal remedies. Patients often do not think of these as medications when asked about their medication use (see also later section in this chapter related to medication reconciliation).

Potentially Inappropriate Drugs

Some drugs are considered to be inappropriate to use in most older persons because of their adverse effects. The drugs considered to be potentially inappropriate usually are referred to as being on the "Beers list" (see pages 142–146). Despite this list, the use of potentially inappropriate medications continues to be of concern and has been found to have serious implications.

Inappropriate use of medications among older adults is highly prevalent with estimates ranging from 12% in community-dwelling elders to 40% in nursing home residents (Mansur, Weiss, & Beloosesky, 2009). In a study of older patients seen in the emergency department, 32% were taking at least one potentially inappropriate medication. The most common were propoxyphene/acetaminophen, muscle relaxants, and antihistamines (Hustey, Wallis, & Miller, 2007).

The use of inappropriate medications has been associated with an increased risk of falling in older adults, especially in patients receiving long-acting benzodiazepines and other inappropriate psychotropics or medications with anticholinergic properties (Berdot, Bertrand, Dartigues et al., 2009).

Beers Criteria

The Beers Criteria for Potentially Inappropriate Medication Use in Older Adults (American Geriatrics Society [AGS], 2012) has had several revisions over the more than 20 years of its existence. The most current is the 2012 version in which an evidence-based approach was used in its development. "The role of the 2012 criteria should be to inform clinical decision making, research, training, and policy to improve the quality and safety of prescribing medications for older adults" (Resnick, 2012). The nurse can use the list as a basis of questioning the prescribing clinician about the appropriateness of a drug being used in a particular patient. There may be instances when the drug is used appropriately in a specific patient. The list also is useful in helping the nurse to be aware of the adverse effects that should be monitored if an older patient is receiving these drugs. There are three lists: medications that are potentially inappropriate (Table 6-6), medications that may be inappropriate in patients with certain conditions or other drug therapies (Table 6-7), and medications that should be with caution (Table 6-8).

TABLE 6-6	2012 AGS Beers Criteria for Potentially Inappropriate Medication Use in Older Adults
Organ System/Therapeutic Category/Drug(s)	**Recommendation, Rationale, *Quality of Evidence (QE) and Strength of Recommendation (SR)***
Anticholinergics *(excludes TCAs)*	
First-generation antihistamines (as single agent or as part of combination products) • Brompheniramine • Carbinoxamine • Chlorpheniramine • Clemastine • Cyproheptadine • Dexbrompheniramine • Dexchlorpheniramine • Diphenhydramine (oral) • Doxylamine • Hydroxyzine • Promethazine • Triprolidine	**Avoid.** Highly anticholinergic; clearance reduced with advanced age, and tolerance develops when used as hypnotic; increased risk of confusion, dry mouth, constipation, and other anticholinergic effects/toxicity. Use of diphenhydramine in special situations such as acute treatment of severe allergic reaction may be appropriate. *QE = High (Hydroxyzine and Promethazine), Moderate (All others); SR = Strong*
Antiparkinson agents • Benztropine (oral) • Trihexyphenidyl	**Avoid.** Not recommended for prevention of extrapyramidal symptoms with antipsychotics; more effective agents available for treatment of Parkinson disease. *QE = Moderate; SR = Strong*
Antispasmodics • Belladonna alkaloids • Clidinium-chlordiazepoxide • Dicyclomine • Hyoscyamine • Propantheline • Scopolamine	**Avoid except in short-term palliative care to decrease oral secretions.** Highly anticholinergic, uncertain effectiveness. *QE = Moderate; SR = Strong*
Antithrombotics	
Dipyridamole, oral short-acting* *(does not apply to the extended-release combination with aspirin)*	**Avoid.** May cause orthostatic hypotension; more effective alternatives available; IV form acceptable for use in cardiac stress testing. *QE = Moderate; SR = Strong*
Ticlopidine*	**Avoid.** Safer, effective alternatives available

TABLE 6-6   2012 AGS Beers Criteria for Potentially Inappropriate Medication Use in Older Adults (continued)

Organ System/Therapeutic Category/Drug(s)	Recommendation, Rationale, Quality of Evidence (QE) and Strength of Recommendation (SR)
Anti-Infective	
Nitrofurantoin	**Avoid for long-term suppression; avoid in patients with CrCl < 60 mL/min.** Potential for pulmonary toxicity; safer alternatives available; lack of efficacy in patients with CrCl < 60 mL/min due to inadequate drug concentration in the urine. *QE = Moderate; SR = Strong*
Cardiovascular	
Alpha$_1$-blockers • Doxazosin • Prazosin • Terazosin	**Avoid use as an antihypertensive.** High risk of orthostatic hypotension; not recommended as routine treatment for hypertension; alternative agents have superior risk/benefit profile. *QE = Moderate; SR = Strong*
Alpha agonists • Clonidine • Guanabenz* • Guanfacine* • Methyldopa* • Reserpine (>0.1 mg/day)*	**Avoid clonidine as a first-line antihypertensive. Avoid others as listed.** High risk of adverse CNS effects; may cause bradycardia and orthostatic hypotension; not recommended as routine treatment for hypertension. *QE = Low; SR = Strong*
Antiarrhythmic drugs (Classes Ia, Ic, III) • Amiodarone • Dofetilide • Dronedarone • Flecainide • Ibutilide • Procainamide • Propafenone • Quinidine • Sotalol	**Avoid antiarrhythmic drugs as first-line treatment of atrial fibrillation.** Data suggest that rate control yields better balance of benefits and harms than rhythm control for most older adults. Amiodarone is associated with multiple toxicities, including thyroid disease, pulmonary disorders, and QT interval prolongation. *QE = High; SR = Strong*
Disopyramide*	**Avoid.** Disopyramide is a potent negative inotrope and therefore may induce heart failure in older adults; strongly anticholinergic; other antiarrhythmic drugs preferred. *QE = Low; SR = Strong*
Dronedarone	**Avoid in patients with permanent atrial fibrillation or heart failure.** Worse outcomes have been reported in patients taking dronedarone who have permanent atrial fibrillation or heart failure. In general, rate control is preferred over rhythm control for atrial fibrillation. *QE = Moderate; SR = Strong*
Digoxin > 0.125 mg/day	**Avoid.** In heart failure, higher dosages associated with no additional benefit and may increase risk of toxicity; decreased renal clearance may increase risk of toxicity. *QE = Moderate; SR = Strong*

Note: *Infrequently used drugs.

Abbreviations: ACEI, angiotensin converting-enzyme inhibitors; ARB, angiotensin receptor blockers; CNS, central nervous system; COX, cyclooxygenase; CrCl, creatinine clearance; GI, gastrointestinal; NSAIDs, nonsteroidal anti-inflammatory drugs; QE, quality of evidence; SIADH, syndrome of inappropriate antidiuretic hormone secretion; SR, strength of recommendation; TCAs, tricyclic antidepressants.

Source: American Geriatrics Society Updated Beers Criteria for Potentially Inappropriate Medication Use in Older Adults. © 2012 in *Journal of American Geriatrics Society, 60*(40): 616-631. Retrieved from http://www.americangeriatrics.org/files/documents/beers/2012BeersCriteria_JAGS.pdf. Copyright holder: American Geriatrics Society. Used with permission.

TABLE 6-7	2012 AGS Beers Criteria for Potentially Inappropriate Medication Use in Older Adults Due to Drug–Disease or Drug–Syndrome Interactions That May Exacerbate the Disease or Syndrome	

Disease or Syndrome	Drug(s)	Recommendation, Rationale, *Quality of Evidence (QE) and Strength of Recommendation (SR)*
Chronic constipation	Oral antimuscarinics for urinary incontinence • Darifenacin • Fesoterodine • Oxybutynin (oral) • Solifenacin • Tolterodine • Trospium Nondihydropyridine CCB • Diltiazem • Verapamil First-generation antihistamines as single agent or part of combination products • Brompheniramine (various) • Carbinoxamine • Chlorpheniramine • Clemastine (various) • Cyproheptadine • Dexbrompheniramine • Dexchlorpheniramine (various) • Diphenhydramine • Doxylamine • Hydroxyzine • Promethazine • Triprolidine Anticholinergics/antispasmodics • Antipsychotics • Belladonna alkaloids • Clidinium-chlordiazepoxide • Dicyclomine • Hyoscyamine • Propantheline • Scopolamine • Tertiary TCAs (amitriptyline, clomipramine, doxepin, imipramine, and trimipramine)	**Avoid unless no other alternatives.** Can worsen constipation; agents for urinary incontinence: antimuscarinics overall differ in incidence of constipation; response variable; consider alternative agent if constipation develops. *QE = High (For Urinary Incontinence), Moderate/Low (All Others); SR = Strong*
History of gastric or duodenal ulcers	Aspirin (>325 mg/day) Non–COX-2 selective NSAIDs	**Avoid unless other alternatives are not effective and patient can take gastroprotective agent (proton-pump inhibitor or misoprostol).** May exacerbate existing ulcers or cause new/additional ulcers. *QE = Moderate; SR = Strong*

TABLE 6-7	2012 AGS Beers Criteria for Potentially Inappropriate Medication Use in Older Adults Due to Drug–Disease or Drug–Syndrome Interactions That May Exacerbate the Disease or Syndrome (*continued*)

Disease or Syndrome	Drug(s)	Recommendation, Rationale, *Quality of Evidence (QE) and Strength of Recommendation (SR)*
Kidney/Urinary Tract		
Chronic kidney disease stages IV and V	NSAIDs Triamterene (alone or in combination)	**Avoid.** May increase risk of kidney injury. May increase risk of acute kidney injury. *QE = Moderate (NSAIDs), Low (Triamterene); SR = Strong(NSAIDs), Weak (Triamterene)*
Urinary incontinence (all types) in women	Estrogen oral and transdermal (excludes intravaginal estrogen)	**Avoid in women.** Aggravation of incontinence. *QE = High; SR = Strong*
Lower urinary tract symptoms, benign prostatic hyperplasia	Inhaled anticholinergic agents Strongly anticholinergic drugs, except antimuscarinics for urinary incontinence	**Avoid in men.** May decrease urinary flow and cause urinary retention. *QE = Moderate; SR = Strong (Inhaled agents), Weak (All others)*
Stress or mixed urinary incontinence	Alpha-blockers • Doxazosin • Prazosin • Terazosin	**Avoid in women.** Aggravation of incontinence. *QE = Moderate; SR = Strong*

Note: Abbreviations: AChEIs, acetylcholinesterase inhibitors; CCBs, calcium channel blockers; CNS, central nervous system; COX, cyclooxygenase; NSAIDs, nonsteroidal anti-inflammatory drugs; QE, quality of evidence; SR, strength of recommendation; SSRIs, selective serotonin reuptake inhibitors; TCAs, tricyclic antidepressants.

Source: 2012 AGS Beers Criteria for Potentially Inappropriate Medication Use in Older Adults Due to Drug-Disease or Drug-Syndrome Interactions That May Exacerbate the Disease of Syndrome. © 2012 in *Journal of American Geriatrics Society, 60*(4): 616-631. Retrieved from http://www.americangeriatrics.org/files/documents/beers/2012BeersCriteria_JAGS.pdf. Copyright holder: American Geriatrics Society. Used with permission.

Appropriate Use of Psychotropics

The use of psychotropic drugs in older persons, especially those in institutional settings, is of concern due to potential use of these drugs for less than optimal therapeutic reasons. Some uses of these drugs may be considered **"chemical restraints,"** that is, being used to quiet a person or subdue certain behaviors rather than using other nonmedication measures.

In one study nearly one third of nursing home residents with dementia received antipsychotic medications, primarily atypical agents (Kamble, Chen, Sherer et al., 2009). Another study found a similar result and also found that 32% of those receiving these mediations had no clinical indication for them (Briesacher, Soumerai, Field et al., 2010). The 1987 Omnibus Budget Reconciliation Act (OBRA 87) legislated the appropriate use of medications in institutionalized older persons, especially as their use may constitute a chemical restraint. "Chemical restraints" may

only be used to ensure the physical safety of older patients in emergency situations, but these medications have the potential to be used inappropriately to quiet a person or subdue certain behaviors in place of other nonpharmacologic measures. Overuse of psychotropic medications is of concern because of the chance of serious adverse events and syndromes associated with these medications (Box 6-8). Use of these medications without careful nursing assessment can mask serious symptoms such as depression, pain, and exacerbation of chronic illness.

A 2007 study found that many (51%) atypical antipsychotic drugs for older nursing home residents were either not actually administered or were not used for medically accepted conditions (Office of Inspector General, 2011).

Nurses working in long-term care facilities should be knowledgeable about the policies and regulations of the facility, the state, accreditation standards, and Medicare and other federal agencies. Many Medicare regulations can be

TABLE 6-8	2012 AGS Beers Criteria for Potentially Inappropriate Medications to Be Used With Caution in Older Adults
Drug(s)	**Recommendation, Rationale, *Quality of Evidence (QE) and Strength of Recommendation (SR)***
Aspirin for primary prevention of cardiac events	**Use with caution in adults ≥ 80 years old.** Lack of evidence of benefit versus risk in individuals ≥ 80 years old. *QE = Low; SR = Weak*
Dabigatran	**Use with caution in adults ≥ 75 years old or if CrCl < 30 mL/min.** Increased risk of bleeding compared with warfarin in adults ≥ 75 years old; lack of evidence for efficacy and safety in patients with CrCl < 30 mL/min *QE = Moderate; SR = Weak*
Prasugrel	**Use with caution in adults ≥ 75 years old.** Greater risk of bleeding in older adults; risk may be offset by benefit in highest risk older patients (e.g., those with prior myocardial infarction or diabetes). *QE = Moderate; SR = Weak*
Antipsychotics Carbamazepine Carboplatin Cisplatin Mirtazapine SNRIs SSRIs TCAs Vincristine	**Use with caution.** May exacerbate or cause SIADH or hyponatremia; need to monitor sodium level closely when starting or changing dosages in older adults due to increased risk. *QE = Moderate; SR = Strong*
Vasodilators	**Use with caution.** May exacerbate episodes of syncope in individuals with history of syncope. *QE = Moderate; SR = Weak*

Note: Abbreviations: CrCl, creatinine clearance; QE, quality of evidence; SIADH, syndrome of inappropriate antidiuretic hormone secretion; SNRIs, serotonin–norepinephrine reuptake inhibitors; SR, strength of recommendation; SSRIs, selective serotonin reuptake inhibitors; TCAs, tricyclic antidepressants.

Source: 2012 AGS Beers Criteria for Potentially Inappropriate Medications to Be Used with Caution in Older Adults. © 2012 in *Journal of American Geriatrics Society, 60*(4): 616-631. Retrieved from http://www.americangeriatrics.org/files/documents/beers/2012BeersCriteria_JAGS.pdf. Copyright holder: American Geriatrics Society. Used with permission.

found on the Medicare website. The CMS *State Operations Manual,* which is used by states in their surveys of long-term care facilities, provides a great deal of information about medications as well as other aspects of patient care in long-term care facilities.

Long-term care facilities must ensure that residents who have not used antipsychotic drugs are not given these drugs unless antipsychotic drug therapy is necessary to treat a specific condition, as diagnosed and documented in the clinical record. Residents who use antipsychotic drugs must receive gradual dose reductions, drug holidays, or behavioral programming, unless clinically contraindicated, in an effort to discontinue these drugs. See Box 6-6 on unnecessary drugs and Box 6-7 on gradual dose reduction (page 141).

Conditions that are considered to be inappropriate as the sole basis for the use of antipsychotic drugs are wandering, poor self-care, restlessness, impaired memory, mild anxiety, insomnia, unsociability, inattention or indifference to surroundings, fidgeting, nervousness, uncooperativeness, or verbal expressions or behavior that are not due to approved indications (Box 6-9) and do not represent danger to the resident or others (CMS, 2011).

Another important aspect in the use of psychotropic drugs in the older person is the daily dose. Table 6-9 lists the Medicare (CMS) maximum daily doses for anxiolytics and sedative-hypnotics. See Box 6-10 for a list of indications for use of anxiolytic medications. Unless an attempt at gradual dose reduction has been unsuccessful, the daily use of both long- and short-acting benzodiazepines should be limited to less than 4 continuous months; dose reductions should be considered after 4 months of continuous use (CMS, 2011).

A **medication regimen review (MRR)** is a process required by Medicare that involves a thorough evaluation of an individual's medication regimen by a pharmacist, in collaboration with other members of the interdisciplinary team. It is intended to promote positive outcomes

BOX 6-8 **Syndromes and Adverse Effects of Psychotropic Drugs**

Neuroleptic malignant syndrome (NMS) is a syndrome related to the use of medications, mainly antipsychotics, that typically presents with a sudden onset of diffuse muscle rigidity, high fever, labile blood pressure, tremor, and notable cognitive dysfunction. It is potentially fatal if not treated immediately, including stopping the offending medications.

Serotonin syndrome is a potentially serious clinical condition resulting from overstimulation of serotonin receptors. It is commonly related to the use of multiple serotonin-stimulating medications (e.g., selective serotonin reuptake inhibitors [SSRIs], serotonin–norepinephrine reuptake inhibitors [SNRIs], triptans, certain antibiotics). Symptoms may include restlessness, hallucinations, confusion, loss of coordination, fast heart beat, rapid changes in blood pressure, increased body temperature, overactive reflexes, nausea, vomiting, and diarrhea.

Tardive dyskinesia refers to abnormal, recurrent, involuntary movements that may be irreversible and typically present as lateral movements of the tongue or jaw, tongue thrusting, chewing, frequent blinking, brow arching, grimacing, and lip smacking, although the trunk or other parts of the body may also be affected.

Extrapyramidal symptoms (EPS) are neurologic side effects that can occur at any time from the first few days of treatment to years later. EPS includes various syndromes such as:

■ *Akathisia*, which refers to a distressing feeling of internal restlessness that may appear as constant motion, the inability to sit still, fidgeting, pacing, or rocking.

■ *Medication-induced parkinsonism*, which refers to a syndrome of Parkinson-like symptoms including tremors, shuffling gait, slowness of movement, expressionless face, drooling, postural unsteadiness, and rigidity of muscles in the limbs, neck, and trunk.

■ *Dystonia*, which refers to an acute, painful, spastic contraction of muscle groups (commonly the neck, eyes, and trunk) that often occurs soon after initiating treatment and is more common in younger individuals.

Source: Centers for Medicare and Medicaid Services (CMS). (2011). *State operations manual appendix PP: Guidance to surveyors for long-term care facilities.* Retrieved from http://www.cms.hhs.gov/manuals/Downloads/som107ap_pp_guidelines_ltcf.pdf.

BOX 6-9 **Indications for Use of Antipsychotic Medications**

An antipsychotic medication should be used only for the following conditions/diagnoses as documented in the record and as meets the definition(s) in the American Psychiatric Association's *Diagnostic and Statistical Manual of Mental Disorders*, Fourth Edition, Text Revision (DSM-IV-TR) or subsequent editions:

■ Schizophrenia
■ Schizo-affective disorder
■ Delusional disorder
■ Mood disorders (e.g., mania, bipolar disorder, depression with psychotic features, and treatment refractory major depression)
■ Schizophreniform disorder
■ Psychosis not otherwise specified (NOS)
■ Atypical psychosis
■ Brief psychotic disorder
■ Dementing illnesses with associated behavioral symptoms
■ Medical illnesses or delirium with manic or psychotic symptoms and/or treatment-related psychosis or mania (e.g., steroids)

Source: Centers for Medicare and Medicaid Services (CMS). (2011). *State operations manual appendix PP: Guidance to surveyors for long-term care facilities.* Retrieved from http://www.cms.hhs.gov/manuals/Downloads/som107ap_pp_guidelines_ltcf.pdf.

TABLE 6-9 **Maximum DAILY ORAL Doses**

Anxiolytic Medications	Sedative-Hypnotic Medications
Alprazolam 25 mg	Chloral hydrate* 500 mg
Chlordiazepoxide 20 mg	Diphenhydramine* 25 mg
Clonazepam 1.5 mg	Estazolam 0.5 mg
Clorazepate 15 mg	Eszopiclone 1 mg
Diazepam 5 mg	Flurazepam* 15 mg
Estazolam 0.5 mg	Hydroxyzine* 50 mg
Flurazepam 15 mg	Lorazepam 1 mg
Lorazepam 2 mg	Oxazepam 15 mg
Oxazepam 30 mg	Quazepam* 7.5 mg
Quazepam 7.5 mg	Ramelteon 8 mg
	Temazepam 15 mg
	Triazolam* 0.125 mg
	Zaleplon 5 mg
	Zolpidem CR 6.25 mg
	Zolpidem IR 5 mg

Note: *Not considered medications of choice for the management of insomnia, especially in older individuals.

Source: Centers for Medicare and Medicaid Services (CMS). (2011). *State operations manual appendix PP: Guidance to surveyors for long-term care facilities.* Retrieved from http://www.cms.hhs.gov/manuals/Downloads/som107ap_pp_guidelines_ltcf.pdf.

and minimize adverse consequences associated with medication. The review includes preventing, identifying, reporting, and resolving medication-related problems, medication errors, or other irregularities (CMS, 2011).

Evaluating Appropriate Prescribing of Medications

The following questions can guide the clinician in reviewing appropriateness of a medication:

1. Is the condition sufficiently problematic to require treatment?
2. Are there nursing or other nonpharmacological treatments that could alleviate the condition, prevent or delay use of a medication, or complement drug therapy?
3. If a drug is indicated for treatment of a specific condition, is the need for the medication documented in the medical record (e.g., an established or working diagnosis for which the drug is approved)?
4. Has informed consent for the prescription been obtained from the patient or legally determined surrogate decision maker?
5. Is the prescription likely to be effective in achieving the prescriber's preset goals for therapy (i.e., objective measures of signs or symptoms)?
6. How long should the drug be used before decreasing a dosage or discontinuing it? Will this be at a specific time or based on a change in the patient's condition?
7. Is there duplication of the specific drug with other drugs the patient is taking or overlap of therapeutic or adverse effects of other drugs being taken?

8. Are the dose and timing correct? Is the drug being administered correctly?
9. Are there potential drug–drug, drug–disease, or drug–nutritional interactions?
10. Is the patient being adequately monitored for common serious side effects (e.g., periodic blood levels, functional and mental status tests, movement disorder scales)?
11. If side effects are present, is there a positive balance of the risks and benefits? Are the negative effects of treatment outweighed by the positive aspects (e.g., improving, maintaining, or slowing decline of resident function or alleviating suffering)?

> **Practice Pearl ▶▶▶** Before administering any medication to an older person, it is important to undertake a risk–benefit analysis. In consultation with the physician, patient, and family, the nurse should discuss the risks versus the benefit of the medication. If the risks are perceived to be too great, a nonpharmacological approach to the patient's problem should be considered.

QSEN Recommendations Related to Pharmacology

The Quality and Safety Education for Nurses (QSEN) project addresses the challenge of preparing future nurses with the knowledge, skills, and attitudes (KSAs) to continuously improve the quality and safety of the healthcare systems in which they work (Cronenwett et al., 2007). See the QSEN table for tips on meeting QSEN standards.

BOX 6-10 ▶ **Indications for Use of Anxiolytic Medications**

Use is for one of the following indications as defined in the DSM-IV-TR or subsequent editions:

a. Generalized anxiety disorder
b. Panic disorder
c. Symptomatic anxiety that occurs in residents with another diagnosed psychiatric disorder
d. Sleep disorders
e. Acute alcohol or benzodiazepine withdrawal
f. Significant anxiety in response to a situational trigger
g. Delirium, dementia, and other cognitive disorders with associated behaviors that:
  Are quantitatively and objectively documented;
  Are persistent;

Are not due to preventable or correctable reasons; and
Constitute clinically significant distress or dysfunction to the resident or represent a danger to the resident or others; or
Evidence exists that other possible reasons for the individual's distress have been considered; and
Use results in maintenance or improvement in the individual's mental, physical, or psychosocial well-being (e.g., as reflected on the MDS or other assessment tools); or
There are clinical situations that warrant the use of these medications such as a long-acting benzodiazepine is being used to withdraw a resident from a short-acting benzodiazepine used for neuromuscular syndromes (e.g., cerebral palsy, tardive dyskinesia, restless leg syndrome or seizure disorders); and symptom relief in end of life situations.

Source: Centers for Medicare and Medicaid Services (CMS). (2011). *State operations manual appendix PP: Guidance to surveyors for long-term care facilities.* Retrieved from http://www.cms.hhs.gov/manuals/Downloads/som107ap_pp_guidelines_ltcf.pdf.

Meeting QSEN Standards: Pharmacology

	KNOWLEDGE	SKILLS	ATTITUDES
Patient-Centered Care	Involvement of patient and family in drug regimen is crucial.	Family assessment Adult learning principles.	Appreciate uniqueness of each patient/family.
	Examine barriers that may lead to medication errors or adverse drug reactions.	Evaluate for depression, vision/hearing, cognitive status.	Provide patient-centered care to improve successful nursing outcomes.
Teamwork and Collaboration	Recognize need for input from interdisciplinary team members including dietitian, pharmacist, physician, advanced practice nurses, and others on the team to reduce risk of adverse drug reactions and medication errors.	Use leadership skills to coordinate team and share knowledge.	Value the contribution of each member of the team to improve outcomes.
	Be aware of organizational problems that can inhibit effective team functioning and establish plan for communication.	System assessment skills.	Be open to input from team members on effective means to improve communication and collaboration.
Evidence-Based Practice	Describe effective interventions to decrease risk factors and improve overall health and function. Utilize Beer's criteria and FDA recommendations as appropriate.	Access current evidence-based protocols to guide interventions.	Possess confidence in necessary skills to evaluate and incorporate nursing interventions from the literature.
Quality Improvement	Recognize the need for patient–family education regarding early recognition of adverse drug reactions.	Skills in data management, technology, and U.S. government and FDA sites describing current incidence and prevalence of ADRs and medication errors.	Value the use of data and outcomes as a key component of QI efforts.
Safety	Describe common medication errors and patient–family characteristics that increase the likelihood of such errors.	Use appropriate strategies to provide written information to compensate for memory loss (if present).	Appreciate the impact of cognitive loss on the occurrence of adverse drug reactions.
Informatics	Provide input into the formation and maintenance of patient databases needed for gathering QSEN data and providing patient care.	Utilize the electronic health record.	Protect patient confidentiality according to HIPAA standards.

Medication Management

The nurse has a major role in promoting the safe and effective management of medications, whether the patient is at home or in an institutional setting. This includes the correct storage, preparation, and administration (right patient, right drug, right dose, right route, and right time).

Identification of patients by ID bracelets is important, especially with older persons who may have hearing or cognitive deficits and may not respond appropriately to a name being called.

In the home setting, the patient or family members assume the responsibilities of medication management. The nurse can help them to do this safely through patient and family teaching. The nurse also is responsible for promoting the intended therapeutic effect or reducing or eliminating the need for the medication (see examples in Table 6-2, page 136). See Box 6-11 for a description of the criteria for successful medication management. Perhaps most important in any setting is to have an understanding of the older person's unique patterns of behavior and physiological functions so that the nurse can detect unusual responses that might result in the need to initiate or discontinue a medication. It is also important to document indications that the therapeutic effect is or is not being achieved. Examples would be reduction of fever in a patient receiving anti-infectives or decrease in blood pressure in a patient receiving antihypertensives.

Monitoring for adverse effects is another important role. This includes observation of the patient for known adverse effects of a medication as well as more general symptoms that might be drug related (e.g., nausea, loss of appetite, cognitive changes). Monitoring laboratory tests such as potassium levels in patients receiving thiazide diuretics or International Normalized Ratio (INR) in patients on warfarin therapy is another important role. Prevention of adverse drug effects involves checking the patient's history for allergies and using knowledge of drug pharmacology to detect potential or actual interactions or contraindications.

In institutional settings, additional precautions are necessary to ensure the safe administration of medications. Institutional policies and practices need to be reviewed periodically to reduce medication errors. If patients are allowed to administer their own medications, policies should be in place that reflect applicable state laws and provide protection for patients. Computerized drug prescribing and the use of bar coding on medications is becoming the standard for reducing medication errors. Medication labels have bar codes similar to those used in grocery stores. When administering the drug, the nurse scans both the patient ID bracelet and the drug label. The computer then determines if the matches are correct in light of the physician's orders.

Delegation of Medication Administration

Whether or not it is legal for the nurse to delegate responsibility for administering medication to an unlicensed person (i.e., unlicensed assistive personnel or UAP) depends on state laws. Some states allow the delegation of medication administration in certain settings or under certain conditions, while others specify that the delegation of administration is specifically not permitted. The nurse needs to be aware of the legal aspects of delegation of medication administration for the state in which he or she practices as well as the policies of the employing agency. Delegation does not remove responsibility from the nurse for assessing and monitoring the patient for therapeutic and adverse effects. In assisted living settings, some states may allow unlicensed assistive personnel to supervise that the resident is taking his or her medications (Mitty & Flores, 2007a, 2007b).

Promoting Adherence

The use of the term *noncompliance* is objectionable to some patients and clinicians since it implies a patient must surrender to the orders of the clinician. Some prefer the term *adherence*. Adherence with a prescribed regimen presumably leads to better patient outcomes (Gould & Mitty, 2010). Nonadherence with medication regimens results in considerable costs to patients, employers, health insurers, and the healthcare system. Estimates of nonadherence usually range from 40% to 60%, depending on the definition used (Wu, Moser, Lennie et al., 2008).

Weblink: Medication List Form

BOX 6-11 ▸ **Medication Management**

Medication management supports and promotes:

- Selection of medications(s) based on assessing relative benefits and risks to the individual resident;
- Evaluation of a [patient's] signs and symptoms, in order to identify the underlying cause(s), including adverse consequences of medications;
- Selection and use of medications in doses and for the duration appropriate to each resident's clinical conditions, age, and underlying causes of symptoms;
- The use of nonpharmacological interventions, when applicable, to minimize the need for medications, permit use of the lowest possible dose, or allow medications to be discontinued; and
- The monitoring of medications for efficacy and clinically significant adverse consequences.

Source: Centers for Medicare and Medicaid Services (CMS). (2011). *State operations manual appendix PP: Guidance to surveyors for long-term care facilities.* Retrieved from http://www.cms.hhs.gov/manuals/Downloads/som107ap_pp_guidelines_ltcf.pdf.

Although medication adherence has been studied, no interventions have been shown to be effective in all patients. The use of pillboxes is a common strategy of older patients and can serve as a reminder to take medications and simplify complicated dosing schedules. Developing personal systems by looking at each patient's life routines and their impact on medication taking may help to improve adherence (Russell, Ruppar, & Matteson, 2011).

> **Practice Pearl** ▶▶▶ Download a free medication list form for patients to use. Encourage patients to use this type of form, keep it updated, and bring it with them on visits to the hospital or physicians.

The nurse can be instrumental in promoting compliance and appropriate management of drug therapy by older patients or their caregivers in the home. Some community-dwelling older adults may reduce their medication dosage or discontinue a drug if they experience side effects that are bothersome or that they felt their prescriber did not address. Nurses can help patients cope with side effects and help them to continue with their medication regimen.

The higher number of drugs usually prescribed for older people makes drug regimens more complex. Cognitive changes resulting from aging processes, pathophysiological alterations, or drug therapy need to be carefully assessed (initially and on an ongoing basis) to determine if the patient is able to understand and remember instructions. Physical limitations may affect the patient's ability to open medication vials and packaging or to administer certain types of medications. The more complicated the dosing regimen, the more pills taken daily, and the more often pills must be taken, the greater the chance of error and adverse drug reactions.

The following nursing diagnoses are useful for describing situations requiring nursing intervention to promote the effective use of medications by patients: *Noncompliance (specify); Therapeutic Regimen Management, Ineffective; or Therapeutic Regimen Management, Family.*

Various levels of cognitive and physical skills are needed by the older person to safely take medications as prescribed. Patients should be asked to perform these tasks for each of the prescription and nonprescription medications that they are taking. Depending on the drug and route of administration, the nurse should assess the following factors: ability to read and comprehend main label (prescription), ability to read and comprehend the auxiliary labels (e.g., warnings), and manual dexterity (open vials, remove correct number of tablets, recap medication) (Hartford Institute for Geriatric Nursing, 1999).

Measures to help older people manage their medications correctly include:

- Simplifying the regimen by decreasing, to the extent possible, the number of drugs and the number of pills to be taken in a day.

- Establishing a routine for taking medications, such as preparing medications for the day in different containers.
- Scheduling medications at mealtime or in conjunction with other specific daily activities (e.g., before brushing teeth at night or before leaving for a daily activity such as exercise or card playing) unless contraindicated. When teaching a patient to take medications in relation to meals, it is important to determine if the patient does indeed have three meals a day and at what time of day to be sure the medication will be taken at the intended time interval.
- Developing a method with the patient for remembering if he or she actually took the medication (e.g., moving the medication to another place).
- Conducting a total assessment of all medications by asking the patient to bring in all medications he or she has at home, including OTC and herbal preparations. These can be checked for outdated preparations, unused or unfinished prescriptions, overlap, or duplication of medications.
- Considering the use of telephone reminders or computer-based or e-mail reminders.

Encouraging patients to obtain all of their medications (prescription and OTC) from the same pharmacy will help the pharmacist to monitor medication use. Patients can request that prescribed drugs be dispensed without the childproof packaging or caps. However, one needs to consider possible dangers to children who might visit the patient's home.

It is important to determine any financial restraints that may affect the patient's ability to actually obtain the medication. Less expensive mail-order options may be available. Some states and the federal government may provide assistance to some older adults with high medication expenses. See further details in the section in this chapter on financial considerations in medication use.

> **Practice Pearl** ▶▶▶ If a medication is not demonstrating the expected therapeutic effect in a patient, the nurse should investigate carefully. The patient may not be taking the medication at all or as prescribed because of cost and may be embarrassed to share this information.

When the nurse suspects that the older patient is not taking medications as prescribed because of financial difficulties, it is suggested that the following steps be initiated:

- Assess the patient's financial situation. It is not necessary to know the actual income of a patient, but rather ask questions such as "Do you have enough money to buy food and medicine without difficulty?" "Do you sometimes put off refilling your medicine because of lack of money?"
- Consult with the physician and pharmacist to see if a generic brand of the medication or lower cost drug is an option.

■ Seek advice from the geriatric social worker who may be aware of government-sponsored, pharmaceutical company–sponsored, and private patient assistance programs. Many of these programs offer medications at low cost, no cost, or significant discounts.

Some patients may experience difficulty in physically obtaining the prescriptions, especially if they are on multiple medications with frequent and different dates for refill. Coordination of refills with the prescribing clinician and the pharmacist may help to alleviate stress on the patient and family as well as help to ensure that the patient has an adequate supply of medications.

Careful instruction should be given, providing written instructions in the language and at a reading level the patient can understand. Most prescriptions are dispensed with written information about the medication. An audiotape could be used for patients with visual impairments. Materials should be written at the fifth-grade level or lower. Instructions should include what adverse effects should be reported and to whom as well as what to do if a dose is missed. The nurse needs to consider possible vision and hearing deficits, decreased attention span, and decline in cognitive function that may affect the learning processes of the older individual. If possible, a family member or home caregiver should also receive instructions.

Health literacy has been found to be associated with poor health outcomes and even increased mortality. Providing information does not necessarily increase patient's knowledge. Health professionals believe that written health information is important for adherence and should be brief and include information about adverse effects. Many patients, however, prefer that the information be individualized to their particular situation and that written information not be a substitute for information provided orally by the prescriber. They want information on the benefits and possible harm so that they can decide on whether or not to take a medication and, if they were taking a medicine, how to manage it and how to interpret any symptoms they may have (Raynor et al., 2007).

★ Drug Safety

Concern for drug safety includes institutional as well as home and other community settings.

Nurses' responsibilities for assuring older patients' safe and effective use of medication occurs in a variety of settings—wherever the patient is located. Medication errors can occur in any setting, including the patient's home. The "five rights" of drug administration are important, but additional aspects, such as organizational policies and procedures designed to prevent errors, need to be included whenever considering the problem of medication errors. Nurses can play a leadership role in looking at the entire medication system, reporting any problems, and recommending improvements for improved safety.

Medication Reconciliation

As many as 50% of all medication errors and up to 20% of adverse drug events in the hospital can be attributed to poor communication of medical information at transition points (Midelfort, 2012). The medication reconciliation process should be used whenever an individual moves from one care setting to another.

Medication reconciliation involves identifying an accurate list of all medications a patient is taking (name, dosage, frequency, route, and patient's medical history), verifying that the medications and dosages are appropriate for the patient and the patient is taking the medications correctly, and then comparing these medications with the physician's admission, transfer, and/or discharge orders and reconciling or resolving any discrepancies. When interviewing a patient about his or her medications use the following tips in order to obtain the most accurate information. Ask a variety of open-ended and yes/no answer questions: avoid medical jargon as it has the potential to increase the chances of error; ask specifically about over the counter medications, herbal remedies, vitamin and mineral supplements, patches, creams, inhalers, and other items as some older people may not include them in their list of medications; make sure to clear up any discrepancies in the medication list and use medical records, medication lists, family member's recollection, and, with the patient's permission, contact previous healthcare providers and all pharmacies from which the patient has obtained current or past prescriptions (in general, it is safer for older patients to obtain all of their medications from one pharmacy to increase the probability that drug interactions could be identified and changes made before an adverse drug interaction can occur); question patients carefully about allergies to make sure that drug side effects or intolerances are not noted to be allergies; inquire as to how/when and why each medication is taken to determine adherence to health care provider's instructions; and urge patients to keep a current list of medications that can be brought to each visit with all health care providers (including specialists) in order to decrease prescription duplication, adverse drug interactions, and omission of key drugs.

Sometimes patient medications may be stored in another container (e.g., pillbox) and it may be necessary to identify the medication. Help in identifying a pill based on its physical characteristics, such as color, shape, and coding, can be found at several websites. *However, in a suspected overdose, a poison control center should be contacted immediately.*

Use of Internet Pharmacies

Medications can be purchased online from legitimate pharmacies. However, some websites may be risky. Sites should require a prescription from a prescriber who is familiar with the patient and should have policies for verifying prescriptions. They also should have policies that ensure privacy and

FDA Tips to Help Protect You If You Buy Medicines Online

Know Your Source to Make Sure It's Safe. Make sure a website is a state-licensed pharmacy that is located in the United States. Pharmacies and pharmacists in the United States are licensed by a state's board of pharmacy. Your state board of pharmacy can tell you if a website is a state-licensed pharmacy, is in good standing, and is located in the United States. Find a list of state boards of pharmacy on the National Association of Boards of Pharmacy (NABP) website at www.nabp.info. The NABP is a professional association of the state boards of pharmacy. It has a program to help you find some of the pharmacies that are licensed to sell medicine online. Websites that display the seal of this program have been checked to make sure they meet state and federal rules. For more on this program and a list of pharmacies that display the Verified Internet Pharmacy Practice Sites™ Seal (VIPPS® Seal), go to www.vipps.info.

Look for Websites With Practices That Protect You. A safe website should:

Be located in the United States and licensed by the state board of pharmacy where the website is operating (check www.nabp.info for a list of state boards of pharmacy)

Have a licensed pharmacist to answer your questions

Require a prescription from your doctor or other healthcare professional who is licensed in the United States to write prescriptions for medicine

Have a way for you to talk to a person if you have problems.

Be Sure Your Privacy Is Protected. Look for privacy and security policies that are easy to find and easy to understand. Don't give any personal information (such as Social Security number, credit card, or medical or health history) unless you are sure the website will keep your information safe and private. Make sure the site will not sell your information unless you agree to let them do so.

Source: U.S. Food and Drug Administration. (2012). *Buying prescription medicine online: A consumer safety guide*. Retrieved from http://www.fda.gov/buyonlineguide.

confidentiality. The legitimacy of a pharmacy can be checked by contacting the state board of pharmacy or the National Association of Boards of Pharmacy (NABP). If a website displays NABP VIPPS (Verified Internet Pharmacy Practice Site), this ensures that the site meets all applicable state and federal requirements. Box 6-12 contains suggestions from the FDA for ordering medications over the Internet.

Practice Pearl ▶▶▶ The nurse should inform older patients and families that medications bought on the Internet or illegally imported from other countries may be counterfeit, expired, or contaminated. Although credentialed Canadian pharmacies are generally safe, there are many bogus providers victimizing older Americans. These illegal drugs may cause more harm than good.

Medication Use During Emergencies

Patients should be assisted in making plans for continuing their drug therapy in emergencies and natural disasters. A basic emergency supply kit (preferably waterproof) should include a first-aid kit, at least a 3-day supply of medications, copies of prescription medication names and doses, and OTC medications for pain (e.g., acetaminophen or aspirin, antidiarrhea medication, and antacid). Box 6-13 outlines considerations for use of medications that have been exposed to flooding or dirty water or have not been refrigerated.

Unsafe Medication Practices

Older patients should be cautioned to avoid certain risky medication behaviors such as these:

- **Sharing others' medications.** Sometimes older persons share their medications with each other. They should be cautioned that this practice is unwise and that they should take only medications prescribed for them.
- **Using imported medications.** The use of medication imported from or obtained in another country is controversial and is considered illegal. Some health professionals are concerned that imported medications may not meet the quality standards of drugs approved for use in the United States. Others claim that some drugs from other countries such as Canada come from the same drug manufacturers as the medications sold in the United States.
- **Using outdated medications.** The use of medications that are outdated is risky. The medications not only may be ineffective but also can actually cause injury to the heart, liver, or kidneys. It is unwise to use old medications in an attempt to save money.

Drug Safety After Natural Disasters

Flood and Unsafe Water

Discard all exposed drugs (including pills, oral liquids, drugs for injection, inhalers, skin medications). Reconstitute drugs only with purified or bottled water.

Drugs Requiring Refrigeration (e.g., Insulin and Reconstituted Drugs)

If electrical power has been off for a long time, the drug should be discarded. However, if the drug is absolutely necessary to sustain life (insulin, for example), it may be used until a new supply is available.

Unopened insulin products may be left unrefrigerated (between 59° and 86°F) for up to 28 days and still maintain potency.

Source: U.S. Food and Drug Administration. (2012). *Information regarding insulin storage and switching between products in an emergency*. Retrieved from http://www.fda.gov/Drugs/EmergencyPreparedness/ucm085213.htm.

Safe Storage and Disposal of Medications

If older persons request that they receive their prescription medications without childproof caps, they need to take special precautions if young children are present in the home, even for a short duration. Medications should be routinely reviewed to be sure that they have not reached their expiration date. Generally medications should not be kept longer than a year. Because sewage treatment facilities may not be able to remove all medicines from the water and thereby harm fish and wildlife, flushing medicines down the toilet is no longer recommended by the Environmental Protection Agency (EPA). There are programs for safe disposal at some pharmacies (e.g., Walgreens, RiteAid, CVS) where patients purchase a mailing envelope and send their unused medications to a place where they are disposed of safely. In addition, the Nationwide Safe Medication Disposal Program usually has a special day for disposing of medications in various communities. Patients may also contact their city or town or ask their pharmacist about the best way to dispose of medications. Some communities have specials days for residents to bring in expired or unused medications.

Obtaining Medications Outside of the United States

Patients may consider obtaining medications in another country when they are traveling or to obtain medications less expensively. In addition to concerns about the purity of drugs in some countries, confusion may occur about drug brand names. Patients should be cautioned about buying drugs outside of the United States because different drug brand names may lead to issuing of a drug with different ingredients than the U.S. drug. The FDA has identified 103 U.S. brand names that look or sound similar to those in other countries but have different ingredients. For example, Urex in the United States has methenamine, which is used to treat urinary tract infections. Its active ingredient has the same brand name in Australia but its active ingredient is furosemide, a diuretic. Rubex is a brand name for doxorubicin for treatment of cancer in the United States but is the name for ascorbic acid in Ireland (FDA, 2006).

Healthcare Fraud

Healthcare fraud is a major problem for the older person because many older people have chronic conditions such as arthritis and cancer, and they are more likely to be susceptible to claims of unproven remedies. In addition to wasting money, unproven remedies pose two major dangers: (1) from the preparation itself, which may be impure, toxic, or incompatible with the patient and ongoing therapy; and (2) from delay in or rejection of accurate diagnosis and treatment.

Clinicians should be able to answer questions patients may have about health products advertised in the media. They can provide guidelines to patients about how to evaluate claims. Some red flags to watch for include celebrity endorsements, inadequate labeling, claims that the product works by means of a secret formula, and promotion of the treatment only in the back pages of magazines, over the phone, by direct mail, in newspaper ads in the format of news stories, or in 30-minute infomercials (Kurtzweil, 1999). Other clues are claims that a product is all natural or effective for a wide variety of disorders (e.g., cancer, arthritis, and sexual dysfunction), or that it works immediately or completely, making visits to the doctor unnecessary.

Assessing Older Patients' Appropriate Use of Medications

Nurses should assess the medications used by older patients in all settings: acute care, long-term care, or at home. Assessment of drug effects is a nursing responsibility whether or not the nurse administers medications to the patient. The nurse should follow these guidelines:

1. Review the patient's medical conditions and allergies. Ask about the use of grapefruit juice since this can dramatically increase the absorption of some medications. Ask for details about an allergy: "What happened when you took this drug?" Sometimes the patient uses the word *allergy* to describe an intolerance such as upset stomach. Be sure the patient's records have appropriate alerts warning of any allergies. Check patients for MedicAlert jewelry or cards indicating that they are taking certain medications or have certain allergies.
2. Review each drug. If patients are living at home, have them assemble all medications for review whether prescribed or OTC, including vitamins and herbal remedies. This is sometimes called a "brown bag" review because patients often bring their medications in a brown bag.
   a. Has it been prescribed? If not prescribed, does the physician prescribing other drugs for the patient know the patient is taking this OTC or herbal preparation? When was it prescribed? Has continued need for it been reviewed by the physician?
   b. Is the drug considered to be inappropriate for use in older persons?
   c. Is the patient taking it as prescribed with regard to the dose, route, frequency, and timing in relation to food or other medications, method (e.g., with fluid or food), and duration?

d. Is the medication producing the intended therapeutic effect? Are appropriate observations or laboratory tests being used to determine this and are they documented in the patient record (e.g., blood pressure readings to evaluate effects of antihypertensives)?

e. Is the medication outdated? Is it being stored properly (e.g., refrigerated, away from sunlight or heat, away from reach of small children)?

f. Does the patient understand what condition the drug is treating and the signs and symptoms that should be reported to a physician immediately?

g. Does the patient have any cognitive or physical condition affecting the ability to safely administer the medication (i.e., remembering to take the medication, ability to read labels, ability to physically handle and administer the medication)?

h. Does the patient have financial resources for the costs of the medication? Is there a generic version of this drug (or another that is equally effective for the patient's condition) available that would be less expensive? Is the patient able to manage obtaining and renewing prescriptions?

i. Does the patient have any cultural or ethnic beliefs or practices that might impact compliance? A person from a culture that believes in balancing "hot" and "cold" or yin and yang may not take certain prescribed medications that do not fit these beliefs. Sometimes a different medication or another brand of the same medication is acceptable.

j. Does the patient have a family member or friend who can help with medication management on a regular basis if needed (e.g., if the patient becomes ill)?

k. Review each drug for:
   - Interactions with other drugs
   - Interactions with herbal medicines
   - Interactions with vitamins or foods
   - Allergies
   - Duplicate therapy (from more than one prescriber or from patient's use of OTC medications containing the same or similar ingredients as prescribed medications)

Financial Considerations in Medication Use

Medications can be costly for the older person and may be a factor in nonadherence to prescribed drugs. Financial pressures may result in people taking dangerous actions related to prescription drugs. The Consumer Reports National Research Center (2011) reports that in 2011 the percentage of those skimping on their medications rose from 39% to 48%. This includes not filling prescriptions, taking expired medications, skipping a scheduled dose, splitting pills in half inappropriately, and sharing prescription medications with someone else.

Medicare Part D

In January 2006, Medicare Part D prescription drug coverage went into effect and has assisted many with their drug costs. However, many older adults' drug costs are not completely met by this plan. Some individuals have difficulty paying monthly premiums, copayments, and/or the full costs of prescription drugs once they have reached the coverage gap (often referred to as the "donut hole"). The "donut hole" coverage gap is when enrollees have had to assume total costs for their prescription drugs after a certain amount has been spent in a calendar year. In January 2011 Medicare began a transition to closing this coverage gap during the next 10 years until it is closed in 2020. At that point after an individual has paid a certain amount for prescription drugs, he or she will qualify for catastrophic coverage and only be responsible for 5% of his or her prescription drug costs for the rest of the calendar year.

Extensive information about each Part D drug plan available in the patient's state can be found on the Medicare website, including performance ratings for each plan.

Although participation in Medicare Plan D is voluntary, an individual who does not participate and later wishes to enroll must pay a financial penalty on his or her monthly premium. Some individuals who have "creditable" prescription drug coverage through their employer's retirement plan would not be subjected to the extra charge. Creditable coverage means that the employer's retirement plan offers prescription drug coverage equal to or superior to that offered through the independent prescription drug plans. Each plan varies by the medications covered and a list is included in the plan's formulary along with the amount of monthly premiums, deductibles, and copayments. Most plans have a lower copayment (or even waive the copayment) for generic drugs. The covered drugs (i.e., the drugs in each plan's formulary) can be changed by the plan with 60 days notice. For some more expensive drugs, the patient must obtain prior approval and/or have step therapy, which means that generic drugs or another drug to treat the patient's condition must be tried first. Individuals can change or re-enroll in a plan each year during the preceding 3-month period. The website for Medicare Part D allows individuals to enter information about their drugs and their preferred pharmacy. The older person then receives information about the costs and coverage of each plan offered in their area.

Medicare Part D coverage reduces medication costs for many but not all patients. Since Medicare Part D coverage does not cover the cost of all prescription drugs, the nurse should encourage patients to contact a SHINE (Serving the Health Information Needs of Elders) counselor or go to the BenefitsCheckUpRx website, which will tell an individual about governmental programs and subsidies that he or she may not be aware of. SHINE is a program that provides free, unbiased information about Medicare and other health insurance benefits. Please refer to individual state websites related to aging and older adults for information about how to contact a counselor or how to volunteer to become a certified counselor.

Additional suggestions to patients to reduce costs of medications include the following:

- Ask the physician if the drug is really necessary or if there is a less expensive substitute.
- Ask the physician about free samples.
- Do not order a large amount of a newly prescribed medication until you know that it is effective and that you can tolerate it.
- Ask if there is a generic version of the medication.
- Contact different pharmacies; shop around.
- Ask the pharmacist about store-brand substitutes for more expensive brand-name OTC medications.
- Ask for senior citizen discounts.

- Contact the American Association of Retired People (AARP) or disease organizations for information about drugs that might be available at a discount.
- Go to the BenefitsCheckUpRx website at the National Council on the Aging to determine eligibility for help from community, state, or federal programs, or from drug companies.
- Try mail-order prescriptions. Copayments are usually less when obtained through mail-order pharmacies.
- Try Internet pharmacies.
- Apply for help. Contact Social Security at 800-772-1213.
- Try national and community-based charitable programs.
- Look for pharmaceutical assistance programs and patient assistance programs offered by drug manufacturers.

Patient and Family Teaching

Gerontological nurses require skills and knowledge related to teaching patients and families about the key concepts of gerontology and gerontological nursing. The patient–family teaching guidelines in the following feature will assist the nurse to assume the role of teacher and coach. Educating patients and families is critical so that nurses can interpret scientific data and individualize the nursing care plan.

Patient–Family Teaching Guidelines

The following are guidelines that the nurse may find useful when instructing older persons and their families about medications and drug safety.

MEDICATIONS AND THE OLDER ADULT

1 **I am taking a lot of medications prescribed by my doctor. How do I know if they are all safe?**

Medications can be lifesaving and promote health and quality of life. However, you enter into a partnership with your doctor when you agree to take a medication he or she prescribes for you. Here are some suggestions for taking medication safely:

- Inform your doctor of all allergies, medical problems, drug reactions, OTC medications, herbal remedies, and recreational drugs (including tobacco and alcohol) that you use.
- Ask about how to take the drug. Possible questions might include: Does "two tablets a day" mean two in the morning?

One in the morning and one at night? Should it be taken with water? Should I sit up after taking the medication? Can I take it at the same time as my other medications? What should I do if I am ill and cannot take the medication?

- Ask about alternatives to the medication. Are there dietary or lifestyle changes that might decrease the need for, or dose of, the medication?

- What are the common side effects? What should be reported immediately?

- If you are on multiple medications, go over the schedule with your nurse. Write it down so you can keep the schedule in your wallet or pocketbook.

Patient-Family Teaching Guidelines *(continued)*

- Take the exact amount as prescribed.
- Do not share medications with others.
- Ask if you can drink alcohol. If so, ask how much is safe.
- Check for expiration dates on your medicine and throw away expired bottles. The medications may be unsafe to take.
- Take all medications as prescribed, even if you are feeling better. Check with your doctor or nurse before stopping a medication in the middle of the treatment.
- Adhere to lab tests, blood pressure checks, and ongoing monitoring so that your doctor can keep track of the effectiveness and safety of your medications.

RATIONALE:

Empowering the patient to ask questions and teaching about appropriate use of medications can help to decrease anxiety about the prescribed medications and the therapeutic regimen.

Any drug or substance used by the patient may interfere with or interact with prescribed medications. This also can avoid duplicative therapy such as when a patient uses an OTC drug that may contain an ingredient in a prescribed drug (e.g., caffeine, aspirin).

Answers to these questions can help the patient develop an appropriate and convenient schedule for taking medications. Promotes patient involvement in the therapeutic regimen.

Helps the patient to be aware of measures he or she can take to manage medications and his or her condition.

Helps patient to know when a symptom is urgent and which can be delayed in reporting to physician.

Helps patient to remember when and how to take medications. Provides a visual reminder.

Emphasizes that dose is prescribed in order to have full therapeutic effect and to avoid adverse effects.

Sharing medications is dangerous and may be illegal. Another person may have a different condition, have an allergy to the medication, or may take other medications that may interact.

Cautions the patient that alcohol is also a drug and can interact with other medications.

Drugs beyond the expiration date may have deteriorated and are no longer effective; some may be toxic if used.

If drug therapy is stopped, the patient may have a relapse of symptoms. Adverse effects can occur with some drugs if they are discontinued abruptly. Antibiotics may cause resistance in microorganisms if the patient discontinues the antibiotic before the end of the prescribed time. Promotes involvement of the patient in the overall therapeutic regimen.

2 **As my nurse, how can you help me to take medications safely?**

As your nurse, I would like to review your medications with you at every clinic visit. This should be done on a regular basis and after every acute care hospitalization because many medicines are changed when you go to the hospital. I will also make sure that you have not started taking any new OTC medications or herbal remedies that could interact with your prescription medicine. I will ask you questions regarding dizziness, rashes, constipation, dry mouth, or other changes to make sure you are tolerating your medications without side effects. I will also let you know if there are any warnings or changes regarding the safety or interactions of your medications. If you would like, I will write out medication instructions for you after you have seen the doctor so that you can refer to the instructions at home if you have questions.

RATIONALE:

Reviewing patients' medications can further enhance the nurse–patient relationship, provide opportunities for teaching, and can help the patient to see the nurse as a helpful resource.
Alerts patient to topics that the nurse will cover.

3 **What is the pharmacist's responsibility?**

Tell your pharmacist if you have trouble reading small labels or opening the childproof prescription bottles. If you request bottles without childproof caps, store them in a safe place if grandchildren or neighborhood children are visiting your home. Try not to store medications in a bathroom medicine cabinet if you take long, steamy showers. The humidity can cause the medication to break down and become ineffective.

Be sure to ask questions about the name of the medication, and go over instructions regarding dosage and how to take it. Check the label before you leave the pharmacy. Make sure you have the correct prescription. If the medication looks different, check with the pharmacist to verify there is no error. Medication safety is a team effort, and you and your family are the key players on the team. Remember, medicines that are strong enough to cure you can also hurt you if they are not used correctly. Do not be afraid to ask questions and advocate for your own safety.

RATIONALE:

Including the pharmacist as part of the therapeutic team provides the patient with an additional and valuable resource for help in medication management.

CARE PLAN A Patient Experiencing a Possible Adverse Drug Reaction

Case Study

Mrs. Nash is a 75-year-old widow. She lives alone and has two children and five grandchildren ages 2 through 12 who visit regularly. Her prescribed medications are "baby aspirin," a beta-blocker, a thiazide diuretic, and warfarin. Her non-prescribed OTC medications are a multivitamin, vitamin C, vitamin E, calcium tablets, and Bayer PM for sleep. For an upset stomach she takes Tums, and for a headache either aspirin or acetaminophen. She also has been taking a laxative for some constipation she has developed recently. She is concerned about feeling "washed out," sleeping poorly,

and feeling chronic fatigue. Within the last 2 weeks, she has not been able to do her usual daily half-mile walk.

Her 24-hour diet recall revealed the following:

- Breakfast: grapefruit juice, blueberry muffin, coffee with cream
- Lunch: grilled cheese, tea
- Late afternoon: glass of milk with cookies
- Dinner: cheese with crackers and wine, broiled chicken, peas, carrots, mashed potato, butter, chocolate ice cream
- Bedtime snack: coffee-flavored yogurt

Applying the Nursing Process

Assessment

Several factors may be contributing to Mrs. Nash's fatigue. A holistic assessment is needed. The nurse should consider malnutrition, constipation, depression, adverse drug effects, and polypharmacy.

Constipation may be a side effect of beta-blockers, and also can be caused by her calcium intake from calcium tablets, Tums, ice cream, yogurt, and cheese.

Beta-blockers can cause depression with long-term use and also may affect a person's ability to exercise due to a "braking" effect on cardiac response. Hypnotics could be causing a "hangover" effect. Mrs. Nash also may be experiencing hypokalemia from thiazide diuretics, especially since she has not had potassium-rich foods such as oranges, apricots, bananas, or prune juice.

Her use of grapefruit juice may increase the absorption of some of her drugs, causing toxic effects. Vitamin C may be affecting the renal excretion of some of her medications.

She is on the oral anticoagulant warfarin, and a major concern would be the level of anticoagulation. It would be important to know when the last INR was checked and the results. It also would be important to check on whether

she has been taking the correct dose. The nurse should assess Mrs. Nash for other indications of bleeding such as hematuria, blood in stools, decreased blood pressure, and postural blood pressure. The nurse should also inquire about recent headaches that might suggest bleeding.

Mrs. Nash is taking nonprescribed OTC medications that should be avoided in patients taking warfarin. She has been prescribed a small daily dose of aspirin, but on her own she has been taking aspirin for headaches and Bayer PM, which also contains aspirin. Vitamin E prolongs bleeding. Acetaminophen also can affect her INR reading. Many drugs that affect the INR of patients on warfarin can be used if they are given daily on a regular basis and the warfarin dosage is established while the patient is taking the same daily dose of the medications.

The patient's total caffeine intake (coffee, tea, and chocolate) should be reviewed and may be contributing to her sleeping difficulty. Caffeine should be avoided in the evening. The nurse can suggest that she use decaffeinated coffee and tea and that she have a glass of warm milk to produce a hypnotic effect from the natural tryptophan content.

Diagnosis

The current nursing diagnoses for Mrs. Nash include the following:

- *Sleep Pattern, Disturbed*
- *Imbalanced Nutrition: Less Than Body Requirements*
- *Activity Intolerance*
- *Constipation*
- *Poisoning: Risk for* (through polypharmacy)
- *Ineffective Coping* (possible depression)

NANDA-I © 2012.

CARE PLAN | **A Patient Experiencing a Possible Adverse Drug Reaction** *(continued)*

Expected Outcomes

Expected outcomes for the plan of care specify that Mrs. Nash will:

- Become aware of the harmful effects of poor diet on overall health and function.
- Utilize sleep hygiene measures to improve sleep.
- Develop a more trusting relationship with her physician to schedule monitoring of her physical and psychological status (including monitoring her INR and dose adjustment of warfarin).
- Agree to establish a therapeutic relationship with the nurse and develop a mutually acceptable plan to work toward these outcomes.

Planning and Implementation

The following nursing interventions may be appropriate for Mrs. Nash:

- Establish a therapeutic relationship.
- Educate Mrs. Nash regarding eating a balanced diet.
- Increase fluid and fiber intake to ease constipation. Measures to offset the constipation would be to decrease cheese intake, increase bulk in diet (e.g., bran muffins or cereal, adding a salad to her lunch and dinner), increasing fruit intake (e.g., apple), and increasing her fluid intake and level of exercise.
- Encourage Mrs. Nash to begin her daily walking regimen.
- Encourage a family meeting to talk about health issues in general with the patient's permission.
- Begin a sleep assessment to establish the underlying cause of Mrs. Nash's sleep disturbance.
- Begin a values clarification to establish long-term goals and facilitate end-of-life planning.

Evaluation

The nurse hopes to work with Mrs. Nash over time and to form a therapeutic relationship with her. The nurse will consider the plan a success based on the following criteria:

- Mrs. Nash will continue to engage in her daily walk.
- A family meeting will be held to discuss her overall health.
- Mrs. Nash will begin to report improved sleep based on relief of constipation and engagement in daily exercise.
- She will resume her normal bowel function with daily or every other day bowel movements that are passed without strain.
- She will visit her primary care provider and cooperate with monitoring her INR and titration of her daily warfarin dose.

Ethical Dilemma

You are working in a long-term care facility. A patient's daughter wants to know why her mother is not receiving anything to make her "calm down." She says that when she was caring for her at home, she would give her mother diazepam (Valium) to keep her quiet even when her mother did not want it. She said she disguised it in applesauce.

It would be important to know if the mother was mentally competent to make decisions. If she is, then she has the ethical right (principle of autonomy) and the legal right to refuse this or any other medication. Disguising medications suggests deception and lying to the patient. Patients have the right to be free from "chemical restraints" (unless they are necessary for the safety of the patient or others).

In response to the daughter, the nurse might explore other nondrug measures to calm her mother that were successful in the past and that may be appropriate for use at this time.

(continued)

CARE PLAN **A Patient Experiencing a Possible Adverse Drug Reaction** *(continued)*

Critical Thinking and the Nursing Process

1. Go to a local pharmacy or consult an online pharmacy and compute the cost of medications for one of your older patients who is taking five or more medications. Notice how the prices differ from various sources. Discuss the difference in costs of medications with your classmates. Are you surprised by the degree to which prices vary? How does this affect your older patient?

2. Identify an older patient you are caring for in your clinical practicum. Review the number and types of prescription, OTC, and herbal medications that your patient is taking. Compare to the medical record. Are there differences? Is the record an accurate reflection of the patient's report?

3. Assess an older patient's knowledge about adverse side effects of a medication he or she is taking on a regular basis. Analyze the patient's knowledge base and try to describe factors that increase or decrease an older person's knowledge about medication safety.

4. As a classroom exercise, purchase a large bag of colored M&M candies. Instruct your classmates to take four orange pills three times a day, two red in the morning, one blue at hour of sleep, and so on. Check with them the next day to see if they were able to follow your oral instructions without error.

■ Evaluate your responses in Appendix B.

Source: Adapted from Hartford Institute for Geriatric Nursing, *Best nursing practices in care for older adults,* 1999.

Chapter Highlights

■ Older persons receive considerable benefit from the many drugs available that can cure or control diseases and improve longevity and the quality of life.

■ As people age they develop unique physiological responses and patterns of behavior that can impact their responses to medications.

■ The prevention and management of adverse drug effects and drug interactions are major concerns of the nurse.

■ The medication needs of older persons pose special challenges to the nurse and other clinicians. Healthcare professionals should provide the appropriate type and dose of medication to optimize the intended therapeutic effects and avoid or reduce the possibility of adverse outcomes of drug therapy. The aging process and other characteristics of each older person dictate his or her unique drug regimen.

■ The nurse can play a major role in the successful use of medications to enhance the quality of life of older adults and to decrease the need for medications in all settings.

Pearson Nursing Student Resources
Find additional review materials at
nursing.pearsonhighered.com
Prepare for success with additional NCLEX®-style practice questions, interactive assignments and activities, web links, animations and videos, and more!

References

American Geriatrics Society. (2012). Updated Beers criteria for potentially inappropriate medication use in older adults. *Journal of the American Geriatrics Society, 60*(4), 616–631.

Ang-Lee, M. K., Moss, J., & Yuan, C.-S. (2001). Herbal medicines and perioperative care. *Journal of the American Medical Society, 286*(2), 208–216.

Bent, S., & Ko, R. (2004). Commonly used herbal medicines in the United States: A review. *American Journal of Medicine, 116* (7), 478–485.

Berdot, S., Bertrand, M., Dartigues, J.-F., Fourrier, A., Tavernier, B., Ritchie, K., & Alpérovitch, A. (2009). Inappropriate medication use and risk of falls—A prospective study in a large community-dwelling elderly cohort. *BMC Geriatrics, 9,* 30. doi:10.1186/1471-2318-9-30

Berry, S. (2011). Antidepressant prescriptions: An acute window for falls in the nursing home. *Medscape.* Retrieved from http://www.medscape.com/viewarticle/742843

Briesacher, B., Soumerai, S., Field, T., Fouayzi, H., Gurwitz, J. (2010) Medicare part D's exclusion of benzodiazepines and fracture risk in nursing homes. *Archives of Internal Medicine,* 170:693–698.

Budnitz, D., Lovegrove, M., Shehab, N., & Richards, C. (2011). Emergency hospitalizations for adverse drug events in older Americans. *New England Journal of Medicine, 365,* 2002–2012.

Centers for Medicare and Medicaid Services (CMS). (2011). *State operations manual appendix PP: Guidance to surveyors for long-term care facilities.* Retrieved from http://www.cms.hhs.gov/manuals/Downloads/som107ap_pp_guidelines_ltcf.pdf

Cherniack, E. P., Ceron-Fuentes, J., Florez, H., Sandals, L., Rodriguez, O., & Palacio, J. C. (2008). Influence of race and ethnicity on alternative medicine as a self-treatment preference for common medical conditions in a population of multi-ethnic urban elderly *Complementary Therapies in Clinical Practice, 14*(2), 116–123.

Cockcroft, D. W., & Gault, M. H. (1976). Prediction of creatinine clearance from serum creatinine. *Nephron, 16,* 31.

Consumer Reports National Research Center. (2011, September 27). Risky prescription drug practices are on the rise in a grim economy. *Consumer News.* Retrieved from http://news.consumerreports.org/health/2011/09/risky-prescription-drug-practices-are-on-the-rise-in-a-grim-economy.html

Cronenwett, L., Sherwood, G., Barnsteiner, J., Disch, J., Johnson, J., Mitchell, P., Sullivan, D., & Warren, J. (2007). Quality and safety education for nurses, *Nursing Outlook, 55*(3) 122-131.

Eisenhauer, L. A., Hurley, A., & Dolan, N. (2007). Nurses' reported thinking during medication administration. *Journal of Nursing Scholarship, 39*(1), 82–87.

Farrell, B., Szeto, W., & Shamji, S. (2011). Drug related problems in the frail elderly. *Canadian Family Physician, 57*(2), 168–169.

Food and Drug Administration [FDA]. (2006, January). Public health advisory: Consumers filling U.S. prescriptions abroad may get the wrong active ingredient because of confusing drug names. Retrieved from http://www.fda.gov/oc/opacom/reports/confusingnames.html

Food and Drug Administration (FDA). (2011, August). Guidance for Industry: E2F, Development update safety report. Retrieved from http://www.fda.gov/downloads/Drugs/.../Guidances/ucm073109.pdf.

Fox, C., Richardson, K., Maidment, D., Savya, G. M., Matthews, F. E., Smithard, D., Coulton, S., Katona, C., Boustani, M., & Brayne, C. (2011) Anticholinergic medication use and cognitive impairment in the older population. *Journal of the American Geriatric Society, 59*(8), 1477–1483.

Glassock, R., & Winearls, C. (2009). Ageing and the glomerular filtration rate: Truths and consequences. *Trans American Clinical Climatology Association, 120,* 419–428.

Gould, E., & Mitty, E. (2010). Medication adherence is a partnership, medication compliance is not. *Geriatric Nursing, 31*(4), 290–298.

Grissinger., M. (2007). Cultural diversity and medication safety. *Pharmacotherapy and Therapeutics.* Retrieved from http://www.nipcweb.com/Medication_Errors.pdf

Handler, M., & Hanlon, J. T. (2010). Detecting adverse drug events using a nursing home specific trigger tool. *Annals of Long-Term Care, 18*(5), 17–22.

Hartford Institute for Geriatric Nursing. (1999). *Best nursing practices in care for older adults.* Retrieved from http://www.hartfordign.org

Hustey, F. M., Wallis, N., & Miller, J. (2007). Inappropriate prescribing in an older ED population. *American Journal of Emergency Medicine, 25*(7), 804–807.

Hutchison, L. C., & O'Brien, C. E. (2007). Changes in pharmacokinetics and pharmacodynamics in the elderly patient. *Journal of Pharmacy Practice, 20*(1), 4–12.

Joint Commission. (2007). *Sentinel event glossary of terms.* Retrieved from http://www.ashp.org/DocLibrary/Policy/QII/IBJointCommission.aspx

Kamble, P., Chen, H., Sherer, J., et al. (2009). Use of antipsychotics among elderly nursing home residents with dementia in the U.S.: An analysis of National Survey Data. Drugs & Aging, 26(6), 483–492.

Kemper, R. F., Steiner, V., Hicks, B., Pierce, L., & Iwuagwu, C. (2007). Anticholinergic medications: Use among older adults with memory problems. *Journal of Gerontological Nursing, 33*(1), 21–31.

Kongkaew, C., Noyce, P., Ashcroft, D. (2008). Hospital admissions associated with adverse drug reactions: A systemic review of prospective observational studies. *Annals of Pharmacotherapy, 42*(7), 1017–1025.

Kurtzweil, P. (1999). How to spot health fraud. *FDA Consumer, 33*(6).

Lenz, T. (2010). Pharmacokinetic drug interactions with physical activity. *American Journal of Lifestyle Medicine, 4*(3), 226–229.

Low, L. F., Anstey, K. J., & Sachdev, P. (2009). Use of medications with anticholinergic properties and cognitive function in a young-old community sample. *International Journal of Geriatric Psychiatry, 24*(6), 578–584.

Mansur, N., Weiss, A., & Beloosesky, Y. (2009). Prescription drug use and adherence in discharged elderly patients. *Annals of Pharmacotherapy, 43*(2), 177–184.

McClennon, P. A., Owlsey, C., Rue, L. W., III, & McGwin, G., Jr. (2009). *Older adults' knowledge about medications and their impact on driving.* Washington, DC: AAA Foundation for Traffic Safety.

Meuleners, L. B., Duke, J., Lee, A. H., Palamara, P., Hildebrand, J., & Ng, J. Q. (2011). Psychoactive medications and crash involvement requiring hospitalization for older drivers. *Journal of the American Geriatrics Society, 59*(9), 1575–1580.

Midelfort, L. (2012). *Medication reconciliation review.* Institute for Health Care Improvement. Retrieved from http://www.ihi.org/knowledge/Pages/Tools/MedicationReconciliationReview.aspx

Mitty, E., & Flores, S. (2007a). Assisted living nursing practice: Medication management: Part 1: Assessing the resident for self-medication ability. *Geriatric Nursing, 8*(2), 83–89.

Mitty, E., & Flores, S. (2007b). Assisted living nursing practice: Medication management: Part 2: Supervision and monitoring of medication administration by unlicensed assistive personnel. *Geriatric Nursing, 28*(3), 153–160.

National Center for Complementary and Alternative Medicine. (2010). *Homeopathy: An introduction* (NCCAM Publication No. D439). Retrieved from http://nccam.nih.gov/health/homeopathy#overview

Office of Inspector General. (2011). Medicare atypical antipsychotic drug claims for elderly nursing home residents. Retrieved from http://oig.hhs.gov/oei/reports/oei-07-08-00150.pdfDHHS

Qato, D. M., Alexander, C., Conti, R. M., Johnson, M., Schumm, P., & Lindau, S. T. (2008). Use of prescription and over-the-counter medications and dietary supplements among older adults in the United States. *Journal of the American Medical Society, 300*, 2867–2878.

Raynor, D. K., Blenkinsopp, A., Knapp, P., Grime, J., Nicolson, D. J., Pollock, K., Dorer, G., Gilbody, S., Dickinson, D., Maule, A. J., & Spoor, P. (2007). A systematic review of quantitative and qualitative research on the role and effectiveness of written information about individual medicines. *Health Technology Assessment, 11*(5), iii, ix–xi, 1–173.

Resnick, B. (2012). 2012 Beers criteria. *Journal of the American Geriatrics Society, 60*(4), 612–613.

Reyes, C., Van de Putte, L., Falcón, A. P., & Levy, R. A. (2004). *Genes, culture, and medicines: Bridging gaps in treatment for Hispanic Americans*. Washington, DC: National Alliance for Hispanic Health and the National Pharmaceutical Council.

Russell, C. L., Ruppar, T. M., & Matteson, M. (2011). Improving medication adherence: Moving from intention and motivation to a personal systems approach. *Nursing Clinics of North America, 46*(3), 271–281.

Shiel, W. (2009). Herbs: Toxicities and drug interactions. Retrieved from http://www.medicinenet.com/script/main/art.asp?articlekey=7506

Tache, S., Sonnichsen, A., & Ashcroft, D. (2011). Prevalence of adverse drug events in ambulatory care settings: A systematic review. *Annals of Pharmacother*apy, *45*(7–8), 977–989.

Woodruff, K. (2010). Preventing polypharmacy in older adults. *American Nurse Today, 5*(10).

Woolcott, J., Richardson, K., Wiens, M., Patel, B., Mann, J., Khan, K., Marra, C. (2009). Meta-analysis of the impact of 9 medication classes on falls in elderly persons. *Archives of Internal Medicine, 169*(21), 1952–1960.

World Health Organization. (2008). Safety of medications: A guide to detecting and reporting adverse drug reactions. Retrieved from http://www.who.int/mediacentre/factsheets/fs293/en

Wu, J.-R., Moser, D., Lennie, T., & Burkhart, P. V. (2008). Medication adherence in patients who have heart failure: A review of the literature. *Nursing Clinics of North America, 43*(1), 133–153.

Psychological and Cognitive Function

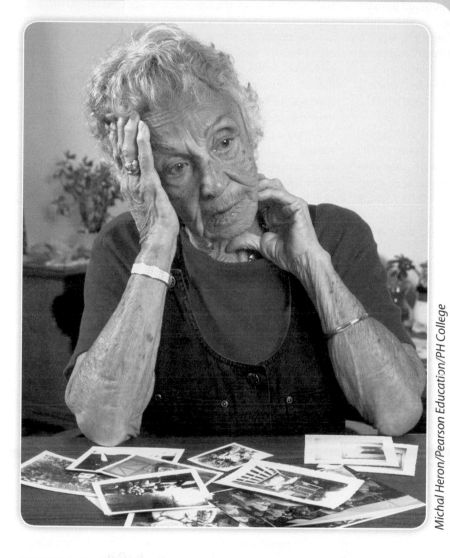

Michal Heron/Pearson Education/PH College

LEARNING OUTCOMES

On completion of this chapter, the reader will be able to:

1. Describe age-related changes that affect psychological and cognitive functioning.
2. Explain the impact of age-related changes on stress and coping.
3. Detect risk factors for high levels of stress, poor coping, and impaired mental health, including alcoholism, stress-related disorders, and depression.
4. Examine risk factors that influence cognitive functioning in older adults.
5. Define appropriate nursing interventions directed toward assisting the older adult to develop coping resources, use effective coping mechanisms, and minimize the functional consequences of stress.
6. Identify means to strengthen social support groups and healthy aging.
7. Formulate interventions directed toward alleviating risk factors for late-life depression, treating depression in older adults, and preventing suicide.

The well-being of older adults is a major concern to healthcare providers in the United States and to society in general. Undiagnosed and untreated mental disorders such as **depression** or despondent mood marked by decreased energy, feeling worthless and guilty, problems with concentration, and thoughts of death or suicide can lead to increased disability, premature death, increased morbidity, cognitive decline, increased risk of institutionalization, and a significant decrease in an older person's quality of life (National Institute of Mental Health [NIMH], 2010).

Many factors can affect the psychological and cognitive function of older adults. Some problems of older adults are the same as those experienced by people of other ages while others are more likely to emerge in the later years of life. Special challenges faced by older adults include accomplishing life-cycle developmental tasks, achieving positive psychological growth in later years, and coping with change.

As with physical problems, the older adult may experience multiple psychological symptoms or syndromes that make recognition and diagnosis challenging for the gerontological nurse and other healthcare providers. Additionally, psychological problems can result from and coexist with physical problems. For instance, an older person with heart failure may complain of symptoms of lethargy, inability to eat, and falling. This older person may be taking several medications. These symptoms may be the result of a drug–drug interaction, a physical response to chronic illness, a new-onset psychological problem, or a combination of all of these factors.

The expanding older population will place increasing demands on mental health services and create greater demands for mental health care (American Psychological Association [APA], 2011). Healthcare professionals, including nurses, should aggressively work to improve the quality of mental health services delivered to older adults in order to meet the mental health goals established in *Healthy People 2020,* to improve mental health through prevention, and to ensure access to appropriate, quality mental health services (U.S. Department of Health and Human Services [USDHHS], 2012).

Major population-based surveys find that the overall prevalence of mental disorders for older adults is lower than for any other age group. Only cognitive impairments such as Alzheimer's disease (AD) show a definite age-associated increase (see Chapter 22 ⬤▭ for a complete discussion of AD and dementia). About 20% of older people suffer from mental health problems including **anxiety** (a state of apprehension, uneasiness, or distress), severe cognitive impairments, and mood disorders; however, many feel that this number should be higher because of underreporting. The rate of suicide is highest among older adults when compared to other age groups and the suicide rate is highest of all in non-Hispanic white men over age 85 with a rate of twice the national average (NIMH, 2010). Yet, when older adults experience mental health problems, they may be denied access to mental health services for a variety of factors, including missed diagnosis of psychological problems, denial of problems, funding issues, lack of coordination between mental health and aging care providers, shortages of health professionals with geriatric mental health expertise, and the perceived stigma many older people attach to having a psychological problem. The rate of utilization of mental health services is lower in older people than in any other age group and it is estimated that only half of those older adults with mental health problems receive mental health services (American Association for Geropsychiatry, 2012). As a result of this unfortunate situation, an older person may find their **competence,** or ability to care for themselves and make decisions, questioned. An older adult whose competence is questioned may suffer losses of autonomy and independence such as having a legal guardian appointed or being prematurely institutionalized in a nursing home or long-term care facility when in fact, with appropriate mental health services and support, the person may have been able to live in a less restrictive community-based environment.

Normal Changes in Aging

Normally, an older person's mental health and cognition remain relatively stable. For those functions that do change, usually the change is not severe enough to cause significant impairment in daily life or social ability. Severe changes and sudden loss of **cognitive function** are usually symptoms of a physical or mental illness such as Alzheimer's disease, stroke, or serious depression. Following are some general cognitive changes considered to be normal age-related changes:

- Information-processing speed declines with age, resulting in a slower learning rate and greater need for repetition of information.
- The ability to divide attention between two tasks shows age-related decline.
- The ability to switch attention rapidly from one auditory input to another shows age-related decline (visual input switching ability does not change significantly with age).
- Ability to maintain sustained attention or perform vigilance tasks appears to decline with age.
- Ability to filter out irrelevant information appears to decline with age.

- Short-term or primary memory remains relatively stable.
- Long-term or secondary memory exhibits more substantial age-related changes, with the decline greater for recall than for recognition. (Cueing improves performance of long-term memory.)
- Most aspects of language are well preserved, such as use of language sounds and meaningful combinations of words. Vocabulary improves with age. However, word finding, naming ability, and rapid word list generation decline with age.
- Visuospatial task ability such as drawing and construction ability declines with age.
- Abstraction and mental flexibility show some age decline.
- Accumulation of practical experience, or wisdom, continues until the very end of life.

American Psychological Association, 2011.

> **Practice Pearl** ▶▶▶ Normal healthy older persons who forget where they put the keys can be assured there is no significant memory problem. But if they forget what a key is for or how to use it, they should be referred for further evaluation and treatment.

Decrements in intellectual function are generally greater in older people who develop disease and disability than in those who remain healthy. Many decrements in cognitive capacity, mood, and performance that formerly were attributed to "normal aging" are now known to be associated with psychiatric illness or physical disease. Contrary to the stereotype of increasing rigidity and inflexibility with age, healthy older people maintain stable personalities and psychological adaptation throughout their lives. **Personality** stability across the second half of the adult life span may be stronger than across the first half because during youth and early middle age, personality and personal identity are still evolving.

Late adulthood is no longer seen as a period of growth cessation and arrested cognitive development, but rather a continued period of growth with the opportunity for development of unique capacities (Stanford Center on Longevity, 2011). Education, pulmonary health, general health, and activity levels all influence cognitive activity in later life. Older adults often have a positive outlook and seek challenges and activities that maintain their well-being. Many older people take classes, participate in elder hostels, exercise, study new subjects, travel, and maintain healthy interpersonal and sexual relationships.

Cognition is a complicated process by which information is learned, stored, retrieved, and used by the individual.

Cognitive processing supports reasoning, problem solving, remembering, interpreting, and communicating. Normal, healthy aging is not characterized by cognitive and mental disorders (National Alliance on Mental Illness [NAMI], 2011). Some cognitive abilities may decline with age, some may improve, and some stay relatively stable. These changes are highly variable from one person to another as they age and may even vary within a given person over time. Most older people will not suffer significant memory impairment, but many may experience mild problems with word finding and remembering names. Usually, however, these problems are mild in scope and the older person can compensate for these deficits. (For a complete discussion of Alzheimer's disease, see Chapter 22 ⊂⊃.) Older adults cope with normal aging changes in a variety of ways. Since most changes of aging are gradual in onset, the older person gradually adjusts to the changes. Methods for coping with age-associated cognitive changes include:

- Making lists, posting appointments on calendars, and writing "notes to self"
- Learning memory training and memory enhancement techniques (for instance, when meeting a new person for the first time, trying to link his or her name to a common object or easily remembered item)
- Playing computer games that emphasize eye/hand coordination and memory of shapes, colors, and objects
- Keeping the mind challenged and mentally active (e.g., reading daily, completing a crossword puzzle, or playing bridge)
- Using assistive devices such as pillboxes and reliance on habit such as preprogrammed telephones, parking in the same place in the mall parking lot, and so on, to reduce chances of forgetting vital information
- Seeking support and encouragement from others
- Staying positive and hopeful for the future, including laughing at oneself when appropriate ("You won't believe what I did today. I showed up for my doctor's appointment with one brown and one black shoe! Oh well, at least I'm not a slave to fashion!")

Older adults must be able to monitor their cognitive abilities and adapt to changes in their memory skills to function safely in their everyday lives. Some people with severe cognitive deficits may continue to engage in behaviors that are unsafe for them such as driving, cooking, and trying to live independently. Others with good memories may continuously live in fear that they are developing Alzheimer's disease whenever they forget a name or an appointment. It is difficult to predict whether an older person who has mild problems with memory will go on to develop more severe memory loss. Some older people try to hide or cover up memory problems because they fear restrictions on their freedoms and living situation. Memory changes may result from a variety of causes, including Alzheimer's disease, depression, underlying psychiatric illness, physical illness, medications, vitamin deficiencies, and sensory impairments. Any alteration or concerns over cognitive abilities should be assessed to identify reversible causes of memory loss and institute appropriate safety measures in a supportive environment.

HEALTHY AGING TIP

Mental Health

▶ Maintain an active social life and engage in plenty of interesting conversations.

▶ Read newspapers, magazines, and books.

▶ Play "thinking" games like Scrabble, computer games, cards, and Trivial Pursuit.

▶ Take a course on a subject that interests you.

▶ Develop a new hobby.

▶ Learn a second language or how to play a musical instrument.

▶ Watch "question-and–answer" game shows on TV, and play along with the contestants.

▶ Keep stress under control with meditation, exercise, and relaxation, because stress hormones like cortisol can damage neurons.

▶ Stay healthy and active.

Stanford Center on Longevity, 2011.

Psychological changes and chronic illness associated with older adulthood may affect a person's functional abilities; however, the psychosocial changes are often the most challenging and demanding. Some of the psychosocial challenges arise from physical changes, but many are attributable to changes in roles, relationships, losses, and living environments. Like many age-related psychological changes, some psychosocial changes are inevitable and somewhat predictable. Therefore, older adults can prepare for, and respond to, psychosocial changes by developing and using effective coping strategies they have developed in their earlier lives. With each day that passes, the opportunity for change, both positive and negative, presents itself. A rich, full life usually encompasses joyous and sad events. Some older people experience multiple and significant losses as they age. The positive **coping mechanisms** (methods used by older adults to adjust to or accept a threat or challenge) that a person developed and used earlier in life may be inadequate in later life, and depression or another serious mental health problem may result from inadequate coping ability such that additional services and support may be needed.

Practice Pearl ▶▶▶ Most older adults successfully adjust to the challenges of aging, but nurses must be alert for the symptoms of depression that will present differently in the older person. Vague physical decline and somatic complaints may be the only clues of underlying depression.

Drug Alert ▶▶▶ Certain medications like sleeping pills, tranquilizers, and some pain medications can cause symptoms similar to dementia (confusion, lack of interest, memory impairment) but are not true dementia. These symptoms are called false dementia or pseudodementia.

Educational attainment within the older population has increased significantly and is projected to continue to increase during the next decade. Higher education levels are linked to better health outcomes and a higher standard of living in retirement. The percentage of Americans completing high school continues to rise with an 89.9% graduation rate in 2008 (Chapman, Laird, & KewalRamani, 2011). The proportion of older Americans with at least a bachelor's degree grew fivefold from 1950 (3.4%) to 2003 (17.4%) and by 2030 it is estimated that 25% of the older population is expected to have an undergraduate degree. Higher levels of education are associated with increased travel, recreation, income, and opportunities for personal growth and development. However, even though older people share similar generational experiences, there may be considerable diversity among them. Life experiences, health status, race, culture, sexual orientation, and a variety of other factors can make an older person who is a high school dropout think and act more like a college professor and vice versa.

Positive mental health is a necessary component of successful aging. Box 7-1 lists the key components of mental health as defined by the Surgeon General of the United States. Positive mental health can last a lifetime and support growth, creativity, sense of humor, and zest for life until the moment of death. For instance, Georgia O'Keeffe and Pablo Picasso painted into their 90s and were considered by many to do their best work in their old age. Jeanne Calment of Arles, France, took up fencing lessons at the age of 85 and rode a bicycle at age 100. At Mme. Calment's 120th birthday party, a journalist hesitantly told her, "Well, I guess I'll see you next year." Instantly she replied, "I don't see why not. You look to be in pretty good health to me!" Her life ended on August 4, 1997, at age 122 years, 5 months, and 14 days. She is believed to have lived longer than any person in recorded history (National Institute on Aging, 2002).

| BOX 7-1 | Mental Health: Themes |

- Mental health is fundamental to health.
- Mental illnesses are real health problems.
- The efficacy of mental health treatments is well documented.
- Mind and body are inseparable.
- There is a serious shortage of trained mental health professionals to meet the need for services.
- Stigma is a major obstacle preventing older people from getting help.

Source: Centers for Disease Control and National Association of Chronic Disease Directors (2009).

Cultural Considerations

The older population is highly heterogeneous and includes a diverse mix of immigrants, refugees, and multigenerational Americans with vastly different histories, languages, spiritual practices, demographic patterns, and cultures. Currently, the typical older person is a Caucasian; however, by 2030 the number of older African Americans will triple, increasing their proportion of the total older adult population from 8% to 14%. The number of older Asians will increase to 6%, and Hispanics will increase from less than 4% to nearly 20% of the older population (U.S. Census Bureau, 2008). Generations within the same minority family may represent different racial or cultural orientation, religious affiliation and practices, societal values, and attitudes toward the larger society. The unique life experiences, values, and beliefs of these diverse older persons may be very different from those of the larger cohort of older adults. Racial and ethnic minorities bear a greater burden of unmet mental health needs and thus suffer greater losses that negatively impact their overall health and productivity at all ages.

To reach the *Healthy People 2020* goal of equal access to health care, the mental health needs of minority elders, who are at highest risk of death and disability, should be addressed. Poor income and low literacy, often associated with minority status, are important risk factors for major chronic illness (APA, 2011). Minority elders may be considered especially vulnerable and at risk for mental health problems because of **ageism** (negative stereotypes toward older adults) and cultural bias.

Several factors should be acknowledged regarding health status and minority aging:

- The onset of chronic illness is usually earlier than in Caucasian older adults.
- There are frequent delays in seeking health treatment.

- Health problems may be underreported because of lack of trust in healthcare workers.
- Mental health services are underutilized.
- There are higher rates of treatment dropout and medical noncompliance.
- Although longevity for African American men is shorter than that for Caucasian men, African American men and women surviving to the age of 75 live longer than Caucasians.
- There is a higher incidence of obesity and type 2 diabetes mellitus.
- A large number of minority elders possess no health insurance.

Additional factors contributing to poor mental health in minority elders include poverty, segregated and disorganized communities, poor quality of education, few role responsibilities, sporadic and chronic unemployment and underemployment, stereotyping, discrimination, and poor health status and health care (APA, 2011).

Most minority groups are less likely than Whites to use services, and they receive poorer quality mental health care, despite having similar community rates of mental health problems. Especially at risk are racial and ethnic minorities and older gay men and lesbians (Warner et al., 2004). Similar prevalence, combined with lower utilization and poorer quality of care, means that minority communities have a higher proportion of individuals with unmet mental health needs. Because of preventable disparities in mental health services, a disproportionate number of minority older persons are not fully benefiting from the opportunities that others have to enjoy their older years. The major barriers include the cost of care, societal stigma, and the fragmentation of services. Additional barriers include healthcare providers' lack of awareness of cultural issues, bias, or inability to speak the older person's language, and the older person's fear and mistrust of treatment (Leong & Kalibatseva, 2011). The use and refinement of culturally sensitive instruments to assess mental status, depression, dementia, and pain are encouraged.

Personality and Self-Concept

Erik Erikson's original theory (1963) about the eight stages of life has been used widely in relation to older adulthood. Erikson defined the stages of life as trust versus mistrust, autonomy versus shame and doubt, initiative versus guilt, industry versus inferiority, identity versus identity diffusion, intimacy versus self-absorption, generativity versus stagnation, and ego integrity versus despair. Each of these stages presents certain conflicting tendencies that must be balanced before the person can move successfully from that stage. In 1982, when Erikson was 80 years old, he described the task of old age as balancing the search for integrity and wholeness, thus avoiding a sense of despair. He believed that successful accomplishment of this task, achieved primarily through life review activities, would result in wisdom.

Havighurst (1972) concentrated his studies of developing life course theories on middle or later adulthood. He defined tasks of later life as (1) adjusting to decreased physical strength and health, (2) adjusting to retirement and reduced income, (3) adjusting to death of a spouse, (4) establishing an explicit association with one's group, (5) adapting to social roles in a flexible way, and (6) establishing satisfactory physical living arrangements.

These and many other personality type theories attempt to question whether personality changes or remains the same throughout the life course. Although most researchers agree that personality remains relatively stable over the life span, they disagree about the extent and causes of personality change. Neugarten and Hagestad (1976) conducted studies and identified three basic personality characteristics occurring in older people: (1) a change of focus from the outer world to the inner world, (2) a movement from active mastery of the environment to a more reactive or accommodating approach, and (3) establishing patterns of isolation from the outside world. This last group included people with psychological problems, those with irrational behavior, and those who failed to cope with the demands of daily living.

When rigidity and excess cautiousness are apparent in an older person, the underlying explanation may be generational or cohort differences rather than a normal change of aging. Older people have been brought up with different expectations, have had different life experiences, and possess different generational values. As a result, they may be hesitant to make decisions in areas where they feel less comfortable and the outcome is uncertain. For instance, some older people may be hesitant to invest in the stock market, preferring instead to put their money into low-interest-rate bank accounts or safety deposit boxes. Others may prefer to invest their money in riskier ventures to gain higher returns and may even become victims of scam artists and others who take advantage of older adults. Like younger people, older people assess risk in very different ways.

Self-concept is a component of personality (APA, 2011) that can be viewed as an attitude toward the self. Usually this self-concept is developed during one's life and depends on how a person is treated by others, the successes and failures one experiences, and how an older person incorporates these events into his or her existence. For instance, an older person may suffer a foot injury and develop a permanent limp. A person with a strong self-concept might say, "Well at least I can still get around on my own" while another with a more negative self-concept might say, "Look at me limping and walking just like an old man."

An older person's self-concept can be eroded or enhanced over time as a result of circumstance and life experiences. Additionally, an older person's personality influences self-concept and adaptation to role transitions, such as widowhood or retirement. Research related to personality traits and self-concept indicates that individuals can maintain continuity and coherence in the course of adult life. People do not necessarily become depressed, isolated, and rigid with older age, and well-adjusted and happy individuals are likely to remain so in late life. Those who are less happy with themselves can take steps such as counseling or engage in self-help groups to improve their self-concept and change their lives.

Life Satisfaction and Life Events

Life satisfaction is an attitude toward one's own life; it may be defined as a reflection of feelings about the past, present, and future. Life satisfaction and morale are closely related to well-being. George et al. (1985) posited that life satisfaction is the cognitive assessment of well-being, and happiness is the affective assessment. The two major components of well-being are affect (happiness) and satisfaction (realized expectations). These components may reflect a changing balance with age. Thus, age-related declines in positive affect may be countered by increases in the sense of satisfaction with life accomplishments (Maddox, 1994). Less than one third of older people report feelings of boredom or loneliness, and they express more life satisfaction when their social networks include friends as well as relatives (NAMI, 2011). Some researchers have found that greater independence in instrumental activities of daily living and greater perceived control of events significantly attenuate the adverse effects of stress on psychological well-being.

Life satisfaction usually does not decrease as one ages. Recent studies document that life satisfaction increases until about the age of 65 and then begins to decrease. However, while that was the average, there is huge variation between individuals, with older persons diagnosed with serious illness showing the greatest decreases and those who were relatively healthy showing slower declines (NAMI, 2011). Significant changes in mood, cognitive ability, and personality should never be dismissed as normal aging, but always aggressively assessed and referred for treatment.

Life events demand an emotional adjustment on the part of the person experiencing the event, and different challenges are likely to occur during different periods in life. Some of these life events might be unexpected, unwanted, or feared. Others, such as coping with the loss of a spouse, might be more or less expected. Some examples of events requiring psychological adjustments in older adults are widowhood, confronting negative attitudes of aging, retirement, chronic illness, functional impairments, decisions about driving a car, death of friends and family, and relocation from home to assisted living or long-term care. Although not all older people will experience these events, every person who is privileged to live a long life may experience significant events that require psychological adjustment and mobilization of coping mechanisms. The longer a person lives, the more likely it is that events will occur that require coping and adaptation. Older adults may encounter losses of significant magnitude, such as losses of people or objects that have been part of their lives for many decades. Older adults with troubled pasts are less likely to adjust to losses and may develop chronic health problems and experience negative feelings such as anxiety or powerlessness. For example, people who fled from Europe to escape persecution before and during World War II, people who suffered great losses such as tsunamis or other natural disasters, or people who have been victims of serious crime may be at risk for anxiety or depression when attempting to cope with an adverse life event. These older people may experience pain and loss much differently than the older person who has had a stable life without major trauma or fear. It is always valuable to consider how the events of history and past experience can affect the orientation and personality of the older person.

Stress and Coping

Stress is a universal phenomenon that all people experience in their daily lives. **Stress** is the response to demand or pressure. However, excessive and persistent stress has been linked to the development of illness (Selye, 1965). Gerontological nurses should recognize and understand stress and its influence on older persons. Chemically, stress mimics the fight-or-flight response that can preserve life in the short term, but threaten life if allowed to persist for long periods of time. The fight-or-flight response stimulates epinephrine release and increases in pulse, blood pressure, blood glucose, and muscle tension. The person may feel alarm, and thinking usually becomes narrow and concrete, focusing on the threat at hand. Ability to communicate decreases as all the emphasis is on mobilization of body defenses. If left untreated, persistent stress can result in exhaustion, adrenal cortex hormone depletion, and even death.

Conditions most likely to produce stress-related health problems include accumulation of stressful situations that a person cannot easily control; persistent stress following a traumatic event such as death of a loved one; and acute stress following a serious illness such as cancer or heart disease

(University of Maryland Medical Center, 2011). Risk factors for high levels of stress and poor coping are diminished economic resources, immature developmental level, many hassles at the same time in one day, poor health status, and many major life events occurring in a short period of time. Unrealistic appraisal of a situation also may increase risk for poor coping because the individual has to recognize the need for change in a given situation. High levels of stress and poor coping can cause mental and physical health impairments.

Stressors are highly individual. The event that one older person perceives as challenging may be stressful for another. Stressors may be physical, emotional, biological, or developmental. One older person may dread the thought of moving into an assisted-living facility. He or she may fear loss of privacy or independence, loss of cherished possessions, or even separation from loving memories of family events. Another older person may eagerly anticipate the move and feel joy at the thought of living in a secure environment with proximity to others. He or she may have felt lonely in a large family home and inadequate to cope with the demands of maintaining the home and yard. How the older person appraises an event depends on the individual's personality, values, and past experiences. With aging comes diversity as persons reflect on their past histories, their present circumstances, and their hopes for the future.

The way an older person copes with excessive stress has been associated with poor health outcomes. Higher rates of heart disease, cancer, and other illness have been cited in the literature (McCance & Huether, 2010). Symptoms that indicate the older person may be suffering negative effects of stress include the following:

- Sleep problems and insomnia
- Chronic high anxiety levels
- Use or abuse of alcohol, prescription or recreational drugs, or tobacco
- Jumpiness and inability to remain still for long periods of time
- New-onset hypertension, tachycardia, tremors, or irregular heartbeat
- Depression, chronic fatigue, or lack of pleasure in life
- Chronic pain or physical complaints

Nurses working with older people with high stress levels sometimes start to feel stressed themselves. It is important to understand the concept of stress and to break the cycle before long-term negative effects can occur. Suggested nursing actions include:

- Assist older persons to identify stressors and rate their levels of stress.
- Educate the older person and family about stress theory and the stress cycle.

- Help the older person identify successful coping mechanisms used in the past during periods of high stress.
- Assist the older person to examine current coping mechanisms and behaviors and to alter or eliminate negative or maladaptive mechanisms.
- Reinforce and strengthen positive coping mechanisms.
- Monitor and maintain physical health by urging health promotion activities and practices.
- Investigate community resources, support groups, stress-reduction clinics, and other stress relievers that may be useful to the older person.

> **Practice Pearl ▶▶▶** Ask your older patients to tell a short story about themselves or a significant event in their life. By analyzing the content of the story, you can learn if an older patient is a survivor, a victim, or a person who relies on the help and guidance of others. This brief story can reveal a lot about the older person's self-concept.

Personality Disorders

The incidence and prevalence of most personality disorders decline with age. Narcissistic, borderline, histrionic, and antisocial personality disorders generally peak in the younger years. However, personality disorders may present differently in the older adult. Any selfish or impulsive behavior toward family or caregivers should be carefully investigated by the gerontological nurse and others on the healthcare team and referred for further evaluation and treatment if indicated.

Psychiatric symptoms that should be investigated and not written off as normal changes of aging include:

- **Memory and intellectual difficulties. Pseudodementia** or cognitive changes due to underlying anxiety, chronic pain, depression, or other potentially treatable psychiatric disorders can masquerade as Alzheimer's disease.
- **Change in sleep patterns.** Drastic changes in sleep patterns such as early morning awakening, declines in total sleep time, and increased sleep latency (longer time to fall asleep) may be signs of underlying anxiety or depression. Physical problems such as pain, respiratory disease, and cardiac disease can also interfere with sleep. Underlying psychiatric problems can exaggerate and intensify sleep disturbances in the older adult.
- **Changes in sexual interest and capacity.** Healthy older adults with a history of and interest in normal sexual function should be evaluated when sudden changes in sexual interest and capacity occur. In men, erectile dysfunction can have physical and psychological

correlates. In women, libido and ability to reach orgasm can likewise be affected by a variety of factors. Common medical causes, medications, and underlying psychiatric problems can all contribute to sexual dysfunction in both genders. See Chapter 17 ⬜ for further information on the evaluation of sexual dysfunction.

- **Fear of death.** For healthy older people, fear of death is uncommon. While older people do think about death and their own mortality, excessive focus on death and high death anxiety is uncommon. When older people focus excessively on death, they may be exhibiting signs of depression or anxiety, or they may be struggling to cope with a diagnosis of a terminal illness.
- **Delusions. Delusions** are false beliefs that persist and exert a negative influence on behavior or attitude (e.g., the belief that all food is poison and eating food will cause death).
- **Hallucinations. Hallucinations** are false perceptions and sensations such as hearing voices (auditory hallucinations) or seeing people (visual hallucinations) who are not there.
- **Disordered thinking.** Disordered thinking is characterized by lack of logical thought processes. As a result, thoughts and communications become disorganized and fragmented. Serious problems such as legal situations can result from poor judgment and an inability to communicate basic needs and safety concerns.
- **Problems with emotional expression.** Sudden or prolonged gradual loss of emotional responsiveness and expression may indicate the presence of psychiatric illness in the older adult. Failure to show emotion, laugh, cry, or make eye contact, or withdrawal from opportunities for human interaction, may be signs of severe depression. This is sometimes called the **flat affect** (NAMI, 2011).

Psychotic Disorders

Schizophrenia rarely occurs for the first time in old age. Only about 10% of people with diagnosed schizophrenia experience the onset of symptoms after the age of 40 (NIMH, 2011). Therefore, it is likely that the older person with schizophrenia will have a long history of hospitalization and psychotropic drug use. Some symptoms of schizophrenia such as hallucinations and delusions appear to decline with age, but other symptoms such as apathy and withdrawal may place the older person at high risk for social isolation and neglect.

The most common form of psychosis in later years is paranoia (NIMH, 2011). Hearing loss may place older persons at risk for developing paranoia because they may, for example, misinterpret the casual conversation of others and believe they are the focus of the conversation. Other risk factors include social isolation, underlying personality disorder, cognitive impairment, and delirium. Older persons with early dementia may blame others for hiding or stealing their belongings when, in reality, they have simply forgotten where they have been left. These delusions can be hurtful to family and friends who are attempting to assist the older person and may result in increased social isolation.

Adjustment Disorder

The most common stressor that leads to adjustment disorder in later life is physical illness. Other stressors that may precipitate adjustment disorders among older adults include forced relocation, financial problems, family problems, and lengthy hospitalizations (NIMH, 2010).

Bereavement and Depression

Bereavement

Most older adults experience the loss or death of loved ones, including spouse, family members, and friends. While bereavement is considered a normal reaction to loss and death, pathological grief may occur in some older adults. Symptoms of pathological grief among older adults are essentially the same as those of younger adults. They include preoccupation with death, extensive guilt, an overwhelming sense of loss and worthlessness, marked psychomotor retardation, and functional impairment. The length of time spent in grieving is culturally determined and is also a function of the individual's resources and the circumstances of death. In the United States, grief in the older adult is considered normal within a 2-year time frame, but grief persisting longer than 2 years is considered pathological. However, establishing preconceived time frames and judging others according to various theories quickly becomes problematic. In some cultures, bereavement lasts for the lifetime of the survivor. Traditional Greek widows wear black for the rest of their lives. The professional standard of care regarding the grieving older person should not be time related, but rather focus on the prevention and early recognition of grief-related psychiatric disorders, profound depression, medical illness, and social incapacitation (NIMH, 2010).

> **Practice Pearl ▶▶▶** Some define grief as sadness turned outward, including public crying and talking about the loss, while depression is sadness turned inward and a feeling of isolation or separation from others.

Factors that can affect the duration and course of grieving include:

- **Centrality of the loss.** If the person who has died occupied a central place in the survivor's life (either physically or emotionally), the loss will be harder to bear. An older person with psychological attachments to others will receive support and assistance with grieving after the loss.
- **Health of the survivor.** An older person with robust mental and physical health will be better able to cope with loss of a loved one and complete the work of grieving. Unresolved issues from the past, feelings of ambiguity toward the one who has died, and unresolved or incomplete coping with previous losses can all complicate the grieving process and prolong the time required to perform the grief work.
- **Survivor's religious or spiritual belief system.** Personal religion or spirituality can be deeply integrated into the older person's perspective and positively influence the grieving process. When an older person believes a loved one has lived a meaningful life and has passed into the care of a Higher Power, a sense of self-worth and acceptance of the death may occur. However, the gerontological nurse should be aware that older persons who are religious are not necessarily spiritual, and vice versa. Some people attend churches or temples for the social or recreational opportunities and can find very little comfort from their religion when it is most needed. Other older people may have grown away from organized religion but still may possess a deep and abiding faith in God and the meaning of life.
- **History of substance abuse.** Older people who have used drugs or alcohol to cope with unpleasant life events and serious losses in the past may experience a desire to use these substances again. Careful monitoring and support of these older adults is warranted.
- **Nature of the death.** Sudden deaths that are a result of trauma, natural disaster, or violent acts may be more difficult to bear and prolong the grieving process. These deaths, in addition to the great personal loss felt by the survivor, may also trigger more symbolic losses such as loss of trust, security, and control. These older adults may experience the double psychological burden of bereavement and post-traumatic stress reaction. Symptoms include feelings of shock, horror, and numbness. Recurrent violent and frightening dreams may disrupt sleep and cause daytime anxiety. These older adults may focus exclusively on retelling the horrific events of the death, return to the scene of the old crises, overidentify with the deceased, and focus on pictures and objects. The gerontological nurse can assist older people with their grief work and help them gain mastery and control over the trauma by urging them to seek mental health services and counseling while providing support. (See Chapter 11 for a further discussion of grief and grieving.)

Practice Pearl ▶▶▶ Some older people will grieve the loss of a pet to the same extent as the loss of a family member. The centrality of the loss is the predictor of the depth and duration of grief, not the societal value of the being who has died.

Depression

Depression is the mental health problem of greatest frequency and magnitude in the older population. Depression is defined as a clinical syndrome characterized by low mood tone, difficulty thinking, and somatic changes precipitated by feelings of loss or guilt. The risk of depression in the older person increases with other illnesses and when ability to function becomes limited. Estimates of major depression in older people living in the community range from less than 1% to about 5%, but rises to 13.5% in those who require home health care and to 11.5% in older hospitalized patients (NIMH, 2010). Symptoms of depression are often associated with chronic illness and pain. While the rates of major depression are lower in the older population, 27% of older adults (or about 6.5 million older people) experience some depressive symptoms (Kurlowicz & Greenberg, 2007; NAMI, 2011).

Depression in older adults is often undetected and untreated. Therefore, it is difficult to determine prevalence rates. Primary healthcare providers are often not vigilant or consistent in their diagnosis of depression and may fail to make the diagnosis. One approach is to distinguish between the psychiatric diagnosis of major depression and the depression-related affective disturbances (minor depression) of daily life. Using these categories, the rate of major and minor depression in community-living older adults is approximately 13%, and 43% among institutionalized older adults. The symptoms of depression are often associated with chronic illness and pain.

Symptoms of depression may be emotional and physical. Emotional symptoms include sadness, diminished ability to experience joy in life, inability to concentrate, recurrent thoughts of death, and excessive guilt over things that happened in the past. Physical symptoms can include body aches, headaches, pain, fatigue, change in sleep habits, and weight gain or loss. The economic cost of this disorder is high, but the cost in human suffering associated with caregiver burden and distress is significant. The burden of illness with depression is thought to cost the United States $43.7 billion per year. This cost includes lost productivity, the cost of direct treatment and medications, household and social difficulties, and limitation in functional ability (Mental Health America, 2011). Serious depression can destroy family life as well as the life of the ill person.

Depression is best understood as a group of disorders with variable severity. Depression can include mild sadness over long periods of time, brief periods of sadness, intense reaction to loss, severe psychotic depression with hallucination and bizarre behavior, or the profound regression of pseudodementia where the older person "tunes the world out" and appears to be cognitively impaired. During the early phases of dementia, the older person may be aware that something is wrong. These feelings may trigger the onset of depressive symptoms, and depression and dementia may coexist. These patients may barely cooperate with mental status testing. When asked questions, they may respond, "I don't know." They often appear hopeless and respond slowly. They may have a flat affect and put little effort into performing any requested task. Referral to a skilled clinician (neuropsychologist, geriatric psychiatrist, or gerontological mental health nurse) is usually indicated to diagnose and treat these complicated coexisting morbidities.

Some older people may have persistent mild feelings of sadness called **dysthymia,** yet may not meet the criteria for diagnosis of clinical depression with few accompanying physical symptoms. This less severe type of depression involves long-term, chronic symptoms that do not disable, but instead keep the older person from functioning well or from enjoying life to the fullest. Many older people with dysthymia also experience major depressive episodes at some time in their lives. Older people with dysthymia may benefit from increased socialization and involvement with others. They are less likely to benefit from traditional psychotherapy. However, they require close monitoring to ensure they do not develop symptoms of major depression.

Signs of Depression

The major signs of depression in the older person include multiple somatic complaints and reports of persistent chronic pain. Many older people with depression tend not to consider themselves depressed and therefore complain more of physical symptoms than emotional ones. There is a stigma among many older people toward the diagnosis or acknowledgment of mental illness or psychiatric problems. Some older people find it more socially acceptable to seek advice and support from a physician or nurse for a physical reason rather than seek out a psychiatrist for mental health problems. Only about 20% of older depressed patients seek advice and counseling from a mental health professional (NAMI, 2011).

Older women experience depression about twice as often as men, are more likely to remain depressed, but are less likely to die while depressed (NIMH, 2010). Although men are less likely to suffer from depression, 3 to 4 million men in the United States are affected by the illness. Men are less likely to admit to depression, and doctors are less likely to suspect it. Gender differences in the prevalence of depression may be explained by social risk factors. More than 50% of older women live alone compared to 25% of older men. Older women may be more prone to loneliness, financial difficulties, and loss of independence due to functional disability. Marriage has been shown to be protective against the development of depression, and married older people have a lower suicide rate than others. Further, older women are more likely to be institutionalized in a nursing home. Stress and coping styles may differ by gender with older women developing depression in response to a stressful life event at a rate three times higher than that of older men (Stanford Center on Longevity, 2011). Some people have the mistaken idea that depression is a normal occurrence in older adults. However, most older people feel satisfied with their lives. When depression develops, it is sometimes dismissed as a normal part of aging. Undiagnosed depression in the older person causes unnecessary suffering for the family and for the individual. Depressive symptoms can be side effects of medications the older person is taking for a physical problem; therefore, it is important for the nurse to become familiar with medications that can cause or exacerbate symptoms of depression. Patients with symptoms of depression taking these medications should be urged to seek consultation with their primary care provider to see if the medication can be safely discontinued or switched to another medication without this troubling side effect. Box 7-2 lists some of the medications that can cause depressive symptoms.

Nursing Assessment of Depression

Various instruments are used to assess depression in the older adult. Each instrument has advantages and limitations. The symptoms of depression can be so vague and unique to each individual that the gerontological nurse is urged to use various methods and multiple observations when assessing depression. Sometimes after spending time with a depressed older patient, the nurse will also feel a little "down" or "blue." Because nurses are caring and empathetic individuals, we often pick up on subtle cues the patient is transmitting and become aware of the patient's sadness. Careful and systematic assessment can lead to a definitive diagnosis and early treatment.

The Geriatric Depression Scale (GDS) is a screening instrument used in many clinical settings to assess depression in older people. The GDS is a 30-item (long version) or 15-item (short version) instrument with questions that can be answered "yes" or "no." An older person can complete the GDS alone by circling the correct answer, or it can be read to an older person. When tested in various groups of older people, the GDS was found to successfully distinguish between depressed and nondepressed older people (Yesavage et al., 1983). The GDS can be used for screening physically

---

BOX 7-2 | **Medications That Can Cause Symptoms of Depression**

Analgesics
    Narcotics (e.g., codeine, morphine)
    Nonsteroidal anti-inflammatory agents (ibuprofen, naproxen, indomethacin)
Antihypertensives/cardiac
    Clonidine, methyldopa, propranolol, reserpine, thiazide diuretics, digitalis
Antipsychotics
    Chlorpromazine, fluphenazine, haloperidol, thioridazine, thiothixene
Anxiolytics
    Chlordiazepoxide, diazepam, lorazepam, oxazepam
Chemotherapeutics
    L-asparaginase, cisplatin, tamoxifen, vincristine
Sedative-hypnotics
    Ethchlorvynol, flurazepam, pentobarbital sodium, phenobarbital, secobarbital sodium, temazepam, triazolam
Other
    Antiulcer medications—cimetidine, ranitidine hydrochloride
    Anticholesterol medications/statins
    Corticosteroids—dexamethasone, prednisone
    Alcohol

Source: Adapted from Epocrates.com, 2011; McPhee, Papadakis, & Rabow, 2011; Reuben et al., 2011.

---

healthy or ill individuals, and those with cognitive impairment (Mini-Mental State Examination [MMSE] score above 15) (Kurlowicz & Greenberg, 2007). Older people scoring above 10 should be referred for further assessment. The Cornell Depression Scale (CDS) can be used to screen for depression in older adults with severe cognitive impairments (MMSE below 15). The CDS does not rely on patient responses, but rather observations of behaviors and functional measures. People who score 12 or above on the CDS should be referred for further assessment. Because the CDS requires patient observations, it takes slightly longer to administer than the GDS. (See Best Practices: Geriatric Depression Scale: Short Form for the GDS.) A geropsychiatrist or mental health expert such as an advanced practice nurse or social worker can often treat depression successfully. Different therapies seem to work for different people. For instance, support groups can provide new coping skills or social support if an older person is dealing with a major life change. Several kinds of talk therapies are useful as well. One method of talk therapy is focusing on life successes and strengths and might help older people think in a more positive way. Always being negative and thinking about the sad things in life or what has been lost can lead to depression. Another method works to improve social relationships with others so depressed older people can have more hope about the future. Talk therapies can often serve as effective treatments for depression on their own or as useful adjuncts to pharmacological treatments with antidepressants (National Institute on Aging, 2009).

> **Practice Pearl** ▶▶▶ Chronic depression has been shown to decrease immune function and therefore depressed older persons are more at risk for the development of acute illness or exacerbation of chronic illness.

The criteria for diagnosis of a major depression as manifested by the *Diagnostic and Statistical Manual of Mental Disorders,* Fourth Edition, Text Revision (*DSM-IV-TR*) (American Psychiatric Association, 2004) include verification of a unique set of symptoms that go beyond an older person's statement that they are experiencing feelings of sadness. Older persons will often express somatic or physical complaints such as sleep disorders, changes in appetite, feelings of guilt, inability to concentrate, and perhaps thoughts of suicide. Usually these symptoms must persist for at least two consecutive weeks. A mental health clinician will take the time to carefully assess an older person and gather the needed information to confirm the diagnosis of depression. The assessment usually includes:

- a medical evaluation
- a clinical interview
- a medication review, and
- neuropsychological testing, as needed.

For further information, consult the DSM-IV-TR manual. The DSM-V is currently in the planning stage and is due for publication in 2013.

Bipolar Disorder

Another type of depression is bipolar disorder, also called manic-depressive illness. This disorder is not as prevalent as other forms of depressive disorders in the older person. Bipolar disorder is characterized by cycling mood changes with severe highs (mania) and lows (depression). Sometimes the mood switches are dramatic and rapid, but most often they are gradual. When in the depressed cycle, an individual can have any or all of the symptoms of a depressive disorder (American Psychiatric Association, 2004). The individual in the manic cycle may be overactive and have a great deal of energy. Mania often affects thinking, judgment, and social behavior in

---

BOX 7-3 ▶ **Symptoms of Mania in Bipolar Depression**

- Abnormal or excessive elation
- Unusual irritability, high levels of energy and activity
- Decreased need for sleep
- Grandiose notions
- Increased talking
- Racing thoughts
- Increased sexual desire
- Markedly increased energy
- Poor judgment, going on spending spree, using recreational drugs
- Inappropriate social behavior

Source: National Institute of Mental Health. (2009). *Bipolar disorder.* Retrieved from http://www.nimh.nih.gov/health/publications/bipolar-disorder/what-are-the-symptoms-of-bipolar-disorder.shtml

ways that cause serious problems and embarrassment. The symptoms of mania in bipolar depression are listed in Box 7-3.

Some types of depression appear to be familial and occur generation after generation. However, depression can also occur in older people who have no family history of the disorder. Depressive disorders are often associated with changes in brain structure or brain function. People who have low self-esteem, who consistently view themselves and the world with pessimism, or who are readily overwhelmed by stress are prone to depression. In recent years, researchers have shown that physical changes in the body can be accompanied by mental changes as well. Physical illnesses such as stroke, heart attack, cancer, and Parkinson disease can be accompanied by disabling symptoms of depression. These symptoms can cause older persons to be apathetic and unwilling to care for their physical needs, thus prolonging the recovery period. It has been estimated that up to 57% of patients with Alzheimer's disease, 40% of patients with Parkinson disease, 30% to 60% of those who have had a stroke, and 25% of those with cancer and diabetes suffer from disabling symptoms of major depression (Cigna, 2011).

Those older persons with depression who also have been diagnosed with chronic illness are less likely to participate in rehabilitation activities and more likely to neglect self-care, thus delaying healing and resulting in loss of function and perhaps premature institutionalization in a long-term care facility.

Additional physical diagnoses associated with depression include endocrine disorders (hypo- and hyperthyroid), neoplastic disorders (brain tumors, pancreatic cancer, metastatic bone cancer), epilepsy, multiple sclerosis, congestive heart failure, vitamin B_{12} deficiency, and viral illness. Serious losses, difficult relationships, financial problems, and unwelcomed stressors such as changes in life patterns can trigger depressive episodes. Changes in social roles require adjustment and can affect the identity of the older person involved. Retirement, widowhood, or an unplanned move from the home may precipitate a role change that can be perceived as positive or negative by the older person. If much of the older person's identity is based on the lost role, coping problems and depression can follow. For instance, if the older woman primarily thinks of herself as Mrs. John Smith or the wife of John Smith, the death of her husband may be difficult and more likely to negatively affect her mental health.

Suicide

Older persons age 65 and over have the highest suicide rates of all age groups. A major risk factor for suicide is depression. Older Caucasian men have the highest death rates from suicide of all groups of older people. Older men, but not women, with serious neurologic, vascular, and heart diseases were found to be at increased risk for suicide (NIMH, 2010). Approximately 70% of older adults who commit suicide had visited their primary care physician within the previous month (USDHHS, 2012). Caucasians have the highest suicide rates, followed by Asians, Hispanics, and non-Hispanic blacks (NIMH, 2010).

older men – guns
older women – overdose on meds

Gerontological nurses can play a key role in the identification and referral of those older people who are depressed and at risk for suicide. When the gerontological nurse is interacting with an older patient who seems sad or depressed, the nurse should ask about suicidal intent. Many nurses are hesitant to do this because of fear of placing the idea in the older person's mind. However, this is rarely, if ever, the case. Most older people, when asked this question gently by a caring nurse, will respond openly and appreciate the gesture. The nurse may ask, "Mr. Jones, you seem sad today. Over the past 2 weeks have you felt down, depressed, or hopeless? Have you felt little pleasure in doing things?" If the older person answers affirmatively, further assessment is warranted. An older patient is considered to be in a major depression with the presence of four of the following symptoms that persist for at least 2 weeks along with changes in social relationships and daily function:

- Significant weight loss or gain/changes in appetite
- Disturbances in sleep patterns
- Noticeable agitation or slowness
- Fatigue or loss of energy
- Inappropriate feelings of worthlessness or guilt
- Inability to concentrate or make decisions
- Recurrent thoughts of suicide or death

National Institute of Mental Health, 2010.

Best Practices　Geriatric Depression Scale: Short Form

Choose the best answer for how you have felt over the past week:

1. Are you basically satisfied with your life? YES / **NO**
2. Have you dropped many of your activities and interests? **YES** / NO
3. Do you feel that your life is empty? **YES** / NO
4. Do you often get bored? **YES** / NO
5. Are you in good spirits most of the time? YES / **NO**
6. Are you afraid that something bad is going to happen to you? **YES** / NO
7. Do you feel happy most of the time? YES / **NO**
8. Do you often feel helpless? **YES** / NO
9. Do you prefer to stay at home, rather than going out and doing new things? **YES** / NO
10. Do you feel you have more problems with memory than most? **YES** / NO
11. Do you think it is wonderful to be alive now? YES / **NO**
12. Do you feel pretty worthless the way you are now? **YES** / NO
13. Do you feel full of energy? YES / **NO**
14. Do you feel that your situation is hopeless? **YES** / NO
15. Do you think that most people are better off than you are? **YES** / NO

Answers in **bold** indicate depression. Score 1 point for each bolded answer.
A score > 5 points is suggestive of depression.
A score ≥ 10 points is almost always indicative of depression.
A score > 5 points should warrant a follow-up comprehensive assessment.

Source: "Proposed factor structure of the geriatric depression scale," Author: J. I. Sheikh, Author: J. A. Yesavage, Author: J. O. Brooks. Copyright © 1991 *International Psychogeriatric Association*, pp. 23–28, http://www.epocrates.com. Reprinted with permission from Cambridge University Press.

In the older population, the ratio of attempts to completed suicides is 4 to 1. An older person who contemplates suicide is more likely to complete the act than a younger person. There are several reasons for this fact. First, older people often employ lethal methods when attempting suicide. Second, older people experience greater social isolation (NIMH, 2010). Finally, older people generally have poorer recuperative capacity, which makes them less likely to recover from a suicide attempt. A way to decrease the rate of suicide in older people is to educate healthcare providers about the signs and symptoms of depression and suicide, because many older people have seen a primary care provider in the month before their death. Improving outreach programs to identify, protect, and treat older adults at risk for suicide is a major challenge for our healthcare system.

> **Practice Pearl** ▶▶▶ Suicide attempts are expressions of extreme distress, not harmless bids for attention. An older person who appears suicidal should not be left alone and needs emergency mental health services (NIMH, 2010).

A direct relationship exists between alcoholism, depression, and suicide. Studies indicate that the risk of suicide in alcoholics is 50% to 70% greater than in the general population. Studies show that individuals suffering from a major affective disorder have a greater than 50% higher suicide rate than the general population. Lifetime risk for suicide in the general population is 1%, compared with 15% for persons suffering from depression and 15% for alcoholics. Studies of alcoholics reveal that between 30% and 60% suffer from depression, and a significant proportion of alcoholics have other persons in their families suffering from depression.

Risk factors for suicide that may be determined from the past health history include a previous suicide attempt, alcohol or substance abuse, presence of a psychiatric illness, history of a psychiatric illness, presence of auditory hallucinations (sensory misperceptions such as hearing voices commanding action), living alone, presence of firearms in the home, and exposure to suicidal behavior of others such as family member, peers, or celebrities in the media (NIMH, 2010). Older men are more likely to have access to and use guns as a means to suicide, whereas older women are more likely to overdose on medications. Once the suicide intent is verbalized, the means to carry out the plan should be assessed. Older patients who have the means to carry out a suicide attempt should be immediately referred for evaluation. Those perceived to be at risk for suicide will probably be hospitalized for a short period to protect their lives and provide for intensive observation and treatment.

Patients hospitalized with suicidal ideation will be placed on "suicide precautions" that include one-to-one monitoring by an observer, locked windows, and removal of items that have potential for self-harm such as belts, sharp knives, and medications. Therapy and treatment of the underlying depression will most often improve the older patient's situation. By providing a safe and supportive environment and listening therapeutically to the older patient, the nurse has the opportunity to prevent suffering and the needless loss of human life. Counseling and cognitive psychotherapy have been shown to be effective in reducing the rate of repeated suicide attempts during a year of follow-up therapy (NIMH, 2010).

Some nurses confuse an older patient's desire to have a natural death with suicidal intent. A seriously ill patient who cries and states "I'm ready to go when God calls me" is probably not expressing suicidal thoughts. Any patient who receives bad news of serious illness or failed treatment has the right to be sad and overwhelmed. Serious chronic illness imposes heavy physical, social, emotional, and economic burdens on patients, families, and society (NIMH, 2010). Each older person who is diagnosed with a life-threatening illness may react differently and begin the work of preparing for death as the gerontological nurse and the healthcare team are providing care. However, patients who request assistance from the nurse with suicide and active euthanasia should be informed that the nurse cannot participate, as these acts are in direct violation of the American Nurses Association's (2010) *Code of Ethics for Nurses*. Active euthanasia or "mercy killing" means that someone other than the patient commits an action with the intent to end the patient's life. According to the ANA *Code of Ethics for Nurses*, mercy killing is immoral and illegal, even when a suffering patient requests assistance from the nurse to hasten death. An example may be the injection of a lethal dose of morphine into a patient, not to relieve suffering, but to end life. Active euthanasia is distinguished from assisted suicide in that with active euthanasia someone not only makes the means of death available, but also serves as the direct agent of death. The ANA statement advances that assisted suicide and active euthanasia are inconsistent with the code for nurses and are ethically unacceptable. There are many ways to support older patients and their families at the end of life without participating in assisted suicide or active euthanasia. Gerontological nurses should aggressively investigate depression and advocate for effective pain control to prevent needless suffering at the end of life (see Chapter 11 ▭ for further information on end-of-life care).

Alcohol Abuse/Substance Abuse

The prevalence of **alcohol abuse** (use of alcohol to excess) and **alcohol dependence** (craving or reliance on alcohol) despite problems resulting from continued use

in older adults ranges from 2% to 5% for men and about 1% for women. There is a decline in substance abuse for older adults after the age of 60. There are several reasons, however, why drinking alcohol may negatively impact the physical and mental health of the older person. Age-related physical changes, diagnosed physical illness, and prescription drugs can combine with relatively low levels of alcohol to produce negative outcomes in older people. Older persons experience higher blood levels per amount of alcohol consumed due to decreased lean body mass and total body water. Older patients are hospitalized as frequently for alcohol-related problems as they are for heart attacks (Blazer & Wu, 2009). It is recommended that alcohol consumption for older adults be limited to one standard drink per day or seven standard drinks per week. A standard drink is defined as 12 oz of beer, 4 to 5 oz of wine, or 1½ oz of distilled spirits (National Institute of Alcohol Abuse and Alcoholism, 2008). However, red wine consumed in small to moderate amounts has been shown to decrease risk of cardiovascular disease. As the number of older people increases, so will the absolute number of older people who have alcohol abuse problems.

Risk factors for alcohol abuse include genetic predisposition, being male, limited education, poverty, and a history of depression (APA, 2011). Men over age 65 are five times more likely to suffer from alcoholism than their female counterparts; however, older women with drinking problems are more likely to go undetected (Chou, Liang, & Mackenzie, 2011). Older women are more likely to become dependent on prescription drugs, such as benzodiazepines, than their male counterparts (Moore et al., 2011). Older widowers have the highest prevalence rates of alcohol abuse among older adults (APA, 2011). Problems related to excessive or regular alcohol consumption include:

- **Malnutrition.** Failure to prepare and eat an adequate diet.
- **Anxiety**, or state of apprehension, uneasiness, or distress. Increases in baseline levels.
- **Falls.** Consistent and recurrent bruises and fractures.
- **Social isolation.** Avoidance of friends who do not drink or who are judgmental.
  - **Headaches.** Often occurring at night or early morning.
  - **Sleep disorders.** Early morning awakening and daytime sleepiness.
- **Cirrhosis of the liver.** One of eight leading causes of death for the older person.
- **Osteomalacia.** Thinning of the bones.
- **Decreases in gastric absorption.** Failure to absorb key minerals and vitamins from ingested food.
- **Decline in cognitive function or ability to think, reason, remember, and communicate.** Impairment of memory and information processing.

- **Interactions with medications.** Interaction with benzodiazepines greatly increases risk of falls and hip fractures.

APA, 2011; Moore et al., 2011.

Unlike other psychoactive drugs, alcohol has a generalized effect on the central nervous system. Alcohol seems to impair learning and memory because of its ability to inhibit acetylcholine action. Judgment and reasoning are also adversely affected, with degree of impairment related to blood alcohol level or duration of consumption. Additionally, alcohol can lead to loss of social inhibition and problems in regulation of emotion. Higher levels of consumption lead to drowsiness, stupor, and motor coordination problems (Moore et al., 2011). Alcohol consumption in excess of three drinks per day increases the risk of hypertension, some cancers (esophagus and breast in women), and possibly injury (World Health Organization, 2011). Alcohol may interact with certain drugs and cause adverse systemic effects. These drugs include antihypertensives, nonsteroidal anti-inflammatory drugs (NSAIDs), H_2-blockers, sedatives, and antidepressants (Reuben et al., 2011).

The criteria for possible alcohol dependence include:

- establishing that the older adult has developed tolerance to alcohol over time
- may suffer withdrawal effects when intake is stopped
- a history of unsuccessful attempts to stop drinking
- continuing to drink despite physical or psychological problems, and
- spending a great deal of time using alcohol and recovering from its effects.

Signs of alcohol abuse may include:

- drinking because of feelings of failure
- drinking in situations where it is physically dangerous (e.g., driving),
- drinking despite social problems resulting from alcohol use, and
- presence of legal problems as a result of drinking.

Screening for alcohol use not only is a means for detection, but also provides the opportunity for intervention to reduce adverse consequences (APA, 2011).

The Hartford Institute of Geriatric Nursing's *Best Practices in Nursing Care to Older Adults* (Naegle, 2012) recommends the Short Michigan Alcoholism Screening Test–Geriatric Version (SMAST-G). A score of 2 or more "yes" responses suggests an alcohol problem (see Best Practices: Short Michigan Alcoholism Screening Test–Geriatric Version [SMAST-G]).

Older persons who are dependent on or abusing alcohol should be referred for further evaluation and treatment.

The gerontological nurse plays a key role in educating the older person about the potential health problems associated with continued alcohol use. Self-help groups such as Alcoholics Anonymous, professional counseling, social support, and drug therapy have all been shown to be effective in treating alcohol problems in older people. Disulfiram (Antabuse) is not recommended for use in older people because of the potential for serious cardiovascular side effects and multiple drug interactions (Reuben et al., 2011).

Older people who are hospitalized or institutionalized in long-term care facilities may become delirious during acute alcohol withdrawal. Acute agitation and hallucinations may occur (delirium tremens). Nonpharmacological measures to protect patient safety include keeping the room as quiet as possible, avoiding excessive light and stimulation, encouraging family visitation for comfort and reassurance, providing orientation to time and place, communicating directly and succinctly, and providing frequent observation and monitoring of vital signs. Usually the physician will prescribe lorazepam (Ativan) 0.5 to 2.0 mg every 4 to 6 hours to prevent alcohol withdrawal seizures.

Adequate hydration and nutrition will ease the withdrawal process (Reuben et al., 2011).

Older people receive about 75 million prescriptions for sedative and tranquilizer medications each year (National Institute on Drug Abuse, 2011). Often these medications can interact with each other or with alcohol. Signs and symptoms of alcohol or medication-related problems include:

- Memory problems after having a drink or taking a medication
- Ataxia or loss of muscle coordination (may be frequent faller or have multiple bruises)
- Changes in sleep or eating patterns
- Irritability, sadness, or depression
- Trouble concentrating or finishing projects
- Chronic pain
- Smell of alcohol or frequent mouthwash on breath
- Keeping bottles of prescription drugs/tranquilizers close by and taking them for minor reasons throughout the day
- Wanting to be alone or avoiding friends and family
- Lack of interest in usual activities

National Institute on Drug Abuse, 2011.

Best Practices **Short Michigan Alcoholism Screening Test–Geriatric Version (SMAST-G)**

	YES (1)	NO (0)
1. When talking with others, do you ever underestimate how much you drink?		
2. After a few drinks, have you sometimes not eaten or been able to skip a meal because you didn't feel hungry?		
3. Does having a few drinks help decrease your shakiness or tremors?		
4. Does alcohol sometimes make it hard for you to remember parts of the day or night?		
5. Do you usually take a drink to relax or calm your nerves?		
6. Do you drink to take your mind off your problems?		
7. Have you ever increased your drinking after experiencing a loss in your life?		
8. Has a doctor or nurse ever said they were worried or concerned about your drinking?		
9. Have you ever made rules to manage your drinking?		
10. When you feel lonely, does having a drink help?		
TOTAL SMAST-G SCORE (0–10) _____		
SCORING: 2 OR MORE "**YES**" RESPONSES IS INDICATIVE OF AN ALCOHOL PROBLEM.		

Source: The Regents of the University of Michigan, 1991. University of Michigan Alcohol Research Center. Reprinted with permission.

Nurses who suspect an older person is taking prescription drugs in an inappropriate way or has become overly reliant on them should discuss this with the older person directly and state concerns in an open manner. Often, older adults will need education regarding the harmful side effects of taking sedating drugs for long periods of time and may not realize the potential harmful side effects that they are risking over time. Often, older people receive health care and prescription medications from several healthcare providers. If their providers do not communicate with each other, duplicate or interacting prescriptions may be written, resulting in overmedication or drug interactions. Lack of awareness on the part of healthcare providers, failure to obtain accurate drug and alcohol histories, fear of asking questions about drug and alcohol use, and lack of knowledge about how to treat substance abuse problems can all contribute to the problem.

Nursing actions that may be appropriate include teaching the patient to:

- Review all medications and instructions for use on a routine basis.
- Urge older persons not to drink alcohol if they are taking medications for sleep, pain, anxiety, or depression.
- Keep track of all side effects or changes in cognition or function (especially when new medications are started).
- Clean out the medicine cabinet every year.
- Ask your primary healthcare provider to review all medications each year.

National Institute on Drug Abuse, 2011.

Older patients with a history of long-term benzodiazepine dependency may need to be hospitalized and closely monitored while the drug is being discontinued. Abrupt discontinuation of many sedative and narcotic medications can result in seizures, muscle pain, anxiety, and depression.

Basic Principles for Psychological Assessment

Because of the physical and sensory changes of aging, the testing environment must be appropriate to ensure optimal performance by the older adult. Specially trained neuropsychologists can administer a battery of neuropsychological tests to provide specific and detailed information about the older person's cognitive and psychological status. The gerontological nurse may be the first to notice signs and symptoms of psychological change and recommend the referral to the geriatric mental health specialist. Psychological testing should be done under the following circumstances:

- When considering admission to a geropsychiatric inpatient unit or long-term care facility

- When considering need for, and benefit of, outpatient geropsychiatric services
- To assist in the diagnosis of dementia versus depression
- To provide information for the legal determination of competency
- When evaluating sudden or severe changes in mood, personality (personal characteristics attitudes and beliefs that influence how an older person interacts with the world), or psychological function
- To initiate, evaluate, and/or monitor response to therapy or psychotropic medication

The nurse's interpersonal skills will facilitate the clinical interview and the gathering of information in an individualized, comprehensive, and holistic assessment. Some suggestions for improving the quality of information gathered at the clinical interview include the following:

- Make sure the older patient is not in pain, has been to the bathroom, and has water or juice to sip on during the assessment. If the older person wears glasses or hearing aids, make sure they are in place and functioning.
- Educate the older adult about the purpose and procedure for the testing. The nurse may say, "I'm going to ask you some questions about your mood. Some of these may seem silly to you, but we ask these questions of most of our clinic patients." Older adults may not be used to testing procedures or questions about their feelings and relationships and may need some reassurance.
- Try to make the testing environment as quiet as possible. Turn off the paging system and any beepers. Make sure there is adequate lighting.
- Speak slowly and clearly. Make sure the older adult understands the testing instructions. If vision is impaired, use a magnifying lens or large-print testing materials.
- Observe the older patient carefully. If the patient becomes tired and has difficulty concentrating, take a break and resume testing at another time.
- If English is the second language for the older patient, request assistance from a translator rather than asking a family member to translate. The translator has been trained in the precise use of medical terminology.

The gerontological nurse should assess the older patient's current mental status and obtain informed consent before beginning mood testing. The older patient's education, culture, ethnicity, religion, health status, and comfort should form the context for the nurse's assessment. The older person's social situation should also be considered. Financial stressors, active grieving, living situation, social support, and degree of loneliness will greatly affect the older person's responses. Mood is evaluated by observation of the patient (e.g., facial expressions, posture, speed of movements, and thoughts), use of standardized assessment tools such as the GDS, and of verbal responses to questions. Although patients sometimes spontaneously express feelings of helplessness, hopelessness, worthlessness, shame, or guilt, they should be asked directly about such feelings (e.g., "Do you feel that you are a good person?" "Do you feel guilty about things you have done?") and about mood (e.g., "Are you in good spirits?" or "How is your mood?").

Current and past medical history is needed to assess the impact of physical illness on psychological status. Chronic pain is a known correlate of depression, and a careful pain assessment should be done whenever depression is suspected. The patient should be asked about changes in energy, appetite, or sleep that are related to mood disturbances. Additional assessment information includes use of prescription and over-the-counter medication, as well as current and past use of alcohol, tobacco, and recreational drugs. The nurse should ascertain whether the older patient is taking the medication as directed, whether the prescription is current and not expired, and whether the conditions under which the medication is taken are appropriate (e.g., on an empty stomach, before bed, only when needed). It is important to pay special attention to sudden changes in mood or personality, because these may be signs of delirium related to recent changes in medication, onset of undetected illness, or exacerbation of chronic illness. When the older patient's cognitive status appears to be impaired, the nurse should request the patient's permission to include a family member or caregiver in the assessment to supplement and verify the information reported by the patient.

> **Practice Pearl ▶▶▶** When a family member reports that an older person's behavior or attitude has changed, always listen carefully to this information. Family members are often the first to notice subtle changes that may not become apparent to others for weeks or months.

Depression presents differently in older adults and may manifest itself as a sense of dread or impending doom, as apathy, or as irritability without a specific cause. Depression may also be suggested by vague complaints of pain, tiredness, or other physiological changes; by slow speech; by anxiety (sometimes as panic attacks with shortness of breath, palpitations, and sweating); by phobias, obsessions, or compulsions; or by abnormal perceptions (e.g., delusions, hallucinations). When the nurse suspects an underlying anxiety disorder, the patient should be asked about all medications and phobias or irrational fears of particular places, things, or situations.

Older patients should also be asked about obsessions (recurrent, unwanted ideas that cannot be resisted, although they may seem unreasonable) and compulsions (repeated, unwanted behaviors such as hand washing or rechecking a locked door). Obsessions in the older person may be due to severe depression. Obsessions can be elicited by asking, "Do you have thoughts that keep coming to your mind and are difficult to get rid of?" Compulsions can be elicited by asking, "Do you feel that you do certain things (e.g., wash your hands) repeatedly, more than you need to?" Sometimes older adults who are aware that they have memory deficits become obsessed with certain objects for fear of losing them. For instance, an older woman may hold onto her pocketbook and refuse to give it up because if it is out of her sight, she is afraid she will not be able to find it.

Additionally, older persons with depression and cognitive impairments may exhibit signs of delusions. Delusions are false, fixed, and idiosyncratic ideas. Patients may reveal delusional thoughts when questioned (e.g., "Are people treating you kindly?" "Is anyone trying to harm you?"). Delusions of harm (e.g., of food poisoning) or of harassment may occur in older people with paranoid schizophrenia or *paraphrenia* (late-life schizophrenia). Delusions also occur frequently in persons with dementia. Delusions of poverty or of fatal illness may occur in depressed persons, who may verbalize multiple somatic complaints and become overly focused on body functions. *Delusions of persecution* (e.g., belief that someone is out to get them) or of *misidentification* (e.g., belief that family members are strangers or that persons long dead are alive) may occur in persons with cognitive impairment. Furthermore, the nurse should be able to detect hallucinations in the form of false visual, auditory, olfactory, or tactile perceptions. The presence of visual or auditory hallucinations may be elicited by asking, "Do you hear voices or see visions? If you hear voices, are they telling you what to do?" Further questioning is needed to determine whether the phenomena are really perceived (e.g., "Do you hear the voices even when you do not see anyone talking? Do you hear them through your ears, or are they in your thoughts?" The nurse should respond with sympathy (e.g., "That must have frightened you"), not with surprise or disbelief. Visual and tactile (feeling bugs crawling on skin when none are present) hallucinations are prominent in delirium, and auditory hallucinations may occur when the older person is cognitively impaired and in paraphrenia. Auditory hallucinations (e.g., hearing one's name called) also may occur in late-life depression. Hallucinations may occur in persons with sensory deficits, especially profound blindness, at which time the condition is called Charles Bonnet syndrome. In addition, hallucinations may occur during bereavement, when the patient sees or hears the deceased person.

> **Practice Pearl** ▶▶▶ An older person may appear to be paranoid when he or she says that a family member has stolen a wallet or purse, but further investigation may reveal the presence of a cognitive impairment that has caused the older person to forget where the wallet or purse was placed.

When all the information from the older patient has been gathered, the nurse and other members of the health-care team will integrate the findings with relevant social and health variables. Strengths and weaknesses should be identified so the gerontological nurse can begin to formulate nursing interventions that build on areas of strength and compensate for areas of weakness. Older patients in acute psychological distress such as those who are severely agitated, depressed, or in danger of harming themselves or others should be referred to an emergency mental health worker for initiation of protective services including psychotherapy and/or psychotropic medication. If underlying health problems are thought to be negatively influencing psychological function, a referral to an internist or geriatrician may greatly benefit the older person. Complete assessment of health problems includes a head-to-toe physical examination and a variety of laboratory tests, including a complete blood count (CBC), a chemistry panel (SMA-18), test of thyroid function (TSH), and assessment of serum levels of medications taken on a regular basis (e.g., digoxin, warfarin). Additional testing may be needed based on the older patient's unique personal and health history.

Nursing Interventions

Treatment of mental health problems in the older person can use nonpharmacological approaches, pharmacological approaches, or a combination of the two. Information on these techniques follows.

Nonpharmacological Treatments

Many older adults referred for psychological services will feel embarrassed or ashamed of the need for psychotherapy or psychotropic medication. The gerontological nurse can reassure the older person and the family that mental health problems can be effectively treated. This treatment will enhance the chances of returning to former levels of psychological function.

No single psychological intervention is preferred for older adults. The treatment of choice is guided by the nature of the problem, therapeutic goals, preferences of the older adult, and practical considerations (APA, 2011). Both individual and group psychotherapy have been shown to be effective in treating the older adult's psychological problems.

Family or couples therapy may be appropriate when marital or family relationship problems occur within the context of late-life illness or stress. Often, a family member may feel stress by the burden of caring for a spouse or parent and may need support and respite from the responsibility of care. Behavior modification, self-help groups, educational sessions, and changes in the social or physical environment may lead to improved emotional health and functioning.

Some older people find it beneficial to engage in reminiscence or a "life review" of the present, the past, and the future. Both successes and failures should be considered in an effort to identify the older person's life themes with the goal of attaining greater psychological integration and emotional strength. Geriatric social workers and advanced practice psychiatric–mental health nurses can greatly assist with this process.

Support group attendance can help the older person and the family cope with problems by identifying with others who are in the same situation. The Alzheimer's Association, the American Cancer Society, and other groups focusing on specific illnesses in late life (e.g., Parkinson disease, arthritis, cardiac or lung problems) provide a forum for conversation, social interaction, education, and problem solving. Grief or bereavement groups can also assist the older person dealing with multiple or serious losses or unresolved grief. Additional helpful interventions include travel with senior citizens' groups, taking classes at the local college, elder hostels, volunteer work, regular exercise, hobbies and crafts, and increased family involvement.

For older persons experiencing caregiver stress, attendance at self-help groups can be especially helpful. There are an estimated 25 million family caregivers in the United States who deliver care to a frail older person (spouse, parent, sibling), including help with daily activities and around-the-clock supervision. Caregivers can experience enormous stress from the added responsibility of caring for a loved one and may become depressed or anxious, or develop physical illness as a result of the stress of caregiving. In addition to concrete suggestions to improve safety in the home, education about stress-reducing techniques emphasizes mutual support and caring. The following suggestions for caregivers may help to reduce stress:

- Share the responsibility for care. Do not take on more than you can handle, and involve others who can help out.
- Meditate, listen to music, or take a brief walk every day. Caregivers who do not care for themselves will be of no use to anyone.
- Set priorities. Work on one problem at a time. Trying to do too much will cause you to feel distracted, frustrated, and "at loose ends." Make a list and cross one problem off before moving to the next.

- Maintain your own physical health. Get regular check-ups, take medications, eat nutritious meals, avoid alcohol and caffeine, and get regular exercise. Should something happen to you, your loved one may be at risk for institutionalization.
- Seek love and support from your family, friends, clergy, and others. Do not be afraid to seek additional help and recognize when professional counseling is needed to cope with difficult decisions.
- Educate yourself about your loved one's condition. Knowledge is power.
- Join a local support group. Contact your local aging resource center for phone numbers.
- Accept yourself for who you are. Do not strive for perfection. You are a human being doing the best you can to cope with a difficult situation. Self-acceptance and nurturing will go a long way.

Light therapy has been shown to be effective for older patients diagnosed with **seasonal affective disorder,** a cyclic depression that occurs when hours of daylight are short, usually in the fall and early spring. Older patients who respond to light therapy will sit before specially designed lights for several hours during the shortened daylight periods. Biochemical changes are thought to be stimulated in the brain by various blue and red hues in the spectrum of light. Medications can also be used to augment light therapy in older patients with seasonal affective disorder.

Older persons with substance abuse problems (drug or alcohol) may attend Alcoholics Anonymous meetings. They may benefit from professional treatment and counseling or age-specific inpatient or outpatient treatment during the withdrawal period. Many late-life mental health problems are recurrent. The goals of treatment should be flexible and emphasize improving function, managing disabling symptoms, preventing relapse, and building a safety net for quick recognition of recurring problems.

COMPLEMENTARY AND ALTERNATIVE THERAPIES

Ginkgo biloba originates in Asia and is used to improve memory and cognition. Although widely used, there are few double-blind placebo-controlled studies that demonstrate clinical effectiveness in humans. Older persons taking ginkgo biloba should stop taking this herbal supplement about a week before surgery, because it inhibits clotting and may result in excessive bleeding. Additional cautions include the recommendation to avoid taking ginkgo biloba with warfarin, aspirin, ibuprofen, ergotamine, or other anticoagulants as it will increase the International Normalized Ratio (INR) and may result in subdural hematoma or other cranial bleeds (National Center for Complementary and Alternative Medicine [NCCAM], 2010).

Valerian is another commonly used herbal supplement and is used as a sleep aid and antianxiety agent. It can be taken during the day or at bedtime and is usually well tolerated. Side effects include gastrointestinal upset, nervousness, and sleep disturbances. It should not be taken with alcohol, sedating drugs, or benzodiazepines because excess sleepiness or drowsiness may occur (NCCAM, 2010).

St. John's wort is used for a variety of mental health problems including depression, anxiety, insomnia, and neurogenic pain. Clinical studies indicate it can be used effectively in patients with mild to moderate depression, but clinical effectiveness has not been demonstrated in patients with severe depression. St. John's wort may interact with many other medications including antiretrovirals used to treat HIV infections, acid-suppressing drugs, anticonvulsants, antihypertensives, cyclosporine, hormonal contraceptives, antidepressants (some selective serotonin reuptake inhibitors), and warfarin. All older patients taking herbal supplements should be monitored for improvement, side effects, and interactions with other medications (NCCAM, 2010).

Pharmacological Treatments

The pharmacological treatment of depression begins with a careful diagnosis and ongoing assessment of suitable medications with ongoing monitoring and adjustments as needed. When the older patient experiences only a partial response or no response at all after 6 to 12 weeks of therapy and nonpharmacological interventions for depression, use of antidepressant medication is usually warranted. As with all drugs prescribed to an older person, the risks and benefits should be carefully analyzed. Many antidepressant drugs, especially the tricyclic antidepressants, have troublesome anticholinergic side effects and can cause orthostatic hypotension.

Because many of the antidepressants take 6 to 12 weeks to achieve therapeutic effects and ease depression, the older person and the family should be patient and realistic in their expectations regarding antidepressant therapy. For mild, moderate, or severe depression, the duration of therapy should be at least 6 to 12 months following remission for older patients experiencing their first depressive episode. Most older patients with a history of major depression require lifelong antidepressant therapy (Reuben et al., 2011). As with all medications, the initial dose should be about one half the usual adult dose, in order to decrease the severity of any adverse side effects. Careful monitoring is needed during the first few days of treatment so that any adverse side effects can be quickly noted and the medication changed or discontinued if needed. Falls, sedation, urinary retention, constipation, drowsiness, visual changes, appetite changes, tachycardia, and photosensitivity have all been reported as side effects of antidepressants and may pose a significant health and safety risk for older adults. Some antidepressants can increase the therapeutic effects and interact with warfarin, anticholinergics, antihistamines, opioids, and sedative-hypnotics. Older patients taking warfarin should be closely monitored during the first few weeks of the initiation of antidepressant therapy.

Antidepressants can decrease the effects of certain drugs, including some anticonvulsant medications (phenytoin) and some antihypertensives. Postural blood pressure should be carefully monitored during the first few weeks of antidepressant therapy in older patients with hypertension. Older patients should be strongly urged to avoid alcohol while taking antidepressant medications.

Because many of the tricyclic antidepressants (TCAs) are associated with anticholinergic side effects such as constipation, urinary retention, dry mouth, hypotension, and tachycardia, some geriatricians prefer to use the selective scrotonin reuptake inhibitors (SSRIs) as first-line drugs for many older patients, especially those with the following conditions:

- Heart conduction defects or ischemic heart disease
- Benign prostatic hypertrophy
- Difficult-to-control glaucoma

In general, the SSRIs are well tolerated in the older person. Side effects include nausea, diarrhea, headache, erectile dysfunction, insomnia, or somnolence. Table 7-1 lists the SSRIs commonly used with older people.

The TCAs have been the most widely used antidepressants in the older population. In general, those who respond best to these medications are older people with loss of appetite, psychomotor agitation or retardation, history of previous use and response to TCAs, and family history of depression that responded to TCA treatment (Kane, Ouslander, & Abrass, 2008). All of the tricyclics have the potential to produce bothersome and potentially dangerous side effects including serious cardiac arrhythmias. Careful nursing assessment is indicated during the initial dosing period. Divided dosages can help minimize side effects. For older patients with sleep disturbances, a single bedtime dose can be used to take advantage of the sedative side effects; however, these patients are at risk for postural hypotension and may fall if they get out of bed to use the bathroom in the middle of the night. Many prescribers avoid the use of imipramine and amitriptyline because they can cause severe orthostatic hypotension, placing the older person at risk for fall and injury. To decrease the development of symptoms of tardive dyskinesia such as dystonia and parkinsonism, amoxapine should be avoided. Table 7-2 lists the TCAs commonly used in older people.

Additional drugs sometimes used to treat depression in the older person include bupropion (Wellbutrin). This drug may lower the seizure threshold, so it is contraindicated in older patients with seizure disorders. It is usually started at 37.5 mg bid and titrated to 75–100 mg bid. It has been used successfully in some older patients who have failed to respond to SSRI and TCA therapy (Reuben et al., 2011). Side effects include agitation, dry mouth, tremor, headache, nausea, and insomnia (McPhee et al., 2011). Mirtazapine (Remeron) has been shown to increase appetite in older adults and may be helpful in those with poor food intake. Beginning dose is 15 mg at bedtime and may be titrated to 45mg/day (Reuben et al., 2011).

TABLE 7-1	SSRIs Used in Older Adults		
Drug	**Initial Dose**	**Usual Dose**	**Comments**
Citalopram (Celexa)	10 mg	20–30 mg daily	Hyponatremia in renal failure
Escitalopram (Lexapro)	10 mg	10–20 mg daily	Dry mouth, sweating, cardiac arrhythmias, withdrawal effects when abruptly stopped
Fluoxetine (Prozac)	5 mg	10–50 mg q a.m.	Long half-life; raises levels of haloperidol, diazepam, valproate, alprazolam, and carbamazepine
Sertraline (Zoloft)	25 mg	50 mg q a.m.	Short half-life; raises levels of warfarin
Paroxetine (Paxil)	5 mg	10–20 mg daily	Short half-life; raises levels of digoxin

Source: Adapted from Epocrates.com, 2011; Reuben et al., 2011.

TABLE 7-2	Commonly Used TCAs in Older People			
Drug	Initial Dose	Usual Dose	Comments	
Desipramine (Norpramin)	10 mg a.m.	50–100 mg a.m.	Activating agent	
Nortriptyline (Pamelor)	10 mg hs	75–100 mg hs	Long half-life	

Source: Adapted from Epocrates.com, 2011; Reuben et al., 2011.

Lithium carbonate has been used to treat recurrent bipolar illness and some atypical cases of depression. The half-life of lithium is prolonged in the healthy older person (more than 36 hours) and greatly prolonged in older persons with chronic renal failure. Side effects include bradycardia, hypothyroidism, dry mouth, nausea, vomiting, diarrhea, hypotension, nystagmus, tremor, mental status changes, and seizures (Drugs.com, 2011a). This drug must be used with caution, and blood levels and patient function must be carefully monitored during the initial dosing period.

Monoamine oxidase inhibitors (MAOIs) are sometimes used in older people with dementia and depression and in those who have not responded to other drug therapies. Orthostatic hypotension is common and peaks 4 to 5 weeks after beginning therapy. Additional side effects include drowsiness, dizziness, increased sun sensitivity, and blurred vision (Drugs.com, 2011b). Because these drugs inhibit the metabolism of norepinephrine, hypertensive crisis can occur if they are administered with other drugs or food that raise blood pressure such as anticholinergics, stimulants, and foods containing tyramine (e.g., red wine, cheese, beer, bologna, pepperoni, liver, raisins, bananas). These restrictions apply during use and for 14 days following discontinuation of the MAOIs. Older patients and their families should be well informed about the adverse effects and drug and dietary restrictions necessary for safe administration.

Electroconvulsive Therapy

Electroconvulsive therapy (ECT) is indicated in older patients who do not respond to other antidepressant medications, are diagnosed with delusional depression, or have life-threatening behaviors (e.g., suicidal ideation, catatonic). ECT involves the use of a brief, controlled electrical current to produce a seizure within the brain. This seizure activity is believed to bring about certain biochemical changes that may cause an older person's symptoms to diminish or even disappear. A series of seizures is required to produce such a therapeutic effect (McPhee et al., 2011).

The ECT process has been greatly improved since the 1950s, and the ECT procedure is relatively quick and simple. In most cases, the patient is responsive in 15 minutes, and fully recovered and ready for discharge within 1 to 2 hours. Patients should avoid driving, operating heavy machinery, and drinking alcohol during the treatment period. Short-term memory loss is common for up to 2 weeks after the treatment, so older patients should forgo making important decisions during this period. ECT is contraindicated for patients with increased intracranial pressure, space-occupying brain lesions, severe heart disease, recent myocardial infarction and/or stroke, and aortic aneurysm because of the increased risk of arrhythmia and death (Reuben et al., 2011). The mortality rate is low (less than 1 in 10,000) and the relapse rate is 50% to 70% without maintenance with antidepressant drugs or maintenance ECT therapy.

Nursing Diagnosis

Gerontological nurses soon come to recognize the cardinal symptoms of depression in the older person. Older people who look sad, experience functional decline, and seem to have no enjoyment in life will alert the nurse to carry out a complete depression assessment and evaluation. Physical diagnoses that may be used based on somatic symptoms related to depression include *Constipation, Fatigue, Social Isolation, Nutrition, Imbalanced, Self-care Deficit,* and *Sleep Pattern, Disturbed.* Nursing diagnoses addressing the older person's psychological state may include *Anxiety, Coping, Ineffective, Self-esteem Situational Low, Powerlessness, Hopelessness, Caregiver Role Strain, Spiritual Distress,* and *Suicide, Risk for.* Some experts recommend that NANDA develop a nursing diagnosis for depression based on the *DSM-IV-TR* criteria, etiologies, and defining mood characteristics so that advanced practice nurses can be reimbursed for psychiatric services (Maas et al., 2001). The nurse should be familiar with the *DSM-IV-TR* criteria published and regularly updated by the American Psychiatric Association, because these criteria provide for a categorical approach to the diagnosis and treatment of depression.

The following nurse-sensitive outcomes are identified in the *Nursing Outcomes Classification (NOC)* (Johnson, Maas, & Moorhead, 2000):

- **Suicide self-restraint.** Indicated by establishing and maintaining a contract to not harm himself or herself, seeks help with feeling self-destructive tendencies, maintains connectedness in social relationships, expresses feelings in therapeutic counseling.
- **Mood equilibrium.** Exhibits appropriate affect, maintains self-care including grooming and hygiene, complies with medication regimen, reports adequate sleep, shows interest in surroundings.

- **Hope.** Expresses optimism, looks forward to and plans future events, expresses joy in life, appears to have inner peace.
- **Coping.** Identifies and uses effective coping strategies, modifies lifestyle with behaviors to minimize **stress** (an internal or external event that creates a nonspecific response in the older person), seeks out and uses social and professional support, reports decreased severity and number of stress-related physical symptoms.

Because all older patients are different and unique in their mental health needs, the nurse should choose the most appropriate nursing outcomes to establish the effectiveness of the nursing care plan.

Provision of quality mental health services to older adults includes:

- Awareness of developmental issues in late life
- Identification of cohort or generational effects

- Recognition of the impact of physical illness
- Identification of the effects of taking multiple medications
- Assessment of cognitive or sensory impairments
- Documentation of past history of medical and emotional disorders.

QSEN Recommendations Related to Mental Health

The Quality and Safety Education for Nurses (QSEN) project addresses the challenge of preparing future nurses with the knowledge, skills, and attitudes (KSAs) to continuously improve the quality and safety of the healthcare systems in which they work (Cronenwett et al., 2007). Review the QSEN table for tips on meeting QSEN standards.

Meeting QSEN Standards: Mental Health

	KNOWLEDGE	SKILLS	ATTITUDES
Patient-Centered Care	Involvement of patient and family in psychologic care is crucial.	Family assessment Mood, suicide, substance abuse skills.	Appreciate uniqueness of each patient/family.
	Examine barriers that may lead to errors in mood assessment and treatment of psychological problems.	Evaluate values, attitudes, and cultural norms relating to counseling and psychotropic medication use.	Provide patient-centered care to improve successful nursing outcomes.
Teamwork and Collaboration	Recognize need for input from interdisciplinary team members including dietitian, pharmacist, physician, advanced practice nurses, and others on the team.	Use leadership skills to coordinate team and share knowledge. Consult with social worker to assess insurance status and financial resources to obtain mental health services.	Value the contribution of each member of the team to improve outcomes.
	Be aware of organizational problems that can inhibit effective team function and establish plan for communication.	System assessment skills Safeguard private mental health information according to current HIPAA standards.	Be open to input from team members on effective means to improve communication and collaboration.

(continued)

Meeting QSEN Standards: Mental Health (continued)

	KNOWLEDGE	SKILLS	ATTITUDES
Evidence-Based Practice	Describe effective interventions to decrease risk factors and improve overall health and function. Utilize Beer's criteria and FDA recommendations as appropriate if pharmacological treatment is indicated.	Access current evidence-based protocols to guide interventions.	Possess confidence in necessary skills to evaluate and incorporate nursing interventions from the literature.
Quality Improvement	Recognize the need for patient–family education regarding early recognition of signs of improvement in mood or expression of suicidal ideation.	Skills in data management, technology, and U.S. government and FDA sites describing current incidence and prevalence of ADRs and medication errors.	Value the use of data and outcomes as a key component of QI efforts.
Safety	Describe common medication dosing errors and side effects of psychotropic drugs. Assess patient/family characteristics that increase the likelihood of ADRs.	Use appropriate educational strategies to provide written information to compensate for memory loss (if present) individual learning style. Provide repeat information in high stress situations.	Appreciate the impact of cognitive loss, stress, and attitudes toward psychological problems in order to provide patient-centered care.
Informatics	Provide input into the formation and maintenance of patient databases needed for gathering QSEN data and providing patient care.	Utilize the electronic health record and standardized patient assessment instruments to follow progress and effectiveness of interventions.	Protect patient confidentiality according to HIPAA standards.

Patient and Family Teaching

Gerontological nurses require skills and knowledge related to teaching patients and families about the key concepts of gerontology and gerontological nursing. The patient–family teaching guidelines in the following feature will assist the nurse to assume the role of teacher and coach. Educating patients and families is critical so that nurses can interpret scientific data and individualize the nursing care plan.

Patient–Family Teaching Guidelines

The following are guidelines that the nurse may find useful when instructing older persons and their families about mental health.

MENTAL HEALTH AND THE OLDER ADULT

Many older people think it is normal to have a variety of physical and mental problems. However, mental health problems, including depression and anxiety, are not part of the normal aging process. If you, a family member, or friend experience a sudden change in mood, the way you think, or your memory, see your healthcare professional as soon as possible.

1 What causes mental health problems?

Some mild memory or mood problems can occur in healthy older adults, but serious problems can be a sign of underlying mental health disease.

RATIONALE:

Chronic unrelieved pain, some physical illnesses, problems with eyesight and hearing, certain medications, and use of alcohol can cause mental health problems. To further complicate things, serious physical illnesses can cause delirium or acute mental status changes that will usually resolve when the underlying cause is treated. Late-life psychosis or paraphrenia is a serious mental condition in which a person loses touch with reality and has difficulty telling fact from fantasy.

2 What tests are needed to tell if I have a serious mental health problem?

Your healthcare provider will probably conduct a complete physical examination, ask about your daily function, survey your medications (prescription and over the counter), and obtain some laboratory tests to make sure you are not anemic, to make sure you have adequate levels of B_{12} and folate, or to determine if you are having trouble with your thyroid. Your healthcare provider will also ask a lot of questions about your mood and memory. Sometimes a CT scan of the brain or other tests such as a PET scan or MRI are necessary to detect the source of mental health problems. If further information is needed, you may be referred to a neuropsychologist for more in-depth testing that can give more detailed information about your memory and mood. The results of this test can help your healthcare provider decide if additional testing is needed to diagnose your mental health problem.

RATIONALE:

Mental health problems in the older person can be caused by a variety of factors. A complete holistic assessment of physical, social, and psychological function is indicated.

3 How do I know if I have depression?

If you experience feelings of sadness, fatigue, lack of enjoyment of life, sleep problems, feelings of being helpless and hopeless, loss of interest in sex, or difficulty concentrating and making decisions, you may be depressed. Some older people say that they just do not feel like their old self. Others gain or lose weight because they change the way they eat. Others may avoid going out to social events and prefer to stay home alone. Everyone is different, so it is important to think broadly and look for a variety of symptoms.

RATIONALE:

Recognition of depression in the older person is a key skill for every clinician working with older patients. Depression is a treatable disease and may masquerade as a symptom of illness or be falsely attributed to normal aging.

4 Is suicide a problem with older people?

Yes, some groups of older people (especially older Caucasian men) have high suicide rates. If you have persistent thoughts of death or harming yourself or others, seek help immediately. Mental health professionals are available to protect your life and help you return to mental health. Do not risk ending your life prematurely.

RATIONALE:

Older people with suicidal ideation need immediate help and preventive services. Inform your patients and their families that help is available if needed.

5 Is treatment available and effective for older people with mental health problems?

Yes, there are a variety of pharmacological and nonpharmacological methods to treat mental health problems. The newer antidepressants have fewer side effects and are just as effective in treating depression in older people as they are in treating middle-aged and younger people, so do not be afraid to try them if your doctor thinks it will help you. Mental health professionals such as social workers, psychologists, psychiatrists, and psychiatric–mental health nurses can also provide counseling to help you identify the source of, and appropriate intervention for, your mental health problems. Nonpharmacological ways to ease depression include exercise, increased social activity, alcohol avoidance, light therapy, and a variety of other methods unique to each older person.

RATIONALE:

Many older people and their families are afraid to acknowledge a mental health problem. They may see it as a sign of weakness, or be fearful of institutionalization in a mental hospital. Be sure to stress the benefits and possibilities of treatment for mental health problems.

CARE PLAN   A Patient With Depression

Case Study

Mrs. Drew is an 80-year-old woman who lives alone in a senior citizens' housing project. She is quite functional and manages very well with the assistance of a weekly homemaker and her daughter. Mrs. Drew has several stable chronic illnesses such as type 2 diabetes mellitus, hypertension, age-related macular degeneration, insomnia, and mild depression. She had a myocardial infarction several years ago and had a stent inserted in a partially occluded coronary artery. Since then she has done quite well and engages in social activities with her family and friends in her housing complex.

Recently, Mrs. Drew began to complain to her physician and nurse that she has been increasingly irritated with her upstairs neighbor. She relates, "She stomps around all night. I think she was rearranging furniture the other night at 2 a.m. I've called the apartment manager to complain but they don't do a thing. Now my neighbor doesn't speak to me and I think she's telling everyone who lives in our complex." In addition, the nurse notes that Mrs. Drew's blood pressure is elevated, her blood sugar is higher than normal, and she looks disheveled. Normally she is well dressed and well groomed. Mrs. Drew reports that she has not bothered to refill her blood pressure medication. When asked about this she just sighs and says, "Why should I bother to fix up and take so many pills? I just sit in my apartment all day. No one really cares about me anyway."

Applying the Nursing Process

Assessment

Mrs. Drew is exhibiting a change in function and mood. While she has been mildly depressed in the past, she has always cared for herself and exhibited an enjoyment of life. Recently, she has become more irritable and has become noncompliant in taking her medications. Should the trend continue, she could suffer another heart attack, further complications from uncontrolled diabetes, and increasing social isolation. The nurse should carefully assess Mrs. Drew's current situation and determine the following:

■ Has any recent event or significant loss occurred?
■ Has there been any change in financial situation or family structure?
■ Has any significant decline in her physical condition or chronic illnesses occurred that could be causing or exacerbating this mood disorder?

Diagnosis

Appropriate nursing diagnoses for Mrs. Drew may include the following:

■ *Social Isolation*
■ *Sleep Deprivation*

■ Does she ever think of harming or ending her own life?
■ Does she have insight into her situation and have any ideas as to why she is feeling hopeless?

The complete nursing assessment should include the following:

■ Cognitive testing—the MMSE
■ Depression screen—the GDS
■ Suicide screen—to rule out the risk of suicide
■ Further assessment of physical condition—assessment of all vital signs, pain screen, and physical examination
■ Medication survey—review of all prescribed and over-the-counter medications, compliance with medications, and presence or absence of medication side effects

■ *Self-Esteem, Situational or Chronic Low*
■ *Loneliness, Risk for*
■ *Health Maintenance, Ineffective*

NANDA-I © 2012.

CARE PLAN   **A Patient With Depression** (continued)

Expected Outcomes

Short-term goals might include that Mrs. Drew will:

1. Return to taking medications as ordered by the physician.
2. Have normal blood pressure and blood sugar levels at her next scheduled clinic visit.
3. Return to daily self-care and grooming activities.

Long-term goals might include that Mrs. Drew will:

1. Resume former sleep patterns and social activities.

Planning and Implementation

The following nursing interventions may be appropriate for Mrs. Drew:

- Establish a therapeutic relationship.
- Assess ability to obtain and pay for needed medications.
- Consult with the social worker colleague for information on socialization and community linkages that may increase Mrs. Drew's daily contact with other persons and are appropriate for someone with limited vision.
- Establish a schedule to monitor her ability to manage her chronic illnesses and care for herself.

Evaluation

The nurse hopes to work with Mrs. Drew over time and realizes the chronic nature of mood problems in older people. The nurse will consider the plan a success based on the following criteria:

- Mrs. Drew will resume attending social activities within her capabilities and exhibit improved function and social skills.

2. Comply with recommendations for antidepressant medication, counseling, or nonpharmacological recommendations to improve her mood and ease her symptoms of depression.
3. Identify and appraise past adaptive coping mechanisms and implement them to maintain her mood improvement and prevent further depressive episodes.

- Begin a values clarification to establish long-term goals and facilitate end-of-life planning; for example:

  Mrs. Drew has a history of appropriate self-care and independence. She has family support and is cognitively intact (scored a 28 on the MMSE). Her score on the GDS was 8, indicating her mild depression has progressed in severity. She is nonsuicidal and expresses faith in God and a reason for living. Her physical illnesses appear to be stable, and her blood pressure and blood sugar should return to normal limits when she begins to take her medication.

- She will resume taking medications to manage her health problems.
- She will engage in counseling and take antidepressant medications if indicated and report improved sleep and mood as a result of these interventions.

Ethical Dilemma

Mrs. Drew informs the nurse that she is suspicious that her homemaker, Ms. Miller, is stealing money and jewelry from her apartment. Within the past few weeks she has been unable to find her bankbook, some gold jewelry, and some coins she has saved for her great-grandchildren. When the nurse asks Mrs. Drew if she has reported this to the agency providing the homemaker's services, she replies, "Oh no. I don't want her to get fired. I'm afraid she would try to get back at me if I did that." What are appropriate nursing actions?

Mrs. Drew should be encouraged to seek her family's assistance to carry out a systematic search and ascertain the items are truly missing and not merely misplaced. Because Mrs. Drew has macular degeneration and a visual impairment, she may be unable to see clearly into the back of drawers or other poorly lighted storage areas. If the items are truly missing, persons other than Ms. Miller (if any) who may have taken these items should be identified. If it is fairly clear that Ms. Miller is a potential thief, Mrs. Drew

(continued)

CARE PLAN **A Patient With Depression** *(continued)*

should be encouraged to report this to the agency. Although she may not have her items returned, she may be able to stop Ms. Miller from stealing from others and causing further distress. Further investigation as to why Mrs. Drew is afraid of retribution is needed. Has she ever been threatened or intimidated by Ms. Miller? If so, it may constitute elder abuse and

should be reported and investigated by state officials. The principle of Mrs. Drew's autonomy (she is cognitively intact and expressing clearly her wishes) is weighed against the principle of justice (doing the right thing to prevent Ms. Miller from hurting others) and beneficence (the nurse's desire to do the right thing and help Mrs. Drew to report Ms. Miller's crime).

Critical Thinking and the Nursing Process

1. List the 10 major causes of depression in the older person from your perspective.
2. Describe how common sensory impairments can cause an older person to have delusions or become paranoid.
3. What factors make alcohol use and abuse more difficult to detect in an older person?
4. In your opinion, what factors make the assessment and treatment of an older person with mental health problems challenging for the gerontological nurse and other members of the healthcare team?
5. What actions can society take to improve the mental health of all Americans and older people in particular?

■ Evaluate your responses in Appendix B.

Chapter Highlights

■ The gerontological nurse can educate other professionals about the facts regarding normal aging, mental health problems the older adult may encounter, and the various options for addressing those problems.

■ Education takes place not only in the classroom, but also at professional meetings, at community gatherings, and by serving as a role model to other nurses in the workplace.

■ Gerontological nurses should seek opportunities to volunteer and consult with self-help groups because 80% of long-term care is provided by family members (APA, 2011). Many older persons, families, and even healthcare professionals are unaware of the issues involved with the assessment and treatment of mental health problems in the older adult.

■ Although depression is not necessarily more common in the older adult, the presence of functional disability, numerous losses, and physical illness all predispose the older person to develop depressive symptoms that if left untreated may progress to a major depression. Older persons suffering from major depression are more likely to develop serious illness, are less likely to recover and cooperate with rehabilitation after illness, and have a lower life expectancy.

■ Gerontological nurses along with other healthcare providers can engage in a wide variety of advocacy efforts on behalf of older adults in need of mental health services. Providing local and state lawmakers with information about the mental health needs of older people can facilitate the development of public policy to support and encourage appropriate mental health services.

■ The nurse can support and augment the efforts of professional nursing organizations to advocate and encourage legislation and policy to improve the intellectual, social, and emotional well-being of older adults.

Pearson Nursing Student Resources
Find additional review materials at
nursing.pearsonhighered.com
Prepare for success with additional NCLEX®-style practice
questions, interactive assignments and activities, web links,
animations and videos, and more!

References

American Association for Geropsychiatry, (2012). Positive aging fact sheet. Retrieved from http://www.aagponline.org/index.php?src=gendocs&ref=FactSheetPositiveAgingAct&category=Advocacy

American Nurses Association. (2010). *Code of ethics for nurses with interpretive statements.* Retrieved from http://www.nursingworld.org/MainMenuCategories/EthicsStandards/CodeofEthicsforNurses/Code-of-Ethics.pdf

American Psychiatric Association. (2004). *Diagnostic and statistical manual of mental disorders* (4th ed., text revision). Retrieved from http://allpsych.com/disorders/mood/majordepression.html

American Psychological Association. (2011). *Psychology and aging: Addressing mental health needs of older adults.* Retrieved from http://www.apa.org/pi/aging/resources/guides/aging.pdf

Blazer, D. G., & Wu, L. (2009). The epidemiology of at-risk and binge drinking among middle-aged and elderly community adults: National survey on drug use and health. *American Journal of Psychiatry, 166,* 1162–1169.

Centers for Disease Control and Prevention and National Association of Chronic Disease Directors. (2009). *The state of mental health and aging in America. Issue Brief 2: Addressing depression in older adults: Selected evidence-based programs.* Atlanta, GA: National Association of Chronic Disease Directors. Retrieved from http://www.cdc.gov/aging/pdf/mental_health_brief_2.pdf

Chapman, C., Laird, J., & KewalRamani, A. (2011). *Trends in drop-out and high school completion rates in the United States: 1972–2008.* Retrieved from http://nces.ed.gov/pubs2011/2011012.pdf

Chou, K. L., Liang, K., & Mackenzie, C. S. (2011). Binge drinking and Axis I psychiatric disorders in community-dwelling middle-aged and older adults: Results from the National Epidemiologic Survey on Alcohol and Related Conditions (NESARC). *Journal of Clinical Psychiatry, 72*(5), 640–647.

Cigna. (2011). *As we age: Depression and suicide among older adults.* Retrieved from

http://www.cignabehavioral.com/web/basicsite/bulletinBoard/olderAdultsSuicide.jsp

Cronenwett, L., Sherwood, G., Barnsteiner, J., Disch, J., Johnson, J., Mitchell, P., Sullivan, D., & Warren, J. (2007). Quality and safety education for nurses, *Nursing Outlook, 55*(3), 122–131.

Drugs.com. (2011a). *Lithium side effects.* Retrieved from http://www.drugs.com/sfx/lithium-side-effects.html

Drugs.com. (2011b). *Parnate.* Retrieved from http://www.drugs.com/cdi/parnate.html

Epocrates.com. (2011). *Drug information.* Retrieved from http://www.epocrates.com

Erikson, E. H. (1963). *Childhood and society.* New York, NY: Norton.

George, L., Okun, M., & Landerman, R. (1985). Age as a moderator of the determinants of life satisfaction. *Research on Aging, 7,* 209–233.

Havighurst, R. J. (1972). Nurturing the cognitive skills in health. *Journal of Health, 42*(2), 73–76.

Johnson, M., Maas, M. L., & Moorhead, S. (Eds.). (2000). *Nursing outcomes classification (NOC)* (2nd ed.). St. Louis, MO: Mosby.

Kane, R., Ouslander, J., & Abrass, I. (2008). *Essentials of clinical geriatrics* (6th ed.). New York, NY: McGraw-Hill.

Kurlowicz, L., & Greenberg, S. (2007). The geriatric depression scale (GDS). *Try this: Best nursing practices in care for older adults* (No. 4). Hartford Institute for Geriatric Nursing. Retrieved from http://consultgerirn.org/uploads/File/trythis/try_this_4.pdf

Leong, F. T. L., & Kalibatseva, Z. (2011). *Cross cultural barriers to mental health services in the United States.* The Dana Foundation. Retrieved from http://www.dana.org/news/cerebrum/detail.aspx?id=31364

Maas, M. L., Reed, D., Specht, J. P., Swanson, E., Tripp-Reimer, I., Buckwalter, K. C., . . . Kelly, L. S. (2001). Family involvement in care: Negotiated family-staff partnerships in special care units for persons with dementia. In S. G. Funk, E. M. Tornquist, J. Leeman, M. S. Miles, & J. S. Harrell (Eds.). *Key aspects of preventing and managing chronic illness* (pp. 330–345). New York: Springer.

Maddox, G. (1994). Lives through the years revisited. *Gerontologist, 34*(6), 764–767.

McCance, K., & Huether, S. (2010). *Pathophysiology: The biologic basis of disease in adults and children.* New York, NY: Mosby.

McPhee, S., Papadakis, M., & Rabow, S. (2011). *Current medical diagnosis and treatment* (50th ed.). New York, NY: McGraw-Hill.

Mental Health America. (2011). *Ranking America's mental health: An analysis of depression across the states.* Retrieved from http://www.nmha.org/go/state-ranking

Moore, A., Blow, F., Hoffing, M., Welgreen, S., Davis, J., Lin, J., Ramirez, K., Liao, D., Tang, L., Gould, R., Gill, M., Chen, O., & Barry, K. (2011). Primary care-based intervention to reduce at risk drinking in older adults: a randomized controlled trial. *Addiction, 106*(1), 111–120.

Naegle, M. (2012). Alcohol use screening and assessment. *Try this: Best practices in nursing care to older adults* (No. 17). Hartford Institute for Geriatric Nursing. Retrieved from http://consultgerirn.org/uploads/File/trythis/try_this_17.pdf

National Alliance on Mental Illness [NAMI]. (2011). *Depression in older persons fact sheet.* Retrieved from http://www.nami.org/Template.cfm?Section=By_Illness&template=/ContentManagement/ContentDisplay.cfm&ContentID=7515

National Center for Complementary and Alternative Medicine. (2010). *Herbs at a glance.* Retrieved from http://nccam.nih.gov/health/herbsataglance.htm

National Institute on Aging. (2002). *Aging under the microscope: A biological quest* (NIH Publication No. 02-2756). Bethesda, MD: National Institutes of Health.

National Institute on Aging. (2009). *Age page: Depression.* Retrieved from http://www.nia.nih.gov/healthinformation/publications/depression.htm

National Institue of Alcohol Abuse and Alcoholism. (2008). Older adults and alcohol problems. Retrieved from http://pubs.niaaa.nih.gov/publications/Social/Module10COlderAdults/Module10C.html

National Institute on Drug Abuse. (2011). *Prescription drugs: Abuse and addiction.* Retrieved from http://www.nida.nih.gov/researchreports/prescription/prescription5.html

National Institute of Mental Health [NIMH]. (2009). *Bipolar disorder.* Retrieved from http://www.nimh.nih.gov/health/publications/bipolar-disorder/what-are-the-symptoms-of-bipolar-disorder.shtml

National Institute of Mental Health [NIMH]. (2010). *Older adults: Depression and suicide facts.* Retrieved from http://www.nimh.nih.gov/health/publications/older-adults-depression-and-suicide-facts-fact-sheet/index.shtml

National Institute of Mental Health [NIMH]. (2011). *Schizophrenia.* Retrieved from http://www.nimh.nih.gov/health/publications/schizophrenia/complete-index.shtml

Neugarten, B., & Hagestad, G. (1976). Age and the life course. In R. Binstock & E. Shanas (Eds.), *Handbook of aging and the social sciences* (pp. 35–57). New York, NY: Van Nostrand Reinhold.

Reuben, D., Herr, K., Pacala, J., Pollock, B., Potter, J., & Semla, T. (2011). *Geriatrics at your fingertips* (13th ed.). New York, NY: American Geriatrics Society.

Selye, H. (1965). *The stress of life.* New York, NY: McGraw-Hill.

Stanford Center on Longevity. (2011). *Expert consensus on brain health.* Retrieved from http://longevity.stanford.edu/brain-health/expert-consensus-on-brain-health

University of Maryland Medical Center. (2011). *Stress-risk factors.* Retrieved from http://www.umm.edu/patiented/articles/who_at_risk_chronic_stress_or_stress-related_diseases_000031_6.htm

U.S. Census Bureau. (2008). *Projected population of the US by race and Hispanic origin: 2000 to 2050.* Retrieved from http://www.census.gov/population/www/projections/usinterimproj

U.S. Department of Health and Human Services [USDHHS]. (2012). *Healthy people 2020: Mental health and mental disorders.* Retrieved from http://www.healthypeople.gov/2020/default.aspx

Warner, J., McKeowan, E., Griffin, M., Johnson, K., Ramsay, K., Cort, C., & King, M. (2004). Rates and predictors of mental illness in gay men, lesbians and bisexual men and women. *British Journal of Psychiatry, 185,* 479–485.

World Health Organization. (2011). *Action needed to reduce health impact of harmful alcohol use.* Retrieved from http://www.who.int/mediacentre/news/releases/2011/alcohol_20110211/en/index.html

Yesavage, J., Brink, T., Rose, T., Lum, O., Huang, V., Adey, M., & Leirer, V. O. (1983). Development and validation of a geriatric depression screening scale: A preliminary report. *Journal of Psychiatric Research, 17,* 37–49.

Sleep and the Older Adult

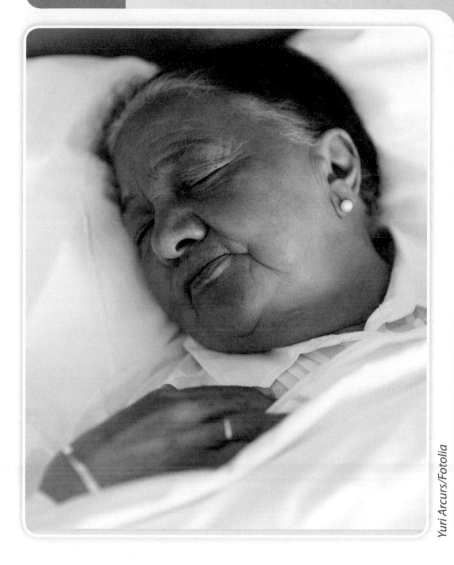

Yuri Arcurs/Fotolia

KEY TERMS

abnormal sleep behaviors *196*
bedtime rituals *203*
circadian rhythms *194*
insomnia *194*
sleep *194*
sleep apnea *196*
sleep architecture *194*
sleep hygiene *194*

LEARNING OUTCOMES

On completion of this chapter, the reader will be able to:

1. Discuss the importance of obtaining adequate sleep and the sleep cycle.
2. Describe normal changes in sleep occurring with aging.
3. Identify potential causes of sleep disruption in older people.
4. List the risks and benefits of pharmacological and nonpharmacological interventions for sleep disturbance.
5. Formulate appropriate nursing interventions to improve or restore sleep.

Sleep is a natural periodic state of rest for the mind and body that is necessary for health and human function. Sleep complaints are common among older people, and the incidence of sleep problems increases with age. Older adults experience age-related changes in the nature of their sleep, including greater difficulty falling asleep, more frequent awakenings, decreased amounts of nighttime sleep, and more frequent daytime napping. Proper **sleep architecture,** or cycles and phases that comprise the underlying physiological sleep mechanisms, and adequate total sleep time are necessary for proper functioning. In order for sleep to be restful and restorative, the sleeper must progress through non–rapid eye movement (NREM) stages of slow-wave sleep, and about every 90 minutes throughout the night cycle into rapid eye movement (REM) stages. With the exception of shift workers (e.g., evening and night nurses, policemen, firefighters), most people sleep in the dark portion of the 24-hour cycle and carry out activities during the light portion. Sleep and wakefulness fall into a circadian pattern of periodicity meaning about one cycle per 24-hour period. This sleep–wake distribution pattern is regulated by the suprachiasmatic nucleus located in the hypothalamus and forms the basis for **circadian rhythms,** or the 24-hour cycle of rest–activity patterns that is based on environmental cues. This rhythmic pattern can be disrupted by isolation from the normal light–dark cycle, isolation from environmental stimuli, and rapid travel to differing time zones (jet lag).

The exact purpose of sleep is unclear, but sleep deprivation can result in harmful physical and psychological changes, including daytime fatigue, irritability, impaired learning ability, delayed healing, and visual and auditory hallucinations. Sleep disturbances can exacerbate behavioral problems in older people with Alzheimer's disease and other cognitive impairments.

To assist people with sleep disturbances, nurses need scientific knowledge about sleep. NANDA (2012) recognizes sleep pattern disturbance as an alternation in an individual's habitual pattern of sleep and wakefulness that causes discomfort or interferes with a desired lifestyle. Defining characteristics according to NANDA criteria include the following:

- Complaints of difficulty falling asleep (sleep latency greater than 30 minutes)
- Awakening too early in the morning
- Three or more nighttime awakenings
- Changes in behavior and function, including lethargy, listlessness, and irritability
- Decreased ability to function
- Dissatisfaction with sleep and not feeling well rested

- Presence of related factors including:
  - Physical discomfort/pain
  - Psychological discomfort
  - **Sleep hygiene** problems (spending too much time in bed and lack of consistent bedtime and awakening time with excessive napping)
  - Environmental factors

Sleep problems can be classified as transient (short term), intermittent (on and off), and chronic (constant). Transient sleep problems may be caused by short-term health problems, stress, worry related to a situational event like a move to a new residence, or changes in sleep schedules such as those due to travel and jet lag. Intermittent sleep problems may be related to exacerbations of chronic illness or recurrent anxiety.

Insomnia is a condition defined as having trouble falling or staying asleep occurring on most nights and lasting for 3 weeks (short term) or long term (chronic) (National Institutes of Health [NIH], 2011a). Some older people with insomnia may fall asleep easily and wake up too soon while others have the opposite problem. The result is poor-quality sleep that causes daytime drowsiness and detracts from adequate daytime concentration and function.

Sleep Architecture

For sleep to be restorative and restful, the sleeping person must cycle through several sleep stages. Normal sleep physiology is composed of four distinct stages when measured by electroencephalography. Sleep ranges from stage 1 (light sleep) to stage 4 (deep sleep) and can be classified as either REM sleep or NREM sleep (Figure 8-1 ▶▶▶).

During NREM sleep, growth hormone, prolactin, and thyroid-stimulating hormones are released, aiding in physiological restoration. Deep sleep appears to stimulate physical restoration through the release of growth hormone while decreasing blood pressure and respiratory function (McCance & Huether, 2012). With aging, the amount of time spent in deep sleep decreases as the night progresses. In a healthy older adult, deep sleep comprises 33% of the first sleep cycle, 17% of the second, 6% of the third, 2% of the fourth, and 1% of the fifth. Stage 1 is light sleep in which people feel as if they are drifting in and out of sleep and can be accompanied by a feeling of falling with sudden muscle contractions. In stage 2, brain waves slow and eye movements stop. Stage 3 sleep is characterized by slowing brain waves and sleep spindles, which are bursts of electrical activity. In stage 4, the brain produces mostly delta waves characterized by large, slow patterns of brain activity. During stages 1 and 2, sleepers are easily aroused from sleep, whereas sleepers in

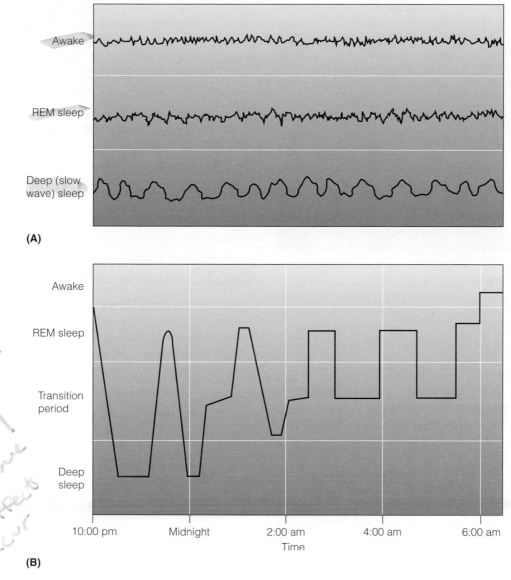

Figure 8-1 ▶▶▶ Sleep stages. A. Electroencephalograph tracings of awakeness, REM, and non-REM sleep. B. Sleep cycles during nighttime sleep.

stages 3 and 4 sleep are more difficult to arouse. As the sleep stages progress, it becomes increasingly difficult to awaken the sleeper, and the more frequent nighttime awakenings observed in older people may be related to the reduced amount of slow-wave sleep in this cohort. This process of slow-wave sleep reduction begins at about age 20 with the deepest sleep occurring in childhood (Figure 8-2 ▶▶▶). The abundance of slow-wave sleep in childhood lends support to the expression "sleeping like a baby."

REM sleep is characterized by intense brain activity resulting in small, brief muscle contractions. REM sleep is accompanied by an increase in heart rate and blood pressure. Breathing is irregular and shallow, eyes dart quickly from side to side, and limbs become temporarily paralyzed. REM sleep is sometimes referred to as "dream sleep" because dreaming occurs during REM sleep and is thought necessary for psychological restoration. REM sleep is necessary for learning, memory consolidation, and daytime concentration. REM sleep occurs cyclically every 90 to 120 minutes throughout the night. As the night progresses, sleep becomes lighter and the person spends more time in REM sleep.

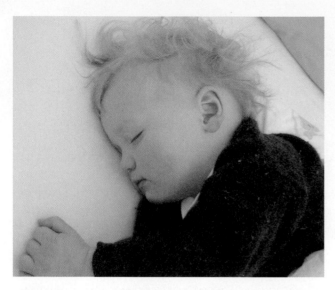

Figure 8-2 ▶▶▶ The deepest slow-wave sleep occurs in childhood.

Source: Carolin Hansa/Pearson Education/PH College.

NORMAL CHANGES OF AGING

Age-related changes in the nervous system can affect sleep. These changes may be at the chemical, structural, and functional levels and may result in a disorganization of sleep and disruption of circadian rhythms (McCance & Huether, 2012). The neuromechanisms for sleep are distributed in the brain stem, basal forebrain, and subcortical and cortical regions. Neurotransmitters such as serotonin and norepinephrine keep some parts of the brain on alert during sleep. Sensory inputs such as loud noises and bright lights can stimulate the reticular activating system and cause an older person to awaken. Other neurons at the base of the brain send signals to disregard stimuli that would normally keep a person awake. Normal sleep depends on the integrity of these complex mechanisms. Declines in the cerebral metabolic rate and cerebral blood flow, reductions of neuronal cell counts, and structural changes such as neuronal degeneration and atrophy can all occur with aging (U.S. National Library of Medicine [NLM], 2010). The amount of time spent in deeper levels of sleep diminishes with aging. There is an associated increase in awakenings during sleep and an increase in the total time spent in bed trying to sleep as sleep becomes less efficient.

HEALTHY AGING TIPS

▶ Stay busy during the daytime. Staying active and engaged keeps you from napping and expends positive energy.

▶ Stay positive. If you're depressed, seek treatment and talk to someone. Getting worries and cares off your shoulder can improve your sleep.

▶ Exercise regularly. Exercise early in the day. Exercise releases endorphins and other helpful biochemicals that reduce stress and anxiety.

▶ Limit caffeine, alcohol, and other stimulants. These substances can disrupt sleep and stay in the body for many hours.

▶ Get a few minutes of sunlight every day. Bright sunlight helps regulate melatonin and coordinates your sleep–wake cycle.

Robinson, Kemp, & Segal, 2012.

Sleep Disruption

Abnormal sleep behaviors are a category of events that can occur at any time throughout the life cycle but become more common with advancing age. These behaviors may include the following:

- Myoclonus or sudden contractions of muscles and tingling feelings in the legs, also called *restless leg syndrome*. Complaints may include tingling, creeping, crawling, or aching sensations in the legs.
- Habitual loud snoring, choking, or gasping, periods of **sleep apnea** or disturbed or interrupted breathing during sleep.
- Unusual behaviors that may occur during sleep such as vivid dreams or sleepwalking.

National Heart, Lung, and Blood Institute [NHLBI], 2011.

Older people exhibiting these sleep problems will experience daytime sleepiness as a result of poor quality and insufficient quantity of sleep. This group of abnormal sleep behaviors requires evaluation from neurologists or sleep specialists and is usually treated with a variety of lifestyle modifications and medications.

Some healthy older adults continue to have satisfactory sleep throughout advanced age (Figure 8-3 ▶▶▶). A common myth held by many nurses and laypersons is that a person's need for sleep decreases with age. In general, the amount of sleep needed in old age is about the same as was needed in youth and middle age. However, it may be more difficult for many older adults to obtain the quality and quantity of sleep that supports health and well-being because sleep efficiency declines with age and older adults may find that they have to spend more time in bed to obtain the amount of sleep needed in order to feel refreshed in the morning. Adverse health outcomes associated with

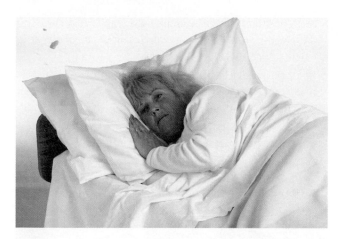

Figure 8-3 ▶▶▶ Healthy older people require 6 to 10 hours of sleep nightly.
Source: Dorling Kindersley.

sleep problems in older adults include poor self-reported health status, cognitive decline, depression, disability in basic ADLs, poor quality of life, and institutionalization (McPhee & Papadakis, 2011).

Most older adults require 6 to 10 hours of sleep nightly. Less than 4 or more than 8 hours of sleep is associated with higher mortality rates than those sleeping 8 hours (McPhee & Papadakis, 2011). Often, the time it takes to fall asleep serves as a good indicator of whether a person is getting enough sleep. Those who fall asleep almost immediately upon placing their head on the pillow may be sleep deprived. When an older person's sleep requirements are not met, a sleep deficit accumulates with resulting loss of overall daytime function. When a person regularly loses 1 to 2 hours of sleep each night, the lack of sleep can accumulate leading to chronic excessive sleepiness. Lifestyle factors such as irregular sleep schedules; use of caffeine, tobacco, and alcohol; excessive time spent in daytime napping; and certain medications can make sleep problems worse. Driving while drowsy can be just as dangerous as driving under the influence of alcohol. It is estimated that up to 60% of motor vehicle accidents involve sleep-deprived drivers (Six Ways, 2012).

Older people may nap more often during the day, thus further disrupting normal circadian patterns. While one "cat nap" a day of 30 minutes or less in the early afternoon was found not to disrupt the nighttime sleep of older people, more frequent daytime napping can be disruptive (Brannon, 2012). If an older person normally requires 8 hours of sleep in a 24-hour period and 2 to 3 hours of sleep occur during the daytime hours, the person cannot expect to enjoy 8 hours of uninterrupted sleep at night. The older person may toss and turn, become frustrated with the inability to sleep, and suffer further disruption in his or her sleep–wake patterns.

For good sleepers, the bed and bedroom are strong cues for drowsiness and sleep; for poor sleepers, these places signal alertness, frustration, and sleeplessness.

> **Practice Pearl** ▶▶▶ Changing problematic sleep behaviors is a long-term process. Goals that are set too high or too quickly will discourage the nurse and the patient. Realistic goals are the key to success.

Sleep disruption is common among older people with psychosocial problems. Life stresses when combined with predisposing emotional factors such as depression and anxiety may be related to the onset of sleep problems (McPhee & Papadakis, 2011). Many studies identify anxiety, stress, and depression as major deterrents to falling and staying asleep in people of all ages. Psychosocial influences that may disrupt sleep include social isolation, caregiving stress and strain, and grief and bereavement.

Mental health problems associated with poor sleep include anxiety, depression, and substance abuse disorders (Reuben et al., 2011). Sleep problems identified in depressed older people include difficulty falling asleep, increased frequency of early morning awakenings, and frequent daytime napping. For some older women, sleep problems begin during menopause. Menopause, the cessation of menstruation resulting from declines in estrogen levels, is associated with a variety of behavioral changes, including hot flashes and mood swings. Hot flashes that occur routinely during sleep can lead to fatigue, irritability, and chronic sleep disruption, establishing a poor sleep pattern that persists into old age for many women (McCance & Huether, 2012). Older adults who are depressed are more likely to report somatic complaints like sleep problems and changes in appetite rather than feeling "sad" or "blue." Younger people are more likely to acknowledge the connection between sleep disturbances and emotional problems; therefore, the nurse should be aware of this connection.

Health Problems and Sleep Disruption

Approximately 5 million older adults in the United States have a serious sleep disorder (NLM, 2010). Sleep problems in older adults may result from personal characteristics, environmental characteristics, or a combination of these factors. Personal characteristics include advanced age (generally considered over 60), female gender, and history of depression. Further, older women are more likely than older men to experience sleep disruption, with 35% of older women reporting moderate to severe insomnia compared to 13% of older men (Brannon, 2012).

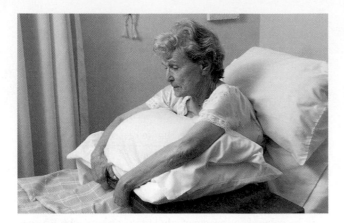

Figure 8-4 ▶▶▶ Sleep may be difficult for older adults with heart and lung disease.

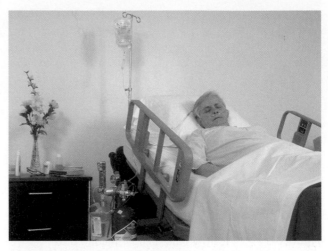

Figure 8-5 ▶▶▶ Sleep disturbances in institutional settings are common.

Various health problems and the medications used to treat them are associated with sleep disruption in older people. Pulmonary disease, heart disease, arthritis, dementia associated with Alzheimer's disease, and depression may cause sleep disruption. Diseases of the cardiac and respiratory system are often associated with orthopnea and shortness of breath. People with heart failure are often asked "the pillow question" as an indicator of the stability and progression of their disease. The nurse should ask, "How many pillows do you sleep with at night? Is this your usual number of pillows?" Older people with severe heart failure may find it necessary to sleep sitting nearly upright to allow the lungs to clear fluid and breathe, but this position may not offer adequate support for the back and the head during deep sleep (Figure 8-4 ▶▶▶).

Physical discomfort or pain can be a major deterrent for sleep. Older people with pain take longer to fall asleep and have an increased number of nighttime awakenings. Pain makes it difficult to achieve a comfortable sleeping position, may cause tension and muscle spasms, and may keep an older person awake during the night if pain medication wears off (Reuben et al., 2011). A common source of pain in older adults is the chronic pain resulting from osteoarthritis. Because osteoarthritis of the hip and knee is so common in aging, it can result in chronic sleep disruption for large numbers of older people. Further, older adults who experience chronic pain may also limit daytime activities, resulting in physical inactivity, deconditioning or loss of physical strength and function, and further disruption of the sleep–activity cycle. Acutely ill hospitalized patients may also experience pain from surgical incisions, pain from the trauma or injury that was the cause of the hospitalization, or discomfort from intravenous tubing, indwelling urinary catheters, or other instrumentation (Figure 8-5 ▶▶▶).

Dementia

Older people with dementia endure even more sleep disruptions than other older people. Sleep disruptions common in dementia such as those with Alzheimer's disease include breakdown of the normal sleep–wake cycle with short periods of fragmented sleep occurring throughout a 24-hour period, reduced stage 3 and REM sleep, and no stage 4 sleep (Alzheimer's Association, 2012). Older people with dementia may suffer other problems as a result of their impairment such as social isolation, boredom, excessive daytime napping, and periods of agitation or restlessness throughout the evening or night. Sleep disturbances in older people with dementia cause caregiver stress, increase the potential for nursing home placement, and cause serious problems for those providing care in the nursing home or home environment. These behaviors may contribute to caregivers' complaints about their own disrupted sleep, daytime sleepiness, and fatigue (Alzheimer's Association, 2012). If nighttime wandering occurs, serious safety problems can result such as older people leaving their homes, becoming disoriented, and wandering into heavy traffic or remote wooded areas. Every year, there are news reports of older people who die or suffer serious trauma from exposure when they are found several days after wandering from home. The Alzheimer's Association conducts a "safe return" program that encourages older people with Alzheimer's disease to register with the local police department.

In an attempt to promote more normal sleep patterns in those with dementia, psychotropic medications may be administered. These medications are usually indicated for short-term use only. When used for chronic sleep problems, the side effects may become problematic. Typical side effects of hypnotic drugs include falls, swallowing difficulties, constipation, dizziness, and daytime sleepiness (Reuben et al., 2011). Additionally, most psychotropic medications alter sleep architecture, including decreases in REM sleep, decreased levels of arousal, and increases in slow-wave sleep. The older person habitually taking these medications may report feeling "hung over" or lethargic during the daytime as a result of these changes in sleep architecture. For a thorough discussion of dementia in older people, refer to Chapter 22 ⬤.

Snoring

Many older people consider snoring a minor annoyance, but it can signal a potentially serious condition known as sleep apnea, or temporary interruption of breathing during sleep. For those affected by sleep apnea, there can be many temporary interruptions in breathing, each lasting about 10 seconds throughout the sleep period. These interruptions in breathing can occur as often as 20 to 30 times per hour (McCance & Huether, 2012). Symptoms of sleep apnea include the following:

- Heavy snoring, usually on inspiration
- Choking sounds or struggling to breathe during sleep
- Delays in breathing during sleep (usually with a reduction in blood-oxygen saturation), followed by a snort when breathing begins
- Excessive daytime sleepiness
- Morning headaches
- Difficulty with concentration and staying awake during driving or other tasks

Older people who repeatedly suffer repetitive hypoxemic events may be more prone to sudden death, stroke, angina, and worsening hypertension (NLM, 2010). Bed partners are very helpful in providing information about snoring and nighttime breathing difficulties. For older people living alone, a portable tape recorder may be placed by the bed at bedtime. The nurse can later play the recording to hear any snoring or breathing problems on the audiotape.

Sleep Apnea ⬤

Sleep apnea can be caused by problems with the central nervous system and the brain or may be caused by partial obstruction of the airway when the muscles in the throat, soft palate, and tongue relax during sleep (Reuben et al., 2011). This can lead to partial or complete collapse of the airway, making breathing labored (Figure 8-6 ▶▶▶). Apneic episodes are followed by brief awakenings, which usually occur without the sleeper's knowledge but can disrupt sleep and result in daytime drowsiness. If the older person does not fully experience deep sleep, the REM stage will not occur. Risk factors for sleep apnea include obesity (body mass index > 30), hypertension, male gender, atrial fibrillation, and anatomical abnormality to the upper respiratory tract (Reuben et al., 2011). Sleep apnea is further associated with cigarette smoking and large neck size.

If sleep apnea is suspected, the older person should be referred to a sleep center for an overnight sleep study using polysomnography, a specialized method of sleep testing that measures brain and body activity during sleep. The polysomnogram includes the following:

- Electroencephalograms to monitor brain waves and identify sleep stages

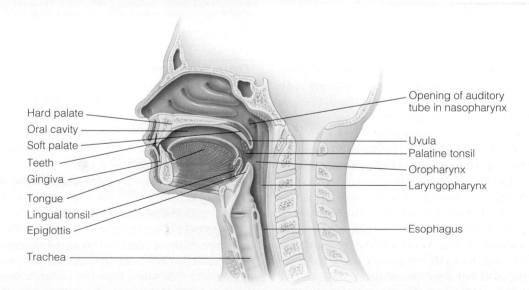

Figure 8-6 ▶▶▶ Structures of the mouth, the pharynx, and the esophagus.

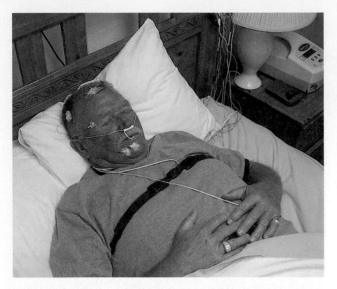

Figure 8-7 ▶▶▶ Polysomnography measures brain and body activity during sleep.
Source: John Childers.

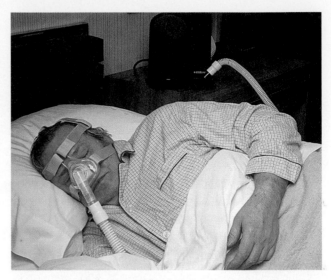

Figure 8-8 ▶▶▶ Continuous positive airway pressure (CPAP) is a noninvasive method for treatment of sleep apnea.

- Electro-oculograms to measure eye movement so that REM sleep can be distinguished from NREM sleep
- Facial and leg electromyograms to measure muscle tone and movement
- Electrocardiograms to monitor cardiac activity
- Measurement of chest movement and oxygen saturation

Unfortunately, many older people find it difficult to sleep with all the wires and monitors attached to them and often must return a second night to achieve any sleep at all (Figure 8-7 ▶▶▶).

Treatment for sleep apnea may begin with simple interventions designed to keep the airway open such as weight reduction for the obese, encouraging sleep on the side rather than the back by wearing a tennis ball in a pocket sewn on the back of a nightshirt, avoiding sleeping pills and alcohol before sleeping, and avoiding smoking (Pace, Lynn, & Glass, 2001). For those with anatomical abnormalities of the upper airway, surgery may be required to restore normal structure and function. The surgery, known as uvulopalato-pharyngoplasty, is usually performed to the pharyngeal walls or the base of the tongue to enlarge the pharyngeal air space (Reuben et al., 2011). However, the most common medical treatment for sleep apnea is continuous positive airway pressure (CPAP). CPAP is a noninvasive treatment administered through a nasal mask (Figure 8-8 ▶▶▶). The pressure keeps the airway open, preventing its collapse and allowing the patient to breathe more normally. When used correctly CPAP is 100% effective for relieving upper airway obstruction, but some estimates indicate that only 50% to 60% of patients use their CPAP on a regular basis as prescribed (Blazek, 2011).

Some of the resistance to use may be due to discomfort associated with the face mask, so it is important to make sure the mask fits correctly. Usually, between 5 and 20 cm of CPAP is needed to prevent apnea and maintain adequate oxygen saturation. Nurses should be aware that sedative-hypnotic medications are contraindicated in patients with untreated sleep apnea, because they raise the arousal threshold to the extent that the patient does not awaken when apneic. Older people with sleep apnea should inform healthcare providers of their apnea before any surgical procedure because of the danger of severe apnea after preoperative medications are administered (Reuben et al., 2011).

> **Drug Alert** ▶▶▶ Older people with untreated sleep apnea should not use alcohol or sedative-hypnotic medications because of their potential to increase the severity of apneic episodes.

Urinary Problems

Older people may be awakened from sleep because of the need to urinate. Common age-related alterations in urinary tract function include urinary frequency, nocturia, and benign prostatic hypertrophy (Reuben et al., 2011). These alterations result from changes in the renal and hormonal systems that control urine production and from decreases in the reservoir capacity of the bladder. In youth, there is a circadian pattern to urine production with nighttime urine production less than daytime production; with aging, nighttime urine flow rates may equal or exceed daytime rates. Voiding frequency, nocturia, and urinary urgency have been shown to increase with age (McCance & Huether, 2012). Many older adults take diuretics, which increase urinary output. Older men may suffer from benign prostatic hypertrophy, which inhibits complete emptying of the bladder and may be associated with the sensation of always feeling the urge to void. Nurses who suspect urinary retention in older men with benign prostatic hypertrophy are encouraged to consult with the physician and receive authorization to check post-void residual by inserting a urinary catheter immediately after the patient voids to ascertain the amount of urine that is retained in the bladder. Older men who retain more than 50 mL of urine should be referred to a urologist for urological evaluation or cystoscopy and cystometric studies. Many older people suffer from recurrent urinary tract infections. Older people who report urgency, frequency, burning on urination, foul odor, and cloudy urine should seek medical evaluation. Sometimes treatment with a simple antibiotic such as sulfamethoxazole–trimethoprim (Bactrim DS) can ease the symptoms of urinary tract infection and help restore restful sleep.

For those who are institutionalized in a hospital or nursing home, nurses may do frequent nighttime checking on those with urinary incontinence in order to prevent skin breakdown. Almost 50% of nighttime awakenings in the nursing home are caused by the staff's incontinence care routines or other activities (Endeshaw, Johnson, Kutner, et al., 2004). Because sleep is so fragmented in those frail, older residents, many of whom have dementia, intensive interventions to improve continence at night may disrupt sleep further. The nurse must individualize nighttime care in this population with the goal of minimizing sleep disruption while maintaining skin integrity and the dignity of the older person (Endeshaw et al., 2004). An alternative approach might involve frequent rounding to observe the nursing home resident or hospitalized patient, but providing care only when the patient appears to be awake or moving about in the bed. For patients who appear to be deep in sound sleep or REM sleep, the nurse may wish to return in 30 minutes to ascertain if the patient requires incontinence care.

Sleep Problems in Hospitals and Nursing Homes

When older people are hospitalized, they frequently complain of sleep disruption. Studies of sleep in the acute care setting indicate that patients have extremely fragmented and disturbed sleep regardless of their diagnosis (Reuben et al., 2011). Ironically, nurses contribute to their patients' sleep disruption, and the frequent repetitive delivery of nursing care in the acute care setting leaves patients little chance to sleep. Factors such as excessive noise levels and switching on of bright lights can further disrupt sleep patterns (Ellenbogen et al., 2011). The lack of restful sleep can slow an older person's recovery to health. Other stressors identified by

patients in a critical care unit include lack of sleep, enforced mobility, pain from procedures, and poor communication with staff members (Fong et al., 2009). Additionally, many older people report the hospital environment is too hot (or cold), the bed may be uncomfortable (hard plastic surface), a sleeping partner or comfort item (e.g., cat or dog) may be missed, or nighttime rituals may be disrupted. It is often difficult to distinguish between sleep pattern disturbances caused by the hospital environment and those caused by the illness itself (Ellenbogen et al., 2011).

> **Practice Pearl** ▶▶▶ When older people are institutionalized in the hospital or nursing home, sleep problems are common and the environment may be part of the problem. Nurses should ask themselves, "Would I like to sleep here tonight? What would bother me if I were sleeping here?" Some care rituals cannot be avoided, but they can be timed to coincide with awakenings naturally occurring during the patient's sleep cycle. Waking a patient from deep sleep to provide routine care can result in sleep deprivation, which can delay healing and recovery.

Alcohol and Caffeine

Alcohol consumed at bedtime, after an initial stimulating effect, may decrease the time required to fall asleep. Because of alcohol's sedating effect, many older people with insomnia consume alcohol to promote sleep. However, alcohol consumed within an hour of bedtime appears to disrupt the second half of the sleep period (NLM, 2010). Further, many older people are on medications that have the potential for serious interactions with alcohol (Reuben et al., 2011). Cardiac medications, diuretics, sedative-hypnotic drugs, and painkillers can have their therapeutic effects heightened and reach toxic levels when combined with alcohol. Older people who consume alcohol at bedtime may be at risk for falls and injury due to increased unsteadiness that may occur when ambulating at night. Additionally, caffeine and nicotine can affect the older adult's ability to initiate and maintain sleep. Nicotine extends the time it takes to fall asleep and reduces total sleep time and REM sleep. Both caffeine and nicotine increase the number of nighttime awakenings and the length of time it takes to fall back to sleep. Because alcohol, caffeine, and nicotine are typically used in conjunction with one another, the sedating and arousal effects frequently interact, creating multiple sleep disturbances.

Sleeping Medications

Prescription drugs have also been shown to affect sleep. It is generally agreed that long-term administration of hypnotics is an inadequate treatment strategy for chronic insomnia in the older adult (Reuben et al., 2011). Hypnotic medications are generally recommended for short-term use: about 2 weeks or less. Long-term use will blunt the effect of these medications. For those with long half-lives, steady states or relatively high constant blood levels will occur, which can cause excessive daytime sleepiness. Older people may also use over-the-counter (OTC) sleep aids without seeking medical advice or attention. The major ingredient in OTC sleep aids is antihistamines, especially diphenhydramine (Benadryl). These drugs have a number of side effects, including daytime sleepiness, dizziness, and blurred vision. These effects can exacerbate an older person's risk of fall and injury.

Drugs used to treat mood disorders such as depression can also affect sleep. Some drugs are sedatives and should be given in the evening, whereas others are stimulants and are best taken in the morning. Sedating antidepressants best taken in the evening include the following:

- Amitriptyline (Elavil)
- Doxepin (Sinequan)
- Trazodone (Desyrel)

Stimulating antidepressants best taken in the morning include the following:

- Desipramine (Norpramin)
- Sertraline hydrochloride (Zoloft)
- Paroxetine hydrochloride (Paxil)

Unfortunately, many medications used to treat sleep problems in older people can result in serious side effects including falls, death, disruption of sleep architecture, worsening of sleep apnea, and increased daytime drowsiness (McPhee & Papadakis, 2011). Drugs used to treat sleep disorders should be used cautiously and on a short-term basis, if at all.

Sleep problems and insomnia can also be caused by use of certain medications including decongestants and antihistamines, diet pills, steroids, beta-blockers, beta-agonists, opioids, some antidepressants, and use of recreational drugs (Pierse & Dym, 2011). A complete medication history is needed.

Diagnosed medical problems that involve pain, itching, inflammation or chronic infection can also adversely affect sleep. Common examples include cancer, parkinsonism, rheumatoid arthritis, fibromyalgia, and diabetes mellitus.

> **Drug Alert ▶▶▶** Some benzodiazepines carry a high risk of addiction. Diazepam (Valium) and alprazolam (Xanax) are not recommended for routine use with older people because of this risk.

When the nurse is asked to advise an older person regarding the discontinuation of sleep medication, the following rule is advised: If the medication has been used at least 5 nights a week for greater than 2 weeks, a taper and withdrawal schedule should be followed. By using a gradual withdrawal schedule (one half the dose for 1 week prior to discontinuation), the chances of inducing rebound insomnia and other withdrawal symptoms are lessened (Reuben et al., 2011).

> **Practice Pearl ▶▶▶** It is difficult to ask an older person to give up part of a nighttime ritual. If taking a sleeping pill is a longtime habit, the nurse can suggest substituting a vitamin pill as an alternative allowing the older person to complete the pill-taking ritual without the risk of medication side effects.

Nursing Assessment

Nursing assessment of sleep problems in older people should utilize a holistic approach. Because of the multifactorial causes of sleep problems in the older person, a thorough evaluation should precede any nursing intervention. The components of a sleep assessment should include a health history, a physical examination, daily sleep diaries, and polysomnography testing if sleep apnea is suspected. Key assessment areas are as follows:

Health History
- Diagnosed acute or chronic illness
- Current medications (including herbal and OTC)
- Chronic pain or pruritus
- Psychological problems
- Change in living conditions or sleep routines
- Current stressors or worries
- Nicotine, alcohol, or caffeine use
- Last complete medical examination

> **Practice Pearl ▶▶▶** Sleep problems arise from a variety of causes. It is poor nursing practice to suggest or offer a therapeutic solution without a complete nursing assessment. A Band-Aid approach may cover up and mask serious underlying problems.

Best Practices

The Pittsburgh Sleep Quality Index (PSQI) is an effective instrument for measuring the quality and patterns of sleep in the older adult (Hartford Institute for Geriatric Nursing, 2012). It differentiates "poor" from "good" sleep by measuring seven domains: subjective sleep quality, sleep latency, sleep duration, habitual sleep efficiency, sleep disturbances, use of sleeping medication, and daytime dysfunction during the past month. A global sum of 5 or greater indicates a poor sleeper. The PSQI can be used for initial assessment

Weblink: The Pittsburgh Sleep Quality Index (PSQI)

and ongoing comparative measurements with older adults in a variety of settings. Please refer to The Sleep Medicine Institute of the University of Pittsburgh's website for futher information on the PSQI.

Nursing Interventions

The nurse is in an ideal situation to intervene with older people with sleep problems. Nursing interventions for sleep promotion should be grounded in an understanding of the relationship between mind and body. Sleep disturbances caused by underlying medical problems should be referred for treatment. Nighttime pain should be investigated for cause and treated. Depression and anxiety disorders likewise require medical intervention and treatment.

The gerontological nurse should carefully measure the older patient's blood pressure, pulse, height, and weight. A nasal/oral examination can rule out nasal obstruction and defects in the oral pharynx. The primary healthcare provider may wish to obtain laboratory tests to examine thyroid function, ferritin levels, and other measurements such as drug levels to rule out drug toxicity if suspected.

Sleep hygiene should be encouraged in any older person with a sleep problem. Emphasis is placed on correcting and improving problem behaviors or inadequate environmental conditions in order to improve sleep efficiency. Inadequate sleep hygiene refers to daily activities that interfere with the maintenance of good quality sleep and daytime alertness. Environmental problems should be corrected if possible. If the nighttime environment is too hot or cold, portable air conditioners or heaters may be appropriate. Earplugs may ease nighttime noise. The timing of medications should be examined for appropriateness. Dietary and lifestyle changes should be recommended after the older person is appropriately educated regarding the harmful effects of nicotine, caffeine, and alcohol on sleep. Activities, hobbies, and special interests should be pursued, and multiple long naps should be avoided because excessive daytime sleep and boredom may interfere with nighttime sleep (NLM, 2010). Appropriate exercise like walking and stretching should be recommended, but not within 3 hours before bedtime. Sleep hygiene measures such as limiting time spent in bed to 8 hours a night, avoiding daytime napping, and using the bed only for sleep and sexual activity have been found to be an effective intervention (Reuben et al., 2011).

Additional Nonpharmacological Measures

Sleep restriction therapy is based on the theory that many older people with sleep problems spend too much time in bed trying

to get 8 hours of satisfactory sleep. Therefore, the nurse can assist the older person to identify how many hours of sleep are needed to feel rested and refreshed in the morning. Prompts can include: "How many hours of nighttime sleep is normal for you?" or "Name a time in your life when you thought your sleep was good. How many hours were you sleeping then?"

After the nurse and the older person have identified an appropriate goal, a schedule is established for time to bed and time to arise. For instance, if an older person wishes to obtain 8 hours of quality sleep and wishes to go to bed at 11 p.m., he or she must arise at 7 a.m. At first, older people with sleep problems will be sleep deprived because they will be spending time in bed trying to sleep, but this helps to consolidate sleep (Peters, 2011). Gradually, older people will increase their sleep efficiency as their bodies learn to become more sleep efficient. Additional rules to be followed in sleep restriction therapy include:

- Use the bed only to sleep. No reading, TV watching, or eating in bed is allowed. Sexual activity is the only exception to this rule.
- If you are unable to sleep, get up and go to another room. Watching the clock is not recommended. When you are sleepy, go back to bed. The goal is to learn to associate the bed with restful sleep.
- Get up at the same time every day, regardless of the amount or quality of sleep obtained the night before.
- Do not nap during the day.

Older people who vigorously adhere to the provisions of sleep restriction therapy may experience improved quality and quantity of sleep.

Cognitive therapy focuses on changing the older person's expectations about sleep. Many older people worry about their inability to sleep and become anxious "trying" to sleep. With instruction and support from the nurse, the older person with sleep problems may be taught to understand that everyone has a sleep problem from time to time and that daytime fatigue usually follows a circadian pattern and can be managed with short rest periods. **Bedtime rituals** such as performing progressive relaxation exercises, listening to nature tapes, praying, reading a few pages of a novel, or other relaxing activities may assist the older person who is anxious at bedtime to sleep. The hour before the older person goes to bed should be considered a "transition" hour in which the daytime cares and activities begin to shut down and the body and mind begin to prepare for the onset of sleep. Loud or violent television programs should be avoided. Even the nightly news can be upsetting to some older people if shootings, car crashes, fires, and other disasters are reported in detail. Once a satisfactory nighttime ritual has been established, it should be maintained to ease the transition from wakefulness to sleep.

Unfortunately, the nonpharmacological interventions mentioned above are not appropriate for the older person living in a long-term care facility or hospitalized in the acute care setting. Sleep fragmentation can occur for several reasons in these settings. The central nervous system is unable to maintain 8 hours of consolidated sleep in the older person with dementia. In addition, environmental factors may disrupt sleep in institutional settings. Environmental noise, light, and care routines can disrupt sleep in many cases. The following recommendations are made to nurses working in institutional settings (adapted from King, Halley, & Olson, 2007; Schnelle, Alessi, Al-Samarrai, et al., 1999):

- Establish consistent nighttime routines and quiet times, which signal to both staff and residents that sleep is to be facilitated.
- Reduce noise and light disruption throughout the night.
- Schedule routine care and examinations in the early evening hours.
- Turn down televisions and radios and ringers on phones.
- Avoid using intercoms and beepers during sleep hours.
- Turn night-lights on at the hour of sleep and turn off overhead lights.
- Keep residents busy and occupied during the daytime with exercise and recreational programs so that long naps are avoided.
- Do not put residents to bed immediately after supper. Try to provide restful evening activities like music or group readings so that gastrointestinal problems such as gastroesophageal reflux disease are avoided.
- If residents are awake and noisy during the night, assist them from bed to a lounge or recreation area where they will not disturb other residents. When they become sleepy, they can return to their beds.
- Prohibit examinations, laboratory procedures, and X-rays except in emergency situations.
- If it is necessary to enter a patient's room to observe a patient, enter quietly using a handheld flashlight instead of turning on a bright overhead light.

A multifaceted intervention to improve sleep hygiene can successfully be implemented in the institutional setting to improve sleep and overall well-being for many of the residents. Educate family members and visitors about the importance of quiet time so that they realize the benefits of sleep and rest to the healing and recovery process.

Pharmacological Treatments for Altered Sleep Patterns

A variety of prescription and nonprescription medications as well as herbal remedies are taken by older people for sleep. When behavioral interventions are not helpful,

pharmacotherapy may be indicated. Many older people with sleep problems are chronic users of sleep medication. Sleep medication use is more prevalent among older adults, particularly older women (NLM, 2010).

Studies have shown that most benzodiazepines are effective for promoting sleep on a short-term basis. However, the nurse should be aware of the lack of evidence that these drugs are effective for long-term use.

> **Drug Alert ▶▶▶** Benzodiazepine therapy is recommended for short-term use not to exceed 2 weeks. If used long term, it is to be given in intermittent courses.

Daytime residual effects include tolerance, psychological dependence, rebound insomnia on discontinuation, and impairment of psychomotor and cognitive performance. It is important to avoid using the benzodiazepines with longer half-lives such as alprazolam and diazepam. These drugs are associated with abuse potential, daytime sedation and falls, and memory impairment (Reuben et al., 2011). Shorter-acting benzodiazepines (half-life 6 hours) such as lorazepam are suggested to be the better choice for older adults. These drugs have the best effect profile and raise the fewest safety concerns. These preparations are metabolized in the kidneys and are less likely than other agents to cause liver damage. As previously mentioned, risks associated with benzodiazepine use include tolerance, dependency, rebound insomnia on discontinuation, daytime drowsiness, and risk for falls.

Sedating antidepressants may also be used if the older person exhibits signs and symptoms of depression. The nurse must carefully monitor the older person for postural hypotension and other anticholinergic side effects such as constipation, dry mouth, tachycardia, and changes in cognitive status. Generally, lower doses of tricyclic antidepressants are needed for sleep disorders than are needed to treat depression, thereby lessening the risk of adverse side effects. Antidepressants may worsen sleep-related movement disorders (e.g., restless leg syndrome), disrupt sleep architecture, and increase the risk for falls (NHLBI, 2011).

Antihistamines such as diphenhydramine (Benadryl) should not be used because of their anticholinergic side effects and the potential to decrease respiratory drive. Barbiturates, sedatives, hypnotics, opiates, and antipsychotics should not be used for the routine treatment of sleep disorders. The use of barbiturates has fallen out of favor because of the potential for abuse, overdose, and severe withdrawal symptoms. Additionally, movement disorders such as tardive dyskinesia are common with antipsychotics.

Zolpidem (Ambien) and zaleplon (Sonata) have been used in low doses for older adults. Unlike other classes of sleep-inducing drugs, these drugs usually do not adversely affect sleep architecture and have not been associated with harmful side effects. Daytime sedation and decreased cognitive performance have been reported in older adults, especially when the medication is taken in the middle of the night and the older person does not remain in bed for a full 8 hours of sleep. A newer drug, ramelteon (Rozerem), works as a melatonin receptor agonist, enabling naturally occurring melatonin in the brain to promote sleep. It is deemed low risk for abuse and dependence and should not be taken immediately after a high-fat meal (Reuben et al., 2011). As with other sleep aids, however, tolerance quickly develops within 2 weeks of use and the drug can cause gastric irritation as well as renal, hepatic, and cardiac toxicity (Reuben et al., 2011). In general, sleep medication should not be taken for more than 3 to 4 weeks.

COMPLEMENTARY AND ALTERNATIVE THERAPIES

Many older people also use herbal or natural remedies. Melatonin is a hormone produced in the pineal gland that plays a role in the regulation of sleep. Melatonin is sold in many pharmacies and health food stores and is effective for some older people with sleep disturbances due to decreased levels of melatonin. Doses of 0.5 to 3 mg have been suggested for sleep. It should be taken approximately 2 hours before bedtime. Melatonin has been found to significantly improve sleep onset in older people with insomnia; however, it has been found not to affect sleep quality, number of awakenings after sleep onset, total sleep time, or sleep architecture (NIH, 2011b). The most commonly reported side effects include nausea, dizziness, and drowsiness. Melatonin is generally considered safe for short-term use and no significant drug interactions are described. Because melatonin has a short half-life (about 40 minutes), a controlled-release formulation is recommended to maintain sleep throughout the entire sleep cycle (Reuben et al., 2011).

Additional natural remedies include herbal chamomile tea (if no allergies to ragweed or daisies), hops, lemon balm, and valerian (NIH, 2011c). Valerian root has been used in Europe for the past several years, and a dose of 400 to 450 mg of the extract will shorten sleep latency in a manner similar to that of a short-acting benzodiazepine. However, the NIH concluded that there is not enough hard evidence to support the effectiveness of valerian in treating insomnia. Common side effects include headache, dizziness, itchiness, and gastrointestinal upset. Older patients taking valerian should be warned that it can have toxic interactions with other medications such as alcohol, sedating drugs, benzodiazepines, and barbiturates. Sometimes a small evening snack such as a glass of milk or a turkey sandwich may promote sleep onset because of the natural tryptophan contained in these foods.

Cognitive–behavioral therapy (CBT), a short-term goal-focused therapy, has been used to improve sleep. CBT interventions include sleep restriction (limiting the time spent in bed), stimulus formation (learning to associate the bed with sleep and rest), biofeedback, and relaxation techniques. CBT has been shown to be effective in improving sleep efficiency and significantly decreasing insomnia symptoms in a majority of older patients studied (McPhee & Papadakis, 2011).

> *handwritten: CAM*
> **Practice Pearl ▸▸▸** When developing interventions to improve sleep, it is important to include the patient. Priorities should be set according to the patient's wishes. It may be difficult for older adults to change their diet, exercise more, avoid caffeine, limit daytime napping, and so on. Making all of these changes at once may be nearly impossible. Approaching each individual behavior with a reasonable plan and appropriate goal setting is key to success.

Patient–Family Teaching Guidelines

The following are guidelines that the nurse may find useful when instructing older adults and their families about sleep problems (adapted from NIH, 2011a).

INSOMNIA OR SLEEP PROBLEMS

1 What is insomnia or disordered sleep?

These disorders are characterized by the perception or complaint of inadequate or poor quality sleep because of:

- Difficulty falling asleep (longer than 20 minutes is considered a problem)

- Waking up often during the night and being unable to fall quickly back to sleep
- Waking up too early in the morning and staying awake
- Waking up in the morning without feeling refreshed

(continued)

Patient–Family Teaching Guidelines *(continued)*

RATIONALE:

Insomnia is not defined by the number of hours of sleep a person gets or tries to get or even how long it takes to fall asleep. Insomnia is the older person's perception and complaint about either the quality or the quantity of sleep.

2 What causes sleep problems?

Certain conditions make some older people more likely to have sleep problems than others. Examples of these conditions include the following:

- Age over 60
- Female gender
- History of or current diagnosis of depression
- Certain medications (diuretics or long-term use of sleep medications)
- Daytime loneliness or boredom in addition to long naps
- Chronic illness with components of pain or difficulty breathing
- Diagnosis of Alzheimer's disease or other neurological problems
- Situational events like moving to a new home or loss of a loved one

RATIONALE:

Everyone has transient sleep problems from time to time. In general, the amount of sleep needed remains stable throughout the lifetime, but periods of stress, illness, travel, or other change in life events can precipitate sleep problems. The goal is to quickly retrain the body and brain to regain normal sleep.

3 What seems to make sleep problems worse?

The following behaviors seem to perpetuate sleep problems and make them more likely to become chronic:

- Worry about sleep and expecting to have problems every night
- Drinking too much caffeine
- Drinking alcohol before bedtime
- Smoking cigarettes before bedtime
- Sleeping longer than 50 minutes during the day
- Being told by a sleep partner that you are snoring and gasping during sleep

- Not seeking medical attention for pain, urinary problems, nighttime gastroesophageal reflux disease, or tingling sensation in the legs

RATIONALE:

These behaviors may prolong transient insomnia or sleep problems or be responsible for causing the problem initially. Stopping these behaviors and investigating the cause of others early on may eliminate the problem completely.

4 Where should the older person go for evaluation and treatment?

An older person who does not have a current healthcare provider should seek evaluation from a primary care physician, geriatrician, or gerontological nurse practitioner. Underlying acute and chronic health problems should always be investigated and ruled out or treated optimally. These providers can then make referrals for polysomnography and sleep laboratory testing if appropriate. It is helpful to keep a sleep diary for a week or so before the medical appointment because this valuable information will encourage better decision making by the healthcare provider.

RATIONALE:

The older person should not be labeled as having insomnia or chronic sleep problems without a thorough evaluation and physical examination. Some older adults are automatically given sleeping pills that can mask the symptoms of underlying health problems such as untreated or diagnosed pain, cardiac disease, or psychological disorders and have the potential for harmful side effects.

5 How are sleep problems treated?

Some sleep problems are transient and intermittent and will resolve spontaneously. For instance, jet lag may last only a few days. Pain from a fractured bone may resolve within a week or 10 days. The strangeness of moving to a new home may resolve within a few weeks. For long-term sleep problems, the treatment will depend on the cause. A thorough assessment of sleep problems will guide the competent clinician toward appropriate treatment.

RATIONALE:

It is important to avoid taking over-the-counter sleep medications or prescription sleep aids for extended periods of time. They suppress normal sleep architecture, perpetuate sleep problems, and have the potential to cause harmful side effects.

CARE PLAN | A Patient With a Sleep Problem

Case Study

A nurse working at an adult day care center notices that Mrs. Johnson, an 84-year-old woman who has attended the center regularly for 1 year, is lethargic, disinterested, and constantly nodding off to sleep during activities. Other older persons at the center have begun to complain about her and have asked the nurse to speak with her and tell her to "stay home if she wants to sleep all day."

Applying the Nursing Process

Assessment

Mrs. Johnson has recently had a complete physical examination and health history, and there is no apparent medical reason for her sleep problems. The nurse requests permission from Mrs. Johnson to visit her at home and she agrees. The next day during the home visit the nurse notices a liquor bottle on the counter. When asked about this, Mrs. Johnson replies, "Oh yes. I take a nip or two every night because I can't sleep at all without it. Don't tell my son because he wouldn't approve and I'm afraid he would think I'm an alcoholic or something like that." She appears angry and defensive as she makes this statement.

Diagnosis

The current nursing diagnoses for Mrs. Johnson include the following:

- *Sleep Pattern, Disturbed*
- *Activity, Deficient Diversional*

NANDA-I © 2012.

Expected Outcomes

The expected outcomes for the plan of care specify that Mrs. Johnson will:

- Become aware of the harmful effects of alcohol on quality and quantity of sleep and be able to discuss them with her nurse within 1 week after receiving instruction from the nurse.
- Use sleep hygiene measures as an alternative to alcohol and report decreased use of alcohol within 1 week after her instruction from the nurse.
- Develop a more trusting and open relationship with her son regarding her health status as evidenced by her report of having a discussion with her son regarding her health status within 2 weeks.
- Agree to establish a therapeutic relationship with the nurse and develop a mutually acceptable plan to work toward these outcomes.

Planning and Implementation

The following nursing interventions may be appropriate for Mrs. Johnson:

- Establish a therapeutic relationship.
- Avoid being judgmental or using "scare" tactics.
- Encourage a family meeting with the son present to talk about health issues in general with Mrs. Johnson's permission.
- Begin a sleep assessment to establish the underlying cause of her sleep disturbance.
- Begin a values clarification to establish long-term goals and facilitate end-of-life planning.

(continued)

CARE PLAN   ## A Patient With a Sleep Problem *(continued)*

Evaluation

The nurse hopes to work with Mrs. Johnson over time and realizes the chronic nature of sleep problems in older people. The nurse will consider the plan a success based on the following criteria:

- Mrs. Johnson will continue to attend the day care center with improved function and social skills.

- A family meeting will be held to discuss her overall health.
- Mrs. Johnson will begin to decrease her alcohol consumption at bedtime and report improved sleep based on positive behavioral changes.

Ethical Dilemma

The ethical dilemma that emerges in this case is the conflict between the nurse's obligation to patient autonomy and confidentiality versus beneficence. Mrs. Johnson is physically frail but cognitively intact. The nurse cannot share confidential information with others who may wish to assist Mrs. Johnson to improve her health status. This includes her family, her physician, and other healthcare providers. However, the nurse wishes to meet her moral and professional obligation to assist this patient to regain her previous function and vigor and realizes the addictive and harmful effects of alcohol use in older people.

Critical Thinking and the Nursing Process

1. What is the physiological basis for Mrs. Johnson's poor quality of sleep after alcohol consumption?
2. Explain possible reasons in addition to alcohol consumption for this patient's poor sleep.
3. Outline a teaching plan with behavioral interventions designed to improve Mrs. Johnson's sleep.
4. Suggest a nursing action if Mrs. Johnson continues to increase her alcohol consumption and still refuses to accept family or professional help for her drinking.

5. Suppose that Mrs. Johnson asks if sleeping medication may be appropriate for her to use. How should the nurse respond?

- Evaluate your responses in Appendix B.

Chapter Highlights

- Older people often report sleep problems. Some are transient in nature, but many are chronic. These problems may be the result of age-related changes, physical or mental health problems, medication use or abuse, or lifestyle issues.

- To be restful and restorative, sleep must cycle through stages and phases. Normal changes of aging and some medications suppress the cyclic changes, making restful sleep harder to achieve.

- Older adults in nursing homes and hospitals may have disrupted sleep because of noise and light interruptions from nursing staff and other residents. Every attempt should be made to minimize nighttime awakenings so that restful sleep may be achieved.

- Alzheimer's disease and other kinds of dementia can further disturb sleep. These disruptions may lead to institutionalization if caregivers become fatigued by their inability to achieve restful sleep.

- Sleep apnea can be a significant problem for older people. Those at high risk—including people who snore, have hypertension, are obese, or have central nervous system problems—should seek polysomnography testing in a sleep laboratory.

- Prescription and OTC sleep aids can have dangerous side effects when taken by older people. These drugs should be used in the smallest doses for the shortest period of time.

- Nurses should carry out a complete sleep history before recommending an intervention for an older person with sleep problems. Sleep problems may result from a variety of causes, and the nursing intervention should be appropriately based on the cause.

Pearson Nursing Student Resources
Find additional review materials at
nursing.pearsonhighered.com

Prepare for success with additional NCLEX®-style practice questions, interactive assignments and activities, web links, animations and videos, and more!

References

Alzheimer's Association. (2012). *Treatments for sleep changes.* Retrieved from http://www.alz.org/alzheimers_disease_10429.asp

Blazek, N. (2011). Sleep apnea linked to clinical decline. *Clinical Advisor.* Retrieved from http://www.clinicaladvisor.com/sleep-apnea-linked-to-cognitive-decline/article/209388

Brannon, G. (2012). Geriatric sleep disorders. *Medscape Reference.* Retrieved from http://emedicine.medscape.com/article/292498-overview

Ellenbogen, J., Buxton, O., Wang, W., Carballeira, A., O'Connor, S., Cooper, D., McKinney, S., Solet, J. (2011). *Sleep disruption due to hospital noises.* Retrieved from http://www.aami.org/alarms/Materials/ICBEN2011_Ellenbogen.pdf

Endeshaw, Y., Johnson, T., Kutner, M., Ouslander, J., & Bliwise, D. (2004). Sleep-disordered breathing and nocturia in older adults. *Journal of the American Geriatrics Society, 52*(6), 957–960.

Fong, T., Jones, R., Shi, P., Marcantonio, E., Yap, L., Rudolph, J., Yang, F., Kiely, D., & Inouye, S. (2009). Delirium accelerates cognitive decline in Alzheimer's disease. *Neurology, 72,* 1570–1575.

Hartford Institute for Geriatric Nursing, Division of Nursing, New York University. (2012). The Pittsburgh Sleep Quality Index (PSQI). *Try this: Best practices in nursing care to older adults.* Retrieved from http://consultgerirn.org/uploads/File/trythis/try_this_6_1.pdf

King, K., Halley, N., & Olson, D. (2007). To sleep, perchance to heal: A tale of quiet time and sleep promotion in the ICU. *American Nurse Today, 2*(10), 44–46.

McCance, K., & Huether, S. (2012). *Understanding pathophysiology* (5th ed.). New York, NY: Elsevier Mosby.

McPhee, S., & Papadakis, M. (2011). Sleep disorders. In *Current medical diagnosis and treatment* (50th ed., Chap. 25). New York, NY: McGraw-Hill Medical.

NANDA International. (2011). *NANDA International nursing diagnoses: Definitions and classification, 2012–2014.* Hoboken, NJ: Wiley-Blackwell.

National Heart, Lung & Blood Institute (NHLBI). (2011). *Your guide to healthy sleep.* Retrieved from http://www.nhlbi.nih.gov/health/public/sleep/healthy_sleep.pdf

National Institutes of Health (NIH). (2011a). Insomnia. *Medline Plus.* Retrieved from http://www.nlm.nih.gov/medlineplus/ency/article/000805.htm

National Institutes of Health (NIH). (2011b). *Melatonin for sleep disorders.* Retrieved from http://ahrq.gov/clinic/epcsums/melatsum.htm

National Institutes of Health (NIH). (2011c). *Valerian.* Retrieved from http://nccam.nih.gov/health/valerian

National Library of Medicine (NLM) (2010). Sleep disorders in the elderly. Retrieved from http://www.nlm.nih.gov/medlineplus/ency/article/000064.htm

Pace, B., Lynn, C., & Glass, R. (2001). Breathing problems during sleep. *Journal of the American Medical Association, 285*(22), 2936.

Peters, B. (2011). Sleep restriction is an effective behavioral therapy. *About.com.*

Retrieved from http://sleepdisorders.about.com/od/sleepdisorderstreatment/a/Sleep_Restriction_Insomnia.htm

Pierse, J., & Dym, H. (2011). An update on the treatment of sleep disorders. *Clinical Advisor.* Retrieved from http://www.clinicaladvisor.com/an-update-on-treatments-for-sleep-disorders/article/202451

Reuben, D., Herr, K., Pacala, J., Pollick, B., Potter, J., & Semla, T. (2011). *Geriatrics at your fingertips* (13th ed.). New York, NY: American Geriatrics Society.

Robinson, L., Kemp, G., & Segal, R. (2012). *Insomnia in older adults: Tips for sleeping better as you age.* Retrieved from http://www.helpguide.org/life/sleep_aging.htm

Schnelle, J., Alessi, C., Al-Samarrai, N., Fricker, R., & Ouslander, J. (1999). The nursing home at night: Effects of an intervention on noise, light and sleep. *Journal of the American Geriatrics Society, 47,* 430–438.

Six ways lack of sleep is costing you money. (2012). *U.S. News & World Report.* Retrieved from http://money.usnews.com/money/blogs/my-money/2011/08/15/6-ways-lack-of-sleep-is-costing-you-a-fortune

U.S. National Library of Medicine (NLM). (2010). *Aging changes in the nervous system.* Retrieved from http://www.nlm.nih.gov/medlineplus/ency/article/004023.htm

Pain Management

Katherine Tardiff, MSN, GNP-BC

CLINICAL OPERATIONS MANAGER, SENIOR CARE OPTIONS, TUFTS HEALTH PLAN

KEY TERMS

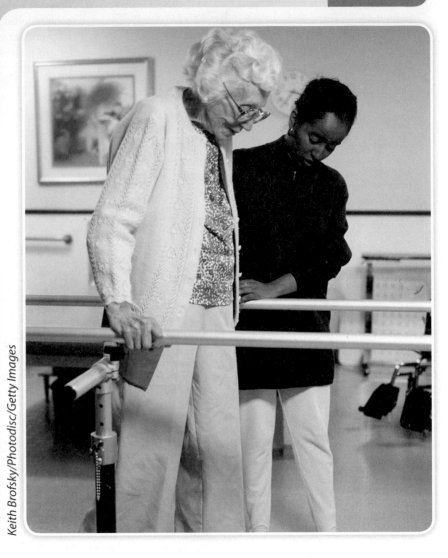

Keith Brofsky/Photodisc/Getty Images

LEARNING OUTCOMES

On completion of this chapter, the reader will be able to:

1. Define pain and the consequences of pain in the older adult.
2. Identify appropriate pain assessment techniques, including those to use with dementia.
3. Describe pharmacological and nonpharmacological approaches useful in treating pain in the older adult.
4. Recognize the nurse's role in treating pain in the older adult.
5. Explain patient–family teaching guidelines for pain management.

Pain is a common unpleasant sensation experienced by all human beings at some point during their lives. This complex phenomenon is both a sensory and emotional experience that impacts many aspects of an older adult's life. Older adults are at particular risk for experiencing both **acute pain,** or pain typically caused by a defined event and occurring for a short period of time, and **persistent pain,** or pain that continues for a prolonged period and may not be associated with a defined event or illness. As people age, they often develop multiple chronic medical issues that may result in several sources of pain (American Geriatrics Society [AGS], 2009). Painful conditions such as arthritis, bone and joint disorders, back problems, cancer, and nerve pain are common in this population. In fact, studies have shown that 57% of older adults in the Untied States often experience pain with 35% to 48% of community-dwelling older adults experiencing daily pain (American Pain Foundation [APF], 2008; Krueger & Stone, 2008; Maxwell et al., 2008).

Pain is not only common, it is also costly. A recent report commissioned by the Institute of Medicine (IOM, 2011) cites pain as a public health challenge due to the significant physical, personal, and financial impact of pain. In 2008, the federal Medicare program, which provides health care for individuals over the age of 65 and younger people with disabilities, spent at least $65.3 billion in costs related to pain, equal to 14% of all Medicare costs (IOM, 2011).

Undertreatment of acute and persistent pain is a serious problem relating to care of older adults. Despite the fact that safe and effective pharmacological and nonpharmacological techniques are available to treat pain, many older adults live with untreated pain on a daily basis. Furthermore, pain is undertreated in the population of older adults with dementia, and research has demonstrated that patients with severe cognitive impairment receive fewer pain medications than those who are cognitively intact (Herr, 2011; Reynolds, Hanson, DeVellis, et al., 2008).

There continues to be increased emphasis on the assessment and treatment of pain in the older adult, and patients and their families are more aware now of the need to treat both acute and persistent pain. However, there are many barriers to effective assessment and **pain management,** or the formulation and implementation of a plan to alleviate or reduce pain to an acceptable level of comfort, in the older adult. Some older adults may be reluctant to report pain for fear of invasive testing or fear of drug **addiction,** defined as having intense need and compulsive dependence on opioids to such an extent that not having these drugs causes severe yearning and triggers physiological withdrawal symptoms. Other older adults may expect pain and believe it cannot be alleviated (AGS, 2002). Many older adults and their families believe that pain is a normal part of aging and fear that complaining is

a sign of weakness (Hadjistavropoulos et al., 2007). Clinical barriers such as inadequate training and use of inappropriate assessment tools by clinicians result in poor pain assessments (McAuliffe, Nay, O'Donnell et al., 2009). Further complicating the issue, many factors affect the experience and report of pain in the older adult. According to Hadjistavropoulos et al. (2007), "biologic aging, prior experiences, attitudes, beliefs, expectations, memory, presence and response of significant others, fear, and social context are among many variables that will influence pain reports" (p. S2).

The high prevalence of pain in older adults as well as the detrimental consequences of undertreated pain make it imperative that nurses working with the older adult population be educated in appropriate pain assessment and management techniques.

> **Practice Pearl ▶▶▶** It is common for older adults to deny pain but acknowledge sensations such as discomfort, hurting, aching, or soreness. Ask "Do you have pain or discomfort today?" and "How about aching or soreness?" (AGS, 2002; Hadjistavropoulos et al., 2007).

Pathophysiology of Pain

Pain and pain transmission involve both the peripheral receptors and sensory pathways and synaptic contacts in the spinal cord and brain stem. Processes within the dorsal horn are essential elements in modulating and facilitating pain transmission and initiating efferent responses. Nociceptors, or pain receptors, are nerve endings in the peripheral nervous system that respond to stimuli that threaten or produce damage to the organism. A person perceives pain when noxious stimuli are transmitted to the central areas of the brain via the dorsal horn of the spinal cord (Helms & Barone, 2008). The sensation of pain occurs at the thalamus; however, the limbic system (emotional center) and cerebral cortex perceive and interpret the pain. Figure 9-1 ▶▶▶ illustrates the configuration of the brain, spinal cord, and peripheral receptors.

When tissue damage occurs, the body releases chemical substances into the extracellular tissue that cause vasoconstriction, vasodilation, or altered capillary permeability. These substances, including histamine, substance P, bradykinin, acetylcholine, leukotrienes, and prostaglandins, activate pain receptors by irritating nerve endings (Helms & Barone, 2008). At the same time, the body initiates an intrinsic pain control response, releasing neuromodulators (endogenous opioids) that inhibit the action of the neurons transmitting the pain response.

Pain can be classified as nociceptive or neuropathic. The **nociceptive pain** sensation may be **visceral** (pain of the

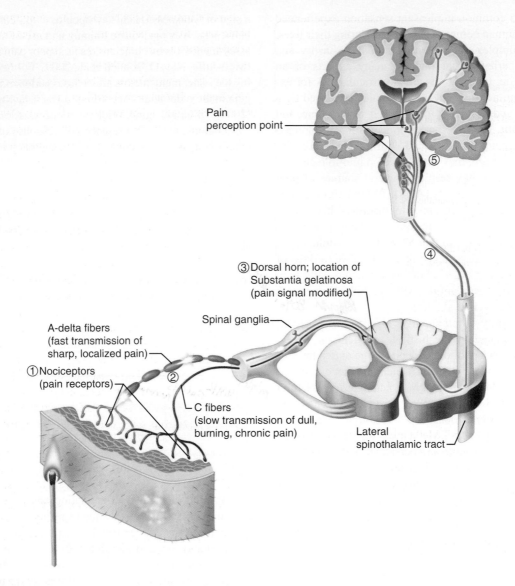

Pain
perception point

⑤

③ Dorsal horn; location of
Substantia gelatinosa
(pain signal modified)

Spinal ganglia

④

A-delta fibers
(fast transmission of
sharp, localized pain)

① Nociceptors
(pain receptors)

②

C fibers
(slow transmission of dull,
burning, chronic pain)

Lateral
spinothalamic tract

Figure 9-1 ▶▶▶ The brain, spinal cord, and peripheral pain receptors.

body's internal organs that is often poorly localized and described as deep or aching) or **somatic** (pain of the muscles, joints, connective tissues and bones that typically is well localized). It is designed to provide a signal that actual or potential tissue damage is occurring somewhere in the body (International Association for the Study of Pain [IASP], 2011). Nociceptive pain is associated with skin, muscle, bone, joint, or other connective tissue trauma or degenerative disease (Hadjistavropoulos et al., 2007). For example, nociceptive pain may be caused by arthritis or chronic tendonitis or it may be related to inflammation of internal organs. **Neuropathic pain** results from damage to the central or peripheral nervous system (IASP, 2011). Painful neuropathic conditions common in the older adult include

diabetic neuropathy and post-herpetic neuralgia. Although acute pain can be protective, undertreated pain can become an intolerable burden and may lead to depression, decreased socialization, reduced functional abilities, malnutrition, and insomnia (Herr, 2011). Box 9-1 lists common conditions that are associated with pain in older adults.

With untreated pain, nociceptors become sensitive and more responsive to stimuli with a lowered pain threshold. This can lead to **hyperalgesia** or an increased sensitivity to pain or enhanced intensity of pain sensation (IASP, 2011). This sensitization can result in an exaggerated pain response to stimuli that usually causes only discomfort or mild pain such as administration of injections, starting an intravenous (IV) line, or even taking a blood pressure. Nurses and other

BOX 9-1 **Conditions Associated With Pain in Older Adults**

- Osteoarthritis
- Rheumatoid arthritis
- Spinal stenosis
- Osteoporosis (with and without spinal fracture)
- Peripheral neuropathy
- Post-herpetic neuralgia
- Fibromyalgia
- Gastroesophageal reflux disease
- Complex regional pain syndrome (CRPS)
- Peripheral vascular disease
- Headache
- Oral problems and gum disease
- Amputation, postsurgical pain
- Pressure ulcers
- Angina and other cardiac disease
- Cancer pain and pain from resulting treatment

Source: National Pain Foundation (NPF). (2011). *Pain causes among older adults*. Retrieved from http://www.nationalpainfoundation.org/articles/245/pain-causes-among-older-adults

healthcare providers may become impatient with older adults exhibiting this exaggerated pain response and feel that it is out of proportion to the procedure being carried out. The older person may be labeled as a "hypochondriac," and further complaints of pain may not be taken seriously.

NORMAL CHANGES OF AGING

Few studies have examined the relationship between pain perception and aging. The AGS (2002) notes that any age-related changes in pain perception are probably not clinically significant. Certain types of visceral pain may be less severe in the older adult, and that may explain the higher incidence of silent myocardial infarction and the less dramatic presentation of peptic ulcer disease (Moore & Clinch, 2004). The younger adult experiencing myocardial infarction will most often report severe, crushing chest pain, often with radiation down the left arm, sweating, and tremor. However, the older person may report vague complaints of pain that can be attributed to heartburn or sour stomach, the presence of nausea and vomiting, or unexplained fatigue or falls.

Acute Pain in Older Adults

Acute pain is pain that results from a harmful or injurious stimulus; the pain is short lived and resolves when the stimulus is removed or the injury has healed. When acute pain occurs, it is important for the nurse to adequately identify the source of the pain and facilitate treatment of the underlying

disease or trauma whenever possible. Conditions that cause acute pain in older adults include exacerbations of degenerative joint disease; flare-ups of chronic conditions such as gout or rheumatoid arthritis; trauma from falls including muscle strain, bone fractures, bumps, and bruises; skin problems such as burns, decubitus ulcers, and skin tears; presence of infection such as urinary tract infection; pleuritic pain in pneumonia and the neuropathic pain of herpes zoster; constipation; and postoperative pain from surgical intervention.

Persistent Pain in Older Adults

Persistent pain that continues over a prolonged period of time affects one in five adults ages 65 and older. This type of pain may not be related to a well-defined disease process. Although the terms *chronic pain* and *persistent pain* may be used interchangeably, it is suggested that the term *persistent pain* be used because it is less associated with negative stereotypes (AGS, 2009). Persistent pain may be related to musculoskeletal disorders (spinal stenosis, osteoporosis with compression fractures, osteoarthritis, degenerative disk disease, and arthritis and related disorders), cancer, or neuropathic disorders. Other common conditions include back pain and the ischemic pain of vascular disease.

Although good coping mechanisms and family support can lower pain levels, depression can exacerbate pain. It is recommended that nurses routinely screen for depression when working with older patients with persistent pain. A comprehensive pain treatment plan is needed to treat the biopsychosocial needs of the older patient. A vicious persistent pain cycle can occur with negative consequences, including decreased socialization, withdrawal from daily life, fatigue, sleep disturbance, irritability and physical deconditioning, and other signs of stress and depression (Bishop & Morrison, 2007).

Pain Assessment Techniques

Pain is measured subjectively according to the patient's self-report or by careful observation in a patient who is nonverbal or who has a severe cognitive impairment. Older people who feel that their reports of pain will be taken seriously are more likely to be open and honest during the pain assessment process. Even patients with mild to moderate cognitive impairments can be assessed with simple questions and screening tools (AGS, 2002). Many residents with cognitive impairment can report pain accurately at the time of interview but have difficulty reporting intensity and duration of previous episodes. The nurse may need to do more frequent assessments to obtain an accurate pain assessment for the patient with a cognitive impairment. Pain assessment is never a single event, but rather part of an ongoing process (Herr, 2011). Box 9-2

BOX 9-2   **Geriatric Pain Assessment**

This form is ideal for clinical use because it is brief and objective. It summarizes pertinent information and quantifies mood, bowel habits, exacerbating and relieving factors, and a plan for pain relief.

Date:

Patient's Name: Date of Birth:

Diagnosis:

Problem List:

Medications:

Pain Description:

Pattern: ❏ constant   ❏ intermittent   ❏ other:

Pain Intensity at Present:

0	1	2	3	4	5	6	7	8	9	10

None   Moderate   Severe

Worst Pain in Last 24 hours:

0	1	2	3	4	5	6	7	8	9	10

None   Moderate   Severe

Best Pain in Last 24 hours:

0	1	2	3	4	5	6	7	8	9	10

None   Moderate   Severe

Acceptable Level of Pain:

0	1	2	3	4	5	6	7	8	9	10

None   Moderate   Severe

Duration:

Location:

How does the patient describe the pain?

❏ stinging   ❏ throbbing   ❏ aching   ❏ pulling   ❏ dull

❏ burning   ❏ prick   ❏ sharp   ❏ radiating   ❏ shooting

❏ tingling   ❏ other:

What causes the pain to increase?

What relieves the pain?

❏ eating   ❏ massage   ❏ relaxation techniques   ❏ prayer

❏ rest   ❏ sleep   ❏ heat   ❏ cold

❏ repositioning   ❏ exercise   ❏ other:

| BOX 9-2 | **Geriatric Pain Assessment** (*continued*) |

Indicate How Pain Affects:

Mood:

Activity:

Sleep Quality:

Bowel Habits:

Nutrition:

Social Interactions:

Self Image:

Sexuality:

Associated Symptoms (patient rates on scale of 0–10)

Nausea:	Vomiting:	Anorexia:	Diarrhea:	Constipation:
Anxiety:	Depression:	Fatigue:	Dyspnea:	Sedation:
Insomnia:	Pruritus:			

Other Assessments or Comments:

Most Likely Cause of Pain:

Plan:

Source: Adapted from AGS, 2009; Dartmouth-Hitchcock Medical Center, n.d.; Otis-Green, S., n.d.; University of Wisconsin Hospitals and Clinics Home Health Agency, n.d.

provides an example of a medical record form that can be used to summarize pain assessment in the older adult.

A comprehensive clinical assessment for pain is multifaceted and should include a medical and pain history, a physical exam, and diagnostic testing if necessary (Herr, 2011). Before proceeding with the assessment, it is important to determine the presence of any sensory impairments and to ensure that assistive devices (e.g., hearing aids) are working properly (Hadjistavropoulos et al., 2007). A thorough pain history characterizes the report of pain in terms of intensity (the descriptive rating of the pain experience), quality (the characteristics of the pain, e.g., sharp, dull, throbbing), location (the anatomical site of the pain, including radiation), pattern (the course of the pain over time, including onset, duration, and frequency), and aggravating and relieving factors. It is important for the nurse to observe and document any nonverbal signs of pain such as guarding, grimacing, or restricted movement (Herr, 2011).

Additional information may be gathered by asking the patient to complete graphic rating scales such as the Faces Pain Scale, the Numeric Rating Scale, and the Verbal Descriptor Scale. According to the Hartford Institute for Geriatric Nursing (2007) all of these scales are appropriate and have been shown to be valid and reliable pain measurement tools. These simply worded, easily understood tools are the most effective for assessing pain in the older adult. The nurse should identify an assessment tool that can be used easily by the older adult patient and consistently use the same scale with each assessment; pain tools are not interchangeable and therefore do not represent comparable findings (Hadjistavropoulos et al., 2007). See Best Practices: Rating Scales for Assessing Pain in the Older Adult.

Box 9-3 illustrates sample questions that may be included in a pain interview. Once the nurse has completed the history, it is important to examine the area for signs of inflammation, such as redness, swelling, and warmth (Herr, 2011). The nurse should then list and prioritize each report of pain. This valuable information will guide the practitioner in the design of a pain management plan that targets the individual needs of the patient. The nurse should also indicate when the next pain assessment will occur and how often pain should be assessed. For patients

Best Practices   Rating Scales for Assessing Pain in the Older Adult

Faces Pain Scale – Revised

The Faces Pain Scale was originally developed to assess pain in children and is now sometimes used with older adults (Hicks, von Baeyer, Spafford, van Kortaar & Goodenough (2001). The Scale is composed of six drawings of a human face beginning with a slight smile and gradually progressing to a face depicting severe pain with an open mouth. The older person is shown the scale and asked to choose the face that best represents his/her level of pain. For further instructions on the correct use of the scale in order to obtain a valid pain rating in the older adult, please go to www.painsourcebook.ca.

Numeric Rating Scale

Please rate your pain from 0 to 10 with 0 indicating no pain and 10 representing the worst possible pain.

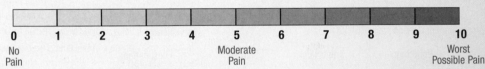

| 0 | 1 | 2 | 3 | 4 | 5 | 6 | 7 | 8 | 9 | 10 |

No Pain   Moderate Pain   Worst Possible Pain

Source: Adapted from Jacox, A., Carr, D. B., Payne, R., et al. (1994, March). *Management of cancer pain: Clinical practice guideline No. 9* (AHCPR Publication No. 94-0592). Rockville, MD: Agency for Health Care Policy and Research, U.S. Department of Health and Human Services.

Verbal Descriptor Scale

Please describe your pain from "no pain" to "mild," "moderate," "severe," or "pain as bad as it could be."

Source: Adapted from Jacox, A., Carr, D. B., Payne, R., et al. (1994, March). *Management of cancer pain: Clinical practice guideline No. 9* (AHCPR Publication No. 94-0592). Rockville, MD: Agency for Health Care Policy and Research, U.S. Department of Health and Human Services.

in severe pain, the reassessment should occur within 24 hours. Documentation should be kept in an accessible location so that there is open communication among the care team members. The nurse can facilitate continuity of care and an empathetic attitude in order to reassure the patient and build a trusting relationship.

Pain Assessment in the Person With Severe Cognitive Impairment

For those unable to verbally communicate their pain experience, pain often goes undertreated or untreated. A hierarchy of techniques for assessing pain in the nonverbal patient has been developed and supported by the American Society for Pain Management Nursing and an interdisciplinary panel of experts (Herr, Coyne et al., 2006). There is no reason to believe that the patient with a cognitive impairment is insensitive or indifferent to pain, and older adults with cognitive impairment should be questioned about the presence of pain. Furthermore, nurses can and should continue to use pain scales like the Faces Pain Scale and the Verbal Descriptor Scale in the population of older adults with mild to moderate dementia (Herr, 2011). Second, an attempt should be made to determine the underlying cause of the pain or discomfort, taking into consideration underlying chronic conditions such as arthritis or neuropathy as well as recent falls or infections.

check vitals

| BOX 9-3 | **Sample Pain Interview Questions** —Don't Rush! |

1. **Pain history.** When did the pain start? Use words such as "discomfort" or "pressure" or "ache." Consult with a family member to gain his or her perspective, with the patient's permission. Try to pinpoint the onset of the pain.

2. **Distinguish acute from persistent pain.** Can you describe your pain? Is it burning, stabbing, throbbing, aching? How does the pain in your hip affect your headache? Older patients in persistent pain are sometimes more sensitive to acute pain and persistent pain can be exacerbated by new-onset acute pain.

3. **Location.** Where is the pain? Many patients have pain in multiple sites. Pain from systemic diseases like rheumatoid arthritis may be felt all over the body. Pain may also be referred from one site to another.

4. **Frequency.** Does the pain occur every day? Does it come and go? Is there a constant level of baseline pain? Is breakthrough pain present and predictable? Many patients will report a pain pattern with pain levels consistently higher or lower at various times of the day.

5. **Intensity.** On a 1 to 10 scale with 10 being the worst pain ever, can you rate your pain? How does the rating vary during the day or night? How does the pain impact your life and mental health? For the patient with a cognitive impairment, observe moaning, limitation of movement, grimacing, physical distress illustrated by increased blood pressure or respiratory rate.

6. **Alleviating and aggravating factors.** What makes it better? What makes it worse? What have you tried that seems to relieve your pain?

Consider nonpharmacological approaches including exercise, massage, warm baths, heat pads, ice packs, topical rubs, acupuncture, and other alternative therapies.

7. **Associated symptoms.** Do you have other symptoms with your pain? Are you having any nausea, vomiting, chills, cramps, or loss of appetite?

8. **Response to previous and current analgesic therapy.** Are you taking pain medication now? Have you ever taken pain medication before? Was it effective? Do you have any medication allergies or intolerances? Are you reluctant to take pain medication? Is the cost of the medication a barrier? Are any side effects such as nausea, constipation, or lethargy associated with the medication regimen? Do you have trouble swallowing pills? Are there important or anticipated events that may occur during a typical day that may interfere with medication dosing? Many older patients and their families are concerned that they will become "drug addicts" or "hooked on narcotics." Reassurance, education, and treatment of side effects may be needed to achieve effective pain relief.

9. **Meaning of the pain.** What does the pain mean to you? How does your culture and religion influence the meaning of pain for you and your family? Some older patients and their families see pain as punishment for previous deeds while others may feel pain is to be expected and courage and fortitude are needed to be a strong person. Refer issues you are uncomfortable dealing with to a priest, minister or rabbi, social worker, or spiritual advisor.

Source: Data from Elliott, T. (2000). *Principles of analgesic use in the treatment of acute pain and cancer pain*. Glenview, IL: Author; McCaffery, M., & Pasero, C. (1999). *Pain: Clinical manual* (2nd ed., pp. 9–17). St. Louis, MO: Mosby; Wells-Federman, 1999; and Wittink, H., & Carr, D. (2008). *Pain management evidence, outcomes and quality of life*. New York, NY: Elsevier.

Next, the nurse should assess for the presence of pain-related behaviors (Herr, Coyne et al., 2006). Based on review of the literature, the AGS (2002) has identified six main types of pain behaviors and indicators in older adults with dementia. These include:

- Facial expression (e.g., frowning, frightened face, grimacing)
- Verbalizations/vocalizations (e.g., sighing, moaning, chanting)
- Body movements (e.g., tense posture, guarding, gait/mobility changes)
- Changes in interpersonal interactions (e.g., aggressiveness, combativeness, withdrawal)
- Changes in activity patterns or routines (e.g., appetite changes, changes in sleep periods, increased wandering)
- Mental status changes (e.g., crying, increased confusion, irritability) (AGS, 2002)

Reports from caregivers are valuable in assessing pain in the nonverbal older adult, though it remains important to use both self-report and nonverbal measures when assessing pain in this frail population.

> **Practice Pearl** ▶▶▶ Patients with late-stage dementia often are unable to advocate for themselves. Nurses in long-term care should be expert in assessing for pain and providing effective pain control in this population.

Ideally, the nurse should conduct a baseline patient assessment prior to a known painful event such as surgery, an invasive medical procedure, or a planned rehabilitation event such as postoperative physical therapy. This baseline assessment will allow the nurse to (1) investigate pain terminology and behaviors typically used by the patient and the patient's attitudes toward pain medication and pain relief techniques, (2) identify sociocultural variables that may influence pain behaviors and expression, (3) obtain a health history that can identify accompanying chronic conditions that could contribute to the anticipated pain experience, (4) investigate past methods of pain relief, (5) identify pain medications used effectively in the past and any medication allergies and intolerance, and (6) select an appropriate pain scale and measurement technique for later use (Ardery, Herr, Titler, et al., 2003; Titler & Mentes, 1999).

> **Practice Pearl** ▶▶▶ Pain intensity and relief must be assessed and reassessed at regular intervals.

The Art and Science of Pain Relief

The goal of ideal pain management is to relieve both acute and persistent pain with appropriate pharmacological and nonpharmacological techniques while minimizing side effects. Nurses often assume responsibility for the assessment of pain, administration of medications, and assessment of the effectiveness of the pain management plan. Each older patient is a unique individual and will respond differently to analgesic medications and other pain control techniques. Therefore, individually tailored pain management plans are necessary for each patient. This requires careful titration of analgesic drugs and consistent monitoring of therapeutic and adverse effects by the nurse and other members of the healthcare team. Patients with severe pain require more rapid titration to get symptoms under control. This is often better accomplished in the acute care setting where nurses can carefully monitor function, vital signs, and renal and hepatic function (AGS, 2002). Generally, older patients are more susceptible to adverse drug reactions, but analgesic drugs can be safely and effectively used with proper monitoring. Older patients usually have more sensitivity to opioid analgesics, and most often these patients are started on smaller doses to avoid toxicity. The dose is then titrated upward until effective pain relief is achieved without adverse effects. The titration process may take several days or even longer, especially when drugs with longer half-lives are used.

According to the AGS Ethics Committee (2005), pain should be treated with a combination of pharmacological and nonpharmacological techniques. The nurse should assess the older patient's beliefs and willingness to use relaxation techniques, heating pads or cold compresses, biofeedback, music, therapeutic touch, or other methods to enhance or replace analgesic drugs. Additionally, the nurse should question the patient about use of over-the-counter (OTC) medications or herbal remedies that may interact with medications taken as part of the pain management plan. Ineffective drugs or drugs that cause troubling side effects should be tapered or discontinued because they do not contribute to a positive therapeutic outcome.

If the nurse first encounters the patient at a time when he or she is experiencing acute pain, such as in the emergency department after a trauma, the first priority after life-sustaining care is provided is to relieve pain through the administration of analgesics. The safe administration of analgesics in the older person is complicated by a number of factors, including potential drug interactions with underlying chronic disorders, potential drug–drug interactions, presence of underlying nutritional deficiencies, and altered pharmacokinetics. Therefore, dosing should be initiated at lower levels and titrated upward carefully. The oral route of administration should be considered first; however, emergency relief of pain may best be provided by administration of analgesics by the intravenous route (AGS, 2009). Slowed intramuscular absorption of analgesics in older patients may result in delayed or prolonged effect, altered analgesic serum levels, and potential toxicity with repeated injections.

Patient-controlled analgesia can be used in older adults and is especially effective following surgical procedures for acute pain management (Herr, Bjoro et al., 2006). However, cognitive and physical ability should be assessed prior to initiation of treatment. Also, the nurse must carefully monitor the patient during the immediate post-trauma or postoperative period. If acute confusion develops, it is important to assess for contributing factors—such as unrelieved pain—before discontinuing analgesic medication.

Dying patients have special pain and symptom control needs that mandate respectful and responsive care. Concern for the patient's comfort and dignity should guide all aspects of care during the final stages of life. Effective pain management is appropriate for all patients, not just the dying; however, preventing needless pain and suffering at the end of life is a key aspect of the nurse's role, no matter what the age of the patient. Given nursing's ongoing presence and care of the dying at the bedside, the nurse has the opportunity not only to assess and manage pain, but also to educate, support, serve as patient advocate regarding end-of-life preferences, and collaborate with others to develop systems-level policies and procedures related to implementation of advance directives. Management of pain in terminal conditions may call for higher doses of opioids; however, pain should be treated aggressively to maximize comfort, even if the unintended effect of treatment results in the hastening of death (AGS Ethics Committee, 2005). (See Chapter 11 for further discussion of death and dying.)

Pharmacological Management

Pain management in the older adult may be more difficult due to age-related changes such as declines in renal and hepatic function and changes in body fat and water distribution (Reisner, 2011). In most cases, it makes sense to progress from nonopioid analgesics such as acetaminophen to anti-inflammatory drugs, and opioids to balance the risk and benefits of treating more severe pain (AGS, 2002). The World Health Organization has developed a "Pain Relief Ladder" to aid in the administration of the appropriate pain management plan. Furthermore, more than one medication may be necessary to achieve pain control. The use of two or more drugs in combination with complementary therapies may result in improved pain control with decreased likelihood of adverse effects (AGS, 2009). This is known as *rational polypharmacy* (AGS, 2009).

Nonopioid Analgesics

Pain medications within this group include nonsteroidal anti-inflammatory drugs (NSAIDs), acetaminophen, and tramadol. These medications are typically used for mild to moderate nociceptive pain; NSAIDs also have anti-inflammatory properties. According to the AGS (2009), older adults often respond well to pain management with acetaminophen and its use is safe in older adults with normal kidney and liver function who have no history of alcohol abuse. It is not associated with significant gastrointestinal bleeding, adverse renal effects, or cardiovascular toxicity. Doses of acetaminophen should not exceed 3,000 mg per day from all sources. The NSAIDs (aspirin, ibuprofen) are more effective at treating chronic inflammatory pain though they have been shown to carry significant risk of gastrointestinal bleeding and impaired renal function in the frail older adult. They should be used with caution in this population (AGS, 2009).

A newer class of NSAIDs, the cyclooxygenase-2 (COX-2) inhibitors, were developed with the belief that the COX-2 selective drugs were safer than the nonselective NSAIDs; however, several studies since have shown that the COX-2 inhibitors are associated with increased risk of adverse cardiovascular events (Bishop & Morrison, 2007). Topical NSAIDs, such as diclofenac or salicylate derivative, have been used in the hopes of providing effective pain relief without the risks of systemic NSAIDs. Some short-term studies have shown safe, positive effects, however, long-term studies are needed (AGS, 2009).

Tramadol is indicated for moderate to severe pain and has been shown to be effective in relieving pain in older adults. Tramadol may be used when nonopioids like acetaminophen and ibuprofen do not control pain, but the patient wishes to avoid an opioid (McPherson & Uritsky, 2011). Because Tramadol is centrally acting, it carries some properties of opioid analgesics, and may cause drowsiness, constipation, and nausea (AGS, 2009). It is not, however, a controlled substance.

Opioid Analgesics

Opioids have become a mainstay for moderate to severe pain management in the older adult population (McPherson & Uritsky, 2011). Both the AGS and an expert panel assembled by the American Pain Society and the American Academy of Pain Medicine recommend the use of opioids for management of moderate to severe pain in carefully monitored patients (AGS, 2009; Chou et al., 2009). The guidelines also recommend consideration of opioid therapy in patients with functional impairments or reduced quality of life related to pain.

The AGS guidelines do not specifically recommend which opioid should be used; rather, the prescribing clinician should select an opioid based on the clinical picture and needs of the patient (Gloth, 2011). Morphine is a commonly used and versatile opioid for the treatment of moderate to severe pain. Short- and long-acting formulations exist, and the drug can be delivered via many routes including oral (tablet or liquid), rectal, or parenteral (intramuscular, intravenous, subcutaneous, epidural, and intrathecal). Morphine is metabolized by the liver, and the primary metabolite may accumulate in patients with reduced renal function, causing central nervous system excitation and myoclonus, nausea, and sedation.

Fentanyl is another commonly used opioid. The transdermal formulation has become more widely used for the management of persistent pain in older adults; it is not indicated for acute pain. The patch is applied to the skin surface and changed every 3 days. Fentanyl should never be used in people who are opioid-naïve and caution should be used with those who have low fat stores (McPherson & Uritsky, 2011). Fentanyl is also available in three short-acting, transmucosal formulations.

Certain opioids should be avoided in older adults including meperidine and propoxyphene (Reisner, 2011). Meperidine has the potential to cause confusion or seizures due to buildup of a toxic metabolite. Propoxyphene, a drug with efficacy similar to aspirin or acetaminophen, also carries the risk for potentially serious or even fatal heart arrhythmias. Additionally, there is the burden of serious side effects (delirium, ataxia, and dizziness) caused by the accumulation of toxic metabolites. Following a request from the U.S. Food and Drug Administration (2010), the manufacturers of the propoxyphene brand drugs voluntarily withdrew them from the U.S. market in 2010; manufacturers of generic propoxyphene-containing products have been asked to remove their products as well. Other drugs are suggested for the treatment of persistent pain in the older person.

Another drug that has received a resurgence of attention in recent years is methadone. Methadone has a long half-life, which may result in toxic accumulation of drug in the person with hepatic or renal impairment. Methadone should be initiated and titrated cautiously, and only prescribed by clinicians experienced in its use (Gloth, 2011). Therefore, caution is warranted when using methadone to manage persistent pain in the older adult. Table 9-1 provides information on pharmacotherapeutic agents that may be used to treat persistent pain in older adult patients.

> **Drug Alert** ▶▶▶ Opioid analgesics should be titrated slowly. Common adverse effects such as constipation, sedation, and nausea should be anticipated until tolerance develops (McPherson & Uritsky, 2011).

Preventing and Managing Adverse Effects

Constipation

Most opioid analgesics will slow the intestinal tract and result in poor bowel elimination. Constipation may contribute to increased pain in older patients, and it is extremely important for the nurse to monitor the bowels carefully. A prophylactic bowel regimen must be initiated when opioid analgesics are utilized. This includes the use of stool softeners (e.g., docusate sodium) and bowel stimulants (e.g., senna). Senna tea and fruits may also be helpful and patients should be encouraged to increase their fluid intake if possible. Bulking agents (e.g., psyllium) should be avoided to prevent fecal impaction.

Sedation

Many older adults will experience sedation when opioid analgesics are initiated or increased; however, this effect

TABLE 9-1	Pharmacotherapeutic Agents and Dosing Suggestions for Management of Persistent Pain in the Older Person			
Drug	**Starting Dose**	**Titration**	**Comments**	
Nonopioids				
Acetaminophen	325 mg q4h	After 4–6 doses	Maximum dose 3 g/24 hr. Reduce dose with hepatic disease or history of alcohol abuse.	
Ibuprofen	400–600 mg q6h	After 2–3 days	Take with food to reduce risk of GI distress.	
Corticosteroids	5 mg daily	After 2–3 doses	Use lowest possible dose to avoid chronic steroid side effects.	
Tricyclic antidepressants	10 mg at bedtime	After 3–5 days	Significant risk of anticholinergic side effects.	
Anticonvulsants				
Carbamazepine	100 mg daily	After 3–5 days	Monitor Liver Function Tests, CBC, BUN/creatinine, electrolytes.	
Gabapentin	100 mg bedtime	After 1–2 days	Monitor sedation, ataxia, edema.	
Opioids				
Morphine sulfate	5–10 mg q4h	After 1 day	Start low and titrate to comfort. Anticipate and treat side effects.	
Oxycodone hydrocodone	5–10 mg q4h	After 1–2 days	Start low and titrate to comfort. Anticipate and treat side effects.	
Hydromorphone	0.5–1 mg q4h	After 1–2 days	Start low and titrate to comfort. Anticipate and treat side effects.	
Transdermal fentanyl	12.5 µg/hr q72h	After 3 days	Apply to clean, dry, hairless skin. Peak effects of first dose take 24 hr, so cover with oral meds the first day of application.	

should subside within 24 to 48 hours. If the patient remains sedated after 24 to 48 hours, and other correctable causes have been accounted for and managed, the patient may require a dose reduction, opioid rotation, or a psychostimulant (McPherson & Uritsky, 2011; Paice, 2010). Although sedation is commonly cited as a reason for avoiding opioids in older adults, evidence is lacking to support this claim (Bishop & Morrison, 2007).

Respiratory Depression

Respiratory depression is often a concern for healthcare providers when using opioids for pain management; however, it is rarely a clinically significant problem for opioid-tolerant patients (McPherson & Uritsky, 2011). If respiratory depression (respiratory rate < 8 breaths/minute or O_2 saturation $< 90\%$) occurs, it usually has a multifactorial etiology. Most patients will develop a tolerance to respiratory depression within 5 to 7 days.

Nausea and Vomiting

Nausea and vomiting are common with the use of opioids in opioid-naïve patients due to the activation of the chemoreceptor trigger zone in the medulla, vestibular sensitivity, and delayed gastric emptying (McPherson & Uritsky, 2011; Paice, 2010). Antiemetics that the patient has used successfully in the past may be scheduled for the first 2–3 days of opioid treatment with a gradual tapering of the dose. Symptoms should subside within a few days if the underlying cause is the opioid analgesic; however, if symptoms do not resolve, the patient may need rotation to a different opioid (McPherson & Uritsky, 2011).

Myoclonus

Myoclonic jerking movements may be associated with high-dose opioid therapy (especially morphine). An alternate opioid should be used if this occurs.

Pruritis

Pruritis is most commonly associated with the use of morphine and is related in part to a release of histamine caused by the drug. Treatment with antihistamines (e.g., diphenhydramine) is effective, but is very likely to cause sedation in the older adult.

Adjuvant Drugs for Older Patients With Pain

Adjuvant drugs are not typically considered pain medicines, but they may relieve discomfort, potentiate the effect of pain medications, and reduce the side effect burden.

Examples of adjuvant drugs that nurses may see used in the clinical setting include the following:

1. **Tricyclic antidepressants (amitriptyline, desipramine, and nortriptyline):** helpful for diabetic neuropathy, trigeminal neuralgia, and post-herpetic neuralgia; significant risk for adverse effects in older adults

2. **Mixed serotonin- and norepinephrine-uptake inhibitors (SNRIs—duloxetine, venlafaxine):** helpful for various neuropathic pain conditions and fibromyalgia; fewer side effects than tricyclic antidepressants

3. **Anticonvulsants (gabapentin, pregabalin):** helpful for various neuropathic pain conditions; fewer side effects than older anticonvulsants and tricyclic antidepressants

4. **Corticosteroids:** may be helpful for a variety of conditions including rheumatoid arthritis, polymyalgia rheumatica, giant cell arteritis, and other autoimmune disorders; may also be helpful in some neuropathic pain syndromes and cancer pain; significant risk for adverse effects and toxicity in short- and long-term use

5. **Topical analgesics (capsaicin, menthol methylsalicylate, EMLA cream, lidocaine patch/gel):** helpful for persistent arthritis pain, herpes zoster, and diabetic neuropathy; may be used in anticipation of painful procedures such as venipuncture for blood draws and IV insertion

6. **Muscle relaxants (baclofen):** helpful when there is a significant muscle spasm component to pain; to be used in addition to, not in place of, analgesic medications.

7. **Antianxiety medications (diazepam, doxepin, oxazepam):** helpful when patient is anxious or agitated or for relief of muscle spasm; however, there is no direct analgesic effect and antianxiety medications present a high-risk profile in older adults

8. **Calcitonin and bisphosphonates:** helpful in various cases of bone pain related to vertebral compression fractures and cancer with bone metastases as well as for some neuropathies (AGS, 2009; McPherson & Uritsky, 2011; Reisner, 2011)

Special Pharmacological Issues

It is becoming more acceptable for clinicians to manage acute and persistent pain with the use of opioid analgesics (Chou et al., 2009). With the increased use of opioids in pain management, there is increased concern among clinicians, families, and patients that older adults will become addicted to these drugs. *Addiction* is defined as a disease with "genetic, psychosocial, and environmental factors influencing its development and manifestations. It is characterized by behaviors that include one or more of the following: impaired control over drug use, compulsive use, continued use despite harm, and craving" (American Academy of Pain Medicine [AAPM], American Pain Society [APS], & American Society of Addiction Medicine [ASAM], 2001, p. 2). Although true addiction to opioid medication in older adults is rare, physical dependency is an inevitable consequence over time, especially when patients experience relief from persistent, debilitating pain. **Physical dependence** is a state of adaptation that is manifested by withdrawal symptoms when the drug is abruptly stopped or decreased (AAPM et al., 2001). Studies indicate that **tolerance,** or the need for more drug to get the same therapeutic effect over time, is slow to develop in the face of stable disease (AGS, 2002). Nurses should urge patients to seek further diagnostic testing and evaluation of persistent illnesses when the need for opioid medication increases suddenly rather than assuming that tolerance to opioids is the underlying issue. Concerns over drug dependency and addiction do not justify the failure to relieve pain (McPherson & Uritsky, 2011).

When mixed drugs containing opioids and acetaminophen or aspirin are used to control pain (acetaminophen with codeine, oxycodone with aspirin, aspirin with codeine), the nurse should be aware that doses are limited by the toxic effect that can occur as a result of high salicylate or acetaminophen levels. Acetaminophen is hepatotoxic above 4 g/day, and aspirin can cause gastric bleeding and abnormal platelet function at doses above 4 g/day. Special caution is advised in older patients with decreased renal and hepatic function and those currently using alcohol or possessing a history of alcohol abuse.

Polypharmacy

Polypharmacy (further discussed in Chapter 6 ⬡) is the excessive or unnecessary use of medications, both prescription and nonprescription. Polypharmacy occurs when multiple medications are used to treat the same disease or condition, medications interact, inappropriate dosages are supplied, and medications are prescribed to treat adverse drug effects. The pain management plan may require the use of more than one pain medication as well as the use of adjuvant drugs to adequately control pain in the older adult. By combining medications that have different mechanisms of action and utilizing adjuvant drugs, the patient may experience less pain while requiring lower doses of pain medication; however, it is important for the nurse to monitor closely for drug–drug interactions. This is especially true for the older adult with multiple comorbidities who is taking several other medications. Furthermore, the expected adverse effects of pain medications (such as constipation, sedation, and nausea) may be exacerbated in the

older adult because of hepatic impairment or age-related declines in renal function, requiring the addition of medication for treatment of these adverse effects.

Pharmacological Principles for Successful Pain Management

The least invasive method of drug delivery should be used, and the oral administration of pain medications is the preferred means of controlling pain in the older adult (AGS, 2009). Even patients who cannot swallow can be given concentrated liquid morphine drops by the sublingual or buccal route. It is the safest, least expensive, and easiest route of administration. When pain medication is given via the IV route, mobility is restricted due to the IV apparatus and needle placement in the arm. Additionally, should the needle be displaced and the solution infiltrate into the surrounding tissue, the IV must be discontinued and restarted, causing the patient to experience some period of time without medication. This may be insignificant in the acute care setting where many nurses are available to restart IVs, but delays may occur in the nursing home, community, and hospice settings if trained nurses are not immediately available.

Pain management is most effective when it is administered around the clock with the goal of preventing the occurrence of pain. The nurse's familiarity with the analgesic's duration of action and appropriate timing of administration contributes to the achievement of this goal. When scheduled and administered appropriately, patients avoid the needless suffering and mental anguish that can occur when medication is given on a PRN (as-needed) basis. Management of pain with PRN medications requires patients to wait until they experience pain, request pain medication, and then wait for the medication to relieve their pain. Older adults with persistent pain should be managed with scheduled long-acting oral medications (e.g., MS Contin) once or twice daily, with short-acting, immediate-release oral preparations (e.g., Roxanol) as needed for breakthrough pain or pain associated with activity or procedures (AGS, 2009).

> **Practice Pearl** ▶▶▶ Avoid the use of PRN medication for pain control, because the patient will learn to expect the return of pain, suffer psychologically and spiritually by dealing with recurrent pain, and need more medication to relieve the recurrent pain.

If the patient experiences breakthrough pain on a consistent basis, the nurse should notify the patient's provider so that the dose of the long-acting, sustained-release preparation can be increased to more effectively control the pain. If the nurse notes that pain is effectively relieved for a period of time but recurs at the end of the dosing interval, end-of-dose failure should be suspected. In this case, the analgesic medication should be dosed more frequently, if possible, depending on the product. For instance, a medication administered every 12 hours may be changed to every 8 hours to provide improved coverage. Breakthrough pain may also include incident pain, caused by activity, and spontaneous pain, common in neuropathic syndromes (AGS, 2009). The nurse should educate the patient and the family to monitor the pain sensation and intensity during the course of treatment to provide ongoing assessment of the success of the pain treatment plan.

> **Drug Alert ▶▶▶** Warn patients that crushing or chewing sustained-release preparations of analgesics destroys their controlled-release properties and causes rapid absorption of the entire dose, resulting in possible overdose (AGS, 2002).

The use of placebos, that is, inert medications, sham injections, and other pain control methods known to be ineffective, is considered to be unethical in clinical practice for management of acute or persistent pain (AGS, 2009). Placebos should be limited to research protocols where patients have given informed consent and are aware that they may receive an inert medication as part of the research protocol.

Patients who experience a poor response to a well-developed pain management plan should be encouraged to speak with their healthcare provider regarding referral to a pain management clinic. These specialty clinics may be housed in larger teaching hospitals and usually utilize the services of pain specialists and a well-trained multidisciplinary team.

COMPLEMENTARY AND ALTERNATIVE THERAPIES

Pain is among the most common reasons that adults use complementary and alternative therapies (National Center for Complementary and Alternative Medicine [NCCAM], 2011). Nontraditional methods to control pain can be effective as stand-alone treatments and adjuncts to traditional pharmacological interventions with the potential to reduce dosages of medications and thus reduce the risk of adverse drug reactions. Nurses can assess older patients' preferences and attitudes toward nontraditional methods of relieving pain and encourage them to use methods appropriate for their needs. Older adults are increasingly using complementary and alternative medicine therapies to manage painful conditions, most commonly back pain, arthritis, and headaches (NCCAM, 2011). These therapies include dietary supplements such as glucosamine, chondroitin, and herbals, acupuncture, guided imagery, hypnotherapy, massage, meditation, relaxation

therapy, chiropractic services, tai chi, and yoga (NCCAM, 2011). Table 9-2 describes several different types of CAM therapies as well as possible adverse effects.

Other types of nonpharmacological methods of pain control include pain education programs; spiritual intervention; socialization or recreation programs (movies, therapeutic use of art and music); psychological approaches (counseling, biofeedback, imagery, hypnosis, relaxation); physical therapy (ultrasound, exercise, hot and cold packs); and neurostimulation (transcutaneous nerve stimulation [TENS]). Patient education programs have been shown to improve pain management significantly (AGS, 2002).

HEALTHY AGING TIPS TO REDUCE ARTHRITIS PAIN

Engage in gentle, regular exercise such as 20 minutes of walking, bicycling, and swimming every day.	Regular exercise strengthens muscles that support painful joints and may help speed recovery, prevent further injury, and reduce disability.
Maintain a healthy weight.	Weight control reduces pain, especially in older adults with knee osteoarthritis.
Avoid positions and activities that may increase or cause pain.	Recognizing avoidable injurious events helps prevent worsening pain symptoms.

Consequences of Unrelieved Pain

Unfortunately, persistent pain has become a label associated with negative images and stereotypes of long-standing psychiatric problems, futility in treatment, malingering, or drug-seeking behavior (AGS, 2002). Depression, anxiety, decreased socialization, sleep disturbance, impaired ambulation, and increased healthcare costs have all been found to be associated with the presence of pain in older people (Herr, 2011). Older patients suffering the psychological burden of pain are less likely to participate in rehabilitation and self-care activities, potentially slowing recovery from illness and decreasing their quality of life.

> **Practice Pearl ▶▶▶** Be alert for patients who report that their pain level is tolerable and that it only hurts when they move. These patients are likely to suffer the negative effects of long-term immobility such as decubitus ulcers, aspiration pneumonia, deep vein thrombosis, dehydration, and constipation. Effective pain relief should be provided to encourage movement and participation in rehabilitation activities.

TABLE 9-2	Complementary and Alternative Therapies for Pain Management in the Older Adult
Therapy	Comments
Acupuncture	Among the oldest forms of CAM in the world and a key component of traditional Chinese medicine. Commonly used to treat back, joint, and neck pain as well as headaches. Pain is treated by inserting thin needles through the skin at specific points. Generally considered safe when performed by skilled practitioners using sterile needles. Rare complications include infection and punctured organs.
Dietary Supplements	Risk for potential interaction with other medications.
Glucosamine/Chondroitin	Natural substances found in and around cartilage cells. Used in patients with osteoarthritis and may provide pain relief to those with moderate to severe pain. Risk for mild GI side effects including epigastric discomfort, heartburn, diarrhea or constipation, and nausea/vomiting.
Topical Capsaicin	A chemical compound derived from cayenne pepper. Effective in the treatment of osteoarthritis. Will cause a burning sensation when first applied, though this subsides when applied frequently. Avoid getting capsaicin in eyes or on open wounds as this will cause burning.
Massage Therapy	Commonly used in older adults for a variety of health-related purposes, including to rehabilitate injuries, reduce stress, increase relaxation, address anxiety and depression, aid general well-being, and relieve pain. May offer pain relief through physical and mental relaxation, blockage of pain signals to the brain, and release of chemicals in the body, such as serotonin or endorphins. Risks are few if performed by a trained massage therapist but may include temporary pain or discomfort, bruising, or swelling. Massage is contraindicated in patients with bleeding disorders or low platelet counts (people taking anticoagulants should avoid vigorous massage), blood clots (DVT), acute inflammation, open wounds, skin infection, fractures, burn areas. Massage is generally safe in people with cancer, but the oncologist should be consulted; direct pressure over the tumor is discouraged.
Relaxation Techniques	Mind–body practices including progressive relaxation, guided imagery, biofeedback, self-hypnosis, and deep-breathing exercises. The goal of relaxation techniques is to induce a "relaxation response" with increased well-being as well as body relaxation, resulting in slowed breathing and lower blood pressure. Generally considered safe for healthy people; people with heart disease should talk with their healthcare provider before doing progressive muscle relaxation.
Spinal Manipulation	Performed by practitioners using their hands or a device to move a joint of the spine beyond its passive range of motion with the goal of relieving pain and improving physical functioning. Practiced by chiropractors, physical therapists, and osteopathic physicians. Commonly used in older adults to treat low back pain. Relatively safe when performed by a trained practitioner. Most common adverse event is short-term discomfort, headache, or tiredness; caution is advised for frail patients.
Tai Chi	Mind–body practice sometimes referred to as "moving meditation" because patients move their bodies slowly in rhythm with deep breathing. Used for its low-aerobic benefits, to improve physical condition, strength, coordination, flexibility, and balance and to improve sleep and overall well-being. Improves musculoskeletal pain, depression, and quality of life and is promising for the treatment of osteoarthritis. Risks include soreness; modifications might be suggested if the patient has a hernia, joint problems, back pain, fractures, or severe osteoporosis.
Yoga	Mind–body practice with origins in ancient Indian philosophy that combines physical postures, breathing techniques, and meditation. Hatha yoga is most commonly used in the United States. Can reduce functional disability, pain, and depression in people with low back pain. Yoga may also improve sense of well-being, reduce stress, improve muscle relaxation, and improve overall fitness. Considered safe when practiced appropriately. Inverted poses should be avoided in some patients including those with extremely high or low blood pressure, retinal detachment, and severe osteoporosis.

Source: Adapted from APF, 2011; Berenson, 2006; Berman, Langevin, Witt, et al., 2010; NCCAM, 2011.

BOX 9-4 Your Rights as a Patient with Pain

As a person with pain, you have a right to:

- Receive a complete assessment of your pain and an opportunity to meet with physicians, nurses, physical therapists, clinical pharmacists and other healthcare professionals.
- Be informed of the opinions of the pain treatment professionals regarding the origin of your pain, and have the opportunity to give input into the treatment plan.
- Be informed of the risks, benefits, treatment options, and cost of treatment for your pain including co-payments and out of pocket expenses.
- Receive timely and effective treatment for your pain.
- Receive ongoing pain assessment with modification of the treatment plan as needed.
- Be referred to a pain specialist if your pain cannot be relieved to your satisfaction.

Although not required by law, these are the rights you should expect for your pain care.

Source: Adapted from American Pain Foundation (2012). *Pain care bill of rights.*

When older people are actively involved in the assessment and management of their pain, the nurse has a better chance of implementing an effective plan for pain relief. Patients have the right to expect humane and expert assessment and treatment of their pain in order to achieve optimum levels of pain relief (Box 9-4).

> *Practice Pearl* ▶▶▶ Many older adults and some healthcare providers believe pain is a normal part of aging. When caring for an older person with unrelieved pain, the nurse should be persistent in assessing and establishing a pain management plan. Effective pain management will allow the patient to maintain dignity, functional capacity, and quality of life (AGS, 2009).

To change the mind-set and culture regarding pain control that exists in some healthcare facilities, the Joint Commission developed new standards for institutional pain assessment that went into effect on January 1, 2001. The pain management standards address the assessment and management of pain. The standards require accredited organizations to:

- Recognize the right of patients to appropriate assessment and management of pain.
- Screen patients for pain during their initial assessment and, when clinically required, during ongoing, periodic reassessments.
- Educate patients suffering from pain and their families about pain management (Joint Commission, 2011).

Analysis of the Pain Management Plan

When pain persists despite the administration of analgesics, the pain treatment plan can be analyzed to refine the treatment and successfully manage the pain for most individuals. The nurse may follow these steps:

1. Review the initial pain assessment. Was anything missed? Was any area incomplete? Where is further information needed?
2. Analyze the alignment of the intensity of pain with the analgesia provided. Are mild analgesics being prescribed for severe pain? Is the patient taking the medication properly? If PRN medications are available, have they been appropriately administered?
3. Determine the patient's medication requirement. Has partial response been achieved at a certain dose? Have side effects occurred?
4. Provide feedback and documentation as needed to refine the plan. Are there indications that stronger medications are needed? Are dosing changes indicated? Should more effective relief of breakthrough pain be available? Are there indications that dosing intervals should be shortened?
5. Use nondrug techniques to complement the analgesic regimen. Have heat and cold packs been tried? Have patients had access to social or recreational activities?
6. Use all available resources in the clinical setting. Have pain experts, if available, been consulted? Can any other members of the interdisciplinary team offer insight? Are there unaddressed spiritual or religious issues?

Adapted from AGS, 2009; Chou et al., 2009; Herr, 2011; Reisner, 2011.

QSEN Recommendations Related to Pain Management

The Quality and Safety Education for Nurses (QSEN) project addresses the challenge of preparing future nurses with the knowledge, skills, and attitudes (KSAs) to continuously improve the quality and safety of the healthcare systems in which they work (Cronenwett et al., 2007). See the QSEN table for tips on meeting QSEN standards.

Patient and Family Teaching

Gerontological nurses require skills and knowledge related to teaching patients and families about the key concepts of gerontology and gerontological nursing. The guidelines in the following feature will assist the nurse to assume the role of teacher and coach.

Meeting QSEN Standards: Pain

	KNOWLEDGE	SKILLS	ATTITUDES
Patient-Centered Care	Involvement of patient and family in plan of care is crucial.	Provide patient-centered care with sensitivity and respect.	Respect patient values, preferences, and expressed needs.
	Examine barriers that may keep patients from being active in formulating their plan of care.	Assess presence and levels of pain, depression, and cognitive impairment.	Provide patient-centered care to improve successful nursing outcomes.
Teamwork and Collaboration	Recognize contributions of interdisciplinary team members.	Integrate contributions of interdisciplinary team as a means of helping the patient/family achieve goals.	Value teamwork and the importance of professional collaboration.
	Identify barriers that can inhibit effective team function.	Follow communication practices to minimize risks associated with handoffs.	Be open to different communication styles of each member of the team.
Evidence-Based Practice	Describe effective assessment techniques and interventions to reduce pain and improve function.	Access current evidence-based protocols to guide care plan development.	Value the need for continuous improvement in the clinical practice of pain assessment and management based on new knowledge.
Quality Improvement	Explain the importance of measuring patient outcomes to improve pain assessment and management.	Use quality measures to understand performance and evaluate the results of improved pain assessment and management.	Appreciate that continuous quality improvement is a key component of good patient care.
Safety	Describe common adverse effects associated with pain treatment plans.	Communicate observations related to adverse effects or errors to patients, families, and the interdisciplinary team.	Value own role in preventing or minimizing risk for adverse effects.
Informatics	Explain why information and technology are essential for safe patient care.	Utilize the electronic health record to support safe processes of care.	Value technologies that support clinical decision making, error prevention, and care coordination.

Patient–Family Teaching Guidelines

The following are guidelines that the nurse may find useful when instructing older adults and their families about persistent pain.

DEALING WITH CHRONIC PERSISTENT PAIN

1 What is chronic persistent pain?

Chronic or persistent pain is discomfort that continues for an extended time. Some conditions that cause pain can come and go over a period of years. In addition to pain, you can also suffer from depression, insomnia, problems walking, and difficulty healing from disease. There are treatments for pain that can make you feel better.

RATIONALE:

Many older people do not report their symptoms of pain because they are afraid to be labeled as complainers. By validating their situation and pain, the nurse gives the older person permission to discuss the pain and the implications it has on health and well-being.

2 How can I tell my doctor and nurse about my pain?

Chronic persistent pain can be reported to your healthcare providers. Be as specific as you can to accurately convey your situation. Keep a diary or pain log for a few days before your visit. Here are things to jot down:

- Where it hurts
- How often it hurts
- What the pain feels like (burning, stabbing, shooting, dull ache, etc.)
- What makes it worse
- What makes it better
- What medications you have tried and which work and which don't
- How the pain affects your life

RATIONALE:

Helping the older patient organize his or her thoughts about pain will help the healthcare provider appreciate the patient's unique situation. A pain diary is a good place to start.

3 Will over-the-counter remedies help?

Acetaminophen (Tylenol) is a good choice for mild to moderate pain caused by osteoarthritis. Check with your healthcare provider about the dose if you take it for more than a few days. Nonsteroidal anti-inflammatory drugs (NSAIDs) such as aspirin and ibuprofen work well also, but are associated with the risk of side effects like stomach upset and ulcer formation. Take NSAIDs with food for a short period of time. If you have or have had ulcers, avoid NSAIDs altogether.

RATIONALE:

Older patients should be carefully and completely informed about the nature of the medications they are taking for chronic persistent pain because in all probability they will be taking them for years. Careful monitoring and support is needed to prevent adverse drug reactions.

4 Will I get addicted to my pain medicine?

Most older people take painkillers, even opioids, safely without becoming addicted. It is important not to drive or engage in tasks requiring your full attention (such as babysitting) when you start a new pain medication.

RATIONALE:

Many older people are fearful they will turn into "drug addicts" and therefore do not take prescribed pain medications. Reassurance is required.

5 Once my pain is treated, will I be back to my old self again?

In addition to treating your pain, you may also need treatment for accompanying conditions such as depression. People with persistent pain often complain of feeling blue, and these feelings sometimes hang on even when the pain is gone. Antidepressants can help older people to deal with certain kinds of pain (from nerve diseases or nerve injury) and treat the depression that can result from living with pain. Using a second medication may allow your healthcare provider to prescribe a lower dose of pain medication, thus lessening the risk of side effects.

RATIONALE:

The older patient should be prepared to think beyond the immediate pain and issues of pain relief. Even though the pain is treated, the underlying chronic illness remains and that may be a cause of concern for the patient. Patients with complicated pain or severe depression should seek a referral to a geropsychiatrist or pain clinic for specialized care.

CARE PLAN A Patient With Chronic Persistent Pain

Case Study

Mr. Adams is a 79-year-old man who suffers from persistent pain in his knees. The physician has diagnosed Mr. Adams with osteoarthritis of both knees and has advised him to take acetaminophen (Tylenol) for the pain. He reports he has been taking it "on and off" with some relief.

Mr. Adams lives by himself in senior citizen housing and has an apartment on the second floor. Recently, he has been unable to walk up the stairs without experiencing severe pain. The building does not have an elevator.

He reports that after walking and stair climbing, the pain is an 8 on a 10-point scale. He usually shops for groceries every other day, but now in order to avoid the stairs, he has been shopping once a week. Additionally, Mr. Adams used to play bridge once or twice a week with friends, but he has stopped that to "conserve energy." He has a daughter to help him out, but she works full-time and has three young children.

Applying the Nursing Process

Assessment

Mr. Adams recently had a complete physical examination and health history and was found to have a chronic degenerative process causing pain in both of his knees. He is at risk for malnutrition and depression because of his inability to get up and down the stairs without experiencing severe pain. It is unlikely that he would be able to shop efficiently and carry the needed groceries up the stairs to his apartment.

It appears that the patient's attempts to manage his pain are ineffective. He reports that after walking and climbing stairs, his level of pain increases. This is unfortunately a common occurrence with many older people, and the natural response is to limit movement. The nurse needs more information about his baseline level of pain, level of pain with other activities, ability to care for himself, and perception of his situation. By limiting his socialization and bridge playing with his friends, he is at risk for social isolation and depression. The nurse should conduct a complete functional health pattern assessment.

Diagnosis

The current nursing diagnoses for Mr. Adams include the following:

- *Loneliness, Risk for*
- *Physical Mobility, Impaired*

- *Activity Intolerance*
- *Pain, Chronic*
- *Nutrition Imbalanced: Less Than Body Requirements*

NANDA-I © 2012.

Expected Outcomes

Expected outcomes for the plan of care specify that Mr. Adams will:

- Keep a pain diary and record pain levels several times a day, systematically noting the effectiveness of acetaminophen on his pain and identifying any nonpharmacological ways to treat his pain that might be appropriate for him.

- Request help from family and friends to assist in obtaining groceries and needed supplies.
- Agree to a physical therapy consultation for strengthening exercises and assistive aids to decrease pain.
- Agree to establish a therapeutic relationship with the nurse and develop a mutually acceptable plan to work toward these outcomes.

CARE PLAN

A Patient With Chronic Persistent Pain *(continued)*

Planning and Implementation

The following nursing interventions may be appropriate for Mr. Adams:

- Establish a therapeutic relationship.
- Explore alternative living situations or other supports.
- Encourage a family meeting to talk about health issues in general with Mr. Adams's permission.
- Begin an in-depth pain assessment of the effectiveness of pharmacological and nonpharmacological techniques to treat pain.
- Begin a values clarification to establish long-term goals and facilitate end-of-life planning.

Generally, osteoarthritis pain responds well to heating pads, OTC topical creams, and mild exercise and physical

therapy. Mr. Adams should be educated about the issues involved with treating persistent pain and the need to take medication on a regular basis. Mr. Adams should be informed that acetaminophen is not habit forming and can be very effective in controlling the pain of osteoarthritis. He should be informed about side effects and dosing recommendations to avoid medication-related problems. If a trial of acetaminophen twice or three times a day for several days does not help to control his pain, he should return to the physician for further advice and evaluation of his osteoarthritis.

Evaluation

The nurse hopes to work with Mr. Adams over time and realizes the persistent nature of pain in older people. The nurse will consider the plan a success based on the following criteria:

- Mr. Adams will report improved function and social skills.
- A family meeting will be held to discuss his overall health.

- Mr. Adams will report decreased levels of pain as a result of pain management techniques.
- He will continue to be well nourished and hydrated by obtaining groceries through the help of family and friends.

Ethical Dilemma

As the nurse gets to know Mr. Adams better, he reports in confidence that his friend has told him the best way to make his knees feel better is to drink a glass of wine with his acetaminophen. He asks the nurse not to tell his daughter about this habit. How should the nurse respond?

Taking acetaminophen with alcohol is a very risky behavior and can cause liver damage. Mr. Adams should be informed that if this practice continues, he is placing

himself at risk for premature institutionalization or injury from falls. Once he is informed of the risk and develops a trusting relationship with the nurse, he may stop taking alcohol with his medication. If he does not, the nurse should recommend that he speak with his physician regarding this practice. Perhaps the physician can prescribe a more effective medication that does not need wine to boost its analgesic effects.

Critical Thinking and the Nursing Process

1. What is the physiological basis for Mr. Adams's pain?
2. Explain possible reasons for this patient's pain in addition to degenerative joint disease.
3. Outline a teaching plan with behavioral interventions designed to improve Mr. Adams's level of pain.

4. Suggest a nursing action if Mr. Adams continues to consume alcohol while taking acetaminophen.

- Evaluate your responses in Appendix B.

Chapter Highlights

- With aging, the probability that the patient will develop a condition that can cause pain increases.

- Many healthcare professionals who care for older patients have not had sufficient education regarding pain control in older adults. Common errors or omissions include inadequate pain assessment and reluctance by clinicians to use appropriate pain medications, including opioids, with older adult patients.

- Older people will often not report pain because they fear hospitalization, worsening of their disease, or being labeled a chronic complainer.

- When a patient has unrelieved pain, many negative effects occur such as depression, anxiety, insomnia, problems of immobility, and nutritional problems. All of these conditions can slow healing and rehabilitation, placing the older person at risk for complications and premature institutionalization.

- In addition to the traditional pain assessment methods, when the patient is nonverbal or suffers from severe dementia, the nurse should gather information from caregivers and behavioral observations.

- The general rule for analgesic medications is to start low and go slow. When analgesic medications are started, the nurse should carefully monitor the patient for adverse events, educate the patient regarding the pain management plan, implement nonpharmacological methods as appropriate to the patient, and keep the lines of communication open through periodic and regular reassessment of the patient's pain.

Pearson Nursing Student Resources
Find additional review materials at
nursing.pearsonhighered.com

Prepare for success with additional NCLEX®-style practice questions, interactive assignments and activities, web links, animations and videos, and more!

References

American Academy of Pain Medicine (AAPM), American Pain Society (APS), & American Society of Addiction Medicine (ASAM). (2001). Definitions *related to the use of opioids for the treatment of pain.* Retrieved from http://www.erowid.org/psychoactives/addiction/addiction_definitions1.pdf

American Geriatrics Society (AGS) Ethics Committee. (2005). The care of dying patients. *Annals of Long-Term Care, 13*(3), 23–25.

American Geriatrics Society (AGS) Panel on Chronic Pain in Older Persons. (2002). The management of persistent pain in older persons. *Journal of the American Geriatrics Society, 50,* S205–S224.

American Geriatrics Society (AGS) Panel on the Pharmacological Management of Persistent Pain in Older Persons. (2009). Pharmacological management of persistent pain in older persons. *Journal of the American Geriatrics Society, 57,* 1331–1346.

American Pain Foundation (APF). (2008). Overview of American pain surveys: 2005–2006. *Journal of Pain and Palliative Care Pharmacotherapy, 22,* 33–38.

American Pain Foundation (APF). (2011). *Complementary and alternative medicine.* Retrieved from http://www.painfoundation.org/painsafe/healthcare-professionals/cam

American Pain Foundation (APF). (2012). *Pain care bill of rights.* Retrieved from http://www.painfoundation.org/learn/publications/pain-care-bill-of-rights.html

Ardery, G., Herr, K., Titler, M., Sorofman, B., & Schmitt, M. (2003). Assessing and managing acute pain in older adults: A research base to guide practice. *Medical-Surgical Nursing, 12*(1), 7–18.

Berenson, S. (2006). Complementary and alternative therapies in palliative care. In F. Ferrell and N. Coyle (Eds.), *Textbook of palliative nursing* (pp. 491–509). Oxford, UK: Oxford University Press.

Berman, B. M., Langevin, H. M., Witt, C. M., & Dubner, R. (2010). Acupuncture for chronic low back pain. *New England Journal of Medicine, 363,* 454–461.

Bishop, T. F., & Morrison, S. (2007). Geriatric palliative care—part I: Pain and symptom management. *Clinical Geriatrics, 15*(1), 25–32.

Chou, R., Fanciullo, G. J., Fine, P. G., Adler, J. A., Ballantyne, J. C., Davies, P., Donovan, M. I., Fishbain, D. A., Foley, K. M., Fudin, J., Gilson, A. M., Kelter, A., Mauskop, A., O'Connor, P. G, Passik, S. D., Pasternak, G. W., Portenoy, R. K., Rich, B. A., Roberts, R. G., Todd, K. H., & Miaskowski, C. (2009). American Pain Society–American Academy of Pain Medicine Opioids Guidelines Panel: Clinical guidelines for the use of chronic opioid therapy in chronic noncancer pain. *Journal of Pain, 10*(2), 113–130.

Cronenwett, L., Sherwood, G., Barnsteiner, J., Disch, J., Johnson, J., Mitchell, P., Sullivan, D.,

& Warren, J. (2007). Quality and safety education for nurses, *Nursing Outlook,* 55(3) 122-131.

Dartmouth-Hitchcock Medical Center. (n.d.). *Initial pain rating tool.* Retrieved from http://prc.coh.org/pdf/initial_pain_rating_dartmouth.pdf

Elliott, T. (2000). Principles of analgesic use for the treatment of acute pain and cancer pain. *Journal of Palliative Care Medicine, 3*(1), 98–99.

Gloth, F. M. (2011). Pharmacological management of persistent pain in older persons: Focus on opioids and nonopioids. *Journal of Pain, 12*(3), S14–S20.

Hadjistavropoulos, T., Herr, K., Turk, D. C., Fine, P. G., Dworkin, R. H., Helme, R., Jackson, K., Parmelee, P. A., Rudy, T. E., Lynn Beattie, B., Chibnall. J. T., Craig, K. D., Ferrell, B., Ferrell. B., Fillingim, R. B, Gagliese, L., Gallagher, R., Gibson, S. J., Harrison, E. L., Katz, B., Keefe, F. J., Lieber, S. J., Lussier, D., Schmader, K, E., Tait, R. C, Weiner, D. K., & Williams, J. (2007). An interdisciplinary expert consensus statement on assessment of pain in older persons. *Clinical Journal of Pain, 23,* S1–S43.

Hartford Institute for Geriatric Nursing. (2007). Pain assessment for older adults. *Try this: Best practices in nursing care to older adults.* Retrieved from http://www.hartfordign.org

Helms, J. E., & Barone, C. P. (2008). Physiology and treatment of pain. *Critical Care Nurse, 28*(6), 38–49.

Herr, K. (2011). Pain assessment strategies in older patients. *Journal of Pain, 12*(3), S3–S13.

Herr, K., Bjoro, K., Steffensmeier, J., & Rakel, B. (2006). *Acute pain management in older adults.* Iowa City, IA: University of Iowa Gerontological Nursing Interventions Research Center, Research Translation and Dissemination Core.

Herr, K., Coyne, P. J., Manworren, R., McCaffery, M., Merkel, S., Pelosi-Kelly, J., & Wild, L. (2006). Pain assessment in the nonverbal patient: Position statement with clinical practice recommendations. *Pain Management Nursing, 7*(2), 44–52.

Hicks, C., von Baeyer, C., Spafford, P, van Korlaar, I. & Goodenough, B. (2001). The Faces Pain Scale-Revised: Toward a common metric in pediatric pain measurement. *Pain, 93*(2), 173–183.

Institute of Medicine (IOM). (2011). *Report from the Committee on Advancing Pain Research, Care, and Education: Relieving pain in America, a blueprint for transforming prevention, care, education and research.* Washington, DC: National Academies Press.

International Association for the Study of Pain (IASP). (2011). *IASP taxonomy.* Retrieved from http://www.iasp-pain.org/Content/NavigationMenu/GeneralResourceLinks/PainDefinitions/default.htm

Joint Commission. (2011). *Facts about pain management.* Retrieved from http://www.jointcommission.org/assets/1/18/Pain_Management.pdf

Krueger, A. B., & Stone, A. A. (2008). Assessment of pain: A community-based diary survey in the USA. *Lancet, 371,* 1519–1525.

Maxwell, C. J., Dalby, D. M., Slater, M., Patten, S. B., Hogan, D. B., Eliasziw, M., & Hirdes, J. P. (2008). The prevalence and management of current daily pain among older home care clients. *Pain, 138,* 208–216.

McAuliffe, L., Nay, R., O'Donnell, M., & Fetherstonhaugh, D. (2009). Pain assessment in older people with dementia: Literature review. *Journal of Advanced Nursing, 65,* 2–10.

McPherson, M. L., & Uritsky, T. J. (2011). Pharmacotherapy of pain in older adults: Opioid and adjuvant. In F. M. Gloth, III (Ed.), *Handbook of pain relief in older adults: An evidence-based approach* (pp. 83–95). New York, NY: Springer.

Moore, A., & Clinch, D. (2004). Underlying mechanism of impaired visceral pain perception in older people. *Journal of the American Geriatrics Society, 52,* 132–136.

National Center for Complementary and Alternative Medicine (NCCAM). (2011). *Chronic pain and CAM: At a glance.* Retrieved from http://nccam.nih.gov/health/pain/D456.pdf

National Pain Foundation (NPF). (2011). *Pain causes among older adults.* Retrieved from http://www.nationalpainfoundation.org/articles/245/pain-causes-among-older-adults

Otis-Green, S. (n.d.). *Psychosocial pain assessment form.* Retrieved from http://prc.coh.org/pdf/PSPAF.pdf

Paice, J. A. (2010). Pain at the end of life. In B. R. Ferrell & N. Coyle (Eds.), *Textbook of palliative nursing* (pp. 161–185). Oxford, UK: Oxford University Press.

Reisner, L. (2011). Pharmacological management of persistent pain in older persons. *Journal of Pain, 12*(3), S21–S29.

Reynolds, K. S., Hanson, L. C., DeVellis, R. F., Henderson, M., & Steinhauser, K. E. (2008). Disparities in pain management between cognitively intact and cognitively impaired nursing home residents. *Journal of Pain and Symptom Management, 35,* 388–396.

Titler, M., & Mentes, J. (1999). Research utilization in gerontological nursing practice. *Journal of Gerontological Nursing, 25*(6), 6–9.

University of Wisconsin Hospital and Clinics Home Health Agency. (n.d.). *Pain management flow sheet.* Retrieved from http://prc.coh.org/pdf/HH-pain-mgmt.pdf

U.S. Food and Drug Administration. (2010). *Xanodyne agrees to withdraw propoxyphene from the U.S. market. FDA News Release.* Retrieved from http://www.fda.gov/NewsEvents/Newsroom/PressAnnouncements/ucm234350.htm

Wells-Federman, C. (1999). Care of the patient with chronic pain: Part I. *Clinical Excellence in Nursing Practice, 3*(4), 192–204.

Wittink, H., & Carr, D. (2008). *Pain management evidence, outcomes and quality of life.* New York, NY: Elsevier.

Violence and Elder Mistreatment

Terry Fulmer, PhD, RN, FAAN, and Patricia Cabrera, MD
BOUVÉ COLLEGE OF HEALTH SCIENCES, NORTHEASTERN UNIVERSITY

KEY TERMS

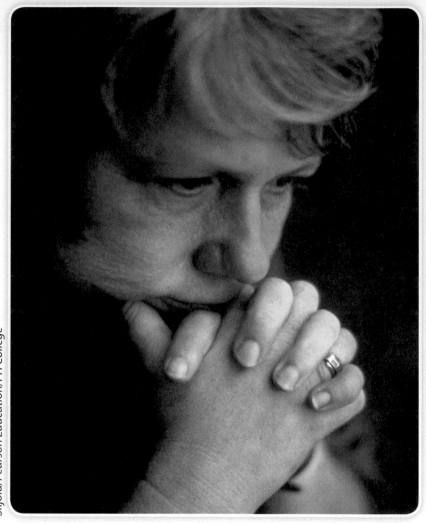

Skjold/Pearson Education/PH College

LEARNING OUTCOMES

On completion of this chapter, the reader will be able to:

1. Discuss current trends in elder mistreatment, including incidence and prevalence.
2. Review key reasons elder mistreatment occurs.
3. Conduct clinical assessment for screening and detection of elder mistreatment.
4. Create a nursing care plan for the ongoing well-being of older patients.
5. Summarize key resources for elder mistreatment information.

This chapter will explore the nursing role in identifying and managing the serious and potentially life-threatening syndrome of **elder mistreatment.** Elder mistreatment is a part of a larger societal problem, **domestic violence.** It has been defined as (a) intentional actions that cause harm or create serious risk or harm (whether or not harm is intended) to a vulnerable elder by a caregiver or other person who stands in a trust relationship to the elder or (b) failure by a caregiver to satisfy the elder's basic needs or to protect the elder from harm (Bonnie & Wallace, 2003). Elder mistreatment is the outcome of abuse, **neglect, exploitation,** or abandonment of older adults and represents some of the most tragic behavior in the area of family violence. Prevalence estimates from a nationally representative study document 9% of older adults as victims of verbal mistreatment, 3.5% as victims of financial mistreatment, and 0.2% as victims of physical mistreatment by family members (Laumann, Leitsch, & Waite, 2008). Acierno and colleagues (2010) used a representative sample obtained through random digit dialing across geographic strata and determined that the 1-year prevalence for emotional abuse was 4.6%, physical abuse 1.6%, sexual abuse 0.6%, and potential neglect 5.1%, with financial abuse at 5.2% by family members. Nurses are in key positions to screen, assess, and intervene for older adults subjected to elder mistreatment (Baker & Heitkemper, 2005; Fulmer, 2008).

Theories of Elder Mistreatment

Several leading theories or conceptual frameworks are used to examine the etiology of elder mistreatment. The first is *psychopathology of the abuser,* which refers to caregivers who have preexisting conditions that impair their capacity to give appropriate care. For example, a caregiver who has a developmental disability or alcohol dependency may not be able to exercise appropriate judgment in caregiving of older adults, which can ultimately lead to abuse or neglect. The next framework is referred to as *transgenerational violence.* Elder mistreatment is thought to be a part of a family violence continuum, which may begin with child abuse and end with elder mistreatment. Little work has been done to generate empirical evidence to support this; however, selected case studies indicate this could be important to the study of elder mistreatment. Another aspect of transgenerational violence relates to adult children who have had a long-standing, contentious relationship with an older parent. For example, a child who is abused by a parent and then grows up to be the caregiver may ultimately become aggressive and abusive toward the older person. Finally, transgenerational violence has been explained in terms of

a *learning theory* in that a child who observes violence as a coping mechanism may learn it and bring it to adult life.

The next is *situational theory,* which is often discussed related to caregiver stress. Amstadter and colleagues (2010) used a random digit dialing survey to study a representative sample of noninstitutionalized older adults. Of the 5,777 participants, poor self-rated health was noted by 23.3% of the sample, further underscoring the importance of analyzing care needs and any resultant elder abuse or neglect. As care burden increases, the caregiver's capacity to meet the needs of the older adult may be inadequate. *Isolation theory* espouses that mistreatment is prompted by a dwindling social network. According to the National Elder Abuse Incidence Study (National Center on Elder Abuse, 1998), about 25% of all older adults live alone and even more interact only with family members and have little social interaction with the outside world. Isolated older adults are at particular risk because there are no "gatekeepers" for them. They may not be identified as at-risk by the healthcare system or reporting agencies until it is too late. It is difficult to determine whether isolation is the result of mistreatment (family members or caregivers may be trying to hide the mistreatment from the outside world) or a precipitating factor for mistreatment.

The identification of elder mistreatment is most often done by healthcare professionals. A review of elder mistreatment measurements showcased the advances made in screening and assessment, providing a summary of their utility within specific settings and situational contexts (Fulmer, Guadagno, Bitondo Dyer, et al., 2004); these will be discussed later in the chapter.

National Incidence and Prevalence of Elder Mistreatment

The *2004 Survey of State Adult Protective Services* (APS) builds on previous efforts to describe a national picture of elder mistreatment by combining state data. These data have been collected since 1986, and the 2004 survey provides data to identify trends (Teaster, Dugar, Mendiondo, et al., 2006). Key findings include the following:

- There was a 19.7% increase in total reported elder abuse and neglect since the 2000 survey.
- There was a reported 15.6% increase in proven elder abuse and neglect since the 2000 survey.
- The vast majority of abuse and neglect (89.3%) occurred in the domestic setting.
- The typical elder who is abused is a Caucasian woman over the age of 80.
- The typical abuser was an adult child (32.6%) or family member (21.5%); spouses accounted for only 11.3%.

Furthermore, cases of elder mistreatment have been shown to be largely unreported, and most **adult protective services (APS)** programs (social services organized to protect vulnerable older adults who may be abused, neglected or exploited) have severe staff and funding shortages (Appleseed, 2011). It is estimated that for every case reported to authorities, approximately five more cases of abuse or neglect go unreported. Allen (2006) documented a decline in the prevalence of elder mistreatment in nursing homes when relatives and friends are regularly present. This has implications for nurses working in long-term care who need to be vigilant for any mistreatment in their settings.

Definitions for Elder Mistreatment

The Panel to Review Risk and Prevalence of Elder Abuse and Neglect (Bonnie & Wallace, 2003) defined emotional/psychological abuse, sexual abuse, financial/material exploitation, neglect, **self-neglect**, abandonment, and institutional

mistreatment as subtypes of elder mistreatment. Table 10-1 lists the types of elder mistreatment reflected in current scientific literature.

Cultural Perceptions of Elder Mistreatment

Elder mistreatment needs to be understood in the context of individual cultures. Researchers and clinicians have documented differences in the way people from different cultural groups experience elder mistreatment, as well as in the behaviors that they perceive as abusive or neglectful (Dong & Simon, 2010; Moon & Benton, 2000). For example, in elder mistreatment studies involving older Chinese adults, researchers have found that loneliness (Dong, Simon, Gorbien, et al., 2007) and disrespect (Tam & Neysmith, 2006) are risk factors for elder mistreatment or abuse that perhaps are not assessed directly by instruments developed by Western researchers. Furthermore, others

TABLE 10-1   **Types of Elder Mistreatment**

Type	Definition	Examples	Signs and Symptoms
Physical abuse	Intentional infliction of physical injury or pain	Hitting, shaking, pushing, improper use of physical restraints	Bruises, black eyes, bone fractures, injuries in various stages of healing
Psychological/emotional abuse	Infliction of anguish, pain, distress	Yelling, swearing, name calling	Emotional upset or agitation, extreme withdrawal
Sexual abuse	Any form of nonconsensual sexual intimacy	Rape, molestation, sexual harassment	Genital bruising, unexplained sexually transmitted disease
Financial exploitation	Taking advantage of an older person for monetary or personal benefit	Unexplained monetary expenditures, lack of money for personal necessities	Unexplained inability to pay bills or purchase necessity items such as food
Caregiver neglect	Intentional (active) or unintentional (passive) failure to meet needs necessary for elder's physical and mental well-being	Failure to provide adequate food, clothing, shelter, medical care, hygiene, or social stimulation	Dehydration, malnutrition, unattended or untreated health problems, listlessness, decubitus ulcers, urine burns, history of being left alone
Self-neglect	Personal disregard or inability to perform self-care	Poor hygiene, unkempt home environment	Malnutrition, fungal skin and nail infections, insect and rodent infestation in the home
Abandonment	Desertion or willful forsaking of an elder	Dropping off an older adult in the emergency department	An older adult left inappropriately alone
Institutional mistreatment	When older adult has a contractual arrangement and suffers abuse or neglect	May be any combination of the aforementioned	See above column entries

inappropriate use of restraints + seclativas
chemical restraints

have found that members of some minority groups may not define abusive behavior the same way that professionals do and that when cultural norms and legal regulations are in conflict, there is a need to educate and intervene to protect the vulnerable older person (Teaster et al., 2006).

Elder mistreatment cannot be tolerated, despite differing cultural perceptions. In a review paper, Patterson and Malley-Morrison (2006) summarized recent thinking related to culture, human rights, and elder abuse and examined family structure as well as social systems as essential underpinnings for research in this area. They noted how important it is to consider the cultural background and family beliefs in families where elders are being mistreated, because different cultures have different accepted behaviors, especially related to conflict management. Nurses need to be aware of the cultural differences; however, mistreatment cannot be tolerated and education related to societal norms is important.

Discrepancies across cultural and ethnic subgroups may be linked to the fact that subgroups have different expectations about the responsibility that grown children and other relatives have for caring for older adults (Tam & Neysmith, 2006; Tomita, 1999). Some researchers speculate that cultural-specific approaches to interventions based on these differences in perception would be more effective than a general approach (Dong, 2008; Dong & Simon, 2010; Moon & Benton, 2000). However, the findings from studies on elder mistreatment and culture are less than conclusive, and no studies examining different interventions for cultural subgroups have been completed to date. At the very least, nurses and other clinicians should be aware of the possibility of differences in perceptions about what constitutes mistreatment based on culture and should take this into account during assessment and care planning in patient education sessions. The Institute of Medicine stresses the importance of understanding the physical, cultural, and community environments in order to adequately address family violence. Cultural and linguistic competences are important for successful intervention in cases of elder mistreatment (Bonnie & Wallace, 2003). See Chapter 4 🔗 for a detailed discussion on culture and older adults.

Legal Issues

All states have some mechanism, whether mandatory or voluntary, for reporting elder mistreatment. State-by-state variations exist in terms of definitions, mechanisms for reporting, and appropriate governmental intake agencies (Jogerst, Daly, Dawson, et al., 2006). In most cases, long-term care reporting is distinct from community-based reporting because the standards of care for nursing homes are based on policy stipulated in the Nursing Home Reform Act of 1987 (Omnibus Budget Reconciliation Act of 1987). This law was promulgated to prevent substandard care and mistreatment of older adults. Elder mistreatment mandatory reporting laws exist in all but four states, and those four states provide mechanisms for voluntary reporting. These reporting processes provide support to clinicians who are worried that mistreatment may be present, but are unsure what to do and how to act in a professional manner to address the concern. In some states, failure by clinicians to report suspected incidents of mistreatment is a misdemeanor, punishable by fine or penalty (Otto, 2005; Jogerst et al., 2006). The *National Elder Mistreatment Study* documents the need for better education for all healthcare providers in reporting elder mistreatment (Acierno et al., 2010).

Current Evidence

Elder mistreatment generally affects disadvantaged older adults. A study that compiled a representative sample by random digit dialing across geographic strata analyzed 5,777 respondents and noted that 45.7% of the respondents had low household income, 80.9% were unemployed or retired, 22.3% had poor health, and 62% had experienced a previous traumatic event. Further, 43% indicated that they had low social support, 40% used some form of social services, and 37.8% needed assistance with activities of daily living (Acierno et al., 2010). This would indicate that nurses would have a higher level of sensitivity to elder mistreatment signs and symptoms if they noted any of these characteristics in their older patients. Obviously, with an 11% prevalence of elder mistreatment in all older adults, most patients are not victims of elder mistreatment but it is imperative that nurses have a high level of appreciation and remain vigilant for those who may be victims. Older adults who have chronic, disabling illnesses that impair function and create care needs that exceed their caregiver's capacity to meet these needs are at higher risk of being mistreated. The likelihood of verbal mistreatment is higher for women and those with physical limitations and is lower for Latinos than for Caucasian adults. Financial mistreatment was found to be higher for African Americans and lower for Latinos than for Caucasians. Verbal mistreatment was reported as lower for spouses and romantic partners than for those without partners (Laumann et al., 2008). The risk of self-neglect is increased with older age, female gender, African American race, lower income, lower cognitive and physical function, and lower social engagement (Dong, Simon, & Evans, 2010). See Table 10-2.

Low household income, unemployment, poor health self-report, prior family violence, and poor social support have consistent contextual factors for the outcome of elder mistreatment (Acierno et al., 2010; Fulmer et al., 2005;

TABLE 10-2	Elder Mistreatment Characteristics	
Older Adult Characteristics	**Abuser Characteristics**
Over 75 years old*	Mental illness
Dependent functional status*	Substance abuse
Poor social network (less than three significant others)*	History of family violence
Poverty+	Legal or financial issues
Minority+	Poor social network
Cognitive impairment+	Dependency on older adult
Living with one individual+	
Less than 8th-grade educational level	
Female	
Older adult living alone or living with abuser	
History of family violence	

Source: *Lachs, M. S., Berkman, L., Fulmer, T., & Horwitz, R. (1994). A prospective community-based pilot study of risk factors for the investigation of elder mistreatment. *Journal of the American Geriatrics Society, 42*(2), 169–173.
+Lachs, M. S., Williams, C., O'Brien, S., Hurst, L., & Horwitz, R. (1996). An 11-year longitudinal study of adult protective service use. *Archives of Internal Medicine, 156*(4), 449–453.

Lachs & Pillemer, 1995; Laumann et al., 2008). It has been documented that fewer older adults report mistreatment by family members, which may be a protective act (Laumann et al., 2008). Caregivers of older adults should be assessed at each primary care visit for caregiver stress, substance abuse, and a history of psychopathology (Nadien, 2006; Swagerty, 1999). The Modified Caregiver Strain Index has been recommended by the Hartford Institute of Geriatric Nursing as a best practice in the nursing care of older adults. This instrument is a valid and reliable screening tool and can identify caregivers in need of support (see the Best Practices feature on page 258). In summary, older adults who are disadvantaged socioeconomically or by disability are more at risk for elder mistreatment.

Institutional Mistreatment

Most of the elder mistreatment research to date focuses on mistreatment in the domestic setting; there is a dearth of information about mistreatment in nursing homes and other residential care facilities (Payne & Fletcher, 2005). Research

that does exist suggests abuse and neglect of nursing home residents by staff may be a widespread phenomenon (Hawes, 2002). The types of mistreatment that occur in nursing homes likely mirror those that occur in domestic settings, such as physical abuse, sexual abuse, neglect, financial abuse, and psychological abuse. One survey of nursing home staff members revealed that 36% had witnessed at least one incident of physical abuse by another staff member in the previous year and 81% had observed at least one incident of psychological abuse. Ten percent of the staff members reported actually committing an act of physical abuse against a resident in the previous year, and 40% admitted to having committed an act of psychological abuse (Pillemer & Moore, 1989). Patient aggressiveness was found to be a predictor of physical and psychological abuse by staff members and that abusers are more likely to be younger than nonabusers (Pillemer & Moore, 1989). Those researchers have also speculated that shortages of staff, inadequate staff training, and staff burnout may be precipitating factors in mistreatment of nursing home residents.

A federal report revealed large delays in the reporting of incidents of elder mistreatment in nursing homes (*Elder Justice*, 2002). One of the issues highlighted in this report is that there currently exists no federal law requiring criminal background checks of nursing home employees, although many states require them. Furthermore, although the U.S. Centers for Medicare and Medicaid Services requires that incidents of abuse and neglect be promptly reported to law enforcement or state survey agencies, approximately 50% of the notifications to state survey agencies reviewed in the report had been submitted two or more days after the alleged incident occurred. In addition, great delays were reported in the length of time it takes for state survey agencies to follow up and make determinations about reports of mistreatment. These delays hamper efforts of state survey agencies and, ultimately, put other nursing home residents at risk of being mistreated by nursing home staff members against whom complaints have been made (*Elder Justice*, 2002). Burgess, Dowdell, and Prentky (2000) reported several reasons for delay in reporting incidents of mistreatment in nursing homes. Residents may be afraid of retribution, and family members may fear having to find a new nursing home for the resident. Staff members may fear losing their jobs or facing recrimination by other staff members and management if they report abuse. Finally, managers of nursing homes may want to avoid adverse publicity.

It is important to note that an emerging area of elder mistreatment research examines violence perpetrated by residents of nursing homes, or resident-to-resident mistreatment. In a population-based cohort study, Lachs and colleagues (2007) found that of 79 incidents reported to police for investigation, 89% surrounded a violent episode initiated by a resident, directed toward another resident. The researchers highlighted that additional study regarding this phenomenon is warranted, and should include ways to prevent these potentially violent resident-to-resident encounters. Data gleaned from nurses in focus groups is further helping to explain this phenomenon (Rosen et al., 2008).

Assessment

Screening for elder mistreatment has been an ongoing recommendation by the American Medical Association (AMA) for more than two decades (AMA, 2008; Aravanis et al., 1993). See Figure 10-1 ▶▶▶ for a sample of an Elder Mistreatment Assessment Instrument. Nurses should complete this assessment with older adults and recognize any unusual responses that might indicate elder mistreatment and need intervention.

Interdisciplinary comprehensive geriatric assessment of the older adult's cognitive and psychosocial function is essential in identifying elder mistreatment, and the nurse's role is of utmost importance (Baker & Heitkemper, 2005; VanderWeerd, Firpo, & Fulmer, 2006). Some institutions have elder mistreatment teams comprised of interdisciplinary members to assist staff in evaluating elder mistreatment cases. These teams, which may consist of geriatricians, nurses, social workers, and perhaps representatives from APS agencies, have been very effective in managing cases of elder mistreatment (Fulmer, 2008). Researchers and clinicians recognize the need to incorporate an interdisciplinary team approach into APS systems to use comprehensive geriatric assessment to best identify and serve mistreated older adults (Dyer & Goins, 2000; Wiglesworth, Mosqueda, Burnight, et al., 2006). The nursing history should include questions for older adults about the presence of violence in their lives. Research has demonstrated that nurses can effectively screen for elder mistreatment across a variety of practice settings (Fulmer, 2008; Fulmer, Paveza, Abraham, et al., 2000). Sample screening questions are listed in the case study on page 246.

Various screening instruments have been developed that support nursing assessment of elder mistreatment. The Hartford Institute for Geriatric Nursing (2007) recommends the Elder Assessment Instrument (EAI) for use in the clinical setting. Screening can facilitate accurate assessment, risk categorization, referral for services, and ultimately protection of the older person who is being mistreated or abused.

The EAI (Anthony, Lehning, Austin, et al., 2009; Fulmer, 2008; Fulmer & Cahill, 1984; Fulmer et al., 2005; Fulmer, Street, & Carr, 1984) assesses signs and symptoms of elder mistreatment. First, nurses should observe the general appearance of the older adult and make a determination based on the context of the clinical encounter whether or not there are any signs and symptoms of elder mistreatment. For example, an older adult appearing disheveled with poor hygiene should be evaluated for potential neglect if there is a responsible caregiver who may be having trouble meeting the caregiving needs of the older patient. Signs of mistreatment include bruising, malnutrition, burns, excoriations, and fractures. Clinical manifestations of neglect might include dehydration, malnutrition, decubitus ulcers, and contractures. Additionally, the healthcare professional can look for signs and symptoms of elder mistreatment, which include delays in seeking medical treatment for an injury or illness, frequent visits to the emergency department, and diagnostic testing results inconsistent with the history given (Bonnie & Wallace, 2003; Fulmer, 2008; Lachs & Pillemer, 1995). See Table 10-3.

Ideally, the older adult and any suspected abuser should be interviewed separately. Maintaining a nonjudgmental approach will enable the nurse to obtain more accurate data. A caregiver's refusal to allow for separate interviews should increase suspicion of elder mistreatment (Fulmer et al., 2005; Nadien, 2006).

Assessing caregiver stress and burden is a key element in an elder mistreatment review. Various caregiver burden questionnaires are available in the literature.

Physical Examination

The physical symptoms of elder mistreatment are often difficult for clinicians to discern because older adults may suffer from chronic and acute illnesses that mask or mimic the presence of mistreatment (Collins, 2006). Older adults with cognitive impairment provide an additional challenge. Their self-reporting may be questioned for accuracy or they may be unable to express the mistreatment situation due to amnesia, *aphasia* (total or partial loss of ability to speak or understand language), *agnosia* (inability to recognize common people and things), or *apraxia* (inability to perform simple tasks), which commonly occur with dementia. It is often difficult to determine whether the older adult's worsening physical condition is a result of the natural progression of illness or mistreatment on the part of a caregiver. Because some frail older individuals are prone to underlying conditions that give rise to trauma, such as instability of gait and poor vision resulting in falls, it may be difficult for clinicians to differentiate accidental from willful injuries. The presence of both fresh and healing injuries may suggest ongoing episodes of trauma and represent the need for further investigation to determine whether abuse or neglect may be a contributing factor.

TABLE 10-3	Elder Mistreatment Assessment Tools	
Measures/Author	**Characteristics**	**Source**
Adult Protective Service Reports (APS)	No specific format. Intake forms used to document calls of suspected elder mistreatment from public hotlines and state agencies.	Varies from state to state.
AMA Assessment Protocol	Checklist to use if abuse is suspected.	AMA, 1992; Aravanis et al., 1993
Brief Abuse Screen for the Elderly—BASE	Five standard questions.	Reis & Nahmiash, 1995
Case Detection Guidelines	Reference list of risk factors and physical findings.	Rathbone-McCuan & Voyles, 1982
Conflict Tactic Scale (CTS)	A 19-item self-report, e.g., "Has anyone threatened you with a knife or gun?" Perception of upsetting and injurious circumstances in a person's life.	Straus & Brown, 1978
Elder Abuse and Neglect Protocol	Comprehensive outline describing an approach to abuse.	Tomita, 1982
Elder Assessment Instrument (EAI)	A 40-item screening tool with both subjective and objective items to determine if an older person should be referred for suspected elder mistreatment. Provides information to clinicians to better inform judgments about risk of elder mistreatment.	Fulmer et al., 1984
Fulmer Restriction Scale (FRS)	A 34-item scale designed to elicit information regarding unnecessary restriction of the older adult. Assessment of physical, psychological, and financial restriction of older adults.	Fulmer & Gurland, 1996
Health Attitudes to Aging & Living Arrangements Finances (H.A.L.F.)	Checklist requiring interview and period of observation.	Ferguson & Beck, 1983
Hwalek-Sengstock Elder Abuse Screening Test (H-S/EAST)	A 15-item assessment screen for detecting suspected elder abuse and neglect. Assessment of physical, financial, psychological, and neglectful situations.	Hwalek & Sengstock, 1986; Neale, Hwalek, Scott, et al., 1991
Indicators of Abuse Screen (IOA)	A 29-item set of indicators for use by social service agency practitioners to identify elder mistreatment. Developed specifically for use by social service agency practitioners likely to visit the older adult in the home.	Reis & Nahmiash, 1998
Pathophysiological signs and symptoms	Subjective and objective clinical observations as documented by healthcare clinicians. Uses items such as unexplained bruising, dehydration, urine burns, and fractures.	Dyer, Pavlik, Murphy, et al., 2000; Fulmer, 1984; Lachs & Fulmer, 1993; Haviland & O'Brien, 1989; O'Brien, 1986
The QUALCARE Scale	A 53-item observational rating scale designed to quantify and qualify family caregiving. Assessment of six areas: physical, medical management, psychosocial, environmental, human rights, and financial.	Phillips, Morrison, & Chae, 1990a; Phillips, Morrison, & Chae, 1990b
Screening Protocols for the Identification of Abuse and Neglect in the Elderly	Checklist requiring interview and period of observation.	Johnson, 1981
Screening Tools and Referral Protocol Stopping Abuse Against Older Ohioans: A Guide for Service Providers—STRP	A combination of several tools; includes a referral protocol.	Anetzberger et al., 2000

Source: Adapted from Elder mistreatment. In J. Fitzpatrick, P. Archbold, B. Stewart, & K. S. Lyons (Eds.), *Annual review of nursing research: Focus on geriatric nursing* (Vol. 20, pp. 369–394).

ELDER MISTREATMENT ASSESSMENT

TYPE OF MISTREATMENT SUSPECTED	YES	NO	UNSURE
Physical—Hitting, pushing or slapping			
Sexual—Forcing or coercion into sexual activity			
Emotional—Yelling, threatening, denying access to friends and enjoyable activities			
Financial—Income and belongings are stolen or diverted without the older adult's consent to pay for things that do not benefit the older adult			
Abandonment—Leaving the older adult alone without access to care			
Caregiver Neglect—Needs of older adult ignored by caregiver			
Physical/Sexual Signs and Symptoms			
Bruises, abrasions, cuts, fractures, scars			
Heat burns			
Pressure ulcers, urine burns			
Poor hygiene, dirty clothing, mouth ulcers			
Signs of vaginal or rectal penetration or trauma			
Uncut fingernails and toenails			
Weight loss or malnutrition			
Excessive use of medication (over-sedated)			
Failure to monitor/treat/assess illness			
Rehab services and supportive therapies discontinued without explanation			
Statement by older person regarding physical/sexual mistreatment			
Emotional Signs and Symptoms			
Excessively fearful or anxious			
Appears depressed or withdrawn			
Acts agitated or violent			
Shows signs of trauma: rocking back and forth			
Experiences difficulty sleeping			
Does not take part in activities enjoyed in past			
Statement by older person regarding emotional mistreatment			
Financial Signs			
Recent name changes on a will, bank account or title to a house			
Indications that checks have been forged			
Credit cards used without consent/knowledge of older person			
Social security checks taken and used to pay for things not benefitting the older adult			
Money, jewelry, or valuables reported stolen or missing			
Statement by older person regarding financial mistreatment			

Figure 10-1 ▶▶▶   Sample elder mistreatment assessment.

Source: Adapted from National Institute on Aging, 2011. *Elder Abuse: Age Page.* Retrieved from http://www.nia.nih.gov/sites/default/files/elder_abuse.pdf.

(continued)

Abandonment/Neglect Signs			
Caregivers often reported absent and older adult left unattended			
Older adult found alone in unsafe circumstances on more than one occasion			
Older adult unable to obtain needed food, medical care, rehab services due to absence or unavailability of caregiver			
Statement by older person regarding caregiver abandonment			
Caregiver Assessment			
Does the caregiver have a positive relationship with the older person?			
Is the older person difficult to care for and/or demanding?			
Has the caregiver been pressured or forced into assuming the role of caregiver by others?			
Does the caregiver receive help and support from others in the family/community?			
Does the caregiver have the financial resources to adequately care for the older person?			
Are there services or other options that could assist the caregiver to care for the older person?			
Is the burden of care very high for the caregiver (over 8 hours/day)?			
Final Assessment: Sufficient Evidence Suggests Presence of:			
Physical/Sexual mistreatment			
Emotional mistreatment			
Financial mistreatment			
Abandonment or neglect			
Caregiver strain			
None of the above			
Action Taken:			
Immediate help needed-Call 911 or notify proper authorities			
Family members notified			
Health care team members notified (e.g., physician, social worker)			
Outcome unsure-continue to closely monitor			
Other:			
Signature & Date:			

Figure 10-1 ▶▶▶ (*continued*)

> **Practice Pearl** ►►► If you suspect elder mistreatment or abuse, a complete visual examination of the older person without clothing is necessary. Abusers may strike where clothing hides the resulting bruises. You can protect privacy by assessing the older person's body one area at a time from head to toe.

Laboratory findings that support the presence of dehydration and malnutrition without medical causes also increase suspicion for elder mistreatment. The nurse may anticipate the need for diagnostic studies such as a complete blood count to evaluate for anemia; chemistry studies to detect dehydration; and levels of vitamin B_{12}, folate, total protein, and albumin to evaluate nutritional status; and toxicological screening to assess for evidence of illicit drug use. If sexual abuse is suspected, the nurse may need to assist with a pelvic examination that will likely include a Papanicolaou test (Pap smear) and cultures for sexually transmitted diseases. Radiological testing may also be anticipated if there is suspicion of fractures or internal injuries.

Nursing Diagnoses

Elder mistreatment may be addressed by the following nursing diagnoses from NANDA International (2012):

- *Caregiver Role Strain*
- *Coping Family: Compromised*
- *Coping Family: Disabled*
- *Coping, Ineffective*
- *Protection, Ineffective*
- *Rape-Trauma Syndrome*
- *Self-Care Deficit* (Bathing, Dressing, Feeding, Toileting)
- *Self Esteem, Situational Low*
- *Social Isolation*

NANDA-I © 2012.

These nursing diagnoses do not specifically address elder mistreatment, with the exception of *Rape-Trauma Syndrome*. Cowan (2001) has suggested the need for research and practice to further develop specific classifications for elder mistreatment to facilitate data collection and interpretation in data sets. Doing so may assist in tracking elder mistreatment trends to facilitate policy initiatives.

Interventions

Nurses working with older adults must be aware of the elder mistreatment reporting laws in their state. As previously mentioned, many states have mandatory reporting laws, and healthcare professionals must report suspected cases. Nurses and other healthcare professionals should make themselves familiar with the contact information for local departments on aging and APS agencies. State contact numbers for reporting suspected elder abuse cases are available online at the National Center on Elder Abuse website.

> **Practice Pearl** ►►► When beginning employment in a new clinical agency, it is important to ask about the protocol for reporting elder mistreatment. Identify members of the interdisciplinary team who can be of assistance, identify and record appropriate phone numbers, assemble forms that should be completed in the reporting process, and familiarize yourself with any other institutional procedures involved in the reporting process. Later on, you can report suspected mistreatment in an accurate and timely manner if the situation should arise.

Elder mistreatment requires an interdisciplinary team approach. Some forms of elder mistreatment, such as caregiver neglect, may benefit from interdisciplinary interventions. Educational interventions that may assist a stressed informal caregiver include disease management, maximizing healthcare services, respite services, behavioral management, or caregiver support groups. Informing families about Medicaid benefits and home care services can often alleviate caregiver burden (Parks & Novielli, 2000).

In cases where mistreatment is suspected, an older adult may benefit from a respite admission to allow the healthcare team to carefully assess and formulate a plan of care. Some institutions have ethics committees that evaluate cases of elder mistreatment. This strategy may be particularly helpful if legal action, such as seeking **guardianship** for an older adult, is necessary.

For the older adult living in long-term care facilities, the California Advocates for Nursing Home Reform (2008) recommend the following steps in preventing elder abuse in long-term care settings:

- Residents and significant others should join or form a resident's council.
- Residents and their significant others must stay informed by being active participants in care plan meetings and monitoring care.
- Significant others should stay connected to long-term care residents and visit at varied times.

Documentation

Excellent documentation is extremely important in elder mistreatment cases. Older adults who appear fearful when in the presence of a suspected abuser will need careful

Screening and assessment for elder mistreatment should follow a routine pattern. Assessment of each case should include the following:

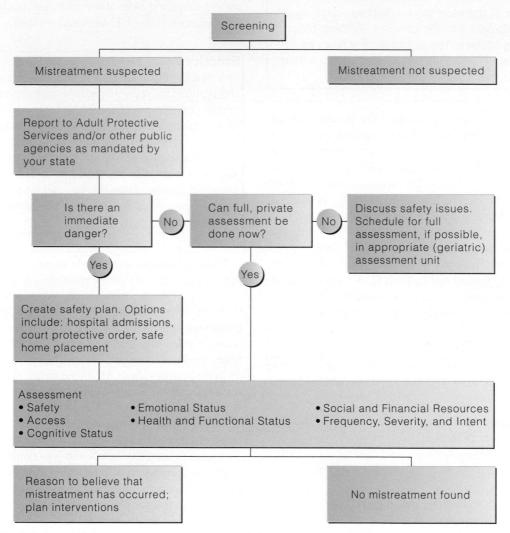

Figure 10-2A ►►► Intervention and case management: part 1.

Source: Reprinted with permission of the American Medical Association (1992). Diagnostic and treatment guidelines on elder abuse and neglect, 14. All rights reserved.

assessment as this may be a warning sign of mistreatment. Physical indicators of elder mistreatment that are clearly described will assist interdisciplinary members with diagnosis as well as with planning goals of patient care. Photographic documentation is especially helpful in cases where there is observable evidence.

Implications for Gerontological Nursing Practice

The Joint Commission recommends the American Medical Association's *Diagnostic and Treatment Guidelines on Elder*

Abuse and Neglect (AMA, 1992; Aravanis et al., 1993). These guidelines are presented in Figures 10-2A and 10-2B ►►►.

Future Considerations

Barriers to detecting and treating elder mistreatment include denial, cultural issues, and lack of education of healthcare professionals. Accurate and uniform data must be continuously collected at state and national levels so that elder mistreatment trends can be monitored

Case management should be guided by choosing the alternatives that least restrict the patient's independence and decision-making responsibilities and fulfill state-mandated reporting requirements. Intervention will depend on the patient's cognitive status and decision-making capability and on whether the mistreatment is intentional or unintentional.

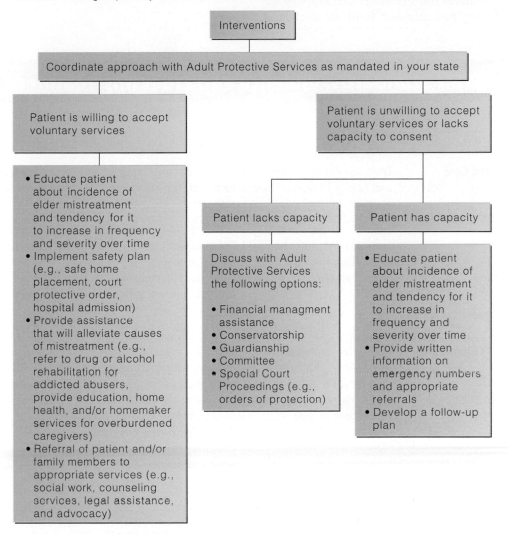

Figure 10-2B ▶▶▶ Intervention and case management: part 2.

Source: Reprinted with permission of the American Medical Association (1992). Diagnostic and treatment guidelines on elder abuse and neglect, 14. All rights reserved.

(Teaster et al., 2006). There is a paucity of evidence-based interventions to offer victims and their families, and there is a need to increase community and professional education and interventions nationally. Future research focusing on evidence-based interventions to prevent elder mistreatment is needed. The patient–family teaching guidelines at the end of the chapter will help the nurse assume the role of teacher and coach in detecting elder mistreatment.

QSEN Recommendations Related to Elder Mistreatment

The Quality and Safety Education for Nurses (QSEN) project addresses the challenge of preparing future nurses with the knowledge, skills, and attitudes (KSAs) to continuously improve the quality and safety of the healthcare systems in which they work (Cronenwett et al., 2007).

See the QSEN table for tips on meeting QSEN standards.

Patient and Family Teaching

Gerontological nurses require skills and knowledge related to teaching patients and families about the key concepts of gerontology and gerontological nursing. The guidelines in the following feature will assist the nurse to assume the role of teacher and coach.

Meeting QSEN Standards: Violence and Elder Mistreatment

	KNOWLEDGE	SKILLS	ATTITUDES
Patient-Centered Care	Involvement of patient and family in plan of care is crucial.	Provide patient-centered care with sensitivity and respect.	Respect patient values, preferences, and expressed needs.
	Examine barriers that may keep patients from being active in formulating their plan of care.	Assess presence and levels of potential abuse or neglect by carefully documenting bruises, injuries, pain, depression, and cognitive impairment.	Provide patient-centered care to improve successful nursing outcomes. Establish a therapeutic relationship in order to gain trust.
Teamwork and Collaboration	Recognize contributions of interdisciplinary team members. Be aware of reporting policies and procedures in your state of practice.	Integrate contributions of interdisciplinary team members as a means of helping the patient/family achieve goals. Consult with medicine, pharmacy, dietary, social work and advocate as needed.	Value teamwork and the importance of professional collaboration.
	Identify barriers that can inhibit effective team function. Schedule team meetings as needed.	Follow communication practices that minimize risks associated with handoffs.	Be open to the different communication styles of each member of the team.
Evidence-Based Practice	Describe effective assessment techniques and interventions to reduce opportunities for abuse and neglect and advocate for services to improve patient safety.	Access current evidence-based protocols to guide care plan development.	Value the need for continuous improvement in the clinical practice of pain assessment and management based on new knowledge.
Quality Improvement	Explain the importance of measuring patient outcomes to improve patient safety and decrease abuse potential.	Use quality measures to understand performance and evaluate the results of patient safety plan.	Appreciate that continuous quality improvement is a key component of good patient care.

	KNOWLEDGE	SKILLS	ATTITUDES
Safety	Describe common adverse effects associated with elder abuse/neglect treatment plans.	Communicate observations related to adverse effects or errors to patients, families, and the interdisciplinary team.	Value own role in preventing or minimizing risk for adverse effect and negative outcomes.
Informatics	Explain why information and technology are essential for safe patient care.	Utilize the electronic health record to support safe processes of care.	Value technologies that support clinical decision making, error prevention, and care coordination.

Patient-Family Teaching Guidelines

The following are guidelines that the nurse may find useful when instructing older adults and their families about elder mistreatment.

EDUCATING ABOUT ELDER MISTREATMENT

1 **I am worried about my older aunt who I suspect is being abused by her son. What is elder mistreatment?**

Any action or inaction that harms or endangers the welfare of an older adult may be considered elder mistreatment. Approximately 2.1 million cases of elder mistreatment occur in the United States each year (Acierno et al., 2010).

Types of Abuse

- Physical abuse is an intentional infliction of physical injury or pain such as slapping or hitting.

- Psychological or emotional abuse is infliction of anguish such as repeatedly scolding an older individual who cannot perform personal hygiene tasks.

- Sexual abuse is any form of nonconsensual sexual intimacy.

- Financial exploitation is when an older individual is taken advantage of for monetary or personal benefit.

- Neglect may be on the part of a caregiver who intentionally or unintentionally does not provide adequate care or services for an older adult (i.e., not seeking health care when

needed or withholding prescribed medications). Neglect may also be on the part of the older adult (self-neglect) who exhibits personal disregard or inability to perform self-care.

- Institutional mistreatment occurs when an older adult has a contractual arrangement and suffers abuse or neglect.

- Abandonment is desertion or willful forsaking of an older person. An example of this is when an older individual is dropped off and left alone at the emergency department.

RATIONALE:

Most people are unaware of the broad definition and scope of caregiver activities that are legally considered abuse, neglect, and mistreatment of older people. A complete description is needed when abuse is suspected.

2 **If she is being abused, how can I help? I am only a niece.**

If you suspect elder mistreatment, contact your local adult protective services office or the department of human services in your

(continued)

Patient-Family Teaching Guidelines (continued)

state, county, or local jurisdiction. A caseworker will visit your aunt and assess the situation. If help and support for her caregivers is needed, additional services will be brought into the home and the situation will be monitored to protect your aunt's safety.

RATIONALE:

Many people are unsure of how to proceed when they suspect abuse or mistreatment of an older person. Education and identification of resources will empower them to act responsibly.

3 **What if abuse or neglect of my aunt is found? Will she be put in a nursing home?**

The goal of the caseworker's first assessment is to determine whether your aunt is in immediate danger. Older people in immediate danger from abuse are removed from the home and

temporarily protected in hospitals or safe havens with the authority of a court order. If the abuser needs mental health treatment or detoxification from drugs or alcohol, this will be facilitated. The goal is to improve the situation if possible and return the older person to the home environment when safe. If your aunt is not in immediate danger, resources will be brought into the home to ease the caregiver strain and improve your aunt's safety.

RATIONALE:

Many people are hesitant to make referrals regarding possible abuse because they fear the older person will be placed permanently in a long-term care facility. Reassurance and education regarding all of the possible outcomes are needed.

CARE PLAN   A Patient With Signs of Self-Neglect

Case Study

Mrs. Baker is brought to the emergency department by ambulance attendants. Her mail carrier noticed that her mail had not been collected for 2 days and called 911. She is in a diabetic coma.

Mrs. Baker's past medical history is significant for heart failure, hypertension, diabetes, peripheral vascular disease, and depression.

A review of her social history reveals that Mrs. Baker is a 70-year-old widow whose only living relatives are her 95-year-old mother who lives in a nursing home 500 miles away and a daughter who lives 70 miles away. She lives alone in a lower-middle-class neighborhood in a modest but run-down home. She has a protective services caseworker who has tried to arrange help, but Mrs. Baker refuses. Her usual routine consists of eating an occasional meal (soup, a sandwich, or cereal), smoking two packs of cigarettes a day, drinking a pint of alcohol every 2 days, and lying on the sofa watching television. She rarely sees her neighbors and does not respond to her physician's request to see him. On occasion, she may answer her telephone or doorbell. Last year she was the victim of fraud

by two men claiming to protect her home from termites and water damage. She realizes she cannot fully maintain her home or herself on her own, but she refuses in-home assistance and is determined to stay in her home, manage her own money and affairs, and die there.

Mrs. Baker remains in the emergency department, receives her insulin, and is stabilized for admission. The nurse is unable to get an accurate history of her medications and cannot tell what she is taking. She refuses to answer any questions about a caregiver. She says she is completely independent and refuses to discuss her financial support. She denies being left alone for long periods of time and says she has all the contact she wants. She says she is able to express her needs and have them met.

Mrs. Baker's vital signs are as follows:

- Temperature: 98°F, oral
- Pulse: 70, regular
- Respiratory rate: 20
- Blood pressure: 210/100

CARE PLAN   ## A Patient With Signs of Self-Neglect (continued)

Applying the Nursing Process

Assessment

A complete assessment of Mrs. Baker's health status and self-care is needed. Some appropriate questions the nurse may ask include:

1. Has anyone tried to hurt you in any way?
2. Do you feel safe at home?
3. How can I help you to feel safer when you are home alone?

Diagnosis

The current nursing diagnoses for Mrs. Baker might include the following:

- *Caregiver Role Strain, Risk For*
- *Coping, Family: Compromised or Disabled*
- *Coping, Ineffective*
- *Protection, Ineffective*

- *Self-Care Deficits*
- *Self-Esteem, Situational Low*
- *Social Isolation*
- *Poisoning, Risk for: Alcohol and Tobacco Abuse*

NANDA-I © 2012.

Expected Outcomes

The expected outcomes for the plan of care specify that Mrs. Baker will:

- Become aware of the harmful effects of alcohol and tobacco on overall health status.
- Identify family and community supports that might allow her to return home and achieve her goal of spending the rest of her life there.

- Develop a more trusting and open relationship with her physician regarding her health status.
- Agree to establish a therapeutic relationship with the nurse and develop a mutually acceptable plan to work toward these outcomes.

Planning and Implementation

The following nursing interventions may be appropriate:

- Establish a therapeutic relationship.
- Avoid being judgmental or using scare tactics.
- Encourage a family meeting with the daughter present to talk about health issues in general with Mrs. Baker's permission.

- Begin a mental status and mood assessment to establish the underlying cause of Mrs. Baker's self-neglect.
- Begin a values clarification to establish long-term goals and facilitate end-of-life planning.

Evaluation

The nurse hopes to work with Mrs. Baker over time and realizes the sensitive nature of self-neglect in older people. The nurse will consider the plan a success based on the following criteria:

- During hospitalization, Mrs. Baker's condition will become stable and physical indicators of health status will improve (e.g., dehydration, nutrition, skin integrity).
- A family meeting will be held to discuss Mrs. Baker's overall health and values.

- She will accept counseling and discuss beginning to decrease her alcohol and tobacco consumption.
- Ongoing assessment of Mrs. Baker's cognitive status, mood, and resources will be conducted as her condition stabilizes.
- Appropriate discharge planning will take place, and safe living arrangements will be identified and used at the time of hospital discharge.

(continued)

CARE PLAN

A Patient With Signs of Self-Neglect *(continued)*

Ethical Dilemma

On physical examination, the nurse notes Mrs. Baker is 5'5", 101 lbs. Her cognition is abnormal, she is extremely dirty, and she has evidence of greater than 15% dehydration. She has a small blister on her left thigh, which looks like a burn. She also has a sacral pressure ulcer 2 cm in diameter. She has no bruising, contractures, diarrhea, impaction, or urine burns.

Mrs. Baker says the burn is from a cigarette and that she often falls asleep while smoking on the couch. She asks the nurse not to inform the others on the team that she has burned herself. Ignoring the older person's request not to share information with others is usually considered a violation of the right to privacy; however, Mrs. Baker is at immediate and high risk for injury due to self-neglect. Her dehydration, pressure ulcers, uncontrolled diabetes, low body weight, and impaired cognitive status are all indicators that her situation must be reported to a caseworker for investigation. The nurse is bound by law and ethics to intervene on behalf of this patient and advocate for her safety. A report should be filed immediately with the appropriate government agency or police.

Critical Thinking and the Nursing Process

1. What is your emotional response to the thought of caring for an older person who has been mistreated?
2. Can you identify some unique reasons for elder mistreatment in your community?
3. Have you ever witnessed elder mistreatment during your clinical experiences as a student nurse?
4. Identify actions that can help relieve stress in family caregivers.

■ Evaluate your responses in Appendix B.

Chapter Highlights

■ Elder mistreatment is a general term for both abuse and neglect.

■ The prevalence of elder mistreatment is difficult to ascertain because many cases go unreported.

■ Family violence is a significant public health issue for all of society, and the rates of elder mistreatment are expected to increase in the coming years.

■ Elder mistreatment may include physical abuse or neglect, psychological abuse or neglect, financial or material abuse or neglect, or self-abuse or neglect.

■ Indicators of mistreatment are subtle and vary according to the situation. Complete assessment of possible mistreatment and contributing factors is needed.

■ Nearly all states require designated healthcare professionals, including nurses, to report suspected elder mistreatment to a state authority. Calls are confidential.

Note: The authors wish to acknowledge a previous version of this chapter authored by Sheryl M. Strasser, PhD, MPH, MSW, and Annemarie Dowling-Castronovo, RN, MA, GNP. We also wish to acknowledge the administrative assistance of Melissa Crocker.

Pearson Nursing Student Resources
Find additional review materials at
nursing.pearsonhighered.com

Prepare for success with additional NCLEX®-style practice questions, interactive assignments and activities, web links, animations and videos, and more!

References

Acierno, R., Hernandez, M. A., Amstadter, A. B., Resnick, H. S., Steve, K., Muzzy, W., & Kilpatrick, D. G. (2010). Prevalence and correlates of emotional, physical, sexual, and financial abuse and potential neglect in the United States: The National Elder Mistreatment Study. *American Journal of Public Health, 100*(2), 292–297. doi:AJPH.2009.163089 [pii] 10.1177/0886260510383037

Allen, P. D. (2006). Long-term care ombudsman volunteers: Making a measurable difference for nursing home residents *International Journal of Volunteer Administration, 24*(2), 5–14.

American Medical Association (AMA). (1992). *Diagnostic and treatment guidelines on elder abuse and neglect.* Chicago, IL: Author.

American Medical Association (AMA). (2008). *American Medical Association National Advisory Council on Violence and Abuse Policy compendium 2008.* In N. A. C. o. V. a. Abuse (Ed.).

Amstadter, A. B., Begle, A. M., Cisler, J. M., Hernandez, M. A., Muzzy, W., & Acierno, R. (2010). Prevalence and correlates of poor self-rated health in the United States: the national elder mistreatment study. *American Journal of Geriatric Psychiatry, 18*(7), 615–623. doi:10.1177/0886260510383037

Anetzberger, G. J., Palmisano, B. R., Sanders, M., Bass, D., Dayton, C., Eckert, S., & Schimer, M. R. (2000). A model intervention for elder abuse and dementia. *Gerontologist, 40*(4), 492–497.

Anthony, E. K., Lehning, A. J., Austin, M. J., & Peck, M. D. (2009). Assessing elder mistreatment: Instrument development and implications for adult protective services. *Journal of Gerontological Social Work, 52*(8), 815–836. doi:915858527 [pii] 10.1080/01634370902918597

Appleseed Foundation. (2011). *Strengthening APS and informing implementation of Elder Justice Act: A nationwide survey of APS administrators.* Lifelong Justice. Retrieved from http://appleseeds.net/LinkClick.aspx?fileticket=cuvxlBcxzwQ%3D&tabid=157

Aravanis, S. C., Adelman, R. D., Breckman, R., Fulmer, T., Holder, E., Lachs, M. S., O'Brien, J. G., & Sanders, A. B. (1993). Diagnostic and treatment guidelines on elder abuse and neglect. *Archives of Family Medicine, 2*(4), 371–388.

Baker, M. W., & Heitkemper, M. M. (2005). The roles of nurses on interprofessional teams to combat elder mistreatment. *Nursing Outlook, 53*(5), 253–259. doi:S0029-6554(05)00082-5 [pii] 10.1016/j.outlook.2005.04.001

Bonnie, R. J., & Wallace, R. B. (2003). *Elder mistreatment: Abuse, neglect and exploitation in an aging America.* Washington, DC: National Academy Press.

Burgess, A. W., Dowdell, E. B., & Prentky, R. A. (2000). Sexual abuse of nursing home residents. *Journal of Psychosocial Nursing, 38*(6), 10–18.

California Advocates for Nursing Home Reform. (2008). A citizens guide to preventing and reporting elder abuse. Retrieved from http://ag.ca.gov/bmfea/pdfs/citizens_guide.pdf

Collins, K. A. (2006). Elder maltreatment: A review. *Archives of Pathology & Laboratory Medicine, 130*(9), 1290–1296. doi:RA-5-878 [pii] 10.1043/1543-2165(2006)130[1290:EMAR]2.0.CO;2

Cowan, P. S. (2001). Elder mistreatment. In M. L. Mass, K. C. Buckwalter, M. D. Hardy, T. Tripp-Reimer, M. G. Titler, & J. P. Specht (Eds.), *Nursing care of older adults: Diagnoses, outcomes, & interventions.* St. Louis, MO: Mosby.

Cronenwett, L., Sherwood, G., Barnsteiner, J., Disch, J., Johnson, J., Mitchell, P., Sullivan, D., & Warren, J. (2007). Quality and safety education for nurses, *Nursing Outlook, 55*(3) 122-131.

Dong, X.-Q. (2008). A descriptive study of sex differences in psychosocial factors and elder mistreatment in a Chinese community population. *International Journal of Gerontology, 2*(4), 206–214.

Dong, X., & Simon, M. A. (2010). Is impairment in physical function associated with increased risk of elder mistreatment? Findings from a community-dwelling Chinese population. *Public Health Rep, 125*(5), 743–753.

Dong, X. Q., Simon, M., & Evans, D. (2010). Cross-sectional study of the characteristics of reported elder self-neglect in a community-dwelling population: Findings from a population-based cohort. *Gerontology, 56*(3), 325–334. doi:000243164 [pii] 10.1159/000243164

Dong, X., Simon, M. A., Gorbien, M., Percak, J., & Golden, R. (2007). Loneliness in older Chinese adults: A risk factor for elder mistreatment. *Journal of the American Geriatrics Society, 55*(11), 1831–1835. doi:JGS1429 [pii] 10.1111/j.1532-5415.2007.01429.x

Dyer, C. B., & Goins, A. M. (2000). The role of the interdisciplinary geriatric assessment in addressing self-neglect of the elderly. *Generations, 24*(2), 23–27.

Dyer, C. B., Pavlik, V. N., Murphy, K. P., & Hyman, D. J. (2000). The high prevalence of depression and dementia in elder abuse or neglect. *Journal of the American Geriatric Society, 48*(2), 205–208.

Elder justice: Protecting seniors from abuse and neglect. (2002, June 18). Hearing before the Committee on Finance, U.S. Senate, 107th Congress, Second Session.

Ferguson, D., & Beck, C. (1983). H.A.L.F.—A tool to assess elder abuse within the family. *Geriatric Nursing, 4*(5), 301–304.

Fulmer, T. (1984). Elder abuse assessment tool. *Dimensions of Critical Care Nursing, 3*(4), 216–220.

Fulmer, T. (2008). Screening for mistreatment of older adults. *American Journal of Nursing, 108*(12), 52–59; quiz 59–60.

Fulmer, T., & Cahill, V. M. (1984). Assessing elder abuse: A study. *Journal of Gerontological Nursing, 10*(12), 16–20.

Fulmer, T., Guadagno, L., Bitondo Dyer, C., & Connolly, M. T. (2004). Progress in elder abuse screening and assessment instruments. *Journal of the American Geriatrics Society, 52*(2), 297–304.

Fulmer, T., & Gurland, B. (1996). Restriction as elder mistreatment: Differences between caregiver and elder perceptions. *Journal of Mental Health and Aging, 2*, 89–98.

Fulmer, T., Paveza, G., Abraham, I., & Fairchild, S. (2000). Elder neglect assessment in the emergency department. *Journal of Emergency Nursing, 26*(5), 436–443.

Fulmer, T., Paveza, G., VandeWeerd, C., Fairchild, S., Guadagno, L., Bolton-Blatt, M., & Norman, R. (2005). Dyadic vulnerability and risk profiling for elder neglect. *Gerontologist, 45*(4), 525–535.

Fulmer, T., Street, S., & Carr, K. (1984). Abuse of the elderly: Screening and detection. *Journal of Emergency Nursing, 10*(3), 131–140.

Hartford Institute for Geriatric Nursing. (2007). *Elder mistreatment course: Vital guidance in identifying and stopping elder abuse.* Retrieved from http://hartfordign.org/education/elder_abuse_course

Haviland, S., & O'Brien, J. (1989). Physical abuse and neglect of the elderly: Assessment and intervention. *Orthopedic Nursing, 8*(4), 11–19.

Hawes, C. (2002). *Elder abuse in residential long-term care facilities: What is known about prevalence, causes, and prevention.* Testimony before the U.S. Senate Committee on Finance.

Hwalek, M., & Sengstock, M. (1986). Assessing the probability of abuse of the elderly: towards the development of a clinical screening instrument. *Journal of Applied Gerontology, 5*, 153–173.

Jogerst, G. J., Daly, J. M., Dawson, J. D., Peek-Asa, C., & Schmuch, G. (2006). Iowa nursing home characteristics associated with reported abuse. *Journal of the American

Medical Directors Association, 7(4), 203–207. doi:10.1016/j.jamda.2005.12.006

Johnson, D. (1981). Abuse of the elderly. *Nurse Practitioner, 6*(1), 29–34.

Lachs, M., Bachman, R., Williams, C. S., & O'Leary, J. R. (2007). Resident-to-resident elder mistreatment and police contact in nursing homes: Findings from a population-based cohort. *Journal of the American Geriatrics Society, 55*(6), 840–845.

Lachs, M. S., Berkman, L., Fulmer, T., & Horwitz, R. (1994). A prospective community-based pilot study of risk factors for the investigation of elder mistreatment. *Journal of the American Geriatrics Society, 42*(2), 169–173.

Lachs, M. S., & Fulmer, T. (1993). Recognizing elder abuse and neglect. *Clinical Geriatric Medicine, 9*(3), 665–681.

Lachs, M. S., & Pillemer, K. A. (1995). Abuse and neglect of elderly persons. *New England Journal of Medicine, 332*(7), 437–443.

Lachs, M. S., Williams, C., O'Brien, S., Hurst, L., & Horwitz, R. (1996). Older adults. An 11-year longitudinal study of adult protective service use. *Archives of Internal Medicine, 156*(4), 449–453.

Laumann, E. O., Leitsch, S. A., & Waite, L. J. (2008). Elder mistreatment in the United States: Prevalence estimates from a nationally representative study. *Journals of Gerontology Series B: Psychological Sciences and Social Sciences, 63*(4), S248–S254. doi:63/4/S248 [pii]

Moon, A., & Benton, D. (2000). Tolerance of elder abuse and attitudes toward third-party intervention among African American, Korean American and White elderly. *Journal of Multicultural Social Work, 8*(3/4), 283–303.

Nadien, M. B. (2006). Factors that influence abusive interactions between aging women and their caregivers. *Annals of the New York Academy of Science, 1087,* 158–169. doi:1087/1/158 [pii] 10.1196/annals.1385.019

NANDA International. (2012). *NANDA International nursing diagnoses: Definitions and classification, 2012–2014.* Philadelphia, PA: Wiley-Blackwell.

National Center on Elder Abuse at The American Public Human Services Association in Collaboration with Westat, I. (Ed.). (1998). *The National Elder Abuse Incidence Study: Final report.* Washington, DC: National Aging Information Center.

Neale, A., Hwalek, M., Scott, R., Sengstock, M., & Stahl, C. (1991). Validation of the Hwalek-Sengstock Elder Abuse Screening Test. *Journal of Applied Gerontology, 10*(4), 406–418.

O'Brien, J. G. (1986). Elder abuse and the physician. *Mich Med, 85*(11), 618, 620.

Otto, J. M. (2005). *Abuse and neglect of vulnerable adult populations.* Kingston, NJ: Civic Research Institute.

Parks, S., & Novielli, K. (2000). A practical guide to caring for caregivers. *American Family Physician, 62*(12), 2613–2620.

Patterson, M., & Malley-Morrison, K. (2006). A cognitive-ecological approach to elder abuse in five cultures: Human rights and education. *Educational Gerontology, 32*(1), 73–82.

Payne, P., & Fletcher, L. (2005). Elder abuse in nursing homes: Prevention and resolution strategies and barriers. *Journal of Criminal Justice, 33,* 119–125.

Phillips, L. R., Morrison, E. F., & Chae, Y. M. (1990a). The QUALCARE Scale: Developing an instrument to measure quality of home care. *International Journal of Nursing Studies, 27*(1), 61–75.

Phillips, L. R., Morrison, E. F., & Chae, Y. M. (1990b). The QUALCARE Scale: Testing of a measurement instrument for clinical practice. *International Journal of Nursing Studies, 27*(1), 77–91.

Pillemer, K. A., & Moore, D. W. (1989). Abuse of patients in nursing homes: Findings from a survey of staff. *Gerontologist, 29*(3), 314–320.

Rathbone-McCuan, E., & Voyles, B. (1982). Case detection of abused elderly parents. *American Journal of Psychiatry, 139*(2), 189–192.

Reis, M., & Nahmiash, D. (1995). When seniors are abused: An intervention model. *Gerontologist, 35*(5), 666–671.

Reis, M., & Nahmiash, D. (1998). Validation of the indicators of abuse (IOA) screen. *Gerontologist, 38*(4), 471–480.

Rosen, T., Lachs, M. S., Bharucha, A. J., Stevens, S. M., Teresi, J. A., Nebres, F., & Pillemer, K. (2008). Resident-to-resident aggression in long-term care facilities: insights from focus groups of nursing home residents and staff. *Journal of the American Geriatrics Society, 56*(8), 1398–1408. doi:JGS1808 [pii] 10.1111/j.1532-5415.2008.01808.x

Straus, M. A., & Brown, B. (1978). Family measurement techniques: The Conflict Tactic Scale. In J. Touliatos & B. Perlmutter (Eds.), *Handbook of family measurement techniques* (pp. 417). Newbury Park, CA: Sage.

Swagerty, D. L. (1999). Elder mistreatment. *American Family Physician, 59*(10), 2804–2808.

Tam, S., & Neysmith, S. (2006). Disrespect and isolation: Elder abuse in Chinese communities. *Canadian Journal on Aging, 25*(2), 141–151.

Teaster, P., Dugar, T., Mendiondo, M., Abner, E., Cecil, K., & Otto, J. M. (2006, February). *The 2004 survey of state adult protective services: Abuse of adults 60 years of age and older.* Washington, DC: National Center on Elder Abuse.

Tomita, S. (1982). Detection and treatment of elderly abuse and neglect: A protocol for health care professionals. *Physical Therapy and Occupational Therapy in Geriatrics, 2*(2), 37–51.

Tomita, S. (1999). Exploration of elder mistreatment among the Japanese. In T. Tatara (Ed.), *Understanding elder abuse in minority populations* (pp. 119–139): New York, NY: Taylor & Francis.

VanderWeerd, C., Firpo, A., & Fulmer, T. (2006). Recognizing mistreatment in older adults. In J. J. Gallo, H. R. Bogner, T. Fulmer, & G. J. Paveza (Eds.), *Handbook of Geriatric Assessment* (4th ed.) (pp. 78–101). Sudbury, MA: Jones & Bartlett.

Wiglesworth, A., Mosqueda, L., Burnight, K., Younglove, T., & Jeske, D. (2006). Findings from an elder abuse forensic center. *Gerontologist, 46*(2), 277–283. doi:46/2/277 [pii]

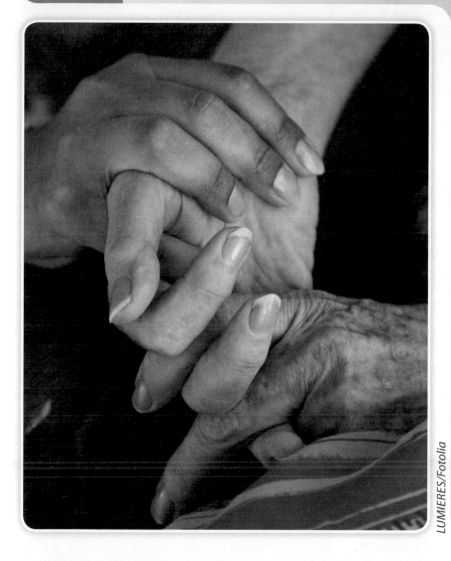

LUMIERES/Fotolia

KEY TERMS

adjuvant drugs *260*
advance directives *266*
bereavement *273*
breakthrough pain *260*
comfort measures only (CMO) *267*
durable power of attorney for
    health care *266*
grief *272*
healthcare proxy *266*
hospice care *255*
living wills *267*
loss *272*
mourning *273*
palliative care *256*
postmortem care *265*

LEARNING OUTCOMES

On completion of this chapter, the reader will be able to:

1. Describe the role of the nurse in providing quality end-of-life care for older adults and their families.
2. Explain changes in demographics, economics, and service delivery that require improved nursing interventions at the end of life.
3. Understand how pain and adverse symptoms affect dying.
4. Discuss the diverse settings for end-of-life care and the role of the nurse in each setting.

5. Explore pharmacological and alternative methods of treating pain.
6. Identify the signs of approaching death.
7. Implement appropriate nursing interventions when caring for the dying patient.
8. Describe postmortem care.
9. Discuss family support during the grief and bereavement period.

he population of older adults in the United States is growing dramatically. Increases in life-limiting illness in this population create an urgent need for nurses with expert knowledge and skill in the care of the older adult at the end of life. Nurses are uniquely qualified to provide comprehensive, effective, compassionate, and cost-effective care to people at the end of life because of their holistic focus. The Hospice and Palliative Nurses Association (HPNA) (2011d) has issued a position statement declaring that professional nursing care is critical to achieving goals of care at the end of life and that support of hospice and palliative care research and education is necessary to ensure delivery of such care.

Among the members of the healthcare team, nurses spend the most time and have the most frequent and continuous contact with patients and families at the end of life (American Nurses Association [ANA], 2010; HPNA, 2011d). Older adults and their families look to their nurse to educate, support, and guide them throughout the dying process. This intimate position allows the nurse to advocate for improved quality of life for the person with serious illness. According to HPNA (2011d), "when faced with serious illness, people turn to professional nurses for education, support, and guidance" (p. 1). Informed understanding of the patient's values, wishes, and goals allows the nurse to attend to the patient's physical, emotional, psychosocial, and spiritual needs.

Death is as natural a part of life as is birth. Although birth is embraced with joy and celebration, death is frequently denied and often prolonged for the sake of the living. Nurses have a unique opportunity and an obligation to help patients and their families through the dying process. Student nurses learn to do this by confronting their own feelings about death and seeking guidance and mentorship when confronting death during clinical experiences. The student nurse learns how to acknowledge and accept death as part of life and realizes that nurses, too, grieve the loss of patients. Viewing death as a natural process—not a medical failure—is of utmost importance. The nurse who helps the patient die comfortably and with dignity provides the following benefits of good nursing care:

- Attention to pain and symptom control
- Relief of suffering
- Coordinated care across settings with high-quality communication between healthcare providers
- Preparation of the patient and family for death
- Clarification and communication of goals of treatment and values
- Support and education during the decision-making process, including the benefits and burdens of treatment

National Consensus Project [NCP] for Quality Palliative Care, 2009.

To achieve these goals, the nurse must be well educated, have appropriate supports in the clinical setting, and develop a close collaborative partnership with hospice and palliative care service providers.

Nurses must be confident in their clinical skills when caring for the dying, and aware of the ethical, spiritual, and legal issues they may confront while providing end-of-life care. Many feel that the first step in the process is confronting their own personal fears about death and dying. By addressing their own fears, nurses are better able to help patients and families when they are confronted by impending death. The nurse may then be more objective in recognizing and respecting the patient's and family's values and choices that guide their decisions at the end of life.

Facing one's own mortality may help to clarify beliefs and values. As death nears, the meaning of hope shifts from striving for cure to achieving relief of pain and suffering. There is no "right" or "correct" way to die, and each person will face death in his or her own unique and individual way. To prepare to work with the dying, the student nurse may wish to consider the questions in Table 11-1. The purpose of this exercise is to increase nurses' awareness of their own feelings about death and dying so that they are better prepared to comfort and care for others.

By coming to terms with their own feelings surrounding death, nurses can better meet the emotional, spiritual, social, and physical needs of their patients. Often, it is the caregiver who forms the bonds with the dying patient and is present when the last breath is taken. The nurse provides a presence as a way of expressing compassionate caring. In this way, nurses enter into another's reality and use all of their skills of compassionate care. This is a humbling and beautiful privilege. It, too, is a celebration of a life lived (Figure 11-1 ▶▶▶).

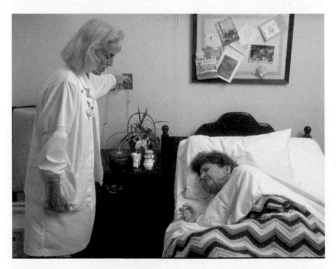

Figure 11-1 ▶▶▶ Providing compassionate and holistic end-of-life care allows the nurse to apply a wide range of skills.

TABLE 11-1	Questions and Critical Thinking in Preparation to Care for Dying Patients
Question for Consideration	**Critical Thinking Application**
Have I ever seen a dead body?	Identify and overcome feelings regarding the lifeless body of another.
What are my own views of death?	Recognize feelings that death indicates a failure of the medical model.
Have I experienced the death of a close friend or relative?	By contemplating the death of a loved one, different emotions emerge including feelings of sadness and perhaps relief or joy for a life well lived.
How would I like to be remembered by my family and friends?	The way we hope to be remembered often adds purpose and meaning to our lives.
What age do I think I will be when I die?	Death in old age is often seen as a natural end to a long and productive life.
How do I think I will die?	The fear of death is often accompanied by fear of pain, suffering, and isolation from family and friends. These fears may be greater than the fear of death itself.

The Changing Face of Death

Many older people grew up with death as a real and inevitable part of life. Some may have cared for their parents or grandparents for extended periods of time and remember holding wakes or funerals in the living room of the home where death occurred. During the mid-1900s, technological advances dictated that sick people should go to hospitals where they could safely receive high-tech care. Surgery, antibiotics, and advanced testing techniques became the focus of health care, shifting away from the provision of

care to the pursuit of cure. Table 11-2 illustrates some of the changing demographic and social trends surrounding death in the years 1900 and 2010.

Many older adults now live into advanced age with chronic illness, and most deaths in this population are the result of chronic disease. The 10 leading causes of death in the United States in 2009 were heart disease, cancer, chronic lower respiratory disease, cerebrovascular disease, accidents (unintentional injury), Alzheimer's disease, diabetes mellitus, influenza and pneumonia, renal disease, and suicide (Kochanek, Xu, Murphy et al., 2011). Considering the burden of advancing chronic illness, the nurse

TABLE 11-2	Cause of Death and Demographic/Social Trends	
	1900	**2010**
Focus of care	Comfort	Cure
Primary cause of death	Infectious diseases—e.g., tuberculosis, influenza	Chronic illnesses—e.g., heart disease, lung disease, cancer
Average life expectancy	46.3 years (males) 48.3 years (females)	76.0 years (males) 80.9 years (females)
Number of older adults (>65 years)	3.1 million	40.3 million
Place of death	Home	Institutions
Caregivers	Family	Professional healthcare providers
Disease trajectory	Short, downward trend	Prolonged, variable, peaks and valleys
Functional decline at the end of life	Short term—expected and surprise	Lingering expected—frailty

Sources: Adapted from Administration on Aging, 2010; Arias, 2011; National Center for Health Statistics (NCHS), 2011.

must consider what their older adult patients want at the end of life.

When surveyed, most Americans express a preference to die in their own homes; however, most die in the institutional settings (Grunier et al., 2007). The past 20 years have seen a shift in the trends in place of death; however, with increasing numbers of people dying in their homes and long-term care settings and decreasing numbers of people dying in the hospital. In 2007, 36% of Americans died in hospitals (down from 49% in 1989), 25% died in long-term care facilities, and 25% died at home (up from 17% in 1989) (NCHS, 2011). Race and ethnicity influence decisions about end-of-life care and place of death among the older adult population. Non-Hispanic White older adults are more likely to die in the nursing home, while older adults in other racial and ethnic groups are more likely to die in the hospital (Grunier et al., 2007; NCHS, 2011).

Not only are fewer people dying in the hospital, older adults are spending less time in the hospital at the end of life. A recent report of the Dartmouth Atlas Project revealed that the average number of days older adults spend in the hospital before death, as well as the percentage of deaths associated with an intensive care stay, has declined in recent years (Goodman, Esty, Fisher et al., 2011). The report also demonstrated that increasing numbers of older adults are choosing hospice care at the end of life.

Data from several landmark studies demonstrate high degrees of distress from unrelieved symptoms in hospitalized patients and long-term care residents, high use of burdensome technologies among people who are seriously ill, caregiver burden on families, and problems with communication between patients, families, and caregivers about the goals of care and medical decisions that should follow (Last Acts, 2002; NCP, 2009; SUPPORT Principal Investigators, 1995). When a national survey asked how the current healthcare system rates in caring for dying people, only 3% of respondents answered excellent, 8% responded very good, 31% responded good, 33% responded fair, and 25% responded poor (Last Acts, 2002). Most professionals agree that there is much room for improvement in view of these results.

Many barriers to the provision of excellent end-of-life care exist and include failure of healthcare providers to acknowledge the limits of medical technology, lack of communication among decision makers, disagreement regarding the goals of care, and failure to implement a timely advance care plan (End of Life Nursing Education Consortium [ELNEC], 2008). Furthermore, existing provider-specific barriers include lack of understanding about palliative care, an unwillingness to be honest about a poor prognosis, discomfort telling bad news, and lack of institutional standards for end-of-life care (Doyle & Woodruff, 2008).

Practice Pearl ▶▶▶ Although not all deaths involve pain and suffering, there are deficiencies in the way end-of-life care is currently provided in the U.S. healthcare system. Barriers include lack of knowledge regarding pain and symptom control. Challenge yourself to develop expert skills in these areas to improve the dying process for your patients.

All healthcare providers, including nurses, are challenged to address and overcome these barriers to improve the quality of care provided to those who are dying and their families. Acknowledgment of the existence of these barriers when caring for the older adult at the end of life allows the nurse to implement more effective plans of care. Some techniques that may be undertaken by the nurse to improve the quality of care at the end of life include scheduled interdisciplinary team meetings to discuss patients' end-of-life concerns, inclusion of key decision makers (e.g., patient, family, primary physician) in care plan discussions, and specialized end-of-life care education and ongoing attendance at continuing education conferences. The nurse with a comprehensive understanding of quality end-of-life care is in a position to advocate for their patients and their families and can help them to improve the quality of their lives during the dying process.

Practice Pearl ▶▶▶ If you are unsure of a person's wishes for care at the end of life, call a team meeting involving key decision makers such as the patient, family members, and the primary care physician. Ongoing open discussion about goals of care will help the patient and his or her family receive the best possible care at the end of life.

Delivery of End-of-Life Care

Relief of suffering, whether physical, emotional, or spiritual, should be made available to all patients from the moment of diagnosis with a life-limiting or debilitating illness (NCP, 2009).

Hospice Care

The hospice movement began in the 1960s when Dame Cicely Saunders introduced the concept of specialized care for dying patients and founded the first modern hospice, St. Christopher's Hospice, in a suburb of London. Soon thereafter, the movement spread to the United States and support for hospice programs in the United States began to grow. Work of nurse leaders such as Florence Wald, Dame Cicely Saunders (also a physician), Jeanne Quint Benoliel, and Betty Ferrell has highlighted the need for competent, evidence-based care to be provided in a way that is compassionate, respectful, and appreciates the needs of the whole person and their family (HPNA, 2011d). Current standards of comprehensive and compassionate hospice and palliative nursing care are built on the foundation of the work of these nurse leaders (HPNA, 2011d). In 2009, approximately 1.56 million Americans received hospice services and an estimated 41.6% of all deaths occurred while the patient was receiving hospice services (National Hospice and Palliative Care Organization [NHPCO], 2010).

Hospice care provides support for people in the last phase of life-limiting illness through expert medical care, pain and symptom management, and emotional and spiritual support so that they may live as fully and comfortably as possible (NHPCO, 2010). When it has been determined by two physicians that the patient has 6 months or less to live, and the dying person and family prefer care and comfort over aggressive medical intervention, hospice is often sought. Hospice care focuses on the whole person by caring for the body, mind, and spirit. The goal is for the patient to live their last days as fully and comfortably as possible. To achieve this goal, an interdisciplinary team of physicians, nurses, therapists, home health aids, pharmacists, pastoral counselors, social workers, and trained lay volunteers assist the family and caregivers in providing care. The hospice nurse assumes the role of specialist in the management of pain and control of symptoms and assesses the patient's and family's coping mechanisms, available resources to care for the patient, the patient's wishes, and the support systems in place.

Hospice personnel may work with caregivers and patients in the home, long-term care facilities, other long-term care settings, and hospitals. Also available in some regions are freestanding hospices that provide a homelike atmosphere in which care is provided by trained staff at the hospice facility. Reimbursement for hospice services is provided by Medicare, Medicaid, private health insurances, and some health maintenance organizations. Some hospices accept donations for care; others may have access to charitable foundations. All hospices encourage family involvement and promote death with dignity. Because the experience of the dying and death of a loved one deeply affects the family, supportive care is provided to family and caregivers throughout the illness trajectory and for a period after the death has occurred.

There are many misconceptions concerning hospice care. Table 11-3 illustrates common myths and facts regarding hospice.

TABLE 11-3   Myths and Facts Regarding Hospice

Myth	Fact
Medicare provides only 6 months of hospice care, so enrollment should be delayed as long as possible.	Medicare law does not limit the hospice benefit, but Medicare regulations often discourage a longer length of stay. Patients may enroll when their physician judges their life expectancy to be 6 months or less.
All hospice care is the same.	Hospices vary widely in the services they provide. Visit and observe services before choosing or recommending one for care.
Patients cannot receive curative treatments while on hospice.	Patients must sign a statement choosing hospice care instead of curative therapies to treat their terminal illness. Medicare will still pay for covered benefits for any health problems that are not related to the terminal diagnosis.
Hospice means giving up hope.	Hope for comfort and relief of pain and suffering is always present.
Hospices help people die.	Hospice workers do not hasten death.
Hospice helps only when advice is needed regarding pain medication.	Hospice care is holistic and goes beyond traditional medical care.
You cannot keep your own doctor on hospice.	Most hospices have working relationships with the referring physician.
Hospice is only for cancer patients.	Hospice is available to all patients with a variety of diagnoses, including those with cancer, dementia, and heart and lung diseases.
Hospice is only for the sick family member.	Hospice supports all family members during the illness and supports the family for 1 year after the death.
Hospice is a place, so you must leave home to go there.	Most hospice care is delivered in the home, although inpatient care is available to those with no in-home caregiver or to those whose families are overwhelmed by providing the care.
Hospice is expensive.	In general, hospice costs less than traditional hospital or long-term care.

Palliative Care *symptom support*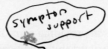

Palliative care began during the hospice movement and is now used widely outside of hospice care. The World Health Organization (WHO) (2011) defines palliative care as "an approach that improves the quality of life of patients and their families facing the problem associated with life-threatening illness, through the prevention and relief of suffering by means of early identification and impeccable assessment and treatment of pain and other problems, physical, psychosocial and spiritual." Nursing interventions that help the patient enhance their quality of life, reduce pain and suffering, optimize functionality, and promote appropriate goal setting and decision making are integral to the provision of excellent palliative care. Regardless of the stage of the disease or the need for curative therapies, palliative care is appropriate for patients with life-limiting, serious illness. It can be delivered concurrently with life-prolonging care or as the main focus of care (NCP, 2009). Although palliative care can be delivered to patients of any age, including children, it is especially appropriate when provided to older people who have:

- Acute, serious, life-threatening illness (such as stroke, trauma, major myocardial infarction, and cancer where cure or reversibility may or may not be a realistic goal but the burden of treatment is high)
- Progressive chronic illness (such as end-stage dementia, heart failure, renal or liver failure, and frailty)

Palliative care may take place across all settings including hospitals, outpatient clinics, long-term care facilities, or the home. The patient and family are supported during the dying process and following the death of their loved one. The care provided emphasizes quality of life until the moment of death.

Stages of the Dying Process

Elisabeth Kübler-Ross, a psychiatrist at the University of Chicago, was also a pioneer for end-of-life care; the early hospice movement was supported by her research. Kübler-Ross (1969) interviewed hundreds of dying patients and published her findings in *On Death and Dying: What the Dying Have to Teach Doctors, Nurses, Clergy, and Their Own Families*. It was through her efforts that healthcare providers began to understand the needs of dying patients. Her work also emphasized the need for pain relief in patients who are terminally ill. The outcome of this research was the development of the "stages of dying" (Box 11-1). Note that a dying person may not exhibit all of these stages, or may move quickly through a stage, only to return to it at a later time.

Kübler-Ross's framework stimulated research and changed practice in the field of end-of-life care. Today,

> **BOX 11-1** ▶ **Kübler-Ross Stages of Grief and Dying**
>
> - **Denial.** They must have the wrong patient or lab results. I can't be dying, I feel so good.
> - **Anger.** I can't believe this. I always took care of others and this is my reward? Why not someone else instead of me?
> - **Bargaining.** OK, doctor. I'll give chemotherapy another try if you can guarantee that I'll live for another year. If God lets me live until my grandson graduates from college, I'll make a large donation to my church.
> - **Depression.** Why should I bother taking my medicine? I'm helpless to fight this cancer. It's stronger than I am and is getting the best of me.
> - **Acceptance.** OK. I'm going to die, so I'd better get my act together. I'd like to leave a few pieces of jewelry to my daughter and my books to my son. I hate to think of leaving this world, but I've had a good life and now my time has come. I'll face this final act with all the dignity and courage I can pull together.

DABDA

however, not all researchers agree with Kübler-Ross and some claim that her research cannot be replicated. Death and dying is a unique experience, and each person and family progresses through the process differently. The nurse should remain objective and not quickly jump to conclusions that "one size fits all."

> ***Practice Pearl*** ▶▶▶ Collaboration of team members is essential for providing end-of-life care to older patients and their families. Effective sharing of information, active listening, and ongoing clarification of the patient's goals and values are critical communication skills.

The Nurse's Role

The nurse providing quality end-of-life care to an older person and their family assumes the role of expert clinician. As an expert clinician, the nurse completes physical, psychological, social, and spiritual assessments, and designs and implements plans of care (in collaboration with the patient, family, and interdisciplinary team) to meet the needs of the patient. Many validated instruments are available for use by healthcare professionals, including instruments for the assessment of pain and symptoms, mental health and mood, meaning in life and spirituality, functional assessment, quality of life, and caregiver strain. See the Toolkit of Instruments to Measure End-of-Life Care (TIME) for online copies and instructions for use of these various instruments.

Core principles for the care of patients at the end of life include the following:

- Communicate effectively with the patient, family, and healthcare team members.
- Display sensitivity and respect for individual, cultural, and spiritual beliefs and customs.
- Recognize one's own attitudes, feelings, values, and expectations about death.
- Alleviate pain and symptoms and promote comfort.
- Assessing, managing, and referring psychological, social, and spiritual problems.
- Collaborate with the interdisciplinary team while promoting the nursing role.
- Provide access to and evaluate the impact of traditional, complementary, and technological therapies that may improve the quality of the patient's life.
- Provide access to palliative care and hospice services.
- Respect the right of patients and families to refuse treatment.
- Promote and support evidence-based clinical research in practice.

Adapted from American Association of Colleges of Nursing, 2004; ELNEC, 2008; NCP, 2009.

NODA

Nurses who regularly assist patients and families to understand changes in their health status and the implications of these changes can alleviate many commonly held patient fears. Common fears and concerns of the dying include the following:

- Death itself
- Thoughts of a long or painful death
- Facing death alone
- Dying in a long-term care facility or hospital
- Loss of body control, such as bowel or bladder incontinence
- Not being able to make decisions concerning care
- Loss of consciousness
- Financial costs and becoming a burden on others
- Dying before having a chance to put personal affairs in order

The nurse can assist the older patient to address some of these fears by ensuring patient comfort and support. Often, the nurse is present for the patient and family and can communicate compassion through caring acts. For instance, the small act of adjusting the patient's position in bed and fluffing the pillow can be greatly appreciated by the patient and family. When an older adult is diagnosed with a serious illness, life continues for an indefinite period of time; many older patients live much longer than their prognosis predicts. It is essential that each person have the opportunity to live life fully each day and engage in living until the moment of death rather than engaging in a long, tedious dying trajectory. Therefore, accurate and timely deliverance of nursing care and addressing potential problem areas is of prime importance. The nurse's assessment guides the interdisciplinary team in providing individualized care with respect for the patient's wishes. The goal of the nurse is to help the older adult achieve the best possible quality of life through relief of suffering, control of symptoms, and restoration of functional capacity while remaining sensitive to personal values, cultural practice, and religious beliefs (Last Acts, 2002).

Best Practices

Caring for a seriously ill older adult can be a stressful experience for the loved ones providing care. According to the Hartford Institute for Geriatric Nursing (2007), informal caregivers, such as family and friends, may be at increased risk for depression, fatigue, and changes in social interaction with prolonged caregiving. It is important for the nurse to assess informal caregivers for caregiver strain and burden throughout the patient's illness trajectory. See Best Practices: Modified Caregiver Strain Index on the next page, which helps the nurse to quickly screen caregivers. By identifying the sources and degree of strain, the Modified Caregiver Strain Index can guide the selection of interventions that might be used to alleviate caregiver strain and improve the lives of caregivers and care recipients. Intervention strategies to reduce the burden of caregiving may include support groups, education, counseling, and respite care. The higher the score, the higher the level of caregiver strain and scores should decline over time if the nurses' intervention strategies are effective.

Pain at the End of Life

The assessment and management of pain in older adults is discussed in detail in Chapter 9 ⬜. Merciful relief of pain is essential for quality end-of-life care in the older patient and nurses have a primary role in assessing and managing pain at the end of life (ANA, 2010). According to the ANA, "nurses, individually and collectively, have an obligation to provide comprehensive and compassionate end-of-life care, including the promotion of comfort, relief of pain, and support for patients, families, and their surrogates when a decision has been made to forgo life-sustaining treatments" (p. 2). Pain during the dying process is feared by patients and families and if unrelieved, creates distress, despair, and suffering; however, through ongoing assessment of levels of pain, administration of pain medication, and evaluation of the effectiveness of the pain management plan, the nurse may help alleviate the distress associated with untreated pain in the older adult (HPNA, 2008).

Best Practices   Modified Caregiver Strain Index

Directions: *Here is a list of things that other caregivers have found to be difficult. Please put a checkmark in the columns that apply to you. We have included some examples that are common caregiver experiences to help you think about each item. Your situation may be slightly different, but the item could still apply.*

	Yes, On a Regular Basis = 2	Yes, Some-times = 1	No = 0
My sleep is disturbed	_____	_____	_____
(For example: the person I care for is in and out of bed or wanders around at night)			
Caregiving is inconvenient	_____	_____	_____
(For example: helping takes so much time or it's a long drive over to help)			
Caregiving is a physical strain	_____	_____	_____
(For example: lifting in or out of a chair; effort or concentration is required)			
Caregiving is confining	_____	_____	_____
(For example: helping restricts free time or I cannot go visiting)			
There have been family adjustments	_____	_____	_____
(For example: helping has disrupted my routine; there is no privacy)			
There have been changes in personal plans	_____	_____	_____
(For example: I had to turn down a job; I could not go on vacation)			
There have been other demands on my time	_____	_____	_____
(For example: other family members need me)			
There have been emotional adjustments	_____	_____	_____
(For example: severe arguments about caregiving)			
Some behavior is upsetting	_____	_____	_____
(For example: incontinence; the person cared for has trouble remembering things; or the person I care for accuses people of taking things)			
It is upsetting to find the person I care for has changed so much from his/her former self	_____	_____	_____
(For example: he/she is a different person than he/she used to be)			
There have been work adjustments	_____	_____	_____
(For example: I have to take time off for caregiving duties)			
Caregiving is a financial strain	_____	_____	_____
I feel completely overwhelmed	_____	_____	_____
(For example: I worry about the person I care for; I have concerns about how I will manage)			

[Sum responses for "Yes, on a regular basis" (2 pts each) and "yes, sometimes" (1 pt each)]

TOTAL SCORE =

Source: Thornton, M., & Travis, S. S. (2003). Analysis of the reliability of the Modified Caregiver Strain Index. *The Journal of Gerontology, Series B, Psychological Sciences and Social Sciences, 58*(2), p. S129. Copyright © The Gerontological Society of America. Reprinted with permission of Oxford University Press.

[handwritten: adjuvant meds - med used for not the primary use]

Pain is associated with many negative outcomes in the dying patient. It has the potential to hasten death and is associated with needless suffering at the end of life. People in pain do not eat or drink well, do not move around, cannot engage in meaningful conversations with others, and often become isolated in order to save energy and cope with the pain sensation. Untreated pain is related to sleeplessness, psychological distress, fatigue, and restlessness, and nurses have a moral obligation to advocate on behalf of their patients so that pain is appropriately managed (ANA, 2010; HPNA, 2008).

Although efforts are under way to improve end-of-life care, there is growing evidence that improvements are not being experienced by all patients. Groups at particular risk for undertreatment of pain at the end of life include older adults (especially those with cognitive impairment), minorities, and women (Broglio & Portenoy, 2011). Inadequate pain relief may stem from the patient's inability to communicate pain; for example, some older patients may be unable to report their pain due to delirium, dementia, aphasia, motor weakness, language barriers, and other factors. Minority patients have been identified as being at high risk for inadequate pain relief at the end of life. Possible barriers for these patients include poor cross-cultural communication on the part of the provider, disparities in access to many treatment options, limited health literacy, and mistrust of the healthcare system (American Pain Foundation [APF], 2011). The provision of culturally sensitive care is a necessary component of effective and comprehensive end-of-life care.

Pain assessment, including a thorough history and physical exam, guides the development of a comprehensive pain management plan. Pain is acknowledged to be a subjective experience with self-report being the gold standard by which pain is measured. When an older adult is unable to speak or self-report the level of pain, the nurse should carefully observe the patient for behavioral symptoms of pain that may include:

- Moaning or groaning at rest or with movement
- Failure to eat, drink, or respond to the presence of others
- Grimacing or strained facial expression
- Guarding or not moving parts of the body
- Resisting care or noncooperation with therapeutic interventions
- Rapid heartbeat, diaphoresis, or change in vital signs

Furthermore, family members and caregivers may be questioned about existence of pain. If a patient has a potential reason for pain at the end of life, the nurse should assume it is present until proven otherwise (Broglio & Portenoy, 2011).

Accurate pain assessment is the basis of pain treatment and should be done in a systematic and ongoing manner. The older adult patient should be questioned as to a person's usual reaction to a painful situation.

Helpful questions may include the following:

- Do you usually seek medical help when you believe something is wrong with you?
- Where does it hurt the most?
- How bad is the pain? (The nurse may use validated pain rating instruments such as the Faces Pain Scale, the Numeric Rating Scale, or the Verbal Descriptor Scale; see Best Practices in Chapter 9 ⬚.)
- How would you describe the pain (e.g., sharp, shooting, dull)?
- Is the pain accompanied by other troublesome symptoms like nausea or diarrhea?
- What makes the pain go away?
- Are you able to sleep when you are having the pain?
- Does the pain interfere with your other activities?
- What do you think is causing your pain?
- What have you done to alleviate the pain in the past?

ELNEC, 2008.

Pain During the Dying Process

Pain at the end of life is complex and multifactorial with prevalence varying by diagnosis and other factors. The concept of "total pain" must be taken into consideration when assessing for and managing pain at the end of life (Broglio & Portenoy, 2011). Total pain recognizes that pain at the end of life is more than just physical suffering; it also includes associated emotional, social, and spiritual suffering. To enhance quality of life, an interdisciplinary team approach is necessary so that all of these domains are adequately assessed and relief of all types of pain may be provided (Jones & Elbert-Avila, 2011). As disease advances and pain worsens, it is important for the nurse to recognize that the patient's goals of care are apt to change (Broglio & Portenoy, 2011). For example, patients may sacrifice being alert in order to better control their pain.

Effects of Unrelieved Pain During the Dying Process *[handwritten: Hospice Pharmacies]*

Unrelieved pain remains a serious problem in the United States (HPNA, 2008). Many healthcare providers, patients, and families believe that pain management with opioids shortens life; conversely, significant evidence exists to the contrary (Paice, 2010). Inadequate pain relief may actually hasten death by increasing physiological stress, potentially diminishing immunocompetency, decreasing mobility, worsening risk of pneumonia and thromboembolism, and increasing the work of breathing and myocardial oxygen requirements (Herr, 2011; HPNA, 2008). Unrelieved pain at the end of life also causes psychological distress and is often associated with negative outcomes such as depression, anxiety, declines in social activities, and decreased quality of life (Herr, 2011).

Principles of Pain Relief During the Dying Process

As discussed in Chapter 9 🔗, pain is common in the older adult population, and it is especially common at the end of life. Pain in patients who are terminally ill may consist of both nociceptive and neuropathic pain. It is important to differentiate among these different types of pain in order for it to be appropriately managed. Nociceptive pain is the signal the brain imparts when there is tissue inflammation or damage. Cardiac ischemia and arthritis are examples of nociceptive pain. Nociceptive pain can be divided into two categories: somatic pain that is characterized by aching, throbbing, or stabbing due to skin, muscle, or bone injury, and visceral pain that is characterized by gnawing, cramping, or aching due to injury of the internal organs. Nociceptive pain usually resolves when the injury is healed. Neuropathic pain occurs when nerves have been damaged and commonly occurs in older adults in the form of diabetic neuropathy, post-herpetic neuralgia, or post-stroke syndrome. The pain associated with these conditions is often described as burning, electrical, or tingling.

Various nonpharmacological and pharmacological methods of pain control may be implemented to control pain in the older person at the end of life. Some nonpharmacological approaches to reducing pain may include providing a glass of warm milk to promote sleep, a back rub, a change of position, a favorite peaceful musical selection, spending time listening to the patient, and visits from a priest, minister, or rabbi to meet spiritual needs.

Pharmacological methods are the mainstay of treatment for pain at the end of life and require close collaboration between the nurse, the prescribing physician or advanced practice nurse, and the pharmacist to ensure the correct medication, dosing regimen, and route of administration are used. There are three categories of analgesic medications: nonopioids (including acetaminophen and nonsteroidal anti-inflammatory drugs [NSAIDs]), opioids, and **adjuvant drugs,** or medications used with analgesics to increase the effectiveness of the pain regimen. Selection of the appropriate treatment plan involves an understanding of the type of pain involved and the pain intensity (Winn, 2010). The WHO (1990) developed a model for pain relief that is the basis for the pharmacological approach to pain management (Figure 11-2 ▶▶▶). It advocates a stepped approach for pain treatment based on the presence of mild, moderate, and severe or unrelenting pain. Mild pain (patient rated as 1 to 3 on the 0 to 10 scale) should be treated

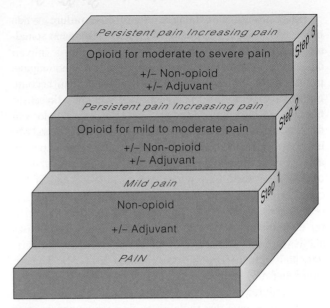

Figure 11-2 ▶▶▶ World Health Organization three-step analgesic ladder.

Source: World Health Organization. (1990). *Cancer pain relief and palliative care* (Technical Report Series, 804). Geneva, Switzerland: Author. Reprinted with permission.

with nonopioid medications or with adjuvant drugs (e.g., antidepressants, muscle relaxants) if the patient has neuropathic pain. Moderate pain (4 to 6 on the pain scale) is treated with low doses of opioids; the use of nonopioids and adjuvants may be continued at this stage. If the pain is severe (7 to 10), higher opioid doses are used. Patients presenting with severe pain should be started at higher doses rather than risking prolonged periods of uncontrolled pain while medications are titrated up from lower doses. Medications should be titrated based on patient goals, requirements for supplemental analgesics, pain intensity, severity of undesirable or adverse drug effects, measures of functionality, sleep, emotional state, and patient's or caregiver's report of the impact of pain on quality of life (ELNEC, 2008).

Studies suggest that many patients, including long-term care residents, are being undertreated for pain (Herr, 2011; HPNA, 2008). Whatever medications are chosen, it is important to administer them routinely and not on an as-needed (PRN) basis in order to prevent the unpleasant experience of the patient perceiving pain and then waiting for pain relief (American Geriatrics Society [AGS], 2009). Long-acting drugs (sustained-release formulations) are ideal because they provide consistent pain relief. Short-acting or immediate-release agents are excellent PRN medications and should only be used to control **breakthrough pain.** Breakthrough pain is defined as the presence of moderate to severe episodes of pain occuring periodically despite adequate levels of baseline pain control. Examples of breakthrough pain include end-of-dose failure, when blood levels of pain medication fall prior to the next scheduled dose; incident pain that occurs with activity (physical therapy, activities of daily living); and spontaneous pain that is common in neuropathic pain and is difficult to predict (AGS, 2009). Breakthrough pain should be treated promptly to avoid the fear or memory of pain, and to prevent decreased functional ability. Older patients who consistently experience breakthrough pain should have the dosage of their regularly scheduled long-acting medications increased.

> **Practice Pearl** ▶▶▶ Anticipate and treat adverse effects such as nausea and constipation. Most patients on opioids will require laxative/stool softener combinations.

Pharmacological Approach to Pain During the Dying Process

After conducting a thorough pain assessment, the nurse shares the information with other members of the healthcare team including the physician, advanced practice nurse, pharmacist, and others. This collaboration is essential to achieve adequate pain control.

The following types of drugs are used to control pain at the end of life:

- **Nonopioids.** Common types of drugs in this category include acetaminophen and NSAIDs. These drugs are very effective for the treatment of mild to moderate nociceptive pain; NSAIDs also have anti-inflammatory properties. They may be used alone or in combination with adjuvant drugs to enhance their effect. *Cautions:* Doses of acetaminophen should not exceed 3,000 mg per day from all sources in patients with normal liver function; exceeding 3,000 mg per day may result in liver damage. It is essential to use acetaminophen with caution in those with liver disease or significant alcohol use. NSAIDs can cause gastric irritation by inhibition of prostaglandin formation. Decreased prostaglandin synthesis results in thinning of the mucous lining that protects the stomach that may result in gastrointestinal bleeding, especially in the older adult. Other common side effects are renal dysfunction and impaired platelet aggregation. A newer class of NSAIDs selectively blocks the cyclooxygenase-2 (COX-2) enzyme, and there appears to be less risk of gastrointestinal bleeding with these drugs; however, this benefit may not extend beyond 6 to 12 months and these drugs have been linked to increased risk of heart attack and stroke.

- **Opioids.** Opioids have become a mainstay for moderate to severe pain management in the older adult population

(McPherson & Uritsky, 2011). These medications block receptors in the central nervous system and prevent the release of chemicals involved in pain transmission. Examples are codeine, morphine, hydromorphone, fentanyl, methadone, and oxycodone. Morphine is considered the gold standard by the WHO for the relief of cancer pain. Adverse effects are rare, and the only absolute contraindication for use is a history of a hypersensitivity reaction (rash, wheeze, edema). Respiratory depression may occur with initiation or titration of opioid analgesics; however, this is rarely clinically significant (McPherson & Uritsky, 2011). Several adverse effects are common in older adults taking opioids for pain management. Constipation should be expected and therefore a plan should be initiated to reduce constipation when an opioid is started. Prevention of constipation may include stool softeners and laxatives. Other troublesome side effects of opioids include sedation, nausea, and vomiting. Further discussion of the adverse effects associated with the use of opioid analgesics can be found in Chapter 9 ⊂⊃. Meperidine is not recommended for use in the older person because of its limited effectiveness in treating pain and association with serious side effects (Reisner, 2011). As disease progresses and organ function deteriorates, the potential for accumulation of toxic metabolites of this drug can lead to seizure, delirium, and tremor.

- **Adjuvant analgesics.** A wide array of nonopioid medications from several pharmacological classes has been shown to improve pain control when used concomitantly with pain medications. Their use may enhance the effectiveness of other classes of drugs, thus allowing improved treatment of pain at lower doses and decreased risk of side effects. They may be used at any step of the "analgesic ladder" developed by the WHO (1990), as presented in Figure 11-2. Medications in this class include muscle relaxants, corticosteroids, anticonvulsants, antidepressants, and topical medications.

Routes of Administration

The oral route of administration is usually preferred because it is the easiest and most comfortable for the patient. However, many routes of administration are available when the patient can no longer swallow at the end of life. Pain medication may be administered by the following routes:

- **Oral.** Tablets, liquids, and capsules are administered orally to control pain. Long-acting or sustained-release tablets can control pain for up to 24 hours. Patients who are able to swallow can use this method until very close to the time of death. Liquid medications can be mixed in juice, and capsules may be opened and the contents mixed with applesauce. Usually a higher dose of medication is needed when given orally because of the first-pass effect (deactivation that occurs when medication passes through the liver). This route may become difficult to utilize near the very end of life when the older person may be unable to swallow.

- **Oral transmucosal.** Some opioids, like fentanyl, are absorbed well by this route. The medication can be delivered even when the patient can no longer swallow because the medication is absorbed from the mucosa and swallowing is not necessary.

- **Rectal.** Some medications are available in suppository form, and the rectal route may be used when the patient can no longer swallow or has problems with nausea and vomiting. The rectal route is invasive and delivering medication by this route may be difficult for family members. If the patient cannot move easily, the positioning required for suppository insertion may be problematic.

- **Transdermal.** The fentanyl patch may be placed on the skin of the upper body every 72 hours for relief of pain. Because of changes in blood flow, metabolism, and fat distribution, some patients do not achieve or maintain stable drug levels and adequate pain relief. Peak onset may be delayed up to 24 hours, necessitating coverage with short-acting agents during the initial day of treatment. Heat should not be applied to the patch because it results in increased absorption and may lead to life-threatening respiratory depression and death.

- **Topical.** Topical capsaicin and local anesthetics (EMLA) can be used for pain associated with post-herpetic neuralgia and arthritis and prior to invasive procedures such as insertion of intravenous medication or injections. Topical medications usually have little systemic absorption when applied in small amounts to confined areas, as is recommended.

- **Parenteral.** The intravenous and subcutaneous routes are used when the patient is unable to swallow. Pain may be associated with these methods of delivery. The IV route provides rapid drug delivery and pain relief, although risks of infection increase due to the need for vascular access. If the intravenous route is used, it is important to use the appropriate fluid delivery system and the smallest amount of fluid possible. This will minimize the risk of volume overload, which can lead to excess secretions and difficulty breathing. Subcutaneous administration is slower to take effect with infusion of 2 to 3 mL/hr the easiest to absorb.

- **Intraspinal.** The administration of drugs into or around the spinal cord via the epidural or intrathecal route is reserved for those patients who cannot achieve pain control in any other manner. Increased costs are related to the complexity of equipment used to deliver medications

in this way, and caregiver burden is a potential risk. Furthermore, risk of infection is a significant concern when these techniques are used.

Patients who are managed with opioid analgesics over a period of time invariably will develop tolerance, the body's normal response to continued exposure to a medication, resulting in less effect over time. Medication dosages that were once effective will no longer be so, especially as disease worsens. It is imperative not to undertreat pain. As pain increases, underlying causes should be explored, the patient should be medicated promptly, response to medication should be monitored, and other team members should be informed about the effectiveness of the pain relief plan. The goal is to reduce pain to a level that is satisfactory to the patient and help the older adult to improve the quality of his or her life through relief of suffering.

> **Drug Alert ▶▶▶** Dying patients may need more pain medication than the normal range for the prescribed drug. Organic changes are occurring rapidly within the body and systems are shutting down; consequently, absorption levels of drugs diminish.

Nursing Care at the End of Life
Mucosal and Conjunctival Care

An older adult's ability to manage secretions and swallowing is reflected by the status of the oral mucosa and general oral hygiene. Painful xerostomia (dry mouth) can contribute to difficulty swallowing and impede clear speech; this is often exacerbated by the use of supplemental oxygen and reliance on open-mouthed breathing at the end of life. Frequent mouth care at this time is crucial to providing comfort. Oral care with soft swabs should be provided several times a day and whenever the mouth has a foul odor or appears uncomfortable for the patient. The nurse may instruct family members to use oral swabs or moistened cloths, allowing the family caregiver to be an active participant in their loved one's care. Alcohol-based products or those that have perfume, lemon, or glycerin can be irritating and drying and their use is discouraged. A salt-soda solution (1 teaspoon salt, 1 teaspoon baking soda, 1 quart tepid water) or artificial saliva used every 30 minutes may minimize dry mouth and the associated sensation of thirst (Emanuel, Ferris, von Gunten et al., 2010). Ice chips to relieve the feeling of dryness may be offered as long as the swallowing reflex is present. To prevent aspiration, the nurse should remind caregivers not to give oral fluids when the patient can no longer swallow. Soothing ointments or petroleum jelly may be applied to the lips to prevent painful cracking or drying. With increasing debility, oral thrush may appear and should be treated with oral antifungal medications (e.g., nystatin swish and swallow).

As death approaches and the patient becomes increasingly sedated, the blink reflex decreases resulting in dry eyes. Opened or half-opened eyelids dry and become irritated. Frequent eye care is provided to promote comfort when this occurs. Artificial tears or ophthalmic saline solutions may be used to prevent drying of the eyes. The appearance of a loved one with half-open eyes, redness, or puffiness may be disturbing to family members and should be reduced and avoided if possible.

Anorexia and Dehydration

Anorexia and dehydration are common and normal in the dying patient; most dying patients stop eating and drinking. If the patient chooses to refuse food and drink, the nurse should consider this a rational decision and offer emotional and psychological support. Most experts believe that dehydration at the end of life does not cause distress and may actually initiate release of endorphins resulting in a sense of well-being (Emanuel et al., 2010). Another benefit of dehydration is the decreased risk of lung congestion due to pulmonary edema, which leads to noisy, labored respirations, the sensation of breathlessness, and cough. By eliminating noisy respirations, the patient is deemed more comfortable and quiet breath sounds decrease anxiety for family members. Oliguria (less than 15 mL of urine produced per hour) is another favorable outcome of dehydration because the patient does not need to be positioned to use the bedpan or urinal frequently. When the patient stops eating, family can be reassured that anorexia may result in ketosis leading to a peaceful state of mind and decreased pain. Furthermore, research has shown that initiation of parenteral or enteral nutrition at this time neither improves symptom control nor lengthens life (Emanuel et al., 2010).

Skin Care

Skin integrity should be monitored carefully because increased fatigue and weakness at the end of life may lead to decreased movement, resulting in pressure over bony prominences. Edema, bruising, dryness, and venous pooling may appear. The patient should be repositioned by using lift or draw sheets, being careful to avoid shearing forces; pressure-reducing surfaces, such as air mattresses or airbeds may help in alleviating pressure without the need to frequently reposition the patient. To promote comfort and reduce the risk of skin breakdown, gentle massage can be provided. The family may feel comfortable applying lotion to the back or hands of their loved one, again allowing participation in the care of their loved one. Areas

of nonblanching erythema and actual breakdown should never be massaged because the pressure exacerbates tissue damage that is already occurring.

Incontinence Care

Bowel and bladder incontinence are frequent occurrences at the end of life. Seepage from body orifices may be uncontrolled and it becomes necessary to have protective pads or briefs. It is extremely important to prevent decubitus ulcers from forming at this time because further breakdown due to contact with urine and feces is common. Barrier creams and change of position may help maintain skin integrity. The nurse should discourage the use of indwelling urinary catheters if at all possible because they often are associated with urinary tract infections that can be distressing and painful to the older patient.

Terminal Delirium

Terminal delirium can be a distressing phenomenon for families and caregivers. It is common at the end of life, occurring in up to 88% of people with a terminal illness in the last days of life (Keeley, 2010). Typically, terminal delirium presents as confusion, restlessness, and/or agitation, with or without day–night reversal. Visual, auditory, and olfactory hallucinations may occur during this time. It is important for the nurse to understand that this condition is often irreversible, and that the patient's experience of the delirium may be very different from what is witnessed by caregivers. In the older adult, delirium is often a presenting aspect of acute illness or exacerbation of chronic illness. Further complicating the issue, delirium may exist concomitantly with dementia in the older adult. Management of delirium includes identification and treatment of underlying causes (infection, electrolyte imbalances), reduction of environmental stimuli, provision of a safe environment, and reduction of anxiety. All nonessential medications (those not needed for comfort) should be discontinued when goals of care so dictate. Pain and other medications used for comfort such as benzodiazepines (lorazepam) and neuroleptics (haloperidol) should be provided.

Complementary and Alternative Therapies

Patients and families may request complementary and alternative medicine (CAM) be provided at the end-of-life to relieve multiple symptoms. Traditional medicine may share the spotlight with such therapies as acupuncture, massage therapy, Reiki therapy, chiropractic care, or herbal medicine. Use of CAM at the end of life is associated with reduction of pain, breathlessness, and anxiety as well as improvement in mood and sense of control (Bercovitz, Sengupta, Jones et al., 2011). Increasing recognition of the benefits of CAM has resulted in increased popularity of its use in palliative and hospice care. A recent report of the National Center for Health Statistics found that in 2007, 41.8% of hospice providers offered CAM to their patients and approximately one third to one half of patients at the end of life use some form of CAM (Bercovitz et al., 2011). The most common types of CAM offered by hospice providers were massage, supportive group therapy, music therapy, pet therapy, guided imagery and relaxation, and therapeutic touch.

HPNA has developed a position statement regarding the use of complementary therapies in end-of-life care. According to HPNA (2011b), nurses working in end-of-life care need to acknowledge the increasing popularity and use of CAM and "recognize that many complementary therapies provide a holistic approach to managing symptoms and promoting wellness at the end of life. The holistic approach is consistent with nursing's historical and philosophical methods of practice" (p. 3). The nurse should be aware of resources about CAM methods so that patients can be guided in making informed decisions about their plan of care (HPNA, 2011b). The National Center for Complementary and Alternative Medicine (NCCAM), the federal government's agency for scientific research on CAM, is one such resource.

Table 11-4 summarizes suggested strategies for the management of common symptoms in older patients at the end of life.

TABLE 11-4 **Suggested Strategies for the Management of Common Symptoms in Older Patients at the End of Life**

Problem	Suggested Nursing Intervention
Constipation	Stimulant such as prune juice, senna, or lactulose. Avoid bulking agents (psyllium) in patients with inadequate fluid intake to avoid impaction. Monitor bowel function. Do not allow the patient to go longer than 3 days without a bowel movement. A mineral oil enema may be necessary to prevent impaction.
Delirium	Treat underlying cause if possible (fever, urinary tract infection, pain). Avoid use of physical restraints, sleep disruption, excessive medications. Urge family to remain with the patient, and have staff frequently visit and speak to and touch the patient. Use alternative interventions such as massage and music.
Dyspnea	Treat underlying cause if known (bronchospasm, hypoxia). Administer opioids to slow respiratory rate. Maintain the patient in a sitting position if possible. Minimize exertion by spreading out interventions and treatments. Provide humidified oxygen for comfort. Use alternative interventions such as massage and music.
Decubitus Ulcers	Use appropriate positioning techniques, changing position every 2 hours. Keep the patient's skin clean and dry. Use special mattress pads to relieve pressure.
Cough	Assess and treat underlying cause such as postnasal drip or obstruction. Use chest physical therapy, cool humidified air, elevate head of the bed, and suction secretions as necessary. Cough suppressants may be used for comfort.
Anorexia and Cachexia	The etiology of cachexia is rarely reversible in advanced disease, and aggressive nutritional treatment does not improve survival or quality of life and may create discomfort for the dying patient whose body is shutting down. Provide excellent mouth care. Treat oral problems such as candidiasis (thrush). Treat constipation, nausea, and vomiting if present as underlying causes. Assess the room for problem odors and try to minimize them as much as possible. Generally, parenteral or enteral nutrition is useful only for patients with an appetite who cannot swallow. Offer the patient's favorite food and fluids as the patient tolerates.
Nausea and Vomiting (N&V)	N&V occurs in up to 70% of patients at the end of life. Causes include metabolic disturbances, visceral disturbances, vestibular problems, medication side effects, emotional upset, and radiation. Assess cause and treat if possible (e.g., remove offending medication). Medications used to treat N&V include anticholinergics, steroids, benzodiazepines, and antiemetics (ondansetron and granisetron). Anticipate N&V and administer medications if needed before symptoms occur. Position the patient to prevent aspiration. Use complementary therapies such as music, relaxation, hypnosis, and acupuncture.
Fatigue	Fatigue is a subjective sense of tiredness or lack of energy that interferes with usual functioning. It may be disease related, treatment related, or psychological. If tolerated, exercise can improve function and sleep. Frequent rest periods and transfusions for very anemic patients may improve quality of life.
Anxiety	Anxiety may be a side effect of many medications such as stimulants and corticosteroids, or a paradoxical reaction to analgesics. Antidepressants and benzodiazepines may be beneficial.

Sources: ELNEC, 2008; Emanuel et al., 2010.

> **Practice Pearl** ▶▶▶ Read a poem, tell a joke, listen to a story about the past, sing a song, report on recent news happenings, linger for a moment, or provide a hug. The nurse should be creative and individualize the care for each patient.

The Dying Process

The nurse's views, knowledge, emotional development, and cultural background help determine how effectively he or she may deal with the death process. Witnessing a death is an intimate experience and a privilege of the nursing profession. Nurses caring for the dying person must be sensitive to the needs of the dying person and the family. Accepting and facing one's own mortality helps nurses deal with the death of others. The fear of watching death needs to be conquered to prevent those responses from being transmitted to the patient and the family.

As terminal illness progresses and the older adult nears death, neurological changes occur and the patient slips from a lethargic state into an unconscious state (which may include periods of lucidness), then coma, and finally death. Family members frequently ask how much longer their loved one will live, and the anxiety and distress of family and friends at this time may be great. The exact time of death cannot be predicted any easier than the time of birth. This may be frustrating to those who are at the bedside.

Before death, there are many physiological processes that must be explained and interpreted to the patient (if possible) and their family and caregivers. An expected set of physiological changes typically occurs when death is imminent related to gradual hypoxia, respiratory acidosis, and renal failure. When these changes are witnessed, the nurse plays an integral role in assisting the family to plan for the actual death (HPNA, 2011c). Some of the physiological changes that the nurse might expect are as follows:

- Lower extremities may become mottled, taking place days or hours before the actual death.
- Saliva and oropharyngeal secretions may build up due to loss of the ability to swallow and lead to gurgling, crackling, or rattling sounds with breathing. This is sometimes referred to as the "death rattle," although this terminology should be avoided as it is often distressing to family members.
- Changes in respiratory patterns (shallow breaths with periods of apnea) may indicate significant neurological declines with Cheyne-Stokes respirations often heralding the impending death.
- Skin may appear dusky or gray, and feel cold or clammy.
- Eyes may appear discolored, deeper set, or bruised.

Witnessing these body changes can be disturbing to family members. Although it is extremely difficult to assure the patient or family that death will happen within a certain time frame, the nurse's approach and explanations of the death process are reassuring to those present. Some family members may want to be present when death happens, and others may want to be nearby but not physically present; it is important for the nurse to support whatever decision is comfortable for the dying person and the family. Furthermore, the older adult may wish to die quietly alone because it may be difficult for the dying person to have loved ones near. Others find comfort in having family or staff present. The dying process is as individual as living.

When respirations cease and the stethoscope does not detect breath sounds or heart sounds, the nurse should use the stethoscope or manually check the patient's carotid pulses. Next, the nurse should check the eyes for pupillary light reflex. If the pupils are fixed and dilated and the heart has stopped beating, the patient can be pronounced dead. Other signs that death has occurred include skin color becoming pale and waxen, cooling body temperature, relaxation of muscles and sphincters, and the release of urine and stool (Emanuel et al., 2010). The nurse should note the time death occurred and chart appropriately, notify the attending physician of the death, and chart the time of notification as well as any directions. In certain settings a nurse may make the death pronouncement, including long-term care. Next, the nurse notifies family members of the death and expresses condolences. Even if the family is expecting the death, the actual notification may be shocking to the family and needs to be handled gently and with empathy. If the family is present, they should be allowed sufficient time to spend with the deceased before having the body removed.

Postmortem Care

One of the most difficult but essential parts of nursing is providing **postmortem care,** or the care provided after the death of a patient. It needs to be done promptly, quietly, efficiently, and with dignity, thereby communicating to the family that the deceased person was valued and respected. Spiritual, cultural, and religious practices of the family should be considered to promote comfort and ease anxiety at a time of stress. The nurse may invite the family to talk about their loved one and encourage the family to touch and hold the person's body as they feel comfortable. If possible, before death occurs, the limbs should be straightened and the head placed on a pillow. If the death is suspicious or occurs outside of a healthcare facility, the coroner may request the body be left undisturbed until an autopsy can be performed. However, most deaths of older people who die in their own homes, hospitals, hospices, and long-term care facilities are not investigated by the coroner.

After the pronouncement, the nurse should glove, remove all tubes, replace soiled dressings, pad the anal area in case of drainage, and gently wash the body to remove any discharges. The body is placed on the back, with head and shoulders elevated on a pillow. The nurse should grasp the eyelashes and gently pull the lids down. Dentures should be inserted. It is important not to tie or secure any body parts because this may cause skin indentations. A clean gown should be placed on the body and a clean sheet pulled up to the shoulders. When the body is moved or the extremities repositioned, the body may produce respiratory-type sounds or the chest may appear to rise and fall. This can be alarming, but is only the sound of air leaving the lungs. The nurse may want to check for respiration sounds again in order to be reassured that the patient is dead. The nurse should gather eyeglasses and prepare necessary paperwork for the removal of the body from the facility; call the funeral home, morgue, or other personnel for the removal of the body; and note the time in the chart as well as who was called and again chart when the body was released and to whom. It is advisable to also note if eyeglasses, dentures, or any personal artifacts were released with the body and to whom they were given. If the facility has a policy to identify the body with an identification tag, it must be secured properly.

Advance Care Planning

Decision making around the time of death raises many legal and ethical questions. Public debate and scrutiny help shape the ethical outcome of medical dilemmas. Healthcare professionals must work within the limits of the law and their professional standards of practice. Established ethical principles and moral norms play a vital role in determining end-of-life healthcare issues.

Advance Directives

Advance directives are legal documents that allow people to convey their wishes for end-of-life care and include living wills, durable powers of attorney for health care, and healthcare proxies. In 1976, the Karen Ann Quinlan case brought life-sustaining medical treatment to the forefront of the U.S. legal system. A medical intervention, procedure, or administration of medicine to prevent the moment of death is seen as life sustaining. This includes cardiopulmonary resuscitation (CPR), renal dialysis, use of ventilators, insertion of feeding tubes, total parenteral nutrition, chemotherapies, and other life-prolonging interventions. When questions regarding the initiation, ongoing use, and removal of life-sustaining technologies arise and there are no advance directives in place, ethical and emotional

issues arise. Many hospitals and long-term care facilities have formed ethics committees to address these issues and provide guidance and advice to the clinician, patient, and family. If the patient lacks a responsible family member, the courts may appoint a legal guardian. This is a cumbersome and difficult process and may be avoided by naming a healthcare proxy or completing a living will.

In 1990, the U.S. Supreme Court declared that all Americans have a right to make healthcare decisions. Even if a patient is deemed incompetent or unable to make his or her own decisions, the patient's previous wishes become the determining factor concerning care. The Patient Self-Determination Act became a federal law in 1991. This act states that the patient must be informed that medical treatment, care, procedures, medicines, and other similar acts may be refused. It also states that patients are to be informed of their right to prepare advance directives.

Most healthcare institutions have developed policies concerning self-determination that comply with specific state laws. The interdisciplinary team needs to form a collaborative relationship with the patient and family in providing proper care as determined by state statutes. When the patient is unable to make decisions, the healthcare team must consider the patient's diagnosis, the benefit or burden of treatment, the effect on the prognosis, and expressed verbal patient preference. Family members or other concerned individuals or surrogates may be involved and should be included in the decision-making process. Reevaluation must be ongoing as the patient's situation changes throughout the entire course of illness and treatment. Although a patient's decision-making capacity may be fluctuating or limited, the patient at times may be able to understand some of the medical situation and even provide or express preferences through nonverbal communication.

Many Americans are fearful of death and hesitate to discuss end-of-life preferences with their families and significant others. This can be problematic when the older person becomes very ill or incapacitated and the family is consulted for medical decision making. People of all ages should begin to discuss these issues with others who may be called on to make decisions if serious illness or injury should occur. This should be done in a noncrisis situation when the older person has time to discuss the issue in depth, ask questions, and think about the risks and benefits of various interventions.

Legal requirements for advance directives vary from state to state; some state laws mandate the use of living wills, others require designation of a healthcare proxy or durable power of attorney for health care. A **healthcare proxy** or **durable power of attorney for health care** is an agent (and an alternate if the primary proxy is not available) designated to make decisions for the older adult if he or she is unable to do so. All of these documents go into effect when the older adult is no longer able to communicate his or her wishes. **Living wills** are legal documents in which older adults describe their wishes regarding treatment at the end of life; this may include acceptance or limitation of life-sustaining treatment in the face of a life-threatening illness. Note, however, that living wills do not allow for selection of a healthcare decision maker should older adults become unable to do so themselves. The older adult should discuss his or her wishes with their identified healthcare proxy or durable power of attorney for health care to ensure appropriate end-of-life care. The healthcare proxy is only responsible for healthcare decisions should the older person be unable to make decisions and does not have legitimate input into any other areas of the older person's affairs, including financial.

Multiple copies of all advance directives should be made and kept in an accessible location by the older adult, a family member or designated healthcare agent, and the older adult's healthcare provider. Often, older adults and their healthcare designee lock the advance directives in a safety deposit box where it is not accessible by others in emergency situations and therefore cannot be honored. The nurse should educate the older adult to keep the documents in a secure but accessible location and to inform their families and healthcare designees of that location. A sample healthcare proxy form is provided in Figure 11-3 ▶▶▶.

Level of Care Designation

Frail older patients and their families face difficult decisions when nearing the end of life. Providing good end-of-life care is often limited by the uncertain prognoses of many chronic illnesses in this population (heart failure, dementia, chronic renal failure). Uncertain prognoses may affect decision making on the part of older adults, their families, and their healthcare providers, leading to overly aggressive intervention and treatments. Older adults have high comorbidity rates and an increased likelihood of dementia, complicating acute illness and aggressive care. For some patients, medical treatments offer little or no benefit and at the same time may be painful or increase the burden of living. Nurses, physicians, social workers, clergy, and others are responsible for counseling patients and families to make decisions regarding the type and level of care they wish to receive for the remainder of their lives. After the decision has been reached, it is usually noted in the patient's chart so that the entire healthcare team will be aware of the patient's wishes. Of course, the patient is always able to reverse these decisions.

An older patient may decide to receive **comfort measures only (CMO),** or allow death to occur naturally

while maximizing comfort. CMO is often the preferred choice when the end of life nears and the time comes to think of care over cure. The use of life-sustaining technologies should be reviewed with the seriously ill older patient and his or her family. If the patient is in an intensive care unit, palliative care and comfort measures may be emphasized and encouraged. Those patients who wish for CMO may receive traditional hospice care with all of the efforts of the healthcare professionals focused on quality of life rather than length of life.

The CMO status is usually ordered by the physician or advanced practice nurse when the patient, family, and staff are in agreement that the best care for the patient is not to prolong the dying process, but to keep the patient as comfortable as possible. Comfort becomes the focus of care when cure is no longer an attainable goal, expected quality of life is unacceptable, and comfort is a priority for the patient and family (Moneymaker, 2005). This does not mean that nursing care or treatments are stopped. Alterations in skin, hydration, continence, activities of daily living, behaviors, and pain control are assessed and managed on a daily basis. Provision of excellent nursing care at the end of life can be a challenge, especially when the family has been told by the physician that "nothing more can be done." The designation of a patient as CMO does not signal the end of care, but rather shifts the focus of care from aggressive treatment of the disease to aggressive nursing interventions to improve function, comfort, and quality of life.

Personal values, past experiences, cultural beliefs, religious preferences, medical knowledge, family orientation, and life experiences all help in determining the end-of-life preferences and development of advance directives. Each older person and his or her family should provide input into treatment decisions based on goals of care, assessment of risk and benefit, best evidence, and personal preferences.

> **Practice Pearl** ▶▶▶ Legally acceptable advance directive documents vary from state to state. Remember to refer to the state law for the state in which the older adult lives to determine the appropriate forms to be completed.

Use of Artificial Nutrition and Hydration at the End of Life

Older adults with multiple comorbidities, cognitive deficits, and life-limiting, progressive illness often experience decreased appetite with loss of interest in eating and drinking and subsequent weight loss (HPNA, 2011b). Dysphagia related to advancing dementia or terminal illness may contribute to this issue. As patients near the end of life, most will be

---

Health Care Proxy

(1) I, _____

hereby appoint

_____

(name, home address and telephone number)

_____

_____

as my health care agent to make any and all health care decisions for me, except to the extent that I state otherwise. This proxy shall take effect only when and if I become unable to make my own health care decisions.

(2) **Optional: Alternate Agent**

If the person I appoint is unable, unwilling or unavailable to act as my health care agent, I hereby appoint

_____

(name, home address and telephone number)

_____

_____

as my health care agent to make any and all health care decisions for me, except to the extent that I state otherwise.

(3) Unless I revoke it or state an expiration date or circumstances under which it will expire, this proxy shall remain in effect indefinitely. *(Optional: If you want this proxy to expire, state the date or conditions here.)* This proxy shall expire *(specify date or conditions):*

_____

_____

(4) **Optional:** I direct my health care agent to make health care decisions according to my wishes and limitations, as he or she knows or as stated below. *(If you want to limit your agent's authority to make health care decisions for you or to give specific instructions, you may state your wishes or limitations here.)* I direct my health care agent to make health care decisions in accordance with the following limitations and/or instructions *(attach additional pages as necessary):*

_____

_____

In order for your agent to make health care decisions for you about artificial nutrition and hydration *(nourishment and water provided by feeding tube and intravenous line),* your agent must reasonably know your wishes. You can either tell your agent what your wishes are or include them in this section. See instructions for sample language that you could use if you choose to include your wishes on this form, including your wishes about artificial nutrition and hydration.

(5) **Your Identification** *(please print)*

Your Name _____

Your Signature _____ Date _____

Your Address _____

Figure 11-3 ▶▶▶ A sample healthcare proxy form.

Source: New York State. (2010). *Healthcare proxy. Information for consumers.* Retrieved from http://www.health.state.ny.us/nysdoh/hospital/healthcareproxy/instructions.htm. Reprinted/posted with permission of the New York State Department of Health.

Health Care Proxy (continued)

[6] **Optional: Organ and/or Tissue Donation**

I hereby make an anatomical gift, to be effective upon my death, of: (check any that apply)

☐ Any needed organs and/or tissues

☐ The following organs and/or tissues _____

_____

☐ Limitations _____

If you do not state your wishes or instructions about organ and/or tissue donation on this form, it will not be taken to mean that you do not wish to make a donation or prevent a person, who is otherwise authorized by law, to consent to a donation on your behalf.

Your Signature _____ Date _____

[7] **Statement by Witnesses** *(Witnesses must be 18 years of age or older and cannot be the health care agent or alternate.)*

I declare that the person who signed this document is personally known to me and appears to be of sound mind and acting of his or her own free will. He or she signed (or asked another to sign for him or her) this document in my presence.

Date   Date

_____   _____

Name of Witness 1   Name of Witness 2

(print) _____   *(print)* _____

Signature _____   Signature _____

Address _____   Address _____

_____   _____

Figure 11-3 ▶▶▶ *(continued)*

unable to or refuse to take food and fluids by mouth (HPNA, 2011b). These changes can cause distress, especially for families and other caregivers, and may lead to questions about initiation of artificial nutrition and hydration (ANH).

The decision to institute ANH should take into account possible benefits and risks. ANH traditionally has been assumed to meet several therapeutic goals: prolong life, prevent aspiration pneumonia and "starvation," maintain independence and physical function, improve nutritional status, assist in healing of pressure ulcers, and decrease suffering and discomfort at the end of life (HPNA, 2011b; Lacey, 2005). These goals, however, are not supported in the literature. Studies have shown that long-term care facility residents living with feeding tubes have similar survival rates as those living without and aspiration rates are higher in patients with feeding tubes (Lacey, 2005). Furthermore, artificial nutrition and nutritional supplements

do not enhance frail elders' strength and physical function (ELNEC, 2008; Hallenbeck, 2005; HPNA, 2011b). Also contrary to expectations, most actively dying patients do not experience hunger even if they have inadequate caloric intake. In fact, risks such as increased infection, sensory deprivation, and restraint use have led researchers and palliative care experts to discourage the use of feeding tubes in dying patients and those with advanced dementia. Collaboration with other healthcare professionals (nutritionists and speech therapists) is indicated to explore alternatives to artificial nutrition techniques.

Older patients who feel strongly that they do not want tube feedings should inform their healthcare proxies and specify this wish in their living wills. Administration of ANH is considered a medical treatment and thus can be accepted or rejected by the patient. This right reflects respect for patient autonomy.

Cardiopulmonary Resuscitation

Cardiopulmonary resuscitation (CPR) is administered to a person experiencing cardiac or respiratory arrest; simply put, it is the process of restarting the heartbeat and/or breathing after one or both has stopped. This intervention is most successful when it occurs in the hospital, specifically in the ICU. However, when the older adult is frail, has multiple chronic conditions, and is nearing end of life, CPR is significantly less effective. Several studies have demonstrated that attempts at resuscitation in long-term care residents are rarely successful. The decision to designate an older person with a do-not-resuscitate (DNR) order is usually made by the older person, his or her family, the nurse, physician, and others on the healthcare team. In most healthcare facilities, the physician or primary healthcare provider must write the DNR order in the chart for it to be legal; if no order is written, CPR must be administered by default if the need arises. It can be very upsetting for the nurse to provide CPR to the ill older adult, and the patient may suffer injury from anoxia, broken ribs, and aspiration.

When the nurse approaches the older patient and the family for clarification of the patient's code status, it is best to discuss the issue as fully and objectively as possible. Facts should be presented with empathy and by conveyance of the idea that the nurse will support whatever reasonable decision is made. This conversation should be part of an ongoing discussion of the patient's wishes and goals for end-of-life care. According to the ANA (2003), "the efficacy and desirability of CPR attempts, a balancing of benefits and burdens to the patient, and therapeutic goals should be considered" (p. 1). The nurse should emphasize that the decision not to resuscitate is not condemning that person to die. Rather, the nurse is helping the person decide whether medical intervention might reverse the death process and even prohibit a peaceful death.

Requests for Assisted Death

Patients with advanced disease who are suffering from physical and emotional pain, functional declines, and multiple losses may express a desire for hastened death (Hudson et al., 2006). Such requests indicate a high degree of suffering, and it is important for the nurse to listen to the person's request and validate his or her suffering. Next the nurse should consult with the patient's medical team so that a comprehensive assessment may be undertaken, preferably by a palliative care or hospice team. Most pain and other causes of suffering can be relieved to acceptable levels with the right treatment plan. If not, however, there are several legally accepted measures the older adult with might take to hasten death, including voluntarily withholding nutrition and hydration, terminal sedation in which a person is sedated to control pain and suffering,

and withdrawal of unwanted life-sustaining therapies (HPNA, 2011a). Although these situations may be distressing to the nurse, the request for assisted death causes the greatest clinical, ethical, and legal dilemma (HPNA, 2011a).

Assisted death refers to a clinician's act of providing a means of suicide, such as medication, a prescription, information, or other intervention, to a patient, knowing the patient's intent to commit suicide. The patient then acts to end his or her own life. There are rare occasions when a medication given for pain relief may have the unintended consequence of shortening the patient's life; however, because the intent of the medication is relief of pain and not the hastening of death, this is not considered assisted death. In 1994, Oregon residents voted to legalize physician-assisted suicide (PAS), which refers to a physician acting to aid a person in ending his or her life. As of 2010, Montana and Washington had also legalized PAS. Terminally ill residents of these three states may receive prescriptions for lethal doses of medications from their physician for self-administration. The ANA (1994) does not endorse the concept of, or participation of nurses in the process of, euthanasia, mercy killing, or assisted suicide.

Cultural Issues

People of many cultural backgrounds reside in the United States. Culture is a group's worldviews and values and encompasses dimensions such as race, ethnicity, gender, age, abilities/disabilities, sexual orientation, religion and spirituality, and socioeconomic status (Bullock, 2011). An ever-changing system, culture is shaped over time as beliefs, values, and lifestyle patterns are passed from generation to generation. Sensitivity and empathy are essential when caring for a dying person from a different culture. Each older person is a unique individual with cultural preferences that influence the specialized needs of the patient, the family, and their caregivers. (See Chapter 4 🔗 for a thorough discussion of culture.)

As the population of ethnic minorities grows in the United States, nurses must be sensitive to the values of the different cultural groups for whom they may care. Care at the end of life is emotionally charged and brings up multiple issues around how different cultural groups wish to receive "bad news," identification of the family decision maker, and "truth-telling" (Searight & Gafford, 2005). For example, in the United States, emphasis and value is placed on "truth-telling," ensuring patients have full understanding of the extent of their disease process so that they can make informed decisions about their care. Outside the United States, this communication may not be as valued and family members may actively protect terminally ill family members from knowledge about their condition.

Some cultures view disclosure of bad news as taking away hope, or that once disclosed, the words may become reality.

Despite efforts to improve access to palliative care to all older adults, improvements are not reaching minority populations. The SUPPORT Principal Investigators (1995) reported that fewer resources were expended on African American patients than on those with similar disease processes; other studies have noted that minority patients are significantly less likely to receive appropriate pain management (APF, 2011). Recent reports reveal that, during the past 5 years, there has been little or no change in the rates of hospice utilization among Black and Latino patients, despite steady increases in the enrollment of patients in hospice (NHPCO, 2010). Disparities result from a multitude of sources including limited access to care, low socioeconomic status, and an underlying mistrust of the healthcare system (APF, 2011) and it is well documented in the literature that African American patients often wish for aggressive life-sustaining interventions in the face of terminal disease (Searight & Gafford, 2005). These patients may choose feeding tubes and CPR because of fears of being denied health care similar in scope to that of Caucasians.

Spirituality and Religion

Spirituality and religion play an important role in the forming of beliefs and practices that are paramount when death is imminent. It is important to note that the terms *religion* and *spirituality* are not interchangeable. Religion typically refers to an organized system of beliefs, practices, and rituals that characterize a community in a particular way (usually based on a belief in a divine being). Spirituality is more broadly defined, and relates to beliefs and practices that give meaning and purpose in an individual's life.

Most patients draw comfort from their spiritual and/or religious beliefs as they face the end of life. Feelings of guilt, remorse, comfort, or peacefulness may all be related to such beliefs. Spiritual and religious customs are extremely important to many dying patients, and concerns or fears may be intensified as death nears. It is helpful to know the preference of an individual, but each patient's spiritual reactions to situations are highly individualized. Requests by family or patients to seek spiritual counseling should be met with respect. Many healthcare facilities have chaplains, clergy, social workers, and others to assist staff. Spiritual care should be individualized and made available to the terminal patient. A consensus panel to improve the quality of spiritual care in palliative care stated that adequate assessment of religious or spiritual needs is necessary to develop a comprehensive care plan at the end of life (Puchalski et al., 2009).

At times, a religious belief may help the patient in determining the type of end-of-life care to request. Nurses must be aware of concerns the patient may have and respond therapeutically. The age-old question "Why is this happening to me?" may take on religious tones or thoughts. Punishment, atonement, God's will, or hope for a miracle may all be discussed or alluded to by the patient. Follow the patient's lead in determining spiritual needs and beliefs. Serious illnesses frequently initiate a search for life's meaning and questions may arise regarding the individual's purpose in life. Even the emotional response to pain may be influenced by religious or spiritual beliefs.

When discussing religion or spirituality with the patient, it is important to assist the patient to seek meaning. Nurses who feel unable to assist older patients in discussions of spirituality should make referrals to others on the team with skills and knowledge in this area. Spiritual care interventions that may be chosen by the older person to affirm life and hope include renewal of vows, faith readings, guided meditation, receiving sacraments, spiritual life review, and discussion of spiritual pain (ELNEC, 2008).

It is common for one of Catholic faith to wish to receive the Sacrament of the Sick to give spiritual strength and prepare for death. A religious item such as a rosary or medal may bring comfort. The Jewish believer may want to see a rabbi and participate in prayers. Burial is performed as soon as possible and before the Sabbath. Muslims may prefer that a family member be notified as soon as death occurs. It is best to wait for the member since there are special washing and shrouding procedures. Islam believers also may prefer that the family wash the body. The body is then placed in a position that faces Mecca. If there is no family member to prepare the body, the staff may do so provided that gloves are worn. Cremation is not accepted, and burial of the body takes place as quickly as possible. Table 11-5 summarizes some religious beliefs and rituals practiced at the end of life.

Preparing for Death

The knowledge or presumption that death is imminent may cause anxiety for the staff, family, and patient. Watching the body shut down life processes can bring feelings of helplessness and anxiety. Questions of an afterlife, unresolved emotional or social issues, concerns centered on family members and their acceptance of death, and financial matters are common issues generated at the end of life. It is part of the nursing role to attempt to allay the fears of patients and families at this time. Nurses must also remember to support themselves through this difficult period, recognizing and accepting an array of personal feelings. Nurses may

redefine hope

TABLE 11-5	Selected Religions and End-of-Life Care	
Religion	**Belief**	**Ritual**
Christian	Christians believe in an afterlife and the resurrection of Jesus Christ.	Catholic • Anointing the sick by a priest. • Reconciliation and communion. • Funeral held 2 to 3 days after death. Protestant • No last rites. • Anointing of the sick by some. Others • Mormons will administer a sacrament. • Jehovah's Witnesses will not receive blood transfusions. • Some sects have hands-on healing techniques.
Judaism	Death confers meaning to life.	Euthanasia is prohibited. Burial usually takes place within 24 hours. The funeral or shivah is held after the burial. Autopsy, organ donation, and cremation are not allowed. A rabbi is usually called when death is near.
Muslim	Muslims believe in an afterlife. The purpose of worldly life is to prepare for eternal life.	As death approaches, the patient is positioned by lying facing toward Mecca. Family members recite prayers and encourage the dying person to repeat the statement of faith. Physician-assisted suicide is prohibited. Discussion of death and grief counseling are discouraged. Organ donation is allowed. Autopsy is discouraged.
Buddhist	Belief in the afterlife through the pursuit of perfection in worldly life.	End-of-life decisions are made with much family consultation. Families often do not want the patient to know diagnosis in order to hide bad news. Older adults do not talk about funeral arrangements and often defer to physicians to make treatment decisions for them.

Sources: Adapted from Burton & Gurevitz, 2010; Puchalski, Dorff, Hebbar et al., 2011.

need individual support as well as team support from outside the healthcare facility in order to express and accept their true feelings. By doing this, burnout may be prevented.

Hope should never be denied the dying patient and family. The nurse should recognize that hope is an ever-changing phenomenon within the context of terminal illness. Hope for a cure is not unusual for both the patient and family throughout the illness trajectory. As disease worsens, the older adult may hope for small things to make the present situation more tolerable such as a favorite meal or a visit from a family member. Living to see a grandchild graduate from college or the birth of a great-grandchild may become a hope of the older adult. Near the end of life, hopes may again transition to include such things as a comfortable death or death in the home. It is not unusual for patients to hope to speak with loved ones before they die. The will to live is extremely strong in many older adults confronting death, especially when there is a sense of unfinished business. Older

patients sometimes need reassurance from their families and caregivers that all is well and it is okay to let go.

Grief, Loss, and Bereavement

Grief refers to the complex emotional reaction that is felt after a **loss,** or a separation from a person, thing, relationship, or situation to which one was emotionally attached. Although loss associated with death may be expected, grief is experienced by the family, friends, and caregivers in many different ways. Factors that may affect the grief experience include the survivor's coping skills, cultural background, belief and faith systems, and past life experiences (ELNEC, 2008). Grief may begin before the death of the patient, as both the patient and their loved ones anticipate and experience losses associated with the dying process. Once the person has died, the grieving process may last for years and affect survivors physically, psychologically, socially, and

TABLE 11-6	Types of Grief	
Type of Grief	**Definition**	**Nursing Considerations**
Normal Grief	Experience of sadness and loss, defined as uncomplicated grief. Feelings, behaviors, and reactions to a loss are consistent with the expectations of a person's experience, culture, social role, and relationship with the deceased. Reactions may include pain, distress, and physical and emotional suffering.	Grieving process may take years. Rates of depression are highest during the caregiving period and during the first few months after death, then decrease over time.
Anticipatory Grief	Also known as preparatory grief. Occurs before a loss associated with a diagnosis, illness, or death and is experienced by the patient, family, and caregivers. Feelings may include fear of actual or potential losses, including loss of health, independence, financial stability, choice, or mental function.	Anticipation and an opportunity to prepare psychologically for death may ease the grieving process after death. Asking questions such as "What are your thoughts about the future?" or "Have you been feeling sad or depressed?" may help the nurse assess for anticipatory grief.
Complicated Grief	Extends beyond the normal grieving process. Survivor may feel hopeless and depressed, and the grief may affect a person's ability to care for him- or herself or others.	Factors that may contribute to complicated grief in older adults include lack of a support network, multiple, concurrent losses, and poor coping skills. Requires the intervention of a physician.

Sources: ELNEC, 2008; MacKenzie, 2011; MacPhee & Bickel, 2008.

spiritually. Table 11-6 describes several types of grief. **Bereavement** includes the inner feelings and outward reactions of the survivor associated with loss. The recovery from the loss is referred to as the period of **mourning.**

> *Practice Pearl* ▶▶▶ Patients, families, and caregivers should be allowed to express their emotions as they cope with loss. Sit quietly with grieving individuals and listen to their concerns, fears, feelings, and emotions. This is a simple, but critical, nursing intervention.

As older adults age, the accumulation of losses they experience may compound the effects of grief and bereavement associated with death. The normal grief process may include these responses:

- **Numb shock.** There is disbelief that death has occurred. This phase is marked by shock, emotional dullness, and restless behavior that may include stupor and withdrawal. It may include physical characteristics such as nausea or insomnia.
- **Emotional turmoil or depression.** Alarm or panic-type reactions occur. Emotional expression may include crying, low mood, sleep disturbance, and anorexia. Anger,

guilt, or longing for the deceased may take place. The bereaved may also become preoccupied with the meaning of the loss.

- **Reorganization or resolution.** Reorganization eventually takes place and coping strategies and positive outlooks emerge. A final resolution phase leads to acceptance of the loss. The bereaved will return to prior levels of functioning.

When the realization of the loss of a loved one sets in, so do regret, self-doubt, and, at times, despair. Life's purpose becomes confusing and mood swings are prevalent. Being alone in the house may be a major problem. The nurse may also encourage the older adult to focus on activities such as volunteer work. While actively participating in such activities, older adults often find the affection and companionship needed at this time.

The nurse should utilize an interdisciplinary team of physicians, nurses, social workers, volunteers, and grief and bereavement counselors to facilitate the grief and bereavement process (ELNEC, 2008). Roles of interdisciplinary team members may include identifying grief, developing strategies to help the bereaved manage grief, and recognizing the need for psychiatric intervention if abnormal or complicated grief develops (MacKenzie, 2011).

Caring for the Caregiver

Most nurses enter the profession to make a difference in others' lives. However, to prevent feelings of stress and burnout, those caring for the dying need support and an opportunity to express emotional responses and grief. A periodic self-assessment might be beneficial to the nurse providing end-of-life care. Some questions may include:

- What have I done to meet my own needs today?
- Have I laughed today?
- Did I eat properly, rest enough, exercise, and play today?
- What have I felt today?
- Do I have something to look forward to?

Caring for oneself prevents anger, frustration, and anxiety. It makes it possible to continue to be a sensitive caregiver. It is important not to neglect personal needs.

The art of healing requires knowing and nourishing oneself. Giving to others, treating patients with dignity and respect, and being compassionate are trademarks of a nurse. Patients give these same gifts back, and help instruct the nurse on how to care. The partnership of caring and receiving becomes gifts given and received.

QSEN Recommendations Related to End-of-Life Care

The Quality and Safety Education for Nurses (QSEN) project addresses the challenge of preparing future nurses with the knowledge, skills, and attitudes (KSAs) to continuously improve the quality and safety of the healthcare systems in which they work (Cronenwett et al., 2007). See the QSEN table for tips on meeting QSEN standards.

Patient and Family Teaching

Gerontological nurses require skills and knowledge related to teaching patients and families about the key concepts of gerontology and gerontological nursing. The guidelines in the following feature will assist the nurse to assume the role of teacher and coach.

Meeting QSEN Standards: End-of-Life Care

	KNOWLEDGE	SKILLS	ATTITUDES
Patient-Centered Care	Possess an understanding of the dimensions of patient-centered care including communication preferences, physical comfort, and emotional support.	Elicit and communicate patient and family values, preferences, and needs.	Support patient-centered care for individuals and groups whose values differ from one's own.
	Demonstrate understanding of the concepts of palliative care and hospice.	Assess levels of physical and emotional comfort.	Appreciate the role of the nurse in relieving pain and suffering.
Teamwork and Collaboration	Recognize contributions of interdisciplinary team members.	Integrate contributions of interdisciplinary team as a means of helping the patient/family achieve goals at the end of life.	Value teamwork and the importance of professional collaboration.
	Describe own strengths, limitations, and values as a member of the interdisciplinary team.	Initiate plan for self-development as a team member caring for patients at the end of life.	Respect the differing strengths and values that members bring to a team.
Evidence-Based Practice	Explain the role of evidence in determining best clinical practice.	Access current evidence-based protocols to guide care plan development.	Value the need for continuous improvement in the clinical practice of end-of-life care.
Quality Improvement	Describe strategies for learning about the outcomes of care in end-of-life care.	Seek information about quality improvement projects in end-of-life care, including pain and symptom management.	Appreciate that continuous quality improvement is a key component of good patient care.
Safety	Discuss potential and actual impact of national patient safety resources and initiatives.	Use national patient safety resources for professional development.	Value relationship between national safety campaigns and their implementation in local practice settings.
Informatics	Describe how technology and information management are related to quality and safety.	Use information management tools to monitor outcomes.	Value nurses' involvement in design, selection, implementation, and evaluation of information technologies.

Patient-Family Teaching Guidelines

The following are guidelines that the nurse may find useful when instructing older adults and their families about their choices at the end of life.

CHOICES AT THE END OF LIFE

1 **I am seriously ill. My physician has recommended a palliative care program. Does that mean I am dying?**

No. Palliative care is a program of care that can be delivered to any person who is seriously ill. Palliative care programs have been developed to provide for pain and symptom control, to help with patient-centered communication and decision making, and to coordinate care across settings. Aggressive care and palliative care can be delivered at the same time by your healthcare provider, thus ensuring your comfort during the treatment process.

RATIONALE:

Older patients and their families may require reassurance when they are considering choosing palliative care programs, because they are relatively new and may not be completely understood. The principles of palliative care should be clearly delineated to prevent misunderstanding and confusion.

2 **How is palliative care delivered?**

The main approach is the relief of suffering through the management of pain and distressing symptoms such as nausea, bowel function, sleep, and nutrition. A team of healthcare experts will address your needs, including physicians, nurses, social workers, nutritionists, pharmacists, chaplains, and others. Because a person with serious illness has a variety of needs, it takes a team of experts to deliver quality care.

RATIONALE:

Older patients and their families may be unfamiliar with the roles and expertise of various members of the healthcare team. A coordinated team approach with good communication between members is essential to the provision of palliative care.

3 **Does my insurance cover palliative care?**

Many insurance programs cover the delivery of palliative care, and more are beginning to examine the payment of this service as a benefit for patients and families. In the long run, it may actually decrease costs to the healthcare system because it has the potential to decrease hospitalization for many things that can be prevented by the palliative care focus such as pain, dehydration, infections, constipation, and other symptoms.

RATIONALE:

Potential payment sources for palliative care services can include Medicare, Medicaid, private insurance, out-of-pocket payment, and community funds for uninsured patients. It is important to check with social worker colleagues to ensure that patients have accessed all possible funding sources for palliative care.

4 **What is the difference between hospice and palliative care?**

Generally, hospice programs accept patients who are near the end of life and are no longer receiving aggressive disease interventions such as chemotherapy and radiation. However, many hospice programs are expanding services and accepting patients who are not near the end of life but may benefit from the principles of palliative care, including the emphasis on pain and symptom control, while they are still receiving aggressive treatment for their illness. Most palliative care programs will help you and your family to receive the care you need in a variety of settings, including your home, the hospital, the long-term care facility, or a hospice if you need that kind of care.

RATIONALE:

The healthcare system is dynamic and complex. The patient and family may move in and out of various care settings as their condition changes over time. The integration of a palliative care program into a coordinated system is a big plus for patients and families. Most palliative care programs can make referrals to other care providers and coordinate services and movement between settings. These settings may include acute care hospitals, palliative care programs, home care agencies, and hospice programs.

CARE PLAN   An Older Person at the End of Life

Case Study

Mrs. Lodge is a 79-year-old woman who is admitted to the long-term care facility after a 6-day hospitalization for pneumonia and weight loss. She had previously lived at home alone. Her hospital discharge record notes that she has lost 15 lbs during the past 6 months and had complained of abdominal pain while in the hospital. A computerized tomograph (CT) scan noted a pancreatic mass, which was thought to be cancer of the pancreas. Other chronic conditions include hearing loss, type 2 diabetes, cataracts, and osteoarthritis. Today, Mrs. Lodge is lethargic and appears withdrawn. Her 58-year-old daughter is present and seems anxious about her mother's condition. Mrs. Lodge's daughter would like to take her home when her condition improves.

Applying the Nursing Process

Assessment

Mrs. Lodge has been diagnosed with a very aggressive form of cancer that usually carries a high treatment burden and a poor prognosis. In addition to her age, she has diagnoses that indicate frailty, including cataracts, weight loss, osteoarthritis, and diabetes. Based on this information, she could be considered a candidate for palliative care services or a hospice referral (depending on her physician's assessment of her prognosis).

Diagnosis

The current nursing diagnoses for Mrs. Lodge include the following:

- *Nutrition Imbalanced: Less Than Body Requirements*
- *Pain: Chronic (osteoarthritis) and Acute (pancreatic cancer)*
- *Activity Intolerance*
- *Fatigue*
- *Coping: Family, Compromised*
- *Risk for Spiritual Distress*

NANDA-I © 2012.

Expected Outcomes

Expected outcomes for the plan of care specify that Mrs. Lodge will:

- Achieve satisfactory pain relief.
- Be free from disabling symptoms associated with the end-of-life trajectory, including constipation, nausea, and disturbed sleep.
- Overcome her fatigue and lethargy as much as possible so that she has the opportunity to engage in discussion with her healthcare providers, daughter, significant others, and clergy (if appropriate) regarding her end-of-life decisions.
- Receive a hospice referral (if appropriate) so that services can be provided to allow Mrs. Lodge to die in her daughter's home if this is consistent with Mrs. Lodge's wishes.

Planning and Implementation

The following nursing interventions may be appropriate:

- Establish a therapeutic relationship.
- Conduct initial and ongoing pain assessment with use of pharmacological and nonpharmacological relief measures.
- Encourage a family meeting with daughter and other family members present to discuss end-of-life planning and care with Mrs. Lodge's permission.
- Consult with other members of the interdisciplinary team to evaluate safety, nutrition, spiritual needs, psychological status, and other key parameters.
- Begin a values clarification process to establish goals and facilitate end-of-life planning.

(continued)

An Older Person at the End of Life (continued)

Evaluation

The nurse will consider the plan a success based on the following criteria:

- Mrs. Lodge will achieve pain and symptom relief.
- A family meeting will be held to discuss her overall health.

- Mrs. Lodge will have access to appropriate services and family support in order to achieve a peaceful death in the setting of her choice.

Ethical Dilemma

As you are preparing to institute a hospice referral, another daughter who lives in a distant state telephones you and says that she feels her mother should receive aggressive chemotherapy to fight the cancer and possibly extend her life. The oncologist has agreed to begin chemotherapy, although he advises that the regimen will be quite toxic with little chance of success. Mrs. Lodge and the daughter who is involved in her care are unsure of what to do, but based on the advice of the palliative care nurse, and others on the healthcare team, they decide to refuse further chemotherapy. The nurse and the palliative care team support the decision to refuse treatment based on the oncologist's recommendation and Mrs. Lodge's preferences. She is competent to make her own decisions regarding treatment, and her refusal of treatment is appropriate to her unique circumstance and immediate family situation.

Critical Thinking and the Nursing Process

1. Speak to nurses and nursing assistants who work in one of your clinical rotations about the assessment of pain in the older patient. What factors do they identify as important?
2. Explain possible reasons caring for older patients at the end of life may be difficult. Tell a story in a small group of fellow students and observe their reactions.

3. Keep a clinical journal of your feelings and experiences as you begin to become proficient in providing end-of-life care to older people and their families.
4. Identify a few key people in your life who can help you as you struggle to become proficient in the provision of end-of-life care.

- Evaluate your responses in Appendix B ⊂▭⊃.

Chapter Highlights

- Studies have documented that the American healthcare system exhibits substantial shortcomings in the care of seriously ill patients and their families.
- Many older patients die in pain or suffering from adverse symptoms.
- Aggressive care that carries a high burden of treatment is often delivered inappropriately to older people because of communication barriers and lack of planning.
- The gerontological nurse can play a key role on the interdisciplinary team and serve as patient advocate, educator, care provider, and planner of quality end-of-life care.

- Pain and symptom control are crucial to the delivery of quality end-of-life care.
- Cultural and ethnic variations are key factors to be considered when providing end-of-life care.
- Palliative care and hospice programs can assist the nurse in the delivery of quality end-of-life care to older patients and their families.
- Families often rely on the nurse for support and assistance during the dying process and afterwards in the mourning and grieving period.

Pearson Nursing Student Resources
Find additional review materials at
nursing.pearsonhighered.com
Prepare for success with additional NCLEX®-style practice
questions, interactive assignments and activities, web links,
animations and videos, and more!

References

Administration on Aging. (2010). *A profile of older Americans: 2010*. Retrieved from http://www.aoa.gov/AoARoot/Aging_Statistics/Profile/2010/docs/2010profile.pdf

American Association of Colleges of Nursing. (2004). *Peaceful death: Recommended competencies and curricular guidelines for end of life nursing care*. Retrieved from http://www.aacn.nche.edu

American Geriatrics Society (AGS) Panel on the Pharmacological Management of Persistent Pain in Older Persons. (2009). Pharmacological management of persistent pain in older persons. *Journal of the American Geriatrics Society, 57*, 1331–1346.

American Nurses Association. (1994). *Position statement: Assisted suicide*. Retrieved from http://www.nursingworld.org/MainMenuCategories/Policy-Advocacy/Positions-and-Resolutions/ANAPositionStatements/Position-Statements-Alphabetically/prtetsuic14456.html

American Nurses Association. (2003). *Position statement on nursing care and do-not-resuscitate (DNR) decisions*. Washington, DC: Author.

American Nurses Association (ANA). (2010). *ANA position statement: Registered nurses' roles and responsibilities in providing expert care and counseling at the end of life*. Washington, DC: Author.

American Pain Foundation. (2011). *Topic brief: Pain management & disparities*. Retrieved from http://www.painfoundation.org/learn/publications/files/Disparities.pdf

Arias, E. (2011). *United States life tables, 2007: National vital statistics reports* (DHHS Publication No. PHS 2011-1120). Hyattsville, MD: National Center for Health Statistics.

Bercovitz, A., Sengupta, M., Jones, A., & Harris-Kojetin, L. D. (2011). Complementary and alternative therapies in hospice: The National Home and Hospice Care Survey: United States, 2007. *National Health Statistics Reports, 33*. Hyattsville, MD: National Center for Health Statistics.

Broglio, K., & Portenoy, R. K. (2011). End-of-life care: Pain management. *UpToDate*. Retrieved from http://www.uptodate.com

Bullock, K. (2011). The influence of culture on end-of-life decision making. *Journal of Social Work in End-of-Life & Palliative Care, 7*(1), 83–98.

Burton, E. C., & Gurevitz, S. A. (2010). *Religions and the autopsy*. Retrieved from http://emedicine.medscape.com/article/1705993-overview#showall

Cronenwett, L., Sherwood, G., Barnsteiner, J., Disch, J., Johnson, J. (Mitchell, P., Sullivan, D., & Warren, J. (2007). Quality and safety education for nurses, *Nursing Outlook, 55*(3) 122–131.

Doyle, D., & Woodruff, R. (2008). *The International Association for Hospice & Palliative Care (IAHPC) manual of palliative care* (2nd ed.). Retrieved from http://www.hospicecare.com/iahpc-manual/lahpc-manual-08.pdf

Emanuel, L., Ferris, F. D., von Gunten, C. F., & Von Roenn, J. H. (2010). *The last hours of living: Practical advice for clinicians*. Retrieved from http://www.medscape.com

End of Life Nursing Education Consortium (ELNEC). (2008). *Promoting palliative care nursing*. Duarte, CA: City of Hope National Medical Center and Washington, DC: American Association of Colleges of Nursing.

Goodman, D. C., Esty, A. R., Fisher, E. S., & Chang, C. (2011). Trends and variation in end-of-life care for Medicare beneficiaries with severe chronic illness. *A Report of the Dartmouth Atlas Project*. Retrieved from http://www.dartmouthatlas.org/downloads/reports/EOL_Trend_Report_0411.pdf

Grunier, A., Mor, V., Weitzen, S., Truchil, R., Teno, J., & Roy, J. (2007). Where people die: A multilevel approach to understanding influences on site of death in America. *Medical Care Research and Review, 64*(4), 351–378.

Hallenbeck, J. (2005). *Fast facts and concepts #11: Tube feed or not tube feed?* (2nd ed.). End of Life Physician Education Resource Center. Retrieved from http://www.eperc.mcw.edu

Hartford Institute for Geriatric Nursing, Division of Nursing, New York University. (2007). The Modified Caregiver Strain Index (CSI). In M. Boltz & S. Greenberg (Eds.), *Try this: Best practices in nursing care to older*

adults. Retrieved from http://www.hartfordign.org

Herr, K. (2011). Pain assessment strategies in older patients. *Journal of Pain, 12*(3), S3–S13.

Hospice and Palliative Nurses Association (HPNA). (2008). *HPNA position statement: Pain management*. Retrieved from http://www.hpna.org

Hospice and Palliative Nurses Association (HPNA). (2011a). *HPNA position statement: Artificial nutrition and hydration in advanced illness*. Retrieved from http://www.hpna.org

Hospice and Palliative Nurses Association (HPNA). (2011b). *HPNA position statement: Complementary therapies in palliative care nursing practice*. Retrieved from http://www.hpna.org

Hospice and Palliative Nurses Association (HPNA). (2011c). *HPNA position statement: Role of the nurse when hastened death is requested*. Retrieved from http://www.hpna.org

Hospice and Palliative Nurses Association (HPNA). (2011d). *HPNA position statement: Value of the professional nurse in palliative care*. Retrieved from http://www.hpna.org

Hudson, P. L., Schofield, P., Kelly, B., Hudson, R., O'Connor, M., Kristjanson, L. J., Ashby, M., & Aranda, S. (2006). Responding to desire to die statements from patients with advanced disease: Recommendations for health professionals. *Palliative Medicine, 20*(7), 703–710.

Jones, C. A., & Elbert-Avila, K. (2011). Palliative care in advanced cancer in older adults: Management of pain, fatigue and gastrointestinal symptoms. *Clinical Geriatrics, 19*(11), 23–29.

Keeley, P. (2010). Delirium at the end of life. *American Family Physician, 81*(10), 1260–1261.

Kochanek, K. D., Xu, J., Murphy, S. L., Miniño, A. M., & Kung, H. (2011). *Deaths: Preliminary data for 2009: National vital statistics reports* (DHHS Publication No. PHS 2011-1120). Hyattsville, MD: National Center for Health Statistics.

Kübler-Ross, E. (1969). *On death and dying: What the dying have to teach doctors, nurses, clergy, and their own families.* New York, NY: MacMillan.

Lacey, D. (2005). Tube feeding, antibiotics, and hospitalization of long-term care facility residents with end-stage dementia: Perceptions of key medical decision-makers. *American Journal of Alzheimer's Disease and Other Dementias, 20*(4), 211–219.

Last Acts. (2002). *Means to a better end: A report on dying in America.* Retrieved from http://www.rwjf.org/pr/product.jsp?id=20938

MacKenzie, M. A. (2011). Preparatory grief in frail elderly individuals. *Annals of Long-Term Care: Clinical Care and Aging, 19*(1), 22–26.

MacPhee, E., & Bickel, K. (2008). Palliative care for patients with dementia: From diagnosis to bereavement. *Annals of Long-Term Care: Clinical Care and Aging, 15*(6), 41–47.

McPherson, M. L., & Uritsky, T. J. (2011). Pharmacotherapy of pain in older adults: Opioid and adjuvant. In F. M. Gloth, III (Ed.), *Handbook of pain relief in older adults: An evidence-based approach* (pp. 83–95). New York, NY: Springer.

Moneymaker, K. (2005). Comfort measures only. *Journal of Palliative Medicine, 8*(3), 688.

NANDA International. (2011). *NANDA International nursing diagnoses: Definitions and classification, 2012–2014.* Hoboken, NJ: Wiley-Blackwell.

National Center for Health Statistics. (2011). *Health, United States, 2010: With special feature on death and dying.* Retrieved from http://www.cdc.gov/nchs/data/hus/hus10.pdf

National Consensus Project (NCP) for Quality Palliative Care. (2009). *Clinical practice guidelines for quality palliative care* (2nd ed.). Retrieved from http://www.nationalconsensusproject.org

National Hospice and Palliative Care Organization (NHPCO). (2010). *NHPCO facts and figures: Hospice care in America.* Alexandria, VA: Author.

New York State. (2010). *Healthcare proxy. Information for consumers.* Retrieved from http://www.health.state.ny.us/nysdoh/hospital/healthcareproxy/instructions.htm

Paice, J. A. (2010). Pain at the end of life. In B. R. Ferrell & N. Coyle (Eds.), *Textbook of palliative nursing* (pp. 161–186). Oxford, UK: Oxford University Press.

Puchalski, C., Ferrell, B., Virani, R., Otis-Green, S., Baird., P, Bull, J, Chochinov, H., Handzo, G., Nelson-Becker, H., Prince-Paul, M., Pugliese, K., & Sulmasy, D. (2009). Improving quality of spiritual care as a dimension of palliative care: The report of the consensus conference. *Journal of Palliative Medicine, 12,* 885–904.

Pulchaski, C. M., Dorff, R. E., Hebbar, B. N., & Hendi, Y. (2011). Religion, spirituality, and end of life care. *UpToDate.* Retrieved from http://www.uptodate.com

Reisner, L. (2011). Pharmacological management of persistent pain in older persons. *Journal of Pain, 12*(3), S21–S29.

Searight, H. R., & Gafford, J. (2005). Cultural diversity at the end of life: Issues and guidelines for family physicians. *American Family Physician, 71*(3), 515–522.

SUPPORT Principal Investigators. (1995). A controlled trial to improve care for seriously ill hospitalized patients. The study to understand prognoses and preferences for outcomes and risks of treatment. *Journal of the American Medical Association, 274*(20), 1591–1598.

Winn, P. A. (2010). Palliative care in LTC: Essentials of pain management. *Annals of Long Term Care, 18*(9), 28–35.

World Health Organization (WHO). (1990). *Cancer pain relief and palliative care* (Technical Report Series, 804). Geneva, Switzerland: Author.

World Health Organization (WHO). (2011). *WHO definition of palliative care.* Retrieved from http://www.who.int/cancer/palliative/definition/en

Physiological Basis of Practice

CHAPTER

12

The Integument
Rita Olivieri, RN, PhD
RETIRED ASSOCIATE PROFESSOR, WILLIAM F. CONNELL SCHOOL OF NURSING AT BOSTON COLLEGE

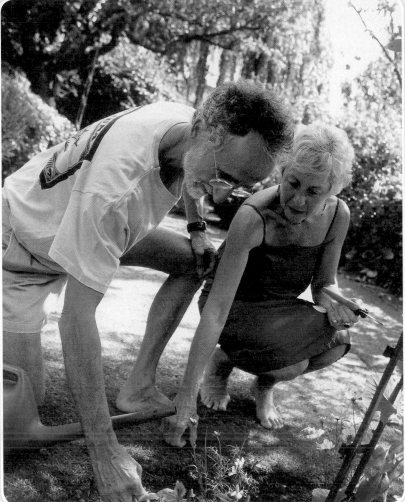

Trish Gant/Dorling Kindersley

KEY TERMS

LEARNING OUTCOMES

On completion of this chapter, the reader will be able to:

1. Describe normal skin changes associated with aging.
2. Identify risk factors related to common skin problems of older adults.
3. Delineate skin changes associated with benign and malignant skin changes.
4. List nursing diagnoses related to common skin problems.
5. Discuss the nursing responsibilities related to pharmacological and nonpharmacological treatment of common skin problems.
6. Explain the nursing management principles related to the care of pressure ulcers.

The skin is the body's largest organ, comprising between 15% and 20% of a person's total body weight. It has three layers, the epidermis, dermis, and subcutaneous layers. Epidermal accessory structures, or appendages, are downgrowths of the epidermal layer and include the hair, nails, and sweat glands. Along with the accessory structures, the skin comprises the integumentary system. The skin covers the entire body and protects it from external forces such as microorganisms, traumatic injury, and sun exposure. In addition, it prevents loss of body fluid, synthesizes vitamin D, regulates normal body temperature, and provides both touch and pressure neuroreception. The overall health of a person is often reflected by an assessment of skin color, texture, warmth, general appearance, and overall grooming. Obvious changes in the skin and hair are an inevitable part of aging that may lead to changes in a sense of self as well as how the individual is perceived by others. When these changes, such as graying of hair and wrinkling of the skin, are viewed as negative, considerable time and money may be spent on efforts to alter outward appearances by using cosmetics, hair coloring, and cosmetic surgery. An important part of the nurse's role is to educate the older adult about the normal skin changes that are expected with aging, maintaining a lifestyle that promotes healthy skin, and minimizing exposure to environmental hazards.

Usual Structure and Function of Skin Layers

The skin can be divided into three major layers: the epidermis, the dermis, and the subcutaneous layer. These layers perform many functions, including protection from the external environment and infection, maintenance of normal fluid and electrolyte balance, and thermal regulation.

Epidermis

The epidermis of the skin has up to five layers, depending on the part of the body, with the palms of the hands and the soles of the feet having five layers and most of the rest of the body having three layers. The skin is continually regenerating and shedding in a process called **desquamation.** The major cells of the epidermis, the keratinocytes, produce keratin, which provides the tough outer barrier of the skin. Langerhans cells reside in the keratinocytes and provide immune protective function. Ultraviolet radiation may damage Langerhans cells, decreasing their ability to protect the skin against cancer. At the junction of the epidermis and dermis are **melanocytes.** These produce melanin, which gives the skin its color and shields the body from the

harmful effects of the sun. Skin tone results from the size and quantity of melanosomes (granules in the melanocyte) and the melanin activity rate. People with dark skin have larger melanosomes and more active melanin production than those with lighter skin. Skin also derives a reddish tone from the vascular bed that is located in the dermis (Browder-Lazenby, 2011; Ignatavicius & Workman, 2010).

Dermis

The dermis, the second layer of the skin, is made up of connective tissue and is rich in blood supply, lymph, and neurosensory receptors. The dermis provides nourishment and support for the epidermis, which does not have its own blood supply. This is the thickest skin layer and contains fibroblasts, mast cells, and lymphocytes. The white elastin fibers and yellow fibrous collagen produced by the fibroblasts provide strength to the skin and give it the ability to stretch during movement. Dermal ground substances retain water and play a role in skin turgor. Sensory nerve endings in the dermis provide responses to temperature, touch, pressure, and pain.

Subcutaneous Layer

The subcutaneous layer, or superficial fascia, is specialized connective tissue that lies beneath the dermis and attaches to the muscles below. This layer also contains blood vessels, lymphatic channels, hair follicles, and sweat glands that extend from the dermis as well as adipose or fat tissue. Fat tissue gives shape to the body and provides cushioning for the bones, protection for delicate internal organs, and insulation from extremes in temperature. Subcutaneous fat is most abundant on the lower back and buttocks and is absent on areas such as the eyelids and tibia. The amount of fat tissue is dependent on age, gender, and hereditary factors.

Dermal Accessory Structures

Accessory structures of the skin include the hair, nails, and glands; each accessory structure has a unique purpose and function.

Hair

Hair color, distribution, thickness, and texture vary greatly based on age, gender, and race as well as overall health. Hair is located on all skin surfaces except the soles of the feet and the palms of the hands. Each strand of hair grows independently in a cyclic fashion and can differ in its rate of growth depending on its location on the body. At any given time, about 10% of the hair on the scalp is in the resting phase. Hair develops from the mitotic activity of the hair bulb that is located in the dermal layer of the skin. As hair grows up the follicle, it becomes differentiated and is fully hardened by the time it reaches the skin surface. Hair growth occurs up the dermis at an angle. When the body temperature drops, the erector pili muscles contract and hair "stands up on end," creating "goose bumps." Hair color, like skin color, is related to the melanin production in the hair follicle.

Nails

Nails are rapidly dividing extensions of the keratin-producing epidermal layer of the skin. The crescent-shaped portion of the nail that is located at the proximal end of the nail plate is the nail matrix. In the nail matrix, specialized, nonkeratinized cells differentiate into keratinized cells, which form nail protein. Fingernail protein grows up the nail from the nail matrix at about 0.1 mm per day. Toenails grow at a slower rate.

Glands

Sebaceous glands are found on most skin areas with the exception of the palms of the hands and the soles of the feet. They are most abundant on the face, head, and chest. Sebaceous glands are usually associated with a hair follicle, forming a pilosebaceous unit. These glands secrete **sebum,** an oily substance that keeps hair supple and lubricates the skin. Sebum protects the skin from water loss and provides protection against infection.

Apocrine sweat glands are large glands that produce a milky substance that, when acted on by bacteria present on the skin, causes odor. These glands begin functioning after puberty and require a high level of sex hormone activity for functioning. They are found primarily in the axilla, perineum, and breast areolae.

Eccrine glands produce sweat, a dilute form of plasma. Sweat production from the eccrine glands is stimulated by exercise, heat (forehead, neck, chest), and psychic origins (palms of the hands, soles of the feet, axillae). Thus, they play an important role in regulating the heat and cooling of the body.

Usual Functions of the Skin

Current research shows the skin to be a "highly active biological factory" (Fore, 2006). It is exposed to and responds to continual environmental hazards. It regulates temperature, contributes to the immune function, and provides the vehicle for vitamin synthesis and sensory reception for the central nervous system.

Regulation of Body Fluids and Temperature

The skin contains epithelial cells that provide a barrier that prevents insensible loss of body fluids from the deeper layers of the skin and the internal organs. The epithelial cells also provide selective transport of nutrients and body wastes, and have a semiregulated permeability to water. Damage to the skin, due to injuries such as burns, may result in life-threatening loss of this protective function.

The epidermis of the skin provides the vehicle for radiation, conduction, and convection of heat from the body. Blood vessels in the dermis help to regulate body temperature by dilating during warm temperatures and constricting during cold. The hypothalamus plays a role in maintaining an approximate core temperature of 37°C by regulating dermal blood flow to the extremities, as well as some facial areas. During periods of intense exercise, or periods of increased external temperature, additional cooling mechanisms are needed. At these times, the eccrine glands produce large volumes of sweat that contribute greatly to the overall ability of the body to regulate temperature. The subcutaneous tissue provides insulation to retain body heat.

Regulation of the Immune Function

Intact skin is an important barrier to prevent infection from bacterial invasion and other microorganisms. Skin is not only a physical barrier, but also an important part of the body's immune response against various antigens. The cells that provide this specialized function are Langerhans cells and keratinocytes in the epidermis, and lymphocytes in the dermis. These cells make it possible for a healthy skin surface to neutralize an attack against various antigenic substances. However, if the skin is damaged or diseased, it may be possible for an antigen to induce an immune response and cause inflammation or infection (Browder-Lazenby, 2011; Zator Estes, 2010).

Production of Vitamin D

The epidermal layer of the skin provides the vehicle for the synthesis of vitamin D. A complex steroid called a sterol is present in the malpighian cells (7-dehydrocholesterol) and is activated by ultraviolet light to produce vitamin D. Vitamin D is important in the absorption of calcium and phosphorus from food.

Sensory Reception

General sensory receptors located in the skin provide the central nervous system with information about changes in the external environment. When stimulated, these specialized receptors detect touch, pressure, temperature, and pain. For example, Merkel disks in the epidermis detect

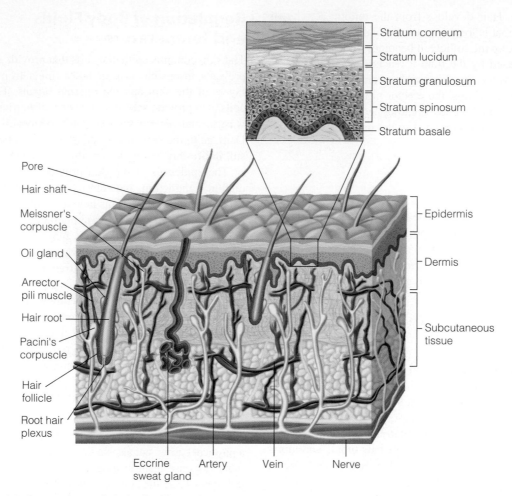

Stratum corneum
Stratum lucidum
Stratum granulosum
Stratum spinosum
Stratum basale

Pore
Hair shaft
Meissner's corpuscle
Oil gland
Arrector pili muscle
Hair root
Pacini's corpuscle
Hair follicle
Root hair plexus

Epidermis
Dermis
Subcutaneous tissue

Eccrine sweat gland   Artery   Vein   Nerve

Figure 12-1 ▶▶▶ Corpuscles and their distribution in the skin.

light pressure, Meissner's corpuscles in the dermis detect light and discriminative touch as well as vibration, and Pacini's corpuscles in the subcutaneous tissue detect deep pressure. Figure 12-1 ▶▶▶ illustrates these corpuscles and their distribution in the skin.

NORMAL CHANGES OF AGING

Multiple age-related changes occur in the skin of older adults. There is a decrease in the thickness and elasticity of the skin, which, by the seventh and eighth decade of life, contributes to the appearance of wrinkled and sagging skin on the face, neck, and upper arms. Although changes occur in all of the body systems throughout life, skin and hair changes are the most visible and may affect a person's self-perception and self-esteem. Age-related changes in the skin's appearance correlate with changes in function; there is an overall decline in the function of the skin with the aging process.

Skin aging may be divided into two types: intrinsic aging, which is caused by **intrinsic factors** such as genetic makeup and the normal aging process, and extrinsic aging, which is the result of **extrinsic factors** such as ultraviolet light exposure, smoking, and environmental pollutants. Exposure to and damage by the sun, known as *actinic damage,* affect the aging appearance of the skin, while the development of wrinkles is also accelerated by smoking. It is important for the older adult to understand the normal changes and to be aware of environmentally induced damage so he or she can work to decrease risk factors and minimize negative consequences. Figure 12-2 ▶▶▶ illustrates normal changes of aging in the integumentary system.

Epidermis

Throughout the normal aging process, the epidermis thins. Furthermore, epidermal cells in the older adult contain less moisture, which contributes to a dry, rough appearance. After 50 years of age, epidermal mitosis slows by 30%,

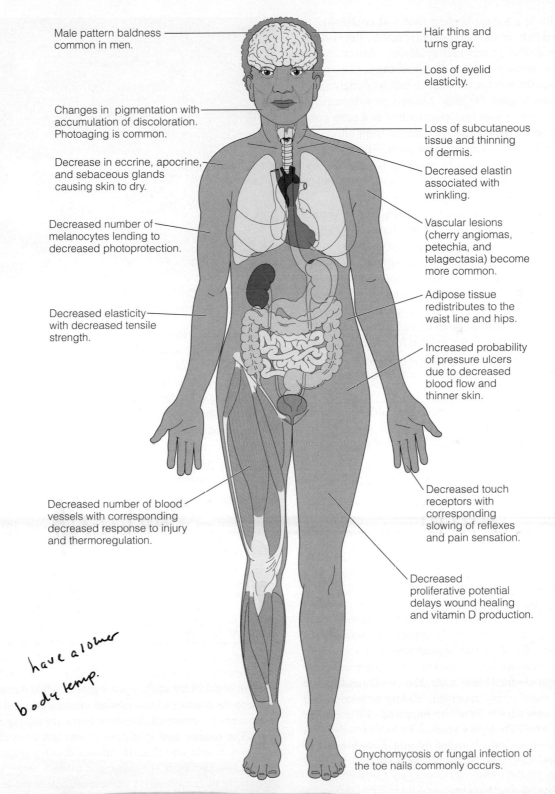

Male pattern baldness common in men.

Hair thins and turns gray.

Loss of eyelid elasticity.

Changes in pigmentation with accumulation of discoloration. Photoaging is common.

Loss of subcutaneous tissue and thinning of dermis.

Decrease in eccrine, apocrine, and sebaceous glands causing skin to dry.

Decreased elastin associated with wrinkling.

Decreased number of melanocytes lending to decreased photoprotection.

Vascular lesions (cherry angiomas, petechia, and telagectasia) become more common.

Adipose tissue redistributes to the waist line and hips.

Decreased elasticity with decreased tensile strength.

Increased probability of pressure ulcers due to decreased blood flow and thinner skin.

Decreased number of blood vessels with corresponding decreased response to injury and thermoregulation.

Decreased touch receptors with corresponding slowing of reflexes and pain sensation.

Decreased proliferative potential delays wound healing and vitamin D production.

have a lower body temp.

Onychomycosis or fungal infection of the toe nails commonly occurs.

Figure 12-2 ▶▶▶ Normal changes of aging in the integumentary system.

which results in a longer healing time and contributes to the increased risk for infection in older adults. Rete ridges, which connect the dermis and epidermis, flatten, which results in fewer contact areas between these two layers. This increases the risk for skin tears when seemingly slight friction occurs against the skin. Melanocytes decrease in number and activity with age, contributing to a paler complexion and an increased risk for damage from ultraviolet radiation for the light-skinned older adult. The remaining cells may not function normally, resulting in scattered pigmented areas such as nevi, age spots, or liver spots and an increase in the number and size of freckles.

With aging the manufacture of vitamin D from natural sunlight becomes less efficient. Further, many older adults should not engage in prolonged sun exposure due to the risk of photodamage, increased sun sensitivity due to certain medications, and risk for hyperthermia. Many older adults living in long-term care facilities and those residing in geographic areas with long, cold winters often cannot get the needed sunlight to produce sufficient vitamin D. Adequate vitamin D levels are needed for calcium absorption, prevention of certain cancers, and reduction of fall risks in older adults (Reddy & Gilchrest, 2010).

> **Practice Pearl** ▶▶▶ Recommend that older adults ask their primary care provider to check their vitamin D blood level to maintain adequate calcium absorption. If the older person resides in a colder climate, check this level during the winter months when sunlight exposure is more likely to be minimal.

Dermis

The dermis decreases in thickness and functionality beginning in the third decade. Elastin decreases in quality but increases in quantity, resulting in the wrinkling and sagging of the skin. Collagen become less organized and leads to a loss of turgor. Men have a thicker dermal layer than women, which explains the more rapidly apparent age-associated changes in the female facial appearance. The vascularity of the dermis decreases and contributes to a paler complexion in the light-skinned older adult. The capillaries become thinner and more easily damaged, leading to bruised and discolored areas known as **senile purpura** as depicted in Figure 12-3 ▶▶▶. There is a gradual decline in both touch and pressure sensations, causing the older adult to be at risk for injury such as burns and pressure sores.

Subcutaneous Layer

With increasing age, there is a gradual atrophy of subcutaneous tissue in some areas of the body, and a gradual increase in others. Subcutaneous tissue becomes thinner in the face,

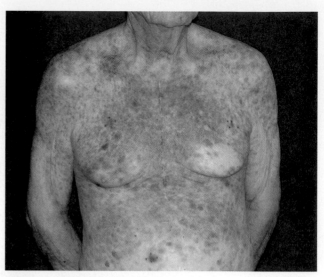

Figure 12-3 ▶▶▶ Senile purpura.
Source: Appears with permission from Logical Images, Inc.

neck, hands, and lower legs, resulting in more visible veins in the exposed areas, and skin that is more prone to damage. Some other areas of the body have a gradual hypertrophy of subcutaneous tissue that leads to an overall increase in the proportion of body fat for the older adult. Overall, with aging, fat distribution is more pronounced in the abdomen and thighs in women, and in the abdomen in men.

HEALTHY AGING TIP

The Integument

Limit showers and bath time. Use warm not hot water and do not rub skin.	Hot water dehydrates the skin and rubbing increases dryness and pruritus.
Avoid soap products that contain harsh chemicals.	Many products can cause sensitization of the skin and lead to a rash.
Pat skin dry gently. Apply moisturizers liberally.	Moisturizers will help retain water and prevent dry skin.

Hair

The hair of the older adult appears gray or white due to a decrease in the number of functioning melanocytes and the replacement of pigmented strands of hair with nonpigmented ones. The texture and thickness of the hair also change, becoming coarse and thin. Hormones decline, resulting in gradual loss of hair in the pubic and axillary areas and the appearance of facial hair on women and hair in the ears and nose of men. By age 50, many older men have experienced a gradual loss of hair and often develop a symmetrical W-shaped balding pattern. Women have less pronounced hair loss than men. The actual age when graying and hair loss begins, as well as the pattern of baldness, is determined in part by a person's genetic makeup. However, many 50-year-old adults have gray, or partly gray, scalp hairs.

Nails

The nails of the older adult become dull, and yellow or gray in color. Nail growth slows, which results in thicker nails that are more likely to split. Longitudinal striations also appear due to damage at the nail matrix. **Longitudinal pigmented bands** are single or multiple brown or black bands on the nail of the thumb and index finger. These bands are common in dark-skinned races and are more visible in the older adult. However, in some cases these pigmented bands may be a sign of melanoma of the nail and a biopsy should be done to rule it out (Zhang, 2011).

Glands

With aging, there is a decrease in the size, number, and function of both eccrine and apocrine glands. The decrease in eccrine or sweat glands results in a decrease in the older adult's ability to regulate body temperature through perspiration and evaporation from the skin. As the ability to sweat decreases, the older adult may be unable to control body temperature by the normal sweating mechanism, and therefore is at a high risk for heat exhaustion. Sebaceous glands increase in size with age, but the amount of sebum produced is decreased. Men experience a minimal decrease in sebum production, typically after 80 years of age, while women begin to produce less sebum following menopause.

Xerosis or dry skin occurs more frequently as a person ages. Long-term care studies have found that xerosis affects between 30% and 60% of the older population (Hurlow & Bliss, 2011). The exact etiology of xerosis is not totally understood. For many years it was thought that the changes in sebum production and water content that occur in the older adult were the basis of the problem. New research suggests that changes in the keratinization process and lipid content in the stratum corneum are more likely the cause of flaking appearance and dry sensation of the skin (Foy White-Chu & Reddy, 2011). Xerosis is found most commonly on the lower legs of older adults, though may also be present on the hands and trunk, and has the appearance of "cracked porcelain." Xerotic skin may be extremely pruritic, leading to scratching and broken skin and putting the older adult at increased risk for infection. Typically, xerosis is worse during dry winter months.

Practice Pearl ▶▶▶ The older person should be alerted to the environmental factors that contribute to xerosis: hot water bathing, use or overuse of soaps and personal cleansers, skin powders, and dry conditions such as winter, a desert climate, or air conditioning (Foy White-Chu & Reddy, 2011).

Sun Damage

A tan is often admired as an attractive and healthy attribute; however, a tan is a protective response of the body to damage caused by the sun. Tanning is a sign of skin damage. The skin never "forgets" the damage done by exposure to ultraviolet radiation (UVR). In fact, a person's risk for melanoma, the most serious of skin cancers, doubles if he or she has had five or more sunburns (Skin Cancer Foundation, 2011c). A tan may be attractive, but the cumulative effect of sun exposure throughout a lifetime leads to premature aging and increases the risk for skin cancer. More than 90% of nonmelanoma skin cancers are caused by sun exposure (Skin Cancer Foundation, 2011c).

The combination of normal age-related changes and UVR-related damage is a complex issue and not entirely understood. However UVR-related skin damage is thought to be distinct from the normal aging process. Because it happens gradually, premature aging is often considered an inevitable part of growing old. In fact, up to 90% of the visible changes in skin that are often attributed to aging are caused by the sun (U.S. Environmental Protection Agency [EPA], 2010).

There are two important types of UVR: ultraviolet A (UVA) and ultraviolet B (UVB). Both have been implicated in skin cancer. UVA rays are responsible for deep skin penetration, cause premature aging, and may also decrease immune system function (Skin Cancer Foundation, 2011d). UVA rays can easily penetrate car windows, making both drivers and passengers susceptible to skin damage and skin cancer (Skin Cancer Foundation, 2010). A recent study revealed that 53% of skin cancers occur on the left or driver's side of the body, linking UV radiation exposure to driving. Windshields are usually treated to block some UVA, but side windows let in about 63% of the sun's UVA.

The older adult who has spent a lot of time outdoors, either working or at leisure, may have long-term UVR damage known as **photoaging,** the damage that is done to the skin from prolonged exposure, over a person's lifetime, to UV radiation. These changes occur on exposed areas such as the face, neck, arms, and hands and include freckling, loss of elasticity, damaged blood vessels, and a general coarse and weathered appearance. Older people whose pigmentation or lifestyle protect them from photodamage, often look younger than their chronologic peers. These changes differ clinically and physiologically from aging itself. Continued damage may result in the development of a precancerous lesion, **actinic keratosis**, which can progress to skin cancer (Skin Cancer Foundation, 2011a).

Drug Alert ▶▶▶ Many medications can cause sun sensitivity. See the following table for some of the most commonly prescribed drugs.

Brand Name	Generic Name	Therapeutic Class
Motrin	ibuprofen	NSAID, antiarthritic
Crystodigin	digitoxin	Antiarrhythmic
Sinequan	doxepin	Antidepressant
Cordarone	amiodarone	Antiarrhythmic
Bactrim	trimethoprim	Antibiotic
Diabinese	chlorpropamide	Antidiabetic (oral)
Feldene	piroxicam	NSAID, antiarthritic
Vibramycin	doxycycline	Antibiotic
Phenergan	Promethazine	Antihistamine
Lasix	Furosemide	Diuretics
Biaxin	co-trimoxazole	Antibiotic
Capoten	captopril	Antihypertension

Source: U.S. Food and Drug Administration, 2010.

Common Skin Conditions in Older Adults

Due to the many age-related changes that occur, older adults are at increased risk for the development of skin-related conditions. Furthermore, older adults may be subject to functional limitation, multiple chronic conditions, and adverse drug effects that may further increase the risk for skin diseases. These changes leave the older person increasingly susceptible to skin injuries such as pressure ulcers and skin tears with a steadily decreasing ability to effect skin repair (Farage, Miller, Berardesca, et al., 2009). Some of the common skin conditions of the older adult include skin cancer, skin tears, pressure ulcers, delayed skin healing, cellulitis, and fingernail and toenail problems.

Practice Pearl ▶▶▶ The prevalence of polypharmacy in the older person increases the risk of drug reactions, which often mimic skin diseases. This greatly complicates the accurate diagnosis of dermatologic problems (Farage et al., 2009). Remind older adults to bring a complete list of all drugs (and the drugs, if possible) to appointments with their primary care provider.

Skin Cancer

Skin cancer is the most common type of cancer in the United States with a million cases diagnosed each year (National Cancer Institute, 2010). As a person ages, the incidence of skin cancer increases, especially for those between 50 and 80 years of age. A North American who lives to age 65 has a 40% to 50% chance of having a nonmelanoma skin cancer (NMSC) at least once. Most of these cancers as well as melanoma skin cancer can be prevented. Enlarging pigmented spots that bleed easily characterize these carcinomas.

Skin cancers that primarily result from sun exposure are basal cell carcinoma, squamous cell carcinoma, and malignant melanoma. The risks for skin cancer seem to be associated with the total amount of time spent in the sun and epidemiologic data suggest that skin cancers can be prevented if children, adolescents, and adults are protected from UVR (National Cancer Institute, 2010). Although older adults with lighter skin are more likely to be at risk for sun damage, darker skinned people including African Americans and Hispanics can also be affected (American Cancer Society [ACS], 2010), indicating the need for sun protection measures for older adults of all skin tones.

The most common precancerous lesion is actinic keratosis, also known as solar keratosis and senile keratosis. Actinic keratoses are more common in men than women and it is estimated that 1 in 1,000 will progress to skin cancer (usually squamous cell carcinoma) in a 1-year period. Erythematous actinic keratosis is the most common type and appears as a sore, rough, scaly, erythematous papule or plaque. Other types of actinic keratoses include hypertrophic and cutaneous horns. The most common sites for all types of actinic keratoses are sun-exposed areas such as the back of the hands, forearm, face, V of the neck, nose, tips of the ears, and bald scalp (EPA, 2010).

Basal cell carcinoma is the most common form of skin cancer in Caucasians and accounts for about 80% of nonmelanoma skin cancers (ASCO, 2012). About 2.8 million people are diagnosed annually in the United States. Basal cell carcinoma can extend below the skin to the bone, but metastasis is rare. This cancer originates in the lowest layer of the epidermis and appears as small fleshy bumps (Figure 12-4 ▶▶▶). Basal cell carcinoma can occur on any exposed skin surface but is frequently found on the face, head, neck, nose, and ears. About 95% of cases occur between 49 and 79 years of age.

Squamous cell carcinoma is the second most common form of skin cancer in Caucasians and represents the remaining 20% of nonmelanoma skin cancers. It is the most common form of skin cancer in people with dark skin. Squamous cell carcinoma originates in the higher levels of the epidermis. It appears as flesh colored to erythematous,

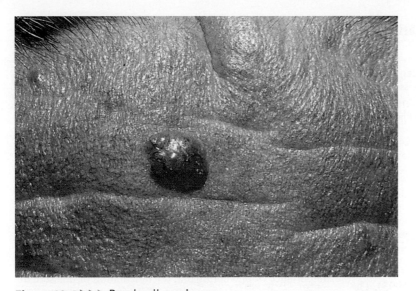

Figure 12-4 ▶▶▶ Basal cell carcinoma.

Source: Reprinted with permission from the American Academy of Dermatology. Copyright © 2012. All rights reserved.

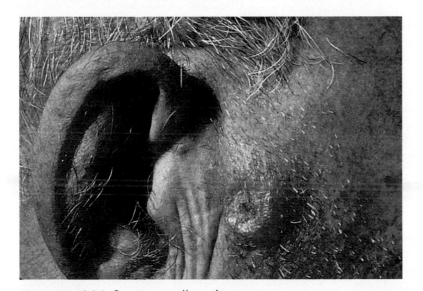

Figure 12-5 ▶▶▶ Squamous cell carcinoma.

Source: Reprinted with permission from the American Academy of Dermatology. Copyright © 2012. All rights reserved.

indurated scaly plaques, papules, or nodules and may have ulceration or erosions in the center (Figure 12-5 ▶▶▶). Metastasis can occur and is more common in lesions of the mucous membranes, such as the lips, and in individuals with a history of inflammatory disease, immune suppression, or exposure to chemicals and other hazardous substances.

Melanoma is the most serious of skin cancers. It is estimated that about 120,000 cases of melanoma are diagnosed each year (ACS, 2011). In 2010, about 68,130 were invasive melanomas, killing approximately 8,700 people annually (Skin Cancer Foundation, 2011c). Melanoma is responsible for more than three quarters of all skin cancer deaths (National Cancer Institute, 2010). About one half of melanomas occur in those over 50 years of age. Melanoma originates in the melanocytes and may grow from an existing mole or a new lesion (Skin Cancer Foundation, 2011b). Melanocytes are cells that are located in the epidermis and are responsible for producing melanin, a brown pigment that helps screen against the harmful effects of UV light. The melanoma begins with a mole or lesion that may enlarge; become brown, black, or multicolored; develop nodules or plaques; and have a black, irregular outline that spreads. The lesions may crust or bleed and are usually greater than 6 mm in diameter. The most common type of melanoma, the superficial spreading type, accounts for 70% of the melanomas (ASCO, 2012) and is commonly found on the upper back on men and women and the lower legs of women. The risk factors for melanoma include a family or past history of melanoma, light skin and hair, a history of severe sunburns, or numerous atypical moles.

Skin Tears

A skin tear is a wound caused by shear, friction, and/or blunt force resulting in separation of skin layers. A skin tear can be partial thickness or full thickness (LeBlanc & Baranoski, 2011). The nurse caring for a frail older adult may, for example, remove an adhesive dressing from an intravenous insertion site and cause a skin tear on the thin vulnerable epidermis. These painful injuries can also occur with simple activities such as dressing, transferring, turning, or lifting. Independent older adults frequently sustain skin tears on the lower legs by bumping into chairs, beds, tables, or open dresser drawers in their home environment. Skin tears may be accompanied by dark purple ecchymosis (senile purpura) and edema because of subcutaneous tissue atrophy. This is particularly true in those areas of the skin at risk such as the face, hands, shins, and feet. Senile purpura is more common in areas of increased sun exposure.

In 2011, an expert panel was convened to provide consensus for the care of patients with skin tears. A three-category system, the Payne-Martin Classification for Skin Tears, was developed and recommended for use by nurses to assess, plan, and document outcomes of skin tear care

TABLE 12-1	Payne-Martin Classification for Skin Tears
Category I	(a) Skin tears ranging from a linear or flap-type tear without tissue loss. (b) Epidermal flap completely covers the dermis within 1 mm of the wound margin.
Category II	Skin tears with partial tissue loss. Considered scant with (a) 25% or less tissue loss, and (b) tissue loss of more than 25%.
Category III	Skin tears with full-thickness complete tissue loss, epidural flap absent.

Source: Adapted from Payne-Martin Skin Tear Classification Tool (1993). See LeBlanc and Baranoski (2011) for additional guidelines.

(LeBlanc & Baranoski, 2011; Payne & Martin, 1993). The categories, which are based on the amount of epidermal loss, are described in Table 12-1.

Pressure Ulcers in the Older Adult

Pressure ulcers affect between 1 million and 3 million people each year in the United States. The majority of pressure ulcers occur on people over 70 years of age. In a quarterly study of pressure ulcer in acute care patients, the prevalence of pressure ulcers was between 12% and 19% of the patient population (Jenkins & O'Neal, 2010). Prevalence rates increase dramatically for high-risk groups of hospitalized patients including patients with quadriplegia, orthopedic patients with fractures, patients admitted to the critical care unit, and older patients admitted with a fracture of the neck of the femur. The estimated prevalence of pressure ulcers among older adults who need long-term acute care is 29.3% (Ayello, 2012). In all patient care environments, individuals more than 65 years old are considered at high risk for developing pressure ulcers.

Healthy People 2020 provides science-based, national objectives for improving the health of all Americans and is an initiative of the U.S. Department of Health and Human Services (USDHHS) to create a healthier nation. One of *Healthy People 2020*'s older adult national objectives focuses on the problem of pressure ulcer–related hospitalizations. The objective states "Reduce the rate of pressure ulcer–related hospitalizations among older adults" (OA-10) (USDHHS, 2010). The baseline data is "958.8 pressure ulcer–related hospitalizations per 100,000 people ages 65 years and older occurred in 2007." The target of "887.3 pressure ulcer–related hospitalizations per 100,000 people ages 65 years and over" is a reduction of 10% by the year 2020. *Healthy People 2020* is an important initiative to keep abreast of national initiatives and provides a wealth of information to support this agenda (USDHHS, 2010).

In 2008, the Centers for Medicare and Medicaid Services (CMS) announced that hospitals will no longer be reimbursed for treatment of pressure ulcers that developed during the hospital stays of Medicare patients. This announcement changed the payment process for pressure ulcers. Stage III and IV pressure ulcers that were present on admission must be documented in the chart within 2 days of admission to qualify for reimbursement; however, pressure ulcers occurring after that time will not be eligible for reimbursement (CMS, 2011). Pressure ulcers are considered a "never event," or an event that CMS asserts could "reasonably" have been prevented through the application of evidence-based practice. There is no recourse for any additional reimbursements related to the care of a hospital-acquired pressure ulcer by Medicare. (For additional information, see Miller, 2009.) This mandate put a new focus, albeit a financial one, on the importance of prevention and documentation of pressure ulcers for nurses and all caregivers in healthcare facilities.

Controversy Regarding Pressure Ulcers as Never Events

The CMS mandate regarding pressure ulcers as a "never event" has met with controversy from various experts in the field. Some reasons for the dialogue are:

1. *Inconsistent policy.* CMS has maintained that not all pressure ulcers are preventable in their long-term care standards. CMS policy states that "In long-term care, where all standards of practice are met, but the residents or patient's condition demonstrates that the pressure ulcers were *unavoidable*, the cost of care will be reimbursed" (Stokowski, 2010). This raises the question of why there are exceptions to the never event of pressure ulcers in long-term care, but there are no such exceptions to the never event pressure ulcer policy in acute care? Furthermore, in acute care the patient will often be sicker due to multiple acute and chronic factors.
2. *Clinical issues.* Clinical issues can make pressure ulcers unavoidable, for example, a preexisting deep tissue injury (no visible ulceration), the end-of-life patient, other patients for whom the preventive care is medically contraindicated (patient cannot be flat in bed due to cardiac or respiratory issues), or the patient who is nonadherent to the nursing plan (see Stokowski, 2010, for further discussion).

Definition and Stages of Pressure Ulcers

The National Pressure Ulcer Advisory Panel (NPUAP), a group of experts in the prevention and management of pressure ulcers, recently redefined a **pressure ulcer** as "localized injury to the skin and/or underlying tissue, usually over a bony prominence, as a result of pressure, or pressure in combination with shear/or friction." A number of contributing or confounding factors are associated with pressure ulcers that have not yet been totally described (NPUAP, 2009, p. 1). The European Pressure Ulcer Advisory Panel and National Pressure Ulcer Advisory Panel (EPUAP-NPUAP) recently suggested the use of the term *category* to replace or explain the former terms *staging* or *grading*. *Category* implies a neutral term that is a nonhierarchical designation. Staging and grading may have implied a mistaken notion of a pressure ulcer "progressing from I to IV and/or healing from I to IV (EPUAP-NPUAP, 2009, p. 4). The most important result from the work of the panel is an international consensus on the definitions of the levels of skin tissue injury even though groups may be using various labels (*staging*, *grade*, *category*).

Category/staging of pressure ulcers is used to describe the physical appearance of the pressure ulcer at a given point in time, like a snapshot. There are four traditional stages of pressure ulcers (I, II, III, and IV) with two additional stages described as deep tissue injury and unstageable pressure ulcer (NPUAP, 2009). Deep tissue injury is an injury caused by damage of underlying tissue from pressure and/or sheer that leads to a purple or maroon localized area of discolored intact skin or blood-filled blister. It may be difficult to detect in older adults with dark skin tones. An unstageable pressure ulcer involves full-thickness tissue loss; however, the base of the ulcer cannot be visualized due to the presence of dead tissue (slough or eschar) in the wound bed (NPUAP, 2009). The traditional stages of pressure ulcers and the general guidelines for nursing management are presented in Table 12-2. The actual layers of the skin and depth of each stage are shown in Figure 12-6 ▶▶▶.

The purpose of defining the specific stages of pressure ulcers is to have a standard for the documentation of clinical data in order to study the best practices and outcomes. Although the stages of a pressure ulcer describe a lesion that begins on the external surface of the skin and progresses inward, this is not always the case in clinical practice.

A review of the research literature by Nixon et al. (2005) clarified the three different types of pressure ulcers and three different pathophysiological mechanisms that lead to pressure ulcers. The three types of pressure ulcers are:

1. A necrosis of the epidermis or dermis, which may or may not progress to a deep lesion
2. A deep or malignant pressure ulcer where necrosis is observed initially in the subcutaneous tissue and tracks outward
3. Full-thickness wounds of dry black eschar (Nixon et al., 2005)

The three types of pressure ulcers are thought to be distinct. The first, necrosis of the epidermis or dermis, may be

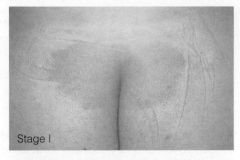
Stage I

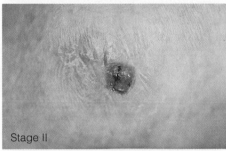
Stage II

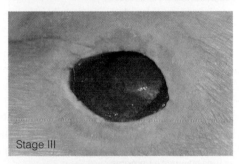
Stage III

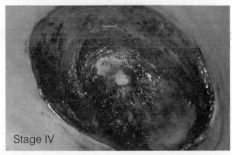
Stage IV

Figure 12-6 ▶▶▶ Layers of the skin and depth of each ulcer.

Source: Karen Lou Kennedy-Evans, RN, CS, FNP. Used with permission. http://www.kennedyterminalulcer.com

I. Skin does not blanch but is intact.
II. Partial-thickness skin loss of the dermis and epidermis.
III. Full-thickness skin loss involving damage or necrosis of the subcutaneous tissue that may extend down to but not through the underlying fascia.
IV. Full-tissue skin loss with extensive destruction extending to muscle, bone, or supporting structures.

TABLE 12-2	Pressure Ulcer Stages/Categories and Management			
Stage	Wound Cleaning/Definition	Debridement	Change Dressing Choices	Frequency*
I	Nonblanchable erythema of intact skin over a bony prominence (compared with adjacent or opposite side) Color: nonblanchable redness on light-skinned person: dark-skinned person skin shows as red or bluish hues. Further assessment: Check for temperature changes (warmness or coolness), tissue consistency (may be boggy), and sensation (may be painful).		Transparent film; adherent hydrocolloid	Based on amount of drainage and rate of healing. See product instructions.
II	Partial-thickness skin loss involving epidermis, dermis, or both, includes abrasions, blisters intact or ruptured. Red pink wound bed. No exposure of subcutaneous. Do not use this category to describe skin tears, tape burns, incontinence-associated dermatitis, maceration, or excoriation.	Normal saline or approved cleaner	Transparent film, hydrogel, hydrocolloid	
III	Full-thickness skin loss (fat visible) involving damage or necrosis of subcutaneous tissue that may extend down to, but not through, underlying fascia. In areas without underlying fat (subcutaneous tissue) to fascia, perichondrium, or periosteum (example malleolus). Undermining and tunneling may or may not be present.	Normal saline or approved cleaner If necrotic tissue is present, debridement must be done.	1. Use calcium alginate, hydrocolloids, or foam. 2. Cover with gauze or foam wafer. 3. Use least irritating taping method.	
IV	Full-thickness skin loss with extensive destruction, tissue necrosis, or damage to muscle, bone, or supporting structures. Often includes undermining and tunneling. May have eschar and slough tissue. Possible extensive destruction and risk of osteomyelitis.	Same as stage III	Same as stage III	

*Change frequency depends on the amount and type of drainage present. Read specific product instructions.

Source: Adapted from the National Pressure Ulcer Advisory Panel (2009). Available at www.npaup.org.

caused by friction against the skin. An example might be if a sheet is pulled from under a patient, causing damage to the epidermis. The second type of pressure ulcer, malignant or deep pressure ulcers, occurs as a result of unrelieved pressure over a long period of time. This type of ulcer begins deep in the subcutaneous tissue and tracks outward toward the dermis. The third type of pressure ulcer, full-thickness wounds of dry black eschar, appears in areas that were previously normal and occurs as a result of chronic arterial narrowing and inadequate tissue perfusion. When a stage IV pressure ulcer occurs, it is not clear which tissue layer has the primary ischemic injury (Nixon et al., 2005).

Pathophysiological Mechanisms Three mechanisms lead to tissue breakdown, although research in this area is limited because of the difficulty in replicating the clinical situation. The first mechanism is the occlusion of blood flow to the skin and the subsequent injury when the occlusion is removed and there is an abrupt reperfusion of the ischemic vascular bed. The second mechanism is caused by damage to the lining of the arterioles and smaller vessels due to the application of disruptive and shearing forces. This mechanism seems to be consistent with the most common body sites affected by pressure ulcers, the sacrum and trochanter. Sliding down in the bed from a sitting position causes disruptive shearing forces and results in damage to the underlying subcutaneous muscle or deep dermis in the sacral area. The trochanter site may be exposed to long periods of external pressure if the patient has not been moved or turned at appropriate times or is in the same position for a long time during surgery. The third cause of pressure ulcers is direct occlusion of the blood vessels by external pressure for a prolonged time period, resulting in cell death. The development of black eschar is usually seen in the lower limbs of patients where the skin is thin, and close to a bony prominence. These individuals usually have a history of arterial narrowing over a long period of time (Nixon et al., 2005).

Etiology of Pressure Ulcers
The general etiology of a pressure ulcer is the intensity and duration of pressure as well as the tolerance of the skin and its supporting structures to pressure. Changes in the skin and supporting structures due to the aging process are significant predictors for a pressure ulcer. In addition to normal age-related skin changes, older people have to cope with a myriad of both acute and chronic illnesses. More than 80% of people over age 65 have one or more chronic diseases (Centers for Disease Control and Prevention, 2011). Chronic health problems such as immobility, malnutrition, or declining mental status increase the risk for pressure ulcers. However, the particular variables that determine the actual development of a pressure ulcer are unique to each person.

Tissue Tolerance: Extrinsic Factors
Extrinsic factors that affect the skin tolerance to pressure forces include shear, friction, moisture, and skin irritants. Pressure is the primary force that occludes blood flow and causes tissue damage, but shearing forces are also an important factor in the development of pressure ulcers. Shearing, the sliding of parallel surfaces against each other, occurs most commonly when the patient slides down in the bed. Shearing forces reduce the amount of pressure needed to occlude the blood vessels by up to 50%. Friction, which occurs with the lateral movement of pulling sheets or clothing from under a person's weight, may remove the stratum corneum, which could disrupt the epidermis and lead to a pressure ulcer. Various skin irritants, such as starch, soaps, and detergents, affect tissue tolerance by removing sebum, which normally protects the skin. The skin then may become dehydrated, decreasing its resistance to other irritants and bacteria.

> **Practice Pearl** ►►► Shear injury happens under the skin so you will not see it occur. Raising the head of the bed increases the risk for shear injury.

Tissue Tolerance: Intrinsic Factors
Intrinsic factors that affect tissue tolerance and lead to skin breakdown include two major areas. The first is the structure and function of the skin and surrounding structures, and the second is the ability of the vascular system to provide circulation to the skin. Intrinsic factors that affect skin integrity include changes in collagen, advancing age, poor nutrition, and steroid administration. Factors that affect the ability of the vascular system to provide adequate perfusion to the skin include blood pressure, smoking, skin temperature, and vascular disease. Collagen seems to play an important role within the skin structure by protecting microcirculation and preventing damage from pressure. The total collagen content of the skin falls gradually after the age of 30, with a dramatic loss of collagen after 60 years of age. Nutritional factors associated with pressure ulcer development include decreased body weight, dehydration, decreased serum albumin, and anemia.

> **Practice Pearl** ►►► The heel is the second most common site for pressure ulcers and the most common site for deep tissue injury. Check the older person's heel for color frequently and document and report any changes immediately:
>
> - Red color signals hyperemia and ischemia
> - Purple color suggests infarction
> - Black color indicates necrosis

Salcido, Lee, & Ahn, 2011.

Wound Healing

The process of wound healing is complex and continuous. It involves three major phases or stages:

1. Inflammation and destruction
2. Proliferation
3. Maturation

Inflammatory Phase

The inflammatory phase of healing in partial- and full-thickness wounds lasts about 5 days and is characterized by the classic symptoms of inflammation: redness, heat, pain, and edema or swelling. The damaged tissues release histamine and other chemicals, resulting in vasodilation. This enhances blood supply to the area, provides additional nutrients, and promotes tissue rebuilding. Neutrophils and macrophages control bacteria and remove debris from the wound. Macrophages also secrete growth factors, such as growth factor beta, that are essential for the initiation and control of wound repair.

Proliferation Phase

Proliferation, the second phase of healing, begins soon after injury and continues for up to 3 weeks. This phase is responsible for rebuilding the damaged tissue by three processes: epithelialization, granulation, and collagen synthesis. In a shallow or partial-thickness wound, viable hair follicles often provide the main source for epidermal regeneration. Epidermal cells migrate across the wound surface and cover and protect it from bacteria. This process of reepithelialization continues to cover the wound base in layers until the area has a normal epidermal thickness. For deeper wounds, healing takes much longer because hair follicles are lost and the wound margins provide the only source for epidermal cell regeneration.

In full-thickness wounds, granulation tissue is formed by new blood vessels and collagen strands. The support matrix of collagen provides strength to the new tissues. Oxygen, vitamin C, dietary amino acids, and trace elements are essential in this process. Granulation tissue becomes beefy red and grainy in appearance as the capillary bed builds. Wound healing usually fills in from the wound bottom so the depth decreases before the wound width is decreased.

Maturation Phase

The last phase of healing for a full-thickness wound is maturation. This phase begins about 3 weeks after the injury and may last for up to 2 years. The process of collagen synthesis continues and the wound becomes thicker and more compact. Another part of the healing process, called contraction, results in a healed scar much smaller in size than the original wound. This process, initiated by myofibroblasts, is an important healing mechanism for wounds with tissue loss because it decreases the area to be healed. The wound is initially dark red in color and, over time, fades to a silver-white color. The scarred area never reaches the strength of the prewound tissue and is therefore more prone to reinjury than normal tissue. The width of the scar of wound healing by secondary intention will be about 10% of the original defect (Baranoski & Ayello, 2007).

Delayed Healing

The following are signs of delayed healing:

- Wound size is increasing.
- Exudate, slough, or eschar is present.
- Tunnels, fistula, or undermining has developed.
- Epithelial edge is not smooth and continuous and does not move toward the wound.

A wound that does not heal within 6 weeks is considered a chronic wound. Common problems that often lead to chronic wounds are diabetes, peripheral vascular disease, and pressure ulcers. Normal aging and chronic disease factors that are often present in older adults will affect their ability to heal.

Some of the considerations related to delayed or impaired wound healing for the older adult are:

- Subclinical bacterial contamination
- Foreign bodies
- Inadequate blood supply
- Inadequate nutrition
- Immunocompetence
- Damage to the wound

Adequate blood volume and cardiac output are the most important components of wound blood flow and oxygen delivery. Oxygen is needed for every phase of the healing process. Chronic cardiac disease, smoking, dehydration, hypovolemia, and the vascular complications of diabetes cause a decrease in blood supply to the tissues, which delays wound healing. Age-related decreases in the number of dermal vessels may predispose the patient to ischemic injury.

Wound healing cannot take place without large amounts of energy (glucose) and protein (amino acids) as well as other substances. Many older adults have protein energy malnutrition, in which the intake of protein and energy is inadequate to meet the body's demands. In the malnourished person, the amino acids must come from muscle and other stores. The body can deal with this demand until there is a loss of 15% of lean body mass. After that, the supply of protein is inadequate to provide muscle replacement and wound healing, thus compromising the healing process.

Older adults have delayed immune function, which impairs the natural ability to fight infection. This delays the normal inflammatory response. Wounds cannot heal without the inflammatory process. Medications that further diminish the immune response include steroids and anti-inflammatory drugs. Weight loss due to an acute and chronic illness results in loss of body protein (lean body mass) and also compromises immune function. Decreased ascorbic acid levels due to age may increase blood vessel fragility.

The wound can be damaged by both excessive or inadequate moisture. A dry wound surface impairs epithelial migration and leads to tissue injury and necrosis. The buildup of tissue exudates is toxic to new growth and leads to tissue hypoxia, which impairs healing. The older adult may also be subject to wound maceration due to urine or fecal contamination, which will further damage the wound. Nursing interventions used to treat the pressure ulcers or chronic wounds can also cause damage. Topical antibiotics, cleansing solutions, and mechanical trauma during dressing changes may all contribute to damage to the wound bed.

Cellulitis

Cellulitis is an acute bacterial infection of the skin and subcutaneous tissue that may cause an older adult a great deal of pain and distress. Cellulitis, which occurs most frequently on the lower legs and face, is characterized by symptoms of inflammation, which include intense pain, heat, redness, and swelling. It may appear in a localized area as a complication of a wound infection, or it may involve an entire limb. Cellulitis often occurs in areas where there is no apparent injury. This occurs in dry and irritated skin where microscopic breaks in the skin allow the bacteria to penetrate (Fleck, 2010). In severe infections, fever may be present, as well as an increase in white blood cells (WBCs) and tender lymph nodes (lymphadenopathy). An elevated WBC count and temperature, although common signs of infection, may not be present in the frail older adult. The organisms most commonly responsible for cellulitis in older adults with normal host defenses are hemolytic streptococci (group G streptococci and *Streptococcus pyogenes*) and *Staphylococcus aureus*. The incidence of more serious staphylococcus infection called methicillin-resistant *Staphylococcus aureus* (MRSA) is increasing. In immunocompromised hosts, gram-negative rods may cause cellulitis (Fleck, 2010). Older adults at risk for cellulitis include those with any break in the skin such as a leg ulceration or pressure ulcer. In addition, those with predisposing factors such as diabetes, obesity, a previous history of cellulitis, peripheral vascular disease, or tinea pedis are at risk. Many normal changes of aging increase the older adult's risk for developing cellulitis. Changes in the thickness of the skin make the older adult more susceptible to breaks in the skin. After the skin is broken, the older adult is at higher risk for infection since wound healing is often delayed.

Fingernail and Toenail Conditions

The distal phalanges are protected from injury and trauma by the nails. Changes in the nail plate occur with aging, and are also affected by trauma, systemic diseases such as diabetes and circulatory disorders, as well as dermatological conditions.

Onychomycosis, a fungal infection (i.e., *Trichophyton rubrum, T. mentagrophytes*) of the toenail, most commonly occurs on the big toe. This condition is often ignored because it can be present for years without causing any pain. The toenail appears thick, discolored, and protruding from the nail bed (American Podiatric Medical Association, 2012). Older adults may complain of severe pain when their shoe presses on the deformed toe, often causing them to reduce their activity or wear open shoes and sandals. The older adult should see their healthcare provider for treatment to prevent the condition from spreading to the other parts of the foot.

Onychia is inflammation of the nail matrix; paronychia is inflammation of the matrix, plus the surrounding and deeper structures. This is a common condition in older adults and is caused by bacteria or fungus. Older adults who have been exposed to wet work such as dishwashing, cleaning, or fishing for many years are at high risk. Trauma caused by tight shoes may also be the source of the problem. This disorder is characterized by separation of the cuticle from the nail, which allows organisms to enter. The organisms may cause swelling, redness, and tenderness of the nail fold, accompanied by purulent drainage.

Onychogryphosis is a chronic hypertrophy of the nail plate characterized by a hooked or curved nail. Any pressure on the nail may cause severe pain. The deformed nail may cause pressure on an adjacent toe, leading to a dangerous pressure necrosis in a vulnerable older adult. Diabetes and circulatory conditions are predisposing factors for these complications.

Nursing Diagnoses

Nursing diagnoses appropriate to the older adult with problems of the skin may include any of the following (North American Nursing Diagnosis Association, 2012):

- *Skin Integrity, Impaired*
- *Skin Integrity, Risk for Impaired*
- *Infection, Risk for*
- *Pain, Acute*
- *Pain, Chronic*

NANDA-I © 2012.

The major nursing diagnoses related to integumentary problems are *Tissue Integrity, Impaired* and *Skin Integrity, Impaired* and *Skin Integrity, Risk for Impaired*.

Tissue Integrity, Impaired is defined as "a state in which an individual experiences, or is at risk for damage to the integumentary, corneal, or mucous membrane tissues of the body." Defining characteristics (major) that must be present include "disruptions of integumentary tissue or invasion of body structure (incision, dermal ulcer)" (Carpenito-Moyet, 2007). *Skin Integrity, Impaired* is defined as "a state in which the individual experiences, or is at risk for damage to the epidermal and dermal tissue" (Carpenito-Moyet, 2007). The major defining characteristic that must be present is disruption of epidermal and dermal tissue. There is both overlap and possible confusion as to when to use these diagnoses. According to Carpenito-Moyet, *Tissue Integrity, Impaired* is the broad category under which more specific diagnoses fall. *Skin Integrity, Impaired* should be used to describe pressure ulcers that have damaged the epidermal and dermal tissue only. *Tissue Integrity, Impaired* would describe pressure ulcers that are deeper than the dermis (i.e., connective tissue, muscle).

Laboratory and Testing Values

Total body photography, skin surface microscopy, machine vision, and skin biopsy are the current modalities that can be used to diagnose malignant melanoma.

Total Body Photography

A series of 24 slides is taken of high-risk patients and used during subsequent visits to identify changes in nevi. Skin surface microscopy uses a handheld instrument to provide a 10× illuminated review of the skin. This process is very time intensive to learn and requires training (Penn Medicine, 2011).

Skin Biopsy with Histologic Examination

A skin biopsy is indicated for all skin lesions that are suspected of being neoplasms. A variety of techniques are available for the examination of the tissue, including immunofluorescence and electron microscopy. A biopsy is indicated for any lesion that has been present for longer than a month. A skin biopsy is also sometimes used to diagnose infections of the skin.

Wound Cultures to Determine Infection

Wound cultures and microscopic examination can identify infectious organisms. Wound cultures should be obtained by the aspiration method or a tissue biopsy. The swab method is not considered useful for obtaining a wound culture since it examines bacteria present on the wound surface, not in the wound bed itself. The tissue that is obtained must be healthy, viable tissue to ensure capturing the greatest number of microorganisms. If eschar or exudate is visible, it must be removed so that the healthy tissue is accessible. The wound is then washed with saline and dried gently with sterile gauze.

The wound biopsy is considered the gold standard for culture. This is done by the removal of a small piece of tissue from the ulcer, which is then sent to the laboratory. The disadvantages of the wound biopsy, however, are that the removal of tissue from the ulcer will delay healing and the procedure is skill intensive and unavailable in many settings.

The aspirate method requires inserting a needle with a 10-mL syringe into the wound and aspirating fluid from the site while moving the needle around the wound base. All air must be removed from the syringe before injecting it into the container. The container must be labeled clearly with the location of the ulcer (e.g., sacral area). The final results are available in 48 hours, but preliminary results can

identify if an infection is present and whether it is gram negative or gram positive. This will allow antibiotic treatment to begin if indicated. Some of the common organisms found in wounds are *Staphylococcus pyogenes, Proteus mirabilis, S. aureus,* group A streptococci, *Escherichia coli*, gram-negative bacilli, and fungi. *Clostridium perfringens*, a bacteria found in soil and stool, can cause gangrene (Thompson & Colby, 2010). The most common type of fungus that causes infection in wounds is *Candida albicans*. Fungi grow very slowly and may take several weeks to show up in a culture.

Laboratory Values to Determine Risk for Pressure Ulcer

Serum albumin, prealbumin, serum transferrin, and a lymphocyte count are useful values that will help to determine nutritional status. These values will be decreased in protein-energy undernutrition. They may also be affected by other illnesses.

Serum albumin indicates the level of protein stores. A normal serum albumin level is 3.5 to 5.0. A level below 3.5 g/dL is considered mild undernutrition, below 3.0 g/dL is considered moderate undernutrition, and below 2.5 g/dL indicates severe undernutrition.

Prealbumin is a sensitive indicator of protein deficiency and improvement of protein status with refeeding. When looking at prealbumin levels, use the "rule of 5s." Greater than 15 mg/dL is normal, less than 15 mg/dL is a mild deficiency, less than 10 mg/dL is a moderate deficiency, and less than 5 mg/dL is a severe deficiency (Lajoie, 2006).

Serum transferrin is considered an accurate indicator of protein stores because it is responsive to acute changes. A normal serum transferrin level is 220 to 400 mg/dL. A serum transferrin level between 201 and 219 mg/dL is considered mild undernutrition, between 150 and 200 mg/dL is moderate undernutrition, and less than 150 mg/dL indicates a serious depletion in protein or severe undernutrition.

The synthesis of lymphocytes is depressed when protein-energy malnutrition exists, which contributes to the decreased ability of the white blood cells to fight infection. A total lymphocyte count of 2,000 to 3,500 μL is normal. Measurements of 1,501 to 1,999 μL are considered mild undernutrition. Results of 800 to 1,500 μL indicate loss of energy to skin and moderate undernutrition. Levels of 800 μL or below are considered to be indicative of severe undernutrition.

Pharmacological Treatment of Skin Problems in Older Adults

Pharmacological treatment of skin problems may include topical or systemic administration of medications. The following agents are used extensively in the clinical setting for management of dermatological problems in the older adult.

Topical and Oral Antifungal Agents

Antifungal agents such as itraconazole are used in the treatment of onychomycosis of the toenails and fingernails. The topical preparation is applied to the affected area and has few side effects. A combination of systemic and topical treatment increases the cure rate. The suggested dosage for treatment of onychomycosis of the toenails is itraconazole 200 mg po daily for 12 weeks. Adverse effects include renal and hepatic damage. The rate of recurrence remains high even with newer agents and the older person should be educated about the costs and risks involved.

Topical Antibiotics

The use of topical antibiotics on local pressure ulcers has met with some debate. In general, topical antibiotics are not recommended for pressure ulcers. Reasons include inadequate penetration if the wound is deep, development of antibiotic resistance, hypersensitivity reactions, and local irritation. All of these can further delay wound healing. If the wound has foul-smelling exudate and is not healing after 2 to 4 weeks of optimal care, a short course of topical antibiotics should be instituted. Some other wounds without local signs may have a high level of bacteria and may also benefit from topical antibiotic therapy.

The topical antimicrobial of choice for the nonhealing ulcer, or one with high bacterial levels (10^5/g of tissue), is silver sulfadiazine. Nanocrystalline silver dressings have been found to be effective against gram-negative, gram-positive, and anaerobic organisms. Cadexomer iodine dressings provide a slow-release form of iodine; these dressings have effective antibacterial action and do not harm granulation tissue. Other options include triple antibiotic and metronidazole (for anaerobic bacteria that is foul smelling). Topical antibiotics are indicated for short-term use and are reevaluated in 2 weeks. Patient teaching includes limiting the product to the number of applications and the condition prescribed (EPUAP-NPUAP, 2009).

Systemic Antibiotics

If a wound shows signs of infection, such as cellulitis, osteomyelitis, or septicemia, appropriate systemic antibiotics should be instituted. Common offending organisms of bacteremia and sepsis include *S. aureus,* gram-negative rods, and *Bacteroides fragilis.* A blood culture will allow the causative organisms to be identified, and antibiotics can be directed at the offending organisms. These are very serious complications and immediate medical attention is advised.

Selected Antimicrobials

Penicillinase-resistant penicillins (methicillin, nafcillin, oxacillin) are indicated against staphylococcal and beta-hemolytic streptococci infections of soft tissue. These drugs have a high degree of safety, but the dose should be adjusted for older adults with renal impairment to prevent nephrotoxicity.

Aminoglycosides

Gentamicin, tobramycin, and streptomycin are rapidly bactericidal against staphylococci and gram-negative aerobic bacteria. The age-related physiological decline in kidney function influences the excretion of numerous antibiotics. This puts the older person at risk for adverse events. Specific examples of adverse antibiotic-related events that seem to appear more commonly in the older person are aminoglycoside-induced nephrotoxicity and ototoxicity and acute liver injury related to prolonged amoxicillin therapy.

Prescription Creams and Lotions for Dry Skin

Often corticosteroids are prescribed as topical treatment for dermatological problems in older people. These creams should be applied sparingly in thin layers to maximize therapeutic outcome and minimize the risk of side effects.

Hydrocortisone 1% or 2.5% is a low-potency topical corticosteroid that can be applied for short-term treatment of inflamed dry skin. Long-term use may cause systemic absorption.

Over-the-counter emollients may contain skin sensitizers for the older person. A **skin sensitizer** is a substance that will induce an allergic response following skin contact (Altox, 2008). Skin sensitization is a skin response to a hapten (allergen). Some individuals experience a type IV delayed hypersensitivity response of the skin after contact with the substance. In the sensitization phase, the substance penetrates the skin and produces an immune response, but there are no clinical symptoms at this time. A later exposure to the allergen will produce an allergic response and is called the *elicitation phase.* Symptoms may include erythema (redness) and pruritus (itching). This condition is also known as allergic contact dermatitis and can occur with exposure to metals, chemicals, and latex gloves. Several skin sensitizers have been identified in emollients. The following skin sensitizers should be avoided by the older person with xerosis because these sensitizers can more easily invade dry, cracked skin:

- Balsam of Peru
- Lanolin
- Aloe vera
- Vitamin E

- Fragrance
- Parabens
- Formaldehyde
- Propylene Glycol
- Polysorbate 60 and 80

Adapted from White-Chi & Reddy (2011); Environmental Working Group (2011).

> **Drug Alert** ▶▶▶ Older adults have a high rate of adverse reactions to corticosteroids and antihistamines, both of which are frequently prescribed for skin problems. Older adults should be reminded not to buy over-the-counter preparations of these drugs without specific instructions from their primary care provider. If these medications are prescribed, directions should be strictly followed and any unusual symptoms reported promptly.

Nonpharmacological Treatment of Skin Problems in Older Adults

Prevention and early treatment of skin problems in older people may also include nonpharmacological interventions and patient education. Identification and correction of factors that may contribute to pathological skin changes is a key nursing responsibility.

Skin Cancer and Precancer Conditions

The nurse's role in the nonpharmacological treatment of skin cancer focuses on giving the older adult and family members the correct knowledge they need for the prevention and early diagnosis of this disease. Teaching the family and older adult the correct methods for self-assessment, as well as practices for daily life, will empower them to focus on self-care and primary prevention.

> **Practice Pearl** ▶▶▶ Wang and Lim (2011) recently discovered that in addition to protecting the skin from UV exposure, broad-spectrum sunscreen products with SPF 30 offer protection from free radicals, molecules that cause skin damage and aging. This is important for older adults since their defense system may no longer be able to absorb free radicals. As of June 2012 the U.S. Food and Drug Administration was requiring all sunscreen products to follow special testing and labeling rules (American Academy of Dermatology, 2011).

Older adults should be taught the ABCDEs of skin cancer, as listed in Box 12-1. If they have any skin changes, such as moles or pigmented lesions, the ABCDEs should be noted.

Patients should also be taught the guidelines on protection from the sun, as listed in Box 12-2. The nurse should emphasize the importance of adhering to these guidelines and assist older adults in adapting the guidelines to their daily lives.

When assessing the skin of people of color, the nurse should become familiar with the characteristics of darker skin. Nurses and other healthcare professionals may find

> **BOX 12-1** ▶ **ABCDEs of Skin Cancer**
>
> **A**symmetrical. One half of the lesion is different from the other half.
> **B**orders are ragged, irregular, notched, or blurred.
> **C**olor is varied within the same lesion. May be shades of brown, black, or red.
> **D**iameter is larger than 6 mm (and size is enlarging).
> **E**volving. Any change in size, shape, elevation, or new symptoms such as itching, bleeding, or crusting.
> Some melanomas do not fit ABCDE rules, so it is important to notice any skin changes.
>
> *Source:* American Cancer Society (2011); Skin Cancer Foundation (2011c).

> **BOX 12-2** ▶ **Guidelines on Sun Protection Year-Round and Wearing Protective Clothing**
>
> These guidelines apply to all outdoor activity from walking to waiting for a bus.
>
> - Use a broad-spectrum sunscreen (UVA and UVB) with a sun protection factor of SPF 30 or above.
> - Use sunscreen while driving or riding in a car. Glass does not protect from sun exposure.
> - Use 1 to 2 oz of sunscreen and reapply after leaving the water, sweating, or drying off.
> - Wear UV blocking sunglasses with wraparound or large frames. This will protect your eyelids and skin around your eyes and decrease risk for cataracts.
> - Avoid the sun during midday (10 a.m. to 4 p.m.).
> - Seek shade during midday (trees, umbrella, hats).
> - Wear hats that protect the face:
>   - Hats with at least a 3-in. brim
>   - Legionnaire hats (baseball hat with ear and neck flaps)
> - Wear protective clothing:
>   - Fabrics with tighter weave transmit less UVR.
>   - If you can see through the fabric, the UV rays can get through, too.
>   - Darker colors transmit less UVR than lighter ones.
>   - Wet or stretched fabrics transmit more radiation.
>
> *Source:* Adapted from American Cancer Society (2011); Skin Cancer Foundation (2011c).

BOX 12-3 **Considerations for Skin Assessment for People of Color**

- Some dark-skinned people have bluish lips or gums.
- Dark-skinned people may have freckle-like pigmentation of gums, buccal cavity, and borders of the tongue.
- A dark-skinned person may lose reddish tones if pallor is present.
- Cyanosis is difficult to assess in a dark-skinned person. The nurse should check soles and heels for color.
- Erythema is an area of inflammation on the skin. On a dark-skinned person, the skin assumes a purplish color when inflammation is present. To assess erythema in a dark-skinned person, the nurse should palpate for warmth and check for hardness and smoothness.
- Ecchymotic lesions are large bruises. Purple or dark color usually can be seen.
- To determine if an area of concern is erythema or ecchymosis, the nurse should use a glass slide and press gently over the area. If the color changes and becomes lighter, it is an erythema. If no change occurs, it is an ecchymotic area.
- Dermatosis papulosa nigra is a type of seborrheic keratoses that occurs only in African Americans. It is characterized by the appearance of many dark, small papules on the face. (Merck Manuals, 2011).

the assessment of darker skin to be more challenging because the traditional hallmarks of redness and color changes may be obscured by the darker skin tone. Box 12-3 illustrates guidelines for assessment of darker skin.

Skin Cancer

The treatment of skin cancers may include any of the following techniques and are appropriate interventions for older people.

Basal Cell Carcinoma and Squamous Cell Carcinoma

The diagnosis of basal cell carcinoma and squamous cell carcinoma must be confirmed by biopsy. Treatment options for basal cell carcinoma and squamous cell carcinoma depend on the size, depth, and location of the tumor. Electrodesiccation and curettage can be used for small tumors. Surgical excision has the highest cure and can be done on an outpatient basis. Margins of 5 cm are considered desirable. Mohs surgery, a microscopically controlled surgical technique, is used for high-risk or large basal cell carcinoma, especially of the head and neck, and has a cure rate of 95% to 97%. The cure rate for other methods used to treat local recurrences of basal and squamous cell carcinoma is only 50% to 60% (Skin Cancer Foundation, 2011b). Mohs surgery helps to prevent tissue loss by sparing uninvolved tissue

while totally removing the cancer. Less common treatment includes cryosurgery and radiotherapy. Radiotherapy may be chosen for the older adult who cannot tolerate surgery. After tumor removal, the older adult should be seen annually for 5 years for follow-up and total skin evaluation.

Malignant Melanoma

Excisional biopsy is done to confirm diagnosis, and prognosis depends on the vertical (depth) thickness of the lesion in millimeters. Treatment of melanoma is excision, with surgical margins dependent on tumor thickness. Recently, Mohs micrographic surgery is increasingly being used as an alternative to standard excision for some types of melanoma. Special stains that highlight melanoma cells have made this technique possible (Skin Cancer Foundation, 2011b). Adjuvant therapies may be offered depending on the stage of the tumor. Therapy for metastatic disease may include chemotherapy, chemo-immunotherapy, and regional radiation therapy. Morbidity rates for older men are especially high, most likely due to delayed diagnosis. Advanced melanoma with metastasis is usually incurable, thus supportive care is offered. Focus should be on determining the wishes of the patient in relation to end-of-life care and pain management.

Prevention and Management of Skin Tears

Skin tears are common in the older adult, with 1.5 million occurring each year. A preventive approach is therefore the key to decrease the risk for skin tears. Older adults, caregivers, and family members should be aware of the following preventive interventions:

- Use a lift sheet to prevent shearing injury.
- Do not use any pulling or sliding movements when assisting older adults with a change in their position.
- Protect the older adult by padding any surfaces that come in contact with leg and arm movements such as side rails, wheelchair arm and leg supports, and table corners.
- Keep the environment free of obstacles and well lit.
- Avoid harsh soaps.
- Keep skin moist with adequate fluids.
- Keep fingernails and toenails cut short and filed to remove rough edges and prevent self-inflicted skin tears.
- Apply skin-moisturizing creams to arms and legs twice daily.
- Use paper tape and remove it cautiously, or substitute for tape with gauze or stockinette.
- Wear long sleeves and long pants to add a layer of protection over the skin.
- Use shin guards for those who have repeat tears to the shin.

LeBlanc & Baranoski, 2011.

The depth of the skin tear, and the agency protocol, will determine the management of skin tears. Unlike chronic wounds, skin tears are acute and have the potential to heal by primary intention. Recommended clinical care of a skin tear would include the following goals: control bleeding, prevent infection, control pain, restore skin integrity, and promote a healing environment (LeBlanc & Baranoski, 2011).

Wound protocol would include:

1. Pat or air dry.
2. Gently place the torn skin in its approximate normal position.
3. Place an arrow to designate the direction of the tear.
4. Apply dressing (saline, foam, gels) and change per protocol or product requirements.
5. Trace the wound.
6. Document the assessment and intervention. Photograph if permitted.

Pressure Ulcers

The nonpharmacological treatment of pressure ulcers has evolved during the past two decades. Research that supports practice has provided nurses and other healthcare workers with evidence-based practice guidelines as well as a synthesis of current expert opinion. The Agency for Healthcare Research and Quality's clinical practice guideline titled *Treatment of Pressure Ulcers* (Bergstrom et al., 1994) was the first attempt to provide the clinical community with a synthesis of research and expert opinion on the treatment options for pressure ulcer and wound healing. Since that time a variety of nursing and healthcare groups have reviewed, developed, and updated the pressure ulcer guidelines. Areas of nursing responsibility that will be addressed for pressure ulcers include risk assessment for pressure ulcers, prevention and modification of pressure ulcer risk factors, and treatment of pressure ulcers.

Risk Assessment for Pressure Ulcers

More than 100 risk factors for pressure ulcers have been identified in the literature. Because pressure ulcers have been associated with quality of care, nurses and others are responsible for preventing or healing them; failure to do so could lead to litigation. Risk assessment and institution of prevention strategies cannot be delayed. Pressure ulcers can develop within 4 to 6 hours in some patients depending on the personal history and severity of illness. Because of the overwhelming number of risk factors, pressure ulcer prediction tools are widely used. Several organizations, including the John A. Hartford Foundation and the Wound, Ostomy, and Continence Nurses Society, recommend use of the Braden Scale for Predicting Pressure Sore Risk (National Guideline Clearinghouse, 2009). The Hartford Institute for Geriatric Nursing recommends this scale be used for risk assessment in the following categories of older patients:

- All bed- or chair-bound patients, or those whose ability to reposition is impaired
- All at-risk patients on admission to healthcare facilities and regularly thereafter
- All older patients with decreased mental status, incontinence, and nutritional deficits

Accepted risk factors that form the basis of this scale generally include mobility, incontinence, nutrition, and mental status. Some of the variables used to develop this scale are expert derived and not based on accepted research evidence. See Best Practices: Braden Scale for Predicting Pressure Sore Risk that follows.

Prevention and Modification of Pressure Ulcer Risk Factors

Mobility and activity are important considerations in preventing and modifying risk factors as well as allowing healing to occur. Interventions include positioning schedules, activities, and bed surface devices. All of these interventions will protect against external mechanical forces, including friction, shearing, and pressure. The older adult who is at risk for a pressure ulcer should have a turning and activity schedule. Nurses and nurse assistants should consistently document their interventions in the flow sheet or progress notes. Mobility and activity considerations for preventing pressure ulcers include the following:

- Reposition q2h. Use a pull sheet to prevent shear and friction. If redness occurs, consider a 1½-hour turning schedule. The older adult should be turned in a 30° angle position to the mattress when on his or her side.
- Ensure proper positioning. Use pillows or wedges to prevent the skin from touching the bed on trochanter, heels, and ankles (Figure 12-7 ▶▶▶). Do not use rings or donuts.

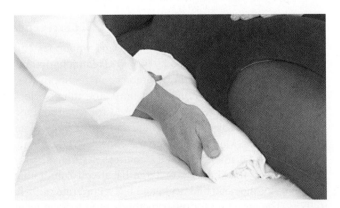

Figure 12-7 ▶▶▶ It is important to use pillows or wedges to prevent the skin from touching the bed on trochanter, heels, and ankles.

Best Practices Braden Scale for Predicting Pressure Sore Risk

The Braden Scale (Braden & Bergstrom, 1994) is a widely used tool that assesses mobility, activity, sensory perception, skin moisture, friction, shear, and nutritional status. Each dimension is rated from 1 to 4 on a Likert-type scale, and the total score range is from 6 to 23. A score of 16 or less indicates a pressure sore risk and the need for a prevention plan. The Braden Scale has been subjected to several validation studies and is considered the most valid of the available risk assessment tools. Once a risk assessment has been completed, and a deficit exists, the nursing care plan should reflect ongoing prevention as well as complete documentation of the older adult's progress. Although the Braden Scale is useful and reliable, it should be used as an adjunct to nursing assessment and clinical judgment (National Guideline Clearinghouse, 2009).

Patient's Name _____   Evaluator's Name _____   Date of Assessment

SENSORY PERCEPTION ability to respond meaningfully to pressure-related discomfort	**1. Completely Limited** Unresponsive (does not moan, flinch, or grasp) to painful stimuli, due to diminished level of consciousness or sedation OR limited ability to feel pain over most of body.	**2. Very Limited** Responds only to painful stimuli. Cannot communicate discomfort except by moaning or restlessness OR has a sensory impairment which limits the ability to feel pain or discomfort over ½ of body.	**3. Slightly Limited** Responds to verbal commands, but cannot always communicate discomfort or the need to be turned OR has some sensory impairment which limits ability to feel pain or discomfort in 1 or 2 extremities.	**4. No Impairment** Responds to verbal commands. Has no sensory deficit which would limit ability to feel or voice pain or discomfort.				
MOISTURE degree to which skin is exposed to moisture	**1. Constantly Moist** Skin is kept moist almost constantly by perspiration, urine, etc. Dampness is detected every time patient is moved or turned.	**2. Very Moist** Skin is often, but not always moist. Linen must be changed at least once a shift.	**3. Occasionally Moist** Skin is occasionally moist, requiring an extra linen change approximately once a day.	**4. Rarely Moist** Skin is usually dry, linen only requires changing at routine intervals.				
ACTIVITY degree of physical activity	**1. Bedfast** Confined to bed.	**2. Chairfast** Ability to walk severely limited or non-existent. Cannot bear own weight and/or must be assisted into chair or wheelchair.	**3. Walks Occasionally** Walks occasionally during day, but for very short distances, with or without assistance. Spends majority of each shift in bed or chair.	**4. Walks Frequently** Walks outside room at least twice a day and inside room at least once every two hours during waking hours.				

(continued)

Patient's Name _____   Evaluator's Name _____   Date of Assessment

MOBILITY ability to change and control body position	**1. Completely Immobile** Does not make even slight changes in body or extremity position without assistance.	**2. Very Limited** Makes occasional slight changes in body or extremity position but unable to make frequent or significant changes independently.	**3. Slightly Limited** Makes frequent though slight changes in body or extremity position independently.	**4. No Limitation** Makes major and frequent changes in position without assistance.
NUTRITION usual food intake pattern	**1. Very Poor** Never eats a complete meal. Rarely eats more than 1/3 of any food offered. Eats 2 servings or less of protein (meat or dairy products) per day. Takes fluids poorly. Does not take a liquid dietary supplement OR is NPO and/or maintained on clear liquids or IVs for more than 5 days.	**2. Probably Inadequate** Rarely eats a complete meal and generally eats only about 1/2 of any food offered. Protein intake includes only 3 servings of meat or dairy products per day. Occasionally will take a dietary supplement OR receives less than optimum amount of liquid diet or tube feeding.	**3. Adequate** Eats over half of most meals. Eats a total of 4 servings of protein (meat, dairy products) per day. Occasionally will refuse a meal, but will usually take a supplement when offered OR is on a tube feeding or TPN regimen which probably meets most of nutritional needs.	**4. Excellent** Eats most of every meal. Never refuses a meal. Usually eats a total of 4 or more servings of meat and dairy products. Occasionally eats between meals. Does not require supplementation.
FRICTION & SHEAR pressure forces applied parallel to the skin disrupting skin anchors and circulation	**1. Problem** Requires moderate to maximum assistance in moving. Complete lifting without sliding against sheets is impossible. Frequently slides down in bed or chair, requiring frequent repositioning with maximum assistance. Spasticity, contractures or agitation leads to almost constant friction.	**2. Potential Problem** Moves feebly or requires minimum assistance. During a move skin probably slides to some extent against sheets, chair, restraints or other devices. Maintains relatively good position in chair or bed most of the time but occasionally slides down.	**3. No Apparent Problem** Moves in bed and in chair independently and has sufficient muscle strength to lift up completely during move. Maintains good position in bed or chair.	
				TOTAL SCORE

- Avoid sitting. The sitting position, either in bed or in the chair, should be limited to 2 hours. Time in the chair should be scheduled around mealtimes. The person in bed should not be left in the 90-degree position except during meals.
- Increase activity. Encourage older adults to change positions by making small body shifts. This will redistribute weight and increase perfusion. Range-of-motion exercises should be done every 8 hours, and the techniques should be taught to family and patients.

> **Practice Pearl** ▶▶▶ Support surfaces alone neither prevent nor heal pressure ulcers but should be used as part of a total program of prevention and treatment of pressure ulcers.

Choose a mattress surface based on the assessment and diagnosis:

- Support surfaces may be described as static or dynamic, and further described as pressure reducing or pressure relieving. A static device relies on distribution of pressure over a large area and does not require electricity. Dynamic surfaces require electricity.
- Pressure-reducing devices do not consistently keep pressure below capillary pressure but are better than a standard mattress. Pressure-relieving devices are those that reduce pressure below capillary pressure and therefore are valuable in helping to prevent pressure ulcers.
- Static devices include air, foam, gel, or water overlay mattress. These devices are considered pressure-reducing devices. These mattresses are indicated for older people who are at high risk for a pressure ulcer or who have a stage I pressure ulcer. At present there is insufficient evidence to support the use of one of these static devices over another but it is important that high-risk older adults not be placed on a standard mattress.

National Guideline Clearinghouse, 2009.

- Dynamic surface specialty beds include low-air-loss beds and air-fluidized beds and they are considered to be pressure-relieving devices. Low-air-loss beds use separate air-filled cushions that are individually monitored to reduce the pressure below capillary closing pressure. Air-fluidized therapy uses warm forced air through silicone beads to simulate a fluid environment. Both of these devices are pressure-relieving devices (Salcido & Lorenzo, 2012). A dynamic air-fluidized bed is indicated for high-risk older people, those with stage III and IV pressure ulcers and for those having grafts or surgery. They are costly, but provide more pressure reduction than other pressure-relieving devices (Merck Manual for Healthcare Professionals, 2011).

> **Practice Pearl** ▶▶▶ High-risk older adults should not be placed in a 90-degree side-lying position. This position places intense weight on the femoral trochanter. Older adults at risk should be turned from supine to the right or left 30-degree oblique position. This position relieves pressure on the bony prominences of the trochanter and lateral malleolus.

Skin care practices for older adults include correct bathing procedure, prevention of injury, and dietary support. These skin care interventions are important to maintain healthy tissue as well as to improve tissue tolerance to decrease further risk of injury. Adequate skin care should be considered a high priority for all patients at risk for pressure ulcers. Older adults and their families should be given educational materials and demonstrations when appropriate. Skin care considerations to prevent pressure ulcers in older adults at risk include the following:

- Keep the skin clean and dry.
- Lubricate the skin with a moisturizer. Massage the area around the reddened area or bony prominence. (Do not massage any reddened area.) Then apply a thin layer of a petroleum-based product, followed by a baby powder–cornstarch product, to reduce friction and moisture.
- Evaluate and manage incontinence. A bowel and bladder management program should be in place. If soiling occurs, skin should be cleansed per routine. Underpads that absorb moisture and present a quick-drying surface to the skin should be used. Plastic-lined bed pads should not contact the person's skin. Use minimal pads and cover them with a sheet or pillowcase.
- Monitor nutrition. Determine factors that might cause inadequate nutrition. Obtain laboratory data. Provide additional canned supplements, vitamin C, and zinc to promote skin healing. Consider alternative methods such as total parenteral nutrition as needed (see Chapter 5 ▭ for further information).

> **Practice Pearl** ▶▶▶ The area at risk for pressure sores should be washed gently with tepid water, with or without minimal soap. Soap removes natural oils from the skin, and cleaning the soap off may cause additional friction damage.

Treatment of Pressure Ulcers

The nursing care related to pressure ulcers is an important part of nursing practice. Therefore, many agencies have established protocols that offer specific nursing care guidelines for each stage of the ulcer. If an ulcer is covered by eschar, it is usually removed. An ulcer cannot be staged until the eschar is removed. Stable dry intact eschar on the heels serves as the body's natural biological cover and should not be removed. The following are the components of the nursing care of a pressure ulcer:

- Assessing and staging the wound
- Debriding necrotic tissue
- Cleansing the wound
- Applying dressings to provide a moist wound bed
- Preventing and treating infection

Assessing and Staging the Wound

The first step in effective pressure ulcer care is to assess the wound. This assessment should include the history of the wound, the pressure ulcer size and depth, and any evidence or signs of tunneling, undermining, exudate, and infection. Once the wound has been assessed and documented, an effective pressure ulcer care plan should be established. The specific treatment of pressure ulcers is determined by the ulcer stage. As previously stated, a four-stage set of criteria for the assessment of pressure ulcers is widely used in healthcare institutions in the United States. The international EPUAP-NPUAP (2009) pressure ulcer classification system retained the original four stages and added two more for the United States: suspected deep tissue injury and unstageable. See *Pressure Ulcer Treatment Quick Reference Guide*, a 47-page, 4-year international effort to provide the latest summary of evidence-based guidelines (EPUAP-NPUAP, 2009).

Practice Pearl ▶▶▶ For a pressure ulcer to heal, the wound must be free from infection and necrotic tissue. Moist, devitalized tissue supports the growth of bacteria, delaying the healing process. Necrotic tissue is avascular; therefore, treatment with systemic antibiotics is not effective.

Debriding of Necrotic Tissue

Debridement is the removal of devitalized necrotic (black) tissue or yellow slough tissue. Debridement is complete when necrotic tissue is gone and the wound surface is covered with granulation tissue. Four methods are available for debridement: sharp, mechanical, chemical, and autolytic debridement.

Sharp debridement involves the use of a scalpel or other sharp instrument to remove necrotic tissue. It is the quickest form of debridement and is indicated when a dangerous sepsis or cellulitis is imminent. Large extensive ulcers, such as stage IV ulcers with thick adherent eschar, often require sharp surgical debridement in the operating room.

Mechanical debridement is the removal of stringy exudate by the use of topical force. Wet-dry dressings, an example of a historical method of mechanical debridement, have fallen out of favor with wound care specialists. Reasons include patients' complaints of pain, and the fact that healthy tissue is removed with necrotic tissue. Wound irrigations are done using gentle pressure, about 4 to 5 psi, to clean the wound and soften eschar. The nurse should use a 35-mL syringe with an 18-gauge angiocatheter to deliver the cleaning agent. A bulb syringe does not deliver adequate pressure for debridement. Urgent debridement in the operating room is required for advancing cellulitis or sepsis.

Chemical debridement is the use of topical enzymatic agents to break down devitalized tissue. It is recommended that the skin be crosshatched with a scalpel before using to improve penetration of the agents. It can be used alone, after sharp debridement, or with mechanical debridement. Collagenase is especially effective because collagen comprises 75% of the dry weight of the skin.

Autolytic debridement involves the use of a moisture-retentive dressing to cover the wound and allow the enzymes in the wound bed to liquefy selective dead tissue. Autolytic debridement may be used for small wounds or wounds that need to be sealed off and protected (because of contamination by urine or feces). DuoDERM or Contreet (contains silver and thus has antimicrobial advantage) are two commonly used autolytic debridement products. This method of debridement is contraindicated if a wound is infected as infected wounds should not be occluded. Occlusion of infected wounds can promote the growth of certain bacteria in the wound and lead to cellulitis and possibly sepsis (Merck Manual for Healthcare Professionals, 2011).

Practice Pearl ▶▶▶ The purpose of debridement is to remove dead, devitalized tissue from the wound bed to allow healing to progress. Therefore, debridement is discontinued once all of the dead tissue has been removed and the wound cleaned (no necrotic tissue). Continuing debriding of any kind will cause damage to delicate new tissue.

Cleansing the Wound

The purpose of cleansing the wound is to remove bacteria, debris, and small amounts of devitalized tissue to allow optimal healing. Cleansing should not be confused with disinfection or antisepsis, both of which relate to the killing of microorganisms. Topical antiseptics such as povidone-iodine, acetic acid, hydrogen peroxide, and Dakin's solution should not be used on a wound because these products have been found to be toxic to the wound fibroblasts and macrophages. The safest, most cost-effective, and most common cleansing agent for wounds is isotonic saline (0.9%). Wound cleansing can be done by (1) pouring a saline solution over the wound, (2) applying saline-soaked gauzes to clean the debris, or (3) squeezing a saline-filled bulb syringe over the wound. For a wound that requires the removal of small areas of nonadherent devitalized tissue, irrigation may be needed. To irrigate for the purpose of cleansing, the nurse should use saline in a catheter tip syringe (60 mL) and apply gentle pressure (4 psi). Wounds with large adherent areas of necrotic tissue or yellow slough should be irrigated (debrided) with a higher pressure stream between 8 and 15 psi. Pressure should not exceed 15 psi, or tissue damage and edema can result.

Applying Dressings to Provide a Moist Wound Bed

To heal a pressure ulcer, a clean, moist environment must be maintained. A moist wound environment promotes cellular activity in all phases of wound healing, provides insulation, increases the rate of epithelial cell growth, and reduces pain. A dry wound environment has been found to result in further tissue death, or dry necrosis, beyond the cause of the wound. Because scientific research demonstrated that a moist wound bed provided the best environment for wound healing, a thriving industry has emerged with hundreds of products developed to promote moist wound healing. Although many of these advanced products are appropriate, many common conventional dressing materials have the advantage of being readily available, effective, and less expensive.

The frequency of dressing change will be determined by the manufacturer's recommendations for the product selected and by the type and amount of exudate and drainage. The amount of wound moisture may change during the healing stages, so the wound may need added absorption during one period, and added moisture during another.

Preventing and Treating Infection

One of the most complex and controversial aspects of wound care has been the use of antibiotics. The presence of an infection is determined by the microbial state of the wound. To apply clinical reasoning to the treatment of wound infection, it is important to understand and differentiate between the three microbial states of a wound:

1. *Contamination* is the presence of microorganisms on the wound. All open wounds are contaminated. The human body has various organisms living both on and in it. Thus, the skin is never sterile.
2. *Colonization* is the presence and proliferation of organisms (bacteria) in the wound but with no signs of local infection, thus no host response. Stage II, III, and IV pressure ulcers are generally considered to be colonized. Therefore, wound cleansing and debriding are instituted to prevent the development of infection.
3. *Infection* is the proliferation of bacteria in healthy cells that produces symptoms of local redness, pain, fever, and swelling. Examples of serious infections that can be complications of pressure ulcers are bacteremia, sepsis, osteomyelitis, and advancing cellulitis.

Use of Topical and Systemic Antibiotics

Urgent care is required for older adults with systemic signs of infection. This care includes obtaining wound cultures and blood cultures, and providing treatment with appropriate systemic antibiotics that will cover the offending organism. All of these conditions could cause delayed healing or further complications from tissue destruction, and may result in death.

Certain local conditions would warrant the use of topical antibiotics:

- A clean pressure ulcer that has not shown signs of healing over a 2-week period
- A pressure ulcer that has increased local discharge but shows no visible signs of infection (See Chapter 6 ⊂⊃ for additional antibiotic information.)

Surgery

Large ulcers with exposure of musculoskeletal structure will need to be surgically closed. Skin grafts are considered useful for large areas but because they do not add adequate circulation to the grafted area, the graft may not heal and remain viable causing further breakdown at the site. Myocutaneous flap is the surgical closure of choice over large bony prominences such as the sacrum and trochanters (Collison, 2010–2011). A rotated myocutaneous flap is a mass of tissue (skin and muscle) with adequate vascularity to permit sufficient tissue to be transferred from one area of the patient's body to another site to be stitched in place to promote healing. This technique allows the grafted tissue to retain its blood supply while it heals and can improve outcomes for the older person. The older person will not have sensation in the area since nerve tissues cannot be grafted.

Management of Cellulitis

Interventions for cellulitis focus on the immediate treatment of the acute infection and prevention of further complications such as abscess formation and tissue damage. The treatment includes appropriate antibiotics, prevention of further infection, immobilization and elevation of the affected limb, pain relief, and possibly anticoagulant therapy (Mayo Foundation for Medical Education and Research, 2010).

Appropriate antibiotics are the priority of treatment. They are usually given intravenously until the infection begins to resolve, and then they are changed to an oral route. Any existing wounds should be assessed, and a wound culture obtained if an infection is suspected. Bed rest should be maintained. If the cellulitis is on the lower extremities, the foot of the bed should be elevated to decrease swelling and allow the leg(s) to be fully supported. The nurse should encourage active foot exercises and calf pumping to decrease pain and swelling and allow the older adult to maintain normal function. Pain should be assessed on a 0-to-10 visual analog scale and medicated with appropriate analgesics. Sheets and blankets must not be allowed to rub against the affected area and cause friction and added pain.

Treatment of Fingernail and Toenail Conditions

Nonpharmacological treatment of fingernail and toenail problems focuses on the immediate treatment of the problem and prevention of further complications.

The treatment of onychomycosis will include relief of pain, patient education, and oral antifungal agents as appropriate. As a temporary measure, older adults should be advised to reduce the pressure on the toe by cutting a hole in their slipper or shoe. In addition, the podiatrist should be consulted periodically for reduction of the nail plate. Patient education includes frequent treatment to prevent the condition from spreading to other parts of the foot. Oral antifungal agents may provide a cure.

The treatment of chronic paronychia will include keeping affected nails dry and perhaps antibiotics. The older adult should be advised to keep the affected nails out of water and to keep the area protected. Drainage is sometimes needed. A physician or nurse practitioner should be consulted for appropriate antibiotic treatment.

The treatment of onychogryphosis will include a podiatry consultation and perhaps surgical intervention for refractory problems. The podiatrist should trim thickened toenails with an electric drill and burrs or a carbon dioxide laser. Nails should be kept short. Proper foot care and hygiene are essential (Rehmus, 2009). If all conservative measures fail, the older adult who is disabled by this disorder should consider surgery.

Nursing Management Principles

Nursing care and documentation of the older adult with a skin problem should focus on careful assessment of the risk factors, provision of nursing interventions to minimize the risk of skin breakdown, documentation of care, and evaluation of the older patient's status.

Nursing Process and Documentation

Nursing care of the older patient should focus on the prevention of pressure ulcers. This goal is difficult to achieve, but research has shown that a large majority of pressure ulcers can be prevented. For the older adult who has a pressure ulcer, the nursing care plan should be a guide for nursing interventions. Ongoing nursing process and best practices should be reflected in each step. Documentation is necessary to ensure that the care plan is appropriate.

The wound is assessed initially, and an evaluation is done with each dressing change. If the nurse assesses that the wound has improved, documentation should reflect the actual changes that the nurse evaluated to make that decision. Wound healing is a process. As the wound changes and evolves, there may be a need to make changes in the dressing protocol. If the wound does not show signs of healing in 2 weeks, the treatment should be reevaluated.

Knowledge-Based Decision Making

To make knowledge-based decisions, the nurse should have access to all appropriate current knowledge regarding research on pressure ulcer care, pressure-relieving devices, and current products for topical treatment. Access to current literature will support decision making and provide information for families and other staff. Product information is helpful, but independent controlled trials of the product provide the needed unbiased results.

The following questions are useful when assessing wound care products:

1. What is the wound assessment? What is the stage, drainage, moisture, eschar?
2. What does the wound need? (This will depend on the assessment and is ongoing.) Does it need absorption, debridement, moisture?
3. What products are available in the setting? Many similarities exist between products, and agencies will not have every product. It is important to understand what the product does.
4. What is the evaluation of the product? What materials are available? Is there a resource manual at the agency that will assist with this process? If not, the nurse should begin the process.
5. What is practical? If the nurse is in the home or if a family member has to do the dressing, the process will have to be as simple as possible to ensure correct technique.

Evaluation and Revision of Nursing Care Plan

Critical evaluation of the care plan is the key to excellence in nursing practice. It is important to determine what practices were successful for the individual patient and what practices need to be modified. Careful, ongoing evaluation of nursing care is the key to a practice base that is constantly being changed to update skills and education that will benefit the older patient. The evaluation step of the nursing process provides the opportunity to determine if the patient goals were met. Possible outcome criteria for an older adult with a pressure ulcer are the prevention of further tissue damage and the promotion of normal wound healing.

The goals and outcome criteria are individualized for each older adult. In the evaluation and revision of the care plan, the needs and opinions of the older adult should always be considered. The nurse should evaluate if the goals were realistic for the older adult's age and condition. If the older adult was at home, were resources sufficient to make success possible? The evaluation of the family situation, resources available, and needs and desires of the older adult will determine the revision of the care plan and the goals and outcome criteria that can be successful. Suggested patient–family teaching guidelines are provided below to assist the nurse in the process of educating patients and families.

QSEN Recommendations Related to the Integument

The Quality and Safety Education for Nurses (QSEN) project addresses the challenge of preparing future nurses with the knowledge, skills, and attitudes (KSAs) to continuously improve the quality and safety of the healthcare systems in which they work (Cronenwett et al., 2007).

See the QSEN table for tips on meeting QSEN standards.

Meeting QSEN Standards: The Integument

	KNOWLEDGE	SKILLS	ATTITUDES
Patient-Centered Care	Teach older person techniques that will help him or her to prevent further injury.	Review skin care and prevention principles.	Be inclusive and give family literature for review.
	Teach the family so that they can support and reinforce the plan of care.	Assess skin daily and keep careful records.	Give encouragement to patient and family.
Teamwork and Collaboration	Care of pressure ulcers requires a team. Incorporate entire team and share views.	Form a group to evaluate new products and keep careful records of use.	Write a short article about your group to show appreciation and get recognition.
	Be aware that a team approach may take time and patience.	Develop short-term goals for the team.	Be open to others' ideas and discussions even if not in agreement.
Evidence-Based Practice	Know pressure ulcer assessment and research-based interventions.	Check NPUAP website for the latest updates. Check National Guideline Clearinghouse for updates.	Advocate for change if current therapy does show healing progress.
Quality Improvement	Document nursing assessment and interventions in a clear and descriptive manner. This will help the patient and team to provide quality care.	Develop skills in data management. Review current practice guidelines at government websites.	Value the use of data and outcomes as a key component of QI efforts.

(continued)

Meeting QSEN Standards: The Integument   *(continued)*

	KNOWLEDGE	SKILLS	ATTITUDES
Safety	Provide older adults with current information on drugs that cause photosensitivity.	Teach the older adult the risks of photosensitivity and how to prevent it.	Relate the importance of safety and prevention and be responsive to questions.
Informatics	Provide input into the formation and maintenance of patient databases needed for gathering QSEN data and providing patient care.	Utilize the electronic health record.	Protect patient confidentiality according to HIPAA standards.

Patient-Family Teaching Guidelines

The following are guidelines that the nurse may find useful when instructing older adults and their families about prevention of skin cancer.

PREVENTION OF SKIN CANCER

1 **What can older adults do to decrease their risk of skin cancer?**

■ Remember that the sun penetrates through clouds, water, and shade throughout the year.

■ Use the appropriate sunscreen protection, at least 15 SPF. It is never too late to protect yourself against further damage.

■ Do a total body check, using a mirror if needed, and record any spots so that change can be noted.

■ Be aware that many drugs can cause increased photosensitivity and accelerate damage to the skin.

■ Reapply sunscreen when needed. Be aware of ears and bald scalp areas when applying sunscreen. These areas are often the sites of skin cancer.

RATIONALE:

*Education is the key to decreasing the older adult's risk of skin cancer. On a cloudy day, 80% of the damaging UVR still penetrates to the skin. Sand and snow are equally risky, reflecting 85% to 95% of the sun's rays. It is important to know one's skin type and apply the appropriate sunscreen so that burning is avoided. If **actinic keratotic lesions** have developed, avoidance of the sun may be sufficient therapy for*

the regression of mild cases. Self-examination is the key. Any precancerous lesions should be checked every 6 months.

Older adults often take multiple medications. All drug labels should be checked for photosensitivity precautions. Examples of common medications that can cause photosensitivity include Bactrim, tetracycline, and ibuprofen.

2 **What causes dry skin (xerosis) in the older adult?**

The exact etiology is not entirely understood, but factors that are thought to contribute to dry skin include age-related changes:

■ Age-related changes in keratinization process and lipid content in stratum corneum (Foy White-Chu & Reddy, 2011)

■ Systemic variables such as vitamin A deficiency, hormones, and stress

Environmental factors include:

■ Dry and/or cool temperatures, such as those experienced in winter; air conditioning, and desert conditions

■ Hot water bathing, harsh cleansers or soaps, and skin powders

Patient–Family Teaching Guidelines *(continued)*

RATIONALE:

The main source of skin hydration or moisture is provided from the underlying vasculature of the tissues. The lipid barrier helps to maintain hydration by adding a protective layer to the skin and prevents loss of water through the epidermis. The changes of aging slowly decrease these features. The result is dry skin from a lack of moisture in the stratum corneum, resulting in less pliable epidermis. This decrease in pliability results in the rough texture and flaking of dry skin.

3 **What treatment is most effective for dry skin?**

The best treatment for dry skin has not been studied so care is based on expert opinion. Personal practices to improve or relieve dry skin include the following:

- Bathe once a day with warm water, using superfatted soaps such as Dove or Caress. Avoid any drying agents such as alcohol.
- Avoid the use of oils for older people since they are at risk for falls.
- Dry with a soft towel, including between the toes.

- Apply prescription creams and lotions liberally to the skin immediately after bathing, while skin is moist. Reapply frequently.
- Use white petroleum for an effective emollient for dry skin treatment. It is inexpensive and does not contain irritating additives such as perfumes.
- Use a humidifier during the winter when humidity levels are 45% to 60%.
- Wear soft, nonirritating clothing next to the skin.
- Prescription creams may also be useful (see the pharmacological interventions section).

RATIONALE:

Research findings indicate that dry skin increases with age and is more severe in winter. Excess bathing depletes the older adult's skin of moisture and increases dryness. The use of superfatted soap for bathing helps to retain moisture in the older adult's skin. The skin should not be rubbed with a towel; it will increase irritation. Applying emollients after bathing retains moisture in the skin. It also helps to keep the home temperature low and use a humidifier, especially in the winter.

CARE PLAN | A Patient With a Pressure Ulcer

Case Study

A registered nurse who works for a home health agency has been assigned to Mrs. Krebs, a 75-year-old patient with a chronic stage III ulcer on her heel that has not shown any progress in the last 3 months. The nurse notes that Mrs. Krebs has a smoking history of 40 years and has not followed her diet instructions. The supervisor of the home health agency has warned the nurse that if Mrs. Krebs does not improve, the insurance company will not continue to provide payment for the visits and treatment. Mrs. Krebs has refused to be admitted to the hospital for ulcer care and feels the nurses and physician do not understand her situation.

Applying the Nursing Process
Assessment

On the first visit, the nurse did a complete assessment and discussed the patient's history, which includes peripheral vascular disease and hypertension. Mrs. Krebs's physical examination showed blood pressure 140/82, pulse 76, respirations 20, and temperature 98°F. On examination of the heel ulcer, the nurse noted a 4-cm by 6-cm stage III ulcer with a minimal amount of serous drainage and no local signs of inflammation.

(continued)

CARE PLAN **A Patient With a Pressure Ulcer** *(continued)*

Mrs. Krebs is eating poorly, mostly frozen and canned foods with little protein and high sodium. She admits that she is smoking and not following her diet. She states, "I lost my husband 6 months ago and have not been able to take care of things. I tried to quit smoking but it only lasted 5 days. I have been smoking for 40 years and it is just too hard to stop. I'm doing the best I can."

Diagnosis

The current nursing diagnoses for Mrs. Krebs include the following:

■ *Skin Integrity, Impaired* stage III ulcer, related to prolonged pressure, inadequate nutrition, decreased vascular perfusion
■ *Health Maintenance, Ineffective* related to complex regimen, limited resources, and impaired adjustment

■ *Nutrition, Imbalanced: Less Than Body Requirements* related to lack of physical and economic resources, and increased nutritional requirements related to ulcer

NANDA-I © 2012.

Expected Outcomes

The expected outcomes for the plan specify that Mrs. Krebs will:

■ Describe measures to protect and heal the tissue, including wound care.
■ Report any additional symptoms such as pain, redness, numbness, tingling, or increased drainage.

■ Demonstrate an understanding of nutritional needs, including the need for supplemental protein drinks and vitamins.
■ Collaborate with the nurse to develop a therapeutic plan that is congruent with her goals and present lifestyle.

Planning and Implementation

The following nursing interventions may be appropriate for Mrs. Krebs:

■ Establish a trusting relationship with Mrs. Krebs.
■ Begin to explore what the patient's goals are in relation to her health care.
■ Determine her daily habits and schedule and find some small measures that can be started for health improvement.

■ Begin to determine ways to work with Mrs. Krebs's family to motivate her toward a healthy lifestyle (i.e., nutrition, smoking, foot care).
■ Set priorities of care that Mrs. Krebs will agree to such as (1) ulcer improvement, (2) diet adjustments, and (3) smoking reductions.

Evaluation

The nurse hopes to develop a long-term relationship with Mrs. Krebs and make an impact on her health and well-being. The nurse will consider the plan a success based on the following criteria:

■ Mrs. Krebs will develop a trusting relationship and develop a plan with the nurse to improve her health.

■ A family member or friend will agree to assist Mrs. Krebs with her wound care and shopping issues.
■ Mrs. Krebs will begin a smoking reduction effort.
■ Mrs. Krebs will agree that if the ulcer is not healing in 4 weeks, she will seek inpatient treatment.

CARE PLAN   A Patient With a Pressure Ulcer *(continued)*

Ethical Dilemma

The primary ethical dilemma that evolves from this situation is the conflict between the moral obligation of the nurse to respect the autonomy of the patient and the principle of beneficence. The patient has a right to self-determination, independence, and freedom. It is important to allow patients to make their own decisions, even if the healthcare provider does not agree with them. However, the nurse has a responsibility to "do good" and "do no harm" based on the principles of beneficence and nonmaleficence. These ethical obligations are outlined in the American Nurses Association's Code for Nurses. A second ethical dilemma is the conflict between the nurse's obligation to the patient and to the home health agency.

The nurse hopes to work with Mrs. Krebs and the supervisor to set new goals and priorities and make progress toward them. The nurse understands that the patient has a right to make any final decisions.

Critical Thinking and the Nursing Process

1. What are the intrinsic and extrinsic factors that can cause skin problems in older adults? Make a list with two columns and see how many factors you can identify.
2. How important is nutrition to the health of your skin?
3. What type of dressings do you see used in your clinical rotations with older people? Are they consistent with current guidelines and recommendations?
4. What positioning techniques have you seen used in your clinical rotations?

■ Evaluate your responses in Appendix B.

Chapter Highlights

■ The most common precancerous lesion is actinic keratosis, also known as solar keratosis and senile keratosis. Erythematous actinic keratosis is the most common type and appears as a sore, rough, scaly, erythematous papule or plaque. The most common sites for all types of actinic keratosis are sun-exposed areas such as the hands, face, nose, tips of the ears, and bald scalp.

■ Basal cell carcinoma is the most common form of skin cancer in white people and accounts for about 80% of nonmelanoma skin cancers.

■ Melanoma is the most serious of skin cancers. Encourage older adults to check their skin frequently for any changes, and ask a friend to check areas that they cannot see. Report changes at once.

■ A wound that does not heal within 6 weeks is considered a chronic wound. Common problems of older adults that often lead to chronic wounds are diabetes, peripheral vascular disease, and pressure ulcers.

■ The wound can be damaged by both too much and too little moisture. A dry wound surface impairs epithelial migration and leads to tissue injury and necrosis. The buildup of tissue exudates is toxic to new growth and leads to tissue hypoxia, which impairs healing.

■ Wound cultures should be obtained by the aspiration method or a tissue biopsy. The swab method is not considered useful for obtaining a wound culture, since it examines bacteria present on the wound surface, not in the wound bed itself.

■ Skin care practices for older adults include correct bathing procedure, prevention of injury, and dietary support. These skin care interventions are important to maintain healthy tissue as well as to improve the tissue tolerance to decrease further risk of injury.

■ The nurse should encourage older adults to change or shift positions by making small body shifts. This will redistribute weight and increase perfusion.

- Range-of-motion exercises should be done every 8 hours and the techniques should be taught to family and patients.

- Topical antiseptics such as povidone-iodine, acetic acid, hydrogen peroxide, and Dakin's solution should not be used on a wound, since they have been found to cause damage.

- To heal a pressure ulcer, a clean, moist environment must be maintained. A moist wound environment promotes cellular activity in all phases of wound healing, provides insulation, increases the rate of epithelial cell growth, and reduces pain. A dry wound environment has been found to result in further tissue death.

- Colonization is the presence and proliferation of organisms (bacteria) in the wound but with no signs of local infection, thus no host response. Stage II, III, and IV pressure ulcers are generally considered to be colonized. Therefore, wound cleansing and debriding are instituted to prevent the development of infection.

- Infection is the proliferation of bacteria in healthy cells that produces symptoms of local redness, pain, fever, and swelling. Examples of serious infections that can be complications of pressure ulcers are bacteremia, sepsis, osteomyelitis, and advancing cellulitis.

Pearson Nursing Student Resources
Find additional review materials at
nursing.pearsonhighered.com
Prepare for success with additional NCLEX®-style practice questions, interactive assignments and activities, web links, animations and videos, and more!

References

Altox. (2008). Non-animal testing methods for toxicity testing. *Skin Sensitization.* Retrieved from http://alttox.org/ttrc/toxicity-tests/skin-sensitization

American Academy of Dermatology. (2011). *New study supports recommendation to use broad-spectrum sunscreen for protection against skin cancer and early aging.* Retrieved from http://www.aad.org

American Cancer Society (ACS). (2010). *Skin cancer prevention and early detection.* Retrieved from http://www.cancer.org

American Cancer Society (ACS). (2011). *Melanoma.* Retrieved from http://www.cancer.org/melanoma

American Podiatric Medical Association, (2012). *Nail problems: Toenails.* Retrieved from http://www.nlm.nih.gov/medlineplus/naildiseases.html

American Society of Clinical Oncology (ASCO). (2012). Cancer in older adults. Retrieved from http://www.cancer.net/coping/age-specific-information/cancer-older-adults

Ayello, E. (2012). Predicting pressure ulcer risks. *Try this: Best nursing practices in care for older adult* (No. 5). Hartford Institute for Geriatric Nursing.

Baranoski, S., & Ayello, A. (2007). Wound care essentials: Practice principles. Philadelphia, PA. Lippincott. Williams & Wilkins.

Bergstrom, N., Allman, R., Alvarez, O., Bennett, M., Carlson, C., & Franz, R. (Eds.). (1994). *Treatment of pressure ulcers: Clinical practice guideline No. 15* (AHCPR Publication No. 95–0652). Rockville, MD: Agency for Health Care Policy and Research, Public Health Service, U.S. Department of Health and Human Services.

Braden, B., & Bergstrom, N. (1994). Predictive validity of the Braden scale for pressure sore risk in a nursing home population. *Research in Nursing and Health, 17,* 459–479.

Browder-Lazenby, R. (2011). *Handbook of pathophysiology* (4th ed.). Philadelphia, PA: Lippincott Williams & Wilkins.

Carpenito-Moyet, L. J. (2007). *Nursing diagnosis: Application to clinical practice.* Philadelphia, PA: Lippincott.Williams & Wilkins.

Centers for Disease Control and Prevention. (2011). Chronic disease prevention and health promotion. *Heathy aging at a glance.* Retrieved from http://www.cdc.gov/chronicdisease/resources/publications/aag/aging.htm

Centers for Medicare and Medicaid Services (CMS). (2011). Hospital-acquired conditions (present on admission indicator). Retrieved from http://www.cms.gov/Medicare/Medicare-Fee-for-Service-Payment/HospitalAcqCond/index.html?redirect=/HospitalAcqCond

Collison, D. (2010–2011). Dermatology: Pressure sores. In R. Porter & J. Kaplan (Eds.), *The Merck manual for health professionals.* Whitehouse Station, NJ: Merck & Co.

Cronewett, L., Sherwood, G., Barnsteiner, J., Disch, J., Johnson, J., Mitchell, P., Sullivan, D., & Warren, J. (2007). Quality and safety education for nurses, *Nursing Outlook, 55*(3) 122–131.

Environmental Protection Agency (EPA). (2010). Facts about skin cancer: Florida. Retrieved from http://www.epa.gov/sunwise/doc/fl_facts_print.pdf.

Environmental Working Group. (2011). *Cosmetic database.* Retrieved from http://www.ewg.org/skindeep

European Pressure Ulcer Advisory Panel and National Pressure Ulcer Advisory Panel (EPUAP-NPUAP). (2009). *Pressure ulcers treatment: Quick reference guide.* Washington, DC: National Pressure Ulcer Advisory Panel.

Farage, M., Miller, K., Berardesca, E., & Maibach, H. (2009). Clinical implications of aging skin: Cutaneous disorders in the elderly. *American Journal of Clinical Dermatology, 10*(2), 73–86.

Fleck, L. (2010). Clinical skills: What's your assessment? *Dermatology Nursing, 22*(3), 23–25.

Fore, J. (2006). A review of skin and the effects of aging on skin structure and function. *Ostomy Wound Management, 52*(9), 24–36.

Hurlow, J., & Bliss, D. (2011). Dry skin in older adults. *Geriatric Nursing, 32*(4), 257–262.

Ignatavicius, D., & Workman, M. (2010). *Medical surgical nursing: Patient centered care*. St Louis, MO: Saunders.

Jenkins, M., & O'Neal, E. (2010). Pressure ulcer prevalence and incidence in acute care. *Advances in Skin and Wound Care, 23*(12) 556–559.

Lajoie, J. (2006). Pressure ulcers: An update from the bedside. *ECPN, 114*(9), 30–37.

LeBlanc, K., & Baranoski, S. (2011). Skin tears: State of the science: Consensus statements for the prevention, prediction, assessment, and treatment of skin tears. *Advances in Skin & Wound Care, 24*(9), 2–14.

Mayo Foundation for Medical Education and Research. (2010). *Cellulitis*. Retrieved from http://www.mayoclinic.com/health/cellulitis

Merck Manual for Healthcare Professionals. (2011). Dermatologic disorders. Retrieved from http://www.merckmanuals.com/professional/dermatologic_disorders.html

Miller, A. (2009, May/June). Hospital reporting and "never events." *Medicare Patient Management*. Retrieved from http://www.medicarepatientmanagement.com/issues/04-03/mpmMJ09-NeverEvents.pdf

National Cancer Institute. (2010). *Skin cancer prevention PDQ*. Retrieved from http://www.cancer.gov/cancertopics/Pdq/prevention/skin/HealthProfessional

National Guideline Clearinghouse. (2009). *Guideline for prevention and management of pressure ulcers*. Retrieved from http://www.guideline.gov/content.aspx?id=23868

National Pressure Ulcer Advisory Panel (NPUAP). (2009). Pressure ulcer prevention and treatment: Clinical practice guidelines. Washington, DC: National Pressure Ulcer Advisory Panel.

Nixon, J., Thorpe, H., Barrow, H., Phillips, A., Nelson, E. A., Mason, S., & Callum, N. (2005). Reliability of pressure ulcer classification and diagnosis. *Journal of Advanced Nursing, 50*(6), 613–623.

North American Nursing Diagnosis Association. (2012). *NANDA nursing diagnosis: Definitions and classification 2012–2014*. Retrieved from http://www.nandanursingdiagnosislist.org/

Payne, R., & Martin, M. (1993). Defining and classifying skin tears: Need for a common language. *Ostomy Wound Management, 39*(5), 16–26.

Penn Medicine. (2011). *Whole body photography*. Retrieved from http://www.pennmedicine.org/dermatology/hup/whole_body_photo.html

Reddy, K., & Gilchrest, B. (2010). Vitamin D sufficiency vs. sun protection: Must we choose? *Dermatology Nursing, 22*(6), 2–8.

Rehmus, W. (2009). Paronychia. *The Merck Manual for Healthcare Professionals*. Retrieved from http://www.merckmanuals.com/professional/dermatologic_disorders/nail_disorders/paronychia.html .

Salcido, R., Lee, A., & Ahn, C. (2011). Heel pressure ulcers: Purple heel and deep tissue injury. *Advances in Skin and Wound Care, 24*(8), 374–379.

Salcido, R., & Lorenzo, C. (2012). Pressure ulcers and wound care. Retrieved from Medscape Reference at http://emedicine.medscape.com/article/319284-overview

Skin Cancer Foundation. (2010). *Press release: Sun safety for drivers*. Retrieved from http://www.skincancer.org

Skin Cancer Foundation. (2011a). *Actinic keratosis*. Retrieved from http://www.skincancer.org/actinic-keratosis-and-other-precancers

Skin Cancer Foundation. (2011b). *Mohs micrographic surgery*. Retrieved from http://www.skincancer.org/Mohs

Skin Cancer Foundation. (2011c). *Skin cancer facts*. Retrieved from http://www.skincancer.org

Skin Cancer Foundation. (2011d). *Year-round sun protection guidelines*. Retrieved from http://www.skincancer.org/year-round-sun-protection.html

Stokowski, L. (2010). In this corner: The unavoidable pressure ulcers. *Medscape Nurses*. Retrieved from http://www.medscape.com/viewarticle/715969

Thompson, G., & Colby, D. (2010). Skin and wound cultures. *Healthwise* Retrieved from http://www.webmd.com/a-to-z-guides/skin-and-wound-cultures?page=3

U.S. Department of Health and Human Services (USDHHS). (2010). *Healthy people 2020*. Retrieved from http://www.healthypeople.gov/2020/default.aspx

U.S. Environmental Protection Agency (EPA). (2010). *Sunwise: Health effects of overexposure to the sun*. Retrieved from http://www.epa.gov/sunwise/uvandhealth

U.S. Food and Drug Administration. (2010). *E-medicine drugs photosensitivity*. Retrieved from http://www.medicinenet.com/sun-sensitive_drugs_photosensitivity_to_drugs/page6.htm.emedcine.medscape.com/article/104648-overview

Wang, S., & Lim, H. (2011). Current status of the sunscreen regulation in the United States: 2011 Food and Drug Administration's final rule on labeling and effectiveness testing. *Journal of the American Academy of Dermatology, 65*(4), pp. 863–869.

White-Chu, E., & Reddy, M. (2011). Dry skin in the elderly: Complexities of a common problem. *Clinics in Dermatology, 29*(1), 37–42.

Zator Estes, M. (2010). *Health assessment and physical examination*. New York, NY: Delmar-Cengage Learning.

Zhang, A. (2011). Dermatology. In K. Phelps & C. Hassed (Eds.). *General practice: An integrated approach*. St. Louis, MO: Elsevier Health Sciences.

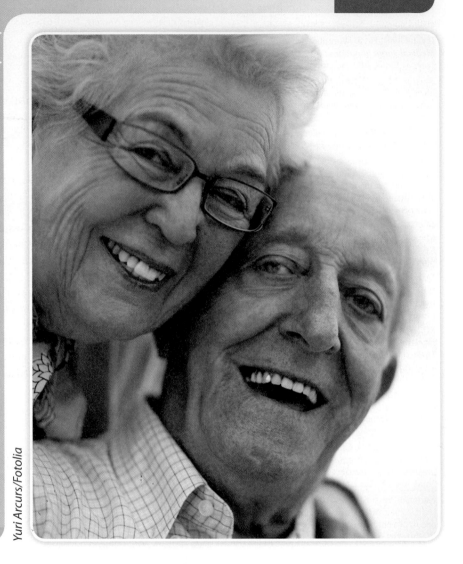

Yuri Arcurs/Fotolia

The Mouth and Oral Cavity

LEARNING OUTCOMES

On completion of this chapter, the reader will be able to:

1. Explain normal changes of aging in the mouth and oral cavity.
2. Identify common diseases of the mouth and oral cavity in older adults.
3. List common nursing diagnoses related to oral problems in older adults.
4. Recognize nursing interventions that can be implemented to assist the aging patient with oral problems.
5. Identify medications that may cause or aggravate oral problems.

Oral assessment and care are important responsibilities of gerontological nurses caring for older adults. The promotion of health through the delivery of good oral hygiene is an essential skill for the gerontological nurse (O'Connor, 2010). The mouth is the beginning of the digestive system and also serves as an airway for the respiratory system. The oral cavity consists of the lips, palate, cheeks, tongue, salivary glands, and teeth. Side effects of medications, illness, and treatment can affect the oral cavity.

NORMAL CHANGES OF AGING

With aging, there is thinning of the epithelium and tissue atrophy in the soft tissue of the oral cavity. The single most important factor relating to oral health in aging is maintaining good oral hygiene. In healthy aging with proper oral hygiene, the teeth and gums appear normal. However, with aging it becomes more difficult to maintain good oral hygiene because of multiple factors, including the number and condition of dental restorations, changing alignment between adjacent teeth due to recession of the gums, impaired visual acuity, possible loss of manual dexterity, restricted range of motion, and the effects of medications on oral health (Victorian Government Health Information, 2011). Figure 13-1▶▶▶ depicts the mouth and oral cavity.

> **Practice Pearl** ▶▶▶ Urge your older patients to brush with soft-bristled toothbrushes and fluoride toothpaste. Stiff bristles lack the flexibility needed to clean curved tooth surfaces and get into crevices between teeth (Treatment of Gingivitis Team, 2011).

The taste buds of the tongue decrease in number with a resulting **hypogeusia,** or loss of ability to taste. Salivary function also decreases over time and results in production of less saliva. The gums may recede, leaving teeth vulnerable to cavities below the gum line. Decreased saliva production may result in an overly dry oral mucosa. Tooth loss may occur in the presence of severe osteoporosis. The enamel on the surface of teeth may be worn away or abraded, leaving teeth open to staining, damage, and cavities. With tooth loss, malocclusion can result as remaining teeth become misaligned with use in chewing. With tooth loss and malocclusion, the older person may avoid eating healthy foods high in fiber such as fruits and vegetables, causing further problems related to poor nutrition. Social isolation may occur when older people lose self-esteem due to cracked or missing teeth.

Older patients with geriatric dental problems are urged to seek care from dentists with training and expertise in the care of older adults and the restorative and preventive skills needed to adequately care for these patients. Dentists

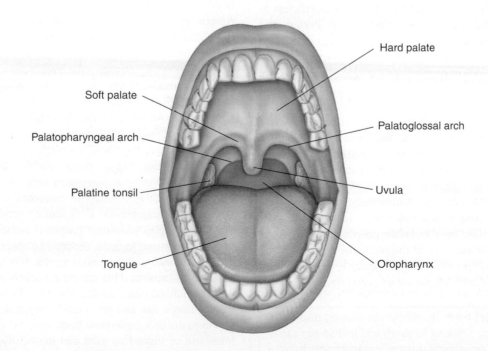

Figure 13-1 ▶▶▶ Normal structures of the oral cavity. Over time, the epithelium becomes thinner and soft tissue atrophies.

skilled in geriatric care have an important role to play in the diagnosis and treatment of oral cancer, soft tissue lesions, salivary gland dysfunction, and taste, smell, and swallowing disorders (National Institute on Aging, 2011).

Common Diseases of Aging Related to the Mouth and Oral Cavity

Oral diseases and conditions are common to those older people who grew up without the benefit of community water fluoridation and other fluoride products. More than 25% of older adults have not seen a dental professional within the past 5 years (Centers for Disease Control and Prevention [CDC], 2011b). About 25% of adults ages 65 and older no longer have any natural teeth and are **edentulous** (without teeth). Rates of edentulism vary, from a high of 37.8% of older Americans in West Virginia, followed by Tennessee and Mississippi, compared to only 13% in Maryland (CDC, 2011b). Having missing teeth can affect nutrition because older adults with no teeth have difficulty chewing and swallowing foods with fiber and texture. Poor oral hygiene and ill-fitting dentures can exacerbate oral problems with an older person's self-esteem and speech, serve as a source of halitosis, increase the risk of aspiration pneumonia, and negatively alter facial appearance (Reuben et al., 2011). Even those with dentures and partial plates may choose softer foods and avoid fresh fruits and vegetables because artificial teeth are not as efficient as natural teeth in the chewing and biting process. **Periodontal disease** (gum disease) or dental **caries** (cavities) most often cause tooth loss. The severity of periodontal disease increases with age. About 20% of people from the ages of 65 to 74 have severe periodontal disease, measured by a 6-mm loss of attachment of the tooth to the adjacent gum (receding gum disease). Men are more likely than women to have more severe gum disease, and older people at the lowest socioeconomic level have the most severe periodontal disease (CDC, 2011a). However, more older adults are retaining their teeth into advanced age and edentulism is no longer considered a normal part of aging (CDC, 2011a). Additionally, the use of fixed dental implants, crowns, and restorations is becoming more widespread in middle-aged and older people and these procedures can improve on some of the problems associated with denture use such as poor chewing efficiency, lowered intake of fresh fruits and vegetables, jaw atrophy, and social isolation.

> **Practice Pearl ▶▶▶** In addition to causing respiratory disease, cigarette smoking in youth and middle age can lead to serious periodontal disease and tooth loss in old age. This is another good reason for nurses to aggressively advocate for smoking cessation in patients of all ages.

Older Americans with the poorest oral health are those who are economically disadvantaged, lack insurance, and are members of racial and ethnic minorities. Being disabled, homebound, or institutionalized also increases the risk of poor oral health. About 7% of older adults report having had tooth pain at least twice during the past 6 months. Older adults who belong to racial or ethnic minorities or who have a low level of education are more likely to report dental pain than older adults who are Caucasian or better educated (CDC, 2011a).

Many Americans lose their dental insurance when they retire, and hence do not have access to regular dental care. The situation may be even worse for older women, who generally have lower incomes and may never have had dental insurance. Medicare does not cover routine dental care or most dental procedures such as cleanings, fillings, tooth extractions, or dentures. Additionally, Medicare does not pay for dental plates or other dental devices (Centers for Medicare and Medicaid Services, 2012). Medicaid, the jointly funded federal–state health insurance program for low-income people, funds dental care in some states, but reimbursement rates are so low that it is often difficult to locate a dentist who will accept Medicaid patients.

Oral and pharyngeal cancers, diagnosed in 30,000 Americans every year, result in about 8,000 deaths annually. Approximately 3% of all malignancies occur in the head and neck. These cancers, primarily diagnosed in older people, carry a poor prognosis. The 5-year survival rate for white Americans is 50% and for African Americans is only 25% (CDC, 2011b). Early detection is the key for increasing the survival rate.

Most older Americans take prescription and over-the-counter medications that can decrease salivary flow and result in xerostomia or dry mouth. It is estimated that 25% to 40% of older Americans suffer from xerostomia (O'Connor, 2010). For example, antihistamines, diuretics, antipsychotics, antidepressants, anticholinergics, chemotherapeutic agents, and antiparkinson drugs can reduce salivary flow. Decreased salivation is associated with increased oral disease because saliva contains antimicrobial components and minerals that help rebuild tooth enamel attacked by decay-causing bacteria. Additional problems associated with salivary dysfunction include dysphagia, difficulty chewing, candidiasis, and denture slippage, which can cause gum irritation and erosion. This can be especially problematic for institutionalized older adults, who take an average of eight medications a day and often drink very little fluid. In addition to maintaining adequate hydration, use of saliva substitutes, use of sugar-free gum and mints, discontinuation of medications that may be causing the problem if possible, and provision of frequent oral care are all nursing interventions to improve patient comfort and preserve oral function.

Painful conditions that affect the facial nerves are more common among older adults and can be severely debilitating. These conditions can affect mood, sleep, and oral-motor functions such as chewing and swallowing. Further, neurological diseases such as Parkinson disease, Alzheimer's disease, and stroke can affect oral sensory and motor functions, limiting the older person's ability for self-care (CDC, 2011a).

Barriers to Mouth Care

Although many older people regularly seek and receive dental care, older adults' use of dental services is the lowest of all adults (CDC, 2011b). Frail or institutionalized older adults may not have the physical or financial resources to travel to the dentist and receive needed care. Older people who are edentulous may erroneously think they no longer need dental services, and they are five times less likely to see a dentist than their peers who still have teeth. Further, many older adults may think that tooth loss is a natural consequence of aging and that dental care is expensive, causes pain, and requires frequent and lengthy visits (CDC, 2011b).

The oral healthcare needs of institutionalized older adults therefore fall to the gerontological nurse and nursing assistants. Many feel that these needs are not being met, and the way nurses provide mouth care has changed little in the past 50 years. Barriers to mouth care include lack of training and knowledge about the importance of oral hygiene, lack of perceived need for oral care, heavy workloads, and resistance by older adults with dementia (O'Connor, 2010). Further, some nurses find cleaning the mouth or handling dentures unacceptable and unpleasant. However, regular and meticulous mouth care decreases the presence of halitosis, difficult-to-clean dentures, and other unpleasant mouth conditions, making the process quicker and more pleasant for the older patient and the nurse providing the care.

Healthy Aging Tips

▶ Drink fluoridated water and use fluoride toothpaste to guard against cavities.

▶ Floss and brush teeth twice daily to reduce plaque and prevent periodontal disease.

▶ Schedule regular dental appointments even if you have dentures. Dentists and dental hygienists conduct oral cancer screenings at each visit.

▶ Avoid tobacco and all tobacco products to decrease the chance of oral or lung cancers.

▶ Limit excessive use of alcohol to decrease the risk of oral, lung, and bladder cancers.

▶ See the dentist before starting chemotherapy or radiation to the head and neck to reduce the risk of mouth ulcers, loss of salivary glands, rampant tooth decay, and destruction of bone.

▶ If you have dry mouth related to medication use, ask your primary care provider to review your drugs and substitute other drugs if possible.

▶ If you receive assistance from others with your oral hygiene, ask your caregiver to follow your established routine, follow the recommendations listed above, and use the products you prefer so that you will more likely be satisfied with your oral care.

Drug Alert ▶▶▶ Sudden changes in food taste and preference may be signs of an adverse drug reaction. Review the medical record for any changes in medications including adding new drugs or increasing the dose of long-prescribed drugs (CDC, 2011a).

A study of oral hygiene practices provided to older people in five long-term care facilities found that a standard protocol consisting of wearing clean gloves, brushing the resident's teeth for at least 2 minutes, flossing, oral assessment, and rinsing with mouthwash was achieved by certified nursing assistants ranging from a low of 0% to a high of 16% in the five facilities included in the study. Additionally, most residents (63%) who received assistance were resistant to receiving oral care (Coleman & Watson, 2006). Clearly, nurses have a responsibility to monitor and supervise nursing assistants to ensure appropriate technique and behavioral approaches so that oral care that meets accepted standards can be provided to those in need of assistance.

Negative Effects of Poor Oral Care

Poor oral care can have serious adverse effects on the physical and psychosocial function and health of the older person. Consequences of poor oral care include the following:

■ Social isolation and depression
■ Systemic illness such as aspiration pneumonia, heart disease, and stroke
■ Periodontal disease, which can negatively affect glycemic control in people with diabetes
■ Malnutrition, vitamin deficiencies
■ Pain, halitosis, tooth loss, dental caries, periodontal disease 'bad breath
■ Denture stomatitis 'sores

CDC, 2011a; Reuben et al., 2011.

> **Drug Alert** ▶▶▶ Calcium channel blockers, chemotherapeutic agents, Dilantin, and immunosuppressants (azathioprine and methotrexate) can cause or exacerbate gingival problems (O'Connor, 2010).

Risk Factors for Oral Problems

All older adults are at risk for oral problems. Normal changes of aging may predispose this population to the development and detection of these problems. Additionally, diseases commonly found in the older person such as diabetes mellitus can suppress neutrophil production, alter the structure of the lining of the blood vessels, and cause decreased circulation to the skin and mucous membranes. This delays healing of oral ulcerations and increases the potential for secondary infections, especially candidiasis (Guo & DiPietro, 2010). Table 13-1 lists risk factors for oral problems.

> **Practice Pearl** ▶▶▶ Virginia Henderson, a noted nurse theorist, stated nearly 50 years ago that the overall standard of nursing care can be judged by the state of the patient's mouth (Henderson, 1960). This statement remains true today.

Nursing Assessment of Oral Problems

Patients should be carefully questioned regarding their oral health history, including date of last dental examination, presence and function of dentures, missing or loose teeth, bleeding gums, dry mouth, presence of sores or lesions, medications, usual oral hygiene routine, altered sense of taste, chewing or swallowing difficulties, and presence of bad breath or halitosis.

A complete oral cavity assessment includes examination of the lips, teeth, interior of the buccal mucosa, anterior and base of the tongue, gums, soft and hard palate, and back of the throat. Careful notation of any cracks, lesions, ulcers, swelling, induration, gingival bleeding, hypertrophy, or dental caries should be made in the patient's record. Patients with **leukoplakia,** or a white patchy coating on the surface of the oral mucosa, should be referred to a dentist or oral surgeon for further evaluation and biopsy. ˜measles

Wearing gloves, the nurse should lift the tongue with a 4 × 4–inch dressing to examine the posterior surface. Extra light will be required to complete visualization. Observe any tremor, coating, or deviation of the tongue.

The lymph nodes of the head and neck should be carefully palpated and any tenderness or enlargement noted. The condition and number of natural teeth should also be noted. Loose or broken teeth should be referred for dental evaluation because the patient is at risk for losing and swallowing the tooth during a meal. Likewise, dentures should be examined for fit and condition. Cracks, poor fit, and missing or broken teeth should be noted.

Common Oral Problems

Common problems of the mouth that occur with aging include xerostomia, oral candidiasis, oral pain, gingivitis and periodontal disease, stomatitis, and oral cancer.

Xerostomia

The most common oral problem occurring in the older adult is xerostomia and may affect as many as 30% of older people (Weiner et al., 2010). Dry mouth can result from mouth breathing, dehydration due to diuretic use, oxygen therapy, oral and systemic diseases, and head and neck radiation. The most common causes appear to be medications, with 80% of the most commonly prescribed medications (about 400 medications) reported to cause xerostomia. The most common offenders are tricyclic antidepressants, sedatives, tranquilizers, antihistamines, antihypertensives (alpha- and beta-blockers), diuretics, calcium channel blockers, ACE inhibitors, cytotoxic agents, antiparkinsonian agents, and anticonvulsant drugs (Reuben et al., 2011). Chemotherapy drugs have also been associated with salivary disorders.

> **Practice Pearl** ▶▶▶ A weight loss of 5% can cause previously well-fit dentures to slip, erode the gums, and cause painful ulcerations. Monitor denture fit on older patients who undergo significant intentional or unintentional weight loss.

Oral symptoms associated with xerostomia include altered taste; difficulty eating, chewing, and swallowing (particularly dry foods); halitosis; chronic burning sensation in the mouth; and intolerance to spicy foods (Academy of General Dentistry, 2012). Difficulty with swallowing leads to increased episodes of choking and aspiration pneumonia.

Nursing interventions to improve xerostomia include the following:

- Urging regular dental evaluation
- Low-sugar diet
- Mouth rinses

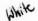
White

TABLE 13-1	Risk Factors for Oral Problems
Risk Factor	**Potential Cause of Oral Problem**
Diseases	Cancer
	HIV/AIDS
	Diabetes mellitus
	Renal failure
	Endocrine disorders
	Dementia
	Stroke
	Psychiatric illness
	Viruses (e.g., herpes simplex, varicella-zoster, coxsackie, HPV16)
Vitamin Deficiencies	
Glossitis (inflammation of the tongue)	Niacin, folic acid, B_6, B_{12}
Glossodynia	B vitamins (riboflavin, niacin, folic acid, B_6, B_{12}, zinc, and iron)
Stomatitis	Niacin, folic acid, B_{12}
Xerostomia	Vitamin A, vitamin B_{12}
Bleeding gums	Vitamin C, vitamin K
Angular cheilosis (cracking at the corners of the mouth)	B vitamins, iron
Medications	Antibiotics
	Antineoplastics
	Biological response modifiers
	Phenytoin
	Antihistamines
	Anticholinergics
	Reserpine and chlorpromazine
	Glucocorticoids (inhaled and oral)
Normal Aging Changes	Thinner enamel on teeth
	Stress lines and cracks in teeth
	Receding gingiva, periodontal ligament, and bone
	Thinner, smoother, and less elastic mucosa
	Decreased salivary production
Functional Problems	Institutionalization
	Caregiver stress/unavailability
	Transportation problems
	Cognitive impairment and resistiveness to care
	Mistrust of healthcare providers
	Poor vision/manual dexterity
Financial Problems	Lack of dental insurance
	Unwillingness/inability to spend money on dental care
Confounding Factors	Oxygen therapy
	Tachypnea/mouth breathing
	G-tube or NPO/decreased level of consciousness or unresponsive
	Oral or nasal suctioning
	Radiation therapy to head/neck
	Tobacco or alcohol use
	Ill-fitting dentures
	Medication toxicity
	Orthopedic replacements or organ transplants

Sources: Guo & DiPietro, 2010; Reuben et al., 2011.

- Sugar-free chewing gum, hard candies, and mints _lemon_
- Artificial saliva and mouth lubricants (Salivart, Xero-Lube)
- Bedside humidifiers
- Dietary modifications including avoidance of foods known to be difficult to chew or swallow and careful use of fluids while eating _avoid salt_

Oral Candidiasis

Oral candidiasis is a frequent complication of dry mouth and is treated with oral antifungal agents. People who have diabetes and have high or elevated glucose levels are at risk for candidiasis (thrush) because the oral flora is altered and the organism *Candida albicans* is encouraged to overgrow. Additionally, those with diabetes have an altered immune response including decreases in leukocyte activity, decreased phagocytosis, and decreased neutrophil production.

> **Drug Alert** ▶▶▶ Older patients using inhaled steroids to treat asthma should rinse their mouths carefully each time the inhaler is used to prevent the formation of oral candidiasis.

The usual treatment is rinsing with topical antifungal agents (nystatin) four times a day for 2 weeks. The nurse should carefully observe older patients to make sure they adequately "swish" for about 2 minutes and then swallow the solution. If an oral troche (a medicated lozenge to soothe the throat) is used, it must be held in the mouth and allowed to slowly dissolve. The troche contains sugar and should not be used with patients who have diabetes (Medicine.net, 2012). Patients with dentures should remove their dentures before rinsing to ensure that the medication reaches all areas of the oral mucosa. One milliliter (or cubic centimeter) of nystatin oral suspension should be added to the water used to soak dentures at nighttime, and dentures should soak for at least 6 hours. If the older person is taking medications associated with xerostomia, the primary care provider should be consulted to see if these drugs might be discontinued. Careful denture cleaning and attention to mouth hygiene are essential.

A small, soft toothbrush is considered the most effective mechanical method to control dental plaque. Teeth or gums should be brushed twice daily for about 3 to 4 minutes. Toothbrushes perform substantially better than foam swabs in the ability to remove plaque from the teeth and gingival margins and from the areas between teeth. Swabs are useful to cleanse and moisten oral mucosa and prevent damage to delicate tissue and may be effectively used when caring for the dying, but a moist toothbrush is more effective in reducing bacterial plaque and cleaning the oral cavity (Coleman & Watson, 2006). _Shingles does not cross midline of body_

> **Practice Pearl** ▶▶▶ Lemon and glycerine swabs are not only ineffective, but are in fact harmful and should not be used (Capezuti, Zwicker, Mezey et al., 2008).

Mouth rinses are available and can serve the purposes of cleansing, moisturizing, or killing germs. Nurses commonly use hydrogen peroxide and sodium bicarbonate although recent evidence suggests that hydrogen peroxide harms the oral mucosa and causes negative subjective reaction in patients. Sodium bicarbonate dissolves mucus and oral debris but has an unpleasant taste and can burn oral mucosa if not diluted properly. Chlorhexidine (Peridex) is used widely to treat gingival and periodontal disease and other oral infections. It can improve oral hygiene in populations with special needs in whom mechanical plaque removal is difficult, such as those with Alzheimer's disease or those who do not possess the dexterity or strength for manual plaque removal.

Oral Pain

Oral pain may indicate an advanced problem in a tooth or the gingival tissues. Although pain may resolve with time, an untreated problem can result in a tooth abscess or serious infection. When older patients complain of mouth pain, the gerontological nurse should carefully inspect the mouth, teeth, and tongue for signs of infection or abscess. Additional information includes checking the patient's temperature, pulse, and respiration to rule out acute infection. Patients with a dental abscess will often have swollen or enlarged lymph nodes under the ear or jaw. Clusters of vesicles with eroded centers and ulcers on the lips and mucosa can indicate the presence of herpes simplex or zoster. Treatment with an antiviral topical ointment or suspension is indicated after referral and assessment by the primary care provider.

> **Practice Pearl** ▶▶▶ Older patients who are unresponsive, NPO, or have G-tubes should receive mouth care every 4 hours including gentle brushing of the teeth, dentures, and tongue and application of lip moisturizer. Elevate the patient's head slightly and position the patient on his or her side to prevent aspiration.

Gingivitis and Periodontal Disease

Inflammation of the gums associated with redness, swelling, and a tendency to bleed are the common presenting signs of **gingivitis.** Gingivitis is a precursor to chronic periodontitis. About 80% of older Americans have some sort of periodontal disease (Perio.org, 2010). Gingivitis results from bacterial

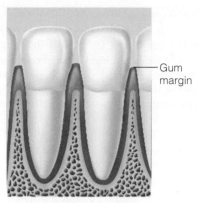

Gum
margin

(a) Normal gum margins
and teeth

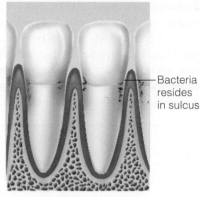

Bacteria
resides
in sulcus

(b) Plaque formation and
early gum erosion

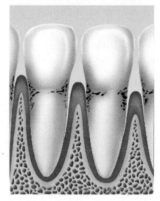

(c) Progressive gum erosion with
early inflammatory response

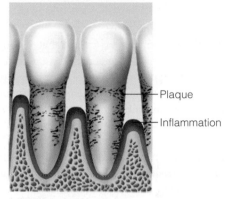

Plaque

Inflammation

(d) Loss of alveolar bone
with full gum erosion

Figure 13-2 ▶▶▶ Gingivitis and resulting gum erosion.

colonization at the gum margin and in the sulcus between the margin and the tooth (Figure 13-2 ▶▶▶). When bacteria are not removed from the mouth, they form a sticky, colorless plaque on the teeth that hardens and forms a sheltered area in which colonies can flourish. The longer plaque and tartar remain on the teeth, the more harmful they become. These bacteria and their products have a direct inflammatory effect and also evoke an immunological response. This response can cause erosion of the gingival sulcus or pocket and resorption of alveolar bone around the tooth, leaving the tooth at risk for a cavity below the gum line. The gums will become red and swollen and bleed easily. Daily flossing and twice-daily brushing with fluoride toothpaste often helps reduce the symptoms of gingivitis. An oral hygienist is needed to remove plaque and tartar with special instruments.

Risk factors for gingivitis include:

- **Smoking.** Smoking cigarettes greatly increases the risk of periodontal disease and lowers the chances of success of dental treatments.

- **Diabetes.** People with diabetes are at higher risk of all forms of periodontal disease.
- **Medications.** Many drugs can reduce saliva production, and thus the protective effect of saliva on the teeth and gums is lost.
- **Poor nutrition.** A poor diet, especially one low in calcium, can lower resistance to gum disease. Eating and drinking foods and drinks high in sugars can damage teeth.
- **Stress.** Older people under stress have more difficulty fighting infection, including gingivitis.
- **Illness.** Diseases like HIV/AIDS and cancer can make fighting any infection more difficult.
- **Genetic susceptibility.** Although not directly inherited, gum disease seems more common in some families (Vardar-Sengul et al., 2007).

Patients with bright red or magenta-colored gums or those complaining of gum bleeding with toothbrushing or eating should be referred to the dentist or periodontist for

floss w/ water

evaluation. The dentist will recommend medications such as antimicrobial mouth rinses, antibiotic gels, and perhaps surgery with bone and tissue grafts to replace lost bone and protect the vitality of the teeth. These treatments are difficult and expensive; therefore, prevention and early intervention is important. As always, meticulous oral hygiene is necessary to prevent tooth loss and progression of the disease.

Practice Pearl ►►► Urge all older patients to engage in self-care activities to prevent gum disease, including daily flossing, twice-daily brushing with fluoride toothpaste, twice-yearly dental cleaning and evaluation, eating a well-balanced diet, and avoiding tobacco products.

Stomatitis

Stomatitis is the inflammation of the mouth that is frequently caused by chemotherapy agents and is a common problem among older patients undergoing cancer treatment. Approximately 40% of patients undergoing cancer treatment will experience this painful condition (WebMD, 2012). Anticancer drugs cause cell destruction throughout the body, and the cells of the mouth can become damaged, leading to erosion, ulceration, inflammation, and secondary infections. Eating and drinking can be painful, and nutritional problems may occur as a result of stomatitis.

Treatments include meticulous oral hygiene, frequent use of a mild saline mouthwash, and avoiding extremes of hot, cold, or very spicy food and liquids. In extreme cases, Super Miracle Mouthwash can be compounded by a pharmacist by prescription from a physician. This is a swish-and-spit solution of Benadryl, lidocaine, hydrocortisone, tetracycline, and nystatin. This solution offers some relief from oral pain and suppresses inflammation, fungal growth, and bacterial overgrowth in the mouth and throat.

Practice Pearl ►►► Older patients should receive oral care a minimum of once every 8 hours while in the acute or long-term care setting. Additionally, the RN should conduct an assessment/evaluation of the oral cavity on patient admission and every shift (Coleman & Watson, 2006).

Oral Cancer

Benign and malignant tumors can occur in the mouth and pharynx. Like other cancers, malignant tumors of the mouth and pharynx can metastasize and invade other parts of the body, making early diagnosis crucial. Oral cancer that metastasizes will usually travel via the lymph nodes in the neck. Squamous cell carcinoma is the most frequent cancer of the

oral cavity and occurs most often in older adults. The 5-year survival rate for treated oral cancer is about 57%, with mortality the highest for cancers of the tongue and lowest for cancers of the lips (Oral Cancer Foundation, 2011).

Oral cancer usually occurs in people over the age of 45 but can develop at any age. Symptoms of oral cancer include the following:

- A sore on the lip or mouth that does not heal within 14 days
- A lump on the lip or in the mouth
- A white or red patch on the gum, tongue, or buccal mucosa
- Unusual bleeding, pain, or numbness in the mouth
- A feeling that something is always caught in the throat
- Difficulty or pain with chewing or swallowing
- Swelling of the jaw that changes the fit and comfort of dentures
- Changes in the voice
- Pain in the ear

Oral Cancer Foundation, 2011.

Patients with these symptoms should seek treatment from their dentist or primary care provider for further assessment and diagnosis. Currently, diagnosis of oral cancer involves checking the histopathology of suspicious cells after biopsy and use of X-ray techniques such as computerized axial tomography scans or magnetic resonance imaging. Treatment involves surgery, radiation therapy, and chemotherapy. A team approach is needed when treating older patients with oral cancer. Key team members usually include an oral surgeon, the gerontological nurse, a medical oncologist, a plastic surgeon, a dietitian, a social worker, and a speech therapist.

Rehabilitation is an important follow-up to treatment for patients with oral cancer. Regular follow-up appointments are needed to check the healing process and monitor for signs of returning cancer. Patients with weight loss should work closely with the dietitian. Most physicians advise patients to stop using tobacco and alcohol to reduce the risk of developing a new cancer (Oral Cancer Foundation, 2011).

Risk factors for the development of oral cancer include:

- **Tobacco use.** Smoking cigarettes, pipes, and cigars accounts for 90% of oral cancers. Cigar, pipe, and chewing tobacco users have the same risk as cigarette smokers.
- **Biologic factors.** Bacterial, viral, and fungal infections of the mouth including the human papilloma virus (HPV16), a common sexually transmitted virus affecting 40 million Americans, has emerged as a serious biologic risk factor.
- **Chronic and heavy alcohol use.** The risks are even greater for older people who smoke and use alcohol.
- **Sun exposure to the lips.** Wearing a brimmed hat and lip balm with sunscreen reduce the risk. Pipe smokers are especially prone to lip cancer.

Race/Ethnicity	Incidence Rate in Males/100,000	Incidence Rate in Females/100,000	Death Rates in Males/100,000	Death Rates in Females/100,000
All Races	16.1	6.2	3.8	1.4
White	16.5	6.3	3.6	1.4
African American	15.4	5.6	5.7	1.4
Asian/Pacific Islander	11.1	5.2	3.0	1.3
American Indian/Alaska Native	10.1	5.0	3.5	1.3
Hispanic	9.1	4.0	2.4	0.7

Figure 13-3 ▶▶▶ Oral cancer incidence and death rates by race and gender.

Source: Howlader, N., Noone, A., Krapcho, M., Neyman, N., Aminou, R., Altekruse, S., Kosary, C., Ruhl, J., Tatalovich, Z., Cho, H., Mariotto, A., Eisner, M., Lewis, D., Chen, H., Feuer, E., Cronin, K. (eds). *SEER Cancer Statistics Review, 1975–2009 (Vintage 2009 Populations)*, National Cancer Institute. Bethesda, MD, http://seer.cancer.gov/csr/1975_2009_pops09/, based on November 2011 SEER data submission, posted to the SEER web site, 2012.

- **History of leukoplakia.** Older people with white patches in the mouth should be closely monitored.
- **Erythroplakia.** People in their 60s and 70s may develop red or magenta patches in the mouth.

African American men have the highest death rates of oral cancer, followed by Caucasian men. African American men tend to be younger at age of diagnosis (peaks at 65 to 69 and at 75 to 79 years of age) than white men (peaks at 80 to 84). This may reflect underlying genetic predisposition and smoking habits. Figure 13-3 ▶▶▶ illustrates oral cancer incidence and death rates by race and gender.

The nursing assessment of the oral cavity includes examination of the lips, oral mucosa, and the tongue. The nurse should also document the presence of natural teeth or dentures and observe the patient's ability to function and speak, chew, and swallow with and without dentures. The Hartford Institute for Geriatric Nursing *Try This* assessment series recommends the Kayser-Jones Brief Oral Health Status Examination (BOHSE) (Morritt Taub, 2012). The BOHSE is a brief screening tool that can be used by nurses and has demonstrated reliability and validity. This 10-item scale can be used to track the progress and treatment of oral health problems and also identifies which patients should be immediately referred for dental evaluation by underlining potentially dangerous symptoms.

Providing Oral Care to Patients with Cognitive Impairments

Many older nursing home residents with cognitive impairments will resist or refuse the nursing staff's attempts to provide mouth care. Some will refuse to open their mouths, resist inserting or removing dentures, try to bite the caregiver or clamp down on the toothbrush, or refuse to swish or swallow mouth rinses. These problems can discourage the nurses and the nursing assistants who are providing mouth care. Nursing research is clearly needed in this area to identify appropriate and effective nursing interventions. Some strategies that may be used and adapted in the nursing home setting when providing mouth care for difficult residents with a cognitive impairment include:

- **Task breakdown.** Time is taken to slowly break down the task into small steps. For instance, "Now I will place some toothpaste on the toothbrush. Does this look like enough to you?" The resident should be involved in each step of the process.
- **Distraction.** Playing music or looking at family pictures may provide some distraction while the caregiver carries out oral care.
- **Hand over hand.** The caregiver places a hand over the resident's hand and guides the activity.
- **Chaining.** The caregiver starts the activity and then asks the resident to complete it. For instance, the nurse may move the toothbrush back and forth a few times and then say, "Now you do it, Mrs. Jones. I may not be doing it exactly how you like it."
- **Protection.** Nurses should never insert their fingers into the mouth of a resident who bites or resists care. Human bites can be painful and infection prone. In extreme circumstances, several tongue blades may be taped together and inserted into the resident's open mouth, providing some small measure of protection should the resident decide to clamp down.

Modified from Jablonski et al., 2011.

Best Practices The Kayser-Jones Brief Oral Health Status Examination (BOHSE)

Resident's Name _____   Date_____

Examiner's Name _____   TOTAL SCORE_____

CATEGORY	MEASUREMENT	0	1	2
Lymph nodes	Observe and feel nodes	No enlargement	Enlarged, not tender	Enlarged and tender*
Lips	Observe, feel tissue and ask resident, family or staff (e.g., primary caregiver)	Smooth, pink, moist	Dry, chapped, or red at corners*	White or red patch, bleeding or ulcer for 2 weeks*
Tongue	Observe, feel tissue and ask resident, family or staff (e.g., primary caregiver)	Normal roughness, pink and moist	Coated, smooth, patchy, severely fissured or some redness	Red, smooth, white or red patch; ulcer for 2 weeks*
Tissue inside cheek, floor and roof of mouth	Observe, feel tissue and ask resident, family or staff (e.g., primary caregiver)	Pink and moist	Dry, shiny, rough red, or swollen*	White or red patch, bleeding, hardness; ulcer for 2 weeks*
Gums between teeth and/or under artificial teeth	Gently press gums with tip of tongue blade	Pink, small indentations; firm, smooth and pink under artificial teeth	Redness at border around 1–6 teeth; one red area or sore spot under artificial teeth*	Swollen or bleeding gums, redness at border around 7 or more teeth, loose teeth; generalized redness or sores under artificial teeth*
Saliva (effect on tissue)	Touch tongue blade to center of tongue and floor of mouth	Tissues moist, saliva free flowing and watery	Tissues dry and sticky	Tissues parched and red, no saliva*
Condition of natural teeth	Observe and count number of decayed or broken teeth	No decayed or broken teeth/ roots	1–3 decayed or broken teeth/roots*	4 or more decayed or broken teeth/roots; fewer than 4 teeth in either jaw*
Condition of artificial teeth	Observe and ask patient, family or staff (e.g., primary caregiver)	Unbroken teeth, worn most of the time	1 broken/missing tooth, or worn for eating or cosmetics only	More than 1 broken or missing tooth, or either denture missing or never worn*
Pairs of teeth in chewing position (natural or artificial)	Observe and count pairs of teeth in chewing position	12 or more pairs of teeth in chewing position	8–11 pairs of teeth in chewing position	0–7 pairs of teeth in chewing position*

Best Practices The Kayser-Jones Brief Oral Health Status Examination (BOHSE) (*continued*)

CATEGORY	MEASUREMENT	0	1	2
Oral cleanliness	Observe appearance of teeth or dentures	Clean, no food particles/tartar in the mouth or on artificial teeth	Food particles/tartar in one or two places in the mouth or on artificial teeth	Food particles/tartar in most places in the mouth or on artificial teeth

Upper dentures labeled: Yes ___ No ___ None ___   Lower dentures labeled: Yes ___ No ___ None ____

Is your mouth comfortable? Yes ___ No ___ If no, explain:_____

Additional comments: _____

<u>Underlined*</u> - refer to dentist immediately

Source: Kayser-Jones, J., Bird, W. F., Paul, S. M., Long, L., & Schell, E. S. (1995). An instrument to assess the oral health status of nursing home residents. *The Gerontologist,* *35*(6), 814–824. Figure 2, p. 823. Copyright © The Gerontological Society of America. Reproduced by permission of Oxford University Press.

Practice Pearl ▶▶▶ Families often judge the adequacy of nursing care by the cleanliness of the patient's mouth. If dried food, stained teeth or dentures, or bad breath are noticed by the family, they often feel their loved one is not getting the required care and needed attention to promote health and function.

As always, timing is key to approaching residents with cognitive impairments. Choose the time of day when the resident is most calm and accepting of care. Should the resident vehemently refuse oral care, it is best to walk away and reapproach the resident at a later time. It is seldom effective to try to force the resident to open the mouth and accept oral care. Even if successful care is achieved during the forced event, the next time oral care is offered, the resident will probably violently refuse again and experience a great deal of distress as a result.

Sometimes the presence of a family member can be reassuring and calming to the resident. A staff member who seems to have a good rapport with the resident should take responsibility for the provision of oral care. Effective and ineffective nursing interventions should be carefully noted in the nursing care plan so that a consistent approach can be used and the resident will come to associate oral care with the pleasant feeling of having a clean mouth.

Nursing Diagnoses

The nursing diagnoses of *Dentition, Impaired* and *Mucous Membrane: Oral, Impaired* may be used for older patients with mouth problems (NANDA, 2012). The presence of acute and chronic pain and nutrition problems would also be noted. The presence of infection, communication difficulties, and self-esteem problems should also be indicated.

COMPLEMENTARY AND ALTERNATIVE THERAPIES

Chamomile is sometimes used topically for stomatitis related to chemotherapy. Anecdotal evidence indicates its effectiveness for soothing these ulcerations, but there are no definitive studies to back up this claim. Allergic reactions including shortness of breath and throat swelling have been noted in some patients especially those with documented allergies to daisies, ragweed, chrysanthemums, and marigolds. No significant drug interactions are described (National Center for Complementary and Alternative Medicine, 2010).

Some research indicates that chewing raw garlic or garlic paste may have antifungal or antibacterial properties (Lynch, 2011). It is noted that there is little evidence to substantiate this claim. Many advocate chewing a sprig of mint or parsley to freshen breath and improve halitosis. A cool, wet tea bag contains tannin, which is a natural pain reliever, and the tea bag may be placed over a canker sore to effectively soothe and relieve the pain. A drop of oil of clove has been documented to temporarily relieve a toothache until a trip to the dentist has been arranged.

QSEN Recommendations Related to the Mouth and Oral Cavity

The Quality and Safety Education for Nurses (QSEN) project addresses the challenge of preparing future nurses with the knowledge, skills, and attitudes (KSAs) to continuously improve the quality and safety of the healthcare systems in which they work (Cronenwett et al., 2007). See the QSEN table for tips on meeting QSEN standards.

The patient-family teaching guidelines in the following feature will assist the nurse to instruct older adults about problems relating to the mouth and oral cavity.

Patient and Family Teaching

Gerontological nurses require skills and knowledge related to teaching patients and families about the key concepts of gerontology and gerontological nursing. The guidelines in the following feature will assist the nurse to assume the role of teacher and coach.

Meeting QSEN Standards: The Mouth and Oral Cavity

	KNOWLEDGE	SKILLS	ATTITUDES
Patient-Centered Care	Involvement of patient and family in plan of care is crucial.	Know family assessment and adult learning principles.	Appreciate the uniqueness of each patient/family.
	Examine barriers that may keep patients from being active in formulating their plan of care.	Evaluate for depression, vision/hearing, manual dexterity, cognitive status.	Understand the importance of oral hygiene and preventive care to overall health.
Teamwork and Collaboration	Recognize scope of practice for interdisciplinary team members.	Use leadership skills to coordinate team members and share knowledge.	Value the contribution of each member of the team to improve outcomes.
	Be aware of organizational problems that can inhibit effective team functioning.	System assessment skills. Serve as a role model and supervisor to certified nursing assistants.	Be open to input from team members on effective means to improve communication and collaboration.
Evidence-Based Practice	Describe effective interventions to decrease risk factors for decline in overall health due to poor oral hygiene.	Access current evidence-based protocols to guide interventions.	Possess confidence in necessary skills to evaluate and incorporate nursing interventions from the literature.
Quality Improvement	Recognize the importance of measuring patient outcomes to improve oral hygiene and mouth care.	Skills in data management, technology, and use of U.S. government and CDC websites describing current incidence and prevalence of mouth and oral disease.	Value the use of data and outcomes as a key component of QI efforts.

Meeting QSEN Standards: The Mouth and Oral Cavity *(continued)*

	KNOWLEDGE	SKILLS	ATTITUDES
Safety	Describe common behavioral interventions appropriate to the patient/family that increase the delivery of mouth care to older adults with cognitive impairment and refusal of care.	Use appropriate techniques to share successful strategies to increase the opportunities and success rate of the provision of oral care to patients with cognitive impairment.	Appreciate the impact of cognitive loss on the refusal of care.
Informatics	Provide input into the formation and maintenance of patient databases needed for gathering QSEN data and providing patient care.	Utilize the electronic health record.	Protect patient confidentiality according to HIPAA standards.

Patient-Family Teaching Guidelines

The following are guidelines that the nurse may find useful when instructing older adults and their families about oral health.

EDUCATION GUIDE TO ORAL HEALTH

Being older does not necessarily mean wearing dentures and being toothless. Older patients should be urged to take these steps to protect their oral health and preserve their teeth.

1 What can I do to protect my teeth now that I am older?

Suggestions for good oral health include:

- Drink fluoridated water and use fluoridated toothpaste; fluoride provides protection against dental decay at all ages.

- Practice good oral hygiene. Brush teeth carefully twice a day with a soft toothbrush and floss daily to reduce dental plaque and prevent periodontal disease. Use an egg timer to ensure that brushing is carried out for at least 2 minutes.

- Get professional oral health care, even if you have no natural teeth. Professional care helps to maintain the overall health of the teeth and mouth, and provides for early detection of precancerous or cancerous lesions. For patients with teeth, see the dentist and dental hygienist twice a year for evaluation, cleaning, and scaling. For the patient without teeth, see the dentist yearly for an oral cancer check.

RATIONALE:

Good oral self-care and professional care are needed to maintain oral health. The presence of gum disease and plaque increases with age. Ongoing yearly or twice-yearly appointments augment self-care practices.

2 Are there substances I should avoid in my daily habits?

- Avoid tobacco. In addition to the general health risks of tobacco use, smokers have 7 times the risk of developing periodontal disease compared to nonsmokers. Tobacco used in any form—cigarettes, cigars, pipes, and smokeless (chewing) tobacco—increases the risk for periodontal disease, oral and throat cancers, and oral fungal infections.

- Limit alcohol. Excessive alcohol consumption is a risk factor for oral and throat cancers. Alcohol and tobacco use together greatly increase the risk.

(continued)

Patient-Family Teaching Guidelines *(continued)*

- Get dental care before, after, and during cancer treatment with chemotherapy and radiation. Careful attention is needed to treat and prevent damage that can destroy teeth and oral tissues.

- Avoid high-sugar foods, soda, and sports drinks. If you do eat or drink these items, brush your teeth immediately to prevent tooth decay.

RATIONALE:

Many older patients and their families are unaware of how important oral health is to their overall health and function. Those without teeth or with dentures may feel that they need

not worry about mouth care. By reinforcing these guidelines, older patients' oral health and general health can be improved (CDC, 2011a).

Caregivers should attend to the daily oral hygiene of older people who cannot care for themselves. This includes older people with cognitive impairments and physical frailty. It is important to note effective techniques and provide a consistent approach.

Sugars stick to tooth surfaces and are likely to cause tooth decay. Many older people feel that tooth decay is only a problem of youth but more than 50% of older adults have new or recurrent dental caries (Morritt Taub, 2012).

CARE PLAN   A Patient With a Problem of the Mouth/Oral Cavity

Case Study

Mr. Graham is a 72-year-old African American man who is admitted to a rehabilitation facility for recovery after falling and breaking his right hip. He is now 3 days postoperative after an open reduction with internal fixation, and had a prosthetic replacement of his hip. He is awake and alert, but the nurse notices that he looks slightly dehydrated and emaciated. His height is 66 inches and his weight is 120 lbs. He reports that his appetite has been poor for the last few months and he has lost some weight. Mr. Graham wears dentures but they seem to move about in his mouth a lot, and he is constantly covering his mouth with his hand. The nurse is concerned that if he does not improve his nutritional intake, his wound might not heal properly and he may be at risk for infection.

Applying the Nursing Process
Assessment

The nurse should assess the dietary history including meal preferences, eating habits, use of tobacco and alcohol, and list of current medications. Also, the gerontological nurse should carefully assess Mr. Graham's mouth to determine his state of oral health, assess skin turgor, and check postural blood pressures. Because he has fallen and fractured a hip, he is at risk for future falls. With dehydration, he may exhibit postural hypotension and become dizzy when rising from a chair.

He seems to have loose-fitting dentures, which is common after a person has weight loss. Weight loss of about 10 lbs (or 5% of body weight) can mean that dentures need to be refitted to provide the tight fit needed for chewing food. He may have ulcerations from ill-fitting dentures, causing pain and discomfort when he ingests food and fluids.

CARE PLAN   A Patient With a Problem of the Mouth/Oral Cavity *(continued)*

Diagnosis

Appropriate nursing diagnoses for Mr. Graham include the following:

- *Nutrition Imbalanced: Less Than Body Requirements,* as evidenced by his weight loss
- *Injury, Risk for* as evidenced by his recent fall and hip fracture

- *Dentition, Impaired* as evidenced by his toothlessness and ill-fitting dentures
- *Mucous Membrane: Oral, Impaired* if evidence exists of gum or mucous membrane ulceration or erosion

NANDA-I © 2012.

Expected Outcomes

The expected outcomes for the plan specify that Mr. Graham will:

- Describe dietary preferences and eat at least 50% of each meal.
- Report any oral symptoms such as pain, redness, swelling, or taste disturbances.

- Demonstrate an understanding of nutritional needs, including the need for supplemental protein drinks and vitamins.
- Collaborate with the nurse to develop a therapeutic plan that is congruent with his goals and present lifestyle situation.
- Suffer no further falls and maintain normal postural blood pressure readings.

Planning and Implementation

The nurse may wish to observe Mr. Graham at mealtime to ascertain his oral intake, chewing ability, and food preferences. Careful documentation regarding the kinds of food and amount of food consumed at each meal is needed. Additionally, family members should be encouraged to bring in favorite foods to stimulate appetite. Pain, if present, should be monitored and treated so that Mr. Graham is

not in pain during mealtimes. Should his dentures need adjustment, temporarily lining them with a gel pad may improve his eating ability. A referral to a dentist will ultimately be needed for a permanent adjustment and realignment for a proper fit. Any ulcers or abrasions to the gums and oral mucosa should be carefully cleaned and monitored to prevent infection and aid healing.

Evaluation

The nurse will evaluate the success of the care plan based on the following:

- Mr. Graham will develop a trusting relationship and work with the nursing staff to improve his nutritional intake.
- He will maintain a stable weight or begin to gain weight slowly over time.

- He will show evidence of recovery from his surgery, including skin and bone healing on X-ray.
- Mr. Graham will report that his dentures fit well and he can chew and swallow without difficulty.

Ethical Dilemma

Mr. Graham states, "I'm hooked on cigarettes. I've smoked a pack a day since I was 15 years old. If I don't have a cigarette I'll crawl out of my skin, and my daughter won't bring me any. Can you get some for me?"

The nurse knows that quitting cigarette smoking "cold turkey" can be very difficult, especially for a patient

who has a long smoking history. However, the nurse also knows that continued smoking will probably further suppress appetite, delay the healing of any ulcerations in the mouth, and increase the risk for many cancers, including oral cancer. The nurse may wish to consult with the patient, family, and primary care

(continued)

A Patient With a Problem of the Mouth/Oral Cavity *(continued)*

provider regarding the use of a nicotine patch or other nicotine substitute. Additionally, some medications (buspirone and varenicline) can ease nicotine withdrawal. It would be unethical to ignore the patient's *request entirely and equally unethical to procure cigarettes for him. By involving Mr. Graham, his family, and the primary care provider, his tobacco addiction can be considered and hopefully addressed.*

Critical Thinking and the Nursing Process

1. How would you feel receiving mouth care from another person? Ask a close friend to brush your teeth, and then brush your friend's teeth. What feelings are elicited? Does your mouth feel fresh and clean afterwards? What suggestions for improvement do you have for your friend?

2. Imagine you are caring for a patient who has smoked cigarettes for many years and now has oral cancer. Are you likely to "blame the patient" for getting the disease because he or she continued to smoke and knew the risks?

3. Your nursing home patient has significant periodontal disease, loose teeth, and many dental caries. He is in pain or discomfort most of the day. The director of nursing cannot locate a dentist who will come to the nursing home, and it is difficult to get the patient to the dentist's office because he has had a stroke and is paralyzed on the right side and is wheelchair-bound. Describe your feelings.

4. You observe a nursing assistant approach a nursing home resident with dementia and say brusquely, "Open your mouth." The resident refuses and the aid walks away, telling you later that the resident refused oral care. What would be an appropriate response?

■ Evaluate your responses in Appendix B. ⬭

- Provision of mouth care and maintenance of oral health are well within the role of the gerontological nurse.

- Normal changes of aging, common diseases affecting older people, and many treatments and medications can negatively affect the teeth and oral cavity.

- There is convincing evidence that oral problems are associated with weight loss, malnutrition, infection, social isolation, depression, and mortality.

- Institutionalized older adults, especially those with cognitive impairments, are completely dependent on nursing staff for oral care and maintenance.

- Conscientious assessment and adherence to promoting oral hygiene and instituting preventive care can improve the quality of life for older patients.

Pearson Nursing Student Resources
Find additional review materials at
nursing.pearsonhighered.com

Prepare for success with additional NCLEX®-style practice questions, interactive assignments and activities, web links, animations and videos, and more!

References

Academy of General Dentistry. (2012). *Dry mouth.* Retrieved from http://www.dental.ufl.edu/patients/Files/oral-health-tips/WhatIsDryMouth.pdf

Capezuti, E., Zwicker, D., Mezey, M., & Fulmer, T. (2008). Evidence based geriatric nursing. Retrieved from http://www.scribd.com/doc/18429147/EvidenceBased-Geriatric-Nursing-Protocols-for-Best-Practice-Third-Edition

Centers for Disease Control and Prevention (CDC). (2011a). *Oral health: Preventing cavities, gum disease, tooth loss, and oral cancer.* Retrieved from http://www.cdc.gov/chronicdisease/resources/publications/aag/pdf/2011/Oral-Health-AAG-PDF-508.pdf

Centers for Disease Control and Prevention (CDC). (2011b). *Oral health resources: Adult indicators.* Retrieved from http://apps.nccd.cdc.gov/nohss/ListV.asp?qkey=5&DataSet=2

Centers for Medicare and Medicaid Services. (2012). *Medicare and you.* Retrieved from http://www.medicare.gov/Publications/pubs/nonpdf/National_508_eBook_v57_TAGGED.pdf

Coleman, P., & Watson, N. (2006). Oral care provided by certified nursing assistants in nursing homes. *Journal of the American Geriatrics Society, 54*(1), 138–143.

Cronenwett, L., Sherwood, G., Barnsteiner, J., Disch, J., Johnson, J., Mitchell, P., Sullivan, D., & Warren, J. (2007). Quality and safety education for nurses, *Nursing Outlook, 55*(3) 122–131.

Guo, S., & DiPietro, L. (2010). Factors affecting wound healing. *Journal of Diabetic Research, 89*(3), 219–229.

Henderson, V. (1960). *Basic principles of nursing care.* Geneva, Switzerland: International Council for Nursing.

Jablonski, R., Kolanowski, A., Therrien, B., Mahoney, E., Kassab, C., & Leslie, D. (2011). Reducing care resistant behaviors during oral hygiene in persons with dementia. *BMC Oral Health.* Retrieved from http://www.biomedcentral.com/1472-6831/11/30

Lynch, A. (2011). What are the benefits of raw garlic for candida? *Livestrong.com.* Retrieved from http://www.livestrong.com/article/445993-what-are-the-benefits-of-raw-garlic-for-candida

Medicine.net. (2012). *Nystatin suspension.* Retrieved from http://www.medicinenet.com/nystatin_liquid-oral/article.htm

Morritt Taub, L.-F. (2012). Oral health assessment of older adults: The Kayser-Jones brief oral health status examination. *Try this: Best nursing practices in care for older adults* (No. 18). Hartford Institute for Geriatric Nursing. Retrieved from http://consultgerirn.org/uploads/File/trythis/try_this_18.pdf

NANDA International. (2012). *NANDA International nursing diagnoses: Definitions and classification, 2012–2014.* Philadelphia, PA: Wiley-Blackwell.

National Cancer Institute. (2009). Cancer of the oral cavity and pharynx for selected subsites (invasive). Retrieved from http://seer.cancer.gov/csr/1975_2009_pops09/browse_csr.php?section=20&page=sect_20_table.02.html

National Center for Complementary and Alternative Medicine. (2010). *Chamomile.* Retrieved from http://nccam.nih.gov/health/chamomile/ataglance.htm

National Institute on Aging. (2011). *Taking care of your teeth and mouth.* Retrieved from http://www.treatmentofgingivitis.com/unveiling-the-causes-and-prevention-of-receding-gum

O'Connor, L. (2010). *Nursing standard of practice protocol: Oral health care in aging.* Retrieved from http://consultgerirn.org/topics/oral_healthcare_in_aging/want_to_know_more

Oral Cancer Foundation. (2011). *Oral cancer facts.* Retrieved from http://www.oralcancerfoundation.org/facts

Perio.org. (2010). *Dispelling myths about gum disease.* Retrieved from http://www.perio.org/consumer/gum-disease-myths.htm

Reuben, D., Herr, K., Pacala, J., Pollock, B., Potter, J., & Semla, T. (2011). Geriatrics at your fingertips. New York, NY: American Geriatrics Society.

Treatment of Gingivitis Team. (2011). *Unveiling the causes and prevention of receding gums.* Retrieved from http://www.treatmentofgingivitis.com/unveiling-the-causes-and-prevention-of-receding-gum

Vardar-Sengul, S., Demirci, T., Sen, B. H., Erkizan, V., Kurulgan, E., & Baylas, H. (2007). Human beta defensin-1 and -2 expression in the gingiva of patients with specific periodontal diseases. *Journal of Periodontal Research, 42*(5), 429–437.

Victorian Government Health Information. (2011). Oral health for older people. *Aged in Victoria.* Retrieved from http://www.health.vic.gov.au/agedcare/maintaining/oralhealth.htm

WebMD. (2012). *Oral health: Stomatitis.* Retrieved from http://www.webmd.com/oral-health/stomatitis-causes-treatment

Weiner, C., Wu, B., Crout, R., Wiener, M., Plassman, B., Kao, E., & McNeil, D. (2010). Hyposalivation and xerostomia in dentate older adults. *Journal of the American Dental Association, 141*(3), 279–284.

Sensation: Hearing, Vision, Taste, Touch, and Smell

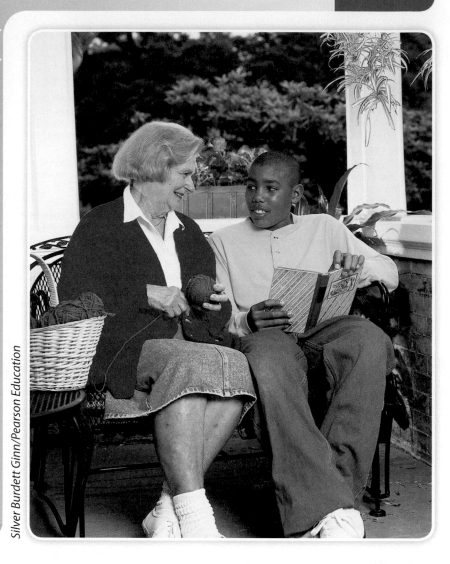

Silver Burdett Ginn/Pearson Education

LEARNING OUTCOMES

On completion of this chapter, the reader will be able to:

1. Explain normal changes associated with the aging process on the five senses—vision, hearing, taste, smell, and touch.
2. List common nursing diagnoses of older adults related to sensory problems.
3. Recognize nursing interventions that can be implemented to assist the aging patient with sensory changes.
4. Identify medications that may cause or aggravate sensory dysfunction.

Changes in vision, hearing, smell, taste, and touch occur naturally throughout the aging process. However, impairments in sensory functioning can greatly alter the capabilities of older adults to complete everyday activities, affecting quality of life and safety. Intact senses allow the older person to accurately perceive the environment and remain appropriately involved with other people, places, and objects. Safety is compromised when the older person cannot see fall hazards on the floor, cannot smell a natural gas leak from a stove, cannot recognize the taste of spoiled milk, cannot hear a signaling fire alarm, and cannot feel a pebble in the shoe that could lead to a blister or foot ulcer. Older adults with sensory dysfunction may suffer functional impairment, injury, social isolation, and depression. This chapter will discuss normal sensory changes, common problems, management, treatment, and nursing interventions for the older adult with sensory disorders.

Vision

Normal age-related changes in vision occur gradually; however, over time these changes can limit the functional ability of the older adult. Approximately 1.8 million community-dwelling older people report some difficulty with basic activities such as bathing, dressing, and walking around the house, in part because they are visually impaired (Kirtland, Zack, & Caspersen, 2012). Unfortunately, visual impairment increases with age. Visual impairment is defined as visual acuity of 20/40 or worse while wearing corrective lenses, and legal blindness or severe visual impairment is 20/200 or more as measured by a Snellen wall chart at 20 feet.

The prevalence of blindness also increases with age, reaching its peak at about the age of 85. Fortunately, the prevalence of blindness in the United States is low, but studies have shown that nursing home residents have a 15-fold increase in blindness over community-dwelling individuals—approximately 15% of residents 60 years old and 29% older than 90 are legally blind (U.S. Equal Employment Opportunity Commission [EEOC], 2011). Visual impairment and blindness in the older person is the result of four main causes: cataracts, age-related macular degeneration, glaucoma, and diabetic retinopathy.

Visual impairment can lead to a loss of independence, social isolation, depression, and a decreased quality of life. Visual impairment increases the risk of falls and fractures, making it more likely that an older person will be admitted to a hospital or nursing home, be disabled, or die prematurely (Ham, Sloane, Warshaw et al., 2007). It is important for the nurse to understand normal versus abnormal changes and how to assist the older adult to improve safety and well-being.

Nurses should urge all older patients to schedule routine eye examinations with an ophthalmologist to maintain and protect vision. Reviews of Medicare beneficiary claims reveal that 30% of older adults have no record of an evaluation by an ophthalmologist or optometrist (American Academy of Ophthalmology, 2012). The healthy older adult should schedule a complete eye examination every other year. During this examination, visual acuity should be evaluated, pupils should be dilated with examination of the retina, and intraocular pressure should be tested. Older adults with diabetes should have this complete visual evaluation yearly (Reuben et al., 2011).

When assessing the vision of an older person, the nurse should first observe the patient's appearance. Older patients with stains on their clothing, older women with too much or poorly applied makeup, or patients with multiple bumps and bruises may be exhibiting signs of visual impairment. Older patients should be questioned regarding adequacy of vision, recent changes in vision, visual problems, and the date of their last complete visual examination. The gerontological nurse should inspect the eyes for any abnormalities, including movement of the eyelids, abnormal discharge, excessive tearing, abnormally colored sclera, and abnormal or absent pupillary response. A Snellen chart (Figure 14-1 ▶▶▶) can be used to measure visual acuity, or the patient can be asked to read from a magazine or newspaper with various print sizes. Acuity tests should also be performed in low light, because many patients may appear to have no visual deficits under the ideal conditions of a brightly lit clinic, but actually suffer from glare and contrast sensitivity in reduced light settings (Ham et al., 2007). Visual field testing can detect blind spots or loss of peripheral vision. Ask the patient to follow your fingers as they move from point to point without changing the head position to check extraocular movements. The older person with glasses should wear them during the vision assessment. For accurate results, ensure lenses are clean and properly aligned prior to starting the visual exam.

In addition to annual or biennial examinations, nurses should urge all older adults who complain of a visual problem to seek a visual evaluation if they experience any of the following problems:

- Red eye
- Excessive tearing or discharge
- Headache or feeling of eyestrain when reading or doing close work
- Foreign body sensation in the eye
- New-onset double vision or rapid deterioration of visual acuity
- New-onset haziness, flashing lights, or moving spots
- Loss of central or peripheral vision
- Trauma or eye injury

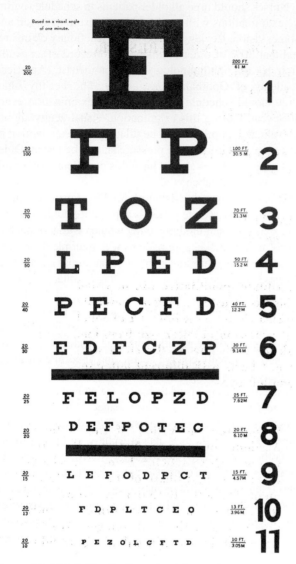

Figure 14-1 ▶▶▶ The Snellen chart is used to measure visual acuity.

Source: National Eye Institute, National Institutes of Health, 2007.

The majority of older people wear some kind of glasses or contact lenses to correct their vision. Ninety-two percent of people over age 70 wear glasses. An additional 18% also use a magnifying glass for reading or close work. Even with glasses, many older people report trouble seeing. Fourteen percent of people ages 70 to 74 report difficulties seeing even with correction, and 32% of those over age 85 offer this complaint (EEOC, 2011).

Although visual aids and suggestions offered by low-vision clinics can assist an older person with visual impairment, fewer than 2% of people over the age of 70 use these services (American Foundation for the Blind, 2012).

Telescopic lenses, books in Braille, computer scanners and readers, tinted glasses to reduce glare, large-print books and magazines, guide dogs, and canes are often rejected because of the stigma attached to them. Because many of these items can be very expensive and are not covered by Medicare, the older person should request the opportunity to try them at home for a few days to see if the visual aid offers improvement of vision and function. Most states offer assistance to people who are legally blind. Older adults who are registered with the Commission for the Blind can borrow books on tape with a tape player, telephones with large numbers, and high-intensity lighting, without cost, if they can furnish a letter from a physician noting that they are legally blind.

Independence may be limited and freedom restricted when visual impairments interfere with the ability to drive, read, and write. Older adults are forced to rely on friends, care-givers, and family to drive them to the grocery store, assist with paying bills, take medications, and do things they were previously able to do on their own. Lack of transportation or the desire not to burden family and friends may leave them socially isolated, with the inability to get places. Leaving home may induce anxiety and fear related to visual difficulties, ultimately leading to voluntary isolation and depression.

NORMAL CHANGES OF AGING

External changes of the eye related to age include graying and thinning of the eyebrows and eyelashes. Wrinkling of the skin surrounding the eyes occurs as a result of subcutaneous tissue atrophy. The eyes may appear sunken as orbital fat decreases and the eyelids sag (U.S. National Library of Medicine [NLM], 2012a). Figure 14-2 ▶▶▶ illustrates the

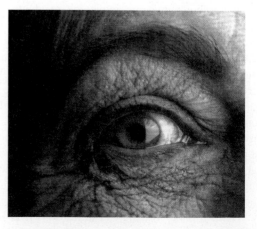

Figure 14-2 ▶▶▶ Normal changes of aging in the eye include a thinning of skin surrounding the eye.

Source: National Eye Institute, National Institutes of Health, 2007.

TABLE 14-1	Age-Related Changes in the Eye and Functional Implications
Age-Related Changes	**Implications**
Thinning of skin surrounding the eye	Cosmetic implications only
Decrease in musculature in eyelids	If severe, may result in drooping eyelids that obscure vision.
Ectropion—the bottom lid sags outward and is no longer in contact with the eye.	Results in chronic eye irritation and bacterial conjunctivitis.
Entropion—the lid turns inward, bringing the eyelashes in contact with the eyeball and causing irritation and abrasion to the cornea.	Results in chronic eye irritation and bacterial conjunctivitis.
Arcus senilis (corneal calcium deposits)	Cosmetic implications only (rare correlation with systemic hyperlipoproteinemia)
Musculature in the iris	Results in smaller pupil size. Use extra light, gradual change from light to dark, avoid glare.
Visual acuity	Decreased reading and color discrimination ability. Wear corrective lenses and use extra light.
Atrophy of lacrimal glands	Results in dry eyes. Saline drops can bring relief.
Intraocular pressure	If untreated, can result in blindness. Regular ophthalmologic evaluation can detect glaucoma and prevent visual loss.

Source: Cacchione, 2010; Reuben et al., 2011.

aging eye, and Table 14-1 describes commonly occurring age-related changes in the eye.

A decrease in endothelial cells on the cornea reduces ocular sensitivity and pain, which may delay awareness for treatment of injuries and infections. Arcus senilis, grayish yellow rings around the peripheral cornea, develop due to lipid deposits; however, this condition is unrelated to hypercholesterolemia or lipid abnormalities except in rare cases.

The lenses thicken and harden with age and appear yellowish and opaque. Thickening of the lenses can cause light to scatter, and opaqueness of the lenses will interfere with color discrimination. This greatly increases the risk for falls and dangerous night driving. Lens thickness also reduces the space for aqueous humor to drain and increases the risk for glaucoma. Hardening impedes **accommodation,** defined as the ability of the lens to change shape and focus images clearly. This loss of pliability in the lens contributes to **presbyopia** or the decrease in near vision, which generally occurs around the age of 40. Visual acuity tends to diminish gradually after the age of 50 and then more rapidly after the age of 70.

Pupils continue to react to light by dilating and constricting; however, this process occurs more slowly with increased age. Accommodation, or the ability to focus on objects at varying distances, declines with age. The greatest declines in accommodation occur between 45 and 55 years

of age, making this more a problem of middle-aged adults than older adults. There is usually no change in accommodation after the age of 60 (Chizek, 2007). A delay in pupillary reaction makes it difficult for older adults to adapt to light changes, putting them at greater risk for falls. Overall pupil diameter is also decreased, which reduces the amount of light reaching the retina, and more light is required to see clearly (Chizek, 2007). The iris loses color and eyes appear gray or light blue.

Light sensitivity, or the ability to adapt to varying degrees of light, declines with age. With increased age, there is a need for increased light (Chizek, 2007). Three functions are associated with light sensitivity:

1. **Brightness contrast.** This is the ability to discriminate between objects in varying degrees of light. Starting at about age 50, more light is needed to see dimly lit objects or objects in shadows on a sunny day.
2. **Dark adaptation.** This is the ability to see objects upon entering a dimly lit room after entering from daylight. An older person will not see objects at first, but with time, outlines will become more discernible.
3. **Recovery from glare.** Glare is excessive light reflected back into the eye. Glare will obliterate normal vision for a period of time (for example, after a flash picture is taken). With age, recovery from glare takes more time.

Nursing Implications for Older Patients With Vision Problems

Understanding the normal changes in vision that occur with age enables the nurse to share appropriate interventions to help the patient adjust and regain confidence. Signs that an older adult may be having difficulty with vision include squinting or tilting the head to see; changes in ability to drive, read, watch television, or write; holding objects closer to the face; difficulty with color discrimination and walking up or down stairs; and hesitation in reaching for objects or not being able to find something (Hsu, Phillips, Sherman et al., 2008).

The gerontological nurse can recommend environmental modifications to assist an older person with visual impairment to maintain independence. The Home Safety Inventory shown in Box 14-1 will assist the gerontological nurse to identify safety problems in the home. Recommendations include the following:

- Provide adequate lighting in high-traffic areas.
- Recommend motion sensors to turn on lights when an older person walks into a room.
- Look for areas where lighting is inconsistent. Dark or shadowy areas can obscure objects.
- Use proper lampshades to prevent glare.
- Use contrast when choosing paint colors so that the older person can easily discriminate between walls, floors, and other structural elements of the environment.
- Avoid reflective floors.
- When designing signs, use bright colors such as red, orange, and yellow. Avoid soft blues, grays, and light greens because the contrast between colors will be poor.
- Use supplementary lamps near work and reading areas.
- Use red-colored tape or paint on the edges of stairs and in entryways to provide warning and signal the need to step up or down.
- Avoid complicated rug patterns that may overwhelm the eye and obscure steps and ledges.

Safety is a major concern with vision changes in the older adult. Because pupillary reaction slows with age, an older adult requires more time to become acclimated to changes in light intensity. Nurses should instruct patients on the importance of walking slowly when entering a room with brighter or dimmer light.

The two leading causes of accidental death in older adults are falls and motor vehicle accidents, respectively. Per mile traveled, fatal crash rates increase starting at age 75 and increase notably after age 80. It is estimated that drivers over the age of 80 have a crash rate per mile driven that is equivalent to that of teenage motorists (Centers for Disease Control and Prevention [CDC], 2011). Therefore, it is very important for older adults to have their vision and driving ability screened

regularly. In the United States, driving is sometimes seen as a right, and many older people are hesitant to relinquish their driver's license because they fear loss of independence.

Many older adults restrict their driving to short distances only during the daytime in an effort to compensate for visual impairment. As a result of recent publicity about older drivers who were involved in fatal pedestrian accidents, many states are struggling to develop systems that can detect older drivers with cognitive and visual impairments on a more timely and accurate basis. Although most states require periodic vision testing for all drivers regardless of age, few require road tests that would simulate actual conditions that an older person may encounter when driving. Such conditions may include driving in the rain and using windshield wipers, encountering oncoming vehicles with headlights on, and driving in bright sunlight with various reflections and solar glare. Safe driving habits, including avoiding drugs or alcohol, wearing seat belts, obeying the speed limit, and limiting driving in poor

---

BOX 14-1 ▶ **Home Safety Inventory— Older Person**

Safety Considerations	Yes	No
1. Lighting adequate on stairs?	[ ]	[ ]
2. Stair rails present and in good repair?	[ ]	[ ]
3. Nonskid surfaces on stairs?	[ ]	[ ]
4. Throw rugs present safety hazard?	[ ]	[ ]
5. Crowded living area presents safety hazard?	[ ]	[ ]
6. Tub rails installed?	[ ]	[ ]
7. Tub has nonslip surface?	[ ]	[ ]
8. Space heaters present safety hazard?	[ ]	[ ]
9. Adequate provision made for refrigeration of food?	[ ]	[ ]
10. Medications kept in appropriately labeled containers with readable print?	[ ]	[ ]
11. Toxic substances have labels with readable print and are stored well away from food?	[ ]	[ ]
12. Home is adequately ventilated and heated?	[ ]	[ ]
13. Neighborhood is safe?	[ ]	[ ]
14. Fire and police notified of older person in home?	[ ]	[ ]

Source: Adapted from Clark, M. J. C. (2002). *Community health nursing: Caring for populations* (4th ed.). Upper Saddle River, NJ: Prentice Hall.

weather conditions, are recommended for all drivers regardless of age. Families with concern over an older person's driving safety are urged to observe firsthand the older person's performance behind the wheel. The American Association of Retired Persons (AARP) offers an 8-hour safe driving course in which older people are taught the effects of aging on driving. There is a nominal charge for the course, and it is taught throughout the United States. Visit the AARP website to find the location of these driver safety courses.

> **Drug Alert ▶▶▶** Nurses should be aware of the potential for visual disturbances as common side effects of the following drugs:
>
> - *Amiodarone (Cordarone):* blurred vision, corneal changes, optic neuropathy, halos
> - *Anticholinergics (asthma medications, decongestants):* blurred vision
> - *Bisphosphonates (Fosamax):* ocular pain, red eye, blurred vision
> - *Digoxin:* yellowish-orange vision, flickering images
> - *Hydroxychloroquine (Plaquenil):* photophobia, blurred vision, and difficulty focusing
> - *Tamoxifen (Nolvadex):* retinopathy and blurred vision
> - *Thioridazine (Mellaril):* blurred vision, impaired night vision, color discrimination problems, dry eye, and glaucoma
> - *Levodopa:* blurred vision, diplopia, and dilated pupils
> - *Propranolol and thiazide diuretics:* dry eyes and visual disturbances
> - *Sildenafil (Viagra):* abnormal vision and vision loss

Sources: MedlinePlus, 2011; Reuben et al., 2011.

If the older person is deemed an unsafe driver, the Department of Motor Vehicles should be notified so the older person will be called in for a road test. If an older adult fails the road test, his or her license will be revoked. Please check the reporting requirements regarding potentially unsafe drivers in your state with the Department of Motor Vehicles.

Visual Problems

ARMD

Age-related macular degeneration (ARMD) is the leading cause of blindness in adults over the age of 65. ARMD is a degenerative disorder of the macula that affects both central vision (scotoma) and visual acuity. The macula is situated in the posterior region of the retina, surrounding the fovea, and is dense with photoreceptor cells (cones and rods) (National Eye Institute [NEI], 2009).

There are two forms of ARMD: dry and wet. The dry form, or atrophic form, occurs as a result of atrophy, retinal pigment degeneration, and drusen accumulations and is the most common form of ARMD. *Drusen* are deposits of cellular debris and appear as yellow spots on ophthalmic examination. Dry ARMD has three stages: early, intermediate, and advanced. Visual loss as a result of this type of ARMD is generally slow in progression, and accounts for only 10% to 20% of severe vision loss. In the wet form, also known as neovascular exudate ARMD, blood or serum leaks from newly formed blood vessels beneath the retina. This seepage of fluid ultimately leads to scar formation and visual problems. Although less prevalent than the dry form, the wet form of ARMD is responsible for about 90% of severe vision loss (McPhee & Papadakis, 2011).

Patients with ARMD often require more light for reading. They often experience blurry vision, central scotomas (blind spots within the visual field), and metamorphopsia, in which images are distorted to look smaller (micropsia) or larger (macropsia) than they actually are.

Another symptom typical of wet ARMD is that straight lines appear crooked or wavy. The Amsler grid was developed as a screening tool to assess for ARMD; patients with this condition experience visual distortions of the lines and central scotomas. A sample grid and the appearance of the grid to a patient with normal vision and one with ARMD are depicted in Figure 14-3 ▶▶▶.

Central vision is mainly affected by this disorder, and peripheral vision remains intact (NEI, 2009). A person with macular degeneration will experience a dark spot in the center of the field of vision and must learn to rely on and interpret peripheral vision in order to function. A person with ARMD might experience vision as depicted in Figure 14-4 ▶▶▶.

Risk factors for ARMD include the following:

- Age above 50
- Cigarette smoking
- Family history of ARMD
- Increased exposure to ultraviolet light
- Caucasian race and light-colored eyes
- Hypertension or cardiovascular disease
- Lack of dietary intake of antioxidants and zinc

NEI, 2009.

Currently, there are no treatments for the dry form of ARMD; however, the wet form may benefit from laser treatments, photodynamic therapy, or injections. Laser therapy can be used to stop neovascularization and leaking vessels. Laser therapy may result in secondary vision loss due to destruction of healthy tissues. Photodynamic therapy involves an intravenous injection of a photosensitive dye medication called verteporfin (Visudyne), which travels through the bloodstream to the capillaries in the eye. Light is directed into the eye for

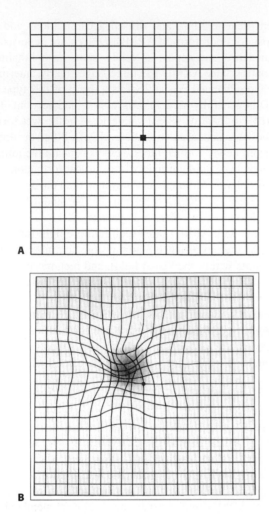

Figure 14-3 ▶▶▶ A. Amsler grid as it appears to a person with normal vision. B. Amsler grid as it appears to a person with macular degeneration.

Source: National Eye Institute, National Institutes of Health, 2007.

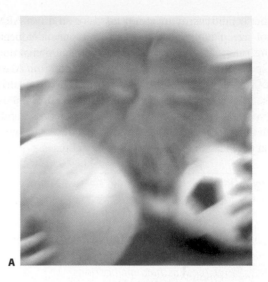

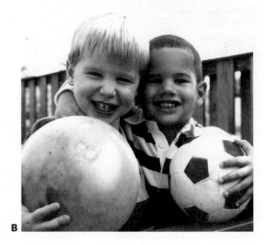

Figure 14-4 ▶▶▶ A. Simulation of vision with macular degeneration. B. Normal vision.

Source: National Eye Institute, National Institutes of Health, 2007.

90 seconds and activates verteporfin. Once activated, the medication destroys new blood vessels by producing "free radicals." The advantage of this procedure is that healthy tissue is not affected and it is relatively painless. Patients must, however, avoid exposure to direct light for 5 days following treatment. Another treatment involves injections of pegaptanib (Macugen), which blocks the effects of growth factor. These injections are administered directly into the eye and interfere with vascular endothelial growth factors (VEGF), which cause abnormal vessels to leak and proliferate. These therapies may slow vision loss, but are temporary and very often need to be repeated (McPhee & Papadakis, 2011).

The Age-Related Eye Disease Study (AREDS) conducted by the National Eye Institute found a 25% risk reduction in the development of age-related macular degeneration by consuming high doses of antioxidants (vitamins C and E and beta-carotene) and zinc. This dietary regimen was shown to slow the progression of ARMD, not cure the condition or restore lost vision (NEI, 2009). More recent studies by the AREDS Research Group (2007) have focused on the role lutein and zeaxanthin play in protecting the eye from ARMD and cataracts. Lutein and zeaxanthin are antioxidant beta-carotenoid pigments that concentrate in the eye. Final results are expected in 2013 but preliminary data suggest that a high dietary intake of lutein and zeaxanthin is associated with a lower risk of ARMD. These nutrients are found in eggs, spinach, romaine lettuce, broccoli, corn, and brussel sprouts.

Due to the severity of vision loss as a result of ARMD, nurses can play an important role in patient education. According to the American Academy of Ophthalmology (2012), people over the age of 65 should be examined every 1 to 2 years. Routine ophthalmic examinations are important to detect early signs of this disease. Nurses should encourage preventive measures such as wearing ultraviolet protective lenses in the sun, smoking cessation, and exercising routinely. In addition, a healthy diet consisting of fruits and vegetables may be helpful not only to increase consumption of antioxidants, but also to reduce the risk of cardiovascular disease (NEI, 2009).

Cataracts

Cataracts are opacities of the lenses. Lenses are normally clear structures through which light passes to reach the retina. Cataracts cloud the lens, decrease the amount of light able to reach the retina, and inhibit vision. Development is slow and painless, and may be unilateral or bilateral. Cataracts are the leading cause of blindness in the world. More than 70% of adults over the age of 75 have visual problems as a result of cataracts (American Academy of Ophthalmology, 2012).

There are four classifications of cataracts based on their location on the lens: nuclear cataracts (central aspect of lens), cortical cataracts (cortex of the lens), posterior subcapsular cataracts (posterior or back of the lens), and mixed cataracts. The most prevalent type of cataracts requiring surgery in older adults is a nuclear cataract (American Academy of Ophthalmology, 2012).

Patients with cataracts may experience blurry vision, glare, halos around objects, double vision, difficulty sensing contrasting colors because colors appear faded or discolored, and poor night vision. They may need more light or illumination when reading, and repeated alterations of their corrective lens prescriptions (NEI, 2009). Figure 14-5 ▶▶▶ depicts normal vision and the vision of a person with cataracts.

Risk factors for the development of cataracts include the following:

- Increased age
- Smoking and alcohol
- Obesity
- Diabetes, hyperlipidemia, hypertension
- Trauma to the eye or history of previous eye surgery
- Exposure to the sun and UVB rays
- Long-term corticosteroid medications
- Caucasian race

Surgery is generally the treatment of choice because there are no medications to treat this problem. Corrective lenses that filter out glare may be effective in managing symptoms in the early phases, but do not stop progression

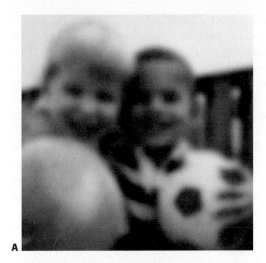

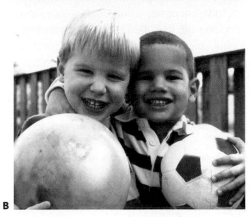

Figure 14-5 ▶▶▶ A. Simulation of vision with cataracts. B. Normal vision.

Source: National Eye Institute, National Institutes of Health, 2007.

of vision loss. As surgical procedures have changed so have the criteria for surgery: surgical recommendations are no longer dependent on visual acuity or allowing a cataract to "ripen" before removal. Recommendations are made when vision problems interfere with daily activities such as reading and driving. The only two instances in which a surgeon may recommend urgent cataract removal is to prevent glaucoma and/or if the cataract is interfering with monitoring of retinal diseases, such as diabetic retinopathy (NEI, 2009).

Surgery can be done on an outpatient basis and requires little systemic medication, because the cornea can be anesthetized locally with topical anesthetic. The procedures available involve removal of the affected lens and insertion of an artificial lens or intraocular lens, laser photolysis, or phacoemulsification (ultrasonic emulsification of the cataract). Phacoemulsification is the treatment of choice today, as the rehabilitation process is significantly shorter: approximately 1 to 3 weeks, compared to 2 to 4 months for cataract extraction. Contraindications for cataract surgery include patients who wish to avoid surgery, satisfactory vision with glasses or visual aides, lack of lifestyle compromise, inability to lie supine for 30 minutes or more, or serious medical problems that make surgery a high-risk procedure (Reuben et al., 2011).

Patient education and support are two important aspects of care that nurses can provide for older adults with cataracts. Cataracts may prevent people from driving and completing their normal daily activities, which can ultimately lead to a loss of independence, feelings of hopelessness, and depression. It is important for patients to understand what cataracts are, cataract symptoms, and cataract treatment options. For patients who undergo surgery, postsurgical education includes reinforcement not to lift any heavy objects, strain at stool, or bend at the waist. Complications of cataract surgery include infection, wound dehiscence, hemorrhage, severe pain, and uncontrolled elevated intraocular pressure (IOP). Patients must be instructed to immediately report the following symptoms to their eye surgeon: pain, conjunctival injection, vision loss, sparks, flashes or floaters, nausea, vomiting, or excessive coughing. Patients with cognitive impairments such as Alzheimer's disease must be carefully supervised for at least 24 hours after surgery to ensure that they do not remove the protective eye patch and do not rub their eye. When surgery is needed in both eyes, one eye is done first and the second procedure is scheduled a month or so later to allow healing and recovery. Adequate home care and support are needed to prevent complications.

Preventive measures to keep eyes healthy should be implemented into teaching. These preventive measures include wearing hats and sunglasses (with UVA and UVB protective coating) when in the sun, smoking cessation, eating a low-fat diet rich in antioxidants and vitamins E and C, and avoiding ocular injury by wearing protective goggles when doing crafts or using power tools. In addition, the nurse can provide patients with information regarding support groups and other resources that offer psychological and emotional support for those adjusting to low vision.

Glaucoma

Glaucoma is associated with optic nerve damage due to an increase in IOP (intraocular pressure), which can ultimately lead to vision loss. In the United States, glaucoma is the second most common cause of blindness (McPhee & Papadakis, 2011).

Aqueous humor or fluid within the eye serves as nourishment for surrounding tissues. Normally, this fluid is produced in the anterior chamber and drains outward via the trabecular meshwork, maintaining an average or normal IOP of 15 mmHg (normal range is 10 to 20 mmHg). If the outflow of aqueous fluid is obstructed, aqueous humor

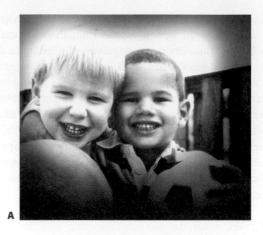

A

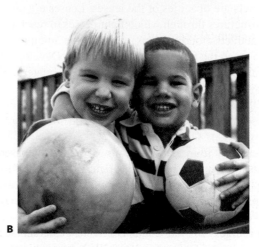

B

Figure 14-6 ▶▶▶ A. Simulated glaucoma vision. B. Normal vision.

Source: National Eye Institute, National Institutes of Health, 2007.

accumulates, increasing the pressure within the eye and damaging the optic nerve. When the IOP is greater than 21 mmHg, the optic nerve has the potential for atrophy and vision loss. The two types of glaucoma are open-angle glaucoma and angle-closure glaucoma (NEI, 2012).

Open-angle glaucoma occurs when the flow of aqueous humor through the trabecular meshwork is slowed and eventually builds up. If the IOP remains elevated, vision may be lost due to damage of the retinal nerve fiber layer. Vision loss is painless and gradual, with midperipheral visual field loss being the classic symptom (NEI, 2012). Simulated vision loss from the effects of glaucoma is pictured in Figure 14-6 ▶▶▶.

Another form of open-angle glaucoma is termed *normal-tension glaucoma*, where the IOP remains within the normal range, but damage to the optic nerve and visual changes still occur. In this circumstance, it is believed that damage to the nerve occurs as a result of ischemia or inadequate blood flow. Damage due to open-angle glaucoma can be visualized in ophthalmic examination by enlargement of the optic cup in relation to the optic disc, nicking of the neuroretinal rim, and small hemorrhages near the optic disc (NEI, 2012).

In angle-closure glaucoma, which is not as common, the angle of the iris obstructs drainage of the aqueous humor through the trabecular meshwork. It may occur suddenly as a result of infection or trauma; symptoms include unilateral headache, visual blurring, nausea, vomiting, and photophobia. Acute-closure glaucoma is an ophthalmic emergency requiring immediate attention by an ophthalmologist to preserve vision (NEI, 2012).

Risk factors for glaucoma include the following:

- Increased intraocular pressure
- Older than 60 years of age
- Family history of glaucoma
- Personal history of myopia, diabetes, hypertension, migraines
- African American ancestry

NEI, 2012.

Patients do not generally report symptoms of glaucoma until advanced stages of the disease, so monitoring of IOP during routine ophthalmic examinations for patients with any of the above risk factors is essential. The American Academy of Ophthalmology (2012) recommends that patients over the age of 65 be examined and screened for glaucoma at least every 1 to 2 years. A complete examination includes the patient's visual acuity with corrective lenses, visual field test to assess peripheral vision, measurement of the IOP noting the time of day because pressures may vary throughout the day, slit-lamp inspection of the iris to assess whether the anterior angle is open or closed, and a complete dilated examination to inspect the optic nerve and retina (American Academy of Ophthalmology, 2012). The image in Figure 14-7 ▶▶▶ illustrates an older patient undergoing IOP testing.

Management of glaucoma involves lowering the IOP to stop damage to the optic nerve and prevent further vision loss. Therapy involves medications (oral or topical) to decrease IOP, and/or laser surgery to increase the flow of aqueous humor, by creating a new drainage exit (McPhee & Papadakis, 2011). Follow-up care with the ophthalmologist is essential to monitor the adequacy of treatment and to ensure that the IOP remains below 20 mmHg. Open-angle glaucoma is usually managed with one or several of the following medications: beta-blockers, miotics, alpha-adrenergic agonists, prostaglandin analogues, and carbonic anhydrase inhibitors. Beta-blockers remain the first-line therapy for glaucoma because they decrease the rate of intraocular fluid production (Reuben et al., 2011).

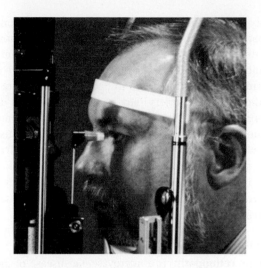

Figure 14-7 ▶▶▶ Intraocular pressure testing.
Source: National Eye Institute, National Institutes of Health, 2007.

Potential adverse effects of ophthalmic solutions include the following:

- **Beta-blockers (Betagan, Timoptic, Ocupress)** *(bottles with blue or yellow caps):* bradycardia, congestive heart failure, syncope, bronchospasm, depression, confusion, and sexual dysfunction
- **Adrenergics (Iopidine, Alphagan, Epinal)** *(bottles with purple caps):* palpitation, hypertension, tremor, and sweating
- **Miotics/cholinesterase inhibitors (pilocarpine, Humorsol)** *(bottles with green caps):* bronchospasm, salivation, nausea, vomiting, diarrhea, abdominal pain, and excessive lacrimation
- **Carbonic anhydrase inhibitors (Trusopt, Azopt)** *(bottles with orange caps):* fatigue, renal failure, hypokalemia, diarrhea, depression, and exacerbation of chronic obstructive pulmonary disease
- **Prostaglandin analogues (Xalatan, Lumigan):** changes in eye color and periorbital tissues, and itching

Epocrates, 2012; Reuben et al., 2011.

When administering eyedrops, it is important for the nurse to first wash his or her hands, ask the patient to tip the head backward and look upward, then pull the lower lid down slightly to make a small pouch. The nurse should try not to drop the medication directly onto the eye but rather into the eyelid pouch to prevent a violent blink reflex and excessive tearing. It is important not to contaminate the dropper by touching it to the eye, and to wait several minutes before administering an additional dose of the same medication or a second medication to allow time for complete absorption and prevent additional medication from simply running out of the eye. The nurse should provide the patient with a facial tissue to blot any medication or tears that may run down the cheek, and when finished, wash the hands carefully again.

If medications are unable to decrease IOP or are contraindicated, then surgery may be an option. Acute angle-closure glaucoma is initially treated with medication (both oral and topical) to decrease IOP, but surgery is usually indicated to improve aqueous fluid drainage. A small opening is made at the base of the iris (iridotomy) to allow the IOP to equalize on either side and prevent the iris from obstructing the outflow channel. Iridotomy with a laser can be performed in the outpatient setting (NEI, 2012).

Diabetic Retinopathy

Diabetic retinopathy is a microvascular disease of the eye occurring in both type 1 and type 2 diabetes. Damage to the ocular microvascular system impairs the transportation of oxygen and nutrients to the eye (Huether & McCance, 2012).

The two forms of diabetic retinopathy are nonproliferative and proliferative. In the nonproliferative form, the endothelium layers of blood vessels within the eye become damaged and microaneurysms develop. These microaneurysms may leak and the surrounding area may become edematous. If swelling occurs near the macula (macular edema), vision is impaired. Proliferative diabetic retinopathy is a more advanced stage and is a result of retinal ischemia due to damaged blood vessels. To increase the blood and nutrient supply to the retina, new blood vessels develop in a process known as neovascularization. The new blood vessels are fragile and tend to leak red blood cells, which can obscure vision depending on the location and degree of hemorrhage. The new blood vessels may also attach themselves to various areas such as the optic disc, retina, vitreous body, and iris. Tension exertion on the retinal surface and vitreous body increases the risk for retinal detachment or further damage to the surrounding blood vessels and hemorrhage. If neovascularization occurs on the iris (rubeosis iridis), drainage of the aqueous humor may be impaired, placing the patient at risk for neovascular glaucoma (Huether & McCance, 2012).

Prevention of diabetic retinopathy is dependent on tight glycemic control in addition to managing hypertension and hyperlipidemia. Goals of treatment for patients with diabetes include maintaining an average preprandial blood glucose of 80 to 120 mg/dL, an average bedtime capillary blood glucose of 100 to 140 mg/dL, and a hemoglobin (HbA_{1c}) of less than 7. (Refer to Chapter 19 ⊂⊃ for additional details on care of the patient with diabetes.) Patients should be referred for ophthalmic examination after diagnosis of diabetes, and recommendations for follow-up will be made at that time (NEI, 2009). Patients with diabetic retinopathy experience

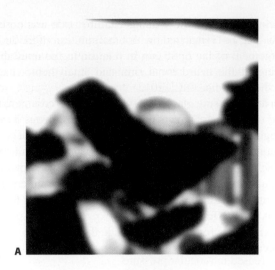

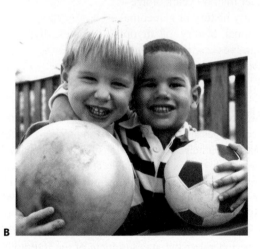

Figure 14-8 ▶▶▶ A. Simulated diabetic retinopathy vision. B. Normal vision.

Source: National Eye Institute, National Institutes of Health, 2007.

gradual vision loss with generalized blurring and areas of focal vision loss. Figure 14-8 ▶▶▶ is a simulation of vision for a person with diabetic retinopathy.

Treatment involves laser therapy for both types of retinopathy. Laser therapy can repair leaking microaneurysms, reducing the amount of ocular edema. Neovascularization may also be halted through the use of laser therapy or panretinal (scatter) laser photocoagulation (PRP). This technique decreases the risk of retinal detachment, hemorrhage, and neovascular glaucoma, but does not reverse vision loss. Secondary visual impairment including peripheral and central vision loss may result from laser therapy if the retina or fovea is damaged. Vitrectomy surgery is indicated for very severe cases of retinopathy, which do not respond to PRP, or if PRP is contraindicated due to severe hemorrhage. A vitrectomy involves removing the gelatinous contents and hemorrhage within the vitreous chamber that was obscuring vision, and replacing it with a salt solution (NEI, 2009).

Nurses can play a major role in educating patients about diabetes mellitus and the importance of glycemic control to prevent retinopathy. Proper nutrition, including a low-carbohydrate and low-cholesterol diet, is imperative to keep blood glucose levels down and decrease the risk not only of cardiovascular disease and hypertension but also to decrease the risk of microvascular damage to the eyes. Exercise helps to lower glucose levels, burns extra calories for weight management, and reduces insulin resistance in people with type 2 diabetes. The nurse should educate patients on how to check serum glucose levels, when and how to administer medications (insulin or oral hypoglycemic medications), and signs and symptoms of hypoglycemia and hyperglycemia.

Nursing Diagnoses Associated With Visual Impairment

Nursing diagnoses associated with visual impairment are diverse and depend on the older person's ability to compensate for visual problems. The gerontological nurse should consider the older patient's functional ability and not just the results of visual acuity testing using the Snellen chart. Appropriate assessments include the older person's ability to perform activities of daily living, including the ability to read medication and food labels, to drive or take public transportation, to ambulate safely in familiar and strange environments, to shop and pay for food and personal items, to prepare food while maintaining a safe and hygienic environment, and to engage in recreational and leisure activities.

The nursing diagnosis *Self-Care Deficit* encompasses a variety of nursing goals and interventions, including communication, safety, mobility, self-care activities, and mood assessment (NANDA International, 2012).

> **Practice Pearl** ▶▶▶ If an older person reports visual problems while wearing glasses, check to see that the glasses are clean and free from scratches. Dirty, scratched lenses can reflect light and distort vision.

Hearing

Auditory problems and hearing loss can severely impact quality of life. Hearing loss can interfere with communication, enjoyment of certain forms of entertainment such as music and television, safety, and ultimately, independence.

Hearing impairments make communication difficult and are often frustrating for both the patient and family. It is difficult for older adults to understand conversations with background noise, and difficulties become apparent at restaurants, stores, and social gatherings. The inability to participate in dialogue with family and friends may result in the lack of desire to attend functions, feelings of social isolation, and depression. The need to repeat oneself or miscommunication can lead to frustrating interactions. Sound distortion may impair the ability to listen to music, hear favorite television shows, or enjoy other forms of entertainment including movies, plays, or concerts. Turning up the volume of the television or radio to a level that one can hear may be unpleasant for others in the room. Hearing impairments also may endanger individuals living alone, due to the inability to hear a smoke detector or security alarm. Crossing the street and driving a car are dangerous if one is unable to hear oncoming traffic, horns, and sirens. As a result of these challenges, independence may be jeopardized because healthcare providers, family, or friends may want to limit activities normally done alone.

Hearing loss is common in older adults. Approximately 314 people in 1,000 over age 65 and 40% to 50% of those over age 75 have hearing loss (American Speech-Language-Hearing Association [ASLH], 2012). Older men of all ages are more likely to be hearing impaired than older women. White men and women are more likely than African American men and women to report hearing problems. Complete deafness in both ears accounts for a little over 20% of all hearing impairments in older people. Although hearing loss in older adults is common, it is estimated that only 25% of Americans who wear hearing aids wear them in both ears (ASLH, 2012). Hearing loss related to normal aging is the most common cause, but other risk factors include the following:

- Long-term exposure to excessive noise
- Impacted **cerumen** (earwax) —might need drops/suction
- Ototoxic medications —gentamycin
- Tumors
- Diseases that affect sensorineural hearing
- Smoking
- Head injury
- History of middle ear infection
- Chemical exposure (e.g., long duration of exposure to trichloroethylene)

Because of the trend toward an aging population in the United States, the number of people with hearing problems will increase significantly, as will the demand for hearing-related services and hearing corrective devices.

NORMAL CHANGES OF AGING

The external appearance of the ear changes with age as the auricle tends to wrinkle and sag. Cerumen or earwax produced by the ceruminous glands is a normal finding. In the older adult, cerumen tends to be drier and harder, and tends to accumulate in the ear canal due to decreased activity of the apocrine glands. Hearing may become impaired if cerumen accumulates to impact the canal. Dryness of the canal can also cause pruritus, and the epithelial lining of the ear canal may be easily irritated and injured if anything is inserted into the ear, increasing the risk of secondary infection (McPhee & Papadakis, 2011).

Changes in the inner ear involve atrophy of the organ of Corti and cochlear neurons, loss of the sensory hair cells, and degeneration of the stria vascularis (Huether & McCance, 2012). Aging produces gradual bilateral hearing loss in many individuals starting as early as age 20 to 30 but appearing more commonly in the 50s and 60s. About one third of all hearing impairments are at least partially attributable to damage from exposure to loud sounds. Sounds that are sufficiently loud to damage sensitive inner ear structures can produce hearing loss that is not reversible. Very loud sounds of short duration, such as an explosion or gunfire, can cause immediate, severe, and permanent loss of hearing. Virtually all of the structures of the ear can be damaged, in particular the organ of Corti, the delicate sensory structure of the auditory portion of the inner ear (cochlea), which may be torn apart. Figure 14-9 ▶▶▶ illustrates the anatomical structure of the ear.

Moderate exposure to loud noise may initially cause temporary hearing loss termed *temporary threshold shift*

(TTS). Many people have experienced TTS after being in a loud environment like a rock concert or sports event. However, TTS can become permanent with continued and longer duration exposure to less intense, but still loud, sounds that erode hearing ability. This danger became apparent several years ago, and legislation was passed to protect workers from hearing loss from loud noise in the workplace. Sounds are measured in A-weighted decibel levels correlating to the perception of loudness in air as heard by the human ear and levels of less than 75 dB(A) are unlikely to cause permanent hearing loss. Sound levels of about 85 dB(A) or greater with exposures of 8 hours per day will produce permanent hearing loss after several years (National Institute on Deafness and Other Communication Disorders [NIDCD], 2010). Some older adults have worked in industrial factories or occupations where loud noises were routinely encountered. The Occupational Safety and Health Administration (OSHA) now regulates the amount of noise that workers can be routinely exposed to and mandates the use of ear protection in noisy environments such as airports and factories where noisy equipment is operated; however, many older adults worked their entire lives in factories that would now be considered unsafe by OSHA standards. Additionally, many veterans who served in active duty during wartime have suffered hearing loss from the firing of heavy artillery.

Types of Hearing Loss

A thorough history and physical examination is important to help determine the cause of the hearing loss. It may be conductive, due to the external aspect of the ear, or sensorineural from inner ear problems.

Conductive hearing loss is related to a problem in the external or middle ear canal, tympanic membrane, bones in the outer and middle ear, or the ossicles (McPhee & Papadakis, 2011). Sound is unable to be transmitted to the inner ear, creating reception and amplification problems. This type of hearing loss may be the result of an external ear infection (otitis externa), impacted cerumen, middle ear infection (otitis media), benign tumors or carcinoma, perforation of the tympanic membrane, foreign bodies, or otosclerosis (a disease affecting the mobility of the middle ear bones) (Reuben et al., 2011).

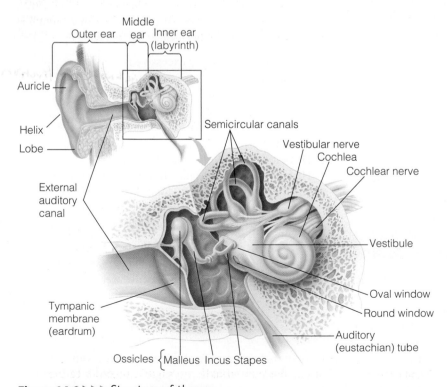

Figure 14-9 ▶▶▶ Structure of the ear.

Cerumen impaction is one of the most common and reversible causes of conductive hearing loss in older adults. Nearly 35% of community-residing older adults have cerumen impaction in one or both ears, and it is estimated that 57% of institutionalized older adults are affected. As described earlier, cerumen becomes harder and drier with age, and may occlude the ear canal. Recommended aural hygiene involves gentle cleansing of the auricles (outside of the ears) while bathing or showering. The use of cotton-tipped applicators to cleanse the ear canal is not recommended because the applicator may push the cerumen deeper into the canal and thus increase the risk of impaction, as well as traumatize the canal wall and tympanic membrane (McPhee & Papadakis, 2011).

An occlusion of cerumen can greatly affect hearing, as sound is unable to reach the inner ear. Examination of the ear canal for cerumen impaction is recommended as part of routine preventive healthcare screening for older adults. The person with cerumen impaction may complain of a feeling of fullness or itching in the ear canal. In addition to hearing loss, cerumen may also cause tinnitus (ringing, buzzing, pulsations, or clicking when no actual sound stimulus is present), ear pain, or vertigo.

> ***Practice Pearl*** ▶▶▶ Contraindications to ear lavage or irrigation include history of ear surgery, ruptured tympanic membrane, and/or otitis externa (swimmer's ear). It is safer to make a referral to an ear, nose, and throat specialist when in doubt.

Two common methods for removal of cerumen from the ear canal are:

- **Curette.** A small instrument with a scoop on the end is inserted into the ear canal while the helix is lifted posteriorly and laterally. The tip of the curette is placed over the top of the impacted cerumen and pulled forward. It is helpful to use both hands and wear a headlamp to provide bright light to visualize the canal as much as possible. The advantage of this method is that no water is needed and therefore there is a lower risk of infection. The disadvantage is that the procedure requires a greater degree of skill, and the risk of injury to the tympanic membrane or ear canal is greater.

- **Lavage or irrigation.** Some nurses like to soften the cerumen for up to 3 days before attempting irrigation with mineral oil or Debrox ear drops up to three times daily. Irrigation is the simpler and more straightforward approach to cerumen removal. However, because it is a blind procedure, the risk exists that water and infectious agents could be pushed through a perforated tympanic membrane into the middle ear space.

> ***Practice Pearl*** ▶▶▶ Contraindications for cerumen removal include perforated tympanic membrane, ear trauma, tumors, and cholesteatoma. Use extreme caution in patients with diabetes due to the increased risk for infection.

To irrigate, the following equipment is needed: a clean bulb syringe, a clean container of warm water or saline solution, an emesis basin, an otoscope, and lots of towels.

The tip of a bulb irrigation syringe is placed into the external canal (Figure 14-10 ▶▶▶). Water should be warmed to 37°C. The nurse can make sure the water is not too hot by testing it on the inside of a wrist. If it feels uncomfortably warm, more cool water is added to avoid burning the patient. Some patients can assist by holding an emesis basin below the ear to catch the water. A plastic cape can be used to protect the patient's clothing. Place gentle pressure on the syringe and angle the water stream posteriorly to wash the impacted cerumen away from the tympanic membrane. It is important to avoid getting air into the syringe as it will

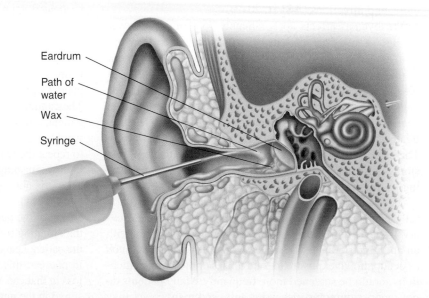

Eardrum

Path of water

Wax

Syringe

Figure 14-10 ▶▶▶ The tip of a bulb irrigation syringe is placed into the external canal.

sound deafening to the patient and will terrify a patient with a cognitive impairment. Pulling the helix of the ear upward and outward will straighten the ear canal. Use the otoscope to check progress and stop the irrigation when you can visualize the tympanic membrane. If the patient experiences discomfort, the nurse should stop. Large pieces of cerumen will be apparent in the emesis basin. Following irrigation, swab and dry the canal carefully to reduce the risk of infection. Some nurses use a water jet dental device, but this is risky because the water pressure cannot be controlled and damage to the tympanic membrane may occur.

Because of the risk of tympanic membrane perforation or damage to the lining of the ear canal, only an advanced practice nurse, physician, or gerontological nurse with specialized training and experience should perform the curette method. Neither the curette nor irrigation method should be attempted if a perforated tympanic membrane is present or suspected.

> **Practice Pearl** ▶▶▶ Use only sterilized equipment to avoid spreading bacteria and possibly infection from one patient to another during ear irrigation for cerumen impaction.

Sensorineural hearing loss is a manifestation of problems within the inner ear. Sound is transmitted to the inner ear, but problems with the cochlea and auditory nerve (eighth cranial nerve) create sound distortion. Causes of this type of hearing loss include **presbycusis** (loss of hearing due to age-related changes in the inner ear), damage due to excessive noise exposure, Ménière's disease, tumors, and infections (ASLH, 2012).

Presbycusis affects approximately 75% of people over the age of 60. Loss of hair cells in the cochlea (sensory loss) and degradation of neurons (neural loss), which occur as part of the normal aging process, result in this form of sensorineural hearing loss. The incidence is greater in men than women and believed to be related to noise-induced hearing loss. Presbycusis occurs gradually and is usually bilateral, impairing the ability to hear high-pitched tones. There are currently no interventions to slow the progression of presbycusis; however, it rarely causes severe hearing loss or deafness (ASLH, 2012).

The American Speech-Language-Hearing Association (2012) recommends asymptomatic adults be screened every 10 years until the age of 50 and then every 3 years with an audiometric battery test. Patients with risk factors such as occupational exposure to loud noises or ototoxic medications should be screened more frequently. Many patients do not report symptoms of hearing loss, and many years may lapse from when patients recognize the problem to the time they report it.

Evaluation of hearing loss is dependent on a thorough history and physical examination. The nurse should inspect the auricle for lumps, lesions, and deformities. Examine the ear canal with an otoscope. It is important to select a speculum for the otoscope that is the appropriate size for the patient. The nurse should hold the otoscope in his or her dominant hand and place the ulnar surface on the patient's occiput to stabilize the instrument and prevent damage to the ear canal should the patient suddenly move his or her head. Most adult ear canals are angled anteriorly and inferiorly, so gently pulling the pinna upward and outward with the opposite hand helps to straighten the canal and allows a better look at the tympanic membrane. Enter the ear canal slowly (only about 1/2 inch) to prevent discomfort to the patient and inspect the canal for cerumen, redness, foreign bodies, swelling, or discharge. If the tympanic membrane is not obstructed it will appear as a smooth, pearly gray object at the end of the ear canal. Some older adults have jagged white scars across the tympanic membrane as a result of ruptured eardrums from infections when they were children before the widespread use of antibiotics. Carefully document all findings. A red, bulging membrane is a sign of a middle ear infection and requires immediate referral to a physician or advanced practice nurse.

Assessing Hearing Loss

Family members may be valuable resources in assessing auditory acuity, because they may have noticed communication problems or social withdrawal. Examination of the ear may reveal an external infection or impaction that can be treated appropriately to resolve the hearing loss. If the problem is not that obvious, a few basic screening tests can be performed: the whisper, Weber, and Rinne tests. The whisper test assesses higher auditory ranges. The examiner instructs the patient to occlude one ear; depending on the patient's physical abilities the examiner may need to assist. The examiner should then stand 1 to 2 feet away from the patient, cover his or her mouth, and whisper a two-syllable word toward the unconcluded ear. The patient should be able to repeat the whispered word. A tuning fork may be helpful in distinguishing conductive versus sensorineural loss; however, it is not appropriate for bilateral hearing loss (Reuben et al., 2011). The Weber test involves placing a tuning fork on top of the patient's head. If the patient hears sound from the vibrating fork equally in both ears, hearing is normal. If the patient hears sound that is lateralized or perceived louder in one ear, this may indicate unilateral conductive hearing loss in that ear. With sensorineural loss, the patient will hear sound in the unaffected ear. The Rinne test involves placing the tuning fork on the mastoid bone to assess bone conduction. The patient is asked to tell the examiner when he or she can no longer hear the sound, and the tuning fork is then placed next to the ear to measure air conduction. Normally air conduction should be longer than bone conduction, so the patient should be able to hear the tuning fork after it is moved alongside the patient's ear. A patient with conductive hearing loss will perceive the bone conduction to be longer and will not hear the tuning fork through the air, as there is an external ear problem (Reuben et al., 2011).

Hearing Aids

Hearing aids amplify sounds and deliver them directly into the ear. Improvements have made them smaller and more discreet. Gerontological nurses should be aware of the cleaning, inserting, and troubleshooting involved with hearing aids. The first priority is to identify patients wearing hearing aids on admission to the hospital or nursing home and make an appropriate notation on each patient's nursing care plan. It is helpful to note the type, model number, and serial number of the hearing aid in case it should become lost. The working condition of the hearing aid is then assessed. Assessment parameters include:

- **Integrity of the ear mold.** Are there cracks or rough areas? Is there a good fit?
- **Battery.** Use a battery tester if one is available. Are the contacts clean? Is the battery inserted correctly with the plus sign (+) on the battery matched to the plus sign in the compartment?
- **Dials.** Are they clean? Easily rotated? Does the patient report variation of volume when the volume dial is moved?
- **Switches.** Do they easily turn on and off? Is there excessive static or feedback?
- **Tubing for behind the ear aids.** Are there cracks? Is there good connection to the earpiece?

Modified from NIDCD, 2010.

Older persons with hearing loss are at risk for communication problems and difficulties relating to the environment. The National Institute on Aging suggests older people use the questions and information described in the feature on the next page to decide if they should discuss their hearing with their health care provider.

All nursing personnel, including nursing assistants, should know how to care for hearing aids. Professional nurses can serve as role models, educators, and instructors for nursing assistants who are unfamiliar with the care of these expensive items. It is also critical to reinforce that patients who wear hearing aids should have them inserted during morning care so that they can effectively communicate throughout the day. Some older people have been labeled as cognitively impaired because they respond inappropriately to questions, while in reality they are hearing impaired.

Even the patient diagnosed with Alzheimer's disease will become more withdrawn, increasingly socially isolated, and more disoriented without the benefit of a hearing aid.

Each evening at bedtime, the hearing aid should be removed and cleansed with warm water or saline and a cotton pad. Harsh soaps or alcohol should not be used, because they will degrade the plastic. Any cerumen should be carefully removed from the earpiece while still soft. The battery should be disengaged from the contacts and the hearing aid stored securely in its case in a safe place. Many nursing home residents and their caregivers routinely misplace hearing aids, eyeglasses, and dentures when they are placed on meal trays or get mixed into bedding and laundry. Frequent inventory and labeling will assist the staff to keep track of these expensive and difficult-to-replace items.

Hearing aids are appropriate for most people with a hearing impairment. To be fitted with the device most appropriate for the individual patient's hearing loss, it is recommended that an independent audiologist be visited for testing and evaluation. Audiologists who do not sell hearing aids have a wider variety of devices to choose from and will not feel pressured to recommend the type of aid sold by their employer. Older hearing aids amplified all noise at the same level, and some older people were not able to tolerate them because of the amplification of loud background noise. Newer aids enhance selected frequencies where the patient exhibits hearing loss and thus are more effective and acceptable to many patients. Amplification in both ears (binaural) achieves the best understanding of speech. Unilateral amplification may be appropriate for those with hearing loss only in one ear, those who cannot afford two aids, or those who may be challenged by the care of two hearing aids.

The U.S. Food and Drug Administration (FDA) has approved implantable hearing devices (cochlear implants) for older adults with moderate-to-severe sensorineural hearing loss. A cochlear implant bypasses the middle ear and directly innervates the auditory nerve. Older adults who may be candidates for a cochlear implant include those with no contraindication to general anesthesia, no external or middle ear pathology, and appropriate family support, motivation, and expectation (Reuben et al., 2011). The device must be implanted into the skull behind the ear. This procedure requires a hospital stay and the administration of anesthesia. After the implantation, significant training is needed with a speech pathologist to recognize and interpret the new electronic sounds produced by the implant. A small battery pack is worn around the waist with a cable that attaches to the implant behind the ear. The device allows many people who were previously unable to do so to speak on the telephone, thus improving safety and quality of life. Positive results in those over age 65 are comparable to those in younger people when the selection criteria are followed (Reuben et al., 2011).

Best Practices Hearing Loss and Older Adults

Do I Have a Hearing Problem?

Ask yourself the following questions. If you answer "yes" to three or more of these questions, you could have a hearing problem and may need to have your hearing checked by your healthcare provider.

	YES	NO
Do I have a problem hearing on the telephone?		
Do I have trouble hearing when there is noise in the background?		
Is it hard for me to follow a conversation when two or more people talk at once?		
Do I have to strain to understand a conversation?		
Do many people I talk to seem to mumble (or not speak clearly)?		
Do I misunderstand what others are saying and respond inappropriately?		
Do I often ask people to repeat themselves?		
Do I have trouble understanding the speech of women and children?		
Do people complain that I turn the TV volume up too high?		
Do I hear a ringing, roaring, or hissing sound a lot?		
Do some sounds seem too loud?		

When you follow-up with your healthcare provider, please make sure to ask the following questions:

1. Do I have a lot of wax or cerumen in my ears that can be harming my hearing?
2. Do I take medications that have side effects that are harmful to hearing?
3. Do I have an ear infection that needs treatment so that my hearing might improve?
4. Should I see an audiologist (special technician who is trained to test hearing) to obtain further information about my hearing?

Can My Friends and Family Help Me?

Yes. You and your family can work together to make hearing easier. Here are some things you can do:

1. Tell your friends and family about your hearing loss. They need to know that hearing is hard for you. The more you tell the people you spend time with, the more they can help you.
2. Ask your friends and family to face you when they talk so that you can see their faces. If you watch their faces move and see their expressions, it may help you to understand them better.
3. Ask people to speak louder, but not shout. Tell them they do not have to talk slowly, just more clearly.
4. Turn off the TV or the radio if it does not have to be on.
5. Be aware of noise around you that can make hearing more difficult. When you go to a restaurant, do not sit near the kitchen or near a band playing music. Background noise makes it hard to hear people talk.

Source: National Institute on Deafness and other Communication Disorders, 2002. Retrieved from http://www.nidcd.nih.gov/health/hearing/pages/older.aspx.

Assistive Listening Devices

Older adults with hearing impairments may also use assistive listening devices. Many theaters are equipped with these devices that amplify the performers' voices by the use of small microphones and then transmit them to headphones or earpieces that are worn in the ear. Wireless transmission, using infrared technology or FM radio listening systems, is useful for people with central auditory processing disorders (Reuben et al., 2011). A telecommunications device for the deaf (TDD) is an assistive device that allows telephone conversation for a deaf person via a keyboard that transmits signals over the telephone wires to another person with a TDD receiver. Special TDD operators can assist with emergency calls when the older person must call someone without a TDD receiver. The use of computers and e-mail has greatly assisted many people with hearing impairments to communicate with the hearing world. Additional hearing assistance devices are available to improve function in many older adults including loud ringing and light flashing telephones, fire alarms, and doorbells; amplified telephones; vibrating watches; wired headsets for television and live-performance attendance; and videophones that allow lip-reading. Many of these devices are costly and not covered by Medicare but can provide peace of mind and promote the safety and function of the older person, so are well worth the investment.

Common Hearing Problems in Older Adults

Tinnitus (abnormal ear or head noises) can occur with or without hearing loss and is associated with increased age. Severe and persistent tinnitus can interfere with sleep and the ability to concentrate and may result in psychological distress. Tinnitus is classified into two categories: objective and subjective. Patients with *objective* tinnitus hear pulsatile sounds caused by turbulent blood flow within the ear; clicking or low-pitched buzzing is indicative of spastic muscles within the ear or spontaneous vibrations of the hair cells. *Subjective* tinnitus is the perception of sound when there is no actual sound stimulus. Causes of this type of tinnitus are medications, infections, neurological conditions, and disorders related to hearing loss (McPhee & Papadakis, 2011).

A thorough history including a complete description of the sound is extremely important to assist in determining the cause. The underlying condition that may be causing the tinnitus must first be addressed (for example, stopping a medication suspected of being the source of the tinnitus or treating the infection). Patients with pulsatile tinnitus need a complete workup because they may have hypertension, anemia, or hyperthyroidism (Reuben et al., 2011).

Treatment for tinnitus first involves preventing exposure to loud noise and ototoxic medications. Pharmacological treatment is quite limited both in effectiveness and duration of symptom relief. Tricyclic antidepressants (i.e., nortriptyline) have been shown to be effective, although they have anticholinergic side effects and caution must be used with the older person. Other therapies include tinnitus retraining therapy, counseling, relaxation, biofeedback, and masking devices (fans and/or white noise machines) to cover up the sounds (Reuben et al., 2011).

Although many feel the urge to shout when they are communicating with older people, in many cases shouting is not helpful. Box 14-2 provides tips for communicating with older adults who have hearing impairments.

> **Drug Alert** ▶▶▶ If a patient on one or more of the following drugs reports a change in hearing, be suspicious of a drug side effect:
>
> - Aminoglycoside antibiotics (gentamicin and erythromycin): ototoxic, tinnitus
> - Antineoplastics (cisplatin): ototoxic
> - Loop diuretics (furosemide): ototoxic
> - Baclofen: tinnitus
> - Propranolol (Inderal): tinnitus and hearing loss

Sources: Epocrates, 2012; Reuben et al., 2011.

BOX 14-2 | **Nursing Interventions to Use When Speaking to an Individual With a Hearing Impairment**

- Eliminate extraneous noise in the room. For example, with the patient's permission turn the television or radio down or off.
- Stand 2 to 3 feet from the patient.
- Gain the patient's attention before speaking. Touch lightly on the arm or shoulder if needed.
- Try to lower the pitch of your voice.
- Pause at the end of each phrase or sentence.
- If the patient has a hearing aid, provide assistance with the device, plus glasses if needed.
- Assess the illumination in the room and make sure that the patient can see you. Face the patient at all times during the conversation.
- The patient may read lips, so it is important not to cover your mouth or chew gum. Do not speak into the chart or converse with someone over your shoulder. The patient will misinterpret your message.
- Speak slowly and clearly in a normal tone of voice—do not shout.
- If the patient does not understand your message, rephrase it rather than repeating the same words.
- Gestures, if appropriate, may help.
- Use written communication if the patient is able to see and read.
- Ask the patient for an oral or written response to determine if the communication was successful.

Sources: Demers, 2007; Reuben et al., 2011.

Nursing Diagnoses Associated With Hearing Impairment

Nursing diagnoses associated with older patients with hearing impairment are diverse and depend on the ability to compensate for hearing problems. The gerontological nurse should consider the older patient's functional ability and not just the results of audiology testing. The nurse should assess the older person's ability to perform activities of daily living, including the ability to communicate, to drive or take public transportation, to hear alarms and doorbells, and to engage in leisure and recreational activities.

The nursing diagnosis *Self-Care Deficit* encompasses a variety of nursing goals and interventions including communication, safety, self-care activities, mood, and leisure activities (NANDA International, 2012).

Taste

The sense of taste allows full appreciation of the flavor and palatability of food and serves as an early warning system against toxins and spoiled food products. Physiologically, taste triggers normal digestion by stimulating gastrointestinal secretions (Mann & Lafreniere, 2007). Taste deficits can result in weight loss, malnutrition, impaired immunity, and worsening of medical illness. Older people sometimes use excessive sugar or salt to compensate for a diminished sense of taste.

A diminished sense of taste, or hypogeusia, is a normal sensory change usually occurring after the age of 70. The exact pathophysiology behind age-related gustatory changes remains unclear but it may be influenced by decreased salivary secretions (Huether & McCance, 2012). However, studies have shown that both taste discrimination and sensitivity significantly change with age. Taste perception of salt and sweetness are most severely affected (Malozemoff, 2007). The sense of taste is mediated by taste buds located on the dorsal surface of the tongue, in the lateral folds on the side of the tongue, on the epiglottis, on the larynx, and even on the first third of the esophagus. Many nerves are responsible for transmitting taste information to the brain, including cranial nerves VII, IX, and X. Taste buds are continually bathed in secretions from the salivary glands, and excessive dryness can distort taste sensation.

Additional factors that may influence alterations in taste include oral condition, olfactory function, medications, diseases, surgical interventions, and environmental exposure (Malozemoff, 2007). Medical conditions that affect the sense of taste are listed in Table 14-2.

Gustatory function may be impaired by poor dentition or improperly fitting dentures that inhibit the ability to chew food properly for flavor release. Dentures covering the soft

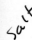

TABLE 14-2	Medical Conditions Affecting Taste
System	**Condition**
Central Nervous System	Head trauma
	Multiple sclerosis
Endocrine	Cushing syndrome
	Hypothyroidism
	Diabetes mellitus
Systemic	Cancer
	Chronic renal failure
	Burns
	Nutritional deficiencies (zinc, niacin, vitamin B$_{12}$)
	Liver disease (cirrhosis)
	HIV/AIDS
Other	Hypertension
	Psychiatric disorders
	Laryngectomy
	Acute infections including the common cold and flu
	Mouth and gum diseases
	Radiation to head/neck
	Candidiasis
	Gingivitis
	Epilepsy

Sources: Malozemoff, 2007; Mann & Lafreniere, 2007; NLM, 2011.

palate obstruct food from reaching the palate and decrease taste perception. Oral infections can release acidic substances, which alter taste. Impaired salivary glands produce less saliva, decreasing the ability for food to dissolve and release flavor (Malozemoff, 2007). Olfactory dysfunction (discussed later in this chapter) can also greatly impair taste sensation because smell stimulates taste and enhances flavor.

Medications can alter taste sensation by affecting peripheral receptors and chemosensory pathways (Mann & Lafreniere, 2007). Drugs known to alter taste are listed in Table 14-3.

Nursing Assessment of the Older Patient With Taste Disturbances

A thorough assessment of the head and neck should be performed to rule out obvious deformity, injury, infection, or obstruction. Mucous membranes should be assessed for

TABLE 14-3	Drugs Affecting Taste		
Class	Drug	Class	Drug
Antibiotics	Ampicillin	**Sympathomimetics**	Amphetamines
	Azithromycin	**Miscellaneous**	Etidronate
	Ciprofloxacin		Iron supplements
	Clarithromycin		Vitamin D
	Griseofulvin	**Antihistamines/Decongestants**	Chlorpheniramine
	Metronidazole		Loratadine
	Ofloxacin		Pseudoephedrine
	Tetracycline	**Cardiac/Antihypertensives**	Captopril
Anticonvulsants	Carbamazepine		Diltiazem
	Phenytoin		Enalapril
Antidepressants	Amitriptyline		Nifedipine
	Desipramine		Nitroglycerin
	Doxepin		Propranolol
	Imipramine		Spironolactone
	Nortriptyline	**Anti-inflammatory Agents**	Colchicine
Antineoplastics	Cisplatin		Dexamethasone
	Doxorubicin		Hydrocortisone
	Methotrexate	**Antiparkinsonian Agent**	Levodopa
	Vincristine	**Muscle Relaxants**	Baclofen
Lipid-lowering Agents	Fluvastatin		Dantrolene
	Lovastatin		
	Pravastatin		

Sources: Ham et al., 2007; Mann & Lafreniere, 2007; NLM, 2011.

dryness, ulceration, or presence of candidiasis. If older patients are noted to have severe gum disease or dental caries, referral to a dentist or oral surgeon is indicated. If the patient wears dentures, they should be removed in order to thoroughly inspect the gums. It is also helpful to question the patient regarding past dietary habits, most enjoyable foods, use of salt and sugar, and preferred beverage at mealtime.

There are no pharmacological treatments to improve taste; however, seasonings and additives to enhance flavor and aroma may amplify taste. Encouraging patients to alternate and eat the different foods on their plate rather than sticking to one food may decrease sensory exhaustion. An intervention used in nursing homes to stimulate gustatory sensation is brewing coffee at mealtimes (Malozemoff, 2007).

Hypogeusia can lead to malnutrition because a decreased ability to sense flavor in foods can lead to lack of motivation and enjoyment in preparing and consuming a

well-balanced diet. The inability to distinguish between salt and sugar can have grave implications for patients with hypertension or diabetes who may not realize that they are consuming too much (Malozemoff, 2007).

Xerostomia, or dry mouth, occurs with salivary gland dysfunction. In the absence of disease and medication effects, salivary function in the older adult generally remains normal. Conditions that may induce xerostomia include systemic diseases (diabetes, HIV, Alzheimer's disease), radiation, medications, and Sjögren's syndrome. The leading cause of dry mouth in the geriatric population is a result of medication. Some examples of medications with xerostomia as an adverse reaction are anticholinergics, antidepressants, antihistamines, diuretics, sedatives, and antipsychotics (Drymouthinfo.com 2012).

Implications of dry mouth include altered taste, difficulty swallowing (dysphagia), periodontal disease (dental caries, gingivitis, oral lesions), speech difficulties, dry lips, halitosis, and sleeping problems. Decreased ability to chew and swallow places those affected at risk for malnutrition and aspiration pneumonia. Dry lips and oral mucosa increases the incidence of infection and dental caries because dry tissues are more easily injured. In addition, dentures can irritate dry oral mucosa (Ham et al., 2007). Speech and eating difficulties may be embarrassing and discourage individuals from wanting to socialize, which can lead to ostracizing themselves from loved ones.

Management of xerostomia involves removal and substitution of offending drugs if possible, good oral care, regular dental examinations, and a diet low in sugar (see Chapter 13 ◖▭◗). Sugar-free candies, mints, and chewing gum may help stimulate salivary secretions. Over-the-counter artificial saliva, oral lubricants, and drinking fluids with meals may help relieve symptoms and dysphagia. Using a humidifier adds moisture to the air and can help with xerostomia that may interfere with sleep. Pilocarpine (Salagen) and cevimeline (Evoxac) are both secretagogues approved by the FDA to relieve symptoms associated with xerostomia, but should be avoided in patients with glaucoma, severe asthma, and COPD ("Anticholinergic drugs," 2011).

Because a large percentage of medications have xerostomia as a side effect, a careful assessment of all medications should be completed to determine if substitutions are possible. Other strategies that may be tried to decrease symptoms include prescribing an anticholinergic medication to be taken during the day instead of at night when salivary secretion normally diminishes, or dividing a larger medication dose from once a day to twice a day to decrease symptoms associated with the larger dose (Ham et al., 2007).

Nurses can assist patients with xerostomia by suggesting these interventions to help relieve symptoms. Understanding which prescriptions cause xerostomia can facilitate discussions with the patient's healthcare provider about a medication review.

Nursing Diagnoses Associated With Taste Impairment

Nursing diagnoses associated with older patients with taste impairment include *Self-Care Deficit*. Additional diagnoses may include *Nutrition, Imbalanced: Less Than Body Requirements* (NANDA International, 2012). Nursing interventions may include appetite enhancement strategies such as adding flavors, checking dentures for fit and cleanliness, inspecting the mouth for ulcers or gingivitis, carefully reviewing medications and identifying any possible offenders

known to affect taste, encouraging fluids, maintaining bowel records, and assessing the palatability of the food. The gerontological nurse working with the institutionalized older person should also survey the dining area with a critical eye and try to ensure that older patients have a pleasant environment in which to eat and are seated with others of their own functional and cognitive levels. Pleasant background music, appetizing smells, clean table settings, and a small bunch of flowers can greatly improve sociability and enjoyment of the mealtime experience.

> **Practice Pearl** ▶▶▶ Gerontological nurses working in long-term care facilities are encouraged to routinely sample the food. Eat with your patients about once a week and you may have additional insights into how to improve the meal service.

Smell

Olfactory dysfunction is more common than taste dysfunction and affects 50% of adults over the age of 60. Normal age-related changes influencing olfactory function are attributed to injury of the olfactory mucosa and reduction in both the number of sensory cells and neurotransmitters. Structural alterations of the upper airway, olfactory tract and bulb, hippocampus, amygdaloid complex, and hypothalamus have also been observed within older adults as contributing factors for diminished sense of smell, or **hyposmia** (NIDCD, 2009).

Although hyposmia may be due to age-related changes, it might also be the result of olfactory nerve damage (cranial nerve I), because this nerve is the sole innervation for smell (Huether & McCance, 2012). Upper respiratory infections (cold, flu, or bronchitis), head trauma, inflammatory conditions (sinusitis or allergic rhinitis), and neurodegenerative diseases (Alzheimer's and Parkinson disease) are the major causes of olfactory damage. Research has shown that unexplained impairments in odor identification, discrimination, and threshold may be an early sign of both Alzheimer's and Parkinson diseases. Other forms of damage may occur as a result of chemotherapy, radiation, and medications. Current or past use of cocaine or tobacco has also been associated with an impaired sense of smell (Mann & Lafreniere, 2007).

Similar to taste disturbances, poor dentition can inhibit olfactory perception if food is not chewed properly because most flavors are perceived retronasally. Dentures covering the soft palate can also block aroma from reaching these receptors (NIDCD, 2009).

Chemosensory impairment can be dangerous because an inability to smell smoke or gas odors increases the potential for fire and explosions. Older adults may also become ill if they lack the ability to smell spoiled food products. Malnourishment is another major implication of hyposmia. Normally, adults experience a decline in metabolic rate with age and consume fewer nutrients. Impaired olfactory function affects appetite, because odor cannot simulate it. Diminished flavor perception makes food less appealing and enjoyable. Loss of sensation can also affect the older adult emotionally and psychologically because the sense of smell triggers memories and pleasurable experiences such as smelling fragrant flowers.

Certain medications have also been known to affect sense of smell. These are listed in Box 14-3.

Nursing Assessment of the Older Patient With Disturbances of Smell

One reason decreased sense of smell fails to be detected is that it is not adequately tested. Most physical examination records state "cranial nerves II–XII intact," completely omitting cranial nerve I. Hyposmia can be related to head trauma, medications, cranial tumors, and upper respiratory infections. The gerontological nurse can examine the mucous membranes of the nares using an otoscope and speculum. The mucous membranes of the nares should be free from polyps, slightly red in color, and without ulceration or copious exudates. The nurse can then ask the patient to occlude one side of the nose, close the eyes, and identify a familiar smell such as vanilla, coffee, or an alcohol swab. This maneuver is repeated on the opposite side using a different odor. Using familiar odors enhances the validity of the test. Commercially prepared scratch-and-sniff tests are available in some smell assessment clinics. These tests contain over 40 odorants and provide more complete information regarding deficits in smell. Patients with obvious deficits in smell should be referred to their primary care provider, an otolaryngologist, and a neurologist of a specialized smell or taste center, usually housed in a large medical center.

Nursing Diagnosis

Nursing diagnoses associated with older patients with hyposmia include *Self-Care Deficit* (NANDA International, 2012). Additional assessment should focus on patient safety and nutrition. Patient education for hyposmia involves safety precautions such as dating and labeling all foods, placing natural gas detectors in the home if the patient has gas heat or a gas stove, placing smoke detectors in strategic locations, and establishing schedules for personal

BOX 14-3	**Medications and Other Factors That Affect Sense of Smell**

- Anesthetics, local
- Antihypertensives
- Antibiotics
- Opioids
- Antidepressants
- Sympathomimetics
- Cocaine hydrochloride
- Diltiazem, nifedipine
- Streptomycin, tyrothricin
- Codeine, hydromorphone, morphine
- Amitriptyline
- Amphetamines
- Other Factors
- Head/neck radiation
- Antihistamines
- Use of medications containing zinc (Zicam nasal gel and swabs)
- Environmental exposure to toxins
- Chemicals and pesticides
- Overuse of antihistamine nasal spray

Sources: U.S. Food and Drug Administration, 2009; NIDCD, 2009.

hygiene and house cleaning. Urge the removal of kitchen waste every evening to prevent a garbage smell from permeating the house, which may be offensive to visitors and go undetected by the older person with hyposmia.

Physical Sensation

As people age, tactile sensation diminishes, due to slower conduction of nerve impulses and diminished function of peripheral nerves. As a result, older adults have decreased perception of pain, vibration, touch, and temperature extremes (NLM, 2012b). Touch is the tactile sense that is perceived by nerve endings and transmits signals to the brain for interpretation. Touch orients a person to the environment and allows the exchange of information and sensation. Psychological benefits to touch include the ability to be soothed, comforted, held, and loved. Some cultures rely heavily on touching others during routine communication and find it difficult to refrain from touching others when they are unable to use their hands. Touch also can be protective by stimulating movement or withdrawal from hot, sharp, or unpleasant stimuli.

Much research has been done to document the importance of touch early in life. Infants in incubators who are not touched will stop eating and fail to thrive. The same may be true for older people, especially those with cognitive or sensory impairments. Institutionalized older adults deprived of caring touch and nurturing physical contact experience a diminishing quality of life, a lessening of their desire to relate to others, and a weakening of what may already be a fragile relationship with physical reality (Kemmet & Brotherson, 2008).

Loss of physical sensation may be harmful for older adults because it increases their risk for injury. Inability to feel the heat of bath or shower water may lead to harmful burns. Injuries or infections may go unnoticed in the lower extremities, delaying needed treatment. Certain medical diagnoses such as diabetes mellitus are associated with peripheral neuropathies that can further decrease touch sensation.

Sedating medications can decrease touch sensation by clouding the sensorium and inducing lethargy. These older patients who may not notice foot ulcers or other injuries require careful monitoring and supervision to prevent injury.

Research in nursing homes has indicated that back rubs, hand and foot massages, and touch therapy sessions can greatly decrease dementia-associated problems such as restlessness, wandering, agitation, and withdrawal (Hirsch, 2011). Gerontological nurses should be well versed in non-pharmacological techniques to improve the quality of life for older adults with dementia. The use of caring touch and massage offers promise as a nursing intervention.

Nursing Assessment of the Older Person With Tactile Impairment

Touch is usually assessed using a wisp of cotton. Patients are asked to close their eyes and nod or say "yes" when they are touched on the face, upper back, and extremities. A cotton swab can also be used with the wooden end pressed lightly against the skin for a sensation of "sharp" and the cotton end for the sensation of "dull." Patients should first be instructed by the nurse with their eyes open so that the sensation can be adequately interpreted. Small

test tubes can also be filled with warm (not hot) and cold water and the tubes pressed to various points on the body for identification with the eyes closed. The patient's ability to discriminate between one and two points can also be assessed using the wooden ends of a cotton swab. Deficits in touch may be referred for further evaluation to the patient's primary care provider or a neurologist.

Nursing Diagnoses Associated With Tactile Impairment

Nursing diagnoses associated with older patients with tactile impairment are diverse and depend on the older person's ability to compensate for tactile problems. Using the diagnosis of *Self-Care Deficit,* the gerontological nurse should assess safety and preventive measures (NANDA International, 2012).

For patients with impaired sense of touch, nursing interventions may focus on continuous monitoring of the intactness of the skin, assessment of safety risks, and the development of a safety plan with instructions to minimize injury. Water heaters should be turned down to 110°F to prevent scalding. Protective padding of upper and lower extremities can prevent bruising and protect skin integrity. Older patients with diabetes mellitus should place a mirror on the wall close to the floor, remove their shoes, and examine the bottoms of their feet daily for blisters, redness, or ulcerations. The use of a good strong light will ease the process and compensate for visual impairment.

> **Practice Pearl ▶▶▶** Advise all older adults to use heating pads on the "low" setting only. Serious burns can result from use of the higher settings.

Patient and Family Teaching

Gerontological nurses require skills and knowledge related to teaching patients and families about the key concepts of gerontology and gerontological nursing. The guidelines in the following feature will assist the nurse to assume the role of teacher and coach.

Patient-Family Teaching Guidelines

The following are guidelines that the nurse may find useful when instructing older adults and their families about sensory changes.

FREQUENTLY ASKED QUESTIONS ABOUT SENSORY CHANGES

1 How can I protect my eyes as I get older?

With aging, vision problems become more common. Some are serious and some are easily treated. The best way to protect your eyes is to:

- Have regular eye examinations every 1 to 2 years.
- Find out if you are at high risk for vision loss (diagnosis of diabetes, family history of eye disease, hypertension).
- Wear sunglasses and a wide brim hat. This will protect your eyes from the sun and prevent cataracts.
- See an eye professional at once if you have loss or dimness of eyesight, eye pain, double vision, swelling, or redness of the eyes.

RATIONALE:

Regular eye examinations and early detection can reduce the risk of vision loss.

2 What are some common eye complaints experienced by older people?

Some common complaints include:

- *Floaters.* These are tiny spots that float across your eyes. They are usually normal but if you see floaters with spots or flashes, call your eye care professional right away.
- *Tearing.* This can result from light sensitivity or dry eye as your body tries to compensate by producing excess tears.
- *Eyelid problems.* Pain, itching, tearing, drooping, or irritation can be corrected with eyedrops or minor surgery.
- *Conjunctivitis.* Also called pink eye, this condition results from allergies or infection. It is easily treated with eyedrops.
- *Presbyopia.* This is the loss of ability to see close objects or small print. Reading glasses can usually correct the problem.

RATIONALE:

Education regarding common complaints can help the older person to evaluate vision changes and decide when to call the eye care professional for more serious problems.

3 What can I do to function better if I have low vision?

Low-vision adaptations can help you to carry out your normal routines. See a low-vision expert for help choosing the right product because they are not all covered by insurance and can be expensive. Most clinics will let you try out some devices to improve your function at home for a week or so before you make the decision to buy them. Simple things you can do at home include:

- Write with bold felt-tip markers.
- Put colored tape on the edge of steps to prevent falls.
- Use contrast whenever possible, like light furniture on dark floors, red dishes on a light-colored table, and so on.
- Use motion lights that turn on by themselves when you walk into a room and timers that turn on lights at dusk.
- Use telephones, clocks, and watches with large numbers.
- Have several pairs of magnifying glasses around the house so that you can set the microwave, adjust the TV, and read the mail easily.
- Use appropriate assistive devices and environmental interventions to improve safety, functional ability, and quality of life. Low-vision clinical evaluation can help you decide what products are right for you. Your primary healthcare provider can help you find a low-vision professional or clinic in your area.

RATIONALE:

Less than perfect vision does not mean that older adults cannot function. The nurse can help them to come up with creative solutions to maximize independence.

4 I think I am getting a little hard of hearing. Is this common at my age?

Yes, about one third of Americans over 60 have hearing problems. It is important to get testing and find out the severity of your problem. See your doctor if:

- You cannot hear on the phone.
- It is hard to keep up with a conversation when several people are talking.
- You need to turn the TV up so loud others complain.
- You have trouble hearing women and children talking.

(continued)

Patient-Family Teaching Guidelines (continued)

RATIONALE:

Older people sometimes gradually adjust to hearing loss and do not recognize they have a problem. Pointing out specific behaviors will help them assess their own situation.

5 What causes hearing loss?

Many things such as earwax, noise exposure over a long period of time, viral or bacterial infections, heredity, certain medications, and other factors cause hearing loss. The only way to know is to see a doctor for examination and testing.

RATIONALE:

Some causes of hearing loss are reversible, and treatment can improve the quality of a person's life. Further testing is always indicated.

6 How can I help myself to overcome my hearing loss?

Some tips include:

- Look at people's faces when they speak.
- Ask people to speak slowly and clearly.
- Read facial expressions such as grins or frowns.
- Be patient and ask people to repeat if you do not hear the first time.
- Use a hearing aid if you need it.

RATIONALE:

Some commonsense tips can help an older person to function more effectively.

7 I have a decreased sense of touch and smell. What should I be concerned about?

The main issue is safety. Our sense of touch and smell alert us to dangers in the environment like smoke from a fire or spoiled food in the refrigerator. It is a good idea to see an ear, nose, and throat doctor for further testing if you have problems with smell, and an internist or neurologist for problems with touch. Some of these problems can be treated, which will improve your safety.

RATIONALE:

Special safety and home modifications are needed for older people with problems of touch and smell. Older patients should be urged to seek testing, to correct the problem if appropriate, and to institute a plan of safety. It is essential to have intact and functioning smoke detectors in the home and natural gas detectors if the patient has gas heat or a gas stove.

CARE PLAN   A Patient With Visual Impairment

Case Study

Mrs. Owen is a 78-year-old woman who has just been admitted to the hospital's rehabilitation unit. She is recovering from an open reduction with internal fixation of her right hip. She fractured her hip 5 days ago at home when she fell getting up to go to the bathroom in the middle of the night. The circumstances of the fall were not documented because she lives alone, but Mrs. Owen states, "I got my feet all tangled up in an electrical cord I was using to run the fan because it was so hot in my room. I just didn't see it." Mrs. Owen has a daughter who lives in a nearby town. The daughter states she is unaware of any other falls her mother may have had, but has noticed numerous bumps and bruises on her mother's arms and legs within the past few months. Mrs. Owen denies this, saying, "Oh, I bruise easily. I always have. It's worse since I'm taking an aspirin every day." Additional medications include atenolol for hypertension, imipramine for depression, and pilocarpine eyedrops for glaucoma.

Mrs. Owen has a regular primary care provider, but has not seen her eye doctor for several years. She states, "Oh, he never does a thing for me. He only tests the pressure in my eyes and says OK, you're good."

CARE PLAN **A Patient With Visual Impairment** (continued)

Applying the Nursing Process

Assessment

Mrs. Owen has suffered a fall with resultant serious injury. Falls in the older person can result from a number of factors, so a complete health assessment is needed. However, the nurse should carefully check postural blood pressures because the patient is taking atenolol and imipramine, both of which can contribute to postural hypotension, dizziness, and falls. Additional information that Mrs. Owen uses pilocarpine for glaucoma but has not been vigilant in following up with her eye care provider or monitoring her intraocular pressures should raise a red flag. This patient needs a complete nursing assessment including functional abilities, mental status and mood testing, nutritional assessment, and safety evaluation.

Diagnoses

Appropriate nursing diagnoses for Mrs. Owen might include the following:

- *Self-Care Deficit* as evidenced by her fall at night and possibly because of damage secondary to poorly controlled IOP as the result of glaucoma
- *Fall, Risk for* related to decreased vision and environmental hazards, multiple medications that can affect blood pressure and cause postural hypotension, and decreased safety awareness as evidenced by placing an electrical appliance with a cord in a walkway
- *Health Maintenance, Ineffective* as evidenced by failure to seek ongoing care and evaluation regarding her glaucoma

NANDA-I © 2012.

Expected Outcomes

The expected outcomes for the plan of care specify that Mrs. Owen will:

- Become aware of the need to follow up with her eye care provider to monitor her IOP.
- Utilize risk reduction measures to decrease fall hazards in her home.
- Develop a more trusting and open relationship with her daughter regarding her health status.
- Agree to establish a therapeutic relationship with the nurse and develop a mutually acceptable plan to work toward these outcomes.

Planning and Implementation

The following nursing interventions may be appropriate for Mrs. Owen:

- Urge family to conduct a safety assessment of Mrs. Owen's home environment so that she will not suffer additional falls or injury after discharge from the hospital.
- Educate Mrs. Owen regarding the importance of seeing her ophthalmologist to have her IOP monitored to avoid further visual impairment as the result of poorly managed glaucoma. Encourage Mrs. Owen to arrange an appointment within 1 month of discharge from the hospital.
- Assess the support system and services needed for Mrs. Owen when she completes her rehabilitation and is discharged to home. Meals-on-Wheels, visiting nurse services, physical therapy, shopping, and transportation services can be supplied as needed.
- Begin to explore Mrs. Owen's problem-solving and coping strategies that she has used to solve problems in the past. Mrs. Owen should be aware of the risk of injury and the need to modify her environment for safety.

(continued)

CARE PLAN **A Patient With Visual Impairment** (continued)

Evaluation

The nurse hopes to work with Mrs. Owen over time to increase her functional status, decrease her fall risk, and monitor the management of her chronic illnesses. The nurse will consider the plan a success based on the following criteria:

- Mrs. Owen will return to her home or the least restrictive institutional environment that is acceptable to her, her daughter, and her healthcare providers.

- A family meeting will be held to discuss Mrs. Owen's overall health.
- She will begin to identify fall hazards in her home and make a plan to minimize risk from falls.

Ethical Dilemma

Change the previous scenario slightly to reflect that Mrs. Owen's fall was caused by her dog Muffin, a toy poodle who constantly runs under her feet. Mrs. Owen states, "I don't care if I did fall on Muffin. I can't imagine life without him. I'll never give him up." How should the nurse respond?

Obviously, Mrs. Owen cares deeply for her dog. Pets improve the quality of life of their owners by providing unconditional love and companionship. However, older people with impaired vision may have difficulty ambulating around a quickly moving dog. Assuming Mrs. Owen is cognitively intact, has good judgment (appropriate assessment required), and can adequately care for Muffin and herself, she has the right to keep her pet.

Should the pet be removed against her will, she would probably suffer from depression and grief, both of which can be detrimental to the function and quality of life of an older person. However, there may be interventions appropriate to improving the situation. For instance:

- Ask a neighbor to walk the dog vigorously once or twice a day to provide a release of energy and perhaps calm

Muffin. If a high school student lives nearby, a small payment would ensure the daily walk and provide socialization for Mrs. Owen.
- Ask Mrs. Owen to use a cane when ambulating. If Muffin should run under her feet, she could use the cane to steady herself.
- Place a bell on Muffin's collar so that Mrs. Owen can be alerted when he runs into the room, and change Muffin's collar to a bright red or orange color to improve Mrs. Owen's ability to see him.
- Use motion sensors to turn on lights at night so that when Mrs. Owen has to get up to go to the bathroom, her way will be well lighted.

Mrs. Owen and all involved with her care and support should be aware of the risks and benefits involved with keeping a pet and the chance of another fall. Careful monitoring and ongoing assessment will be needed.

Critical Thinking and the Nursing Process

1. What strategies can the gerontological nurse use when asking an older person to make environmental changes in the home to improve safety?
2. How can nurses become more proactive and improve the environment for safety in the nursing home and hospital settings?
3. Many older people refuse the use of assistive devices like canes and hearing aids because of vanity. What strategies can gerontological nurses use to increase acceptance of assistive devices?

4. How can the mealtime environment be improved in the facilities where you have had clinical rotations?
5. Wear knit gloves for a few hours at home and try to describe the experience of being unable to directly touch and experience your environment.
6. Examine your own habits in your clinical experiences relating to touch. Do you routinely touch older patients? How do you respond when they touch you? Practice touching others in a caring manner, especially if they are vision and hearing impaired. The insights gained will be invaluable.

- Evaluate your responses in Appendix B.

Chapter Highlights

- Sensory impairments occur commonly in older people as a result of normal changes of aging, the side effects of medications, pathology in certain illnesses, and exposure to environmental insults and chemicals.

- Visual changes involve decreased night vision, color discrimination, and lens accommodation, which all inhibit near vision.

- Hearing loss may result from previous occupational exposure to loud noises for prolonged periods of time.

- Taste, smell, and touch perception gradually decrease over time, but large losses may be the result of comorbid diseases and toxic side effects of medication.

- Older adults with one or more sensory impairments are at risk for injury, weight loss, falls, malnutrition, and social isolation. Careful assessment of the duration, extent, and degree of impact on the functional ability of the older person with a sensory impairment is within the role of the gerontological nurse.

- The nurse can urge older people to seek medical evaluation and advice on assistive devices that can improve function, safety, and quality of life.

- Modifications in the older person's environment can be made to improve safety and function.

Pearson Nursing Student Resources
Find additional review materials at
nursing.pearsonhighered.com

Prepare for success with additional NCLEX®-style practice questions, interactive assignments and activities, web links, animations and videos, and more!

References

Age-Related Eye Disease Study Research Group. (2007). The relationship of dietary carotenoid and vitamin A, E, and C intake with age-related macular degeneration in a case-control study (AREDS Report No. 22). *Archives of Ophthalmology, 125*(9), 1225–1232.

American Academy of Ophthalmology. (2012). Who is at risk for cataracts? *Eye Smart.* Retrieved from http://www.geteyesmart.org/eyesmart/diseases/cataracts-risk.cfm

American Foundation for the Blind. (2012). *Technology advances for people with vision loss.* Retrieved from http://www.afb.org/section.aspx?FolderID=2&SectionID=4

American Speech-Language-Hearing Association (ASLH). (2012). *Hearing loss and the audiologist.* Retrieved from http://www.asha.org/careers/professions/hla.htm

Anticholinergic drugs. (2011). In *Nurse practitioners' reference guide.* New York, NY: Prescribing Reference.

Cacchione, P. (2010). Sensory changes. *ConsultGeriRN.org.* Retrieved from http://consultgerirn.org/topics/sensory_changes/want_to_know_more

Centers for Disease Control and Prevention (CDC). (2011). *Older adult drivers: Get the facts.* Retrieved from http://www.cdc.gov/Motorvehiclesafety/Older_Adult_Drivers/adult-drivers_factsheet.html

Chizek, M. (2007). The aging eye. *Advance for Nurses, 9*(12), 17.

Clark, M. J. C. (2002). *Community health nursing: Caring for populations* (4th ed.). Upper Saddle River, NJ: Prentice Hall.

Demers, K. (2007). Hearing screening in older adults: A brief hearing loss screener. *Try this: Best nursing practices in care for older adults* (No. 12). Hartford Institute for Geriatric Nursing. Retrieved from http://consultgerirn.org/uploads/File/trythis/try_this_12.pdf

Drymouthinfo.com. (2012). *Dry mouth— Treatment of drug induced xerostomia.* Retrieved from http://www.drymouth.info/practitioner/treatment.asp

Epocrates. (2011). Glaucoma medications. *Prescription medication information program.* Retrieved from https://online.epocrates.com

Epocrates. (2012). *Ototoxic drugs.* Retrieved from https://online.epocrates.com/search/search.jsp?lang=en&query=ototoxic drugs

Ham, R. J., Sloane, P. D., Warshaw, G. A., Bernard, M. A., & Flaherty, E. (2007). *Primary care geriatrics: A case-based approach* (5th ed.). Philadelphia, PA: Mosby Elsevier.

Hirsch, C. (2011). Systematic pain management reduced agitation in nursing home residents with demential. *Annals of Internal Medicine, 155*(10), JC5–JC9.

Hsu, C., Phillips, W., Sherman, K., Hawkes, R., & Cherkin, D. (2008). Healing in primary care: A vision shared by patients, physicians, nurses and clinical staff. *Annals of Family Medicine, 6,* 307–314. Retrieved from http://www.annfammed.org/cgi/content/full/6/4/307

Huether, S., & McCance, K. (2012). *Understanding pathophysiology* (5th ed.). St. Louis, MO: Elsevier Mosby.

Kemmet, D., & Brotherson, S. (2008). *Making sense of sensory losses as we age.* North Dakota State University. Retrieved from http://www.ag.ndsu.edu/pubs/yf/famsci/fs1378.html

Kirtland, K., Zack, M., & Caspersen C. (2012). State-specific synthetic estimates of health status groups among inactive older adults with self-reported diabetes, 2000–2009. *Preventing Chronic Disease, 9*. doi:http://dx.doi.org/10.5888/pcd9.110221

Malozemoff, W. (2007). When the nose no longer knows: Smell and taste disorders in elders. *Advance for Nurses*. Retrieved from http://www.nurse.com/ce/course.html?CCID=3387

Mann, N. M., & Lafreniere, D. (2007). *Anatomy and etiology of taste and smell disorders*. Retrieved from http://www.uptodateonline.com.

McPhee, S., & Papadakis, M. (2011). Disorders of the eyes and lids. In *Current medical diagnosis and treatment*. New York, NY: McGraw-Hill Medical.

MedlinePlus. (2011). *Older adults' knowledge about medications that can impact driving.* Retrieved from http://www.aaafoundation.org/pdf/ Knowledge About Medications And Driving Report.pdf

NANDA International. (2012). *NANDA International nursing diagnoses: Definitions and classification, 2012–2014*. Philadelphia, PA: Wiley-Blackwell.

National Eye Institute (NEI), National Institutes of Health. (2007). *Eye photos.* Retrieved from http://www.nei.nih.gov

National Eye Institute (NEI), National Institutes of Health. (2009). *Age related macular degeneration: What you should know.* Retrieved from http://www.nei.nih.gov/health/maculardegen/nei_wysk_amd.PDF

National Eye Institute (NEI), National Institutes of Health. (2012). *Glaucoma.* Retrieved from http://www.nei.nih.gov/health/glaucoma/index.asp

National Institute on Deafness and Other Communication Disorders (NIDCD). (2009). *Smell disorders.* Retrieved from http://www.nidcd.nih.gov/health/smelltaste/pages/smell.aspx

National Institute on Deafness and Other Communication Disorders (NIDCD). (2010). *Hearing aids.* Retrieved from http://www.nidcd.nih.gov/health/hearing/pages/hearingaid.aspx#hearingaid_09

Reuben, D. B., Herr, K. A., Pacala, J. T., Pollock, B. G., Potter, J. F., & Semla, T. P. (2011). *Geriatrics at your fingertips* (13th ed.). New York, NY: American Geriatrics Society.

UpToDate. (2007). *Lutein: Natural drug information.* Retrieved from http://www.uptodate.com

U.S. Equal Employment Opportunity Commission (EEOC). (2011). *Questions and answers about blindness and vision impairments in the workplace and the Americans with Disabilities Act.* Retrieved from http://www.eeoc.gov/facts/blindness.html

U.S. Food and Drug Administration. (2009). *Warnings on three Zicam intranasal zinc products.* Retrieved from http://www.fda.gov/ForConsumers/ConsumerUpdates/ucm166931.htm

U.S. National Library of Medicine (NLM). (2011). *Taste—impaired.* Retrieved from http://www.nlm.nih.gov/medlineplus/ency/article/003050.htm

U.S. National Library of Medicine (NLM). (2012a). *Aging changes in the senses.* Retrieved from http://www.nlm.nih.gov/medlineplus/ency/article/004013.htm

U.S. National Library of Medicine (NLM). (2012b). *Aging changes in the skin.* Retrieved from http://www.nlm.nih.gov/medlineplus/ency/article/004014.htm

CHAPTER

15

The Cardiovascular System

Susan K. Chase, EdD, FNP-BC
ASSOCIATE DEAN FOR GRADUATE AFFAIRS AND PROFESSOR
SCHOOL OF NURSING, UNIVERSITY OF CENTRAL FLORIDA

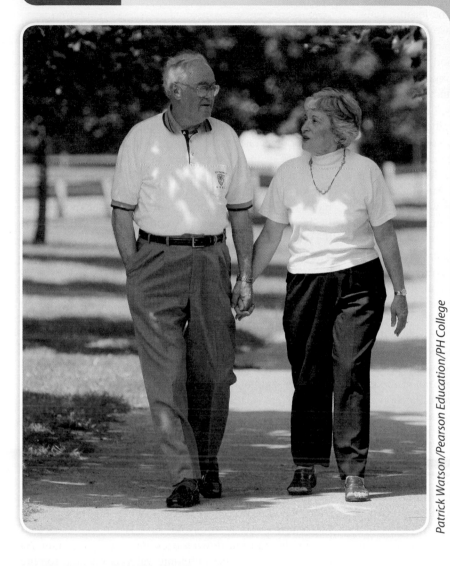

Patrick Watson/Pearson Education/PH College

KEY TERMS

LEARNING OUTCOMES

On completion of this chapter, the reader will be able to:

1. Describe changes in the cardiovascular system that occur with aging.
2. List focus areas of assessment for cardiovascular patients.
3. Relate physiological concepts to the diagnosis and management of common cardiovascular risks and conditions, including hypertension, angina, heart failure, and peripheral vascular disease.
4. Formulate common nursing diagnoses for the cardiovascular patient.
5. Identify specific nursing interventions used with cardiovascular patients.
6. Outline an education plan for cardiovascular patients.

Cardiovascular conditions are the chief cause of death in the United States and other developed countries, particularly as people age. From ages 45 to 64, malignant neoplasms surpass heart disease as the leading cause of death, but from age 65 on, heart disease is the number one cause of death (Murphy, Xu, & Kochanek,, 2012).

The cardiovascular system pumps blood to all parts of the body for the purpose of delivering oxygen and nutrients and removing metabolic waste products. Because its purpose is to supply all parts of the body, the functioning of the system affects functioning of all other systems. In recent years, advanced technology has prolonged the lives of many people with; cardiovascular diseases, but this has resulted in increased numbers of people living with the chronic effects of cardiovascular disease. Any nurse working with older adults will encounter people who are dealing with changes to the cardiovascular system that are a natural part of aging. The Institute of Medicine has called for reform in training and practice of all healthcare providers to provide a healthcare workforce that will be ready to meet the increasing demands of our aging population. Nurses will be key to this endeavor (Committee on the Future of Healthcare Workforce for Older Americans, 2008).

Many people also have specific cardiovascular disorders. By understanding key principles of physiology, the nurse can understand how to assist people in preventing cardiovascular diseases and how new treatment modalities work to reduce symptoms and improve function and quality of life. Nurses need to be able to assess cardiovascular problems, provide effective nursing interventions, and explain conditions and treatments to older patients and their families. Helping older people learn to manage their chronic conditions is very rewarding for the nurse and the patients who are provided the opportunity to enjoy an improved quality of life. Recent studies have led to new treatments and knowledge about diet and exercise that make a difference in patients' ability to function. Working with older adults to improve their ability to manage their cardiovascular health is a rewarding aspect of gerontological nursing.

This chapter reviews the cardiovascular changes related to aging, the pattern of specific cardiovascular conditions, and the medical and nursing interventions used to support older patients who have, or are at risk for, these conditions. As with all health care delivered to older adults, it is important to consider changed response patterns due to age, to preserve function and quality of life, to promote understanding and anticipation of expected changes, to maintain patient dignity, and to promote realistic choices. Changes in cardiovascular function are a feature of every life stage, but this chapter will focus on changes for the young-old (65 to 74 years), the middle old (75 to 85 years), and the old-old (86 and older years). This last age group is the fastest growing segment of the U.S. population.

Structure and Function

The heart is a four-chambered organ positioned slightly left of the sternum. The two upper chambers of the heart are the atria. The two lower chambers of the heart are the ventricles. The ventricles generate power to pump blood through the body systems to which they are connected. The left side of the heart generates greater power to overcome the systemic resistance of the blood vessels of the body. The left ventricle has to send the blood out over the greatest area. The system of chambers and valves allows for one-way flow of blood from the general circulation, through the right side of the heart, to the lungs where blood gases are exchanged for the release of carbon dioxide and the absorption of oxygen. The blood returns to the left side of the heart and then to the general circulation where oxygen is delivered to tissue and carbon dioxide and other wastes are removed. The cardiac cycle is the mechanical sequence and timing of contraction and relaxation in the heart. It is determined by the electrical system of the heart. Figure 15-1 ▶▶▶ illustrates the structure of the heart and the valves.

The inferior and superior venae cavae return blood from the general circulation to the right atrium. Pressures in this chamber are relatively low, which allows for easy return of blood from the peripheral circulation. When the tricuspid valve opens, pressures in the resting right ventricle are lower than in the right atrium and blood flows across the tricuspid valve into the right ventricle. The resting phase of the ventricle is called **diastole.** Atrial contraction forces even more blood into the filling right ventricle. With ventricular contraction, also called **systole,** pressure rises in the ventricle and the tricuspid valve is forced closed, preventing blood from flowing back into the right atrium. As the pressure rises, the pulmonic valve is opened, forcing blood from the now high-pressure right ventricle into the lower pressure pulmonary artery.

The pulmonary artery leads blood into branching vessels of the lungs. During ventricular diastole, the pulmonic valve closes, preventing blood from returning from the pulmonic artery to the right ventricle. Blood flows through the branching vessels and eventually into the lung capillaries where gas exchange takes place. The pulmonary veins return the oxygenated blood from the lungs to the left atrium. On the left side of the heart, the sequence of events is similar and simultaneous with the right-sided events. The opening of the mitral valve allows blood to flow into the relaxed left ventricle. Atrial contraction forces even more blood into the filling left ventricle. When the left

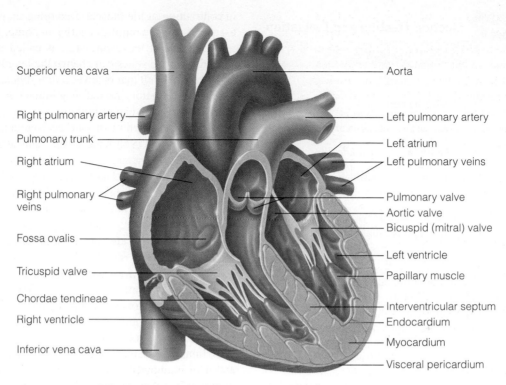

Superior vena cava

Aorta

Right pulmonary artery

Left pulmonary artery

Pulmonary trunk

Left atrium

Right atrium

Left pulmonary veins

Right pulmonary veins

Pulmonary valve

Aortic valve

Bicuspid (mitral) valve

Fossa ovalis

Left ventricle

Tricuspid valve

Papillary muscle

Chordae tendineae

Interventricular septum

Right ventricle

Endocardium

Inferior vena cava

Myocardium

Visceral pericardium

Figure 15-1 ▶▶▶ The structure of the heart and the valves.

ventricle contracts, the mitral valve is forced closed. The aortic valve opens to allow blood to be pumped into the aorta from which it distributes blood to the entire systemic circulation. When the left ventricle relaxes, the aortic valve closes, preventing blood from flowing back into the left ventricle. The pressures generated on the left side of the heart are greater than the pressures generated on the right side of the heart. This greater pressure is necessary to ensure the adequate flow of blood to and from all systems in the body. Over time, and especially when there is increased resistance such as that encountered with peripheral vascular disease and systemic hypertension, this can put stress on the structures of the valves that are associated with the left ventricle, specifically the aortic and mitral valves. The valves can become leaky and damaged, resulting in regurgitation of blood back into the atrium and left ventricular hypertrophy or increased muscle mass to the left ventricle. This can decrease the valuable space needed for blood in the left ventricle.

The amount of blood pumped from the left ventricle with each beat is the **stroke volume.** The amount pumped per minute is the **cardiac output.** This value is reflective of overall functioning of the heart. It can be calculated using the following formula:

$$\text{cardiac output} = \text{heart rate} \times \text{stroke volume}$$

The cardiac output is affected by the heart rate and by the volume of venous blood returned to the heart. The amount of blood filling the left ventricle is reflected in the preload. The afterload reflects the resistance to flow of blood across the aortic valve or through the blood vessels. Cardiac function can be partly regulated by affecting **preload** (amount of blood returning to the heart from the venous circulation), **afterload** (the pressure against which the ventricle ejects blood), and **contractility** (the strength of the cardiac contraction). The body uses neurochemical means, the autonomic nervous system, to regulate factors such as epinephrine, which increases heart rate, and norepinephrine, which increases the force of contraction.

Among the many functions of the autonomic nervous system, the regulation of pressure and volume in the cardiovascular system is of vital importance. Sympathetic receptors can be divided into alpha and beta receptors, which stimulate the heart to work harder or faster. A large group of cardiovascular drugs blocks the alpha and beta receptors, reducing the workload on the heart. The balancing parasympathetic nervous system has neurotransmitters that decrease heart rate. The vagus nerve is one of the major nerves of the parasympathetic system.

Stimulation of receptors of the sympathetic nervous system, sometimes called **adrenergic receptors,** causes increased blood pressure, vasoconstriction, increased heart

TABLE 15-1	Ejection Fraction and Evaluation
Ejection Fraction	Evaluation
55–75%	Normal
40–55%	Below normal
Less than 40%	May support diagnosis of heart failure
<35%	Patient may be at risk for life-threatening cardiac arrhythmias

rate, decreased blood flow to the kidneys, and other effects. This is the fight-or-flight response that is elicited in times of stress.

With aging and the diagnosis of cardiovascular disease, it is important to know how efficiently the heart is able to pump blood throughout the body. The amount of blood pumped from the left ventricle at the end of diastole with each beat is not the complete volume of the blood that filled the ventricle. The proportion of blood that is pumped out in each heartbeat is the **ejection fraction**. Its formula is:

$$\text{ejection fraction} = \text{stroke volume/end diastolic volume of left ventricle}$$

The efficiency of the ventricle's ability to pump is reflected in this volume. The ejection fraction can be affected by the strength of the contraction of the ventricles, the amount of blood contained in the ventricles, the ability of the valves to prevent regurgitation, and the amount of peripheral vascular resistance. The higher the ejection fraction, the more efficiently the heart is able to provide adequate circulation to the body systems (Table 15-1).

Usually a normal ejection fraction is between 55% and 75%; values below 40% indicate poor cardiac output because of an impaired pumping action. Values below 35% may indicate imminent heart failure, whereas values above 75% may indicate a hypertrophic cardiomyopathy when the pumping action and cardiac output are exaggerated (Cleveland Clinic, 2012).

Conduction System

The mechanical events related to heart function are regulated and coordinated by a series of complex electrical events. All cells of the heart are capable of generating and responding to electrical stimulation. The cells of the myocardium are connected in a mesh that allows the transmission of electrical impulses that regulate heartbeat and stimulate coordinated muscle contractions.

When an action potential is generated or transmitted to a cardiac muscle cell, it initiates a chain of events that results in contraction of the muscle. Returning the cell membrane to its resting state requires energy and time. The period before a cell is at its resting state is called the **refractory period.** Disease states can change the length of the refractory period. A cell that receives *and responds* to an impulse during the refractory period may initiate an irregularity of heart rhythm called an arrhythmia.

The normal rhythm of cardiac contraction is initiated by the sinoatrial (SA) node in the right atrium. The cells of this region generate action potential at the fastest rate of all the cells of the heart; therefore, they initiate a new impulse and maintain the ongoing heartbeat. This impulse travels across the atria in a coordinated wave and results in atrial contraction.

A band of nonconductive tissue separates the atria from the ventricles. The slight delay in atrial and ventricular contraction allows for efficient filling of the chambers of the heart and a coordinated heartbeat. This fibrous tissue is where the valves are attached. Only one section of the band that separates the atria from the ventricles allows conduction of impulses. It is called the atrioventricular (AV) node. The impulse through the AV node is delayed somewhat and then is allowed to transmit the action potential wave through the bundle of His and bundle branches, which allow for fast conduction. The bundle branches separate and allow for essential simultaneous activation of the thick ventricular walls. When activated, the ventricles contract at the same time. After the refractory period, the SA node generates a new action potential and the sequence repeats itself.

Electrocardiogram

The electrocardiogram (ECG) can offer valuable information about cardiac function and electrical regulation of the heart. The ideal ECG deflections represent depolarization and repolarization of cardiac muscle tissue in a regular pattern and rhythm. The waves of interest include the P, QRS, and T waves. The P wave represents atrial depolarization. The PR interval represents delay in conduction at the AV node. The QRS complex represents ventricular depolarization. The T wave represents ventricular repolarization. A diagram of a normal ECG is illustrated in Figure 15-2 ▶▶▶.

The Circulatory System

Blood vessels that circulate blood throughout the body include arteries and their smaller branches called arterioles; capillaries, the smallest diameter and thinnest vessels; and veins, which include the smaller venules. Arteries carry blood away from the heart. In the pulmonary circuit, this blood is unoxygenated and is on the way to capillaries in the lungs where gases can be exchanged and the blood is oxygenated. The walls of arteries have several layers of smooth muscle

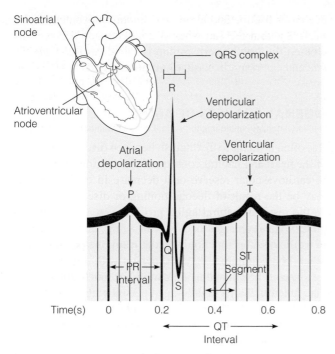

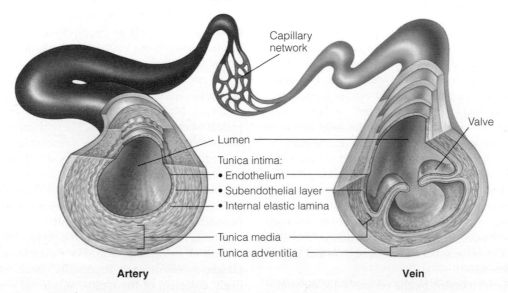

Figure 15-2 ►►► Normal electrocardiogram.

called the tunica adventitia, which is composed of connective tissue. The capillaries have an endothelial layer and a basal lamina. The spacing between the cells of the endothelium varies from one part of the body to another. Serum of the blood, the fluid portion, and the smaller dissolved substances are filtered through the spaces between the endothelial cells of the capillaries. Most of the filtered fluid is returned to the bloodstream in the veins, which have lower pressure than the arteries or capillaries.

Veins have larger diameters than arteries. Because they carry blood under decreased pressure, they have thinner walls. The veins of the legs have valves that assist in returning blood from the lower extremities to the heart. Blood return in the veins relies on skeletal muscle movement. As the muscles of the legs contract, they squeeze the blood upward, facilitating the return of venous blood to the heart. Valves prevent the blood from flowing back due to the pull of gravity. Figure 15-3 ►►► illustrates the capillary network between the arterial and venous blood vessels.

Regulation of Blood Flow

Blood flow in any area of the body is under several types of control. Local control allows for more or less flow of blood due to local conditions—for example, as a result of trauma or inflammation. The endothelial lining of the arteries and veins is metabolically active and capable of the release of nitric oxide, which causes vasodilation or relaxation. Extreme cold in the extremities may shunt blood away from the extremities to vital organs like the heart and brain to prevent loss of essential body heat. This can result in frostbite to fingers and toes. Areas of the circulation that are metabolically active will receive more circulation than

that allow for some local control of diameter and pressure in the system. With contraction of the smooth muscle, the artery becomes smaller, allowing less space for circulating blood and resulting in increased systemic pressure.

The inside layer of the artery is called the tunica intima and includes the endothelium and the basal membrane. The next layer out is the tunica media, which has collagen and fibrous tissue including smooth muscles. The outer layer is

Figure 15-3 ►►► The capillary network between arterial and venous blood.

areas that are at rest. Increased blood flow can be initiated by acidosis. Metabolic activity causes the production of acids as a by-product, so acidosis causes a relaxation of local sphincters and allows more blood to an area. For instance, circulation to the large muscles of the legs will increase during strenuous activity such as jogging or stair climbing. This results in anaerobic metabolism that will cause a local acidosis in the tissue. By increasing blood flow to this area, the circulatory system provides needed oxygen and removes the chemicals that cause acidosis. When the area rests, acidosis decreases and the circulation also decreases. This allows the body to conserve energy and to perfuse those areas that are in greatest need.

The lymphatic system is a separate pathway that collects excess tissue fluid and returns it to the circulatory system. The lymphatic system is a pumpless system and consists of lymphatic vessels and lymph nodes. A series of valves ensures one-way flow of excess interstitial fluid toward the heart. Usually, the lymphatic system drains interstitial fluid (lymph) through a system of nodes where immune system cells screen and protect the body from infection. When the capillary outflow exceeds venous reabsorption, some fluid remains in the interstitium or extracellular space. This fluid must be returned to the blood system to ensure ongoing efficient cardiovascular function. If too much fluid leaves the capillaries because of excessive arterial pressure, or if the pressure in the venous system is too great and the interstitial fluid cannot reenter the venous circulation, then extra interstitial fluid collects and is termed *edema*. This edema often collects in the lower extremities as the result of gravity.

Cardiac Circulation

The heart is supplied with blood by the coronary circulation. The function of the heart muscle depends on adequate circulation to provide oxygenated blood and prevent pain caused by myocardial ischemia or angina. The two coronary arteries arise from the aorta just above the aortic valve. The left coronary artery branches to become the left anterior descending and the circumflex artery. The right coronary artery supplies the right side of the heart. The coronary arteries travel on the outside of the heart, and the branches penetrate to the deeper layers of muscle. Increased cardiac workload such as increases in rate in response to activity and movement requires increased blood flow through the coronary arteries. Atherosclerotic changes in the coronary arteries and the plaque accumulation of coronary artery disease can result in myocardial ischemia, myocardial infarction, and sudden death.

The heart is surrounded by the pericardium, a double-walled sac filled with a small amount of fluid. This fluid decreases friction and allows for smooth movement of the muscle within the sac when it contracts and relaxes. Increased fluid in the pericardium is called *cardiac tamponade* and can result in cardiac compression and death.

NORMAL CHANGES OF AGING

It is often difficult to distinguish between disease processes of the heart and natural consequences of aging. A decrease in cardiovascular reserve or a decrease in cardiac output may be the result of deconditioning or disease or it may be the result of natural aging processes. A wide range of physiological changes occurs with aging, and differences in cardiovascular functioning exist from one person to another. For example, a very old person with a good family history and healthy lifestyle can enjoy much greater cardiac function than a middle-aged person with a family history of cardiovascular problems or a history of smoking. It is important to remember the concept of compensation in cardiovascular function.

Changes in other body systems may occur with aging and can affect the cardiovascular system. Sometimes the compensatory changes in one system correct one problem while others cause problems such as decreased renal functioning. This causes changes in other systems in order to improve function. For example, kidneys that are poorly perfused due to decreased cardiac output produce renin that eventually increases blood pressure, cardiac output, and sodium retention. These compensatory changes are initially benign but can gradually lead to decreased cardiac and renal function and fluid overload. See Figure 15-4 ▶▶▶ for normal changes of aging in the cardiovascular system.

How an individual person ages is determined by genetic factors as well as by physical and social environments. Aging changes are gradual and may not be noticed by the individual or by members of the family. Different body systems age at different rates. One person might have orthopedic problems but relatively few cardiovascular problems. Many cardiovascular functions involve neurological or endocrine systems. These interrelated processes are vulnerable to aging in that a change in one system can affect functioning in many others. Furthermore, physical or emotional stress can cause greater response and require longer time for recovery. Getting the flu can cause greater physical stress and negative consequences for a frail older person than for a middle-aged adult.

Another feature of aging is the atypical presentation of disease in an older person. For example, a middle-aged person experiencing a myocardial infarction will most likely complain of the typical substernal chest pain with radiation down the left arm. However, the older person may

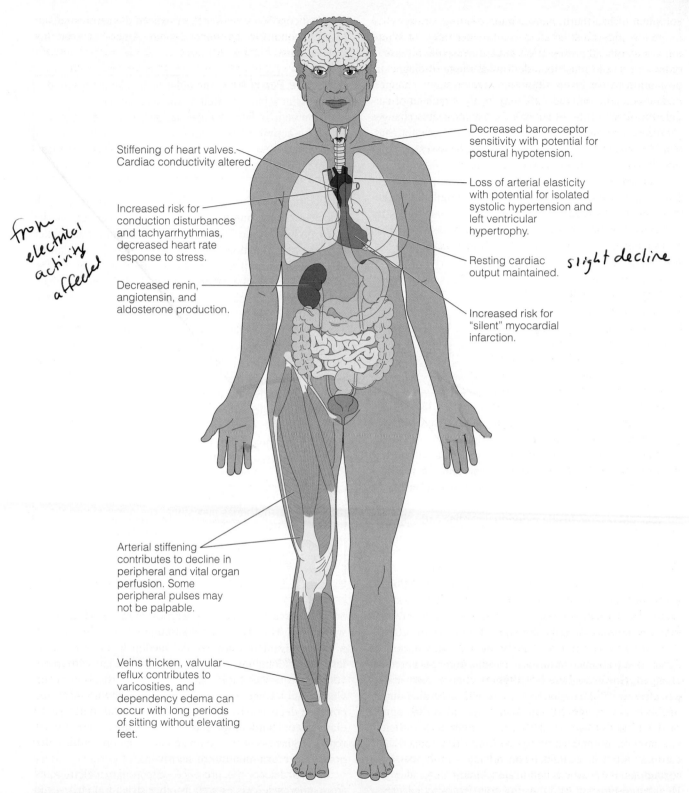

Stiffening of heart valves. Cardiac conductivity altered.

Increased risk for conduction disturbances and tachyarrhythmias, decreased heart rate response to stress.

Decreased renin, angiotensin, and aldosterone production.

Decreased baroreceptor sensitivity with potential for postural hypotension.

Loss of arterial elasticity with potential for isolated systolic hypertension and left ventricular hypertrophy.

Resting cardiac output maintained.

Increased risk for "silent" myocardial infarction.

Arterial stiffening contributes to decline in peripheral and vital organ perfusion. Some peripheral pulses may not be palpable.

Veins thicken, valvular reflux contributes to varicosities, and dependency edema can occur with long periods of sitting without elevating feet.

from electrical activity affected

slight decline

Figure 15-4 ▶▶▶ Normal changes of aging in the cardiovascular system.

complain of heartburn, nausea and vomiting, or excessive fatigue. Nurses must be alert to a broader range of symptoms and atypical presentation of cardiovascular disease in older adults, and must include a wide range of diagnostic possibilities in a given situation. Mental status changes, dizziness, agitation, and falls may be the first sign of cardiac problems in the older person. Mental status changes should never be assumed to be the result of dementia. Sudden changes in cognitive ability should be assessed completely and aggressively (Reuben et al., 2011). Because of compensatory changes in the vascular system that occur with aging, people develop collateral circulation, additional small blood vessels that provide alternate routes for blood to flow. This can change how people experience an acute blockage to major blood vessels such as happens during a myocardial infarction.

> *Practice Pearl* ▶▶▶ Many older women will complain of vague symptoms when having a myocardial infarction, including fatigue, sleep disturbances, and epigastric pain. Be sure to refer older patients with any of these complaints for medical evaluation and teach them to report such symptoms. This is also true of diabetics.

Specific changes in the cardiovascular system with aging include myocardial hypertrophy, an increase in the size of muscle cells of the myocardium. This will change the function of the left ventricular wall and the ventricular septum. The left ventricular wall is 25% thicker for the average 80-year-old person as compared to the average 30-year-old person. Inside individual cardiac cells, lipofuscin and amyloid deposits accumulate and the structure of the myocardium shows increased collagen and connective tissue (McCance & Huether, 2010). Heart valves become stiff with aging as the result of fibrosis and calcification. In addition, changes in the valve rings can contribute to stenosis or incompetence. These changes then have an effect on the heart muscle and chamber sizes (Reuben et al., 2011).

Resting heart rate is relatively unchanged with normal aging. In the absence of disease, cardiac output is not much changed. However, there is a slight decline in cardiac output after age 20. The average man with a cardiac output of 5.0 L/min at age 20 will likely have a cardiac output of 3.5 L/min at age 75. This cardiac output is sufficient to maintain normal adult functioning. The reduction in cardiac output is thought to be related to age-associated reductions in maximum heart rate (American Academy of Health and Fitness, 2011). Aging contributes to a decrease in responsiveness in beta-adrenergic receptors, resulting in a lower or slower response to cardiovascular challenge with the older adult. However, older people in good

physical condition can match or exceed the aerobic capacity of unconditioned younger people (American Academy of Health and Fitness, 2011).

> *Practice Pearl* ▶▶▶ The older heart cannot respond to stressful stimuli as well as the younger heart. Caution your sedentary older patients not to engage in stressful activities like vigorous shoveling of snow or heavy yard work without engaging in a gradual exercise program to build fitness.

Electrical activity of the heart is affected in aging with a decrease in the number of normal pacemaker cells in the sinus node. By age 75, only 10% of original pacemaker cells are still functional, but under normal circumstances this number can still support cardiac function. Similarly, the number of cells in the AV node and in the left bundle branch is lower for the older person. Similar changes have been demonstrated that show a decrease in cells in the bundle of His at age 40 and a decrease in right bundle branch cells by age 50. Other studies show an increase in fat and collagen in these regions. Fibrosis of the AV node can lead to AV block with no other cardiac pathology. The AV node refractory period also increases with aging. The electrocardiogram shows no specific changes with age, although some lengthening of the PR, QRS, and QT interval has been described. The stress of illness can precipitate conduction difficulties for the older person (McPhee & Papadakis, 2011).

> *Practice Pearl* ▶▶▶ New-onset atrial fibrillation and other arrhythmias may signal the onset of serious underlying illness such as hyperthyroidism, electrolyte disturbances, or myocardial infarction. All older patients with complaints of "skipped beats" or "fluttering in the chest" should be referred for medical evaluation.

The vascular system undergoes a range of changes with aging. The layers of the vascular system change with a thickening of the intimal and medial layers. For arteries, the endothelial layer becomes irregular with more connective tissue. Lipid deposits and calcification occur. Calcification can extend to the medial layer with increased collagen deposits. These changes can all lead to decreased elasticity or "hardening" of the arterial walls, or atherosclerosis. High-resolution computed tomography allows for noninvasive examination of narrowing of coronary artery walls and detects the presence of coronary calcification from atherosclerosis as well as other structural changes in the heart. More coronary calcium means more coronary atherosclerosis, suggesting a greater likelihood of significant narrowing somewhere in the coronary system and a higher risk of future cardiovascular events (Cleveland Clinic, 2012). Blood pressure elevation frequently occurs with aging, although it is not considered a normal variant. Isolated systolic hypertension (systolic >140 mmHg) is frequently seen in the older person, although people with less vascular stiffness experience less systolic hypertension (McCance & Huether, 2010). Normally, the arterial wall diameter is controlled by a balance of systems including the autonomic nervous system and beta-adrenergic stimulation. With aging, decreased responsiveness to beta-adrenergic stimulation is noted (McPhee & Papadakis, 2011).

Practice Pearl ▶▶▶ If left uncontrolled, high systolic pressure can lead to stroke, myocardial infarction, heart failure, kidney damage, blindness, or other conditions. Although it cannot be cured once it has developed, isolated systolic hypertension (ISH) can be controlled. Progressive physical activity can reduce vascular wall stiffness and reduce systolic hypertension. Nurses can help patients understand the importance of remaining active in their later years.

Pulmonary changes that occur with aging can affect cardiovascular function. Decreased chest wall compliance is the result of decreased elasticity of lung tissue and stiffness of thoracic and spinal joints. An increase in anteroposterior diameter is seen with aging. This can lead to higher residual volumes. Airway closure in dependent lung areas can occur at higher volumes. This removes portions of the lung from exchange functions. A combination of early airway closure, decreased diffusing capacity, increased lung volumes, and changes in alveolar structure can lead to lower arterial oxygen tension ($Paco_2$). Because carbon dioxide is diffused more readily, no change in $Paco_2$ is noted with aging. Elevated $Paco_2$ would indicate pathology. Ciliary function is decreased with age. This fact, along with decreased immune function, makes the older person more susceptible to pneumonia or other infections (McCance & Huether, 2010).

Renal function declines with age, and the kidneys decrease in size and weight. By age 90, the weight of the kidney is 46% less than the weight of the young adult kidney. Functional decline is also the result of decreased renal blood flow and decreased glomerular filtration. By age 80, the glomerular filtration rate is reduced 30% to 50% compared with that of the 30-year-old person (Glossock & Rule, 2012). Because of a concomitant decrease in muscle mass, serum creatinine levels are not elevated. However, the clearance rate for creatinine and other chemicals, including many medications, is reduced. This results in a longer half-life for drugs administered to the older person. With aging, decreased levels of renin and aldosterone are found in the

plasma. This leads to an increased sensitivity to dietary sodium consumption. Decreased ability to clear sodium from the blood can lead to body water overload. This increased preload can tax the myocardium. Additionally, antidiuretic hormone is less able to be suppressed when serum osmolality is low. This results in further retention of body water. A decreased ability to concentrate urine can result in dehydration. In general, older adults are less able to adapt to fluid volume changes (McCance & Huether, 2010).

In summary, aging brings change to the cardiovascular system. Older people should not expect to become debilitated from normal changes of aging alone. By staying physically active, avoiding obesity, avoiding smoking, and controlling blood pressure and cholesterol levels, many older adults can lead healthy lives without significant cardiovascular problems. However, complaints of fatigue, decreased activity, sleep disturbance, or pain are not normal and should be investigated. Because of normal aging changes, the older person has a decreased capacity to adapt to physiological stressors to the cardiovascular system such as sudden increased metabolic demand due to extreme exercise or serious illness with high fevers and these older adults will need careful monitoring of cardiac function.

Common Cardiovascular Diseases With Older Adults

Cardiovascular disease develops slowly and can take years to develop. Some common conditions such as hypertension, diabetes, and hyperlipidemia are risk factors for developing more serious conditions at any stage in life, and these conditions require ongoing assessment and treatment at any age.

Hypertension

Hypertension is a major risk factor for other cardiovascular conditions, although it does not usually produce symptoms of its own. Since the 1960s, the death rates due to cardiovascular conditions in industrialized nations have decreased, largely due to better control of hypertension with medications. An estimated 1 in 3 adults or 68 million Americans, have hypertension and only 50% of those with hypertension have their hypertension under control (Centers for Disease Control and Prevention [CDC], 2012).

Women are about as likely as men to develop high blood pressure during their lifetimes. However, for people under 45 years old, the condition affects more men than women. For people 65 years and older, it affects more women than men. See Table 15-2 for rates of hypertension by age.

African Americans develop high blood pressure more often, and at an earlier age, than whites and Mexican Americans

TABLE 15-2	Hypertension Rates by Age	
Age	**Men (%)**	**Women (%)**
20–34	11.1	6.8
35–44	25.1	19.0
45–54	37.1	35.2
55–64	54.0	53.3
65–74	64.0	69.3
75 and older	66.7	78.5
All	34.1	32.7

Source: CDC, 2012.

do. Among African Americans, more women than men have the condition. Fortunately, more people with high blood pressure, especially those 60 years and older, have become aware of their condition and received treatment. However, about one in five (20.4%) U.S. adults with high blood pressure do not know that they have it; those not aware of their hypertension and not receiving treatment are at major risk for the development of cardiovascular problems such as heart disease, stroke, heart failure, and kidney disease (CDC, 2012).

> **Drug Alert!** ▶▶▶ Instruct older patients to take blood pressure medication at the same time each day and as prescribed and to never abruptly stop taking a prescribed medication without consulting their primary care provider first. It is important to keep constant drug levels for effective blood pressure control, and rapid discontinuation of medication can result in rebound hypertension.

The definition and cutoff readings for the diagnosis of hypertension are revised as new research is evaluated. The Joint National Committee of the National High Blood Pressure Education Program (JNC) has defined hypertension in stages with recommendations for treatment at each stage. Its most recent version was published in 2004 and is referred to as *JNC 7* (Joint National Committee, 2004) (Table 15-3). This seventh set of guidelines is currently under review and revision to include recent research findings; an eighth version is scheduled to be released in the later half of 2012.

When the systolic and diastolic BP of a particular reading fall in different categories, the higher category should be identified. Isolated systolic hypertension is common in the older person. It is defined as systolic blood pressure greater than 140 mmHg.

TABLE 15-3	Classification of Blood Pressure	
	Systolic Pressure (mmHg)	**Diastolic Pressure Category (mmHg)**
Optimal	<120	and <80
Prehypertension	120–139	or 80–89
Hypertension		
Stage 1	140–159	or 90–99
Stage 2	≥160	or ≥100

Source: Adapted from Joint National Committee (2004).

Highlights from the *JNC 7* report include the following:

- In people older than 50 years, systolic blood pressure greater than 140 mmHg is a much more important cardiovascular disease (CVD) risk factor than diastolic blood pressure.
- The risk of CVD beginning at 115/75 mmHg doubles with each increment of 20/10 mmHg; individuals who are normotensive at age 55 have a 90% lifetime risk for developing hypertension.
- Individuals with a systolic blood pressure of 120 to 139 mmHg or a diastolic blood pressure of 80 to 89 mmHg should be considered as prehypertensive and require health-promoting lifestyle modifications to prevent CVD.
- Thiazide-type diuretics should be used in drug treatment for most patients with uncomplicated hypertension, either alone or combined with drugs from other classes. Certain high-risk conditions (such as diabetes and chronic kidney disease) are compelling indications for the initial use of other antihypertensive drug classes (angiotensin-converting enzyme [ACE] inhibitors, angiotensin receptor blockers, beta-blockers, calcium channel blockers).
- Most patients with hypertension will require two or more antihypertensive medications to achieve goal blood pressure (<140/90 mmHg, or <130/80 mmHg for patients with diabetes or chronic kidney disease).
- If blood pressure is more than 20/10 mmHg above goal blood pressure, consideration should be given to initiating therapy with two agents, one of which usually should be a thiazide-type diuretic.
- The most effective therapy prescribed by the most careful clinician will control hypertension only if patients are motivated. Motivation improves when patients have positive experiences with, and trust in, the clinician.
- A large hypertension study of adults over the age of 80 with no renal or cardiac diagnoses found that stroke, heart failure, and death rates were significantly reduced

in those with BPs of 150/80 mmHg or lower. Thus, a reasonable BP goal for essentially healthy older adults is 150/80 mmHg (Reuben et al., 2011).

■ Empathy builds trust and is a potent motivator (Joint National Committee, 2004).

> **Practice Pearl** ▶▶▶ Older patients with chronic kidney disease or diabetes should be aggressively treated because of additional risk. Their blood pressure goal is below 130/80 mmHg.

Since publication of the Framingham Heart Study, it has been known that blood pressure increases with increased body weight (National Heart, Lung, and Blood Institute [NHLBI], 2004). High blood pressure in genetically related individuals has also been shown to be a risk factor for hypertension (Levy et al., 2009). In the United States, the southern states have been designated the "stroke belt" because of the high incidence of cardiovascular conditions. It is not known if the cause of this higher incidence is genetic or environmental. This part of the country has high rates of obesity, high rates of eating high-sodium and fried food, and lower rates of physical exercise as compared with other areas (Howard et al., 2010).

> **Practice Pearl** ▶▶▶ Identification of cardiac risk factors including smoking, dyslipidemia, obesity, and diabetes mellitus is crucial in treating older adults with hypertension.

The physiological changes associated with hypertension involve an increase in cardiac output or an increase in systemic vascular resistance or both. Baroreceptors in the body constantly assess blood pressure and control blood pressure with a neurohormonal feedback system. Some associated factors include renal regulation of vascular volume. Low-pressure baroreceptors also have an effect on vascular volume. Over long periods of time, high blood pressure results in increased systemic vascular resistance and a decreased cardiac output and stroke volume (McCance & Huether, 2010).

> **Practice Pearl** ▶▶▶ Because changes of aging cause the baroreceptors to be less efficient, it is essential to check postural blood pressures in older patients to detect postural hypotension and teach patients to prevent falls by changing positions slowly.

Etiology and Pathophysiology

The underlying causes of hypertension are not known in most cases and these cases are classified as *primary hypertension*. In a small number of cases, specific causes can be determined and these cases are designated *secondary hypertension*. In general, several mechanisms may be involved, including (1) autonomic nervous system dysfunction with an exaggerated response to autonomic triggers; (2) genetic differences in renal sodium reabsorption, which may be particularly prevalent among non-Hispanic blacks; (3) dysfunction of the renin-angiotensin-aldosterone system, which results in increased body water; (4) impaired endovascular responsiveness; and (5) insulin resistance, noted because hypertension and diabetes frequently occur together. Primary hypertension is diagnosed when no specific cause is known. Secondary hypertension is diagnosed in 5% of cases with specific causes such as renal artery stenosis, sleep apnea, chronic kidney disease, medication side effects, thyroid disease, or adrenal dysfunction (McPhee & Papadakis, 2011).

Untreated hypertension results in several physical changes in the body. The medial layer of artery walls hypertrophies in early stages of hypertension. This results in a narrowing of the lumen of the vessel. Eventually, the endothelium becomes unable to support vasodilation. Hypertension accelerates the rate at which atherosclerosis develops in the aorta and large vessels (McCance & Huether, 2010). Arteriosclerosis occurs when lesions are concentric and dilated. These arteries become stiff as elastin is lost and collagen increases. The heart develops left ventricular hypertrophy and an increased risk for coronary artery disease. In long-term hypertension, the renal afferent arterioles fail to protect the glomerular membrane, resulting in increased filtration pressure. Dissolved proteins, which normally do not cross the glomerular membrane, can be forced across and lost in the urine as proteinuria. Vascular changes in the retina are visible on ophthalmoscopic examination and appear as hemorrhages, exudates, cotton-wool patches, and changes in vascular wall thickness. Arterial-venous nicking results when a thickened artery wall crosses a vein and causes an indentation. Blood vessels to the brain change in long-term hypertension, resulting in narrowing of the internal lumen. Stroke rates are increased in patients with hypertension. Stroke is the number one cause of disability and the number three cause of death in the United States with more than 140,000 Americans suffering a stroke each year (Internet Stroke Center, 2012).

Assessment and Diagnosis

Assessment of the patient with hypertension includes accurate blood pressure monitoring. The Agency for Healthcare Research and Quality (2007) strongly recommends screening adults over the age of 18 for hypertension based on evidence of its effectiveness in identifying people who would benefit from treatment. For people with normal blood pressure, screening every 2 years is sufficient. For those with prehypertension, blood pressure should be assessed annually. For those with hypertension, either stage 1 or 2, more aggressive follow-up is needed (Joint National Committee, 2004). The nurse should record pressures in both upper extremities and in the positions of lying, sitting, and standing. The patient's feet should be firmly planted on the floor and the back should be supported. Diagnosing hypertension requires multiple readings on multiple occasions. Blood pressure can vary widely by time of day and with activity level.

Some people react to the stress of having their blood pressure examined in an office setting by having higher readings than when tested in other settings. This is called *white coat hypertension*. Patients should be taught to monitor their own blood pressure at home, to record the readings, and to bring both the readings record and their equipment to the office to check the validity of their equipment and technique. Because blood pressure levels measured at home may be lower than those measured in a healthcare provider's office due to white coat hypertension, lower target levels may be set for blood pressures measured at home. Assessment should also include looking for evidence of target organ damage with ophthalmic examination and urinalysis for proteinuria. For blood pressure that develops suddenly or is refractory to treatment, secondary hypertension should be considered.

> **Practice Pearl ▶▶▶** Recheck any blood pressure readings taken by nursing assistants or others in your clinical settings to verify abnormally high or low readings. The quality and reliability of blood pressure equipment and techniques vary greatly and when medication or treatment will be changed based on these readings, a second check is always worth the effort.

Treatment

Treatment of hypertension begins with setting blood pressure goals and teaching lifestyle modification. For patients with multiple risk factors such as diabetes and previous myocardial infarction (MI), lower targets are set than for those with fewer risk factors. The target is below 120/80. Lifestyle change is always attempted at every stage of hypertension. Weight loss of even 10 lbs will reduce blood pressure to a certain extent. Even without weight loss, increasing the consumption of fruits, vegetables, and whole grains will lower blood pressure. The Dietary Approaches to Stop Hypertension (DASH) diet was tested in a clinical study and found to be effective in significantly lowering blood pressure in older patients with hypertension (NHLBI, 2004). Beginning an exercise program, stopping smoking, and reducing alcohol intake are also effective measures to lower blood pressure. See Table 15-4 for the

TABLE 15-4	Potential Impact of Lifestyle Modifications	
Modification	Recommendation	Potential Impact of Systolic Blood Pressure
Weight reduction	Achieve/maintain normal BMI between 22 and 25 kg/m²	5–20 mmHg/10 kg
Dietary sodium intake	Reduce sodium intake to 2.4 g/day	2–8 mmHg
Physical activity	30 minutes of aerobic activity per day most days of the week	4–9 mmHg
Moderation of alcohol intake	Limit consumption to no more than 2 drinks/day for men and 1 drink per day in women	2–4 mmHg

Source: Adapted from Joint National Committee, 2004.

potential systolic blood pressure reduction for each lifestyle intervention.

> **Practice Pearl ▶▶▶** When older patients report blood pressure readings taken at home with automatic blood pressure cuffs, ask them to bring their cuffs to the office or clinic setting. The nurse can then compare the readings on the patient's cuff with the readings obtained in the clinic. Widely divergent readings can indicate the cuff used at home may be inaccurate.

Medication management in the older person can be complicated because many different medications are considered appropriate options. In addition, the older person may have coexisting conditions that will affect medication selection. For patients with liver or renal disease, different medications may be required. All medications have side effects, and choosing medications with minimal effects for the particular person is important. The major classes of drugs used in hypertension are listed in Table 15-5. Some oral preparations for hypertension combine more than one medication into a single tablet in order to simplify the dosing regimen. For simplicity, only the single-drug medications are listed in Table 15-5. When administering or teaching about the combination drugs, each component must be addressed separately.

TABLE 15-5 **Medications Used for the Management of Hypertension**

Medication Group	Sample Drugs	Reason to Choose	Side Effects/Precautions
Diuretics Thiazide	hydrochlorothiazide (Microzide, HydroDIURIL) chlorothiazide (Diuril) metolazone (Zaroxolyn)	Good first-line agent, inexpensive, useful with heart failure	Can increase cholesterol and glucose, uric acid, decrease potassium hyperkalemia. Increased adverse drug events noted at doses higher than 25 mg.
Loop	furosemide (Lasix) bumetanide (Bumex) torsemide (Demadex)		Hypokalemia, hyperuricemia
Potassium sparing	amiloride (Midamor) triamterene (Dyrenium)		Hypokalemia, syncope
Aldosterone receptor-blockers	spironolactone (Aldactone) eplerenone (Inspra)		Hyperkalemia
Adrenergic inhibitors, beta-blockers	acebutolol (Sectral) atenolol (Tenormin) betaxolol (Kerlone) bisoprolol (Zebeta) carteolol (Cartrol) metoprolol (Lopressor, Toprol-XL) nadolol (Corgard) nebivolol (Bystolic) (cardioselective) penbutolol sulfate (Levatol) pindolol (Visken) propranolol HCl (Inderal, InnoPran XL) timolol (Blocadren)	Coexisting coronary artery disease, angina, arrhythmias, post-MI	Asthma exacerbation, bradycardia, reduced peripheral circulation, fatigue, decreased exercise tolerance
Adrenergic inhibitors, alpha-blockers	doxazosin mesylate (Cardura) prazosin (Minipress) terazosin HCl (Hytrin)	Dyslipidemia, benign prostatic hypertrophy	Postural hypotension, bronchospasm
Centrally acting alpha$_2$-agonists	clonidine HCl (Catapres; Nexiclon XR) guanfacine HCl (Tenex) methyldopa (Aldomet) reserpine (generic)		Sedation, dry mouth, bradycardia
ACE inhibitors	benazepril HCl (Lotensin) captopril (Capoten) enalapril maleate (Vasotec) fosinopril Na (Monopril) lisinopril (Prinivil, Zestril) moexipril (Univasc) perindopril (Aceon) quinapril HCl (Accupril) ramipril (Altace) trandolapril (Mavik)	Diabetes mellitus, heart failure, renal insufficiency	Dry cough, angioedema, hyperkalemia. Do not give to pregnant women.
Angiotensin receptor blockers (ARBs)	candesartan (Atacand) eprosartan (Teveten) losartan K (Cozaar) olmesartan (Benicar) telmisartan (Micardis) valsartan (Diovan)	Heart failure, diabetes	Angioedema, hyperkalemia. Do not give to pregnant women.

(continued)

TABLE 15-5	Medications Used for the Management of Hypertension (*continued*)			
Medication Group	**Sample Drugs**		**Reason to Choose**	**Side Effects/Precautions**
Calcium channel blockers Nondihydropyridines	diltiazem HCl (Cardizem LA, Dilacor XR, Tiazac) verapamil (Isoptin SR, Calan, Covera HA, Verelan PM)		Angina	Slows conduction, decreased cardiac output Constipation, bradycardia
Dihydropyridines	amlodipine besylate (Norvasc) felodipine (Plendil) isradipine (DynaCirc) nicardipine (Cardene SR) nifedipine (Procardia XL, Adalat CC) nisoldipine (Sular)		Isolated systolic hypertension	Ankle edema, flushing, headache
Direct vasodilators	hydralazine (Apresoline) minoxidil (Loniten)			Headache, tachycardia, fluid retention Hirsutism

Source: Data from Joint National Committee, 2004; *Nurse Practitioner's Prescribing Reference*, 2012; Reuben et al., 2011.

Note: Information pertinent to full group presented first. Specific information on line to right of drug name.

Practice Pearl ▶▶▶ Patients taking antihypertensive medications should be instructed to change positions slowly. Rising too quickly from lying to standing position can result in pooling of blood in the extremities and reduced blood flow to the head. This can cause orthostatic hypotension, which is experienced as light-headedness or syncope.

Nursing Management

The nurse's role in caring for older patients with hypertension is to screen for high blood pressure in a variety of community settings and to promote healthy lifestyles through low-fat and low-sodium diets, weight control, exercise, smoking cessation, and controlled alcohol consumption. Another important role is to teach older patients who are diagnosed with hypertension about the importance of staying on medications even though they do not feel any different, or perhaps feel worse because of side effects. Monitoring the effect of medication and determining barriers to healthy living are important in supporting the patient in self-management.

HEALTHY AGING TIPS

▶ **Urge older adults to be more physically active.** Help your patients decide the type of activities that would be best for them. If possible, set a goal for at least 30 minutes of moderate-intensity activity on most or all days of the week. Every day is best. It doesn't have to be done all at once—10-minute periods will do. Urge activities they enjoy—brisk walking, dancing, bowling, bicycling, or gardening, for example. They may wish to join an exercise group or even a gym. Exercise with others is more fun!

▶ **Urge those who smoke to quit.** Smoking adds to the damage to artery walls. It's never too late to get some benefit from quitting smoking.

▶ **Educate regarding a heart healthy diet.** Educate regarding low-fat foods and those that are low in salt. Eating plenty of fruits, vegetables, and foods high in fiber like those made from whole grains will yield benefits. Men should not have more than two drinks a day and women only one. Limit cholesterol to limit plaque deposits in arteries. Urge older adults to ask their health providers to check a total cholesterol level, LDL level ("bad" cholesterol), HDL level ("good" cholesterol), and triglycerides periodically to make sure dietary changes and medications are not needed and to reward healthy eating habits.

▶ **Keep a healthy weight.** Urge older adults to ask their healthcare provider to check their weight and height to learn their BMI (body mass index). A BMI of 25 or higher means older adults are at greater risk for heart disease as well as diabetes (high blood sugar) and other health conditions. Following a healthy eating plan and being physically active will help control weight.

Hypotension

Low blood pressure, or hypotension, can occur in the older person. It is a frequent side effect of many cardiovascular conditions and many medications. Blood pressure varies widely during the day. As a person ages, the ability to autoregulate blood pressure can decrease. Normally, if there is a transient decrease in cardiac output, the sympathetic nervous system causes an increase in heart rate to maintain cardiac output. With aging, the responsiveness declines. Additionally, decreased muscle tone in the lower extremities can contribute to postural or orthostatic hypotension, which is a rapid decline in blood pressure when the older person rises to a standing or sitting position from a lying position. Diagnosis of orthostatic hypotension can be made by having the patient maintain a supine position for at least 5 minutes. The nurse should check the blood pressure while the patient is supine, and 1 and 3 minutes after sitting or standing. If the pressure drops as much as 20 mmHg systolic or 10 mmHg diastolic after 3 minutes, postural hypotension exists (Bradley & Davis, 2003).

> **Practice Pearl** ▶▶▶ Taking the time to check postural blood pressure readings has the potential to prevent unknown numbers of falls and fractures.

Medications that can cause postural hypotension include alpha-adrenergic blockers, centrally acting antihypertensive agents, psychotropic drugs and tranquilizers, high-dose antibiotics, and nonsteroidal anti-inflammatory drugs (NSAIDs). Patients who experience hypotension can be taught to rise slowly from a lying or sitting position, to use a cane or walker if unsteady, and to drink water, unless restricted, to maintain blood volume (Reuben et al., 2011).

> **Drug Alert** ▶▶▶ People taking angiotensin receptor blockers and ACE inhibitors should be instructed not to share their medications, especially with younger women who may be pregnant.

Hyperlipidemia

The body produces a range of lipid-based chemicals that are useful in cell membrane structure and that form the basis of other chemicals such as steroid hormones. Lipid chemicals circulating in the body come from either dietary sources or from the production of liver cells. Lipids can be classified into several categories, including high-density lipoprotein cholesterol (HDL-C), low-density lipoprotein cholesterol (LDL-C), and triglycerides. High-fat diets, particularly the *trans* fats, and certain hereditary patterns can result in elevated serum lipids. Elevated cholesterol has been shown to be a risk factor for the development of cardiovascular disorders. LDL-Cs have been shown to be the type of lipid associated with increased risk for mortality or morbidity. HDL-Cs have been shown to have a beneficial effect on overall vascular health, probably because they help to mobilize cholesterol from the blood vessels and carry it back to the liver for processing.

The Adult Treatment Panel (ATP III) made recommendations for evaluating and managing elevated cholesterol. They recommended lifestyle and drug therapies based on an individual's cardiovascular risk factors and recommended how aggressive to be in lowering cholesterol levels. Further research was considered in an update on cholesterol management (Coordinating Committee of the National Cholesterol Education Program, 2004). They report that patients with diabetes benefit from lower levels of LDL-C. They also note that older patients benefit from treatment that lowers LDL-C. People with high triglyceride levels or low levels of HDL-C benefit from even more aggressive therapy. The Heart Protection Study (HPS) has also shown that controlling LDL with simvastatin assists in the prevention of coronary heart disease. Risk factors include having other known atherosclerosis such as peripheral arterial disease or abdominal aortic aneurysm, or the presence of diabetes mellitus (Braun & Davidson, 2003). Table 15-6 shows the new recommendations, which include starting medications for people with no evidence of coronary heart

TABLE 15-6	Categories of Risk and LDL Cholesterol Goals	
Risk Category	**LDL-C Goal (mg/dL)**	**Consider Therapy (mg/dL)**
Very high risk: coronary heart disease (10-year risk ≥20%)	<70 for very high risk	≥100
High risk: two or more risk factors, 10-year risk of CHD 10–20%	<100	≥100
Moderate risk: two or more risk factors, 10-year risk of CHD <10%	<130	≥130
Lower risk: zero or one risk factor	<160	≥160 TLC (160–189 drug optional)

Source: Data from Third Report of the NCEP Expert Panel on Detection, Evaluation, and Treatment of High Blood Cholesterol in Adults (ATP III) (Expert Panel, 2004); Reuben et al., 2011.

disease but with positive risk factors. The HMG-CoA reductase inhibitors (also known as statins) have been shown to be the most powerful and best tolerated group of drugs in lowering LDL. The greatest benefit is achieved for the patients most at risk for developing coronary heart disease (CHD). These include people with multiple risk factors for cardiovascular disorders. Research has also shown that reducing LDL with medications reduces coronary events for older adults and for women of all ages. Some have argued that older adults may not benefit from drug therapy to improve lipid profiles because mortality is approaching and the time for prevention of adverse outcomes is shortened. Others have shown that reducing cardiac events decreases morbidity and disability. In addition to lowering LDL cholesterol, statins have such protective effects as being anti-inflammatory and antithrombotic. They also protect intravascular plaque stability. Older patients (ages 70 to 82) who were enrolled in the Prospective Study of Pravastatin in the Elderly at Risk (PROSPER) benefited from statin therapy with reduced rates of MI, but not stroke (Shepard et al., 2002).

It is anticipated that many more patients will be placed on statins in the future, and nurses need to be able to teach patients about their medications. In general, statins are well tolerated, but a small minority of patients experience liver inflammation with elevated liver enzymes or muscle pain and weakness with myopathies.

> **Drug Alert** ▶▶▶ Patients taking statins should be taught to report muscle aches and symptoms to their healthcare provider because new or worsening muscle aches can be a sign of a rare but serious side effect.

Other medications useful in reducing serum cholesterol are most often used to augment the effect of the statins. These have adverse effects that make them less tolerable for many patients, so nurses need to explain their benefits and strategize minimizing unpleasant effects. The first group of drugs also used for cholesterol control is the bile acid sequestrants. They attach to bile in the gut and prevent its return to the liver. Gastrointestinal bloating and constipation are the chief side effects. Secondly, fibrates can be useful in reducing elevated triglycerides. Nausea and abdominal pain are the main side effects. Finally, nicotinic acid is useful in lowering LDL and triglycerides as well as increasing HDL. The major side effect from nicotinic acid is skin flushing, dizziness, and headache (Drugs.com, 2012). Starting with low doses and taking a baby aspirin one-half hour before taking niacin may help to minimize these side effects. Table 15-7 lists medications used for the management of hyperlipidemia.

TABLE 15-7	Drugs Used in the Treatment of Hyperlipidemia		
Medication Group	**Sample Drugs**	**Reasons to Use**	**Side Effects/Precautions**
HMG-CoA Reductase Inhibitors (statins)	atorvastatin (Lipitor) fluvastatin (Lescol, Lescol XL) lovastatin (Altoprev, Mevacor) pravastatin (Pravachol) rosuvastatin (Crestor) simvastatin (Zocor)	Reduce LDL	Gastrointestinal distress, elevation of liver enzymes, myopathies
Bile Acid Sequestrants	colesevelam (Welchol) colestipol (Colestid) cholestyramine (Questran, Questran Light)	Reduce LDL Reduce triglycerides	Constipation, bloating, decreased fat-soluble vitamin absorption
Fibrates	fenofibrate (Antara, Lipofen, Lofibra, TriCor) fenofibric acid (Fibricor, Trilipix) gemfibrozil (Lopid)	Reduce triglycerides	Gastrointestinal distress, abdominal pain
Nicotinic Acid	niacin (Niaspan)	Reduce LDL, elevate HDL, reduce triglycerides	Skin flushing, pruritus, gastrointestinal distress
Lipid Regulator	Omega-3-acid ethyl esters (Lovaza, Omacor)	Reduces triglycerides	Flu syndrome, dyspepsia, taste alteration, infection

Source: Data from *Nurse Practitioner's Prescribing Reference*, 2012; Reuben et al., 2011.

Metabolic Syndrome

Metabolic syndrome is a condition characterized by elevated waist circumference, blood pressure, fasting serum triglycerides, and serum glucose. Patients also have lower than normal HDL cholesterol. Ironically, patients may have relatively low LDL cholesterol levels. Another feature of metabolic syndrome is decreased insulin sensitivity in the cells resulting in elevated serum insulin and glucose. Metabolic syndrome (formerly known as Syndrome X) is associated with an increased risk of cardiovascular disease and diabetes mellitus, and is more likely to be found as people age, particularly women (Adult Treatment Panel [ATP III], 2004). Abdominal fat is a particular component of this condition because the fat cells themselves secrete hormones that promote heart disease and diabetes. Figure 15-5 ▶▶▶ lists the characteristics needed to diagnose metabolic syndrome.

In addition to medications, including cholesterol-lowering drugs and antihypertensives, diet and exercise are important components of the management of metabolic syndrome. A diet high in omega-3 fatty acids (as found in oily fish, walnuts, and certain vegetable oils) and exercise are beneficial. Prescription-strength omega-3 fatty acids are available for dietary supplementation. Simple sugars should be avoided and replaced with more complex carbohydrates. Many processed foods contain a variety of simple sugars including corn syrup. For those who choose to drink alcohol, a moderate intake can be beneficial. A good rule of thumb is one drink per day for women or two for men.

More than that can increase triglycerides. A good exercise guideline is 30 to 45 minutes of moderate-intensity aerobic exercise daily. This can be as simple as walking. Nurses play a large role in helping patients stay motivated to change their lifestyle to promote their health. Even a 10% reduction in weight can result in better cardiovascular profile and increased quality of life.

Chest Pain

Chest pain can occur for a variety of reasons, but the nurse should always consider the possibility of heart-related problems. When the myocardium is deprived of sufficient blood supply and thereby oxygen, ischemia occurs. Ischemia causes pain and loss of function. Acute coronary syndrome (ACS) includes both unstable angina and myocardial infarction. Unstable angina is relieved by nitroglycerin. Chronic ischemic pain is referred to as angina. In addition to coronary artery disease, aortic stenosis and pericarditis are cardiovascular causes of chest pain. Gastrointestinal problems such as heartburn, acid reflux, and ulcers can also cause chest pain. Musculoskeletal causes of chest pain include chondritis. Pulmonary problems such as pulmonary embolus, pneumonia, and pleural effusion are other causes. Herpes zoster (shingles) can cause pain in the skin of the chest. The evaluation of chest pain should be part of a full nursing assessment, which is discussed later in the chapter. The absence of chest pain does *not* indicate the absence of cardiovascular disease. For

---

The American Heart Association and the National Heart, Lung, and Blood Institute recommend that the metabolic syndrome be identified as the presence of three or more of these components:

- Elevated waist circumference:

    Men—Equal to or greater than 40 inches (102 cm)
    Women—Equal to or greater than 35 inches (88 cm)

- Elevated triglycerides:

    Equal to or greater than 150 mg/dL

- Reduced HDL ("good") cholesterol:

    Men—Less than 40 mg/dL
    Women—Less than 50 mg/dL

- Elevated blood pressure:

    Equal to or greater than 130/85 mm Hg

- Elevated fasting glucose:

    Equal to or greater than 100 mg/dL

Figure 15-5 ▶▶▶ Characteristics needed to diagnose metabolic syndrome.

Sources: American Heart Association (AHA). (2012). Statistical fact sheet: 2012 update. Retrieved from http://www.heart.org/idc/groups/heart-public/@wcm/@sop/@smd/documents/downloadable/ucm_319574.pdf

the older person and for women, myocardial infarction can occur with no chest pain. Patients who describe sudden breathlessness or activity intolerance or a feeling of impending doom should be evaluated as aggressively as those who describe chest pain.

Heart Disease

Older Women and Heart Disease

Many people, including some healthcare professionals, still think that heart disease is primarily a health problem for men, but in fact heart disease is the primary killer of women in the United States. After menopause, women are as vulnerable as men to the same risk factors for heart disease, and because the signs and symptoms of heart disease are not as well studied and understood in women as they are in men, more adverse outcomes can result, including the following surprising facts:

- One in 4 women in the United States dies of heart disease, while 1 in 30 dies of breast cancer.
- Twenty-three percent of women will die within 1 year after having a heart attack.
- Within 6 years of having a heart attack, about 46% of women become disabled with heart failure. Two thirds of women who have a heart attack fail to make a full recovery.

NHLBI, 2007.

The symptoms of heart disease in an older women may be vague and often go unreported. Some of these symptoms include sleep disturbance; chest discomfort such as tightness, squeezing, fullness, or pressure that can come and go; discomfort in the back, neck, jaw, or stomach; shortness of breath; and feelings of nausea, light-headedness, or breaking out in a cold sweat. Obtaining treatment quickly within the first hour of onset of symptoms can greatly increase the chance of survival and recognition of the warning signs may save a life. A recent study reported that women wait on average 22 minutes longer than men to seek help when they are having a heart attack (NHLBI, 2007). This delay can postpone the needed emergency department care and testing, including obtaining the ECG and cardiac enzymes needed to diagnose the heart attack and the administration of "clot-busting" drugs and supportive care such as oxygen and intravenous fluids.

Some diagnostic testing, such as exercise tolerance tests, are not as accurate in older women as in older men. Stress tests induced by drugs (dipyridamole, adenosine, or dobutamine) rather than with exercise may be preferable in women who cannot endure the physical demands of treadmill testing and in whom optimal heart rates cannot be achieved. The addition of thallium can improve the accuracy of stress testing. When obtaining care at a facility specializing in treating heart disease in women, stress test results can yield accurate

information comparable to nuclear imaging. The addition of echocardiography and sound wave techniques offers the added advantage of avoiding artifacts or inaccurate readings due to breast tissue. As awareness of the importance of diagnosing and treating heart disease in older women grows, more medical centers are offering specialized cardiac care for women (Massachusetts General Hospital, 2008).

The information shown in Figure 15-6 ▶▶▶ can help older adults (both men and women) calculate their 10-year risk of having a heart attack.

> ***Practice Pearl*** ▶▶▶ The absence of chest pain in the older person does not indicate an absence of ischemic heart disease. Older adults can present with fatigue, weakness, shortness of breath, and gastrointestinal complaints.

Angina

The gradual process of atherosclerosis results in narrowing of the arteries that supply blood to the heart muscle. The incidence of atherosclerosis increases with age. There are two kinds of ischemic heart disease. *Supply ischemia* results from a decreased blood flow to the myocardium, and *demand ischemia* results from increased demand for oxygen related to such conditions as a fast heart rate or thick heart muscle. An inadequate supply of oxygen and nutrients leads to a decrease in adenosine triphosphate production because of a shift to anaerobic metabolism. Anaerobic metabolism is less efficient and produces waste products such as pyruvate and lactate. The acidic condition as well as the loss of adenosine triphosphate results in decreased sodium potassium pump activity and can eventually lead to cell death. Intracellular calcium ion concentration also increases. The accumulation of waste products leads to the release of inflammatory mediators and the activation of white blood cells. Cardiac cells that are stressed can initiate arrhythmias and are less effective in contracting. Is-chemia is a reversible condition and can be improved with lifestyle, medication, or surgical management (McPhee & Papadakis, 2011).

Patients with stable angina report chest pain that is relieved with rest. It is precipitated by activities that increase the workload on the heart. Angina is frequently managed with sublingual nitroglycerin, which causes vasodilatation and increases blood flow to the heart. Patients who need multiple doses of nitrates every day can be placed on long-term nitrate therapy. Many older people do not experience typical chest pain but have anginal equivalent symptoms such as fatigue or weakness, arm or jaw pain, palpitations, sweating, or dizziness. Symptoms that are not relieved with rest or medication can indicate progression of the angina or myocardial

	Points		Points
Age 20–34	−7	Age 55–59	8
Age 35–39	−3	Age 60–64	10
Age 40–44	0	Age 65–69	12
Age 45–49	3	Age 70–74	14
Age 50–54	6	Age 75–79	16

	Points				
Total Cholesterol	Age 20–39	Age 40–49	Age 50–59	Age 60–69	Age 70–79
<160	0	0	0	0	0
160–199	4	3	2	1	1
200–239	8	6	4	2	1
240–279	11	8	5	3	2
≥280	13	10	7	4	2

	Points				
	Age 20–39	Age 40–49	Age 50–59	Age 60–69	Age 70–79
Nonsmoker	0	0	0	0	0
Smoker	9	7	4	2	1

HDL (mg/dL)	Points	HDL (mg/dL)	Points
60	−1	40–49	1
50–59	0	<40	2

Systolic BP (mmHg)	Points		Systolic BP (mmHg)	Points	
	If Untreated	If Treated		If Untreated	If Treated
<120	0	0	140–159	3	5
120–129	1	3	≥160	4	6
130–139	2	4			

Point Total	10-Year Risk %	Point Total	10-Year Risk %	Point Total	10-Year Risk %
<9	<1	14	2	20	11
9	1	15	3	21	14
10	1	16	4	22	17
11	1	17	5	23	22
12	1	18	6	24	27
13	2	19	8	25	30

Figure 15-6 ▶▶▶ Ten-year risk of having a heart attack.

Sources: U.S. Department of Health and Human Services, National Heart, Lung, and Blood Institute (NHLBI). (2007). *The healthy heart handbook for women*. Retrieved from http://www.nhlbi.nih.gov/health/hearttruth/material/NHLBI_3942_HHH_041707.pdf

infarction. This requires immediate medical intervention. Unstable angina occurs when angina is not relieved with rest or medication. It indicates a progression of the coronary artery disease.

Prinzmetal's angina, or atypical angina, is less common and is characterized by chest pain experienced at rest. The pain is not relieved with nitroglycerin, but does not usually progress to myocardial infarction.

It is thought to be caused by transient coronary artery constriction.

The development of coronary heart disease is related to identifiable risk factors, some of which are modifiable. By working on risk factors, patients will decrease their chance of developing heart disease. Even if they have developed heart disease, they can improve their quality of life by following a healthy lifestyle.

[handwritten margin note: ⌀ sedentary adults - no shoveling/yardwork unless building it up gradually]

Nurses can help older patients with angina by supporting lifestyle change and by teaching proper medication usage. Many patients are reluctant to use medications, particularly when prescribed "as needed." The nurse can present scenarios and ask patients what they would do if they have sudden weakness or if they take the medication and it does not help. Cardiac rehabilitation programs can help patients who have not experienced a myocardial infarction increase their exercise tolerance and quality of life.

Myocardial Infarction

Ischemic heart disease is the major cause of death in the United States. It is caused by clot development within the coronary arteries, which causes a blockage in blood flow to the areas normally served by the particular artery. Gradual narrowing of coronary arteries is often not the cause of blockage of blood flow. Rather, rupture of unstable plaque lining coronary arteries is what initiates blood clot development. The development of a myocardial infarction is indicative of a failure of the healthcare system in assisting patients to prevent the development of cardiovascular disease. The blockage in blood flow results in myocardial cell death or myocardial infarction (MI). Ischemia is reversible, but cell death is not. Once the myocardial cell has died, it cannot be resuscitated and the loss of the cell's contraction will decrease the function of the heart itself. Damage to the heart muscle is determined by the size and location of the area of injury and infarct. Left ventricle anterior wall infarcts occur because of a blockage of the left anterior descending coronary artery. Infarcts of the anterior wall result in reduced cardiac output and electrical conduction blockages because the left anterior descending artery also supplies the intraventricular septum. Another type of MI is classified as inferior or posterior. The right coronary artery supplies these areas for most patients. The sinus node and atria are perfused by this artery, and arrhythmias or blocked conduction can occur in these areas. Parasympathetic signs such as nausea, vomiting, or other gastrointestinal complaints are often seen with this type of MI. Lateral wall MIs occur with occlusion of the circumflex branch of the left main coronary artery. This artery also supplies the AV node and ventricular papillary muscles, so dysfunction in these areas can be seen with this type of MI (Zafari, 2012).

The diagnosis of MI involves good history and physical assessment as well as laboratory and electrocardiographic analysis. An MI is an event with several stages, and interpreting these findings requires consideration of the stage of the MI. A history of chest pain may be the major presenting complaint, but in many patients, particularly older women, pain may not be experienced. Accompanying symptoms include nausea or vomiting, weakness, shortness of breath, diaphoresis, confusion, or syncope. The physical examination is often unremarkable (Zafari, 2012).

Electrocardiographic changes associated with MI include ST segment elevation in the leads associated with the area of the infarct. New bundle branch blocks can be seen with widened QRS complexes. The presence of a Q wave (a 1-mm negative deflection before the QRS complex) indicates infarcted tissue. Q waves persist after recovery from MI, so one cannot assume that a Q wave represents a new or recent event (Zafari, 2012).

Laboratory findings consistent with MI include creatine kinase (CK) and the specific enzyme found in heart muscle (CK-MB) elevation 4 to 6 hours after tissue necrosis. Troponin levels rise 6 to 8 hours after infarct. Lactate dehydrogenase is elevated later with a peak at 36 hours after infarct. This is important to remember because patients frequently fail to report significant events when they occur and only mention the problem later or after they feel bad for a day or two (Zafari, 2012).

Other examinations performed in evaluating the patient with suspected MI might include hemodynamic monitoring if heart failure is suspected, and echocardiography to determine wall motion, estimated cardiac output, and valve function.

Immediate complications of MI include arrhythmia and blockages of electrical conduction, heart failure with possible pulmonary edema, and extension of an infarct. Long-term complications from MI include ventricular aneurysms, which are a weakened area of the ventricle wall that has paradoxical motion during systole. Another long-term complication is pericarditis, an inflammation of the pericardial space resulting in pain. Patients are sometimes concerned that they are having another heart attack when they develop the pain of pericarditis. Treatment with anti-inflammatory medications is indicated for this complication.

Newer medications that can dissolve clots in evolution can prevent permanent loss of myocardial cells if they are used within the first several hours of the myocardial event. These clot-dissolving drugs have many precautions because they dissolve all clots in the body and can result in sudden and excessive bleeding. However, they are considered worth the risk and to be lifesavers in certain older adults. Patients with risk factors for MI should be taught to report any change in symptom pattern promptly so that they can receive appropriate therapy. Many cardiologists advise older patients with symptoms of heart attack to chew one aspirin while waiting for the ambulance to arrive.

Some patients benefit from coronary angioplasty procedures, which can be done when unstable angina develops or at the time of MI. This procedure is relatively noninvasive. By threading a balloon-tipped catheter into the coronary artery, the blockage of the artery can be opened. Stents or mechanical supports to keep the artery open can be placed during angioplasty.

If an MI does occur, patients are usually admitted to the hospital for monitoring of hemodynamic status and for arrhythmias. Patients will receive oxygen therapy, pain control, and antiarrhythmic drugs as needed. The nurse's role is to monitor for changes in the patient's condition and treat complications from MI using protocols or to refer to the cardiologist for treatment. The nurse can do much to reduce stress on the myocardium by providing a safe, quiet environment, which reduces endogenous catecholamine release. Research has shown that patients with lower anxiety levels and a higher sense of control have better cardiac outcomes in the post-MI period (Moser et al., 2007). After the patient survives the initial insult, a cardiac rehabilitation program can be designed to offer gradual, supervised increase in activity and to support other healthy lifestyle changes.

Many medications that are important during the evolving MI event and following recovery are useful in other cardiovascular conditions. Beta-blockers are useful during and after MI to reduce the workload of the heart. Patients given beta-blockers have a reduced rate of death and of reinfarction following MI. Beta-blockers can have negative effects on patients with asthma and can reduce the cardiac output, which causes symptoms of heart failure. Calcium channel blockers can be substituted for patients who cannot tolerate beta-blockers, although the research basis for using calcium channel blockers is not as well established as the research for beta-blockers. Calcium channel blockers also reduce workload on the heart and can cause bradycardia. ACE inhibitors can reduce afterload and improve endothelial function. Aspirin or warfarin (Coumadin) therapy can help to prevent new clots from forming.

> **Drug Alert** ▶▶▶ Patients at high risk for falling may not be appropriate candidates for Coumadin therapy. Anticoagulated patients who fall can sustain life-threatening bleeding including the development of subdural hematomas.

Valvular Heart Disease

Because of age-related changes and the long-term effect of conditions such as hypertension, stress on the cardiac valves can result in structural and functional changes. Two categories of disorders affect heart valve function. The first disorder is called **stenosis** or valvular thickening, stiffening, or fusing together of heart valves restricting the flow of blood. Stenosis can occur in all heart valves and results in reduced flow across the valve with a resultant increased pressure required in the chamber from which the blood is being pumped. For example, aortic stenosis results in higher than normal pressure in the left ventricle as well as reduced cardiac output.

The second type of disorder is called **incompetence, regurgitation,** or **insufficiency,** occurring when a valve doesn't close tightly and blood leaks back into the chamber rather than flowing forward through the heart or into an artery. For example, mitral regurgitation results in blood flow from the left ventricle to the left atrium. This stretches the left atrium and also reduces forward pumping of the blood from the left ventricle. Valve disorders can arise in the leaflets themselves, in the fibrous tissue ring to which the leaflets are attached, or in papillary muscles that hold valve leaflets in place. Most valve disease in the older person involves the valves that control flow for the left ventricle, the highest pressure chamber, and the aortic and mitral valves (Cardiosmart, 2011).

In years past, the long-term effects of rheumatic heart disease led to many heart valve problems including mitral stenosis, aortic stenosis, and tricuspid stenosis. Because of the widespread use of antibiotics, the incidence of rheumatic heart disease is decreasing.

The most common valve disorder in the older person is aortic stenosis. It usually involves changes in the valve leaflets, but can also be caused by abnormal tissue in the cardiac septum or aorta. For older adults who develop aortic stenosis, the major cause is calcified degenerative stenosis. Risk factors include hyperlipidemia, diabetes, and hypertension. As the condition progresses, patients tolerate a decrease in cardiac output and an increase in left ventricular hypertrophy quite well. Eventually a critical loss of valve area can lead to symptoms. If the patient develops heart failure, the condition can deteriorate rapidly. Angina can be experienced because blood has difficulty perfusing a thickened myocardium. Syncope can occur because of reduced blood flow to the brain. Orthostatic changes in blood pressure can also reflect a low cardiac output. Increased ventricular and atrial arrhythmias can also occur.

The diagnosis of aortic stenosis is begun during the history and physical examination. Progressive shortness of breath should indicate that aortic stenosis is a possible diagnosis. On physical examination, the murmur of aortic stenosis can be detected as a systolic ejection murmur heard most prominently in the second intercostal space. As the condition progresses, the murmur may decrease as less blood is pumped forward. Jugular venous pressure is normal unless heart failure has developed. The echocardiogram is a good way to evaluate all heart valve function. This test allows the visualization of the valves as they open and close. Using this test, one can determine valve area, cardiac output, and any regurgitant flow. The size of cardiac chambers and movements of the heart muscle can also be tracked. If coronary heart disease is suspected, cardiac catheterization may be performed. This allows direct measurement of chamber pressures and cardiac output (Cardiosmart, 2011).

Definitive therapy for aortic stenosis requires mechanical or surgical intervention. During cardiac catheterization, a balloon device can be used to open the tight valve leaflets. This procedure is less invasive than open-heart surgery but offers less direct control of valve opening. This procedure can improve function but does not correct the underlying problem. Aortic valve replacement is required for true correction of aortic stenosis. However, surgical mortality is higher in the older person with rates ranging from 8% to 20% in older adults with left ventricular heart failure and other markers of poor heart function (WebMD, 2012). Nursing considerations in the care of patients with aortic stenosis are to maintain an index of suspicion with patients who have signs of heart failure, particularly without MI. Nurses should explain the progression of the condition to patients and answer their questions. Monitoring the progression of the disease is important because many patients minimize their symptoms. Caring for patients undergoing cardiac surgery is beyond the scope of this book, but principles of cardiac rehabilitation can be followed during the recovery period.

Heart Failure

Heart failure, formerly referred to as *congestive* heart failure, is a growing problem as baby boomers age and as more people survive damaging cardiac events such as MIs. In the 60- to 79-year-old age group, 9% of men and 5.4% of women have heart failure and in the 80+ age group, 11.5% of men and 11.6% of women have been diagnosed with the disease (American Heart Association [AHA], 2012). One third of all hospital admissions are caused by heart failure, costing the healthcare system $34.4 billion annually (CDC, 2012). The incidence of heart failure is equally divided between men and women. Since the 1950s, the incidence of heart failure for men has remained unchanged, but the incidence for women has declined between 31% and 49%. The mortality rates for both men and women are declining by about 12% every 10 years. Men tend to develop heart failure following MI. Women tend to develop heart failure as a result of long-standing hypertension. Treatment for both hypertension and heart failure is improving through the use of new drugs and technology. However, long-term prognosis is not good. The 5-year survival rate for patients with systolic dysfunction is 50% (AHA, 2012). In addition to being a threat to life, heart failure causes symptoms that have a negative impact on quality of life for the older person. Heart failure is often not recognized because both patients and clinicians often attribute a lack of energy to

perform daily functions as a natural part of aging. This is an error that results in missed opportunities to treat a medical condition that, if controlled, would contribute to improved quality of life.

The loss of contractility of the myocardium results in the inability of the heart to produce a sufficient cardiac output to meet the needs of the body. The muscles do not receive enough blood supply to respond to increased demand, and the person experiences activity intolerance. Heart failure is the number one cause of hospital admissions as patients experience recurring bouts with fluid retention. The body responds to decreased cardiac output using several compensatory mechanisms. One of these compensatory mechanisms is mediated by the sympathetic nervous system and results in increased heart rates and increased vascular resistance. Another compensatory mechanism is mediated by the kidneys, which respond by reproducing renin, which in turn leads to the formation of angiotensin I. This is transformed by enzymes to angiotensin II, a potent vasoconstrictor, elevating both blood pressure and vascular resistance. This increases afterload and further reduces cardiac output. Angiotensin II also promotes the release of aldosterone, which results in sodium and water retention. This further taxes the failing heart. Increased blood volume results in edema of the extremities and can cause pulmonary edema. Another compensatory mechanism involves dilation of the ventricles, a situation that can take advantage of the Frank-Starling response under normal circumstances. In the Frank-Starling response, the stretched myocardial fibers are able to contract with increased force, resulting in increased cardiac output. If fibers become overstretched, however, the force of contraction is decreased, further exacerbating the heart failure.

Heart failure was once thought to be due entirely to pump failure and was diagnosed by the presence of an ejection fraction of less than 40%. Systolic dysfunction can be the result of loss of functional myocardium due to muscle death in MI or from generalized cardiosuppression as found in alcoholic cardiomyopathy. Research has described another facet of heart failure due to diastolic dysfunction. During diastole, the ventricle cannot relax and open enough to allow returning blood to fill it. This is called *noncompliance* and can be due to a thickened muscle or septal wall often resulting from many years of untreated hypertension. Diastolic heart failure with preserved ventricular ejection fraction of greater than 40% can also be diagnosed with echocardiography and Doppler imaging (Reuben et al., 2011).

The most common risk factors for heart failure include coronary artery disease and hypertension. The high prevalence of these conditions makes many people susceptible to heart failure. Other risk factors include family history, cardiotoxic drugs (some cancer chemotherapy drugs), smoking, obesity, pulmonary abnormalities, alcohol abuse, and diabetes mellitus. Reducing modifiable risk factors is important at all stages of heart failure, and the nurse can do much to support patients in making lifestyle changes.

Clinical manifestations of heart failure can be divided into those that are the result of left-sided heart failure and are evidenced by pulmonary symptoms, and those that are the result of right-sided heart failure and are evidenced by systemic signs. Most heart failure symptoms include breathlessness or dyspnea. This can take the form of orthopnea, which is an inability to breathe comfortably while lying flat. Paroxysmal nocturnal dyspnea occurs when edema fluid, which has been collecting in the legs and feet, moves into the circulation when the patient lies down. This extra fluid produces pulmonary edema experienced as dyspnea at night. Crackles detected on lung auscultation are a sign of left-sided heart failure. Physical signs of right-sided heart failure include edema in the extremities, dilated neck veins, and congested liver.

Laboratory and diagnostic tests used to evaluate heart failure include electrocardiogram, which may reveal ST-T wave changes indicating myocardial ischemia, atrial fibrillation, or Q waves from previous MIs. Echocardiograms can reveal chamber size and valve function and can provide an estimated stroke volume, ejection fraction, and cardiac output. Blood tests include the complete blood count to evaluate anemia, which can aggravate heart failure; tests for elevated serum creatinine, which may indicate renal insufficiency; and thyroid function tests. Hyper- or hypothyroid conditions can aggravate heart failure (Reuben et al., 2011). Additionally, B-type natriuretic peptide (BNP) has been used to assess the level of cardiac function. BNP is a peptide released by the ventricles of the heart in response to fluid overload. Elevated levels indicate increased risk of decompensation and death (Reuben et al., 2011).

A recent position statement endorsed by the Heart Failure Society of America and the American Association of Heart Failure Nurses calls for a shared decision-making model when designing care for heart failure patients. A range of providers and patients and families are important when making choices regarding heart failure management (Allen et al., 2012). To guide therapy, a classification for heart failure patients has been proposed by the New York Heart Association. A more recent classification system has been proposed by the American College of Cardiology and the American Heart Association to focus on prevention as well as on treatment (Hunt et al., 2005). Table 15-8 summarizes both sets of classification systems for heart failure patients. The newer guidelines emphasize the progressive nature of heart failure and guide the gradual increase in therapies as the disease advances.

Heart failure patients have a high incidence of sleep disorders. This is a synergistic relationship. Heart failure symptoms disturb sleep, and sleep disturbances cause physiological changes that can exacerbate heart failure. After a complete sleep history, patients may benefit from treatment with low-dose nocturnal oxygen therapy for identified central sleep apnea or Cheyne-Stokes respirations. Obstructive sleep apnea can be treated with continuous positive airway pressure (Parker & Dunbar, 2002).

Patients with stage B heart failure benefit from taking ACE inhibitors for several reasons. ACE inhibitors support healthy endothelial function. That means local areas are less reactive to vasoconstricting factors and fewer structural changes occur. ACE inhibitors prevent the release of aldosterone, thereby allowing sodium to be lost in the urine, maintaining a normal sodium balance. ACE inhibitors decrease the blood pressure, decreasing afterload. They also support healthy renal function for patients with diabetes. The troublesome side effect of dry hacking cough occurs in 10% of patients. These patients may be placed on angiotensin receptor blockers, although the research is not as clear on the long-term helpfulness.

Beta-blockers are helpful in treating patients with heart failure by decreasing the workload on the heart. Some medications (e.g., carvedilol) have been shown to promote healthy remodeling of heart muscle with long-term therapy. Other medications frequently used with heart failure include diuretics. Most stage C patients will require furosemide (Lasix) therapy to keep body water from increasing. Digoxin was once thought to be a major drug used in heart failure therapy. Research has shown that only patients with systolic dysfunction benefit from digoxin therapy; with its narrow therapeutic index, close monitoring is required to detect toxic levels. Women who were randomly assigned digoxin therapy had higher death rates from all causes than women in the placebo control group. The effects of digoxin differ between men and women (AACF/AHA, 2009). Hydralazine and nitrates are vasodilators that can be helpful in stage C patients. Nitrates are useful for patients who also have angina.

Nursing research has shown that a motivational intervention that supported patients in improving self-care abilities using reflective listening, empathy, acknowledgment of cultural beliefs, and negotiation of an action plan resulted in improved reported self-care abilities (Riegel et al., 2006). Patients need to weigh themselves daily to monitor body water. If their weight increases by 2 lbs in a day, they should call their provider to report the change, because this may be the first sign of fluid retention. Waiting to report it until the next appointment could result in an episode of pulmonary edema. Guided exercise is useful for all patients with heart failure except those with an acute exacerbation. Exercise can contribute to better activity tolerance. The chronic nature of heart failure treatment makes it an ideal condition for nurses to manage and support in heart failure clinics. Being able to detect subtle changes

TABLE 15-8   **Functional and Therapeutic Classification Systems**

New York Heart Association Functional Classification (1964)	American College of Cardiology Foundation/American Heart Association Stages of Heart Failure (2005)	Recommendations

	Stage A: Asymptomatic and no evidence of structural problems but high risk for developing heart failure. Risk factors: hypertension, diabetes, obesity, metabolic syndrome	• Manage:
		  • Hypertension
		  • Lipid disorders
		  • Diabetes mellitus
		• Teach:
		  • Smoking cessation
		  • Exercise promotion
		  • Diet modifications
		  • Moderate ETOH
		• ACE inhibitor if indicated

Class I: Evidence of cardiac disease but no limitation in physical activity.	Stage B: Evidence of structural disease but no symptoms of heart failure. Possible past MI, LV hypertrophy, valvular disease, low EF	• All stage A therapies • ACE inhibitor unless contraindicated. (ARB in appropriate patients) • Beta-blocker in appropriate patients
Class II: Evidence of cardiac disease with slight limitation in physical activity. Comfortable at rest. Ordinary activity results in fatigue, palpitations, dyspnea, or angina.	Stage C: Evidence of structural disease with current or prior symptoms of heart failure	• All stage A and B therapies • Sodium-restricted diet • Diuretics for fluid retention ACEIs, beta-blockers • Selected patients: aldosterone antagonist, ARBs, digitalis, hydralazine/ nitrates
Class III: Evidence of cardiac disease with marked activity limitation, comfortable at rest. Less than ordinary activity causes symptoms.	(As above)	
Class IV: Evidence of cardiac disease, symptomatic at rest, any activity causes discomfort.	Stage D: Heart failure refractory to stage C treatment outlined above, requiring specialized interventions	• All therapies as above • Options: mechanical assist devices, biventricular pacemakers, left ventricular assist device • Continuous inotropic IV therapy • Hospice care.

Source: Adapted from American College of Cardiology Foundation/American Heart Association (AACF/AHA) Practice Guidelines: Focused Update, 2009.

in patient function through home visits or phone calls can alert the team that treatment changes are required to prevent hospitalization.

> **Practice Pearl** ▶▶▶ The guidelines for obtaining daily weights include same scale, same clothing, and same time of day. Daily weights can vary by many factors. Adopting these rules will minimize the risk of error.

Arrhythmias and Conduction Disorders

Arrhythmias and conduction disorders are frequently seen in the older person. They can affect function and quality of life and may require medical management. The nurse can assist patients by explaining complicated medical problems, supporting self-care, and monitoring the effects of therapy.

Atrial fibrillation is the most common sustained arrhythmia and is characterized by rapid and disorganized atrial activity. The ECG shows no P wave. The incidence of atrial fibrillation increases with age. Common causes include damaged cardiac musculature after myocardial infarction, hypertension, valvular stenosis that causes stretching of the atria, and ischemic heart disease. Thyroid disorders (especially hyperthyroidism) can also precipitate atrial fibrillation.

The random arrival of impulses to the AV node results in an irregular heart rate. When the atrial fibrillation first begins, the ventricular response can be as high as 160 beats per minute. Atrial fibrillation that is of long-standing duration often slows to a rate in the normal range (60 to 100 beats per minute). Some loss of cardiac output occurs with new-onset atrial fibrillation because of fast rate and short ventricular filling times. A loss of the atrial contraction to fill the ventricles can also decrease the cardiac output. When assessing pulse rates for patients with irregular heart rhythms, the nurse must count the beats for a longer period of time, ideally one full minute. Counting shorter periods such as 15 seconds and multiplying by four can result in over- or underestimating the true pulse rate.

Atrial fibrillation is not a life-threatening arrhythmia, but it can cause morbidity, and mortality increases. One complication of atrial fibrillation is embolic cerebrovascular accidents. This is the result of the failure of the atria to fully empty with an organized atrial contraction. Clots that form in the blood and stagnate in the atria can break loose and follow the circulation to any part of the body. The incidence of stroke is five times baseline for people with atrial fibrillation. Anticoagulant therapy is indicated for any patient with atrial fibrillation for more than 24 hours.

> **Practice Pearl** ▶▶▶ Patients are at risk for ejecting clots from the heart when they are converting from atrial fibrillation to regular sinus rhythm. Coumadin therapy and an INR of about 3.0 are necessary to prevent stroke or thrombus ejection.

Short-term anticoagulation is usually begun with heparin. The blood test that determines the level of anticoagulant activity is the activated partial thromboplastin time. Heparin is given either intravenously or subcutaneously. For long-term therapy, warfarin (Coumadin) is usually prescribed. It can take several days for Coumadin levels to reach a steady state, and patients are usually maintained on heparin until this occurs. The laboratory test that assesses the blood-thinning effects of Coumadin is the international normalized ratio (INR), formerly called the protime.

> **Drug Alert** ▶▶▶ Patients taking Coumadin need to be taught that green leafy vegetables contain vitamin K, which is an antidote to warfarin. Patients should limit or maintain an even intake of green vegetables to prevent fluctuation in warfarin levels. They should also be taught that they are not to take aspirin or NSAIDs as well as to report any change in diet or medication when they are having their INR tested.

Overall treatment goals for atrial fibrillation are to correct hemodynamic instability, control ventricular rate, and restore sinus rhythm if possible. Several medication groups are frequently used for atrial fibrillation. Conversion to sinus rhythm can be achieved by using antiarrhythmic drugs. Ventricular response can be slowed with beta-blockers, calcium channel blockers (particularly verapamil), and digoxin.

If drug therapy is not successful, electrophysiologic studies can be performed to determine whether one particular area of the atria is initiating the irregular rhythm. If an area is located, it can be ablated using radio-frequency waves. This can prevent the recurrence of new atrial fibrillation.

Conduction disturbances can occur with age, as well. These are blocks in the transmission of electrical impulses. First-degree heart block is blockage of the impulse at the AV node, resulting in a prolonged PR interval. First-degree block can progress so that no atrial impulses are transmitted and only the underlying ventricular rate (30 beats per minute) maintains circulation. This is called complete heart block. Heart blocks that result in decreased cardiac output will need to be treated with an internal pacemaker insertion. Patients usually tolerate this procedure well. The nurse will need to monitor functioning of the pacemaker by checking pulse rates and looking for pacemaker activity on the ECG. Pacemakers can support ventricular contraction alone or in combination with atrial and ventricular pacing, therefore improving atrial contraction and ventricular filling simultaneously.

For patients who have experienced life-threatening arrhythmias such as ventricular tachycardia, an implantable cardiac defibrillator (ICD) can be inserted alone or as a combination with a pacing function. The ICD has a battery capacity that allows for enough electrical energy to deliver a cardioversion level of shock. The ICD senses tachycardia and, following internally set protocols, delivers the shock until normal heart rate is returned. Unlike a placed beat, which uses a low energy level, the ICD shock is felt by the patient and is often described as a "kick in the chest." Cases have been reported of patients being repeatedly shocked at end of life. ICDs can be disabled externally at the choice of patient, family, and healthcare provider (Ballentine, 2005). The nurse may be the person who is in a position to initiate the conversation about how the ICD will be used at end of life.

Peripheral Vascular Disease

Over time, disorders can develop in the arterial system, the venous system, or both. Because the etiology of arterial and venous disease is different, the disorders will be described separately.

Arterial Disease

Arterial disease is usually the result of atherosclerosis, which is a diffuse process causing changes in many places in the arterial system. The incidence of peripheral arterial disease (PAD) increases with age. A major risk factor to developing PAD is smoking. Occlusion of specific vessels causes loss of function and symptoms of pain in the areas perfused by the artery. Intermittent claudication is the experience of burning pain in legs or buttocks during exercise, which is relieved by rest. Pain felt in the upper calf indicates superficial femoral artery blockage. Thigh pain indicates common femoral artery disease, and buttock pain indicates aortoiliac disease. Pain occurs at rest as the disease progresses. Patients will frequently allow the affected leg to dangle over the edge of the bed to relieve the rest pain. Without therapy, the disease progresses to cause tissue necrosis and gangrene. This usually occurs in the toes of the affected leg.

A comprehensive history can indicate the extent and location of the blockage, but arteriograms need to be performed to determine the extent of the blockage. Simple pulse palpation is not sufficient to detect PAD. To evaluate circulation of the leg, the ankle brachial index (ABI)—equal to the systolic pressure of the ankle divided by the systolic pressure of the brachial artery, as measured using a Doppler—is useful. In the normal extremity, the ABI is close to 1.0. Decreased arterial flow to the leg is indicated by values of less than 1.0. Intermittent claudication is often seen with ABIs of 0.5 to 0.7. Rest pain, arterial ulcers, or gangrene can occur with ABIs of 9.4 or less (*British Medical Journal*, 2011). Patients may also require exercise treadmill tests, ultrasonography, or more expensive MRI evaluation to fully evaluate their condition.

New classes of drugs can improve peripheral circulation. Antithrombotic agents, prostaglandins, and calcium channel blockers are frequently prescribed. Surgical bypass of the occluded artery is often required to preserve circulation to the leg and prevent amputation. Meticulous care of surgical sites and ischemic extremities can preserve tissue, prevent infection, and preserve function (*British Medical Journal*, 2011).

Vascular rehabilitation programs can improve function and quality of life for patients with arterial occlusive disease. Programs are appropriate for patients who are not in crisis or who are being discharged from revascularization procedures. After a full assessment of risk factors and capacity of exercise, a gradual increase in physical exercise is planned. Patients need support and teaching from the nurse to maintain motivation for lifestyle change, especially smoking cessation.

Venous Disease

Several risk factors predispose the development of venous insufficiency. The most common site is the veins of the leg. Thrombophlebitis sometimes results in damage to the valves of the deep veins. Obesity and occupations that require prolonged standing or sitting can also lead to venous insufficiency. When the valves of the veins are incompetent, higher than normal pressures develop in the veins. This pressure is transmitted to the capillaries of the lower extremities. Over time, a thickening of the tissues around the ankles develops along with a brownish discoloration due to red blood cells that are pressed outside the capillaries. As the cells break down, hemosiderin (a breakdown product of hemoglobin) deposits collect. Eventually, chronic venous insufficiency can lead to nonhealing ulcers. The chronic ulcers caused by venous insufficiency tend to develop over the medial malleolus, the ankle area. The ulcers are different from arterial ulcers in that they are wide and have irregular borders.

Treatment for chronic venous insufficiency often involves wearing external compression hose every day. Because venous insufficiency can co-occur with arterial insufficiency, the ankle brachial index should be measured before beginning external compression. Nonhealing ulcers can be effectively treated with multilayer compression bandages such as the Unna's boot. Occasionally, skin grafts must be performed. Even after ulcers heal, patients need to be instructed that the underlying cause has not been removed and that external compression hose must continue to be worn to prevent ulcer recurrence (Reuben et al., 2011).

Nursing Management

The nurse is in an ideal situation to intervene with older adults with cardiac problems. Nursing interventions for promoting cardiac health should be grounded in an understanding of the relationship between lifestyle modification, judicious use of medications, and ongoing assessment of the older person's cardiac status.

Nursing Assessment

Nursing assessment of cardiovascular function for the older person follows the same principles as health assessment in general. The history is the most important part of the assessment. Taking a history from an older person requires a balance between encouraging the person to share any concerns along with the ability to focus data gathering on the particularly important factors. Older adults may have many physical complaints and a long list of illnesses, surgical procedures, and medications that must be sorted out in building a picture of the health status. Nurses collect information to support medical diagnoses as well as nursing diagnoses to establish treatment and monitoring plans for their patients.

Assessments need to be appropriate to the situation. In an emergency, a focused assessment will streamline care planning, whereas in a long-term or community setting, more extensive assessments can be performed. Comprehensive histories include demographic information, chief complaint, history of the present illness, past health history, a review of systems, family history, social history, and a functional health pattern assessment. When working in a tertiary setting where many providers have access to the patient, the nurse may not need to initiate the medical history. In this setting, the nurse can verify data collected by others and focus on the functional assessment. In the community setting, however, the nurse will need to conduct the entire history and physical to obtain information necessary to plan and monitor care.

The nurse should collect vital demographic information including the patient's date of birth. The source of history other than the patient should be noted. For the older person, a family member or caretaker frequently becomes an important source of information. Sometimes a decrease in function is more obvious to an outside observer than to the patient.

The nurse should carefully note the chief complaint in the patient's own words. The chief complaint is defined as the main reason the person has sought attention by the healthcare provider. The nurse should use quotation marks if possible to record the words of the patient. This minimizes the chance for misinterpretation. Many patients come to a clinic for screening or follow-up and will have no specific complaint. In these cases, the nurse would note the reason for the follow-up or any prompt to the screening. For patients with multiple complaints, a numbered problem list can help to focus assessment and treatment planning. Many patients who come for care unrelated to cardiovascular problems will have a cardiovascular history. For example, the patient who is admitted for a joint replacement may have a history of coronary artery disease and will require monitoring and assistance with rehabilitation.

Next, the nurse should assess the history of the present illness, again using the patient's own words to describe the present health problem. Asking specific questions will help to fill in missing pieces of information. A full description of the symptom will include when and how it began, exactly where it is experienced, how long it has been noticed, associated symptoms, anything that makes it better or worse, and the characteristics of pain. Pain and fatigue can be assessed using numeric scales, although these may be harder for the older person to quantify. The thermometer scale might be more easily understood for some patients. The nurse should pay attention to how serious the patients feel their problems are. Patients frequently know if their problem is serious or life threatening. Laboratory test results can be included in this section for documentation purposes. Tests of interest for cardiac patients include clotting studies, serum electrolytes, and specific indicators such as CK-MB and troponin levels. More indirectly important might be thyroid studies. See Table 15-9 for a list of frequently used cardiovascular laboratory studies.

The next step is to assess the older person's past health history. This section includes health problems other than the present illness, hospital admissions, and surgical procedures. The current medication list is a clue to medical problems. For example, the patient may forget to report thyroid disease, but lists Synthroid on the current medication list. This prompts the nurse to clarify thyroid status. The medication list should include prescription and over-the-counter medications as well as vitamins and supplements. Allergies should be noted in this section. Another way to uncover history of cardiac disease is to ask if cardiac catheterization, stress tests, or other cardiac studies have been conducted. Many patients with serious conditions such as heart failure may never have been told the level of their problem, or may not understand what the diagnostic label means. The nurse must go below the surface to determine the real picture of the patient's medical history.

Assessing family history is important to identify risk factors for cardiovascular disorders. For the older person, asking age and cause of death of parents and health status of siblings and children can offer evidence about genetic risk factors. Such conditions as coronary events, cerebrovascular accidents, peripheral vascular disease, aneurysms, diabetes, alcoholism, and depression all have family patterns of incidence and can affect cardiovascular status.

Next, the nurse should assess the older person's personal or social history. This area contains much information that the nurse will need to plan appropriate care. Each healthcare system will organize this information in different ways. In some systems, a nursing functional health pattern assessment can form the basis of this material and offers broad categories of interest to the nurse. Other settings are structured according to the medical care system. This information can be referred to as current living situation, resources, and supports. The nurse must use the framework that allows essential information to be gathered and report it in this section. Functional health pattern assessments will gather information in 11 pattern areas. The pattern areas

TABLE 15-9	Laboratory Testing Values	
Test	**Normal Geriatric Value**	**Implication**
Hematologic Studies		
Hematocrit	0–45% men	Anemia if too low or diluted
	36–65% women	Polycythemia if too high or dehydrated
Hemoglobin	11.5 g/100 mg/dL	Reflects oxygen-carrying capacity of blood
	11.0 g/100 mg/dL	
Coagulation Studies		
Platelet count	150,000–400,000/mm^3	Thrombocytopenia if too low, can decrease clotting ability
Prothrombin time (PT)	12–15 sec	Prolonged with Coumadin, reflects slower clotting
Partial thromboplastin time (PTT)	60–70 sec	Prolonged with heparin, reflects slower clotting
Electrolytes		
Sodium (Na)	135–145 mEq/L	
Potassium (K)	3.3–4.9 mEq/L	
Chloride (Cl)	97–110 mEq/L	
Carbon dioxide	22–31 mEq/L	
Creatinine	0.9–1.4 mg/dL men	Elevation reflects renal insufficiency
	0.8–1.3 mg/dL women	
Glucose (fasting)	65–110 mg/dL	Elevation reflects diabetes mellitus
Urea nitrogen (BUN)	8–26 mg/dL	Elevation reflects renal insufficiency or dehydration
Uric acid	4.0–8.5 mg/dL men	Elevation can precipitate gout
	2.8–7.5 mg/dL women	
Serum Enzymes		
Creatine kinase-MM	95–100%	Skeletal muscle fraction
Creatine kinase-MB	0–5%	Elevation reflects cardiac muscle damage: peaks day 2, gone day 4
Creatine kinase-BB	0%	Brain fraction
LDH-1	Varies with test system	Reflects muscle damage; elevated in MI: peaks day 4, gone day 12
Myocardial Proteins		
Troponin I	0–2 ng/mL	Elevation reflects cardiac damage
Troponin T	0–3.1 ng/mL	Elevated in muscle damage and renal failure
Myoglobin	10–75 ng/mL	Elevation reflects general muscle damage
Cholesterol		
Total blood cholesterol	<200 mg/dL	Desirable
	200–239 mg/dL	Borderline high
	≥240 mg/dL	High
LDL cholesterol	<130 mg/dL	Desirable
	130–159 mg/dL	Borderline high
	≥160 mg/dL	High
HDL cholesterol	≥35 mg/dL	Desirable
Apoprotein A	120 mg/dL	Elevation reflects increased risk of atherosclerosis
Apoprotein B	134 mg/dL	
C-reactive protein	0–2 mg/dL	Elevation reflects increased risk of coronary disease

Source: Adapted from Reuben et al., 2011; Woods, Froelicher, & Motzer, 2000.

are not rigid categories; information from several can be combined and used as evidence to support problem identification (Gordon, 1994). Table 15-10 lists the best practices for assessing cardiovascular status and functional health pattern areas and pertinent data in older patients.

Finally, the nurse should conduct a complete review of systems. For older patients with cardiovascular problems, the nurse should focus on the presence or absence of chest pain, shortness of breath, syncope, palpitations, edema, nocturnal dyspnea, nocturia, pain in the extremities, cough, and fatigue. It is important to ask if the patient has been less active than previously or seems more easily fatigued. The function of other body systems may point to cardiovascular disorders as well. Peripheral neuropathy may suggest diabetes, which has implications for cardiovascular risk factors. Pulmonary problems may be the result of smoking,

TABLE 15-10	Best Practices for the Assessment of Functional Health Patterns and Cardiovascular Data	
Pattern Area	**Cardiovascular Data**
Health perception/ health management	Do you see yourself as healthy?
	What do you do to stay healthy?
	Do you understand what each of your medications is for?
	Do you have any difficulty getting or taking medications?
	Do you smoke? Did you ever smoke? How much and for how long?
	How much alcohol do you drink in a week?
	If you have a problem, do you call your healthcare provider or do you wait until your next appointment?
Nutrition/metabolic	Have you gained or lost weight in the past (2 months to few days)?
	What do you eat on a typical day?
	Are you able to shop for food that is healthy?
	Do you weigh yourself daily?
Elimination	What is your pattern of urination? How often do you waken at night to urinate?
	How often do you have a bowel movement?
Activity/exercise	How far can you walk before you get short of breath?
	How many flights of stairs can you climb? When was the last time you climbed that many? What is your typical day like? Do you shop for yourself? Do you need help dressing, bathing, toileting, eating, keeping house, or cooking?
Sleep/rest	Do you sleep through the night? Do you feel refreshed? Do you need pillows to sleep comfortably?
	Does your partner say that you snore?
Cognitive/perceptual	Do you have limitations in hearing or seeing? Do you need hearing aids or glasses? Have you noticed a change in your memory? How do you like to receive new information?
Self-perception/self-concept	How would you describe yourself? Are you comfortable with your own life?
Role/relationship	Who do you live with? How many people do you see in a day or week? Where do you see people?
	Do you have one or two good friends you can count on?
Sexuality/reproductive	Are you sexually active? Do you have any concerns about sexuality?
Coping/stress tolerance	What do you do to cope with stresses in your life? Do you feel stressed or worried right now?
Value/belief	What gives your life meaning? Are religious practices important to you? Are there any things about your values that your healthcare providers need to know?

which can also cause cardiovascular problems. The patient may not understand that shortness of breath may have a cardiovascular cause. Indigestion may be a misinterpreted angina symptom. Many cardiac drugs cause constipation, which may be noted on the review of systems. Peripheral edema can indicate fluid retention.

Functional classification of patients with cardiovascular conditions allows for monitoring progress and for planning appropriate support. Table 15-8 on page 386 lists two classification systems that nurses may encounter in use in the practice environment.

An assessment is not complete until the nurse considers and combines patterns of findings from history, physical examination, and laboratory data to arrive at an overall understanding of the patient's situation and condition. Completing the process of assessment will result in an overall clinical judgment. Some conclusions represent medical conditions or complications that must be reported to healthcare providers involved in patient care. Other patterns are recognizable as conditions that the nurse can manage independently. Simply recording data does not complete an assessment. As the nurse gains experience in managing patients with cardiovascular conditions, his or her ability to detect patterns and form accurate clinical judgments will improve.

Pharmacology and Nursing Implications

Many patients have more than one disease and require multiple medications to control cardiovascular conditions. This can lead to a common problem in the older person known as polypharmacy. Many older adults have multiple healthcare providers. The cardiologist may be prescribing medications without knowing what medications the rheumatologist is prescribing. The nurse and the pharmacist are often the only providers to see the full range of medications a patient is taking.

Medications can be both a support and a stress. Because medications cause changes in body systems, the older person takes time to adjust to changes. The general rule of starting with low doses and increasing them slowly is a good practice. The nurse should be alert to side or toxic effects even when the older person is taking medications in the normal adult dosage range.

Nonpharmacological Treatments

One of the most useful methods to help patients adjust to cardiovascular problems is the concept of rehabilitation. Cardiac rehabilitation can be used for patients with angina, recent MI, heart failure, recent revascularization, or other risk factors for heart disease. Most rehabilitation programs include information on exercise and are available while patients exercise in case arrhythmias develop. They also include information on

diet and stress management. Topics such as sexuality can also be addressed in a rehabilitation setting. Having a cardiac diagnosis can cause fear of death or progression of disease. The support of rehabilitation programs can encourage patients to engage in healthy lifestyle patterns.

Nursing Diagnoses

Many cardiovascular conditions require long-term management. Many patients will describe *Fatigue* or *Activity Intolerance,* which are both nursing diagnoses. The nursing diagnosis *Self Health Management, Ineffective* is important for patients with heart failure or angina, and for those with risk factors who do not yet have overt disease. For patients with heart failure, *Cardiac Output, Decreased* and *Fluid Volume: Excess* can direct nursing interventions. For patients with orthopnea or paroxysmal nocturnal dyspnea, *Sleep Deprivation* may be identified (Wilkinson & Ahern, 2009).

Nursing Interventions

Specific nursing interventions are useful in a variety of cardiovascular conditions. Risk factor reduction can be done in a variety of settings from home to hospital to long-term care. Patients can be encouraged to maintain a normal weight, to stop smoking, to moderate alcohol intake, and to exercise. The creativity of nursing is to reach each patient as an individual. Patients who love baseball can be motivated by being in their own "spring training." Feeling well enough to travel to see grandchildren can be a strong motivator for lifestyle change.

Activity and exercise support is an intervention that provides for a supervised increase in activity. Patients should be monitored for changes in vital signs and sudden fatigue. Along with exercise, planning is important for rest.

Diet therapy will involve teaching and may also involve consultation with dietitians. It is best to start with the patient's preferred diet and suggest small changes that are acceptable to the patient.

Smoking cessation is important for cardiovascular patients, and it can be used to prevent cardiovascular problems. Research has shown that healthcare providers often fail to ask patients about their smoking and fail to offer support in stopping smoking. One useful method is to ask patients to record each cigarette daily for a week. Then they select the one time that they think they can comfortably avoid cigarettes and do so for another week. Gradually, the patient is smoking less, which makes stopping more likely. Medication can also assist in smoking cessation.

Medication management is important because so many medications are useful in treating cardiovascular concerns.

Older adults need to be able to open their medication bottles. They need to remember to take medications and when to report side effects.

Caregiver support is important in any chronic condition. Family members need to understand medications and their effect and they need to know what signs or symptoms should be reported to the nurse or doctor. Adult day health programs can offer respite for the caregiver and support for the patient.

Advance directives should be discussed with the patient and family members. Does the patient want aggressive treatment for the condition and understand the burdens of that treatment? Has the patient discussed treatment preferences with a healthcare proxy or with the healthcare provider? These are topics best addressed during a stable time. Crisis is a bad time to begin these discussions. The nurse can assist patients in clarifying their values and wishes and can support them in preparing written advance directives.

Community resources are important in chronic conditions. The American Heart Association has many programs that support healthy living. Many senior centers have cardiovascular programs available. The nurse can become familiar with resources in the community and can refer patients appropriately. Stress and depression increase the risk of cardiovascular disease. Community support through social and religious connections can assist senior citizens in finding meaning in their lives.

COMPLEMENTARY AND ALTERNATIVE THERAPIES

Many complementary and alternative therapies are used for heart disease by older adults and by society in general. Because stress can contribute to the formation and exacerbation of heart disease, nurses have long known that stress reduction techniques are helpful. For instance, meditation, prayer, yoga, massage therapy, listening to music, and engagement in activities that are satisfying or relaxing to the older person can decrease production of enzymes that elevate heart rate and blood pressure. Use of these techniques can delay the need for medication or can decrease the dose needed, thus decreasing the risk of toxic side effects that can occur with higher doses. Many larger healthcare facilities offer stress reduction clinics and the use of biofeedback to patients with stress-related cardiac problems and many health insurance plans will cover the cost of these services. Counseling and nursing presence can help patients who are making decisions about major cardiac interventions or end-of-life care.

Herbal or nutritional substances used to treat heart disease include the use of garlic to reduce blood cholesterol, reduce blood pressure, and provide anticoagulation. Garlic supplements are one of the best-selling herbal supplements sold in the United States. However, garlic may have significant side effects including interactions with medications (aspirin, NSAIDs, and insulin) and prolongation of bleeding or clotting time, so garlic should not be taken with blood-thinning medications such as warfarin and should be discontinued prior to surgery (Cleveland Clinic, 2008).

Soybeans and dietary fiber have been shown to lower LDL blood levels and triglycerides and thus lower the risk of developing coronary heart disease. Soy products can be incorporated into the diet by drinking soy milk, eating tofu, or eating any product made with soybeans. The FDA has allowed the statement that inclusion of soy products in a diet low in saturated fat and cholesterol promotes heart health. Vegetables, fruits, and unrefined grains contain dietary fiber. The fiber found in oat bran, apples, citrus, and whole-grain products is particularly effective in reducing cholesterol. Increasingly, whole-grain pasta, breads, and pulp-added fruit juices have been developed and sold at many supermarkets. If the products alone are not effective in reducing cholesterol to safe levels, they may be combined with cholesterol-lowering medications to enhance the pharmacologic effect (Cleveland Clinic, 2008). Phytosterols (plant sterols) are found in whole grains and many fruits and vegetables and have the ability to interfere with the intestinal absorption of cholesterol. These products have been added to certain margarines and salad dressings and the FDA has approved statements that consumption of these products may reduce the risk of coronary heart disease. Consumption of fish oil and ingestion of omega-3 fatty acids also have been shown to reduce cholesterol levels prompting the recommendation by the American Heart Association that fatty fish (mackerel, lake trout, herring, sardines, tuna, and salmon) be eaten at least two times a week (AHA, 2010).

QSEN Recommendations Related to the Cardiovascular System

The Quality and Safety Education for Nurses (QSEN) project addresses the challenge of preparing future nurses with the knowledge, skills, and attitudes (KSAs) to continuously improve the quality and safety of the healthcare systems in which they work (Cronenwett et al., 2007). See the QSEN table for tips on meeting QSEN standards.

The patient–family teaching guidelines in the following feature will assist the nurse to assume the role of teacher and coach. Educating patients and families is critical so that nurses can interpret scientific data and individualize the nursing care plan.

Patient and Family Teaching

Gerontological nurses require skills and knowledge related to teaching patients and families about the key concepts

of gerontology and gerontological nursing. The guidelines in the following feature will assist the nurse to assume the role of teacher and coach.

Meeting QSEN Standards: The Cardiovascular System

	KNOWLEDGE	SKILLS	ATTITUDES
Patient-Centered Care	Involvement of patient and family in plan of care is crucial.	Know family assessment and adult learning principles.	Appreciate uniqueness of each patient/family.
	Examine barriers that may keep patients from being active in formulating their plan of care.	Evaluate for depression, vision/hearing, and cognitive status.	Provide patient-centered care to improve successful nursing outcomes.
Teamwork and Collaboration	Recognize scope of practice for interdisciplinary team members.	Use leadership skills to coordinate team members and share knowledge.	Value the contribution of each member of the team to improve outcomes.
	Be aware of organizational problems that can inhibit effective team functioning.	System assessment skills.	Be open to input from team members on effective means to improve communication and collaboration.
Evidence-Based Practice	Describe effective interventions to decrease CV risk factors and improve overall health and function.	Access current evidence-based protocols to guide interventions.	Possess confidence in necessary skills to evaluate and incorporate nursing interventions from the literature.
Quality Improvement	Recognize the importance of measuring patient outcomes to improve CV care.	Skills in data management, technology, and use of U.S. government and AHA sites describing current incidence and prevalence of CV disease.	Value the use of data and outcomes as a key component of QI efforts.
Safety	Describe common medication errors and patient/family characteristics that increase the likelihood of such errors.	Use appropriate strategies to provide written information to compensate for memory loss (if present).	Appreciate the impact of cognitive loss on the occurrence of adverse drug reactions.
Informatics	Provide input into the formation and maintenance of patient databases needed for gathering QSEN data and providing patient care.	Utilize the electronic health record.	Protect patient confidentiality according to HIPAA standards.

Patient–Family Teaching Guidelines

The following are guidelines that the nurse may find useful when instructing older adults and their families about hypertension.

HIGH BLOOD PRESSURE OR HYPERTENSION

1 What is high blood pressure?

High blood pressure is a condition of higher than normal pressures inside the blood vessels. It can cause:

- Changes in the thickness of the blood vessels
- Increased risk of heart attack and stroke
- Damage to kidneys

RATIONALE:

Long-term hypertension increases the endothelium of the blood vessels, increases atherosclerosis, and damages renal arteries.

2 What causes high blood pressure?

The cause of most high blood pressure is frequently not known, but is most likely an imbalance in:

- The body's ability to control body water.
- The body's ability to control sodium levels.
- Neuroendocrine controls of blood pressure.

RATIONALE:

Primary hypertension has no direct cause.

3 What can a person do to decrease blood pressure to a healthy level?

It is important to make healthy choices such as the following:

- Maintain a normal body weight.
- Decrease intake of high-fat and high-sodium foods.
- Exercise regularly.
- Stop smoking.
- Limit alcohol intake.
- Take prescribed medications.
- Have blood pressure checked regularly.

RATIONALE:

All of these lifestyle changes will decrease blood pressure. Even losing 10 lbs can significantly lower blood pressure.

4 What is heart failure?

Heart failure happens when the heart is not able to pump enough blood to the body to allow a person to do the things he or she wants or needs to do. People who have heart failure often experience these symptoms:

- Fatigue
- Shortness of breath
- Inability to be comfortable lying flat in bed
- Shortness of breath at night
- Needing to use the bathroom frequently at night
- Swollen ankles

Heart failure patients frequently need to be hospitalized to balance fluid in their body and ease their breathing.

RATIONALE:

Fatigue is caused by inadequate pumping ability of the heart. Shortness of breath and ankle swelling are caused by fluid retention that happens when kidneys do not receive the amount of blood flow that they need. At night, fluid that has collected in the legs is moved into the full circulation, and fluid backs into the lungs.

5 What causes heart failure?

Heart failure is caused by damage to the heart muscle. This can occur from heart attacks (myocardial infarctions) or from long-standing high blood pressure. In some cases, heart valve problems can lead to heart failure. Either the heart cannot pump as well as it should or the workload that the heart is pumping against is increased.

RATIONALE:

Once a heart attack occurs, heart muscle dies and cannot contribute to the pumping function of the heart. Long-standing high blood pressure can cause enlarged heart muscle that prevents blood from entering the heart.

(continued)

Patient–Family Teaching Guidelines *(continued)*

6 **What can a person do to live with heart failure?**

Heart failure patients can improve the quality of their life and reduce hospitalizations by:

- Taking medications as prescribed. If there is any trouble with the medications, either in obtaining them or from side effects, the doctor or nurse should be told.
- Avoiding high-sodium and salty foods.
- Balancing activity and rest.
- Weighing themselves daily to determine if they are holding fluid.

- Reporting any change in weight or how they feel to a doctor or nurse.

RATIONALE:

Medications can assist the body in balancing fluid and sodium. Medications can decrease the workload on the heart. Some patients cannot afford all the medications that they have been prescribed. They should notify their doctor rather than decrease their medication. Salty food causes the body to hold sodium and water, which increases the workload on the heart.

CARE PLAN   A Patient With Heart Failure

Case Study

Mrs. Lockhart lives in senior housing in the small town where she has lived her entire life. She is an 87-year-old widow who was recently hospitalized for exacerbation of her heart failure. She has had two other such admissions already this year. Her son and daughter-in-law live about an hour away.

Applying the Nursing Process

Assessment

When the home care nurse comes to Mrs. Lockhart's apartment the morning after her discharge from the hospital, her vital signs include heart rate of 82, irregular, and blood pressure 138/80. Her lung sounds are clear and she has a mild systolic ejection murmur. Her laboratory values on discharge were normal. She says her medications have not been delivered by the pharmacy yet, but the list from the discharge sheet includes furosemide (Lasix) 20 mg daily, enalapril maleate 5 mg daily, digoxin 0.125 mg, and diclofenac 50 mg twice daily. She seems evasive when questioned about her medications. When asked, she states, "I'm not sure I can afford all these new medications. I hate to ask my son for help." The nurse notes that her kitchen cabinets contain mostly canned and prepared foods such as soup, macaroni and cheese, and beef stew. The nurse asks about where she obtains food, and she says that her son brings things once a week. She has difficulty walking in a store because of her arthritis. When asked, she says that she does not own a bathroom scale.

Diagnosis

The current nursing diagnoses for Mrs. Lockhart include the following:

- *Self Health Management, Ineffective* due to insufficient resources and knowledge
- *Fluid Volume: Excess* due to limited food choices and insufficient knowledge
- *Activity Intolerance* due to pain and deconditioning

NANDA-I © 2012.

CARE PLAN   A Patient With Heart Failure *(continued)*

Expected Outcomes

The expected outcomes for Mrs. Lockhart include that she will:

- Weigh herself daily and record the readings in a chart that she will take to the doctor's appointment.
- Obtain fresh food twice a week from a volunteer church delivery service, including fruits, vegetables, and whole grains that are pleasing to Mrs. Lockhart's tastes and low in sodium.

- Have an organized system for taking medications.
- Gradually increase her activity through participation in senior center activities.
- Discuss more openly with her son what she needs to stay independent.
- Discuss with her doctor the cost of her medications.

Planning and Implementation

The following nursing interventions would be appropriate for Mrs. Lockhart:

- Establish a relationship of trust with the patient.
- Plan a family meeting to discuss obtaining food, a bathroom scale, and medications.

- Plan medication and weight sheet to record medications and daily weight.
- Consult with healthcare providers to coordinate medications that are economical.

Evaluation

The nurse can evaluate the patient plan by reviewing the daily weight record and assessing Mrs. Lockhart's heart, lungs, and peripheral edema. A positive evaluation of the plan will include a reduced rate of hospitalization and improved functional level and quality of life for Mrs. Lockhart.

Ethical Dilemma

The ethical dilemma in this case balances Mrs. Lockhart's wish for autonomy and not being dependent on her son and the principle of beneficence, which motivates care providers to do what is best for the patient. The key to bridging this gap is to help Mrs. Lockhart see that her independence is ultimately supported by accepting some level of care.

Critical Thinking and the Nursing Process

1. Why is cardiac rehabilitation indicated following angioplasty or revascularization with coronary artery bypass grafting?
2. How is knowing and following up with a cardiovascular patient over time important to the caring process?
3. How do you respond when a patient says, "I don't want to run a marathon. Why should I go to rehab?"
4. What supports are necessary to assist older adults who live alone to maintain their independence when they are diagnosed with heart failure?

5. Imagine you are designing an intergenerational program in an inner-city community center. What health issues would benefit both older and younger people?

- Evaluate your responses in Appendix B. ⊂⊐

Chapter Highlights

- Caring for cardiovascular patients is complicated but can be very rewarding. Nearly all older adults have some cardiovascular condition or risk factor. Managing cardiovascular conditions well can add quality and years to a patient's life.

- Most cardiovascular conditions are chronic and require long-term support.

- Assessment skills are important in monitoring cardiovascular conditions.

- Lifestyle factors such as normalizing body weight; choosing foods that include fruits, vegetables, and whole grains; and getting enough exercise can improve quality of life and reduce the risk of further disease.

- Blood pressure should be controlled with lifestyle and with medications to prevent stroke and heart attack.

- Isolated systolic hypertension is frequently seen in older adults, particularly women, and contributes to high rates of stroke.

- African American patients have higher rates of hypertension when compared to Whites and Mexican Americans and may benefit from sodium restriction.

- Heart failure has a poor prognosis, requires frequent expensive hospitalizations, and interferes with quality of life.

- Patient teaching is best conducted in short sessions over time.

- Older adults frequently experience ischemia with symptoms other than chest pain. These include shortness of breath, fatigue, jaw or arm pain, and gastrointestinal distress.

Pearson Nursing Student Resources
Find additional review materials at
nursing.pearsonhighered.com

Prepare for success with additional NCLEX®-style practice questions, interactive assignments and activities, web links, animations and videos, and more!

References

Adult Treatment Panel (ATP III). (2004). *Third report of the NCEP Expert Panel on Detection, Evaluation, and Treatment of High Blood Cholesterol in Adults (ATP III)* (NIH Publication No. 110, pp. 227–239). Bethesda, MD: National Institutes of Health.

Agency for Healthcare Research and Quality. (2007). *Screening: High blood pressure.* U.S. Preventive Services Task Force. Retrieved from http://www.ahrq.gov/clinic/uspstf/uspshype.htm

Allen, L. A., Stevenson, L. W., Grady, K. L., Goldstein, N. E., Matlock, D. D., Arnold, R. M., et al. (2012). Decision making in advanced heart failure: A scientific statement from the American Heart Association. *Circulation, 125*(15), 1928–1952. doi:10.1161/CIR.0b013e31824f2173

American Academy of Health and Fitness. (2011). *Cardiovascular system.* Retrieved from http://www.aahf.info/sec_exercise/section/cardiovascular.htm

American College of Cardiology Foundation/American Heart Association (AACF/AHA).

(2005). AACF/AHA Practice guideline: Retrieved from http://circ.ahajournals.org/content/119/14/e391.full.pdf

American College of Cardiology Foundation/American Heart Association (AACF/AHA). (2009). *AACF/AHA practice guideline: Focused update.* Retrieved from http://circ.ahajournals.org/content/119/14/1977.full.pdf+html

American Heart Association (AHA). (2012). *Statistical fact sheet: 2012 update.* Retrieved from http://www.heart.org/idc/groups/heart-public/@wcm/@sop/@smd/documents/downloadable/ucm_319574.pdf

American Heart Association (AHA). (2010). Fish and omega-3 fatty acids. Retrieved from http://www.heart.org/HEARTORG/GettingHealthy/NutritionCenter/HealthyDietGoals/Fish-and-Omega-3-Fatty-Acids_UCM_303248_Article.jsp

Ballentine, J. M. (2005). Pacemaker and defibrillator deactivation in competent hospice patients: An ethical consideration.

American Journal of Hospice and Palliative Care, 22, 14–19.

Bradley, J., & Davis, K. (2003). Orthostatic hypotension. *American Family Physician.* Retrieved from http://www.aafp.org/afp/20031215/2393.html

Braun, L. T., & Davidson, M. H. (2003). Cholesterol-lowering drugs bring benefits to high-risk populations even when LDL is normal. *Journal of Cardiovascular Nursing, 18*(1), 44–49.

British Medical Journal. (2011). *Best practices: Gangrene.* Retrieved from http://bestpractice.bmj.com/best-practice/monograph/1015/diagnosis/step-by-step.html

Cardiosmart. (2011). *Valve disease.* American College of Cardiology. Retrieved from http://cardiosmart.org/HeartDisease/CTT.aspx?id=112

Centers for Disease Control and Prevention (CDC). (2012). *High blood pressure facts.* Retrieved from http://www.cdc.gov/bloodpressure/facts.htm

Cleveland Clinic. (2008). *Complementary/ alternative medicine (CAM) therapies for cholesterol reduction.* Retrieved from http:// www.cleveland.com/healthfit/index.ssf/2011/08/ complementary_and_alternative.html

Cleveland Clinic. (2012). *Understanding your ejection fraction.* Retrieved from http:// my.clevelandclinic.org/heart/disorders/ heartfailure/ejectionfraction.aspx

Committee on the Future of Healthcare Workforce for Older Americans. (2008). *Retooling for an aging America: Building the health care workforce.* Washington, DC: National Academies Press. Retrieved from http://www.iom.edu/Reports/2008/Retooling- for-an-Aging-America-Building-the-Health- Care-Workforce.aspx

Coordinating Committee of the National Cholesterol Education Program. (2004). Implications of recent clinical trials for the National Cholesterol Education Program Adult Treatment Panel III Guidelines. *Circulation, 110,* 227–239.

Cronenwett, L., Sherwood, G., Barnsteiner, J., Disch, J., Johnson, J., Mitchell, P., Sullivan, D., & Warren, J. (2007). Quality and safety education for nurses, *Nursing Outlook, 55*(3) 122–131.

Drugs.com. (2012). Niacin: Side Effects. Retrieved from http://www.drugs.com/sfx/ niacin-side-effects.html

Expert Panel on Detection, Evaluation, and Treatment of High Blood Cholesterol in Adults (Adult Treatment Panel III). (2004). Executive summary of the third report of the National Cholesterol Education Program (NCEP). *Journal of the American Medical Association, 285,* 2486–2497.

Glossock, R., & Rule, A. (2012). The implications of anatomical and functional changes of the aging kidney: With an emphasis on the glomeruli. *Kidney International, 21*(10), 1038–1042.

Gordon, M. (1994). *Nursing diagnosis: Process and application* (3rd ed.). St. Louis, MO: Mosby.

Howard, V., Woolson, R., Egan, B., Nicholas, J., Adams, R., Howard, G., & Lackland, D. (2010). Prevalence of hypertension by duration and age at exposure to the stroke belt. *Journal of the American Society of Hypertension, 4*(1), 32–41.

Hunt, S. A., Abraham, W. T., Chin, M. H., Feldman, A. M., Francis, G. S., Ganiats, T. G., et al. (2005). ACC/AHA 2005 guidelines update for the diagnosis and management of chronic heart failure in the adult: A report of the American College of Cardiology/ American Heart Association Task force on Practice Guidelines. *Circulation, 112,* e154–e235.

Internet Stroke Center. (2012). *Stroke statistics.* Retrieved from http://www .strokecenter.org/patients/about-stroke/ stroke-statistics

Joint National Committee on Prevention, Detection, Evaluation, and Treatment of High Blood Pressure & National High Blood Pressure Education Program Coordinating Committee. (2004). *The seventh report of the Joint National Committee on Prevention, Detection, Evaluation, and Treatment of High Blood Pressure—Complete report* (National Heart Lung and Blood Institute Publication No. 04-5230). Retrieved from http://www .nhlbi.nih.gov/guidelines/hypertension/ jnc7full.pdf

Levy, D., Ehret, G., Rice, K., Verwoert, G., Launer, L., Dehghan, A., et al. (2009). Genome-wide association study of blood pressure and hypertension. *Nature Genetics, 41,* 677–689.

Massachusetts General Hospital. (2008). *Elizabeth Anne and Karen Barlow Corrigan Women's heart health program.* Retrieved from http://www.massgeneral.org/heartcenter/ services/treatmentprograms.aspx?id=1011

McCance, K., & Huether, S. (2010). *Pathophysiology: The biologic basis for disease in adults and children* (6th ed.). St. Louis, MO: Elsevier, Mosby.

McPhee, S., & Papadakis, M. (2011). *Current medical diagnosis and treatment.* New York, NY: McGraw-Hill Medical.

Moser, D. K., Riegel, B., McKinley, S., Doering, L. V., An, K., & Sheahan, S. (2007). Impact of anxiety and perceived control on in-hospital complications after acute myocardial infarction. *Psychosomatic Medicine, 69*(1), 10–16.

Murphy, S., Xu, J., & Kochanek, M. (2012). Deaths: Preliminary data for 2010. *National Vital Statistics Reports, 60*(4). Retrieved from http://www.cdc.gov/nchs/data/nvsr/nvsr60/ nvsr60_04.pdf

National Heart, Lung, and Blood Institute (NHLBI). (2004). *Your guide to lowering blood pressure: The DASH diet.* Retrieved from http://www.nhlbi.nih.gov/health/ health-topics/topics/dash

National Heart, Lung, and Blood Institute (NHLBI). (2007). *The healthy heart handbook for women.* Retrieved from http://www .nhlbi.nih.gov/health/hearttruth/material/ NHLBI_3942_HHH_041707.pdf

New York Heart Association. (1964). *Nomenclature and criteria for disease* (4th ed.). New York, New York: Little Brown and Company.

Nurse Practitioner's Prescribing Reference. (2012). New York, NY: MPR/Haymarket Media.

Parker, K. P., & Dunbar, S. B. (2002). Sleep and heart failure. *Journal of Cardiovascular Nursing, 17*(1), 30–41.

Reuben, D., Herr, K., Pacala, J., Pollock, B., Potter, J., & Semla, T. (2011). *Geriatrics at your fingertips.* New York, NY: American Geriatrics Society.

Riegel, B., Dickson, V. V., Hoke, L., McMahon, J. P., Reis, B. F., & Sayers, S. (2006). A motivational counseling approach to improving heart failure self-care: Mechanisms of effectiveness. *Journal of Cardiovascular Nursing, 21*(3), 232–241.

Shepard, J., Blauw, G. J., Murphy, M. B., Bollen, E. L., Buckley, B. M., Cobbe, S. M., et al (2002). PROSPER study group. Pravastatin in elderly individuals at risk of vascular disease (PROSPER): A randomized controlled trial. *Lancet, 360,* 1623–1630.

WebMD. (2012). Should I have surgery to replace my aortic valve? *Heart Disease Health Center.* Retrieved from http://www.webmd .com/heart-disease/should-i-have-surgery- to-replace-my-aortic-valve

Wilkinson, J., & Ahern, N. (2009). *Nursing diagnosis handbook* (9th ed.). Upper Saddle River, NJ: Pearson Prentice Hall.

Woods, S. L., Froelicher, E. S. S., & Motzer, S. A. U. (2000). *Cardiac nursing* (4th ed.). Philadelphia, PA: Lippincott.

Zafari, A. (2012). Myocardial infarction. *Medscape Reference.* Retrieved from http://emedicine.medscape.com/ article/155919-overview

The Respiratory System

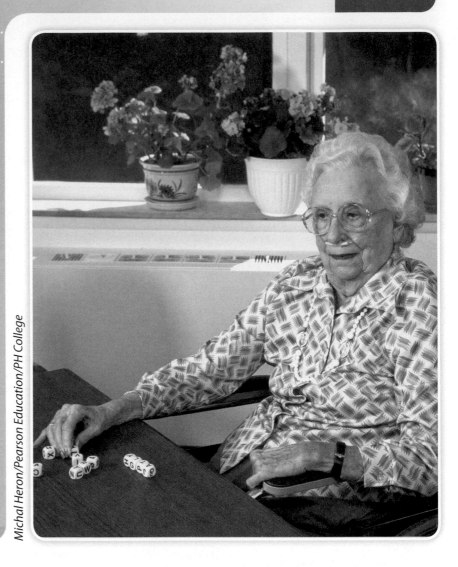

Michal Heron/Pearson Education/PH College

LEARNING OUTCOMES

On completion of this chapter, the reader will be able to:

1. Define normal changes of aging of the respiratory system.
2. Describe appropriate health promotion and disease prevention guidelines relating to the respiratory system.
3. Discuss the nurse's role in caring for older adults with respiratory problems.

4. Classify common diseases of the respiratory system.
5. Identify the nursing assessment process and formulation of nursing diagnoses relating to the respiratory system.

During a normal day, the average person takes 25,000 breaths and inhales more than 10,000 liters of air. The air inhaled is composed mainly of oxygen and nitrogen, but there are also small amounts of other gases, contaminants such as bacteria and viruses, and many environmental pollutants such as tobacco smoke and automobile exhaust.

Most air pollution is simply irritating, but some pollution can lead to permanent injury or death. The lungs have a series of built-in barriers and defenses to protect function and life; however, with aging and disease, damage to the lungs can occur. Over a person's lifetime, the lungs can become damaged by smoking, occupational exposure, the effects of air pollution, and chronic infection and inflammation. These processes may degrade the lung's defenses, and the result is chronic respiratory problems or various lung diseases.

Anatomy and Physiology

The respiratory system is composed of the lungs, the airways leading to the lungs, the blood vessels serving the lungs, and the chest wall. The right lung has three lobes (upper, middle, and lower). To leave space for the heart, the left lung has two lobes (upper and lower). The lobes consist of segments and lobules. They are shaped like cones and they are textured like a fine-grained sponge that can be inflated with air. The lungs occupy the thoracic cage and stretch from the trachea to below the heart. This coordinated system enables the lung to perform its primary function of rapidly exchanging oxygen from inhaled air with the carbon dioxide in the blood. About 10% of the lung is solid tissue, and the remainder is composed of air and blood (National Heart, Lung, and Blood Institute [NHLBI], 2011).

Air enters the body through the nose or mouth, and travels down the throat and trachea into the chest through a pair of tubes called *bronchi*. The bronchi divide and subdivide into successive generations of narrower and shorter tubes of unequal length and diameter. The final destination for inhaled air is the network of about 3 million air sacs, called **alveoli**, located at the ends of the air passages.

The first branching of the trachea divides toward the left and right lung. The two lungs fill most of the chest cavity. The **mediastinum** is the space between the lungs that contains the heart, the esophagus, the trachea, lymph nodes, and large blood vessels. The chest wall with its muscle and skeletal structure supports the lungs. Through the process of expanding and contracting, it allows movement of air in and out of the lungs during ventilation. The chest wall is lined with a membrane called the pleura that adheres to the surface of the lungs. Normally, a small amount of fluid is present in the pleural space between the pleural lining

of the chest wall and the pleural attachment to the lungs. Typically, the pleural space contains only a small amount of fluid and is free of any gas, blood, or other matter. This fluid provides lubrication and permits free and easy movement of the chest wall and lung expansion during respiration. Figure 16-1 ▶▶▶ illustrates the normal anatomy of the lungs and airways.

The first 16 subdivisions of the **bronchi** (larger air passages of the lungs) ending in terminal **bronchioles** (smaller air passages) are called the conducting airways. Terminal bronchioles are the smallest airways without alveoli. They further divide into respiratory bronchioles, ending in alveolar ducts. Respiratory bronchioles have occasional alveoli budding from their walls, and alveolar ducts are completely lined with alveoli, where gas exchange occurs. The lungs have respiratory and nonrespiratory functions. Respiratory functions include gas exchange or the transfer of oxygen from the air into the blood and the removal of carbon dioxide from the blood. Respiration is accomplished by movement of the chest wall, elastic recoil of the lungs, and airway resistance. Normally, breathing is an automatic process that most people take for granted. However, if one of the three conditions is compromised, breathing can become labored, consume a tremendous amount of energy, and cause a great deal of anxiety and stress. While at rest, it takes about a minute for the total blood volume of the body (about 5 liters) to pass through the lungs. It takes a red cell a fraction of a second to pass through the capillary network. Gas exchange is almost instantaneous during this period (NHLBI, 2011).

Movement of the air into the lungs is controlled by the respiratory muscles of the thorax. These muscles, part of the apparatus responsible for ventilation, include the diaphragm (the muscle that separates the chest from the abdominal cavity) and the muscles that move the ribs. The performance of the respiratory apparatus is coordinated and monitored by specific nerve sites called respiratory centers, located in the brain and in the carotid arteries. The respiratory centers respond to changes in blood levels of oxygen, carbon dioxide, and blood pH. The body works to maintain homeostasis or normal levels of these chemicals by altering rate and depth of respiration (NHLBI, 2011).

Once the oxygen has entered the lungs, it must be distributed to the rest of the body. The oxygen in the lungs passes via alveolar pressure through the capillary beds to enter the circulatory system. The heart pumps to continuously perfuse the pulmonary circulation. When ventilation and perfusion are consistent, the arterial blood is saturated with oxygen.

The nonrespiratory functions of the lungs are mechanical, biochemical, and physiological. The lungs provide the first line of defense against airborne irritants and bacterial, viral, and other infectious agents by entrapping and **lysing**

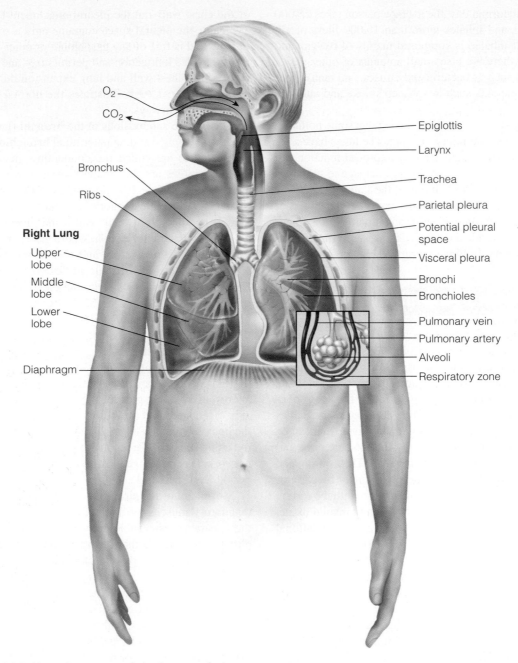

Figure 16-1 ▶▶▶ Normal anatomy of the lungs and airways.

(breaking down) foreign invaders. The lungs also remove volatile and toxic substances generated from metabolism occurring in the body and exhale them with carbon dioxide. Sensitive sensors in the lungs control the flow of water, ions, and large proteins across its various cellular structures. With the liver and kidneys, the lungs remove and control various products of the body's metabolic reactions. Finally, the lungs manufacture a variety of essential hormones and other chemicals that direct and carry out biochemical reactions (NHLBI, 2011).

NORMAL CHANGES OF AGING

The aging process is accompanied by physiological changes to the respiratory system. Differentiating the normal changes of aging from disease-related changes can be difficult. The effects of chronic exposure to tobacco smoke, air pollution, and environmental toxins can further complicate the process of differentiation.

The following changes occur in lung structure and function with normal aging and can limit respiration:

- Stiffening of elastin and the collagen connective tissue supporting the lungs
- Altered alveolar shape resulting in increased alveolar diameter
- Decreased alveolar surface area available for gas exchange
- Increased chest wall stiffness
- Stiffening of the diaphragm

The functional implications of these changes are a decreased elastic recoil of the lung that produces increased residual volume (the amount of air remaining in the lungs at the end of exhalation), decreased vital capacity (the amount of air that moves in and out with inspiration and expiration), and premature airway closure in dependent portions of the lungs, which often traps air in the lower airways. With early airway closure, the mismatch of ventilation and perfusion increases and levels of arterial oxygen decrease. Another factor that can contribute to the decrease in arterial oxygen tension is a decrease in pulmonary diffusion, apparently as a result of the decreased area available for gas exchange. With aging, the amount of oxygen carried by the blood is likely to be lower, and gas exchange will occur more slowly and less efficiently. Figure 16-2 ▶▶▶ illustrates the normal changes of aging in the respiratory system.

> ***Practice Pearl*** ▶▶▶ Lung function in frail older adults is often difficult to assess with your stethoscope because so little air is moved with each inspiration and exhalation that lung sounds are very soft and distant. Always assess lung sounds with your stethoscope directly on the skin (not through clothing), use a good stethoscope with a diaphragm and bell, and seek out a quiet environment.

Changes in Cardiovascular Function

Changes in cardiovascular function that can also affect the pulmonary system include the following:

- Increased stiffness of the heart and blood vessels, rendering these vessels less compliant to increased blood flow demands

- Diastolic dysfunction due to impaired diastolic filling (increased cardiac stiffness)
- Systolic dysfunction due to increased left ventricular afterload (incomplete emptying due to ventricular damage or weakness)
- Decreased cardiac output with rest and with exercise

Changes in Immune Function

The following changes that occur in immune function with normal aging can affect pulmonary function:

- A decrease in the nature and quantity of antibodies produced
- A decrease in effectiveness of the protective cilia of the respiratory tract in removing debris from the airways, allowing more foreign bodies to travel to the lungs
- Decreased production of antibodies after immunization
- Use of medications that can suppress immune function such as corticosteroids, chemotherapeutic agents, and antirejection transplant drugs

Decreased levels of total serum IgE, reduced T-lymphocyte function, and less efficient phagocytosis result in decreased cell-mediated immune function. For older people, the overall decline in immune function results in increased susceptibility to tuberculosis, pneumonia, and influenza. Even after immunization, older people mount a less efficient immune response, and immunity is reduced and of shorter duration (Gerontological Society of America [GSA], 2011). Use of glucocorticoid and antineoplastic medications can suppress immune response and further place an older person at risk for acquiring a respiratory bacterial or viral infection.

> ***Practice Pearl*** ▶▶▶ Smoking paralyzes and damages protective cilia. (During sleep the cilia try to recover and in the morning the smoker may experience relentless coughing, producing large amounts of phlegm.)

Changes in Neurologic, Neuromuscular, and Sensory Functions

Aging results in neuron loss in the brain and central nervous system, which increases reaction time, decreases the ability to respond to multiple complex stimuli, and may impair the ability to adapt and interact with the environment. Changes that can affect pulmonary function include the following:

- Loss of muscle tone, exacerbated by deconditioning, obesity, and sedentary lifestyle
- Increased thoracic rigidity and osteoporotic changes to the spine (kyphosis)

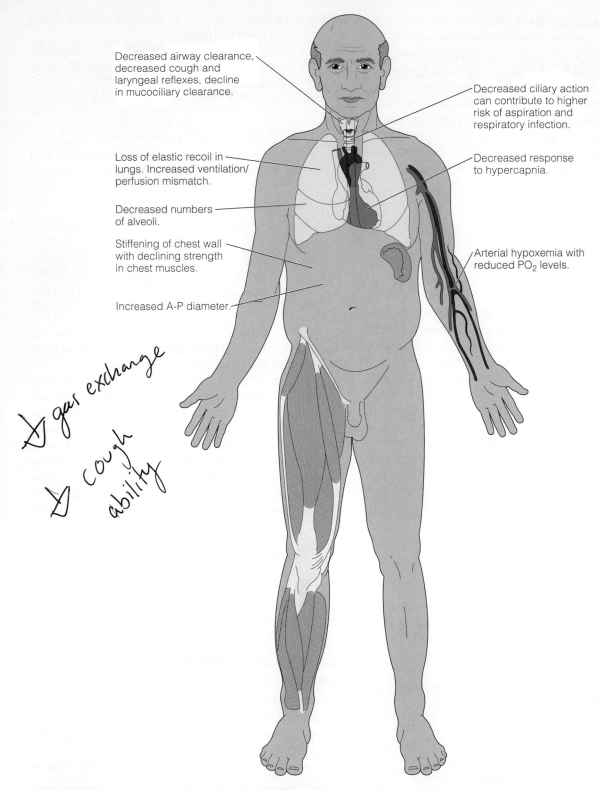

Decreased airway clearance, decreased cough and laryngeal reflexes, decline in mucociliary clearance.

Decreased ciliary action can contribute to higher risk of aspiration and respiratory infection.

Loss of elastic recoil in lungs. Increased ventilation/perfusion mismatch.

Decreased response to hypercapnia.

Decreased numbers of alveoli.

Stiffening of chest wall with declining strength in chest muscles.

Arterial hypoxemia with reduced PO_2 levels.

Increased A-P diameter.

↓ gas exchange

↓ cough ability

Figure 16-2 ▶▶▶ Normal changes of aging in the respiratory system.

- Use of medications such as opioids, diuretics, and beta-blockers that can cause fatigue, depression of the cough reflex, insomnia, dehydration, and bronchospasm
- Diagnosis of neurologic disease or impairment (dementia, Parkinson disease, stroke/cerebrovascular accident)

Older people with decreased muscle tone and osteoporosis of the spine are less able to accomplish complete chest expansion and as a result are more likely to have decreased tidal volumes. Inability to completely fill the lungs with air can lead to atelectasis (areas of the lung that become incapable of expansion and gas exchange) over time, further decreasing respiratory efficiency. Sedative and opioid medications, diuretics, anxiolytics, cough suppressants, and beta-blockers can also decrease neuromuscular function. These medications can contribute to the risk of aspiration pneumonia by suppressing the cough reflex, making oral secretions thicker, decreasing ambulation, and triggering bronchospasm (Reuben et al., 2011).

HEALTHY AGING TIPS

‖‖

▶ Don't smoke. If you do smoke, quit immediately.

▶ Avoid secondhand smoke.

▶ Avoid urban air pollution to the maximum extent possible.

▶ Wear a mask when there is danger of breathing airborne toxins such as spray paint, cleaning solutions, and other hazardous materials.

▶ Eat a healthy diet and maintain a normal weight.

▶ Stay active with daily exercise.

▶ Avoid allergens.

▶ Wash your hands often and avoid direct contact with others suffering from respiratory infections.

▶ Make sure to get a yearly flu vaccination and the pneumonia vaccine at the age of 65 to prevent infection.

Respiratory Diseases Common in Older People

Age-related changes in the lungs, years of exposure to air pollutants and cigarette smoke, and the presence of comorbidities may predispose the older person to respiratory diseases and pulmonary dysfunction. The following diseases are commonly diagnosed pulmonary diseases in the older person.

Asthma

Asthma is a chronic respiratory disease characterized by usually reversible airflow obstruction, airway inflammation, increased mucous secretion production, and increased airway responsiveness (contraction of airway smooth muscles) to a variety of stimuli. Asthma is often overlooked in the older person and can present as a newly diagnosed disease or as a chronic disease that the older person has lived with for many years. Undiagnosed and untreated asthma in the older person detracts from quality of life and contributes to frailty. In older patients, complete reversibility of airflow problems becomes more difficult, especially in those patients with severe and persistent problems, because of the irreversible damage done to the airways by years of inflammatory changes and scarring. Over time, plugging of the bronchioles occurs along with scarring and narrowing of the airways. Normal changes of aging in the lung may interact with asthma-related pathophysiology to further produce irreversible airflow obstruction (Sanassi, 2011). Figure 16-3 ▶▶▶ illustrates a comparison of a normal airway and a scarred and inflamed airway like that typically found in an older patient with asthma, bronchitis, or emphysema.

With asthma, inflamed airways are characterized as "twitchy" and overreact to common irritants like viruses, cigarette smoke, cold air, and allergens. These triggers can activate an inflammatory response including mobilization of mast cells, eosinophils, macrophages, and T lymphocytes. With these inflammatory changes, airway smooth muscle contracts, swells, and produces excessive mucous secretions. With this airway narrowing and inflammation, it becomes difficult for the older person to breathe. The common symptoms of an asthma attack include the following:

- Coughing—may be worse at night
- Wheezing—usually high-pitched whistling sounds on expiration
- Shortness of breath
- Chest tightness

Nurses' Asthma Education Partnership Project, 2003.

These symptoms occur or worsen when the older person experiences:

- Physical exercise
- Viral infection
- Inhaled allergens (animal fur, mold, pollen, dust mites, cockroach or mouse excrement)
- Stress and/or strong emotional expression (laughing or crying)
- Irritants (tobacco or wood smoke, ozone, other chemicals)
- Changes in the weather

NHLBI, 2007.

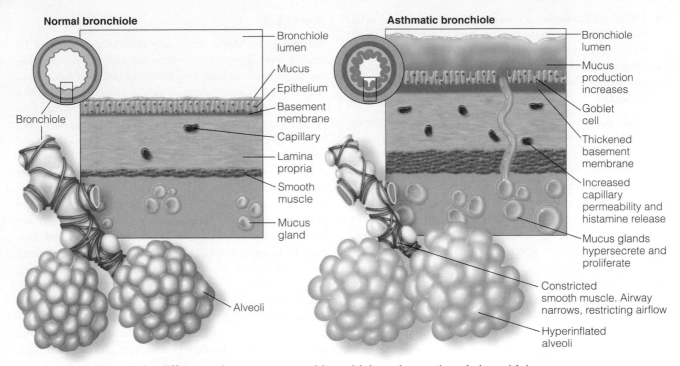

Figure 16-3 ▶▶▶ Note the differences between a normal bronchiole and an asthmatic bronchiole.

Figure 16-4 ▶▶▶ illustrates the relationship between airway inflammation, hyperresponsiveness, airway obstruction, and asthma symptoms.

Mortality from asthma in older adults is reportedly increasing, but it is difficult to define the cause of death in many older people with lung diseases. In 2011, approximately 18.7 million Americans, including 2.6 million older adults, had been diagnosed with asthma. In 2011, more than 1 million older adults had an asthma attack or episode (Centers for Disease Control and Prevention [CDC], 2011d). Every year, asthma puts nearly half a million people in the hospital and kills an estimated 3,500 (CDC, 2011d). Hospital admission rates are 40% to 70% higher for African Americans than Caucasians, and the admission rates for women are approximately 20% to 40% higher than for men in both races. Additionally, the death rate from asthma for African Americans is three times higher than the death rate for other groups. In 2008, 105.5 per 1,000 African Americans had asthma compared to 78.2 per 1,000 Caucasians. The asthma prevalence rate among African Americans was more than 35% higher than the rate for Caucasians (American Lung Association [ALA], 2008).

At any age, the diagnosis of asthma is based on the clinical history, physical examination, and laboratory studies.

When asthma is diagnosed in an older person, other lung and cardiovascular diseases must be eliminated. It is sometimes difficult to distinguish between exacerbations of chronic bronchitis, chronic obstructive pulmonary disease (COPD), and asthma, especially in current and former smokers (McPhee & Papadakis, 2011). The differential diagnosis should also include pulmonary embolism, gastroesophageal reflux disease (GERD), mechanical obstruction of the airway, cough secondary to drugs (angiotensin-converting enzyme [ACE] inhibitors), and vocal cord dysfunction. Additionally, many older people with congestive heart failure will present with signs and symptoms that mimic those of asthma. Table 16-1 presents some of the signs and symptoms of common lung diseases.

Practice Pearl ▶▶▶ Nocturnal dyspnea (feeling of being air starved or short of breath or experiencing labored breathing) occurring with asthma is most likely to take place between 4 a.m. and 6 a.m., whereas nocturnal dyspnea occurring with congestive heart failure typically occurs 1 to 2 hours after retiring. The nurse should try to pinpoint the exact time that breathing difficulties occur.

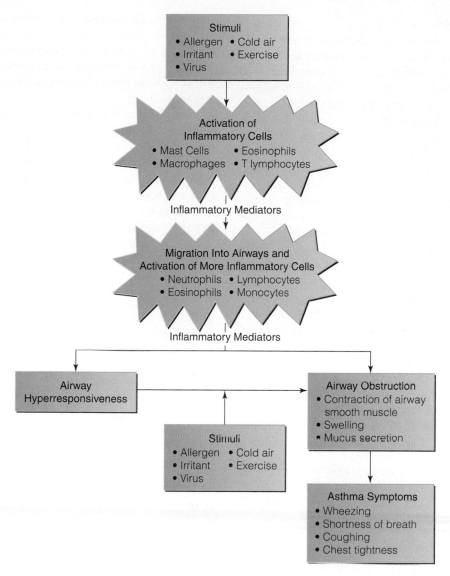

Figure 16-4 ▶▶▶ Relationships between airway inflammation, airway hyperresponsiveness, airway obstruction, and asthma symptoms.

TABLE 16-1 **Signs and Symptoms of Common Lung Diseases**

Symptom	Asthma	Chronic Bronchitis	Chronic Obstructive Pulmonary Disease	Heart Failure
Wheezing	+	+	+	+
Chest tightness	+	+	+	+
Chronic cough with sputum	+	+		+/–
Nocturnal dyspnea	+			+
Smoking history		+	++	+/–

Diagnostic Studies

The physician and/or nurse practitioner will most likely examine the results of pulmonary function tests, chest radiography, electrocardiography, and a complete blood count with differential to confirm the diagnosis of asthma in the older person. The electrocardiogram will help identify the presence of cardiac disease and the risk associated with certain medications that may be used to treat the older patient with asthma and cardiac disease. The chest X-ray in the older person with asthma is usually negative, but the presence of lesions may indicate acute infection, lung tumor, or other abnormalities. Additionally, cardiomegaly and pulmonary congestion would indicate the presence of underlying heart disease. Hyperinflation of the lungs would indicate **emphysema.** The presence of a large number of eosinophils in the blood may indicate an allergic component as a predictor of asthma, but these numbers may be low in some older patients taking corticosteroids or chemotherapeutic agents or in those with a decreased immune response because of the presence of other illnesses.

Pulmonary function tests are the most reliable way to diagnose asthma and differentiate it from other illnesses such as COPD. Spirometry is used to measure the volume of air expired in 1 second from maximum inspiration (FEV_1) and the total amount of air expired as rapidly as possible (forced vital capacity, FVC). The diagnosis of asthma is confirmed by:

- Demonstrated airflow obstruction of FEV_1 less than 80% of predicted and an FEV_1/FVC ratio of less than 70%.
- Evidence that airflow obstruction is reversible (greater than 12% and 200 mL in FEV_1, after the administration of a bronchodilator or over time after a course of corticosteroids).
- Peak expiratory flow (PEF) measurements indicating the maximum flow (expressed in liters per second) that can be generated during a forced expiratory maneuver with fully inflated lungs as measured using a peak flow meter. PEF measurements before and after bronchodilator administration may be useful in confirming the asthma diagnosis. A pattern of greater than 20% variation in PEF from late afternoon to arising the next morning confirms the presence of variable airflow obstructions, often indicative of asthma.

McPhee & Papadakis, 2011; NHLBI, 2007.

Spirometry testing in the older adult can pose practical problems that must be addressed to obtain accurate results. Increasing rigidity of the chest wall, anxiety, weakness or paresthesia in the upper extremities, cognitive impairment, and poor eye–hand coordination can be factors leading to poor results. The gerontological nurse along with the pulmonologist, allergist, and a skilled respiratory therapist may be called on to assist the older patient with spirometry testing. Accurate and reproducible spirometry techniques will provide the necessary information to reach an accurate diagnosis.

Once diagnostic testing is completed, asthma is classified as to severity so that the appropriate treatment and monitoring may be initiated. The four ratings include intermittent, mild persistent, moderate persistent, or severe persistent, and are based on duration of symptoms, presence and severity of nocturnal symptoms, and results of spirometry testing. The goal of treatment is to reduce the frequency and severity of symptoms and improve results of spirometry testing.

Based on the classification of severity, medications are prescribed using the following goals of therapy for asthma control:

- Prevent troublesome symptoms (coughing, breathlessness in the daytime, at night, or after exercise).
- Prevent recurrent exacerbations of asthma and minimize the need for emergency department visits and/or hospitalization.
- Maintain normal activity levels.
- Maintain normal or nearly normal pulmonary function.
- Minimize use of "rescue" short-acting inhaled beta$_2$-agonist (less than 2 days/week).
- Minimal or no adverse effects from medication.

NHLBI, 2007; Nurses' Asthma Education Partnership Project, 2003.

The medications used to treat asthma in the older person do not differ significantly from those used with younger people. However, the risk of adverse effects and the potential for drug interactions are greater because of the use of additional medications to treat coexisting conditions.

Inhaled corticosteroid therapy is the most effective anti-inflammatory treatment for asthma. Use of inhaled corticosteroids has reduced the morbidity and mortality associated with asthma exacerbations (Sanassi, 2011). Adverse effects of inhaled corticosteroids include electrolyte and fluid imbalances in older patients with cardiac or renal disease, the possibility of hypokalemia when the patient is taking a thiazide diuretic, worsening of hypertension, and elevated blood sugar and blood urea nitrogen (BUN) readings in patients with diabetes. Additionally, oral corticosteroids can negatively affect cognitive function, accelerate osteoporosis, cause oral thrush (candidiasis), increase intraocular pressure, and aggravate peptic and gastric ulcers (Partners Health Care, 2010). As with all drugs, the benefits of inhaled corticosteroids must be weighed against their risks. Inhaled corticosteroids are important to facilitate control of asthma in older adults and to avoid the adverse effects of systemic corticosteroids and asthma exacerbations. Although safer than systemic therapy, long-term inhaled corticosteroid use in relatively high doses (>1.6 mg/day) can cause dose-dependent adverse effects similar to those seen with oral doses (Partners Health Care, 2010). Some medication can remain in the mouth after inhalation and be swallowed into the stomach and absorbed systemically. Patients should be urged to use spacers with their metered-dose inhalers and rinse and spit after use of inhaled corticosteroids.

Cromolyn sodium does not appear to be as effective in the older person as it is in children, but this may be related to the presence of additional lung pathology in the older person with asthma. Leukotriene antagonists interfere with the synthesis or action of leukotrienes that can cause bronchospasm, and their use may decrease the need for inhaled steroids in some older people.

Inhaled beta$_2$-agonists are short-acting medications that are effective bronchodilators for all asthma patients. Both long- and short-acting beta$_2$-agonists are available. Only short-acting beta$_2$-agonists (Proventil, Ventolin) should be used for rescue from sudden onset of wheezing, tightness in the chest, or shortness of breath. Long-acting bronchodilators have a duration of action exceeding 12 hours and may reduce asthma symptoms and the frequency of exacerbations. However, long-acting beta$_2$-agonists (Serevent) are not to be used as rescue medications because of their delayed onset and longer duration of action. Side effects from long-acting beta$_2$-agonist therapy include the following:

- Tachycardia, an increased consumption of myocardial oxygen (can induce angina in some older patients)
- Electrocardiographic changes, including ventricular arrhythmias
- Hypokalemia
- Increased blood pressure
- Tremor
- Hypoxemia

NHLBI, 2007; Reuben et al., 2011.

Practice Pearl ▶▶▶ Patients who require the use of rescue inhalers should obtain prescriptions for extra canisters and keep several inhalers in strategic places in the home. It also helps to label them with bright red tape so they can be easily seen if needed quickly.

Methylxanthine (theophylline) is a bronchodilator that may have mild anti-inflammatory effects and is no longer widely used to treat asthma. Currently, many clinical practice guidelines list theophylline as a "not preferred" alternative while recommending newer agents and expressing concerns regarding the risk–benefit ratio of the drug. This has resulted in the drug falling out of favor. Nevertheless, its low cost offers an advantage over other long-term maintenance medications that are added to inhaled glucocorticoids, such as montelukast and long-acting beta agonists and in certain limited circumstances, it may still be used (UpToDate, 2012). It has a narrow therapeutic index and can interact with many other drugs. During therapy serum methylxanthine levels should be measured to prevent toxicity. This drug is associated with the following adverse effects:

- Supraventricular tachycardia, nausea, vomiting, headache, seizures, hyperglycemia, and hypokalemia
- Exercise-induced angina and ST-segment depression
- Toxicity due to metabolic changes in older people

If used, careful monitoring is needed to keep the serum concentrations between 8 and 12 mcg/mL.

Ipratropium bromide is a synthetic atropine-like compound that is sometimes used to treat asthma in the older person. Ipratropium has a lower incidence of tremor and arrhythmia and is associated with the relatively mild side effects of dry mouth and pharyngeal irritation. Older patients on this medication should be carefully monitored for symptoms of xerostomia or dry mouth.

Leukotriene modifiers are powerful mediators that block the release of agents causing inflammation from mast cells, eosinophils, and basophils. These drugs can be used before exercise to block exercise-induced asthma and as an alternative to low doses of inhaled corticosteroids.

A newer class of drugs known as immunomodulators is made from recombinant DNA. These drugs bind with receptors to prevent inflammation by keeping mast cells and basophils from recognizing allergens. The immunomodulators were approved by the U.S. Food and Drug Administration (FDA) for use in 2003 for moderate to severe persistent asthma in those patients who have skin test reactions to allergens and whose symptoms cannot be controlled with inhaled corticosteroids (Sanassi, 2011).

Table 16-2 lists common asthma medications and potential adverse effects.

Some older patients with asthma may prefer nebulizer rather than metered-dose inhaler delivery because of the moisturizing effect of a nebulizer and the decreased need for hand–diaphragm coordination. Nebulizer treatments are an effective way to administer inhaled medications to those with cognitive impairments. Regardless of whether the older patient is using a metered-dose inhaler or nebulizer, proper instruction is needed to administer the medication and care for the equipment. Those choosing a metered-dose inhaler should use a spacer that will allow the medication to be inhaled at a slower rate and be less likely to stimulate a cough reflex. See Figure 16-5 ▶▶▶ for the proper use of a metered-dose inhaler, spacer, and nebulizer.

TABLE 16-2	Asthma Medications and Potential Adverse Effects	
Class of Therapeutic Agent	**Drug**	**Potential Adverse Clinical Effects**
Anti-inflammatory	Oral corticosteroids	↑ Blood pressure, edema, congestive heart failure due to Na$^+$ retention
		Hypokalemia, alkalosis, and resulting arrhythmias due to K$^+$ and H$^+$ excretion
		Worsening diabetes mellitus, cataracts, polyuria with dehydration due to elevated blood glucose
		Thinning of the skin, reduced muscle mass with myopathy, osteoporosis, blood urea nitrogen without change in renal blood flow due to protein catabolism
		Hypoadrenalism due to decreased ACTH
		Cataracts
		Altered cognitive function, depression, delirium
		Joint effusions and articular pain with corticosteroid withdrawal
		Osteoporosis due to decreased calcium absorption
		Glaucoma due to decreased absorption of aqueous humor
		Aggravation of existing peptic ulcer disease
	Inhaled corticosteroids (high doses, e.g., >1.6 mg/day)	Cough, dysphonia, loss of taste, laryngomalacia, oral candidiasis
		Effects on ACTH secretion with hypoadrenalism may be related to the effects on calcium absorption with acceleration of osteoporosis
		Development of cataracts
	Cromolyn sodium	Cough and irritation, unpleasant taste in mouth
	Nedocromil	No significant adverse effect known
Bronchodilator	Short-acting beta$_2$-agonists	Myocardial ischemia due to ↑ myocardial oxygen consumption and mild increase in hypoxemia
		Complex ventricular arrhythmia due to ↑ myocardial irritability
		Cardiac arrhythmias and muscle weakness related to hypokalemia
		Hypotension or hypertension
		Tremor
		With excessive use, ↓ bronchodilator effect and ↑ airway hyperresponsiveness related to down-regulation. of beta receptors
	Long-acting beta$_2$-agonists	Same as for short-acting beta$_2$-agonists
	Theophylline	Cardiac arrhythmias, effect is related to ↑ catecholamine release and is additive with beta$_2$-agonists
		Nausea and vomiting from gastric irritation, gastroesophageal reflux
		Insomnia, seizures related to central nervous system stimulant
		Cardiac arrhythmia due to inotropic and chronotropic effects
		Serum levels increased by heart failure, liver disease, beta-blocker therapy, selected H$_2$-blocker therapy, quinolone therapy, macrolide therapy, ketoconazole therapy
	Ipratropium bromide	Mucosal dryness and other anticholinergic side effects
Leukotriene modifiers	Montelukast	Administer 1 hour before or 2 hours after meals. Monitor liver function tests.
Immunomodulators	Omalizumab	Monitor for anaphylaxis for 2 hours following first three injections

Source: National Asthma Education and Prevention Program, Expert Panel Report 3, 2007, U.S. Department of Health and Human Services, National Institutes of Health, National Heart, Lung, and Blood Institute; McPhee & Papadakis, 2011.

SPACERS: MAKING INHALED MEDICINES EASIER TO TAKE

Unless you use your inhaler the right way, much of the medicine may end up on your tongue, on the back of your throat, or in the air. Use of a spacer or holding chamber can help prevent this problem.

A spacer or holding chamber is a device that attaches to a metered-dose inhaler. It holds the medicine in its chamber long enough for you to inhale it in one or two slow deep breaths.

The spacer makes it easier to use the medicines the right way. It helps you not cough when using an inhaler. A spacer will also help prevent you from getting a yeast infection in your mouth (thrush) when taking inhaled steroid medicines.

There are many models of spacers or holding chambers that you can purchase through your pharmacist or a medical supply company. Ask your doctor about the different models.

HOW TO USE A SPACER

1. Attach the inhaler to the spacer or holding chamber as explained by your doctor or by using the directions that come with the product.

2. Shake well.

3. Press the button on the inhaler. This will put one puff of the medicine in the holding chamber.

4. Place the mouthpiece of the spacer in your mouth and inhale slowly. (A face mask may be helpful for a young child.)

5. Hold your breath for a few seconds and then exhale. Repeat steps 4 and 5.

6. If your doctor has prescribed two puffs, wait between puffs for the amount of time he or she has directed and repeat steps 2 through 5.

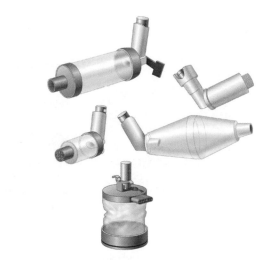

There are a variety of spacers.

YOUR METERED-DOSE INHALER: HOW TO USE IT

Using a metered-dose inhaler is a good way to take asthma medicines. There are few side effects because the medicine goes right to the lungs and not to other parts of the body. It takes only 5 to 10 minutes for inhaled $beta_2$-agonists to have an effect compared to the liquid or pill form, which can take 15 minutes to 1 hour. Inhalers can be used by all asthma patients age 5 and older. A spacer or holding chamber attached to the inhaler can help make taking the medicine easier.

The inhaler must be cleaned often to prevent buildup that will clog it or reduce how well it works.

■ The guidelines that follow will help you use the inhaler the correct way.

■ Ask your doctor or nurse to show you how to use the inhaler.

(continued)

Figure 16-5 ▶▶▶ Instructions for proper use of a metered-dose inhaler, spacer, and nebulizer.

Source: Nurses: Partners in Asthma Care, National Asthma Education and Prevention Program, National Heart, Lung, and Blood Institute, NIH Publication No. 95–3308, 1995.

USING THE INHALER

1. Remove the cap and hold the inhaler upright.

2. Shake the inhaler.

3. Tilt your head back slightly and breathe out.

4. Use the inhaler in any one of these ways. (A and B are the best ways. B is recommended for young children, older adults, and those taking inhaled steroids. C is okay if you are having trouble with A or B.)

   A. Open mouth with inhaler 1 to 2 inches away.

   B. Use spacer (refer to previous section).

   C. Put inhaler in mouth and seal lips around the mouthpiece.

5. Press down on the inhaler to release the medicine as you start to breathe in slowly.

6. Breathe in *slowly* for 3 to 5 seconds.

7. *Hold* your breath for 10 seconds to allow the medicine to reach deeply into your lungs.

8. Repeat puffs as prescribed. Waiting 1 minute between puffs may permit the second puff to go deeper into the lungs.

Note: Dry powder capsules are used differently. To use a dry powder inhaler, close your mouth tightly around the mouthpiece and inhale very fast.

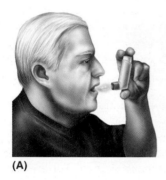 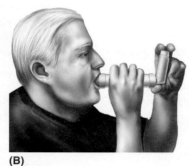 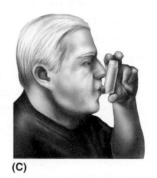

(A) (B) (C)

CLEANING

1. Once a day clean the inhaler and cap by rinsing it in warm running water. Let it dry before you use it again. Have another inhaler to use while it is drying. Do not put the canister holding cromolyn or nedocromil in water.

2. Twice a week wash the L-shaped plastic mouthpiece with mild dishwashing soap and warm water. Rinse and dry well before putting the canister back inside the mouthpiece.

CHECKING HOW LONG A CANISTER WILL LAST

1. Check the canister label to see how many "puffs" it contains.

2. Figure out how many puffs you will take per day (e.g., 2 puffs, 4 times a day = 8 puffs a day). Divide this number into the number of puffs contained in the canister. That tells you how long the canister should last.

   Example:
   Canister contains 200 puffs.
   You take 2 puffs, 4 times a day, which equals 8 puffs/day.
   200 ÷ 8 = 25. The canister will last 25 days.

HOW TO USE AND CARE FOR YOUR NEBULIZER

A nebulizer is a device driven by a compressed air machine. It allows you to take asthma medicine in the form of a mist (wet aerosol). It consists of a cup, a mouthpiece attached to a T-shaped part or a mask, and thin, plastic tubing to connect to the compressed air machine. It is used mostly by three types of patients:

- ■ Children under age 5.
- ■ Patients who have problems using metered-dose inhalers.
- ■ Patients with severe asthma.

A nebulizer helps to make sure you get the right amount of medicine.

Routinely cleaning the nebulizer is important because an unclean nebulizer may cause an infection. A good cleaning routine keeps the nebulizer from clogging up and helps it last longer. (See instructions with nebulizer.)

Directions for using the compressed air machine may vary (check the machine's directions), but generally the tubing has to be put into the outlet of the machine before it is turned on.

Figure 16-5 ▶▶▶ *(continued)*

HOW TO USE A NEBULIZER

1a. If your machine is premixed, measure the correct amount of medicine using a clean dropper and put it into the cup. Go to step 2.

1b. If your medicine is not premixed, measure the correct amount of saline—using a clean dropper—and put it into the cup. Then measure the correct amount of medicine using a *different* clean dropper and put it into the cup with the saline. (Do NOT mix the droppers; use one for saline and another for the medicine.) Put an "S" for saline on one dropper with nail polish.

2. Fasten the mouthpiece to the T-shaped part and then fasten this unit to the cup OR fasten the mask to the cup. For a child over the age of 2, use a mouthpiece unit because it will deliver more medicine than a mask.

3. Put the mouthpiece in your mouth. Seal your lips tightly around it OR place the mask on your face.

4. Turn on the air compressor machine.

5. Take slow, deep breaths in through the mouth.

6. Hold each breath 1 to 2 seconds before breathing out.

7. Continue until the medicine is gone from the cup (approximately 10 minutes).

8. Store the medicine as directed after each use.

CLEANING THE NEBULIZER

Don't forget: Cleaning and getting rid of germs prevent infection. Cleaning keeps the nebulizer from clogging up and helps it last longer.

Cleaning Needed After Each Use

1. Remove the mask or the mouthpiece and T-shaped part from the cup. Remove the tubing and set it aside. The tubing should not be washed or rinsed. The outside should be wiped down. Rinse the mask or mouthpiece and T-shaped part—as well as the eyedropper or syringe—in warm running water for 30 seconds. Use distilled or sterile water for rinsing, if possible.

2. Shake off excess water. Air dry on a clean cloth or paper towel.

3. Put the mask or the mouthpiece and T-shaped part, cup, and tubing back together and connect the device to the compressed air machine. Run the machine for 10 to 20 seconds to dry the inside of the nebulizer.

4. Disconnect the tubing from the compressed air machine. Store the nebulizer in a ziplock plastic bag.

5. Place the cover over the compressed air machine.

Cleaning Needed Once Every Day

1. Remove the mask or the mouthpiece and T-shaped part from the cup. Remove the tubing and set it aside. The tubing should not be washed or rinsed.

2. Wash the mask or the mouthpiece and T-shaped part—as well as the eyedropper or syringe—with a mild dishwashing soap and warm water.

3. Rinse under a strong stream of water for 30 seconds. Use distilled (or sterile) water if possible.

4. Shake off excess water. Air dry on a clean cloth or paper towel.

5. Put the mask or the mouthpiece and T-shaped part, cup, and tubing back together and connect the device to the compressed air machine. Run the machine for 10 to 20 seconds to dry the inside of the nebulizer.

6. Disconnect the tubing from the compressed air machine. Store the nebulizer in a ziplock plastic bag.

7. Place a cover over the compressed air machine.

Cleaning Needed Once or Twice a Week

1. Remove the mask or the mouthpiece and T-shaped part from the cup. Remove the tubing and set it aside. The tubing should not be washed or rinsed. Wash the mask or the mouthpiece and T-shaped part—as well as the eyedropper or syringe—with a mild dishwashing soap and warm water.

2. Rinse under a strong stream of water for 30 seconds.

3. Soak for 30 minutes in a solution that is one part distilled white vinegar and two parts distilled water. Throw out the vinegar water solution after use; do not reuse it.

4. Rinse the nebulizer parts and the eyedropper or syringe under warm running water for 1 minute. Use distilled or sterile water, if possible.

5. Shake off excess water. Air dry on a clean cloth or paper towel.

6. Put the mask or the mouthpiece and T-shaped part, cup, and tubing back together and connect the device to the compressed air machine. Run the machine for 10 to 20 seconds to dry the inside of the nebulizer thoroughly.

7. Disconnect the tubing from the compressed air machine. Store the nebulizer in a ziplock plastic bag.

8. Clean the surface of the compressed air machine with a well-wrung, soapy cloth or sponge. You could never use an alcohol or disinfectant wipe. NEVER PUT THE COMPRESSED AIR MACHINE IN WATER.

9. Place a cover over the compressed air machine.

Figure 16-5 ▶▶▶ *(continued)*

> *Practice Pearl* ▶▶▶ Several medications now
> come prepared as dry powder inhalers and contain no
> propellant. Patients should activate the dispenser, place
> their lips around the mouthpiece, and inhale quickly.
> The dry powder is inhaled into the upper airway when
> done properly.
>
> Older patients using inhaled steroids should rinse
> their mouths with warm water and expectorate after
> medication administration. This will prevent the
> overgrowth of candidiasis or thrush, prevent gum
> disease, and deter tooth decay. The nurse should report
> the presence of painful white lesions in the mouth
> (thrush) to the healthcare provider for treatment.

Certain medications should be avoided when treating patients with asthma because adverse reactions can exacerbate asthmatic problems. These drugs include:

- **Beta-blockers.** Commonly used to treat hypertension in older people, beta-blockers (such as propranolol) can induce bronchospasm. Even ophthalmologic solutions like timolol should be avoided if possible. Hypoxemia can result from bronchospasm and lead to serious consequences.
- **Nonsteroidal anti-inflammatory drugs (NSAIDs).** Sudden, potentially life-threatening bronchospasm has been associated with NSAID and aspirin use in older patients.
- **Diuretics.** Hypokalemia can develop for patients taking thiazide (non–potassium sparing) diuretics. Hypokalemia can be associated with cardiac arrhythmias, especially for those taking digitalis.
- **Antihistamines.** The QT interval can be prolonged in older patients taking beta$_2$-agonists or diuretics. The sedative effect of some antihistamines is also of concern.
- **ACE inhibitors.** Widely used as antihypertensives, ACE inhibitors can produce cough in some patients. This may exacerbate asthma symptoms, causing increases in doses of currently prescribed asthma medications or addition of new medications to achieve control.
- **Antidepressants.** Corticosteroids can worsen underlying depression in the older person and interact with monoamine oxidase (MAO) inhibitors and tricyclic antidepressants.

Table 16-3 lists nonasthma medications with increased potential for adverse effects in older patients with asthma. The gerontological nurse should carefully review the therapeutic effects and side effects,

and monitor for interactions with other medications. Beta-adrenergic blocking agents can trigger acute bronchospasm and hypoxemia, even when administered as ophthalmologic solutions (timolol) and should be avoided if possible.

After the healthcare provider has classified the severity of the asthma and prescribed a treatment plan, it is crucial that the patient be instructed in the use of a peak flow meter. The peak flow meter measures how well air moves in and out of the lungs and will alert older patients to narrowing of the airways hours before the onset of asthma symptoms. By taking medications before the onset of symptoms, the asthma attack may be lessened in severity or stopped completely. Further, the peak flow meter can alert the patient and the healthcare provider by:

- Illustrating the response of various conditions like exercise, exposure to cold weather, and psychological stress
- Monitoring the effect of medications
- Indicating when medication changes are needed
- Indicating that emergency care is needed

The peak flow meter should be used:

- Every day for the first 2 weeks after diagnosis or with change in treatment
- Mornings after awakening and between noon and 2 p.m.
- Before and after taking beta$_2$-agonists to document effect
- When symptoms occur such as wheezing or tightness in the chest
- When the patient feels he or she is coming down with a cold or respiratory infection

Patients should keep a peak flow diary and carefully record readings. At the time of asthma diagnosis, the healthcare provider will inform patients of their "personal best" or highest peak flow number achieved over a 2-week period when asthma is under good control. Good control indicates a feeling of respiratory well-being for the patient and absence of asthma symptoms. Peak flow readings can be classified into three categories:

1. Green zone (80% to 100% of personal best) indicating *good control.* No asthma symptoms are present and medication should be taken as usual.
2. Yellow zone (50% to 79% of personal best) indicating *caution.* An asthma attack may be starting and the patient may not be under control. Medication changes may be needed.

TABLE 16-3	Medications With Increased Potential for Adverse Effects in the Older Patient With Asthma		
Medication	**Comorbid Condition(s) for Which Drug Is Prescribed**	**Adverse Effect**	**Comment**
Beta-adrenergic blocking agent	Hypertension Heart disease Tremor Glaucoma	Worsening asthma • Bronchospasm • Decreased response to bronchodilator Decreased response to epinephrine in anaphylaxis	Avoid where possible; when must be used, use of a highly cardioselective drug is okay.
Nonsteroidal anti-inflammatory drugs	Arthritis Musculoskeletal diseases	Worsening asthma • Bronchospasm	Not all older adults with asthma are intolerant of NSAIDs, but NSAIDs are best avoided if possible.
Non–potassium-sparing diuretics	Hypertension Heart failure	Worsening cardiac function/dysrhythmias due to hypokalemia	Additive effect with antiasthma medications that also produce potassium loss (steroids, beta-agonist); older adults also more likely to receive drugs (e.g., digitalis) where hypokalemia is of increased concern.
Certain nonsedating antihistamines (terfenadine and astemizole)	Allergic rhinitis	Worsening cardiac function/ventricular arrhythmias due to prolonged QT_c interval	
Cholinergic agents	Urinary retention Glaucoma	Bronchospasm Bronchorrhea	Also note that some over-the-counter asthma medications contain ephedrine, which could aggravate urinary retention, glaucoma.
ACE inhibitors	Heart failure Hypertension	Increased incidence of cough	

Source: National Asthma Education and Prevention Program Expert Panel Report 3, 2007. U.S. Department of Health and Human Services, National Institutes of Health, National Heart, Lung, and Blood Institute.

3. Red zone (below 50% of personal best) indicating *danger*. The patient should take a short-acting beta$_2$-agonist immediately and notify the healthcare provider.

Figure 16-6 ▶▶▶ includes instructions for the proper use of a peak flow meter, a sample peak flow diary, and a sample asthma management plan. The gerontological nurse can greatly improve the asthma management plan by teaching the older patient and family members about the peak flow meter and diary so that asthma attacks can be minimized or avoided. Having a written plan and instructions to refer to can improve medication adherence and reduce confusion should the older patient become short of breath or start to wheeze.

Older patients with asthma should be instructed that because of their sensitive airways, they may need to avoid allergens and triggers to asthma attacks. Many times, older patients will undergo allergy testing or report anecdotal evidence that being around certain things can trigger an asthma attack. The common offenders are the following:

■ House-dust mites
■ Animals
■ Cockroaches
■ Tobacco smoke
■ Wood smoke
■ Strong odors and sprays
■ Colds and infections
■ Exercise
■ Weather
■ Pollens
■ Molds

HOW TO USE YOUR PEAK FLOW METER

A peak flow meter is a device that measures how well air moves out of your lungs. During an asthma episode the airways of the lungs begin to narrow slowly. The peak flow meter will tell you if there is narrowing in the airways days—even hours—before you have any symptoms of asthma.

By taking your medicine(s) early (before symptoms), you may be able to stop the episode quickly and avoid a severe episode of asthma. Peak flow meters are used to check your asthma the way that blood pressure cuffs are used to check high blood pressure.

The peak flow meter can also be used to help you and your doctor.

- Learn what makes your asthma worse.
- Decide if your medicine plan is working well.
- Decide when to add or stop medicine.
- Decide when to seek emergency care.

A peak flow meter is most helpful for patients who must take asthma medicine daily. Patients age 5 and older are able to use a peak flow meter. Ask your doctor or nurse to show you how to use a peak flow meter.

HOW TO USE YOUR PEAK FLOW METER

- Do the following five steps with your peak flow meter:
  1. Put the indicator at the bottom of the numbered scale.
  2. Stand up.
  3. Take a deep breath.
  4. Place the meter in your mouth and close your lips around the mouthpiece. Do not put your tongue inside the hole.
  5. Blow out as hard and fast as you can.
- Write down the number you get.
- Repeat steps 1 through 5 two more times and write down the numbers you get.
- Write down in "My Asthma Symptoms and Peak Flow Diary" the highest of the three numbers achieved.

FIND YOUR PERSONAL BEST PEAK FLOW NUMBER

Your personal best peak flow number is the highest peak flow number you can achieve over a 2-week period when your asthma is under good control. Good control is when you feel good and do not have any asthma symptoms.

Each patient's asthma is different, and your best peak flow may be higher or lower than the peak flow of someone of your same height, weight, and sex. This means that it is important for you to find your own personal best peak flow number. Your medicine plan needs to be based on your own personal best peak flow number.

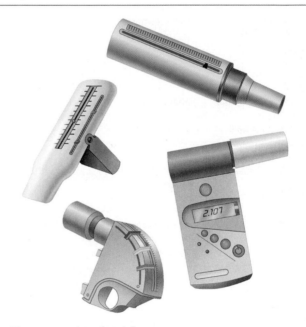

There are a variety of peak flow meters.

To find out your personal best peak flow number, take peak flow readings:

- Every day for 2 weeks.
- Mornings and early afternoons or evenings (when you wake up and between 12:00 and 2:00 P.M.).
- Before and after taking inhaled beta$_2$-agonist (*if* you take this medicine).
- As instructed by your doctor.

Write down these readings in your peak flow diary.

Figure 16-6 ▶▶▶ Instructions for using a peak flow meter.

Source: Nurses: Partners in Asthma Care, National Asthma Education and Prevention Program. National Heart, Lung, and Blood Institute, NIH Publication No. 95–3308, 1995.

THE PEAK FLOW ZONE SYSTEM

Once you know your personal best peak flow number, your doctor will give you the numbers that tell you what to do. The peak flow numbers are put into zones that are set up like a traffic light. This will help you know what to do when your peak flow number changes. For example:

Green Zone (80% to 100% of your personal best number) signals *good control*. No asthma symptoms are present. You may take your medicines as usual.

Yellow Zone (50% to 79% of your personal best number) signals *caution*. You may be having an episode of asthma that requires an increase in your medicine. Or your overall asthma may not be under control, and the doctor may need to change your medicine plan.

Red Zone (below 50% of your personal best number) signals *danger!* You must take a short-acting inhaled beta₂-agonist right away and call your doctor immediately if your peak flow number does not return to the Yellow or Green Zone and stay in that zone.

Record your personal best peak flow number and peak flow zones at the top of "My Asthma Symptoms and Peak Flow Diary."

USE THE DIARY TO KEEP TRACK OF YOUR PEAK FLOW

Write down your peak flow number on the diary every day, or as instructed by your doctor.

ACTIONS TO TAKE WHEN PEAK FLOW NUMBERS CHANGE

■ PEFR goes more than 20% below your personal best (PEFR is in the Yellow Zone).

  ACTION: Take an inhaled short-acting bronchodilator as prescribed by your doctor.

■ PEFR changes 20% or more between the morning and early afternoon or evening (measure your PEFR before taking medicine).

  or

■ PEFR increases 20% or more when measured before and after taking an inhaled short-acting bronchodilator.

  ACTION: Talk to your doctor about adding more medicine to control your asthma better (for example, an anti-inflammatory medication).

Figure 16-6 ▶▶▶ *(continued)*

Figure 16-7 ▶▶▶ provides tips for people who are allergic or bothered by any of these items. Additional items and strategies may be recommended by the pulmonologist or allergist caring for the older patient.

Physical assessment of the older patient with asthma should include observation of the overall shape and movement of the thorax during respiration. The nurse should auscultate the lungs beginning at the apices of one lung and comparing that sound to the same area of the other lung. Usually, auscultation proceeds from posterior to anterior and from the apex downward to the eighth rib. It is important to note the presence of crackles, wheezes, rhonchi, or pleural rub. Wheezing is a sign that air is having difficulty passing through airways narrowed by edema, spasm, or mucus. If wheezing is present, the nurse should note whether it occurs on inspiration or expiration and also note the use of accessory muscles during respiration. Chest excursion is measured by placing the thumbs beside the spine and noting their movement during deep inspiration. Tactile and vocal fremitus, vibrations felt on the surface of the chest, may be slightly decreased in the patient with asthma.

Nursing Diagnoses

Nursing diagnoses associated with the older person with asthma may include *Activity Intolerance* for those with exercise-induced asthma, *Airway Clearance, Ineffective* for those with chronic cough with mucus production, *Breathing Pattern, Ineffective* for those with tachypnea and wheezing with poorly controlled asthma, *Tissue Perfusion; Peripheral, Ineffective* for those with hypoxemia, and *Health Maintenance, Ineffective* for those who are unable or unwilling to monitor the peak flow recordings and adjust medications to prevent asthma attacks and exacerbations (NANDA International, 2012). The nurse should seek advice from the social worker if older patients do not have medication coverage and are having difficulty purchasing the more expensive asthma medications.

Chronic Obstructive Pulmonary Disease

Chronic obstructive pulmonary disease (COPD) is a term used for two closely related diseases of the respiratory system: chronic bronchitis and emphysema. Chronic bronchitis is defined as cough and sputum production

My Asthma Symptoms and Peak Flow Diary

_____ **My predicted peak flow**   _____ **My personal best peak flow**

_____**My Green (Good Control) Zone**	_____**My Yellow (Caution) Zone**	_____**My Red (Danger) Zone**
80–100% of personal best	50–79% of personal best	below 50% of personal best

Date:															
	a.m.	**p.m.**	**a.m.**	**p.m.**	**a.m.**	**p.m.**	**a.m.**	**p.m.**	**a.m.**	**p.m.**	**a.m.**	**p.m.**	**a.m.**	**p.m.**	
Peak Flow Reading															
No Asthma Symptoms															
Mild Asthma Symptoms															
Moderate Asthma Symptoms															
Serious Asthma Symptoms															
Medicine Used to Stop Symptoms															
Urgent Visit to the Doctor															

Directions:

1. Take your peak flow reading every morning (a.m.) when you wake up and every afternoon or evening (p.m.). Try to take your peak flow readings at the same time each day. If you take an inhaled beta$_2$-agonist medicine, take your peak flow reading **before** taking that medicine. Write down the highest reading of three tries in the box that says peak flow reading.

2. Look at the box at the top of this sheet to see whether your number is in the Green, Yellow, or Red Zone.

3. In the space below the date and time, put an "X" in the box that matches the symptoms you have when you record your peak flow reading; see description of symptom categories below.

4. Look at your Asthma Management Plan for what to do when your number is in one of the zones or when you have asthma symptoms.

5. Put an "X" in the box inside "medicine used to stop symptoms" if you took **extra** asthma medicine to stop your symptoms.

6. If you made any visit to your doctor's office, emergency department, or hospital for treatment of an asthma episode, put an "X" in the box marked "urgent visit to the doctor." Tell your doctor if you went to the emergency department or hospital.

No symptoms	= No symptoms (wheeze, cough, chest tightness, or shortness of breath) even with normal physical activity.
Mild symptoms	= Symptoms during physical activity, but not at rest. It does not keep you from sleeping or being active.
Moderate symptoms	= Symptoms while at rest; symptoms may keep you from sleeping or being active.
Severe symptoms	= Severe symptoms at rest (wheeze may be absent); symptoms cause problems walking or talking; muscles in neck or between ribs are pulled in when breathing.

Figure 16-6 ▶▶▶ *(continued)*

Date: _____   Personal Best PEFR _____

Asthma Management Plan for _____

Green Zone = Good Control

Green Zone: _____ to _____ Peak Flow Rate (80–100% of personal best; no symptoms)

To keep your asthma under control: Stay away from things that make your asthma worse (such as animals, smoke, etc.; talk to your doctor about these things). **Take your medicine(s).**

Name of Medicine	How Much to Take	How Often/ When to Take It

Yellow Zone = Caution

Yellow Zone: _____ to _____ Peak Flow Rate (50–79% of personal best)

Take medicine listed below to get your asthma back under control.

Symptoms: Coughing, wheezing, shortness of breath, tightness in the chest, or other symptoms of an asthma episode. Symptoms may be mild.

Early signs your asthma is getting worse: _____

Take your Yellow Zone medication when these early signs occur.

Name of Medicine	How Much to Take	How Often/ When to Take It

- ■ Peak flow rate or symptoms not better in _____ minutes after taking the medicine listed above? Call the doctor.
- ■ Keep taking your Green Zone medicine(s). Keep staying away from things that make your asthma worse.

Figure 16-6 ▶▶▶ *(continued)*

Red Zone = Danger!

Red Zone: Below _____ Peak Flow Rate (below 50% of personal best)

Take the medicine listed below. Then call your doctor.

Symptoms: Coughing, very short of breath, trouble walking and talking, tightness in the chest, other symptoms.

Name of Medicine	How Much to Take	How Often/ When to Take It

- Call your doctor or emergency room NOW, say this is an emergency, and ask what you should do next.
- Go to the doctor or hospital **right away** or call an ambulance without delay if :
  —You are struggling to breathe or your lips or fingernails turn a little blue or grey.
  —Your peak flow remains in the Red Zone level 20 minutes after taking your medicine.
- Keep taking your Green Zone medicine(s).

Doctor: _____

Office Phone: _____

Phone Number After Office Hours: _____

Emergency Room: _____

Notes

Figure 16-6 ▶▶▶ *(continued)*

HOW TO STAY AWAY FROM THINGS THAT MAKE YOUR ASTHMA WORSE

Because you have asthma, your airways are very sensitive. They may react to things that can cause asthma attacks or episodes. Staying away from such things will help you keep your asthma from getting worse.

- ■ Ask your doctor to help you find out what makes your asthma worse. Discuss the ways to stay away from these things. The tips listed below will help you.

- ■ Ask your doctor for help in deciding which actions will help the most to reduce your asthma symptoms. Carry out these actions first. Discuss the results of your efforts with your doctor.

TIPS FOR THOSE ALLERGIC TO OR BOTHERED BY ANY ITEM LISTED BELOW

House-Dust Mites

The following actions should help you control house-dust mites:

- ■ Encase your mattress and box spring in an airtight cover.
- ■ Either encase your pillow or wash it in hot water once a week every week.
- ■ Wash your bed covers, clothes, and stuffed toys once a week in hot water (130°F).

The following actions will also help you control dust mites—but they are not essential:

- ■ Reduce indoor humidity to less than 50%. Use a dehumidifier if needed.
- ■ Remove carpets from your bedroom.
- ■ Do not sleep or lie on upholstered furniture. Replace with vinyl, leather, or wood furniture.
- ■ Remove carpets that are laid on concrete.
- ■ Stay out of a room while it is being vacuumed.
- ■ If you must vacuum, one or more of the following things can be done to reduce the amount of dust you breathe in: (1) Use a dust mask. (2) Use a central vacuum cleaner with the collecting bag outside the home. (3) Use double-wall vacuum cleaner bags and exhaust-port HEPA (high-efficiency particulate air) filters.

Animals

Some people are allergic to the dried flakes of skin, saliva, or urine from warm-blooded pets. Warm-blooded pets include ALL dogs, cats, birds, and rodents. The length of a pet's hair does not matter. Here are some tips for those allergic to animals:

- ■ Remove the animal from the home or school classroom.
- ■ Choose a pet without fur or feathers (such as a fish or a snake).

- ■ If you must have a warm-blooded pet, keep the pet out of your bedroom at all times. Keeping the pet outside of your home is even better.
- ■ If there is forced air-heating in the home with a pet, close the air ducts in your bedroom.
- ■ Wash the pet weekly in warm water.
- ■ Do not visit homes that have pets. If you must visit such places, take asthma medicine (cromolyn is often preferred) before going.
- ■ Do not buy or use products made with feathers. Use pillows and comforters stuffed with synthetic fibers like polyester. Also do not use pillows, bedding, and furniture stuffed with kapok (silky fibers from the seed pods of the silk-cotton tree).
- ■ Use a vacuum cleaner fitted with a HEPA filter.
- ■ Wash hands and change clothes as soon as you can after being in contact with pets.

Cockroaches (Some people are allergic to the droppings of roaches.)

- ■ Use insect sprays; but have someone else spray when you are outside of the home. Air out the home for a few hours after spraying. Roach traps may also help.
- ■ All homes in multiple-family dwellings (apartments, condominiums, and housing projects) must be treated to get rid of roaches.

Tobacco Smoke

- ■ Do not smoke.
- ■ Do not allow smoking in your home. Have household members smoke outside.
- ■ Encourage family members to quit smoking. Ask your doctor or nurse for help on how to quit.
- ■ Choose no-smoking areas in restaurants, hotels, and other public buildings.

Figure 16-7 ▶▶▶ Guidelines for patients with asthma.

(continued)

Source: Nurses: Partners in Asthma Care, National Asthma Education and Prevention Program. National Heart, Lung, and Blood Institute, NIH Publication No. 95-3308, 1995.

Wood Smoke

- Do not use a wood-burning stove to heat your home.
- Do not use kerosene heaters.

Strong Odors and Sprays

- Do not stay in your home when it is being painted. Use latex rather than oil-based paint.
- Try to stay away from perfume; talcum powder, hair spray, and products like these.
- Use household cleaning products that do not have strong smells or scents.
- Reduce strong cooking odors (especially frying) by using an exhaust fan and opening windows.

Colds and Infections

- Talk to your doctor about flu shots.
- Stay away from people with colds or the flu.
- Do not take over-the-counter cold remedies, such as antihistamines and cough syrup, unless you speak to your doctor first.

Exercise

- Make a plan with your doctor that allows you to exercise without symptoms. For example, take inhaled beta$_2$-agonist or cromolyn less than 30 minutes before exercising.
- Do not exercise during the afternoon when air pollution levels are highest.
- Warm up before doing exercise and cool down afterward.

Weather

- Wear a scarf over your mouth and nose in cold weather. Or pull a turtleneck or scarf over your nose on windy or cold days.
- Dress warmly in the winter or on windy days.

Pollens

During times of high pollen counts:

- Stay indoors during the midday and afternoon when pollen counts are highest.
- Keep windows closed in cars and homes. Use air conditioning if you can.
- Pets should either stay outdoors or indoors. Pets should not be allowed to go in and out of the home. This prevents your pet from bringing pollen inside.
- Do not mow the grass. But if you must mow, wear a pollen filter mask.

Mold (Outdoor)

- Avoid sources of molds (wet leaves, garden debris, stacked wood).
- Avoid standing water or areas of poor drainage.

REMEMBER: Making these changes will help keep asthma episodes from starting. These actions can also reduce your need for asthma medicines.

Notes

_____
_____
_____
_____
_____
_____
_____
_____
_____
_____

Figure 16-7 ▶▶▶ *(continued)*

present on most days for a minimum of 3 months for at least 2 successive years or for 6 months during 1 year. In chronic bronchitis, there may be narrowing of the large and small airways, making it more difficult to move air in and out of the lungs. An estimated 9.9 million Americans have chronic bronchitis. In emphysema, there is permanent destruction of the alveoli, the tiny elastic air sacs of the lung, because of irreversible destruction of elastin, a protein in the lung that is important for maintaining the strength of the alveolar walls. The loss of elastin also causes collapse or narrowing of the smallest air passages, called bronchioles, which in turn limits airflow out of the lung. The estimated number of people with emphysema in the United States is over 4.3 million (CDC, 2011e).

In the general population, emphysema usually develops in older people with a long smoking history; however, one form of emphysema tends to run in families. Smoking is believed to be responsible for over 90% of patients diagnosed with COPD. People with familial emphysema have a hereditary deficiency of a blood component, alpha$_1$-proteinase inhibitor, also called alpha$_1$-antitrypsin. It is estimated that only 1% to 3% of all cases of emphysema are due to this deficiency (CDC, 2011e).

In many older patients, chronic bronchitis and emphysema occur together, although one may present more symptoms than the other. Most patients with these diseases have a long history of heavy cigarette smoking. COPD ranks as the third leading cause of death in the United States, with over 124,000 Americans dying from this disease in 2007 (ALA, 2011). Of the top five leading causes of death in the United States, it is the only one on the rise. Caucasian Americans are more at risk for developing and dying from COPD than other racial and ethnic groups; however, African Americans diagnosed with COPD use the emergency department more often for treatment of symptoms (CDC, 2011b).

COPD death rates are also rising in women, exceeding the death rate for men. Over 65,000 women died from COPD compared to 60,000 men in 2005. From 1999 through 2007, COPD hospitalization rates declined for both men and women, but COPD death rates declined only for men (CDC, 2011c).

The symptoms of COPD tend to emerge in the middle years of life, and many people with COPD become disabled with constant shortness of breath. COPD is an important cause of hospitalization in the older adult with approximately 64% of discharges over the age of 65 (ALA, 2011). It is a disease with high individual and societal costs.

Pathophysiology

When COPD develops, the walls of the small airways and alveoli lose their elasticity and thicken, closing off some of the smaller air passages and narrowing larger ones. The lungs contain 300 million alveoli whose ultrathin walls form the gas exchange surface. Enmeshed in the wall of each of these air sacs is a network of tiny capillaries that bring blood to the gas exchange surface. Air can enter the alveoli during inspiration; but on expiration, the air becomes trapped because of collapsing airways. Stale air cannot leave the lungs, and this residual volume adversely affects gas exchange. Over time, pathological changes occur with COPD. Blood flow and airflow to the walls of the alveoli become uneven and mismatched. In some alveoli, blood flow exceeds airflow; in others, the opposite occurs. The end result is that blood is poorly oxygenated and tissue perfusion is less efficient.

Pushing air through the narrow air passageways becomes harder with time, and the respiratory muscles become fatigued. Carbon dioxide cannot be adequately removed from the blood and may accumulate to critical levels, resulting in respiratory acidosis and ultimately respiratory failure.

The ability to efficiently move air into and out of the lungs declines gradually with age, but in most cases lung function remains adequate in nonsmokers, those free from occupational and household exposure to airborne contaminants and secondhand smoke, and those living in geographical areas with relatively clean air. It is never too late to quit smoking because lung function declines much more rapidly in smokers. If smoking stops before serious lung damage occurs, the rate at which lung function declines returns to nearly normal. However, some lung damage cannot be reversed, and over time it is unlikely that lung function will return to normal (ALA, 2011). Figure 16-8 ▶▶▶ illustrates the relationship between smoking and lung function.

COPD also strains the heart, especially the right ventricle, which is responsible for pumping blood into the lungs. As COPD progresses, the amount of oxygen in the blood decreases, causing blood vessels in the lungs to further constrict. As a result, more force is required to circulate blood throughout the lungs. The right ventricle enlarges and thickens, which can result in abnormal rhythms called *cor pulmonale*. Older patients with cor pulmonale suffer from fatigue, rhythm disturbances, and palpitations, and they are at risk for heart failure should additional strain be placed on the heart such as acquiring a respiratory illness.

As COPD progresses, the body tries to boost the amount of oxygen carried in the blood by making extra red blood cells. This condition is *secondary polycythemia* and results in a larger than normal number of red cells in the general circulation. Although these cells are helpful to carry extra oxygen, they clog up small blood vessels and thicken the blood. This results in the formation of a bluish color in the skin, lips, and nail beds called *cyanosis*. Eventually, clubbing of the fingers will become apparent. Too little oxygen

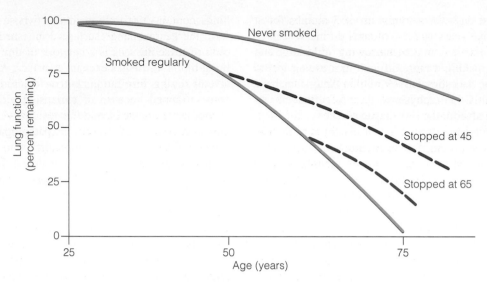

Figure 16-8 ▶▶▶ Age-related change in the lung function and effect of smoking and smoking cessation.

Source: National Heart, Lung, and Blood Institute (2002). The Lungs in Health and Disease.

can also affect the brain, resulting in headache, irritability, impaired cognition, and sleep problems.

Symptoms

The earliest presenting symptom of COPD is early morning cough with the production of clear sputum. The sputum will turn to yellow or green should the older person develop a respiratory infection. Periods of wheezing may occur during or after colds. Shortness of breath on exertion develops later and becomes more pronounced with severe episodes of **dyspnea** occurring during even modest activity like walking or making a bed.

The typical progression of COPD is as follows:

- Usually no symptoms occur for the first 10 years after beginning smoking.
- At about 10 years after beginning smoking, chronic cough with clear sputum develops.
- At about the age of 40 or 50, dyspnea begins to occur.
- At about age 50, increased susceptibility to colds occurs with longer recovery time needed.

Survival of patients with COPD is closely related to the level of their lung function when they are diagnosed and the rate at which they lose their lung function. Mouth breathing, puffing, use of accessory muscles of breathing, and inability to finish a sentence without catching one's breath are signs of dyspnea from air hunger (Huether & McCance, 2012). Patients with severe lung damage sleep in a semisitting position because they are unable to breathe when they lie flat. Dyspnea is the most common reason for emergency department visits and has been associated

with an increased risk of hospitalization in older patients with COPD (CDC, 2011c). Overall, the median survival is about 10 years for patients with COPD who have lost approximately two thirds of their normally expected lung function at diagnosis (ALA, 2011).

> ***Practice Pearl*** ▶▶▶ Older patients with COPD often have calluses on their elbows as a result of leaning over tables to stretch out their torsos so that more air can enter and exit during respiration. It is often referred to as the "tripod" position.

Diagnosis

At present, it is impossible to diagnose COPD before irreversible lung damage occurs. Spirometry is the preferred diagnostic method for testing pulmonary function. The three volume measures most relevant to COPD are forced vital capacity, residual volume, and total lung capacity. Although most of the measured lung volumes change with COPD, residual volume usually increases dramatically resulting in the classic "barrel chest" appearance. This increase is the result of the weakened airways collapsing before all of the normally expired air can leave the lungs. The increased residual volume makes breathing more difficult because the trapped air occupies a large area and impedes the influx of fresh air. COPD is classified into the following stages according to the values obtained with spirometry testing: stage I, mild; stage II, moderate; stage III, severe; and stage IV, very severe.

The FEV_1 (forced expiratory volume in 1 second) also provides valuable information because COPD results in narrowed air passages. When FEV_1 is used as an indicator of lung function, the average rate of decline in patients with COPD is two to three times the normal rate of loss of 20 to 30 mm/year. As COPD progresses, less air can be expelled in 1 second. A greater than expected fall in FEV_1 is the most sensitive test for COPD progression and a fairly good predictor of early disability and death (Reuben et al., 2011).

Because the primary function of the lung is to remove carbon dioxide from the blood and add oxygen, another indicator of pulmonary function is the measurement of blood oxygen and carbon dioxide levels. As COPD progresses, the amount of oxygen in the blood decreases and the amount of carbon dioxide rises. Blood oxygen can be measured by obtaining arterial blood gas levels (the gold standard, but often difficult to obtain in older adults) or by using pulse oximetry (more convenient but less reliable). Pao_2 and $Paco_2$ are measures of arterial oxygen and carbon dioxide. Pulse oximetry is reported in percentage of oxygen in capillary blood. Under normal conditions, the hemoglobin in arterial blood is 97.4% saturated with oxygen while the patient is breathing room air. This level of oxygen saturation is decreased with progressive pulmonary disease.

In most cases, it is necessary to monitor the results of a series of spirometry tests to determine the rate of disease progress or improvement. Measurement of FEV_1 and the FEV_1/FVC ratio should be a routine part of the physical examination of every patient with COPD. The ratio is normally 75% to 85%, depending on the patient's age (ALA, 2011). The ratio is reduced in COPD.

Treatment

Managing patients with COPD focuses on the following broad goals:

- Careful assessment and monitoring of the treatment of the disease
- Reducing risk factors (cigarette smoking and environmental pollutants)
- Managing stable COPD and preventing disease progression
- Assessing and managing anxiety and depression
- Mucolytic therapy
- Rehabilitation
- Managing exacerbations

ALA, 2011; Reuben et al., 2011.

Because cigarette smoking is the most significant cause of COPD, quitting smoking can almost always prevent COPD progression. The goals of treatment are to reduce disability, prevent acute exacerbations, reduce hospitalization, and avoid premature mortality.

Home oxygen therapy (greater than 15 hours/day) has been shown to increase the survival rate of patients with advanced COPD who have hypoxemia, or low blood oxygen levels. This treatment can improve a patient's exercise tolerance and ability to perform on cognitive and physical tests, reflecting improvement in the function of the brain and increased muscle coordination. Oxygen also improves cardiac function and prevents the development of cor pulmonale. Continuous oxygen therapy is recommended for patients with low oxygen levels at rest, during exercise, and while sleeping (ALA, 2011). Many oxygen sources are available for home use including compressed gaseous oxygen or liquid oxygen devices that concentrate oxygen from room air. The patient's insurance may reimburse some of the expense of continuous oxygen therapy, which can be hundreds of dollars a month, once hypoxemia is verified and documented. It is imperative that the older patient not smoke anywhere near oxygen or oxygen equipment because of the danger of fire and explosion.

> **Practice Pearl** ▸▸▸ If an older patient receiving home oxygen states that he or she is smoking but turns the oxygen off before lighting up, please consider discussing complete removal of oxygen equipment from the home. The older patient and the home environment including clothing, furniture, pets, and others living in the home are considered "oxygen enriched" and thus more easily ignited when exposed to a source of fire.

Medications used to treat older patients with COPD are similar to those used to treat older patients with asthma and include the following:

- Bronchodilators help open narrowed airways to improve airflow and gas exchange. The *sympathomimetics* (isoproterenol, metaproterenol, terbutaline, albuterol), and the *parasympathomimetics* (atropine, ipratropium bromide) all can be inhaled or taken by mouth. Scheduled treatment with long-acting bronchodilators is more effective and convenient than treatment with short-acting bronchodilators (McPhee & Papadakis, 2011).
- Inhaled corticosteroids lessen inflammation of the airway. Inhaled steroids include beclomethasone, dexamethasone, triamcinolone, and flunisolide. By decreasing inflammation and swelling, more air can pass through the narrowed airways. Additionally, less inflammation usually means less mucus production and narrowing secondary to scarring. Bronchodilators can be used with inhaled corticosteroids in patients with stage III (severe) and stage IV (very severe) disease. Bronchodilators should be administered before the corticosteroids are inhaled to improve distribution to all parts of the lung. Chronic

treatment with systemic glucocorticosteroids should be avoided because of the risk of systemic side effects (Reuben et al., 2011).

■ Antibiotics (tetracycline, ampicillin, erythromycin, and trimethoprim-sulfamethoxazole combinations) fight infections. Antibiotics are usually prescribed at the first sign of infection or when sputum color changes from clear to yellow or green. The goal is to prevent the development of pneumonia and serious illness requiring hospitalization.

■ Influenza vaccine yearly and pneumococcal vaccine at the age of 65 can reduce the risk of serious illness including pneumonia.

■ Exercise training improves exercise tolerance and symptoms of dyspnea and fatigue.

■ Expectorants loosen mucus and clear the airways.

■ Other drugs can be used to treat associated symptoms, including diuretics for heart failure, analgesics for pain, cough suppressants for cough, and anxiolytics for anxiety and restlessness.

Additional Treatment Options

Bullectomy or lung volume reduction surgery has shown some limited success in selected patients. Portions of the lung that are nonfunctional and filled with stagnant air are removed to make room for the more healthy parts of the lung to expand. However, this is major surgery and many older patients with COPD are poor surgical risks and are prone to life-threatening surgical complications. Lung transplantation has also been used with some COPD patients. The 2-year survival rate in patients with transplanted lungs ranges from 60% to 80% (Moffatt-Bruce, 2011).

Pulmonary rehabilitation is useful in patients with COPD. The goals are to improve overall physical stamina and compensate for the conditions that cause dyspnea and limit functional ability. General exercise training increases performance, improves sense of well-being, and strengthens muscles. Administration of oxygen and nutritional supplements when needed can improve exercise tolerance. Intermittent mechanical ventilatory support relieves dyspnea and rests respiratory muscles in selected patients. **Continuous positive airway pressure (CPAP)** is used as an adjunct to weaning from mechanical ventilation to minimize dyspnea during exercise (see Figure 8-8 ⊂⊃ on page 200). The positive pressure keeps the narrowed airways from collapsing and trapping air. Relaxation techniques may also reduce the perception of ventilatory effort and dyspnea. Breathing exercises and techniques such as pursed lip breathing can improve functional status.

Clearing the air passages of mucus can be difficult in patients with end-stage COPD. **Intermittent positive pressure breathing (IPPB)** may be prescribed for frail and debilitated patients for short-term ventilatory support and delivery of aerosol medications. The IPPB treatment is delivered by a device that assists with intermittent positive pressure inhalation of therapeutic aerosols without a need for the hand coordination required in the use of hand nebulizers or metered-dose inhalers. IPPB can clear secretions and stimulate a cough reflex. Additional methods that may help to loosen and remove troublesome secretions include:

■ **Postural drainage.** The patient lies with the head and chest over the side of the bed. Gravity forces secretions at the bottom of the lungs upward and stimulates a cough reflex. Postural drainage is more effective following inhalation of a bronchodilator.

■ **Chest percussion.** Lightly clapping the chest and back helps to loosen secretions.

■ **Controlled coughing.** The patient can be taught to cough while contracting the diaphragm to maximize the cough response.

■ **Tracheal suctioning.** This method may be needed during the end-of-life phase for frail older patients who are unable to clear their own secretions.

Smoking Cessation

The most important thing a patient with COPD can do is to quit smoking. Older patients and their families may think that if lung damage has occurred, it is too late and therefore not worth the effort. The gerontological nurse can function as educator and change agent for the older smoker.

The NHLBI has developed a smoking IQ test for older smokers that can be used to help start a discussion about smoking cessation with older patients and their families. The nurse should ask the older patient to complete the test and then discuss the correct answers. Box 16-1 lists the questions, scoring, and rationale for each response.

The nurse should investigate community resources and availability of smoking cessation support groups. Many hospitals and community agencies offer programs that stress behavior modification techniques. In addition, nicotine patches and gum with supportive counseling can be effective for some older people. If nicotine replacement transdermal patches are used, they should be applied to clean, nonhairy skin on the upper arm or torso daily. Sites should be rotated to prevent skin irritation. NicoDerm comes in three strengths (21, 14, and 7 mg). It is recommended that older patients begin with the 14-mg strength to prevent possible cardiovascular side effects. After 2 to 4 weeks, the dose should be reduced to 7 mg for 2 to 4 weeks and then discontinued. For older patients reporting sleep difficulties, the patch should be removed 1 hour before bedtime and reapplied first thing in the morning. Patients who smoke while wearing the patch are at risk

If you or someone you know is an older smoker, you may think that there is no point in quitting now. Think again. By quitting smoking now, you will feel more in control and have fewer coughs and colds. However, with every cigarette you smoke, you increase your chances of having a heart attack, a stroke, or cancer. Need to think about this more? Take this older smokers' I.Q. quiz. Just answer "true" or "false" to each statement below.

True or False

1. ○ True ○ False   If you have smoked for most of your life, it's not worth stopping now.

2. ○ True ○ False   Older smokers who try to quit are more likely to stay off cigarettes.

3. ○ True ○ False   Smokers get tired and short of breath more easily than nonsmokers the same age.

4. ○ True ○ False   Smoking is a major risk factor for heart attack and stroke among adults 60 years of age and older.

5. ○ True ○ False   Quitting smoking can help those who have already had a heart attack.

6. ○ True ○ False   Most older smokers don't want to stop smoking.

7. ○ True ○ False   An older smoker is likely to smoke more cigarettes than a younger smoker.

8. ○ True ○ False   Someone who has smoked for 30 to 40 years probably won't be able to quit smoking.

9. ○ True ○ False   Very few older adults smoke cigarettes.

10. ○ True ○ False   Lifelong smokers are more likely to die of diseases like emphysema and bronchitis than nonsmokers.

Test Results

1. If you have smoked for most of your life, it's not worth stopping now.

   False. You have every reason to quit now and quit for good—even if you've been smoking for years. Stopping smoking will help you live longer and feel better. You will reduce your risk of heart attack, stroke, and cancer; improve blood flow and lung function; and help stop diseases like emphysema and bronchitis from getting worse.

2. Older smokers who try to quit are more likely to stay off cigarettes.

   True. Once they quit, older smokers are far more likely than younger smokers to stay away from cigarettes. Older smokers know more about both the short- and long-term health benefits of quitting.

3. Smokers get tired and short of breath more easily than nonsmokers the same age.

   True. Smokers, especially those over 50 years old, are much more likely to get tired, feel short of breath, and cough more often. These

symptoms can signal the start of bronchitis or emphysema, both of which are suffered more often by older smokers. Stopping smoking will help reduce these symptoms.

4. Smoking is a major risk factor for heart attack and stroke among adults 60 years of age and older.

   True. Smoking is a major risk factor for four of the five leading causes of death including heart disease, stroke, cancer, and lung diseases like emphysema and bronchitis. For adults 60 and over, smoking is a major risk factor for six of the top 14 causes of death. Older male smokers are nearly twice as likely to die from stroke as older men who do not smoke. The odds are nearly as high for older female smokers. Cigarette smokers of any age have a 70% greater heart disease death rate than do nonsmokers.

5. Quitting smoking can help those who have already had a heart attack.

   True. The good news is that stopping smoking does help people who have suffered a heart attack. In fact, their chances of having another attack are smaller. In some cases, ex-smokers can cut their risk of another heart attack by half or more.

6. Most older smokers don't want to stop smoking.

   False. Most smokers would prefer to quit. In fact, in a recent study, 65% of older smokers said that they would like to stop. What keeps them from quitting? They are afraid of being irritable, nervous, and tense. Others are concerned about cravings for cigarettes. Most don't want to gain weight. Many think it's too late to quit—that quitting after so many years of smoking will not help. But this is not true.

7. An older smoker is likely to smoke more cigarettes than a younger smoker.

   True. Older smokers usually smoke more cigarettes than younger people. Plus, older smokers are more likely to smoke high-nicotine brands.

8. Someone who has smoked for 30 to 40 years probably won't be able to quit smoking.

   False. You may be surprised to learn that older smokers are actually more likely to succeed at quitting smoking. This is more true if they're already experiencing long-term smoking-related symptoms like shortness of breath, coughing, or chest pain. Older smokers who stop want to avoid further health problems, take control of their life, get rid of the smell of cigarettes, and save money.

9. Very few older adults smoke cigarettes.

   False. One out of five adults age 50 or older smokes cigarettes. This is more than 11 million smokers, a fourth of the country's 43 million smokers! About 25% of the general U.S. population still smokes.

10. Lifelong smokers are more likely to die of diseases like emphysema and bronchitis than nonsmokers.

   True. Smoking greatly increases the risk of dying from diseases like emphysema and bronchitis. In fact, over 80% of all deaths from these two diseases are directly due to smoking. The risk of dying from lung cancer is also a lot higher for smokers than nonsmokers: 22 times higher for males, 12 times higher for females.

Source: NHLBI (2002).

for cardiovascular problems, including heart attack, and should be clearly informed of this risk. If they decide to start smoking during treatment with the patch, they should remove the patch and wait a minimum of 2 hours before having a cigarette (overnight is better).

For patients choosing Nicorette gum, it is recommended that 9 to 12 pieces be used daily. The nurse should instruct patients to chew one piece at a time when they get the urge to smoke. After chewing the gum a few times to soften it, it should be held in the buccal cavity for at least one-half hour to release all the medication.

The healthcare provider can also prescribe bupropion (Zyban) for 7 to 12 weeks to ease tobacco cravings during the cessation process. Bupropion is contraindicated in people with seizure disorder. When it is combined with nicotine replacement, the quit rate doubles to 30% at 12 months (Reuben et al., 2011). Chantix is a medication that is effective when used with behavior modification and counseling to assist patients to stop smoking. Chantix reduces the urge to smoke and the pleasure associated with smoking by releasing dopamine levels in the brain. The most common side effects include nausea (30%); trouble sleeping; vivid, unusual, and increased dreaming; increased depression and suicidal ideation; and constipation, gas, and/or vomiting (Reuben et al., 2011).

Practice Pearl ▶▶▶ Cessation of smoking is the best way to slow the progression of COPD. Nurses should be persistent in educating and urging older patients to quit. The smoking addiction is difficult to beat. Many older people try to quit several times before they are ultimately successful. It is important for nurses not to smoke. Nurses who smoke lose credibility with their patients and put themselves at risk for developing this debilitating disease.

Additional suggestions for patients with COPD include the following:

- Avoid exposure to dust and fumes. Ensure good ventilation when working with solvents, chemicals, and paints. Wear a mask when doing woodwork or sanding furniture. Avoid woodstoves and smoky fires, perfumes, and other indoor pollutants.
- Avoid air pollution, including secondhand smoke. Do not exercise when air pollution or smog levels are high.
- Refrain from close contact with people who have colds or the flu. Be sure to receive a yearly flu shot and pneumococcal vaccine at age 65.
- Avoid excessive heat, cold, and high altitudes. A commercial aircraft maintains a cabin pressure equivalent to an elevation of 5,000 to 10,000 feet. This can result in hypoxemia for some patients with COPD. Supplemental

oxygen may be needed and can be arranged in advance of the flight.
- Drink lots of fluids. Being hydrated can keep sputum loose and secretions easier to clear.
- Maintain good lifestyle habits. Good nutrition, exercise, weight control, and moderation in alcohol consumption can add years and function to the life of a patient with COPD.
- Have spirometry done routinely and get to know the numbers.

Nursing Assessment and Nursing Diagnosis

The gerontological nurse will have the opportunity to work with older patients with COPD over time and get to know them as individuals. Guidelines for care of the patient with COPD are similar to those developed for patients with asthma. It is recommended that each visit include:

- Assessment of the older patient's needs, expectations, and progress
- Introduction or review of actions the older patient should take
- Obtaining an agreement to take specific actions and scheduling a follow-up visit to discuss the patient's progress
- Careful review of the patient's progress toward smoking cessation or continued abstinence from smoking

Physical assessment of the older patient with COPD should include observation of the overall shape and movement of the thorax during respiration. The lungs should be auscultated beginning at the apices of one lung and comparing that sound to the same area of the other lung. Usually auscultation proceeds from posterior to anterior and from the apex downward to the eighth rib, noting the presence of crackles, wheezes, rhonchi, or pleural rub. Wheezing is a sign that air is having difficulty passing through airways narrowed by edema, spasm, or mucus. If wheezing is present, the nurse should note whether it occurs on inspiration or expiration. The nurse notes the use of accessory muscles during respiration, measures chest excursion by placing the thumbs beside the spine and noting their movement during deep inspiration, and notes the presence or absence of lung sounds in the base of each lung. Absence of lung sounds indicates air trapping and lack of air movement. Tactile and vocal fremitus, vibrations felt on the surface of the chest, may be slightly decreased in the patient with COPD.

Nursing diagnoses associated with the older person with COPD may include *Activity Intolerance* for those people with fatigue and air hunger, *Airway Clearance, Ineffective* for those with chronic cough with mucus production, *Breathing Pattern, Ineffective* for those with tachypnea and wheezing with advanced COPD, *Tissue Perfusion: Peripheral,*

Ineffective for those with hypoxemia, and *Health Maintenance, Ineffective* for those who are unable or unwilling to refrain from cigarette smoking and to adjust medications to prevent exacerbations (NANDA International, 2012). The nurse should seek advice from the social worker if older patients do not have medication coverage and are having difficulty purchasing the more expensive medications.

Tuberculosis

Tuberculosis (TB) infects about one third of the world's population, approximately 9 billion people. (It is the third leading cause of death worldwide in people infected with the HIV virus.) *Mycobacterium tuberculosis* is spread through the air and usually infects the lungs, although other organs are sometimes involved. Most people infected with *M. tuberculosis* harbor the bacterium without symptoms but may develop active disease. Each year, 8 million people worldwide develop active TB and 1.4 million die (CDC, 2011h).

In the United States, TB has reemerged as a serious public health problem. A total of 11,182 TB cases (a rate of 3.6 cases per 100,000 people) were reported in the United States in 2010. However, the highest burden of TB continues to be among older adults. In 2010, adults ages 65 years and older had a case rate of 5.5 cases per 100,000, while children ages 14 years or younger had the lowest rate at 1.0 case per 100,000 (CDC, 2011f).

Drug-resistant TB, including extensively drug-resistant TB, presents significant challenges to treatment and control of the disease in the United States and abroad (CDC, 2011f). The number of active cases has been decreasing, mainly due to improved public health control measures. The disease burden is greatest in developing countries where 95% of the cases occur. However, those in the United States who develop TB are often poor, lack access to adequate health care, and often have low cure rates because they have been infected by drug-resistant strains (CDC, 2011f). In addition to those with active TB, an estimated 10 million to 15 million people in the United States are infected without displaying symptoms and are considered to have latent TB. About 10% of these people will develop TB at some time in their lives.

Minorities are disproportionately affected by TB. Since 1993, TB case rates have declined between 54% and 76% in the following racial and ethnic groups: among Hispanic or Latinos from 19.9 to 6.5 cases per 100,000; among non-Hispanic blacks or African Americans from 28.5 to 7.0 cases per 100,000; among American Indian or Alaska Natives from 14.0 to 6.4 cases per 100,000; and among non-Hispanic whites from 3.6 to 0.9 cases per 100,000. In 2010, the TB case rate for Asians remained approximately three times higher than that for Hispanics or blacks or African Americans (CDC, 2011f). The number of new cases

of TB dropped rapidly in the 1940s and 1950s when the first effective antibiotic therapies and treatments were introduced. In 1985, the decline ended and the number of active cases in the United States began to rise. Several factors were behind this resurgence:

- The HIV/AIDS epidemic. People diagnosed with HIV are vulnerable to manifesting active TB when they are exposed to *M. tuberculosis.*
- Increased numbers of foreign-born people entering the United States from parts of the world where TB is indigenous such as Africa, Asia, and Latin America. TB cases among these people account for nearly half of the total number of cases in the United States.
- Increased poverty, injection drug use, and homelessness. Transmission is rampant in crowded shelters and prisons where people weakened by poor nutrition, drug addiction, and alcoholism are exposed to *M. tuberculosis.*
- Failure of patients to take medications as directed, increasing resistant strains of *M. tuberculosis.*
- Increased numbers of residents in long-term care facilities such as nursing homes. Many older people in nursing homes are frail and have weakened immune systems. If exposed to *M. tuberculosis,* they can rapidly develop active TB (CDC, 2011f).

TB in older people can be the reactivation of old disease or a new infection due to exposure to an infected individual. Risk factors for developing or reactivating TB include the following:

- Living in an institution or homelessness
- IV drug abuse
- Exposure to drug-resistant TB
- Previous ineffective TB treatment
- HIV infection
- Diabetes mellitus
- Use of immunosuppressive drugs like corticosteroids or anticancer medications
- Malignancy
- Malnutrition
- Renal failure

Reuben et al., 2011.

Transmission

TB is primarily an airborne disease that is spread by droplets when an infected person coughs, sneezes, speaks, sings, or laughs. Only people with active disease are contagious. It usually takes repeated exposure to someone with active TB before a person becomes infected. On average, most people would have a 50% chance of becoming infected if they spent 8 hours a day for 6 months or 24 hours a day for 2 months working or living with someone with active TB.

The odds of contracting the disease are increased if the person exposed has any of the above risk factors. However, people with TB who have been treated with appropriate drugs for at least 2 weeks are no longer contagious and are incapable of spreading the disease (CDC, 2011f). Adequate ventilation is the most important measure to prevent transmission.

Diagnosis

About 2 to 8 weeks after infection with *M. tuberculosis*, a person's immune system responds by walling off infected cells. From then on the body maintains a standoff with the infection, sometimes for years. Most people undergo complete healing of their initial infection, and the bacteria eventually die off. A positive TB skin test and old scars on a chest X-ray may provide the only evidence of past infection. If, however, resistance is low because of aging, infection, malnutrition, or other reason, the bacteria may break out of hiding and cause active TB (CDC, 2011f).

The risk of developing active TB is greatest in the first year after infection, but it can occur at any time. Early symptoms include weight loss, night sweats, and loss of appetite. One in three patients with TB will die within weeks to months if the disease is not treated. For the rest, the disease either goes into remission or becomes chronic with debilitating cough, chest pain, and bloody sputum.

The hallmarks of TB diagnosis are the skin test and the chest X-ray. People who should be skin tested include:

- Those known to have spent time with someone with active TB
- Those with HIV or malignancy
- Those who think they may have the disease
- Those from parts of the world where TB is common (Latin America, the Caribbean, Africa, Asia, eastern Europe, and Russia)
- Those who use intravenous drugs and alcohol to excess
- Those living in institutions where TB is common (homeless shelters, migrant farm camps, prisons, nursing homes)

The purified protein derivative (PPD) skin test involves the injection of 5 TU (bioequivalent) per dose (0.1 mL) under the skin in the forearm. It should not be given subcutaneously, but rather subdermally. It should barely raise a wheal. If an area of induration results (raised, reddened area) around 72 hours after the PPD has been injected, it should be measured and recorded. Figure 16-9 ▶▶▶ illustrates how to correctly measure the tuberculin skin test. Guidelines for considering the PPD positive are found in Table 16-4.

When performing a PPD test on an older adult, the two-step approach is recommended. If the initial PPD is negative, testing is repeated after waiting 1 to 2 weeks. The

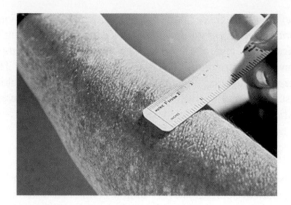

Figure 16-9 ▶▶▶ The tuberculin skin test. Read the tuberculin skin test 48 to 72 hours after injection. Measure only induration, and record reaction in millimeters. *Source:* © CDC/PHIL/CORBIS.

second PPD provides a more accurate reading because the older person's immune system may be sluggish and may not adequately react to the first exposure. It is unclear how

TABLE 16-4	Interpretation of Tuberculin Skin Testing by Risk	
Population		**Area of Induration**
Low-risk, healthy adult		15 mm
Employees of hospitals, nursing homes, prisons, etc.		10 mm
Recent immigrants (<5 years) from high-risk countries		
Intravenous drug users		
People with diabetes, chronic renal failure, leukemia, lymphoma, cancer, gastrectomy or jejunoileal bypass, or weight loss >10% of unexplained origin		
People with recent contact with TB patients		5 mm
Fibrotic changes on chest X-ray consistent with prior TB		
Immunosuppressed (receiving the equivalent of prednisone at >15 mg/day for >1 month), organ transplant recipients, others on drugs causing immunosuppression		
HIV positive		

Source: CDC (2011f); Reuben et al. (2011).

the PPD results should be interpreted for those who have received BCG, the antituberculosis vaccine. The BCG vaccine is not used in the United States but many people coming from other parts of the world have received it in the past. Many healthcare providers recommend that PPD results in patients who have received BCG be interpreted using the same criteria used for nonvaccinated patients. Others do not recommend PPD testing in people who have received BCG because the results will most likely be positive and large areas of induration can result. Either way, these patients should be closely followed up with symptom checklists and chest X-rays if they are in high-risk categories. Patients with a positive test are referred to their healthcare providers for further testing including a chest X-ray and sputum analysis to check for acid-fast bacillus.

Treatment

Successful treatment of TB depends on close cooperation between the patient and healthcare workers. Usually several antibiotics are prescribed and given for between 6 and 12 months. Patients must take their medication at the same time every day to prevent resistance. Treatment of active TB involves the medications listed in Table 16-5.

With appropriate antibiotic treatment, TB can be cured in more than 90% of patients. Serious side effects of isoniazid include loss of appetite, nausea, vomiting, jaundice, fever for more than 3 days, abdominal pain, and tingling in the fingers and toes (CDC, 2011f). Patients taking isoniazid are urged not to drink alcoholic beverages, including wine, beer, and liquor.

When the antibiotic treatment is interrupted because of unpleasant side effects or financial reasons, the TB bacteria may become resistant and be more difficult to eradicate when treatment is started again. Multidrug-resistant tuberculosis (MDR TB) resists eradication with more than one drug. The worldwide problem of MDR TB has been growing and several strains have emerged that are resistant to isoniazid and rifampin, the two most effective mycobacterial drugs available. Treatment of these MDR TB infections involves use of more expensive and less well-tolerated drugs administered over a longer period of time (18 to 24 months). Extensively drug-resistant tuberculosis (XDR TB) is defined as resistance to isoniazid and rifampin plus resistance to any fluoroquinolone and at least one of three injectable second-line anti-TB drugs (i.e., amikacin, kanamycin, or capreomycin). One person was reported to have XDR TB during 2010, compared to no cases in 2009 and five cases in 2008 (CDC, 2011f).

Prevention

TB is largely a preventable disease. In the United States, once people infected with *M. tuberculosis* have been identified, they are treated with isoniazid to prevent active disease. This drug can cause hepatitis in a small percentage of patients and presents a particular risk for those over age 35. Liver function tests should be routinely monitored in the older patient to prevent liver complications.

Hospitals and clinics should take special precautions and isolate patients with active TB. Special filters and ultraviolet light can sterilize the air. Patients with TB should be in special rooms with controlled ventilation and reverse airflow. Healthcare workers should be tested with PPD every year.

Approximately 10 million people worldwide are infected with *M. tuberculosis* and HIV at the same time. The primary cause of death in these patients is TB, not AIDS. In the United States, about 20% of the people who have TB are estimated also to have HIV (CDC, 2011h). TB can be prevented and cured, even in people with HIV. Patients should be referred to clinics where healthcare providers and nurses have experience in the treatment of patients who are HIV positive.

Lung Cancer

Deaths from lung cancer were virtually unknown in the United States until 1900, but the death rate has steadily increased since then. Today in the United States more people die from lung cancer than from any other kind of cancer. This is true for both men and women. In 2007 (the most recent year for which statistics are currently available), lung cancer accounted for more deaths than breast cancer, prostate cancer, and colon cancer combined. In that year, 203,536 people in the United States were diagnosed with lung cancer including 109,643 men and 93,893 women. In that same year, 158,683 people in the United States died from lung cancer, including 88,329 men and 70,354 women (CDC, 2010).

TABLE 16-5	Medications Used to Treat Tuberculosis
Drug	**Dose/Duration**
Isoniazid (INH)	5 mg/kg/day (max 300 mg/day) for 6–9 months
Rifampin plus	10 mg/kg/day (max 600 mg/day)
Pyrazinamide	15–20 mg/kg/day (max 2 g/day) for 2 months
Rifampin	10 mg/kg/day (max 600 mg/day) for 4 months

Source: Reuben, D.B., Herr, K.A., Pacala, J.T., et al. *Geriatrics at your fingertips: 2012*, 14th edition. New York: The American Geriatrics Society; 2012. Reprinted with permission.

Among men in the United States, lung cancer is the second most common cancer among Caucasian, African American, Asian/Pacific Islander, and American Indian/Alaska Native men, and the third most common cancer among Hispanic men. Among women in the United States, lung cancer is the second most common cancer among Caucasian and American Indian/Alaska Native women, and the third most common cancer among African American, Asian/Pacific Islander, and Hispanic women (CDC, 2010). More than 90% of patients with lung cancer are, or have been, cigarette smokers. Quitting cigarette smoking reduces the incidence of lung cancer, but the level of risk reaches that of a nonsmoker only after the person has remained a nonsmoker for 10 to 15 years. However, smoking cessation at any point for a smoker is a good idea and quitting smoking reduces the risk of coronary heart disease, stroke, and peripheral vascular disease. Coronary heart disease risk is substantially reduced within 1 to 2 years of cessation (CDC, 2011g).

Lung cancer and smoking are significant health problems for many Americans. In 2009, smoking was higher among men (23.5%) than women (17.9%). Among racial/ethnic populations, Asians (12%) and Hispanics (14.5%) had the lowest prevalence of smoking; American Indians/Alaska Natives had the highest prevalence (23.2%), followed by non-Hispanic whites (22.1%) and African Americans (21.3%). By education level, smoking prevalence was highest among adults who had earned a General Educational Development (GED) diploma (49.1%) and among those with a 9th- to 11th-grade education (33.6%) and generally decreased with increasing years of education. People ages 65 years and older had the lowest prevalence of current cigarette smoking (9.5%) among all adults. Current smoking prevalence was higher among adults living below the poverty level (31.1%) than among those at or above the poverty level (19.4%) (CDC, 2011g). The mortality rate in African American men is almost 23% higher than that of White men. Women of both races have similar rates (Virginia Department of Health, 2012). Cigarette smoking and exposure to environmental or occupational toxins (air pollution, asbestos, or lead exposure) may have a synergistic effect and speed the production of lung cancer.

Lung cancer deaths are more common in the young-old than in the old-old. Deaths from lung cancer first appear at 35 to 44 years of age, and a sharp increase occurs between the ages of 45 and 55 years. The incidence continues to increase through the ages of 65 to 74 years, after which it levels off and decreases among the very old (Huether & McCance, 2012).

Types of Lung Cancer

At least 12 different types of tumors are included under the broad heading of lung cancer. Cancers of the cells that line the major bronchi or their primary branches are called squamous cell carcinomas. This type of cancer metastasizes mostly to other sites within the thorax. Adenocarcinomas are cancers of the glandular cells that line the respiratory tract. They most often start at the outer edges of the lungs and spread to the brain, the other lung, the liver, and bones. Large cell carcinomas usually begin in the outermost parts of the lung. By the time of diagnosis, they are often large, bulky tumors. Small cell carcinomas, also called "oat cell" cancers, usually begin in the bronchi. Small cell carcinomas metastasize widely to the mediastinum, liver, bones, bone marrow, central nervous system, and pancreas (Huether & McCance, 2012). Growth rate and metastasis rate vary by tumor type. Squamous cell carcinoma grows slowly and metastasizes late, and small cell carcinoma grows rapidly and metastasizes early.

Symptoms

The symptoms of lung cancer are vague and mimic the symptoms of other pulmonary illness, making diagnosis difficult. Chronic cough, **hemoptysis** (coughing up of blood or production of bloody sputum), chest pain, shortness of breath, fatigue, weight loss, and frequent lung infections such as pneumonia and bronchitis that do not resolve with antibiotic treatment could all be warning signs that indicate the older person should be referred to the primary care provider for further testing. The chest X-ray is usually the first examination the healthcare provider will order. Suspicious masses seen on the chest X-ray may signal the need for a computerized axial tomography (CAT) scan, positron emission tomography (PET) scan, or a magnetic resonance imaging (MRI) scan. Both the CAT scan and MRI can provide additional information about soft tissue masses, while the PET scan uses the patient's rapidly dividing cancer cells to validate the diagnosis. Further tests may include pulmonary function tests; bronchoscopy with the collection of lung tissue, cells, or fluids for analysis under the microscope; and biochemical and cellular studies of respiratory fluids removed from the lungs by lavage. Other important tests may include measures of arterial blood gas tensions (Pao_2 and $Paco_2$) (Lungcancer.org, 2012).

Older patients with lung cancer may undergo surgical removal of the tumor or the lung if they are good surgical candidates and are not diagnosed with comorbid conditions. Chemotherapy, ionizing radiation to the thorax, and palliative care are less aggressive approaches used for older patients with comorbid conditions. Newer targeted therapies being developed and tested include bioengineered monoclonal antibodies, anti-angiogenesis agents, growth factor inhibitors, and lung cancer vaccines to stimulate the body's immune system to attack the invading cancer cells (Lungcancer.org, 2012). The 5-year survival rate for people with lung cancer varies according to stage of diagnosis. For those diagnosed with early-stage lung cancer, 53% were alive 5 years later; for those diagnosed with late-stage lung cancer, the 5-year survival rate drops to 4% (Mayo Clinic, 2012).

Respiratory Infections

Infections are a major cause of respiratory illness. They can be caused by bacteria or viruses and can infect the lung, the nose, sinuses, and upper airways. Respiratory infections can also complicate other chronic illnesses and lung disease. Because of the decreased function in the immune system, older people with lung infections may not cough, exhibit an elevated temperature, or show other classic signs of respiratory infection. They may instead become lethargic, fall, exhibit loss of cognitive or physical function, or simply stop eating and drinking. The gerontological nurse must be cognizant of the atypical presentation of respiratory infection in the older person.

Most respiratory tract infections such as the common cold, pharyngitis, and laryngitis affect only the upper airway and require no treatment. These infections, although uncomfortable, are probably viral in nature and will not respond to antibiotics. Supportive care such as rest, cough medication to suppress nighttime cough, throat lozenges, and humidifiers can ease symptoms and improve comfort.

Sinusitis is inflammation of the mucosal lining of the paranasal sinuses that can lead to mucous stasis, obstruction, and subsequent infection. Sinusitis should not be confused with rhinitis, a condition characterized by inflammation of the mucous membranes of the nose, usually accompanied by nasal discharge. Rhinitis can occur in conjunction with an upper respiratory infection or may be allergic in origin.

Sinusitis can also be caused by allergens, air pollution, and irritants such as the use of inhaled recreational drugs. Normally the sinuses will drain up to 2 pints of mucus daily and are self-cleaning through the use of cilia that propel mucus outward to the nose. When bacterial infection occurs, this drainage can be impeded by mucosal swelling induced by the inflammatory response. Sinusitis can also be induced by dental abscess, irritation of nasogastric tubes, and immune deficiency syndromes.

Acute sinusitis may be diagnosed by the presence of dull pain over the maxillary sinuses that is worsened by bending over. Congestion, green nasal discharge, periorbital edema, and fever may also be present. Acute sinusitis often follows an upper respiratory infection. Chronic sinusitis with symptoms lasting longer than 3 months is usually related to allergies. Usually, radiological examinations are not necessary and the symptoms can confirm the diagnosis. Transillumination of the sinuses with a flashlight is seldom effective to confirm the diagnosis of sinusitis in an older person and is difficult to perform in many clinical settings.

Treatment of sinusitis usually involves nasal decongestants (phenylephrine 0.25%), one or two sprays every 4 hours in each nostril for up to 5 days; saline spray to lubricate and moisten the nares; and acetaminophen for discomfort. Humidified air may provide some relief. For acute sinusitis, some clinicians advocate treatment with antimicrobials such as Augmentin 500 mg every 12 hours for 2 weeks. As the sinuses are poorly perfused, longer treatment may be necessary to ensure that all areas of infection receive adequate concentrations of antibiotics and that the responsible bacteria are truly eradicated.

Neti pot irrigation can naturally relieve allergies, sinusitis, breathing problems, nasal congestion, and postnasal drip. It can even help prevent sinus infections. The neti pot has a long spout (Figure 16-10 ▶▶▶). The pot is filled with warm water and 1/4 teaspoon of salt. The nurse should instruct the patient to tilt his/her head to the side and insert the spout into one nostril. The patient should keep the mouth open and breath slowly, letting the water run through the sinus and out the other nostril. When the pot is empty, instruct the patient to lean over the sink and blow out (as if blowing his/her nose). The patient should repeat the process on the other side.

The use of antibiotics to treat upper respiratory infections and simple pharyngitis is not recommended because it encourages antibiotic resistance. Most upper respiratory infections will resolve spontaneously within 7 to 10 days. However, infections of the lower respiratory tract such as bronchitis and pneumonia are more serious in the older person and require aggressive evaluation and treatment.

Infections of the lower respiratory tract are the sixth leading cause of death in the United States and the fourth leading cause of death in Americans over the age of 65 accounting for 40,000 to 70,000 deaths each year. Community-acquired pneumonia (CAP) is responsible for 350,000 to 620,000 hospitalizations in the older adult every year. Older adults have lower survival rates than younger people. Even when older individuals recover from CAP, they have higher than normal death rates during the next several years. Older people who live in nursing homes or who are already sick are at particular risk (Johnstone, Marrie, Eurich, et al., 2007; *New York Times*, 2012).

Pneumonia, or inflammation of the lungs, is the most common type of infectious disease of the lung. Infectious pneumonias are usually identified by naming the cause of the infection or the pattern of infection in the lung (e.g., lobar pneumonia). Mortality rates from pneumonia have not decreased significantly since the 1950s. Among patients with CAP, mortality approaches 20%. Mortality from nosocomial pneumonia, an infection acquired while institutionalized in a hospital or nursing home, can approach 30% and reflects both the underlying frailty of the

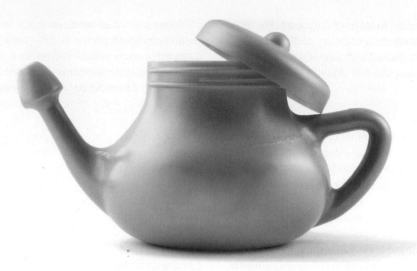

Figure 16-10 ▶▶▶ Neti pot.

Source: blake/Fotolia.

older person and the predominance of virulent pathogens present in institutional settings.

> ***Practice Pearl*** ▶▶▶ Both upper and lower respiratory infections may present atypically in the older person who may exhibit subtle signs and symptoms including mental status changes, falls, new-onset incontinence, or functional decline.

The following risk factors are thought to increase susceptibility to respiratory infection in the older lung and to affect the outcome of pneumonia:

- History of nosocomial pneumonia within the past 6 months to 1 year
- Diagnosed lung disease (COPD)
- Recent hospitalization
- Nursing home residence
- Smoking
- Hyperglycemia
- Use of medications such as immunosuppressants, anticholinergics or other agents that dry secretions, and agents that increase gastric pH
- Alcoholism
- Neurologic disease (dementia, cerebrovascular accident)
- Immunosuppression (corticosteroid use, malignancy)
- Use of oxygen therapy
- Severe protein-calorie malnutrition
- Heart failure
- Antibiotic therapy during the previous month
- Eating dependency
- Enteral feeding by nasogastric tube

Huether & McCance, 2012; Reuben et al., 2011.

Aspiration is a major risk factor for the development of pneumonia and stroke, dementia, and dysphagia. Gastric tube placements are major risk factors for aspiration. Sedative and narcotic use is associated with decreased levels of consciousness, lethargy, and nighttime aspiration. Viral infections, in particular influenza A, are a risk factor for secondary bacterial pneumonia (GSA, 2011).

Pathogens

Bacterial pathogens are the most frequent cause of pneumonia. *Streptococcus pneumoniae* remains the most prevalent bacterial pathogen and is estimated to account for approximately 50% of all infections. In addition, *Haemophilus influenzae, Staphylococcus aureus,* and Enterobacteriaceae cause more pneumonia in the older person than in the young. Atypical agents such as *Legionella* make up a smaller portion of pneumonias in older adults than in younger people, and pneumonia caused by *Mycoplasma pneumoniae* is rare after the age of 55. *H. influenzae* and *Moraxella catarrhalis* bronchial infections are commonly associated with lower respiratory tract infections in patients with COPD (McPhee & Papadakis, 2011; Reuben et al., 2011). Influenza is four times more common in people over 70 years of age than in younger adults. In most years, people over age 65 account for about 90% of influenza-associated deaths in the United States. Epidemics, sometimes associated with high mortality, are a problem in institutional settings. A virus can be spread by airborne droplets, via caregivers, and by exposure to contaminated respiratory equipment.

Symptoms of Pneumonia

The classic symptoms of pneumonia are cough, fever, and sputum production. Fever may be absent because many older people have a lower basal temperature and will not exhibit a fever response in the face of infection. Bacterial pneumonias are commonly preceded by a viruslike prodrome of headache, myalgia, and lethargy. Other symptoms may include abrupt onset of shaking chills (rigors). Nonbacterial pneumonia may be accompanied by substernal chest pain and dyspnea. However, the gerontological nurse must be alert for subtle changes in behavior and baseline physical signs. New-onset tachycardia and tachypnea are important clues to illness with both viral and bacterial pneumonia. Changes in function, appetite, continence, and other subtle symptoms may be the first signs of the onset of illness.

Nursing Assessment

When the gerontological nurse suspects pneumonia, health assessment should include checking vital signs, inspecting the thorax, and auscultating the lungs. The skin should be examined for cyanosis. Cyanosis may be detected around the lips and under the nail beds. Crackles that do not clear with coughing may be suggestive of pneumonia. Signs of consolidation (bronchial breath sounds, dullness to percussion, and egophony) are common findings with late-stage pneumonia.

The primary care provider will probably request a chest X-ray; however, it may be negative in early stages of the disease. Physical findings will probably precede the appearance of an infiltrate by about 24 hours. After resolution of the pneumonia, the chest X-ray will not appear normal for about 6 weeks. Optional testing such as blood cultures and sputum samples may be obtained when there is good reason to suspect the results will change how the patient is managed (Sherman, 2007). It is difficult to obtain sputum for analysis from an older person because a vigorous cough reflex is required to obtain the specimen. Many sputum samples sent for analysis contain mostly saliva or secretions from the upper airways that may reveal "carriage" or "colonization" (the bacteria an older person has living in the upper airway). These organisms may be completely different from the pathogens in the lungs responsible for the pneumonia. Pulse oximetry of arterial blood gases provides valuable information about the patient's status. Hypoxemia is associated with poor outcome. Older patients with severe hypoxemia should be referred to the acute care setting for immediate evaluation. A blood chemistry analysis may reveal marked leukocytosis, indicating that white blood cells are being produced to try to fight off the infection.

Up to 10% of all adult hospitalizations in the United States are due to CAP. Many patients do not need to be hospitalized for pneumonia, and can instead be safely treated at home. Likewise, many patients who are admitted to the hospital could be released sooner, reducing their risk of hospital-acquired infections. A number of strategies are being devised to determine when and which patients can be safely discharged. Studies have shown that low-risk patients with mild to moderate pneumonia do just as well when treated as outpatients and return to work and normal activities faster than those treated in the hospital (Li, Winston, Moore, et al., 2007).

Hospitalization for pneumonia should be considered when:

- Comorbidities are present (lung disease, alcoholism, malnutrition, congestive heart failure).
- Respiratory rate exceeds 30 breaths per minute.
- Hemoptysis is present.
- Diastolic blood pressure is less than 60 mmHg or systolic blood pressure is less than 90 mmHg.
- Temperature exceeds 38.3°C or 101°F.
- Pao_2 is less than 60 mmHg on room air.
- Chest X-ray shows more than one lobe involvement, presence of a cavity, or presence of a pleural effusion.
- There is evidence of sepsis.
- Patient is unable to take oral fluids.

American Thoracic Society, 2002; New York Times, 2012.

The CURB-65 has been endorsed as a simple way to assess need for hospitalization. One point is assigned to each of five easily measured factors: *C*onfusion, *U*remia, *R*espiratory rate (elevated), *B*P (low), and age 65 or older. A score of two points or more suggests the need for hospitalization or intensive home healthcare services (Sherman, 2007).

Treatment of Pneumonia

In the 1940s, widespread use of penicillin helped reduce mortality from *S. pneumoniae* infections. In the 1960s, resistance to penicillin by some organisms began to be reported, with patients dying despite treatment. Resistance was not considered a major problem until the early 1990s. Studies indicate that about 25% of isolates of *S. pneumoniae* are now resistant to penicillin (Reuben et al., 2011). The emergence of drug-resistant pneumococci and the development of new antimicrobials have changed the empirical treatment of pneumonia. Newer fluoroquinolones with activity against *S. pneumoniae* offer alternatives in the treatment of drug-resistant *S. pneumoniae* infection. New macrolides such as azithromycin and clarithromycin may be preferable to erythromycin because of better gastrointestinal tolerance (Epocrates, 2012). Antibiotic treatment should begin as soon as possible after the diagnosis is fairly certain (Sherman, 2007).

The treatment recommendations for older outpatients with community-acquired pneumonia are an oral macrolide (erythromycin, azithromycin, or clarithromycin) or an oral beta-lactam (cefuroxime, amoxicillin, or amoxicillin-clavulanate). For critically ill hospitalized older patients, an intravenous third-generation cephalosporin in combination with a macrolide is recommended.

Additional supportive treatments include chest percussion to clear secretions, inhaled beta-adrenergic agonists to dilate constricted airways, oxygen if needed, and rehydration. Although treatment of pneumonia is the same for all patients regardless of age, the older person requires more careful monitoring. Agents with nephrotoxic potential, like the aminoglycosides, should be used with caution. Hypersensitivity reactions are more frequent in older patients, and risk of antibiotic-associated diarrhea or colitis is common with ampicillin or clindamycin. Drug interactions may also occur between antibiotics and other therapeutic agents commonly used in older adults such as warfarin. Intravenous fluids should be administered slowly in patients with congestive heart failure to prevent overhydration and pulmonary edema.

Prevention

The current 23-valent pneumococcal vaccine was developed in 1983. Although more than 80 serotypes of pneumococci can cause pneumonia, the 23 most common serotypes are covered in the vaccine. The vaccine is approved by the FDA, and Medicare covers the cost of administration.

Vaccination is recommended for all people 65 years of age and older and all adults with immunosuppression or chronic illnesses. It is estimated that only about 25% of older patients with risk factors have received the pneumococcal immunization. The vaccine is approximately 80% effective with decreasing effectiveness over time. Revaccination is recommended 5 years after the first dose for people with renal failure, those who have had splenectomies, those with underlying malignancy, those on high doses of chemotherapy or corticosteroids, and patients with HIV/AIDS. When an older person's immunization status is unknown, the pneumococcal vaccine should be administered (CDC, 2009). Revaccination has minimal side effects, with the most common being a localized reaction at the injection site.

The influenza vaccine should also be received yearly in people who are at risk for pneumonia. The pneumococcal and influenza vaccines may be administered at the same time. The influenza vaccine alone is associated with a 52% reduction in hospitalizations for pneumonia, and the pneumococcal vaccine alone is associated with a 25% reduction in hospitalization for pneumonia. When both vaccines are given, the reduction in hospitalizations for pneumonia is 63% (American Thoracic Society, 2004). Older adults should not receive the live, attenuated influenza vaccine (LAIV) but instead should receive the inactivated influenza vaccine by injection. It is recommended for adults over the age of 50 and those with heart, lung, or kidney disease; those with diabetes, asthma, or anemia; and those with a weakened immune system or those taking drugs that cause immunosuppression. The flu shot is contraindicated in those with a history of Guillain-Barré syndrome, those acutely ill, or those with egg allergies (CDC, 2009). It takes approximately 2 weeks for protection to develop after vaccination.

Influenza may be treated with an antiviral medication if it is begun within 48 hours after the onset of symptoms. The following four antiviral medications are available to treat the influenza virus:

- Oseltamivir (Tamiflu) and zanamivir (Relenza)—effective against types A and B
- Amantadine (Symmetrel) and rimantadine (Flumadine)—effective against type A only (high rates of viral resistance)

McPhee & Papadakis, 2011; Reuben et al., 2011.

> ***Practice Pearl*** ▶▶▶ When an older person has been hospitalized for pneumonia and discharge planning is under way, remind the healthcare provider to order the pneumococcal vaccine before the patient leaves the hospital. Preventing a second episode of pneumonia is a necessary health-promoting intervention that may prevent future disease and hospitalization.

Nursing Diagnoses

The following nursing diagnoses may be appropriate for nursing care plans of older patients with pneumonia: *Infection, Risk for* based on advanced age or immunosuppression; *Health Maintenance, Ineffective* based on poor nutrition, tobacco or alcohol use; *Noncompliance,* based on inability or unwillingness to take medications as prescribed; *Airway Clearance, Ineffective* based on altered cough reflex and excessive secretions; *Aspiration, Risk for* based on diagnosis with neurologic disease such as cerebrovascular accident or dementia; and *Tissue Perfusion: Peripheral, Ineffective* based on the presence of hypoxia (NANDA International, 2012).

Patient-Teaching Guidelines for the Older Patient With Lung Disease

Older patients with pneumonia or influenza should be urged to rest and restrict activities to allow themselves time to heal and completely recover. Many will begin to recover after 5 to 7 days of antibiotic or antiviral therapy. Additional patient education points include the following:

- Stop smoking (permanently if possible, mandatory during acute treatment).
- Take 10 deep breaths an hour to aerate lungs and loosen secretions.
- Drink plenty of fluids to keep secretions moist.
- Take antibiotics or antivirals as prescribed and finish all medication.

- Report any adverse reactions immediately such as diarrhea, gastrointestinal irritation, rash or hives, and difficulty breathing.
- Avoid contact with others who are ill, infants, and frail older adults.
- Avoid coughing in public and practice good hand washing.
- Receive the pneumococcal vaccine as soon as possible after recovery and get a flu shot yearly to minimize the risk of further infection.

Acute Bronchitis

Acute bronchitis is an acute inflammation of the bronchi. It is usually a self-limiting viral illness. The signs and symptoms are similar to those of pneumonia and include productive cough, chills, lethargy, and low-grade fever. Chest X-ray will be negative, showing no active disease or infiltrates. Chest pain may be produced by muscle strain from prolonged and excessive coughing. Treatment consists of rest, humidification of the air, use of cough suppressants, and acetaminophen for aches.

People with COPD will usually be treated for bronchitis with antibiotics because their bronchitis may easily progress to pneumonia. This condition is sometimes called acute exacerbation of chronic bronchitis. Some healthcare providers instruct their COPD patients to phone immediately upon noticing a change in sputum color from clear to white or green.

Pulmonary Embolism

Pulmonary embolism is an occlusion of a portion of the pulmonary vascular bed by an embolus consisting of a thrombus, an air bubble, or a fragment of tissue or lipids. The highly branched network of blood vessels in the lung aerates the blood as it flows through the lungs. When the blockage occurs, gas exchange can no longer take place in this section of the lung. The result is shortness of breath, heart failure, or death. Pulmonary emboli in older people most often originate from deep vein thrombosis in the calf.

Pulmonary emboli are the third leading cause of death in the United States and account for about 100,000 deaths per year (CDC, 2011a). Depending on the size of the embolism, various degrees of hypoxemia can occur. A large occlusion in a major artery will cause severe results such as pain from infarcted lung tissue, decreased cardiac output, hypotension, and death. Smaller emboli may be chronic or recurrent in nature and result in vasoconstriction, pulmonary edema, and atelectasis. If the embolus does not cause infarction, the clot will usually dissolve and the lung will return to normal. If an infarction does occur, scarring will develop and lung function may be permanently lost.

Risk factors for formation of pulmonary embolus include clotting disorders, immobility, dehydration, recent surgery, atherosclerotic changes in the circulatory system, atrial fibrillation, and obesity. As many as 65% of patients with lower extremity trauma or surgery will develop deep vein thrombosis (CDC, 2011a).

Symptoms

Typical symptoms of pulmonary embolus include tachypnea, dyspnea, chest pain, hypoxia, decreased cardiac output, systemic hypotension, and possible shock.

Nursing Assessment

Patients with leg swelling and duskiness are at risk for pulmonary embolus. In people with suspected deep vein thrombosis, the calf of the affected leg should be carefully measured and the size noted and compared to the other leg. Asymmetry of more than 1 cm increases the likelihood of deep vein thrombosis from 27% to 56% in an at-risk individual (Huether & McCance, 2012). Positive ultrasound studies of the leg warrant the initiation of anticoagulation therapy for prevention of pulmonary embolus (Reuben et al., 2011).

Hypoxemia and hyperventilation are suggestive of the diagnosis of pulmonary embolus. A perfusion scan, in which lungs are scanned after injection of a radioactive dye into the venous circulation, can indicate obstruction of pulmonary circulation.

Treatment

Treatment consists of intravenous administration of heparin and other anticoagulant therapy. For large, life-threatening pulmonary obstructions, a fibrinolytic agent such as streptokinase is sometimes used; however, streptokinase cannot be administered within 7 to 10 days after surgery (Reuben et al., 2011). Warfarin therapy may be continued for 3 to 6 months after discharge to prevent the formation of another pulmonary embolus.

The gerontological nurse can play a vital role in the prevention of pulmonary embolus by identifying people at risk and reducing risk factors. Appropriate interventions include minimizing venous stasis by leg elevation, urging passive and active range-of-motion exercises in the immobile older person, encouraging early postoperative ambulation, and placing elastic compression stockings and pneumatic calf compression boots on the postoperative patient. Low-dose anticoagulation therapy with heparin is sometimes beneficial to prevent clots in postoperative patients until they become mobile. Prevention is key because less anticoagulant is needed to prevent a clot than to dissolve one already formed.

Nursing Diagnoses

Nursing diagnoses for older patients with pulmonary embolism may include *Breathing Pattern, Ineffective* when inspiration and/or expiration does not provide adequate ventilation, *Suffocation, Risk for Activity Intolerance* related to hypoxia, and *Pain, Acute* (NANDA International, 2012).

Severe Acute Respiratory Syndrome (SARS)

Within the recent past, an international outbreak of a virus suspected to be a mutated form of the coronavirus occurred. About 26 countries have been affected, with the most severe problems occurring in the Far East and parts of Canada. At this time, there is no definite cure for SARS, but treatment with antivirals and supportive care including oxygen administration and mechanical ventilation has been effective for some SARS patients.

The primary symptoms of SARS are lethargy, muscle aches, dry cough, difficulty breathing, and persistent fever over 38°C or 100.4°F (McPhee & Papadakis, 2011). Older people with these symptoms who have traveled to a high-risk country within the past 10 days, or have been exposed to someone who has, should seek medical attention immediately.

Preventive measures include wearing a face mask when in public areas of high-risk countries, strict isolation of infected people, and careful hand washing. The virus is hardy and has been shown to survive on various surfaces for 24 hours. No new cases have been reported since 2004, indicating the virus may have mutated and become less dangerous (McPhee & Papadakis, 2011).

COMPLEMENTARY AND ALTERNATIVE THERAPIES

Echinacea has been used to treat symptoms of cold, flu, and other respiratory infections and to boost the immune system to help fight off infections. Studies funded by the National Center for Complementary and Alternative Medicine (2011) have shown that echinacea may be helpful in treating upper respiratory infections. Further studies are ongoing to demonstrate effectiveness but to date no study has demonstrated effectiveness. Echinacea has not been documented to have significant side effects or interactions with other medications.

Some believe that there are possible asthma-related benefits associated with increasing the intake of omega-3 fatty acids (found in fish and fish oil). More research is likely needed to definitively answer the question of specific benefit of omega-3 fatty acids and their impact on mediators of inflammation thought to be important in the pathology of asthma; however, intake of high levels of omega-3 fatty acids has been shown to be beneficial for general health and wellness and therefore worthy of recommendation by the gerontological nurse.

In 2008, Airborne, a popular cold and flu remedy invented by a teacher, was advertised as a cure for the common cold or flu. A multimillion-dollar class action suit resulted, and consumers were allowed to file for refunds of up to six purchases. Airborne is compounded from a combination of herbs, vitamins, and minerals, but the FDA does not allow herbal supplements to be marketed as a cure or treatment for disease, thus leading to the claim of false advertising. The main benefit resulting from taking Airborne may be that it does contain 1,000 mg of vitamin C and helps people to stay hydrated because the tablet is a "fizzy" and dissolves in water. Although it may contain no harmful ingredients, it is has not been shown to live up to its claim of curing the cold or flu.

QSEN Recommendations Related to the Respiratory System

The Quality and Safety Education for Nurses (QSEN) project addresses the challenge of preparing future nurses with the knowledge, skills, and attitudes (KSAs) to continuously improve the quality and safety of the healthcare systems in which they work (Cronenwett et al., 2007). See the QSEN table for tips on meeting QSEN standards.

Meeting QSEN Standards: The Respiratory System

	KNOWLEDGE	SKILLS	ATTITUDES
Patient-Centered Care	Involvement of patient and family in plan of care is crucial.	Know family assessment and adult learning principles.	Appreciate uniqueness of each patient/family.

Meeting QSEN Standards: The Respiratory System *(continued)*

	KNOWLEDGE	SKILLS	ATTITUDES
	Examine barriers that may keep patients from being active in formulating their plan of care.	Evaluate depression, vision/hearing, function, tobacco use, and cognitive status.	Provide patient-centered care to improve successful nursing outcomes.
Teamwork and Collaboration	Recognize scope of practice for interdisciplinary team members.	Use leadership skills to coordinate team members and share knowledge.	Value the contribution of each member of the team to improve outcomes.
	Be aware of organizational problems that can inhibit effective team functioning.	System assessment skills.	Be open to input from team members on effective means to improve communication and collaboration.
Evidence-Based Practice	Describe effective interventions to decrease respiratory risk factors and improve overall health and function.	Access current evidence-based vaccination protocols to guide interventions.	Possess confidence in necessary skills to evaluate and incorporate nursing interventions from the literature.
Quality Improvement	Recognize the importance of measuring patient outcomes to improve respiratory care.	Skills in data management, technology, and U.S. government and ALA websites describing current incidence and prevalence of respiratory disease.	Value the use of data and outcomes as a key component of QI efforts.
Safety	Describe common medication and treatment errors and health system characteristics that increase the likelihood of such errors.	Use appropriate strategies to deliver patient/family education and provide written information to compensate for memory loss (if present).	Appreciate the impact of frailty and cognitive loss on the occurrence of adverse drug reactions.
	Recognize the factors that increase the risk of nosocomial infections.	Avoid the use of NG tubes and other interventions that increase the risk of aspiration pneumonia.	Institute infection control practices to decrease the incidence of respiratory infections.
Informatics	Provide input into the formation and maintenance of patient databases needed for gathering QSEN data and providing patient care.	Utilize the electronic health record.	Protect patient confidentiality according to HIPAA standards.

Patient–Family Teaching Guidelines

The following are guidelines that the nurse may find useful when instructing older adults and their families about lung disease.

LUNG DISEASE

1 How can I prevent lung disease?

Because respiratory problems are so often caused or aggravated by environmental exposure to toxins and pollutants, try to avoid these substances if at all possible. Some points to consider are:

- Do not smoke cigarettes or other tobacco products.
- Do not visit or work in areas where dangerous substances or irritants are in the air (oven cleaner, glues, spray paints, etc.).
- Do not go outside or exercise when smog is present or air pollution warnings are in effect.
- Try to avoid contact with ill people and places where illness rates are high.
- Wash your hands often, remove rings, and keep your fingernails short.

RATIONALE:

The prevention of respiratory disease is easier and safer than the treatment and cure. Stress prevention principles whenever appropriate.

2 If I already have lung disease, is there anything I can do to stop it?

Yes. If you smoke, stop immediately! Also carry out all the suggestions listed in question 1. If you are prescribed medication by your doctor, take it exactly as directed. Report any worsening of your condition or new symptoms to your doctor. Have your disease monitored with spirometry testing as often as recommended by your doctor and get to know your numbers.

RATIONALE:

Chronic lung disease requires careful ongoing monitoring to prevent crises and exacerbations. Careful ongoing assessment is needed.

3 Is there anything else I should do to make the most of living with lung disease?

Yes. Exercise to keep your muscles fit and strong, eat a healthy diet, control your weight, get a flu shot every fall, get the pneumonia shot at age 65 and then every 6 years afterward, and visit the dentist regularly. Good oral hygiene can decrease respiratory infections and keep you healthy.

RATIONALE:

Improvement and maintenance of general good health will improve function and quality of life for an older person with respiratory disease. Education regarding health maintenance is always appropriate.

CARE PLAN   A Patient With Lung Disease

Case Study

Mr. Lehman is admitted to the nursing home with the diagnoses of moderate dementia, COPD, and frequent falls. He is 84 years old. He no longer smokes, although he has a 50-year smoking history. He has an involved and loving son who lives nearby and a daughter in California who has not seen her father for several years. He has specified no advance directives.

About 1 week after admission, Mr. Lehman begins to exhibit symptoms of dyspnea on exertion. He had been walking approximately 50 feet to the dining room without difficulty and now finds he has to rest after walking about 20 feet. When questioned, Mr. Lehman states, "I just seem to run out of air when I walk." He has no fever, chills, chest pain, or lower extremity edema. His pulse is 96 and his respiratory rate is 26 at rest.

A Patient With Lung Disease (continued)

Applying the Nursing Process

Assessment

The gerontological nurse faces a dilemma because there is a lack of baseline information regarding Mr. Lehman. However, even with only 1 week of observation and experience, it seems clear that he is having a change from his baseline level of function. The nurse should think broadly and perform a head-to-toe nursing assessment to get further information. Vital signs should be carefully assessed because he presents with tachypnea and tachycardia at rest. Obtaining pulse oximetry at rest and on exertion may yield valuable information. Should hypoxemia be noted, activity should be restricted and oxygen provided to prevent cardiac complications.

Even though Mr. Lehman has a diagnosis of dementia, he should be carefully questioned about any symptoms of chest pain, difficulty breathing at other times, or presence of sore throat or cough that could indicate onset of new illness. It is useful to quantify dyspnea if possible. Sudden and unexpected onset of dyspnea can be associated with pulmonary embolus, pneumonia, or exacerbation of chronic bronchitis. Nocturnal dyspnea may be associated with congestive heart failure. Mr. Lehman should be weighed and his baseline weight compared with the current weight. A change of over 2 or 3 lbs may indicate heart failure with the retention of excessive fluid. Just because he does not have a fever, the gerontological nurse cannot be assured he is not developing a respiratory infection. The medical record should be reviewed to see whether Mr. Lehman received the pneumococcal vaccine within the past 6 years and the flu shot within the past year.

Another possibility is that Mr. Lehman may have an undisclosed swallowing disorder and have aspirated a foreign body that is partially occluding his bronchus. A careful review of his eating habits and preferences will assist the nurse in this area.

Diagnosis

Four possible nursing diagnoses for Mr. Lehman would be:

- *Activity Intolerance* related to hypoxia
- *Memory, Impaired*
- *Fatigue*
- *Gas Exchange, Impaired*

NANDA-I © 2012.

Expected Outcomes

The expected outcomes for the plan of care specify that Mr. Lehman will:

- Return to baseline function with appropriate treatment and monitoring of his chronic lung disease and hypoxia.
- Identify wishes toward treatment and establish advance directives as appropriate to patient and family preferences.

Planning and Implementation

The nurse should contact Mr. Lehman's primary care provider and report the change in condition and the information gathered in the nursing assessment. Because Mr. Lehman has no advance directives and has a diagnosis of moderate dementia, the family should also be contacted. They may be able to provide valuable information regarding his past medical history, including any previous episodes of dyspnea.

Mr. Lehman and his family should also discuss and communicate to the healthcare team regarding the way they would like him to be treated. For instance, they may want him to be sent to the hospital for aggressive assessment and care, they may wish diagnosis and treatment to occur in the nursing home, or they may prefer palliative care be delivered with emphasis on symptom control and patient comfort. This information is crucial and will form the basis for future healthcare decisions.

(continued)

CARE PLAN   ## A Patient With Lung Disease *(continued)*

Evaluation

The nurse hopes to work with Mr. Lehman and will consider the plan a success based on the following criteria:

- Mr. Lehman will exhibit normal pulse and respiratory rates and oxygen saturation readings at rest and on exertion.
- A family meeting will be held to discuss his overall health, values, and advance directives.

- Mr. Lehman will maintain or work toward normal body weight, functional status, and satisfactory quality of life.
- He will receive appropriate immunizations (pneumonia and yearly flu vaccines) to prevent exacerbation of chronic lung disease.

Ethical Dilemma

When Mr. Lehman is questioned about naming a healthcare proxy or someone to make decisions for him if he should become unable, he states, "Yes, I'd like to name my daughter in California. I love my son but I don't trust him to make the right decisions for me." The nurse reports this to the healthcare provider and the appropriate papers are signed.

The next day, the nurse practitioner brings this up in discussion with Mr. Lehman and his son. His son seems offended and states, "Well you know he is ill and sometimes his mind wanders. I think I should be the one to make all healthcare decisions for my dad."

The issue here is the conflict between Mr. Lehman's autonomy (the right to determine his healthcare proxy) and beneficence (what is in his best interest). Clearly, further information and involvement of the healthcare team are

needed. On the surface, it seems to make more sense for Mr. Lehman's son to be the healthcare proxy. He lives locally, is involved in his father's care, visits daily, and keeps track of his progress and health status. However, just because the daughter lives in California and seems less involved does not negate Mr. Lehman's desire to name her as proxy if he has the capacity to make an informed decision.

The nursing code of ethics supports the patient's right to self-determination and believes that nurses will—and must—play a primary role in implementing this right. The nurse should identify and mobilize mechanisms in place within the facility to resolve this conflict. Hopefully, the nursing home has an interdisciplinary ethics team with nursing representation to address and resolve this dispute.

Critical Thinking and the Nursing Process

1. What nursing interventions can you identify to help older adults to quit smoking?
2. What advice would you give to a teenager who is just starting to smoke cigarettes?
3. Imagine that you have to wear a nasal cannula during the day and must keep a portable oxygen tank with you

at all times. Would you feel self-conscious? How would you feel about eating lunch in a restaurant with friends? Write down some of the words that pop into your head as you imagine yourself in these types of situations.

- Evaluate your responses in Appendix B.

Chapter Highlights

- The two major functions of the respiratory system are related to respiration and metabolic function.
- Normal changes of aging, exposure to environmental toxins and pollution, and concomitant illness can affect the structure and function of the respiratory system.

- Because many problems related to respiratory function are a direct result of years of cigarette smoking, the gerontological nurse can function as an educator and change agent to assist the older patient to quit smoking. African

Americans are disproportionately affected by smoking-related respiratory illness.

■ Tuberculosis is a serious problem that can affect older people by reactivation of an old infection or the acquisition of new-onset disease after exposure to others with the disease.

■ Immunosuppression, chronic illness, and living in a long-term care facility are risk factors for developing tuberculosis. Purified protein derivative testing in the older person should involve a two-step approach with another vaccine administered 1 week after the first one with negative results.

■ Respiratory infections like pneumonia and influenza can cause death and disability for the older person, especially in the presence of diagnosed neurologic disease and immunosuppression. Because of the decreased immune response, it may be difficult to diagnose pneumonia in the older person.

■ The gerontological nurse should suspect pneumonia when the older person exhibits changes in behavior, appetite, continence, or function. Tachypnea and tachycardia may be early warning signs of pneumonia.

■ Antibiotic therapy and supportive treatment are necessary to treat pneumonia in the older person. Prevention using the pneumococcal and influenza vaccine is recommended.

■ Pulmonary embolism is a potentially life-threatening blockage of the blood vessels in the lungs and accounts for about 100,000 deaths per year. Preventive measures include minimizing venous stasis through early postoperative ambulation and calf compression. Low-dose anticoagulation may be needed for immobile older adults.

Pearson Nursing Student Resources
Find additional review materials at
nursing.pearsonhighered.com

Prepare for success with additional NCLEX®-style practice questions, interactive assignments and activities, web links, animations and videos, and more!

References

American Lung Association [ALA]. (2008). *Asthma.* Retrieved from http://www.lungusa.org/assets/documents/publications/soldoc-chapters/asthma.pdf

American Lung Association [ALA]. (2011). *Chronic obstructive pulmonary disease (COPD) fact sheet.* Retrieved from http://www.lungusa.org/lung-disease/copd/resources/facts-figures/COPD-Fact-Sheet.html

American Thoracic Society. (2002). *Diagnosis and care of patients with COPD.* Retrieved from http://www.thoracic.org

American Thoracic Society. (2004). *Statement on cardiopulmonary exercise testing.* Retrieved from http://www.thoracic.org

Centers for Disease Control and Prevention (CDC). (2009). *Pneumococcal polysaccharide vaccine.* Retrieved from http://www.cdc.gov/vaccines/pubs/vis/downloads/vis-ppv.pdf

Centers for Disease Control and Prevention (CDC). (2010). *Lung cancer statistics.* Retrieved from http://www.cdc.gov/cancer/lung/statistics

Centers for Disease Control and Prevention (CDC). (2011a). Are you at risk for deep vein thrombosis? Retrieved from http://www.cdc.gov/Features/Thrombosis

Centers for Disease Control and Prevention (CDC). (2011b). *Chronic obstructive pulmonary disease.* Retrieved from http://www.cdc.gov/copd

Centers for Disease Control and Prevention (CDC). (2011c). *Chronic obstructive pulmonary disease among adults aged 18 and over in the United States, 1998–2009.* Retrieved from http://www.cdc.gov/nchs/data/databriefs/db63.htm

Centers for Disease Control and Prevention (CDC). (2011d). *Faststats: Asthma.* Retrieved from http://www.cdc.gov/nchs/fastats/asthma.htm

Centers for Disease Control and Prevention (CDC). (2011e). *Faststats: Chronic obstructive pulmonary disease (COPD) includes: Chronic bronchitis and emphysema.* Retrieved from http://www.cdc.gov/nchs/fastats/copd.htm

Centers for Disease Control and Prevention (CDC). (2011f). *Reported tuberculosis in the United States: 2010.* Retrieved from http://www.cdc.gov/tb/statistics/reports/2010/executivecommentary.htm

Centers for Disease Control and Prevention (CDC). (2011g). *Tobacco use: Smoking cessation.* Retrieved from http://www.cdc.gov/tobacco/data_statistics/fact_sheets/cessation/quitting/index.htm#benefits

Centers for Disease Control and Prevention (CDC). (2011h). *Tuberculosis: Data and statistics.* Retrieved from http://www.cdc.gov/tb/statistics/default.htm

Cronenwett, L., Sherwood, G., Barnsteiner, J., Disch, J., Johnson, J., Mitchell, P., Sullivan, D., & Warren, J. (2007). Quality and safety education for nurses, *Nursing Outlook, 55*(3) 122–131.

Epocrates. (2012). Retrieved from https://online.epocrates.com/noFrame/showPage.do?method=diseases&MonographId=17&ActiveSectionId=42.

Gerontological Society of America (GSA). (2011). Influenza in older adults. *From Publication to Practice.* New York, NY: Author.

Huether, S., & McCance, K. (2012). *Understanding pathophysiology* (5th ed.). St. Louis, MO: Mosby.

Johnstone, J., Marrie, T., Eurich, D., & Majumdar, S. (2007). Effect of pneumococcal vaccination in hospitalized adults with community-acquired pneumonia. *Archives of Internal Medicine, 167,* 1938–1943.

Li, J., Winston, L., Moore, D., & Bent, S. (2007). Efficacy of short-course antibiotics regimens for community-acquired pneumonia: A meta-analysis. *American Journal of Medicine, 120,* 783–790.

Lungcancer.org. (2012). *Diagnosis of lung cancer.* Retrieved from http://www .lungcancer.org/reading/diagnosis.php

Mayo Clinic. (2012). Cancer survival rate: What it means for your prognosis. Retrieved from http://www.mayoclinic.com/health/ cancer/CA00049

McPhee, S., & Papadakis, M. (2011). *Current medical diagnosis and treatment.* New York, NY: McGraw-Hill Medical.

Moffatt-Bruce, S. (2011). Lung transplantation. *Medscape reference.* Retrieved from http://emedicine.medscape .com/article/429499-overview#a05

NANDA International. (2012). *NANDA International nursing diagnoses: Definitions and classification, 2012–2014.* Philadelphia, PA: Wiley-Blackwell.

National Center for Complementary and Alternative Medicine. (2011). *Colds and flu and CAM: What science says.* Retrieved from http://nccam.nih.gov/health/providers/digest/ coldflu-science.htm

National Heart, Lung, and Blood Institute (NHLBI), National Institutes of Health (2002). *The lungs in health and disease* (No. 97-3279). Bethesda, MD. National Institutes of Health, U.S. Department of Health and Human Services.

National Heart, Lung, and Blood Institute (NHLBI), National Institutes of Health. (2007). *Guidelines for the diagnosis and management of asthma* (National Asthma Education and Prevention Program, Expert Panel Report 3). Retrieved from http://www .nhlbi.nih.gov/health/health-topics/topics/ipf/ lungworks.html

National Heart, Lung, and Blood Institute (NHLBI), National Institutes of Health. (2011). *How the lungs work.* Retrieved from http://www.nhlbi.nih.gov/health/health-topics/ topics/ipf/lungworks.html

New York Times. (2012). *Health guide: Pneumonia.* Retrieved from http://health .nytimes.com/health/guides/disease/ pneumonia/prognosis.html

Nurses' Asthma Education Partnership Project. (2003). *Nurses: Partners in asthma care* (NIH Publication No. 95–3308).

Bethesda, MD: National Heart, Lung, and Blood Institute.

Partners Health Care. (2010). *Asthma center.* Retrieved from http://www.asthma.partners .org/newfiles/BoFAChapter44.html

Reuben, D., Herr, K., Pacala, J., Potter, J., Pollock, B., & Semla, T. (2012). *Geriatrics at your fingertip* (14th ed.). New York, NY: American Geriatrics Society.

Sanassi, L. (2011, May). Severe persistent asthma in adults. *ADVANCE for NPs & PAs,* pp. 19–24.

Sherman, C. (2007, October). Navigating the latest pneumonia guidelines. *The Clinical Advisor,* pp. 59–65.

UpToDate. (2012). *Theophylline use in asthma.* Retrieved from http://www.uptodate .com/contents/theophylline-use-in-asthma

Virginia Department of Health. (2012). *African Americans and smoking.* Retrieved from http:// www.vahealth.org/cdpc/TUCP/documents/2011/ pdf/StateFact_Sheets/African%20Americans% 20and%20Smoking.pdf

Wilkinson, J., & Ahern, N. (2009). *Nursing diagnosis handbooks with NIC interventions and NOC outcomes.* Upper Saddle River, NJ: Pearson Prentice Hall.

CHAPTER
17

The Genitourinary and Renal Systems

Tamara L. Zurakowski, PhD, GNP-BC
PRACTICE ASSOCIATE PROFESSOR OF NURSING, UNIVERSITY OF PENNSYLVANIA SCHOOL OF NURSING

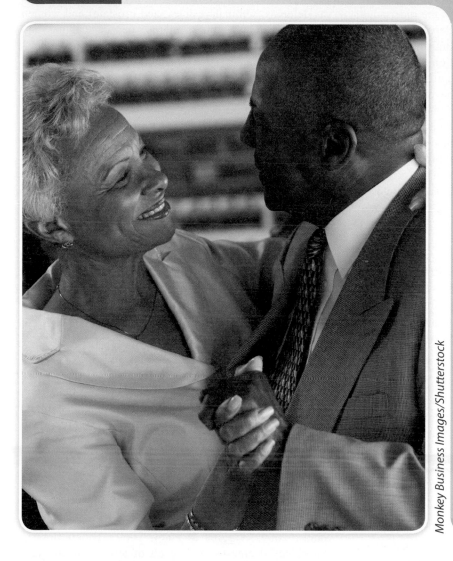

Monkey Business Images/Shutterstock

KEY TERMS

atrophic vaginitis *460*
benign prostatic hyperplasia
  (BPH) *459*
bladder training *458*
detrusor muscles *448*
dyspareunia *466*
erectile dysfunction (ED) *467*
functional incontinence *456*
nocturia *459*
overflow incontinence *455*
pelvic floor exercises (Kegel
  exercises) *458*
renal failure *452*
sexually transmitted diseases *461*
stress incontinence *455*
urge incontinence *455*
urinary frequency *454*
urinary incontinence (UI) *455*
urinary tract infection (UTI) *454*

LEARNING OUTCOMES

On completion of this chapter, the reader will be able to:

1. Describe the normal changes of aging in the physiology of the genitourinary and renal systems.
2. Differentiate among normal and disease-related changes in genitourinary and renal function in the older adult.
3. Identify the impact of changes in urinary function on the quality of life of older adults.
4. Recognize his or her own biases related to sexuality and aging.
5. Discuss the effect of the social and physical environment on genitourinary concerns in older adults.
6. Define appropriate nursing interventions for ameliorating the effect of genitourinary status on quality of life of older adults.

I n Western society, discussions relating to sexuality, the reproductive organs, and elimination of body waste have traditionally been considered socially taboo and may be deeply embarrassing to the older adult. Most older adults have been toileting independently since toddlerhood, and may be reluctant to admit having difficulty in this most private matter. In addition, today's older adults grew up in an era when genitalia, elimination, and sexuality were not discussed, and they have carried these attitudes and values into advanced age. It is unlikely that they discussed any of these topics with their own parents; therefore, they may have very little information about what to expect as they age. In addition, many older people, as well as healthcare professionals, erroneously accept as "normal" such genitourinary phenomena as incontinence, impotence, and dyspareunia.

Some nurses may also find it embarrassing or uncomfortable to discuss sexuality, sexual functioning, and elimination, and may hold unconscious biases about older adults. Some may consider older adults to be asexual, neither desiring nor needing an active sex life. Others may consider incontinence to be a minor annoyance and may overlook the effects it has on the older individual's quality of life. These are issues of both the quality of care that is afforded the older adult, and safety. It is essential to consider the older adult as a full partner in healthcare decisions and interventions, and to collaborate with other healthcare professionals who have expertise in genitourinary concerns of older adults. It is important to be aware of one's own belief system and to identify possible biases. Sensitivity to the emotions, knowledge base, and developmental framework of patient *and* nurse is crucial if the nurse is to intervene effectively to promote or restore the health of people with concerns related to the genitourinary tract.

Compassionate and skillful nursing care for older adults requires scientific knowledge, self-awareness, and strong communication skills. The North American Nursing Diagnosis Association (2012) has identified several nursing diagnoses related to *Urinary Elimination* or *Sexuality Patterns,* and they are as pertinent to older adults as they are to younger people.

NORMAL CHANGES OF AGING

It is difficult to differentiate normal aging of the genitourinary system from changes related to common pathologies found in older people. It is prudent, therefore, to keep an open mind when discussing age-related changes.

The genitourinary system includes the organs of urinary elimination (kidneys, ureters, bladder, and urethra) and reproduction in both men (penis, testis, epididymis, vas deferens, seminal vesicles, and prostate) and women (ovaries, fallopian tubes, uterus, cervix, vagina, and vulva). Hormones, such as testosterone, luteinizing hormone–releasing hormone (LHRH), luteinizing hormone (LH), follicle-stimulating hormone (FSH), estrogens, progesterone, and antidiuretic hormone (ADH), are responsible for regulation of the system (Timiras & Leary, 2007). The urinary system removes wastes from the body and participates in the regulation of fluid and electrolyte balance, acid–base balance, blood pressure, and red blood cell production. The genital system provides for the conception and birth of children, and is integral to expressions of intimacy and self-concept. Figure 17-1 ▶▶▶ illustrates the normal changes of aging in the male and female genitourinary systems. Both men and women undergo physical changes as a result of declines in hormones that regulate fertility and reproduction. This change occurs more gradually in men and more suddenly in women during the perimenopausal period.

Age-Related Changes in the Kidney

Renal function begins to decline around the age of 40, but does not create significant issues for an otherwise healthy individual until the ninth decade of life. At that time, decreased glomerular filtration rate, renal blood flow, maximal urinary concentration, and response to sodium loss are marked. The renal function in an 85-year-old person is only about 50% of that of a 30-year-old person (Timiras & Leary, 2007). Sclerosis may be found in as many as 40% of the remaining glomeruli, and fibrous changes in the interstitial tissues may be found in older adults without kidney disease (Schlanger, Bailey, & Sands, 2009; Wiggins & Patel, 2009). Blood flow to the kidney decreases as a result of atrophy in the supplying blood vessels, particularly in the renal cortex. In addition, the proximal tubules decrease in number and length. Figure 17-2 ▶▶▶ illustrates the anatomy of a nephron. The older adult will usually demonstrate a lower creatinine clearance than a young adult, and will typically excrete lower levels of glucose, acid, and potassium, and more dilute urine (lower specific gravity). As these changes progress, the serum creatinine level and the blood urea nitrogen (BUN) will rise (Esposito et al., 2007). In addition, the kidneys of older adults, in contrast to the kidneys of younger adults, excrete more fluid and electrolytes at night than in the daytime. More urine is formed at night, frequently interrupting sleep patterns.

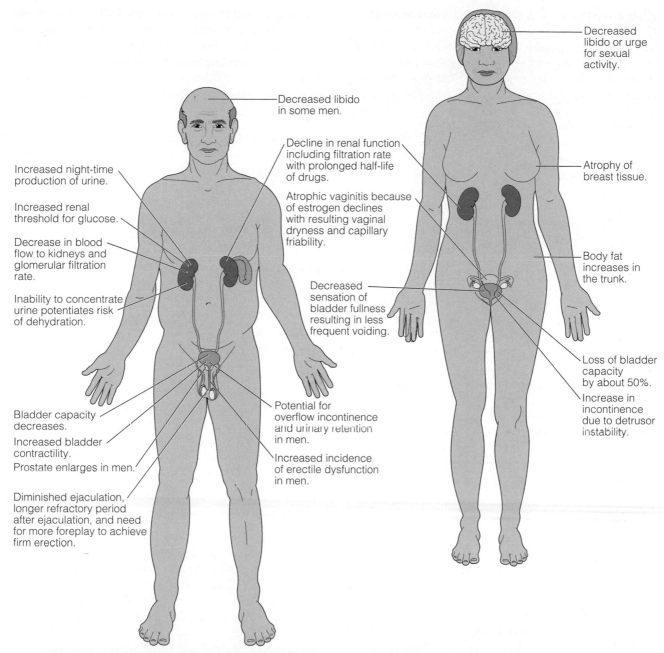

Decreased libido
in some men.

Decreased
libido or urge
for sexual
activity.

Decline in renal function
including filtration rate
with prolonged half-life
of drugs.

Atrophy of
breast tissue.

Increased night-time
production of urine.

Atrophic vaginitis because
of estrogen declines
with resulting vaginal
dryness and capillary
friability.

Increased renal
threshold for glucose.

Decrease in blood
flow to kidneys and
glomerular filtration
rate.

Body fat
increases in
the trunk.

Decreased
sensation of
bladder fullness
resulting in less
frequent voiding.

Inability to concentrate
urine potentiates risk
of dehydration.

Loss of bladder
capacity
by about 50%.

Bladder capacity
decreases.

Increase in
incontinence
due to detrusor
instability.

Increased bladder
contractility.

Potential for
overflow incontinence
and urinary retention
in men.

Prostate enlarges in men.

Increased incidence
of erectile dysfunction
in men.

Diminished ejaculation,
longer refractory period
after ejaculation, and need
for more foreplay to achieve
firm erection.

Figure 17-1 ▶▶▶ Normal changes of aging in the genitourinary system.

One of the consequences of these changes is an impairment in the excretion of drugs and their metabolites, making older adults extremely susceptible to drug overdoses and other adverse medication effects, even within a normal dose range. Another consequence is an increased probability of hyperkalemia, particularly when potassium-sparing diuretics, ACE inhibitors, nonsteroidal anti-inflammatory drugs (NSAIDs), and beta-blockers are used (Timiras & Luxenberg, 2007). A consequence of the older adult's decreased ability to concentrate urine is increased susceptibility to dehydration, a problem that is further complicated by a deficit in the thirst response; therefore, the older person will not feel thirsty even when significantly dehydrated. In addition, an older adult who has concerns about

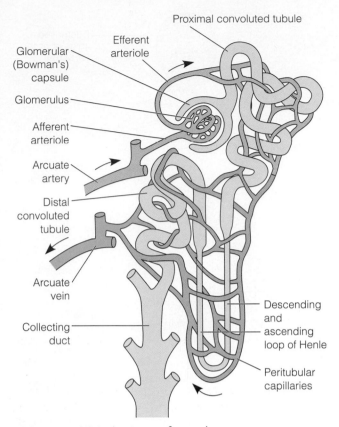

Figure 17-2 ►►► Anatomy of a nephron.

Drug Alert ►►► Because of renal excretion changes, be particularly vigilant for signs of toxicity when older patients are taking antibiotics, digoxin, diuretics, beta-blockers, statin lipid-lowering agents, angiotensin-converting enzyme (ACE) inhibitors, and oral antidiabetic agents. Even in healthy older adults, normal changes of aging affect rates of drug excretion.

Three different methods are used to estimate GFR: the Cockcroft-Gault (C-G) equation, the Modification of Diet in Renal Disease (MDRD) equation, and the Chronic Kidney Disease Epidemiology Collaboration (CKD-EPI) equation. There are significant differences in the GFRs estimated by these three methods when applied to people older than 70 years (Dharmarajan, Yoo, Russell, et al., 2012). The earlier recommendation that the C-G equation be used because the MDRD equation tends to overestimate renal function in elders (Gill, Malyuk, Djurdjev, et al., 2007) is now being called into question. Experts are now recommending that healthcare providers use one formula consistently, and note which formula that is (Dharmarajan et al., 2012).

---

incontinence will choose not to drink for fear of an incontinence accident. A fifth consequence of these changes in older adults is a decline in the ability to respond to a fluid overload by increasing urine production.

Bladder and Urethral Changes With Aging

Changes in the bladder and urethra also occur with aging. The bladder becomes more fibrous, with subsequent decreased capacity and increased postvoiding residuals (McCance & Huether, 2010). Figure 17-3 ►►► illustrates the structure of the bladder and supporting detrusor muscles. Autonomic innervation of the bladder decreases with age, affecting not only contraction of the detrusor muscle, but also the external sphincter. The **detrusor muscles,** three layers of muscle that cover the bladder, become less contractile but also somewhat unstable. This means the older adult is subject to both an inability to completely empty the bladder and involuntary contractions of the bladder (Johnson & Ouslander, 2009). There is age-related weakening of the voluntary pelvic floor muscles that are important to controlling the release of urine from the urethra. There is also evolving evidence that older adults experience neurological changes in the areas of the brain that control the bladder (Griffiths, Tadic, Schaefer, et al., 2009), indicating that there is decreased activation in the brain in response to bladder fullness in older adults. These changes make older adults more likely to have difficulty delaying urination and predispose them to urinary incontinence and urinary tract infection. Even though there are anatomical and physiological changes that make incontinence

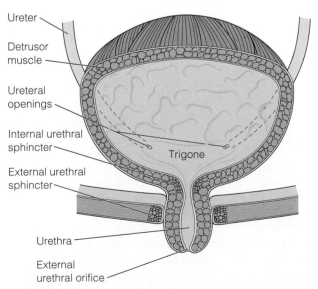

Figure 17-3 ►►► The structure of the bladder and supporting detrusor muscles.

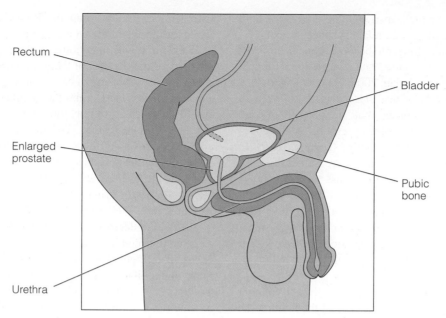

Rectum

Bladder

Enlarged
prostate

Pubic
bone

Urethra

Figure 17-4 ▶▶▶ Enlarged prostate gland and its relationship to the bladder in an older male.

Source: National Institute of Diabetes and Digestive and Kidney Diseases. (2006). Prostate enlargement: Benign prostatic hyperplasia. Available from http://kidney.niddk
.nih.gov/kudiseases/pubs/prostateenlargement/index.htm.

more probable with increased age, urinary incontinence is *not* a normal part of aging.

The urethral changes in women are mostly related to the loss of estrogen following menopause. The external sphincter muscle becomes thinner and less able to resist the pressure of urine from the bladder. In men, there is no muscle thinning, but the enlargement of the prostate may constrict the urethra. Figure 17-4 ▶▶▶ illustrates an enlarged prostate gland and its relationship to the bladder in an older male.

> ***Practice Pearl*** ▶▶▶ Due to estrogen-mediated changes in the perineal area of postmenopausal women, the urinary meatus may be difficult to visualize. When attempting urinary catheterization, you may wish to consider placing the older woman in a side-lying position, and visualize the perineum by lifting the buttock. If you are right handed, assist the woman to lie on her left side, with her back toward you. If you are left handed, assist the woman to her right side. By lifting the buttock, you should be able to visualize the urinary meatus on or near the anterior vaginal wall.

Antidiuretic Hormone and the Aging Process

Older adults tend to have higher basal levels of ADH than younger adults, and the pituitary responds more vigorously to osmotic stimuli by secreting more ADH than in younger

people (Timiras & Leary, 2007). ADH is released as a response to hypotension and hypovolemia; however, its action is blunted in older adults requiring the release of more hormone to achieve the desired antidiuretic effect. In addition, the aging kidney is less responsive to circulating ADH, producing urine that is poorly concentrated and rich in sodium. This puts the older adult at increased risk of hyponatremia, which can be magnified with the use of diuretics.

Male Reproductive System and Advanced Age

The weight of the testes does not decrease in old age, although the testes become less firm. Approximately half of all men continue to produce viable sperm up to the age of 90 years (Veldhuis, Keenan, Iranmanesh, et al., 2007). The number of seminiferous tubules that contain sperm decreases dramatically with age, but the adage "it only takes one" seems to apply here: Older men can father children.

The testes gradually produce less testosterone, starting at approximately age 50 (Veldhuis et al., 2007). Concomitantly, FSH and LH levels increase, probably in response to a decrease in circulating testosterone. The secondary sex characteristics supported by testosterone, such as muscle mass and body and facial hair growth, tend to diminish.

The older man will notice several age-related changes in his sexual response and performance, but it is important for both the patient and nurse to know that sexual response and performance should be present in the older adult. For both men and women, the major age-related change in sexual response is timing. It takes longer to become sexually aroused, longer to complete intercourse, and longer before sexual arousal can occur again (Lindau, 2009; Tenover, 2009).

The decreased levels of testosterone in the older man change the vascular responses that are part of arousal. Arousal in older men occurs more in response to direct penile stimulation than to psychic factors (Lindau, 2009). In general, the older man's libido may decrease but does not disappear. If an older man reports a loss in sexual interest, the nurse should be as concerned as when a younger man reports a loss of interest in sexual activity. Older men achieve an erection that is less firm than in younger men, but still capable of penetration. Ejaculation may take longer to occur, and the older man may have difficulty anticipating or delaying ejaculation.

The orgasm of older men differs from that of younger men in that there are fewer contractions of the urethra, the amount of seminal fluid decreases, and the force of ejaculation lessens. The nipples may not engorge to firm erections, and the rectal sphincter contractions that accompany climax are less frequent. After orgasm, the erection is rapidly lost. The refractory period (time until next erection is possible) is lengthened to several hours, or in some cases, as long as 24 hours (Veldhuis et al., 2007).

Female Reproductive System and Advanced Age

The most obvious change in the female reproductive tract as a woman ages is the cessation of menstruation, although the hormonal changes that bring on menopause are also responsible for a number of other changes in the older woman's body. Menopause is the complete cessation of menstruation secondary to the lack of ovarian function, and the average age of onset varies by geographical region (Palacios, Henderson, Siseles, et al., 2010). Women in Europe and North America have an average age at onset of menopause of approximately 50 to 52 years, whereas women in Latin America may experience menopause as early as age 42 years. African American women enter menopause at the same average age as Caucasian American women (McKnight et al., 2011). During perimenopause, the years leading up to complete cessation of the menses, FSH levels increase, although LH remains constant, and estrogen levels vary widely (Bellino, 2007). Follicles mature irregularly, and ovulation may occur sporadically. Because most of a woman's estrogen is produced by the corpus luteum after ovulation, the fluctuating estrogen levels may be explained by the irregularity of ovulation. Once menopause has occurred, FSH and LH stabilize at levels much higher than in younger women.

Estrogen levels fall off dramatically and remain at very low levels for the rest of the woman's life.

Estrogen affects many other target organs, in particular the mucous membranes of the genitourinary tract. The decreased levels of estrogen cause the vaginal tissues to thin and become less elastic, and the vagina to shorten (Lindau, 2009). There is less vaginal lubrication, potentially making intercourse more painful. The uterus shrinks; the cervix, urethra, and trigone of the bladder also atrophy (Bellino, 2007). When these changes are compounded by the alterations in the bladder and urethra, the older woman is at increased risk for urinary incontinence, urinary retention, and infection.

Just as the decrease of testosterone in the man causes changes in secondary sex characteristics, so does the decrease of estrogen cause similar changes in older women. Pubic and axillary hair may become more sparse. Because women also produce small amounts of testosterone, loss of libido in an older woman may be related to a decrease in testosterone (Lindau, 2009). Breast tissue grows in response to estrogen. As estrogen levels taper off, the breasts become less firm and somewhat pendulous. The glandular tissue in the breast is gradually replaced by fat, and the ligaments supporting the breast (Cooper's ligaments) no longer maintain the lobular shape of the breast. The ducts near the areola become less elastic and may be palpated as firm string-like structures (Bickley & Szilagyi, 2007). The mons and vulva also lose fullness, and the clitoris may become smaller (Lindau, 2009). The level of circulating androgens in the woman, no longer opposed by estrogen, may cause coarsening of the skin and an increase in facial hair.

Older women also experience changes in their sexual responses. It takes longer for the older woman to become sexually aroused and to produce vaginal lubrication. The labia and uterus do not fully elevate, making penetration slightly more difficult. The clitoris remains an important part of orgasm, but may become irritated more easily because the clitoral hood is less protective than in younger women. During orgasm, the uterus will contract less frequently, but the contractions remain vigorous, and orgasm is as intense as in younger women. Box 17-1 summarizes the normal changes of aging related to the genitourinary tract for men and women.

Gay, Lesbian, and Transgendered Older Adults

Sexuality is a multifaceted concept, and includes physical, psychological, and social aspects (Watters & Boyd, 2009). Some of the operant aspects when considering gay, lesbian, or transgendered older adults are sex, sexual orientation, and gender identity (American Psychological Association,

---

BOX 17-1 ▸ **Major Age-Related Genitourinary Changes**

Kidney

↓ Decreased weight, glomeruli, glomerular filtration rate
↓ Decreased concentration of urine
↑ Increased serum creatinine, blood urea nitrogen
↑ Increased nighttime formation of urine
↓ Decreased drug excretion
↑ Increased basal level of antidiuretic hormone

Bladder and Urethra

↓ Decreased autonomic innervation
↓ Decreased capacity
↓ Decreased detrusor contractility
↑ Increased postvoid residual

Male Reproductive Tract

↓ Decreased sperm production
↓ Decreased testosterone
↑ Increased time to arousal, ejaculation, refractory period
↓ Decreased firmness of erection, force of ejaculation

Female Reproductive Tract

Post-Menopausal Changes

↓ Decreased estrogen levels
↓ Decreased thickness, elasticity, lubrication of vaginal tissues
↓ Decreased glandular tissue in breasts
↑ Increased time to arousal

2012). Current scientific evidence posits that sexual orientation and gender identity are biologically based. Sex is the most obviously biological or physical variable, and is based on the chromosomal determination of male or female, the reproductive organs, and external genitalia. Gender is the combination of attributes that a particular social group assigns to people, based on biological sex. For example, in the United States, being a "girl" frequently means wearing pink clothing, being caring toward others, and not being assertive. Sexual orientation is the romantic or erotic attraction of an individual to others of the same or opposite sex, and is not a dichotomous variable. Many people have some level of attraction to both sexes, with attraction to one sex being stronger than to the other. Gender identity is an individual's sense of being a man or a woman. When a person understands him- or herself to be of the gender that is the opposite of that person's biological sex, the individual is considered transgendered. People whose sexual orientation or gender identity is outside of social norms are sometimes referred to as sexual minorities.

Older adult members of sexual minorities experience the same physical changes as do their heterosexual peers. Older gays, lesbians, and transgendered people, however, are affected by many social factors that may exacerbate those physical changes. There is little research on the needs of older adult members of sexual minorities, and research about transgendered elders is almost nonexistent (Addis, Davies, Greene et al., 2009). Nurses must provide excellent care without a well-supported body of knowledge. Some facts, however, are well documented. For example, most gay and lesbian people who are now older adults have experienced blatant hostility toward their sexual orientation

HEALTHY AGING TIPS

▸ Drink plenty of water every day, and don't wait until you are thirsty to get a drink.

▸ Be aware of your response to new medications, because age-related changes in the kidney may lead to over- or underdosing.

▸ Urinary incontinence is never normal, and should be thoroughly evaluated by a healthcare provider.

▸ Screening exams for prostate, cervical, and breast cancers may not provide significant benefits for older adults. Discuss them with your healthcare provider before scheduling these tests.

▸ It is normal to continue to desire sexual activity. It is also normal to have little interest in sex, particularly if that has been a long-term pattern.

▸ If you are going to engage in sexual activity, take appropriate precautions to protect yourself and your partner from sexually transmitted infections.

(Brotman et al., 2007; Haber, 2009; Pope, 1997), and continue to face discrimination in terms of housing, social services, and access to their families when in the hospital (Addis et al., 2009; Haber, 2009). Lack of support from an older adult's biological family may mean that gays and lesbians enter old age with a significant lack of social support and an increased likelihood of living alone (Haber, 2009). Many older members of sexual minorities do not have a reliable source of assistance with the disabilities that may come with aging (Averett, Yoon, & Jenkins, 2011).

They may be even more hesitant than other older adults to discuss sexuality for fear of prejudice or rejection (Addis et al., 2009; Averett et al., 2011; Haber, 2009; Neville & Henrickson, 2010). In addition, older gays and lesbians may be reluctant to seek health care because they fear the response of the healthcare provider (Haber, 2009). An insensitive or judgmental nurse may easily compromise the sexual health of this group of older adults.

Common Genitourinary Concerns

The popular press has brought erectile dysfunction into common discourse, but there are other genitourinary diseases and problems that are also important to older adults. Some, such as malignancies, require effective collaboration among health professionals. The nurse, however, may be the primary healthcare provider for such concerns as urinary incontinence and unsatisfactory sexual activity.

Acute and Chronic Renal Failure

Age-related changes in the kidney, particularly the decrease in glomeruli and glomerular filtration rate, make the older adult particularly vulnerable to renal disease (Schlanger et al., 2009). **Renal failure,** the inability to remove nitrogenous waste from the body and to regulate fluid and electrolytes and acid–base balance, may arise from problems with blood flow to the kidney (prerenal), injury to the glomeruli or tubules (renal), or outflow obstruction (postrenal). The failure may be acute, with a sudden onset; or chronic, in which irreversible damage accumulates, usually over time. Renal failure in the older adult can be difficult to diagnose and treat, in part because of the presentation of symptoms, and in part because of the delicate balance of kidney function in the older adult.

Acute renal failure is a common occurrence among older adults, and can arise from a number of causes (Schlanger et al., 2009). Prerenal causes are common in older adults and lead to poor perfusion of the kidney. Renal causes may be secondary to chronic diseases such as hypertension and diabetes mellitus. One of the most prevalent postrenal causes is prostatic hypertrophy (Table 17-1).

Renal failure has different presentations in older and younger adults. In younger adults, marked oliguria is the most dramatic symptom of acute renal failure, but the older adult may not display this symptom. Postural hypotension is a common finding in prerenal acute renal failure (Schlanger et al., 2009), and the nurse is in a position to monitor for this finding. BUN and serum creatinine levels increase, and dependent edema may be present (Table 17-2). Ultrasound may demonstrate changes in the size of the kidney, or the presence of calculi, in renal and postrenal causes. The complex nature of renal failure in older adults makes an interdisciplinary approach critical. The nurse, nephrologist, and nutritionist are essential members of the care team. A nephrology consult is important in limiting kidney damage and decreasing mortality (Schlanger et al., 2009). Nutritional support is also important, but weight loss of up to 1 lb per day is expected in the older adult with acute renal failure. Any attempt to prevent the weight loss may overtax multiple

TABLE 17-1	Causes of Renal Failure in Older Adults	
Prerenal Causes	**Renal Causes**	**Postrenal Causes**
Dehydration	Acute glomerulonephritis	Benign prostatic hyperplasia
Shock	Aminoglycoside antibiotics	Prostate cancer
Vomiting and diarrhea	Sepsis	Bladder cancer
Surgery	Acute pyelonephritis	Calculi
Cardiac failure	Aneurysms	Fecal impaction
Diuretics	Cholesterol embolus	Urethral strictures
NSAIDs	Allergic response to radiocontrast media	Gynecological cancers
ACE inhibitors	Renal hypertension secondary to renal artery stenosis	
Hypotension	Diabetic nephropathy	

Source: Beers & Berkow (2000); Schlanger et al. (2009); Wiggins & Patel (2009).

TABLE 17-2	**Comparisons of Signs and Symptoms of Renal Failure in Older Adults**	
	Acute Renal Failure	**Chronic Renal Failure**
Onset	Sudden	Gradual
Blood pressure	Postural hypotension	Hypertension
Electrolytes	Increased BUN and serum creatinine	Increased serum phosphate, calcium, BUN, creatinine, potassium Decreased serum calcium Metabolic acidosis
Edema	Dependent	Generalized
Well-being	Fatigue and drowsiness	Fatigue and drowsiness
Urine output	Possible decreased urine output	Volume decrease over time
Gastrointestinal symptoms	Nausea and vomiting Rapid weight loss	Nausea and vomiting Anorexia Weight loss
Other symptoms	Flank pain	Decreased glomerular filtration rate Anemia Pruritus, uremic "bronzing," and uremic odor Altered mental status

Source: Beers & Berkow (2000); Jassal, Fillit, & Oreopoulos (1998); Schlanger et al. (2009).

systems and lead to cardiac failure. For example, the use of nutritional supplements that are high in calories may be contraindicated in the older adult with acute renal failure. Allowing weight loss to occur during this acute phase may better protect the long-term health of the older adult. Dehydration in the older adult is a causative factor in acute renal failure, and it is essential that the older adult with renal failure remain adequately hydrated (Schlanger et al., 2009).

Chronic renal failure is caused by irreversible damage to the kidney and is much more common in older adults than in younger adults (Beers & Berkow, 2000). Diabetes mellitus, benign prostatic hyperplasia, hypertension, and long-term use of NSAIDs all contribute to the higher prevalence of chronic renal failure in older adults. The symptoms and signs are similar to those exhibited by younger people, and include decreased glomerular filtration rate, hyperphosphatemia, hypocalcemia, hyperkalemia, metabolic acidosis, hypertension, and anemia. The assessment of chronic renal failure in the older adult is made more difficult by the age-related decrease in glomerular filtration rate, and the calculations to estimate this rate all tend to *over*estimate kidney function in older adults because of the secretion of creatinine in the renal tubules that is not considered in the formulas (Wiggins & Patel, 2009). As the disease progresses, the older adult may experience pruritus, general lack of well-being, generalized edema, altered

cognition, anorexia, nausea, and weight loss. As with acute renal failure, prompt consultation by a nephrologist is critical to improving the older adult's quality of life and long-term survival (Schlanger et al., 2009).

The treatments for chronic renal failure should be modified for the older adult. The restrictions on fluid intake and dietary protein should be less stringent, since most older adults have already decreased their protein and sodium intakes (Jassal et al., 1998), as well as their fluid intake. Constipation, a concern for many older adults, especially those who curb their own fluid intake, may exacerbate the hyperkalemia that accompanies chronic renal failure. Nursing and medical management for regularity are important contributions to the treatment plan. Thinning, dry skin is a common concern for all older adults, and the pruritus of chronic renal failure can present a real challenge. Careful skin care by the nurse, including moisturizing the skin, will be much appreciated by the older patient.

The definitive treatment for chronic renal failure is renal replacement therapy, either through dialysis or through renal transplant (Schlanger et al., 2009). Older adults in the United States are underrepresented among those receiving any type of dialysis or transplant (U.S. Renal Data System, 2007); however, they are more likely than younger adults to receive in-center hemodialysis, if they are receiving renal replacement therapy at all. This trend is consistent

don't discriminate

with Binstock's (1999) concerns that de facto age-based rationing of expensive healthcare services is being practiced. The nurse must be a strong advocate to ensure that older adults with chronic renal failure are well informed about treatment options and are not discriminated against because of their age in care decisions. It is also important to be realistic about the benefits of renal dialysis. Hemodialysis usually requires 4 hours per day, three or more days per week. Although older adults are living longer after the initiation of renal dialysis than they were 20 years ago, a person who is age 80 or above when they start dialysis will live an average of 2.59 years (Jassal, Trpeski, Zhu et al., 2007). Even among the young-old, those 65 to 69 years of age, the average life expectancy after starting dialysis is only about 4.5 years. The nurse is in an excellent position to help the older adult realistically consider the advantages and disadvantages of this therapy.

Urinary Tract Infection

Changes in the urinary tract of older adults make them more susceptible to urinary tract infections. A **urinary tract infection (UTI)** is the presence of bacteria in the urethra, bladder, or kidney, although the majority of UTIs in older adults are asymptomatic (Nicolle, 2009). Some authors term this condition *asymptomatic UTI,* whereas others apply the term *UTI* only to those older adults with symptoms, and use *bacteriuria* to define the presence of bacteria in the urine with no concomitant symptoms (Nicolle, 2009). (In the following discussion, *UTI* will indicate bacteriuria, symptomatic or not. If indicated, the phrase *asymptomatic UTI* will be used.) Eleven percent of all women experience UTIs annually (Griebling, 2007b), and that number may be almost three times higher in women ages 85 years and above (Eriksson, Gustafson, Fagerström et al., 2010). Older men have about one third the rate of UTIs of older women (Griebling, 2007a). Older adults who have indwelling catheters have a nearly universal rate of asymptomatic UTI, and the rate of symptomatic UTI is much higher than in people without indwelling catheters (McCue, 1999). UTIs in catheterized older adults tend to be polymicrobial and difficult to eradicate. Before using an indwelling catheter, the potential benefits to the older adult must be carefully weighed against the serious risks posed.

Older adults do not present the same symptoms of UTI as do younger adults. Particularly in a long-term care setting, a change in behavior may be the only indicator of a UTI (Woodford & George, 2009). The typical symptoms usually seen in younger adults with UTIs—urgency and frequency—may not be present in the older adult and therefore lack diagnostic usefulness. If, however, an older adult presents with new symptoms of urinary urgency, a shortened period of time between the urge to void and actual urination,

urinary frequency, or more than seven voids per 24-hour period, an investigation of these symptoms is indicated.

> **Practice Pearl** ▶▶▶ It is important to remember the principle of nonmaleficence (do no harm). Although it may seem inappropriate not to treat bacteriuria, if the older patient is not troubled with symptoms, offering an antibiotic will not improve the outcome, and may cause harm.

Asymptomatic UTI does not require treatment. In fact, treatment does not improve the morbidity or mortality in affected older adults (Nicolle, 2009). Routine urinalysis for older adults without symptoms is neither appropriate nor cost effective. In the presence of symptoms, however, treatment decisions should be based on a urine culture and sensitivity test. UTI in an older person with an indwelling catheter is considered to be complicated and may include a variety of microorganisms, such as *Escherichia coli, Proteus mirabilis, Klebsiella pneumoniae, Citrobacter* spp., *Providencia* spp., and *Pseudomonas aeruginosa* (Nicolle, 2009). Even in older adults without indwelling catheters, a wide variety of organisms may be found in the urine. The only way to accurately identify the causative organism, and thus treat the infection effectively, is to obtain a urine culture. If an older adult is able to follow directions and cooperate with the nurse, obtaining a clean-catch urine specimen is done according to standard procedure. Nursing research indicates that cleansing with nonsterile gauze that has been moistened with tap water and soap is as effective for clean-catch specimen collection as prepackaged sterile towelettes (Ünlü, Sardan, & Ülker, 2007), and is gentler to the mucous membranes.

A clean, newly applied condom catheter and collection bag can be used with an older man who cannot participate in specimen collection. Immediately prior to applying the condom catheter, the nurse should thoroughly clean and dry the glans of the penis (Nicolle, 2009). Many experts recommend straight catheterization for collecting an uncontaminated specimen from older women who are unable to cooperate. However, Brazier and Palmer (1995) empirically demonstrated that two other methods also provide an uncontaminated sample. External collection pouches are effective if the labia are properly cleaned and separated. The other method requires an in-toilet collection pan with a sterile bowl placed inside. The nurse assists the older woman to the toilet, separates and cleans the labia with disposable moist towelettes without contaminating the sterile bowl, and then maintains the separation of the labia until the patient voids. The specimen may then be poured from the sterile bowl into a sterile specimen container, and the older woman is assisted to wipe and re-dress herself.

Once the microorganisms have been identified, an appropriate antibiotic is prescribed. The pathogens that cause UTI, particularly *E. coli*, have become increasingly resistant to the usual treatment of trimethoprim-sulfamethoxazole (Bactrim). Fluoroquinolones have been used in its place, raising concerns about diminishing their effectiveness as a broad-spectrum antibiotic. Nitrofurantoin, 100 mg, by mouth, twice a day, for 5 days, has been recommended as an alternative that is effective and appropriate for the treatment of uncomplicated UTI (Gupta, Hooten, Roberts et al., 2007). Gender is a consideration in treatment choices, because men require longer periods of treatment than women. The longer urethra in men makes it less likely that bacteria can ascend into the bladder. When bacteria do reach the older man's bladder, the infection is considered to be complicated and requires a longer course of treatment.

Urinary Incontinence

Urinary incontinence (UI), the involuntary loss of urine, affects over 13 million adults and costs older adults approximately $19.5 billion per year (Hu et al., 2004). Approximately one third of noninstitutionalized older women experience UI (Song & Bae, 2007), and nearly one fifth of community-dwelling older men report UI. These figures

rise to nearly 50% for older men and women in long-term care settings with older women affected twice as often as older men (National Kidney and Urologic Diseases Information Clearinghouse [NKUDIC], 2007a). Symptoms of UI are very bothersome to older adults, and lead to social isolation, skin breakdown, and sleep disturbances (Stenzelius, Westergren, Mattiasson et al., 2006). Nurses are in a key position to decrease these staggering numbers.

> **Practice Pearl** ▶▶▶ Some older adults will not mention incontinence because they consider it embarrassing or just a normal part of aging. It is important to explicitly ask about involuntary loss of urine.

when did it start

UI may be classified by the cause of the involuntary loss (Table 17-3). **Stress incontinence** is defined as the involuntary loss of urine when intra-abdominal pressure is increased, such as during coughing or laughing. Either the pelvic floor muscles or the internal urethral sphincter is not strong enough to counter the pressure on the bladder, and urine is released. **Urge incontinence** occurs when the detrusor muscles contract forcefully and unexpectedly, and the internal sphincter is unable to retain urine in the bladder. **Overflow incontinence** is sometimes known as mechanical incontinence because a blockage of the urethra may be the cause of the bladder overfilling and stretching

Smoke overweight constipation

TABLE 17-3   Types of Urinary Incontinence

Type	Etiology	Examples	Group Most Affected
Stress	Weakened external sphincter/pelvic floor, increased intra-abdominal pressure	Small urine loss during sneezing, laughing, exercise	Women under age 60 Men after prostate surgery
Urge	Detrusor instability, internal sphincter weakness	Overactive bladder and losses or large amounts of urine	Older adults of both sexes, older men somewhat more affected
Overflow	Bladder muscles overextended and have poor tone, overflow of retained urine	Enlarged prostate causes obstruction of the urethra, urine backs up in bladder; diabetic nephropathy affects the contractility of the detrusor muscles. May present as "dribbling" or constant losses of small amounts of urine.	People with diabetes mellitus Men with enlarged prostates People taking calcium channel blockers, anticholinergics, and adrenergics
Functional	Physical or psychological factors impair ability to get to the toilet	An older adult unable to transfer from wheelchair to toilet is unable to obtain needed assistance and often voids large amounts of urine on the floor while walking to the bathroom.	Frail older adults Nursing home residents People with dementias

Source: NKUDIC (2007a).

the bladder muscles beyond the point of contractility. Overflow may also occur if the muscles are unable to contract properly because of lack of innervation, as in spinal cord injury or in diabetes mellitus. Finally, **functional incontinence** is defined as incontinence related to causes external to the urinary apparatus, such that the older adult is unable to get to a toilet to void. For example, a person who is restrained may be aware of the need to void and can control the release of urine (up to a point), but is not assisted to the toilet in a timely manner. Older adults with dementia may experience functional incontinence because they are unable to find the toilet.

Figure 17-5 ▶▶▶ illustrates weakening of pelvic floor musculature as seen in older women with stress incontinence. Lowered estrogen levels after menopause might contribute to stress incontinence by lowering the pressure around the urethra and increasing the chance of leakage.

> **Practice Pearl ▶▶▶** New-onset urinary incontinence is *always* a nursing priority.

The nurse is in an ideal position to collect data to assist in diagnosing and treating UI. Assessment should include the six areas of health history related to UI: mental status evaluation, functional evaluation, environmental assessment,

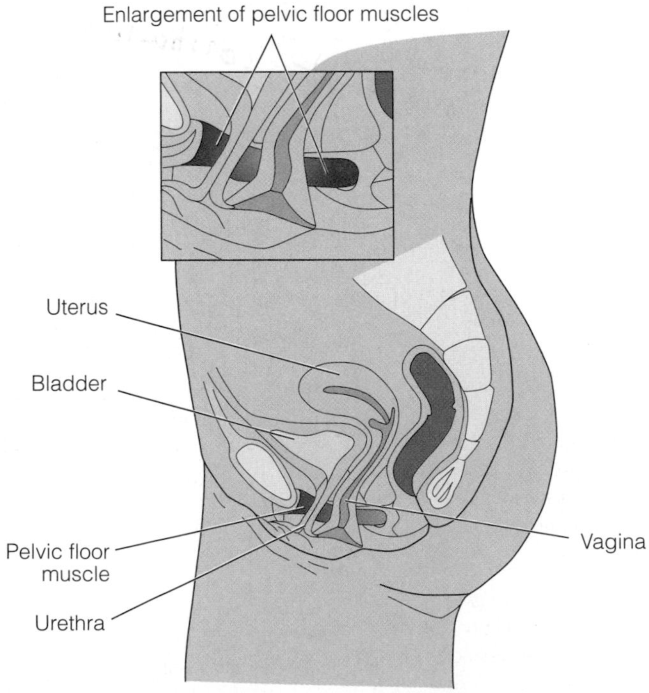

Figure 17-5 ▶▶▶ Pelvic floor muscle weakening in a female with stress incontinence.

Source: NKUDIC (2007a).

social supports, bladder records, and physical examination (Jarvis, 2004). Health history questions related to UI should include the following (Johnson & Ouslander, 2009):

- Is a concurrent medical condition, such as UTI, cerebrovascular accident (CVA), or diabetes mellitus, affecting continence status?
- Has UI occurred before? If so, under what conditions did it occur?
- What is the pattern of UI? The nurse should ask questions that will help categorize the type of UI (see Table 17-3).
- What medications are currently being used?
- What amount, type, and timing of fluid intake are present? It is important to assess fluids that may irritate the bladder or increase urine production (Wyman, Burgio, & Newman, 2009).
- How does the UI affect the older person's quality of life?

In addition to these health history questions, a mental status examination and functional assessment (see Chapter 3⊂⊃) must be completed to evaluate the effect these areas might have on continence. A careful assessment of the environment should include locating the toilet and any obstacles to its use (long distance from where the older adult is, lack of grab bars, poor lighting, lack of room to maneuver, and interior decorating that "disguises" the toilet room) (Lekan-Rutledge & Colling, 2003). The clothing that an older adult wears is also part of the environment and should be evaluated to see if it is impairing continence. For example, can the older person easily remove clothing to use the toilet? The presence of significant others is an important part of the social support that is available to the older adult. The ability and willingness of significant others to assist in toileting should be assessed. Paid assistants, such as certified nurse aides, are also part of this social support evaluation.

> **Practice Pearl ▶▶▶** Although nursing treatments for UTI prevention are important to minimize overuse of antibiotics and medication-related side effects, many of these interventions have not been rigorously tested in clinical trials. Further research is needed to support the effectiveness of these interventions.

New-onset urinary incontinence should be aggressively investigated by the gerontological nurse. The earlier the cause is identified, the sooner nursing interventions can be instituted to correct the problem and improve the patient's situation. The Hartford Institute for Geriatric Nursing (2007) recommends the use of the mnemonic **DIAPPERS** for identifying the cause of new-onset urinary incontinence. This instrument assesses the presence of key causes of incontinence such as infection, mobility restriction and use of certain drugs. See Figure 17-6 ▶▶▶ for an example of a bladder record or diary that may be a helpful tool in evaluating and managing UI.

The primary healthcare provider should perform a physical assessment, focusing on areas that may contribute to incontinence. These include an abdominal examination, particularly looking for distended bowel or bladder; rectal examination, evaluating for impacted stool; and genital examination, observing for skin condition and presence of organ prolapse (Kane, Ouslander, & Abrass, 2004).

Once transient conditions contributing to UI have been identified and treated, and a diagnosis of type of UI has

been made, a treatment plan may be implemented. A certified wound, ostomy, and continence nurse (CWOCN) is a valuable asset to both nurse and patient. The CWOCN is educationally prepared to treat patients with wound, ostomy, or continence concerns, and must pass a rigorous written examination (Wound, Ostomy, and Continence Nursing Certification Board, 2008). They are expert nurses, able to treat patients directly or to offer consultation to nurses who will then implement a plan of care.

Treatments for UI are categorized into five categories: lifestyle modification, scheduled voiding regimens, pelvic floor muscle strengthening, anti-incontinence devices, and supportive interventions (Wyman, 2003). Medications

NAME:					
DATE:					
INSTRUCTIONS: Place a check in the appropriate column next to the time you urinated in the toilet or when an incontinence episode occurred. Note the reason for the incontinence and describe your liquid intake (for example, coffee, water) and estimate the amount (for example, 1 cup).					
Time interval	Urinated in toilet	Had a small incontinence episode	Had a large incontinence episode	Reason for incontinence episode	Type/amount of liquid intake
6–8 A.M.					
8–10 A.M.					
10–noon					
Noon–2 P.M.					
2–4 P.M.					
4 6 P.M.					
6–8 P.M.					
8–10 P.M.					
10–midnight					
Overnight					
No. of pads used today:			No. of episodes:		
Comments:					

Figure 17-6 ▶▶▶ Sample bladder record.

form a sixth category. A combination of interventions from several categories is usually referred to as a toileting program (Lekan-Rutledge & Colling, 2003). The most successful interventions to reduce UI include different combinations of pelvic floor muscle exercises, avoidance of bladder irritants, scheduled toileting, and constipation management (Talley, Wyman, & Shamliyan, 2011). The older adult must be a partner in choosing the interventions (Table 17-4), but the nurse should be aware that an older adult's treatment preferences may be very different from those of care providers (Pfisterer, Johnson, Jenetzky et al., 2007). The Pfisterer et al. study indicated that older adults found "diapers" and medications equally attractive, while care providers were more likely to choose scheduled toileting for the older adult. Nurses should take care to consider the consequences of skin breakdown, pH changes, and hygiene issues if the "diaper" is the older adult's preference. Bradway (2005) also discovered that older women may develop their own interventions, including wearing dark clothing, carrying extra underwear, avoiding public transportation, always locating bathrooms when out, and avoiding sexual intercourse. People with UI can benefit in many ways from good nursing care.

Practice Pearl ▶▶▶ An older adult who is taking diuretics should be helped to identify the onset and peak action of the diuretic, and then aided in developing a toileting schedule to maximize continence.

Several of these interventions merit further discussion, as the nurse may be responsible for a major portion of the actual implementation. Timed voiding has been demonstrated to be effective for older women with stress incontinence and for some older men after prostatectomy (Wyman, 2003).

This intervention, however, requires consistency among caregivers, or an older adult who is independent in toileting, and may be difficult to maintain (Wyman et al., 2009). A schedule is established for toileting, usually every 2 hours, but as long as 3 hours may be acceptable. The older adult is assisted (if needed) to the toilet and encouraged to relax the pelvic floor muscles and attempt to urinate. Because of the importance of adequate sleep (see Chapter 8 ⊂▭), the nurse and older adult should carefully consider whether the schedule will continue throughout the night.

Bladder training is similar to timed voiding, but the intervals between trips to the toilet are gradually lengthened, training the bladder to hold slightly increased amounts of urine. Prompted voiding also uses some of the techniques of timed voiding, but rather than assisting the older adult to the toilet every 2 hours, the nurse reminds the older adult every 2 hours to go to the toilet. Some common foods may act as bladder irritants, and although research findings on them have not been consistent, anecdotal evidence is strong enough to make avoidance of them a reasonable intervention.

Pelvic floor exercises, or **Kegel exercises,** are another UI intervention frequently employed by nurses. The technique works well for urge and stress incontinence. It requires that the older adult be motivated to perform the exercises and be cognitively intact enough to learn them (Wyman, 2003). The older adult is instructed to tighten the muscles of the perineum, without also tensing the muscles of the abdomen, thigh, or buttock (Assad, 2000). It may help to identify the muscles by instructing the older adult to imagine trying not to pass gas. Imagining the perineum as an elevator that goes from floors one through five may help. The "fifth floor" represents a very intense tightening and may produce muscle fatigue, particularly if the contraction is held for more than 10 seconds (Meadows, 2000). Suggest only quick trips to the fifth floor! A recommended

---

TABLE 17-4   Examples of Treatments for Urinary Incontinence

Lifestyle Modifications	Scheduled Voiding Regimens	Pelvic Floor Muscle Strengthening	Anti-Incontinence Devices	Supportive Interventions
Smoking cessation	Timed voiding	Kegel exercises	Pessaries	Elevated toilet seats
Weight reduction	Prompted voiding	Biofeedback	Condom catheter	Gait training
Bowel management	Bladder training	Electrical stimulation	External clamps or urethral plugs	Modified clothing
Caffeine reduction				Absorbent pads or undergarments
Appropriate fluid intake				

Sources: Wyman (2003); Wyman et al. (2009).

pattern is 15 repetitions of rapid contractions, one to three sets, daily (Assad, 2000). Pelvic floor exercises may be combined with a general fitness routine, such as a walking program, to gain even greater control over urinary continence (Kim, Suzuki, Yoshida et al., 2007).

The role of diet in UI is still somewhat controversial, with much anecdotal evidence to support it, and little research either way (Keilman, 2005). Certain foods and beverages may be bladder irritants, and lead to incontinence. Some of the common irritants are carbonated beverages, dairy products, citrus fruits and juices, highly spiced foods, tomatoes, cranberries (yes, you read that correctly), sugar, honey, corn syrup, artificial sweeteners (particularly aspartame), caffeine (coffee, tea, cola, chocolate), and alcohol. Because UI is such a major problem for older adults, the nurse may wish to consider discussing bladder irritants with the patient, even in the absence of consistent evidence. The older adult may want to eliminate irritants from the diet one at a time, and monitor the effect on UI (Wyman et al., 2009).

Several medications are available to assist the person with stress or urge UI. Anticholinergic drugs are generally helpful in reducing symptoms of overactive bladder and urge incontinence (Nabi, Cody, Ellis et al., 2006), but are inappropriate for individuals with glaucoma, high blood pressure, and benign prostatic hyperplasia. They may increase symptoms in older adults with myasthenia gravis, Alzheimer's disease, and Parkinson's disease. Stress incontinence in women may be treated with topical estrogen applications. Medications should be used as an adjunct to other therapies; the risks and benefits should be carefully considered, and discussed with the older adult.

> **Drug Alert** ▶▶▶ Anticholinergic medications, such as those used in treatment of UI, are generally not recommended for use in older adults (American Geriatrics Society Beers Criteria Update Expert Panel, 2012). This class of medications is widely recognized for exacerbating cognitive impairment in older adults, particularly those with Alzheimer's disease, because the neurotransmitter acetylcholine is not produced in the same quantity in older adults as in younger adults. The use of anticholinergic medications, therefore, may further decrease an already limited supply. Within the class of anticholinergic medications, there is a range of potential effect, and it may be possible to select a drug with a milder anticholinergic profile. Most drug handbooks include a table of anticholinergic medications.

Many older adults who experience UI use disposable incontinence pads or protective undergarments. Although these may be helpful in managing the social consequences of UI, they are neither a cure nor without adverse effects. Excellent skin care remains a nursing priority because urine can be very damaging to the skin. That damage can be exacerbated by anything that decreases airflow to the affected area. Pads or undergarments must be changed frequently and after every episode of incontinence. They should be disposed of in ways that minimize environmental impact, especially the patient's immediate surroundings. Used incontinence products can have an unpleasant odor, and care should be taken to keep the older adult's room or home aesthetically pleasing.

> **Practice Pearl** ▶▶▶ It is essential to be considerate of a patient's dignity and self-esteem. The term *diapers* is demeaning to many. The nurse should use the product name (Depends, for example), or *products* or *protective undergarments*. Walk a mile in your patient's shoes: try wearing adult protective undergarments for a few hours. You may find that "diapers" are not as efficacious an intervention as you thought. Not only are they uncomfortable, but they are often visible through the clothing, and can cause damage to the skin.

Benign Prostatic Hyperplasia

Benign prostatic hyperplasia (BPH) affects 50% of men between the ages of 51 and 60 years, and 90% of men over age 80 (National Institute of Diabetes and Digestive and Kidney Diseases, 2001). BPH is classified in three ways. Microscopic BPH is diagnosable only by histologic changes. Macroscopic BPH is characterized by palpable enlargement of the gland during rectal examination (Wei, Calhoun, & Jacobsen, 2007). Clinical BPH refers to observable symptoms related to BPH (Wei et al., 2007). The growth of the prostate is influenced by the interactions among androgens and estrogens (Bushman, 2009). BPH affects older men without regard to race, tobacco use, level of sexual activity, or vasectomy (Chow, 2001), but African American men present more urinary symptoms than other groups (Wei et al., 2007).

The symptoms of BPH are sometimes referred to as "nuisances," although they can have a profound effect on daily living. They include difficulty starting a stream of urine, weak stream, straining to urinate, longer time needed to urinate, and a feeling of incomplete bladder emptying (Bushman, 2009). Collectively, these symptoms are referred to as "lower urinary tract symptoms," or LUTS. As the prostate continues to grow, urinary retention may occur. Symptoms of bladder irritation secondary to the enlarged prostate include urinary urgency, frequency, and **nocturia.** Some men experience urge incontinence as a result of BPH. Nocturia occurs in 83% of men over the age of 70 (Wei et al., 2007), creating serious problems with sleep disturbances (see Chapter 8 ⊂⊃).

> **Drug Alert** ▶▶▶ Urinary retention in men with BPH can be precipitated by several classes of medications, including those with anticholinergic properties and over-the-counter medications for the common cold.

A man presenting with symptoms of BPH should be evaluated with questions about his medical history, presence and severity of LUTS, a physical exam including a digital rectal exam and estimation of the size of the prostate, a urinalysis, and a blood test for prostate specific antigen (PSA) (McVary et al., 2011). Standard treatments include recommendations to lose weight if overweight, increased exercise, appropriate timing of fluid intake, behavioral modification, and use of anticholinergic medications. If symptoms continue at an unacceptable (to the older man) level, additional interventions are recommended. These include alpha-adrenergic blocking medications such as tamsulosin and doxazosin mesylate. If these medications are not effective in reducing symptoms to an acceptable level, or hematuria, pain, UTI, elevated PSA, or abnormal findings on the digital rectal exam are present, further evaluation and intervention are warranted. Interventions may include urodynamic studies, ultrasound imaging or biopsy of the prostate gland, minimally invasive surgical treatments (MIST) to reduce the size of the prostate, or more invasive surgery to remove all or part of the prostate. Other medications are available for the management of BPH symptoms, and include 5-alpha reductase inhibitors, such as finasteride, and antimuscarinics such as darifenacin.

Saw palmetto is an over-the-counter herbal preparation that has been recommended for improving BPH symptoms (Chow, 2001), but empirical studies have not consistently demonstrated its efficacy (McVary et al., 2011). As with any herbal preparation, saw palmetto is not regulated by any organized group. Problems of inconsistent packaging, mixing, and bioavailability should be considered.

When urinary retention becomes refractory to other treatments, or renal insufficiency due to bladder outlet obstruction develops, surgical intervention may be the only treatment option (NKUDIC, 2007b).

Transurethral procedures, such as needle ablation and microwave thermotherapy of the prostate, are Minimally Invasive Surgical Therapies (MIST) recommended for moderate to severe symptoms of BPH (McVary et al., 2011). Surgeries, such as transurethral resection of the prostate (TURP), are now recommended only when there is evidence of BPH-related renal insufficiency, recurrent UTIs, bladder stones, gross hematuria, or LUTS that are not responsive to other treatments. Older men who have the surgery are at risk for erectile dysfunction, retrograde ejaculation, hemorrhage, infection, and incontinence (Chow, 2001; McVary et al., 2011).

Menopause-Related Concerns *Dyspareunia*

Although menopause is an age-related process, not a pathology, some women have troublesome health experiences after the cessation of menses. These include decreased vaginal lubrication, **atrophic vaginitis** (thinning and atrophy of the vaginal epithelium usually resulting from diminished estrogen levels), more frequent UTIs, UI, cognitive changes, vasomotor instability (hot flashes), and sleep disturbances (Palacios et al., 2010). The type and frequency of postmenopausal symptoms varies by racial background, with African American women experiencing more hot flashes than other American women.

Menopause is an emotionally laden subject with many cultural implications. Different societies view aging women differently, and the older woman may internalize some of these views. Women may experience negative changes in their body image, or a feeling that they are no longer sexually viable people (Daniluk, 1998). Some women may celebrate menopause; others attach no significance to it.

The mediating factor in postmenopausal health concerns appears to be estrogen. Until recently, estrogen or hormone replacement therapy (HRT) was commonplace to relieve the problematic effects of menopause. In 2001, however, the American Heart Association strongly advised healthcare providers to stop prescribing HRT to postmenopausal women for cardioprotection (Sitruk-Ware, 2007). The recommendation was based on the Women's Health Initiative study, which demonstrated that HRT was not cardioprotective and could be deleterious to women with concomitant cardiovascular disease (Manson et al., 2003). The International Menopause Society (Sturdee & Pines, 2011) now recommends that the advantages and disadvantages of HRT be considered on an individual basis. It should be part of a menopause management program that includes diet and exercise, smoking cessation, and health promotion. Factors to consider when discussing HRT are the woman's symptoms, concurrent health concerns, and family history. HRT appears to be most effective in managing vasomotor and urogenital atrophy symptoms. HRT is cardioprotective in women who are within 10 years of the onset of menopause, but is associated with increased cardiovascular risk when initiated in women ages 60 and over (Sturdee & Pines, 2011). There are no empirical data on how long HRT should continue, and length of therapy should be based on effectiveness in treating menopausal symptoms, and the estimated risks and benefits for the individual older woman.

Atrophic vaginitis may result in urogenital infection, ulceration, and uncomfortable sexual intercourse. The treatment of choice is topical estrogen as a cream that is applied to the affected tissues (Sturdee & Pines, 2011). Topical creams have not demonstrated the link to adverse effects that systemic HRT has (Sitruk-Ware, 2007; Strandberg, Ylikorkala, & Tikkanen, 2003; Sturdee & Pines, 2011).

Genitourinary Malignancies

Older adults are more susceptible to a number of cancers than are younger adults. Leukemia, lymphomas, lung cancer, and colorectal cancer are all more prevalent in older adults (American Cancer Society [ACS], 2012). Of particular relevance to genitourinary health are cancer of the bladder, breast, prostate, uterus, and ovary (ACS, 2012).

Cancer of the Urinary Bladder

Bladder cancer is one of the more common malignancies that affect older adults. Older men are almost four times more likely to develop bladder cancer than are older women, and approximately 1 in every 27 men over the age of 70 will develop it (ACS, 2012). White, non-Hispanic men are particularly susceptible to the disease, although African American men have a higher mortality rate, probably reflecting the quality of health care available to both groups (Etzioni, Berry, Legler et al., 2002). Common risk factors include cigarette smoking and occupational exposure to certain chemicals known as arylamines.

Some symptoms of bladder cancer are similar to those of other urinary tract diseases: microhematuria, urinary frequency, urgency, and dysuria (Beers & Berkow, 2000). Pyuria, the presence of pus in the urine, may also be a symptom of bladder cancer. There are no recommended screening tests for bladder cancer, although hematuria testing and urinary cytology testing have been evaluated for this purpose (ACS, 2012; National Cancer Institute, 2003). These tests carry a high frequency of false positives, making them too nonspecific for screening. Any patient who presents with the previously listed symptoms, however, should be carefully evaluated. In the absence of UTI, an older adult with either gross or microhematuria should be referred for cystoscopy. In many cases, this procedure can be carried out in a physician's office.

The treatments for bladder cancer are dependent on the anatomical structures involved, the degree of invasiveness, and recurrent status (ACS, 2012). Available treatments range from depositing chemotherapeutic agents into the bladder to removal of the bladder and surrounding organs. If the bladder is removed, a reservoir or an alternative outlet for urine will be created. A loop of intestine may be used to create a continent reservoir or a simple outlet. The urethras are attached to the loop, and a stoma on the abdomen is created. The older adult then wears an external collection device over the stoma. Newer interventions include a reservoir that is capable of storing urine and is catheterized intermittently. More radical interventions include attachment of the ureter to the abdominal wall without the intestinal loop. These surgeries present challenges to the older adult's body image, and the nurse must work with the patient to address these challenges. Specific concerns include the psychomotor skills of managing the urinary reservoir, managing the urinary collection devices, and the ongoing fear of recurrent or metastasizing cancer.

Prostate Cancer

Prostate cancer is even more common in older men than is bladder cancer, and will affect one of every eight men over the age of 70 (ACS, 2012). African American men are more likely to develop prostate cancer, as are men with a family history and those with diets high in animal fats (Pienta, 2009). No reliable links among **sexually transmitted diseases** (diseases contracted through sexual intercourse or intimate sexual contact) and prostate cancer have been found.

The most commonly used screening tests for prostate cancer are digital rectal examination (DRE) combined with prostate-specific antigen (PSA) testing and transrectal biopsy of the prostate with guided ultrasound (NKUDIC, 2007b). A normal PSA level is below 4 ng/mL. Values greater than 10 ng/mL are strongly indicative of prostate cancer, whereas values between 4 and 10 ng/mL are difficult to interpret. During the DRE, the practitioner is able to palpate the prostate, feeling for organ consistency and nodules suspicious for cancer. If either of these screens demonstrates abnormalities, a transrectal ultrasound is usually recommended. In 2008, the U.S. Preventive Services Task Force recommended that men over the age of 75 years not be screened for prostate cancer, creating much discussion in the healthcare community. The same task force reviewed their recommendations in 2011, and concluded that the evidence demonstrated that prostate cancer screening did not decrease mortality from prostate cancer (Lin, Croswell, Koenig et al., 2011). The recommendation remains controversial among some, but both the American Cancer Society and American Urologic Association now recommend that screening for prostate cancer stop when a man has an average life expectancy of 10 years or less (Hoffman, 2011). That essentially means that men over the age of 75 should not be screened, because the average life expectancy for a 75-year-old American man is an additional 10.6 years (Arias, 2011).

Once prostate cancer has been diagnosed, the older man has a variety of treatment options. No one option appears to have significant benefits over the others (NKUDIC,

2007b). Prostate cancer in older men is slow growing, and "watchful waiting" is a realistic option for older men (ACS, 2012). Other options include surgery, external beam radiation, and radioactive seeds implanted into the prostate. All have similar success rates (ACS, 2012). If the cancer is more advanced, external radiation or hormonal treatment may be recommended. The older patient should be offered a thorough discussion of all options with a urologist.

Rates of other genitourinary cancers in older men are low. Testicular cancer is predominantly a disease of young men, and cancer of the penis is rare in all age groups (Howlader, Noone, Krapcho et al., 2011).

Gynecological Malignancies

Ovarian, uterine, and breast cancer are more prevalent in older women than in younger women (Howlader et al., 2011). Cervical cancer, although more prevalent in young and midlife women, remains a concern. Vulvar cancer, signaled by a palpable nodule on the labium and pruritus, is not common in any age group (Brown & Cooper, 1998).

Seventy-five percent of ovarian cancer is diagnosed in women over the age of 55 (Howlader et al., 2011). Approximately one-half of all women diagnosed with ovarian cancer survive for 5 years after diagnosis (Hennessey, Suh, & Markman, 2011). The symptoms are vague, including diffuse abdominal discomfort and gastrointestinal distress. The vagueness of the symptoms may account, in part, for the poor prognosis because women are rarely diagnosed when the tumor is confined to the ovary. More obvious symptoms, such as ascites or a palpable mass, are not frequently present until lymph nodes are involved or metastases are found.

Although there are no screening tests per se for ovarian cancer, there is a blood test for a tumor marker that is both sensitive and specific (Hennessy et al., 2011). However, the CA-125 is not recommended as a screening tool because there is little conclusive evidence that it would decrease the mortality from ovarian cancer (ACS, 2012). Similarly, transvaginal ultrasonography to detect ovarian cancer has not demonstrated a benefit in terms of decreased mortality. Ongoing research holds out the hope for a screening test based on blood proteins (Hennessy et al., 2011).

Treatment options for the older woman with ovarian cancer include surgery to remove the uterus, ovaries, and fallopian tubes, as well as any other affected organs (ACS, 2012). Chemotherapy is important in improving survival, with platinum-containing agents showing the most benefit (Hennessy et al., 2011). Recurrence of the disease is very common.

Cancer of the body of the uterus or endometrium is the most common gynecological cancer in older women (Howlader et al., 2011). Obesity and prolonged estrogen exposure (early menarche with late menopause, nulliparous)

are risk factors for endometrial cancer. HRT, without progestin, is thought to increase the risk of endometrial cancer, although the inclusion of progestin appears to significantly reduce the risk (Taylor & Manson, 2011). The most common symptom is uterine bleeding after menopause, which occurs early in the disease, making early diagnosis and treatment possible. Any older woman who reports postmenopausal uterine bleeding should be assumed to have endometrial cancer until proved otherwise. The diagnosis is usually made by endometrial biopsy, and treatment includes hysterectomy, oophorectomy, and salpingectomy. Chemotherapy after surgery is common. Prognosis is much better if the treatment is begun earlier in the course of the disease.

Cervical cancer in the older woman is primarily a concern because of the confusion around screening for the disease, the Papanicolaou (Pap) smear. The disease itself is more prevalent in younger women. The risk factors of cervical cancer include infection with human papillomavirus, early onset of sexual activity, history of abnormal Pap smears, HIV-positive status, and many sexual partners (National Cancer Institute, 2003). Current recommendations are that women who are over age 65, who have had a regular history of normal Pap smears, and who are not at high risk because of other factors (as previously noted) should *not* receive routine Pap smears (U.S. Preventive Services Task Force, 2012). The American Cancer Society (2012) offers the same suggestion, but recommends women have regular Pap smears until age 70. The most recent update on screening recommendations indicates that either traditional Pap smears or liquid-based cytological exams are equally effective at detecting cancer (Whitlock et al., 2011). Older women who have had a total hysterectomy (cervix removed) for nonmalignant reasons do not need to be screened with Pap smears (Table 17-5).

Breast cancer affects nearly 1 in every 15 women over age 70 (ACS, 2012). Risk factors include advanced age, family history of breast cancer, early menarche and late menopause, estrogen replacement therapy, none or late pregnancy, regular alcohol use, abdominal obesity, exposure to radiation, and personal history of benign breast disease (Gandhi & Verma, 2011). Adequate levels of calcium and vitamin D are protective against the development of breast cancer (Chen et al., 2010). Three specific screening tests are available for breast cancer: mammography, clinical breast examination, and breast self-examination.

Strong evidence exists that yearly mammography for all women over the age of 40 decreases mortality from breast cancer and should be encouraged (U.S. Preventive Services Task Force, 2012). The International Society of Geriatric Oncology suggests that breast cancer screening stop at approximately age 75, because of the increased likelihood of comorbidities that are more deleterious to the older

TABLE 17-5	Pap Smear Recommendations for Women 65 Years and Older				
Risk Factor → Uterine Status ↓	History of Abnormal Pap Smears	HIV-Positive	Human Papillomavirus Positive	Hysterectomy for Previous Cancer	History of Regular, Normal Pap Smears
With intact cervix	Screen	Screen	Screen	Screen	Do not screen
Without intact cervix	Screen	Do not screen	Do not screen	Screen	Do not screen

Note: If "screen" appears under any risk factor for a particular older woman, she should be advised to have an annual Pap smear.

Source: U.S. Preventive Services Task Force (2012).

woman's health than breast cancer (Wildiers et al., 2007). Obviously, the older woman must be a knowledgeable participant in discussions about screening for breast cancer.

The treatment for breast cancer depends on the stage of the tumor when detected. The surgical options are the same as for younger women: breast-conserving lumpectomy or total mastectomy (Wildiers et al., 2007). Axillary lymph node dissection is appropriate if there is clinical evidence of lymph node involvement; otherwise, sentinel node biopsy is adequate. Radiation therapy after breast-conserving surgery is associated with a decreased risk of recurrence, but not with decreased mortality. The use of tamoxifen or anastrozole after surgery appears to increase survival from breast cancer for older women with metastases to the lymph nodes. However, the nurse must carefully monitor the older woman on these drugs, because older women develop higher serum concentrations of tamoxifen per dose than do younger women (Munster & Hudis, 1999). There is evidence that older women frequently do not receive adequate chemotherapy because of fear of side effects (Dellapasqua, Colleoni, Castiglione et al., 2007). Furthermore, older women are underrepresented in clinical trials related to breast cancer treatment. This is completely inappropriate; age alone should not be the determining factor in treatment options offered to the older woman. There is no research evidence that substantiates treating breast cancer based on the patient's age (Dellapasqua et al., 2007). The nurse can be a powerful advocate for the older woman, ensuring that she receives adequate information and access to all treatment options.

Sex and the Senior Citizen

Older adults continue to need intimacy, chosen emotional interconnectedness between two people that includes mutual caring and responsibility, although there may be fewer opportunities and strong social sanctions against this. Sexual desire tends to decline with advancing age, but the major impediment to a satisfying sex life at any age is lack of a partner

(Beutel, Stobel-Richter, & Brahler, 2008; Lindau et al., 2007). Intimacy entails five important aspects: commitment, affective intimacy, cognitive intimacy, physical intimacy, and mutuality (Blieszner & de Vries, 2001). Close friendships, sexual relationships, strong ties to family members, and beloved pets can all contribute to meeting the older adult's need for intimacy but are not always available. Older adults rarely discuss their sexuality concerns with physicians (Lindau et al., 2007). Nursing care may include touching intimate areas of an older person's body, but in a detached and clinical fashion. This may leave the older adult feeling bereft. Awareness on the part of the nurse can be an asset to older adults and their quest for intimacy.

> **Practice Pearl ▶▶▶**
> *The same things that stop you having sex with age are exactly the same as those that stop you riding a bicycle (bad health, thinking it looks silly, no bicycle).*
> Attributed to Alex Comfort (1974)

The age-related changes in sexual response in both men and women do not preclude a satisfying sex life. The prevalence of sexually active older adults varies according to data source. Lindau et al. (2007) determined that 53% of older adults between the ages of 65 and 74 years were sexually active, as were 26% of those ages 75 to 85. Smith and colleagues (2007) found 18% of women and 41% of men over the age of 70 remained sexually active. Because arousal takes longer in both sexes, foreplay is even more important than in younger adults. Hugging, kissing, and caressing are sexual activities that both men and women enjoy. They can be preludes to sexual intercourse or satisfying activities in themselves (Johnson, 1996). The older adults Johnson studied were generally open minded and knowledgeable about sexual matters, but health status was a barrier to sexual expression.

Sexually active older adults reported a high incidence rate of problems with sexual activity (Lindau et al., 2007).

Nearly one half reported at least one difficulty, and nearly one third reported two or more difficulties. Chronic pain and osteoarthritis are two common problems that have deleterious effects on sexual activity and older adults. Arthritis in the hip joint presents the greatest challenge to satisfying sexual activity (Lindau, 2009; Tenover, 2009), but it can be ameliorated by changes in coital position, use of heat applications, and timing during the day when joints are less painful. The "spoon" position, in which partners lie on their sides with the woman in front, allows for penile penetration of the vagina without undue strain to either partner (Monga, Monga, Tan et al., 1999). Warm baths can also help relieve pain and can be incorporated as foreplay.

Many older adults who suffer from cardiovascular disease are concerned about the safety of sex. Men with hypertension are particularly likely to have concerns about sex (Lindau et al., 2007). In general, if an older adult can climb two flights of stairs or walk at a rate of 2 miles per hour without chest pain or shortness of breath, he or she should have no cardiac problems during sexual intercourse (Butler & Lewis, 2003). Consideration should be given to the partner with the less stable vital signs, particularly blood pressure, and that person should not be positioned on top. Sexual intercourse with one partner in a chair, and the other directly in front of the chair, is another variation that may help some older couples (Monga et al., 1999). Figure 17-7 ▶▶▶ illustrates these positions.

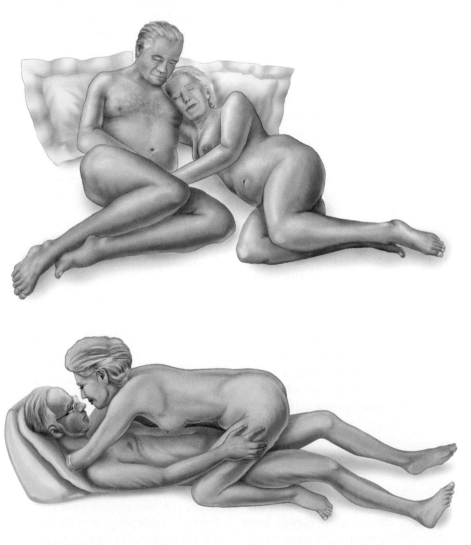

Figure 17-7 ▶▶▶ Coital positions for older adults with cardiovascular disease or painful musculoskeletal conditions.

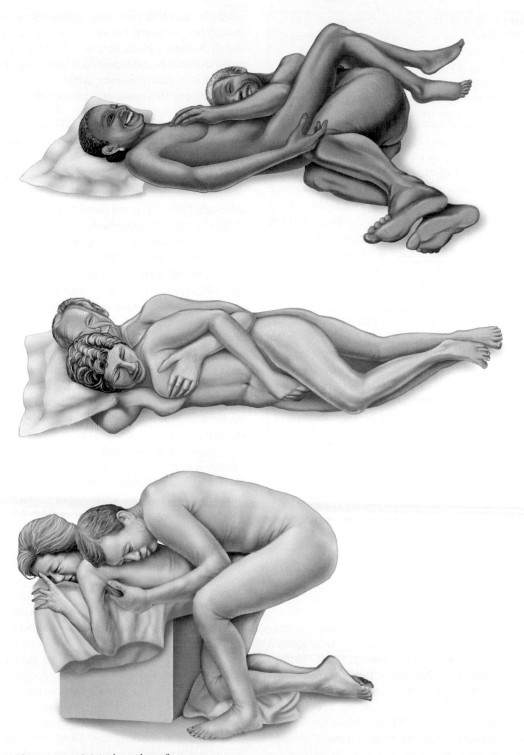

Figure 17-7 ▶▶▶ (continued)

> **Drug Alert** ▶▶▶ A wide range of medications can have negative effects on sexual expression, including many antipsychotics, tricyclic antidepressants, monoamine oxidase inhibitors, diuretics, beta-blockers, ACE inhibitors, and clonidine ("Focus on Effects," 2000).

Dyspareunia, painful intercourse for the older woman, may be related to decreased vaginal lubrication, extension of the labia, and lack of elevation of the uterus during sexual arousal (Monga et al., 1999). Insufficient lubrication may be experienced by over one third of older women (Lindau et al., 2007). Penetration is difficult as the vaginal opening may be partially obscured by the labia, and the lack of lubrication further inhibits entrance of the penis. The older couple might be advised to use a vaginal lubricant as part of their sexual activity and to have the woman use her hand to guide her partner's penis into the vagina.

> **Practice Pearl** ▶▶▶ The nurse should be prepared for nervous giggles or outright laughter when discussing sexuality with an older adult. Many people think that older adults do not and should not have sexual needs or desires. It is important to assure patients that a wide range of feelings about sexuality are appropriate for seniors, just as they are for younger people.

Diabetes mellitus can have negative effects on the sexual expression of both men and women. It is correlated with erectile dysfunction in the man and even greater reduction of lubrication in the woman (Monga et al., 1999). Alternative expressions of sexuality, such as body caressing, manipulation of the partner's genitals with the hand, or mutual masturbation, may be suggested.

Discussing Sexuality With Older Adults

The PLISSIT model of intervention for sexual concerns was developed over 30 years ago, but is still a valid method for nurses to use with older adults (Annon, 1974; Hartford Institute for Geriatric Nursing, 2001). **P** stands for permission, in which the nurse validates the older adult's desire for sexual activity. The nurse may start the conversation with a neutral phrase such as "Many people think older adults aren't interested in sex any more, but that's not true. I wonder if you have questions that I might answer for you." The permission phase is concerned with normalizing the older adult's feelings and concerns.

LI is limited information, and the nurse offers specific, factual information pertinent to the older patient. For example, an older man may appreciate knowing that although his erection is not as firm as it once was, he can still satisfy himself and his partner. **SS** stands for specific suggestions, such as coital positions or timing of pain medication. **IT** is intensive therapy, which requires a referral to an advanced practice nurse or other expert.

Sexuality in Long-Term Care

Meeting the intimacy needs of older adults in long-term care settings can be a challenge to the nurse. A poignant description of the negative view nurses hold of sexuality and older adults in institutions was written by Nay (1992), who concluded, "It is not possible to provide care that aims at maximizing potential, independence, and control, while denying or ridiculing a 'core' aspect of identity. It is not enough to care for the body; recognition of the whole person, including sexuality, must be reflected in nursing care" (p. 314). However, there are both legal and ethical concerns when it comes to sexual activity among residents of long-term care facilities.

Nursing homes have a lack of privacy for residents, and safety is a concern when there are no beds large enough to accommodate two people and sexual activity. Pushing two beds together is not a safe option, unless they are securely fastened together. Privacy for talking without the fear of being overheard, a room with a do-not-disturb sign and a door, and organizational support are all important if a nursing home is going to facilitate sexual expression by residents (Heath, 2011). The attitudes of staff and adult children, however, may be the biggest hurdle sexually active elders have to face (Lichtenberg, 1997; Loue, 2005; Nay, 1992). Adult children may collude with staff members to keep their parent away from a romantic interest.

If one or both of the older adults involved in physical intimacy are cognitively impaired, both legal and ethical responsibilities arise. The nurse must intervene to ensure that both parties are making an informed decision to participate in sexual activity, or at least that there is no exploitation involved (Lichtenberg, 1997). A person with dementia who is unable to make an informed decision should be protected from exploitation. There is no generally accepted standard for when a person with cognitive changes is no longer able to give informed consent, and the nurse will have to assess each situation, although Lichtenberg recommends that a score of at least 14 on the Mini Mental State Exam is a prerequisite. Many individuals may have concerns related to physical intimacy between nursing home residents, including the adult children of the involved residents, the unit staff, governmental agencies, and the administrative team of the nursing home.

meds , penile implants

Some older adults with dementias will engage in sexual activity that is inappropriate, for example, masturbation in public. Although the incidence rate is less than 2% (Alagiakrishnan et al., 2005), it can be very disruptive to the nursing unit. A hormone, medroxyprogesterone acetate, may be effective in managing sexually inappropriate behavior in older men with dementia (Light & Holroyd, 2006). One nursing intervention is to redirect the older adult to a private area or provide distraction (Monga et al., 1999). It is important to consider the motive that may be driving the sexual behavior and attempt to meet those needs (Duffy, 1998). For example, fondling the genitals may be an indication that the older person needs to urinate. At no time should a punitive approach be taken.

Erectile Dysfunction

Impotence, or **erectile dysfunction (ED),** affects nearly 70% of men over the age of 70 (Wessels, Joyce, Wise, et al., 2007), although the Lindau et al. (2007) study found a much lower rate, closer to one third. (The difference in numbers may relate to the methods used to collect the data.) The prevalence rate increases with each decade of age (Wessels et al., 2007). It is defined as the inability to achieve or maintain an erection sufficient for sexual satisfaction (Carbone & Seftel, 2002).

ED may be caused by vasculogenic, neurologic, hormonal, or psychogenic factors. Vasculogenic ED may be caused by poor arterial blood flow into the penis or poor return of blood through the veins. Hypertension, diabetes mellitus, dyslipidemia, and smoking may all cause arterial damage significant enough to lead to ED. ED that has physiological causes is usually accompanied by the absence of nocturnal tumescence, spontaneous erections that occur at night or during the early morning hours. It is important to ask the older man if he continues to have nocturnal tumescence, because this will help determine etiology. A small piece of paper, taped around the penis at bedtime, will be torn if the nocturnal tumescence occurs.

There are no universally recommended diagnostics for ED, and many men are correctly diagnosed based on history and physical exam (Wessels et al., 2007). Treatment is dependent on etiology, so some laboratory studies and specific physical examinations may be conducted. Thyroid-stimulating hormone and serum testosterone may give important information, as may imaging studies (Stern, 1997). A review of the medications an older man takes is critical, because many drugs have ED as a side effect. A neurologic examination and assessment for depression may also be performed (Carbone & Seftel, 2002).

A variety of treatments are available for ED, including oral medication, self-administered injections into the penis, vacuum erection devices, and surgical implants (Carbone & Seftel, 2002). Since the introduction of sildenafil (Viagra) in 1998, fewer men have opted for penile implant surgery. Nearly 6% of all American men take oral ED drugs (Wessels et al., 2007), and the drugs are usually well tolerated. The nurse may act as an advocate to ensure the older man is offered all appropriate treatment options.

Sexually Transmitted Infections

Sexually active older adults are at risk for the same sexually transmitted infections that affect younger adults. They should be offered the same education about safer sex, including the use of condoms. More than 14,000 older adults are now diagnosed with AIDS (Centers for Disease Control and Prevention, 2007), and they face the same stigma as younger adults do, but they experience an additional burden of ageism (Emlet, 2006). The death rate from AIDS in people over 65 years of age was 2.4 per 100,000 in 1997, a small but significant number (National Center for Health Statistics [NCHS], 1999). The incidence of genital herpes among people ages 85 to 94 has doubled since 1994, now affecting 11 of every 100,000 American elders (Chorba, Tao, & Irwin, 2007). Gonorrhea and syphilis are also found in the older population, with Black and Hispanic older adults having higher incidence rates than their White counterparts (NCHS, 1999). This may be a reflection of greater acceptance of sexuality among older adults in these populations. Hillman (2007) discovered that older women did not consider HIV/AIDS prevention as relevant to themselves, and Cooperman, Arnsten, and Klein (2007) found that older men at risk for HIV infection continued to engage in unsafe sex practices. It is clear that nurses should be specific about discussing safer sex practices as they apply to the older adult. Questions related to symptoms of sexually transmitted diseases should be included in the review of systems and nursing assessment of an older adult.

QSEN Recommendations Related to the Genitourinary and Renal Systems

The Quality and Safety Education for Nurses (QSEN) project addresses the challenge of preparing future nurses with the knowledge, skills, and attitudes (KSAs) to continuously improve the quality and safety of the healthcare systems in which they work (Cronenwett et al., 2007). See the QSEN table for tips on meeting QSEN standards.

Patient and Family Teaching

Gerontological nurses require skills and knowledge related to teaching patients and families about the key concepts of gerontology and gerontological nursing. The guidelines in the following feature will assist the nurse to assume the role of teacher and coach.

Meeting QSEN Standards: Genitourinary and Renal Systems

	KNOWLEDGE	SKILLS	ATTITUDES
Patient-Centered Care	Involvement of the older adult is critical in planning nursing care. Older adults may not want adult children involved in discussions of urinary, sexual, or intimacy issues.	PLISSIT model and assessment of family dynamics.	Acknowledge that older adults continue to be sexual beings.
	Examine barriers that may keep older adults from being active in formulating their plan of care.	Evaluate for depression, vision/hearing, cognitive status.	Plan nursing care that is consistent with the needs and desires of older adults, and then determine how to implement it. Barriers should be conquered, not accepted.
Teamwork and Collaboration	Understand the unique contributions each profession can contribute to the genitourinary health of older adults.	Provide process for initiating referrals. Use leadership skills to initiate and coordinate interdisciplinary efforts.	Value each profession's contributions to the care of the older adult. Recognize that the older adult's needs take priority over professional boundaries.
Evidence-Based Practice	Be familiar with the burgeoning body of literature on the genitourinary health needs of older adults.	Know how to access evidence-based guidelines and protocols and best practices from peer-reviewed sources.	Integrate evidence-based practices, even if in conflict with traditional ideas of nursing care.
Quality Improvement	Identify nursing-sensitive outcomes related to genitourinary health in older adults. Identify appropriate measurement strategies.	Design and implement a process for collecting and analyzing data.	Acknowledge the importance of continuously reviewing and improving quality care.

Meeting QSEN Standards: Genitourinary and Renal Systems *(continued)*

	KNOWLEDGE	SKILLS	ATTITUDES
Safety	Describe medication and diagnosis interactions that may have negative influences on the health of older adults. Understand risks and benefits to older adults of various treatment options.	Access reliable data sources on the health of older adults. Edit and individualize published information for each patient to minimize risk of adverse events and maximize chances for successful outcomes.	Advocate for the older adult within the healthcare system.
Informatics	Identify professional computer-based information sources for and about older adults. Discuss attributes of electronic sources, including EMRs, that relate to the health of older adults.	Evaluate the appropriateness of published information for older adults. Identify needs for improvements in EMR systems to safeguard the health of older adults.	Appreciate both the strengths and weaknesses of electronic sources as related to the genitourinary health of older adults.

Patient–Family Teaching Guidelines

The following are guidelines that the nurse may find useful when instructing older adults and their families about urinary tract infections.

INSTRUCTING OLDER ADULTS ABOUT URINARY TRACT INFECTIONS

1 What is a urinary tract infection?

A urinary tract infection is the result of the growth of bacteria (germs) in the kidney or bladder, or in the tubes that connect them. It might also be called a bladder infection, cystitis, or UTI.

RATIONALE:

The older patient may not understand that several different words and diagnoses can specify the same or similar conditions. The nurse should include the terms UTI, cystitis, and bladder infection when educating older patients.

2 Who gets urinary tract infections?

Women who have been through menopause are likely to get urinary tract infections. Men with prostate problems are also likely to get urinary tract infections. Men or women who have a urinary catheter may also get them.

RATIONALE:

UTIs are much less common in men than women because of underlying anatomical differences between the sexes. Men who present with symptoms of UTI and who have not been catheterized should seek advice from a urologist as they may have an undiagnosed prostate problem.

3 What are the symptoms?

Common symptoms of UTI may include:

- Burning or itching during urination
- Feeling of urgency and need to urinate frequently
- Involuntary loss of urine or urinary incontinence
- Back pain, fatigue, nausea, and dull pain or ache in the lower abdomen

(continued)

Patient–Family Teaching Guidelines *(continued)*

- Sometimes mental status changes, especially in those who already have memory problems

RATIONALE:

The symptoms of UTI may be vague and nonspecific. It is important to describe the wide variety of symptoms that may signal UTI in the older person.

4 **How does the healthcare provider know a patient has a urinary tract infection?**

A simple urine test may show white blood cells and the bacteria causing the infection. The healthcare provider will test your urine as a result of your complaints and symptoms. One test can be done quickly in the office or clinic, and the other test (culture and sensitivity) must be sent to the laboratory and takes about 3 days to obtain the final results. If you are very uncomfortable and having severe urinary symptoms, your healthcare provider will probably treat you right away with an antibiotic while awaiting the final test results.

RATIONALE:

Educating older patients and their families about the assessment and treatment process for UTIs will empower patients and facilitate positive outcomes.

5 **What is the treatment for urinary tract infections?**

If you are found to have a UTI with troubling symptoms and bacteria, white blood cells, or blood in your urine, you will probably be given an antibiotic by your healthcare provider. It is very important to take *all* the medicine, even if you start to feel better before it is all gone. Drink at least eight large glasses of water per day.

RATIONALE:

The symptoms of UTI may resolve within the first few days of treatment, but to prevent reinfection the entire 5- to 7-day course of antibiotics should be taken as ordered by the healthcare provider.

6 **How do I prevent another infection?**

Many older people are prone to frequent UTIs. You can help prevent recurrent infections by taking the following steps:

- Make sure you keep drinking at least eight large glasses of water per day.
- Drink a few glasses of cranberry juice if you feel the symptoms of UTI starting to bother you.
- Wear all-cotton underwear, and put on a clean set every day.
- Go to the toilet as soon as you need to urinate—do not wait.
- Make sure to pass a few drops of urine after you have sexual intercourse.

RATIONALE:

These self-care measures can prevent recurrent UTI and are part of a regimen of good urinary health practices.

CARE PLAN   A Patient With a Genitourinary Problem

Case Study

Mr. and Mrs. Brown are 92 and 89 years of age, respectively. They live in their own apartment, with the occasional services of a housekeeper and a visiting nurse. Their adult children and grandchildren live within easy commuting distance. Mr. Brown has osteoarthritis, most significantly in his spine, hands, hips, and knees. He has hypertension that is controlled with hydrochlorothiazide, 25 mg, po, daily; and lisinopril, 20 mg, po, daily. He takes acetaminophen, 1,000 mg, po, tid for his osteoarthritis, and it is moderately effective in controlling his pain.

Mrs. Brown had a CVA 3 months ago. She has no motor deficits, and her speech is intact. Since the CVA, Mrs. Brown has had marked disinhibition, but no other health problems. She does not take routine medications, but has a prescription for Ambien, 10 mg, po, hs, PRN.

At the completion of a home visit, Mr. Brown follows the visiting nurse to the front door of the apartment and asks for a word in private. He appears quite anxious, looks over his shoulder frequently at Mrs. Brown, lowers his voice, and says, "Nurse, I've got a problem. I think my wife is oversexed."

CARE PLAN | **A Patient With a Genitourinary Problem** *(continued)*

Applying the Nursing Process

Assessment

Upon calm, deliberative questioning from the nurse, Mr. Brown reveals that shortly after her CVA, Mrs. Brown began to initiate sexual activity with Mr. Brown every night, sometimes several times a night. Her preferred sexual activity is intercourse. She becomes quite angry when Mr. Brown cannot achieve an erection and has frequently accused him of "fooling around with other women," although Mr. Brown vehemently denies this. Mr. Brown's feelings are hurt by Mrs. Brown's accusations. In addition, sexual intercourse makes his arthritic joints very painful, and he is not getting enough sleep due to nightly intercourse. Mr. Brown loves his wife very much and is concerned about "not satisfying her" as well as "living with a pervert." Mr. Brown tried to discuss this matter with his wife's physician, who told Mr. Brown that he had "never heard of anything as abnormal as an 89-year-old woman wanting sex." Mr. Brown has become increasingly desperate and admits to sometimes giving Mrs. Brown two Ambien tablets "just to keep her from attacking me in the middle of the night." He finishes his tale by poignantly saying, "Fifty years ago she always had a headache, now I'm getting a headache!"

Diagnosis

The current nursing diagnoses for the Brown family include:

- *Sexual Dysfunction*
- *Pain, Chronic* related to Mr. Brown's osteoarthritis
- *Sexuality Pattern, Ineffective*
- *Sleep Pattern, Disturbed*
- *Hopelessness* related to Mr. Brown's perception of his marital and caregiving roles
- *Family Processes, Interuppted*
- *Injury, Risk for* related to use of excessive medication

NANDA-I © 2012.

Expected Outcomes

The expected outcomes for the plan of care specify that the Browns will:

- Achieve a mutually satisfying pattern of intimacy and sexual activity.
- Develop accurate and sufficient knowledge of intimacy and human sexuality.
- Manage Mr. Brown's pain to increase activity tolerance and quality of life.
- Establish productive communication patterns within their marriage, within the constraints of Mrs. Brown's altered cognition.
- Experience adequate rest.
- Identify options and choices in selected situations.
- Agree to establish a therapeutic relationship with the nurse to facilitate these outcomes.

Planning and Implementation

The following nursing interventions may be appropriate for Mr. and Mrs. Brown:

- Establish a therapeutic relationship.
- Provide sources of accurate, appropriate information related to sexuality and older adults:
  - Include information about intimacy as a separate concern from sexual activity.
  - Include information about sexual activities other than intercourse.
  - Include information about positions for sexual intercourse that may be less painful for Mr. Brown.
- Involve Mr. and Mrs. Brown in discussions about their individual concerns and desires for intimacy.
- Assess their sleep and activity patterns:
  - Look for lack of synchronization, for example, does one partner nap from 2 p.m. to 4 p.m., and the other from 1 p.m. to 3 p.m.?
  - Consider the need for additional help with household chores, giving Mr. Brown more rest time.
  - Evaluate the need for occasional respite services for Mrs. Brown, allowing Mr. Brown to have personal time.
- Encourage Mr. Brown to share his concerns with the nurse or other health professional.

(continued)

CARE PLAN   **A Patient With a Genitourinary Problem** *(continued)*

- Approach Mr. and Mrs. Brown in an open, nonjudgmental manner.
- Explore Mr. Brown's need for additional support in caring for Mrs. Brown.

- Explore Mrs. Brown's need for increased meaningful activity.

Evaluation

The nurse will consider the plan a success based on the following outcomes:

- Mr. and Mrs. Brown will verbalize a satisfying level of intimacy, which may or may not include sexual activity.

- Mr. Brown will report that he is able to maintain a satisfactory level of physical activity without pain.
- Mr. and Mrs. Brown will demonstrate open and effective communication about their needs and feelings to each other.

Ethical Dilemma

An ethical dilemma exists when two equally compelling ethical principles are in conflict. The ethical dilemma in this situation is the conflict between beneficence for Mrs. Brown and nonmaleficence for Mr. Brown. Beneficence is the moral duty to do good, and nonmaleficence is the imperative to do no harm. The nurse has to work toward optimal outcomes for both family members, but their needs appear to be in opposition to each other. For example, Mr. Brown needs adequate sleep, but giving extra sleeping medication to Mrs. Brown may be dangerous. Similarly, Mrs. Brown needs to have her sexual and intimacy needs met, but Mr. Brown needs to be free from pain.

Critical Thinking and the Nursing Process

1. Are you comfortable talking with your older patients about sexuality?
2. What are some responses nurses can provide to those who say that older adults interested in sex are abnormal or "dirty old men or women"?

3. What resources do you have in your clinical setting for referral of older people with sexual problems if they need further assistance?
4. What environmental modifications might enhance sexual activity and satisfaction for older adults?

- Evaluate your responses in Appendix B.⊂⊃

Chapter Highlights

- Many age-related changes occur in the genitourinary systems of older men and women.
- Sexuality continues to be a human need throughout the life span.
- Understanding the changes in renal, urinary, and reproductive functions will help the nurse provide safe, effective nursing care that is holistic in nature.
- The kidney becomes less efficient in old age, producing urine that is less concentrated and making the older person more susceptible to fluid and electrolyte disorders.

- Urinary incontinence is not a normal part of aging, but age-related changes make the older adult more vulnerable to it. Urinary incontinence should always be carefully evaluated, and an individualized treatment plan developed.
- Both older men and older women have age-related changes in sexual function, but are fully able to have satisfying sexual experiences.
- Renal failure and genitourinary cancers become more common with increasing age.
- Nursing care for genitourinary concerns requires self-awareness on the part of the nurse and sensitivity to the dignity of the older adult.

Pearson Nursing Student Resources
Find additional review materials at
nursing.pearsonhighered.com

Prepare for success with additional NCLEX®-style practice
questions, interactive assignments and activities, web links,
animations and videos, and more!

References

Addis, S., Davies, M., Greene, G., MacBride-Stewart, S., & Shepherd, M. (2009). The health, social care and housing needs of older lesbian, gay, and transgender older people: A review of the literature. *Health and Social Care in the Community, 17*(6), 647–658.

Alagiakrishnan, K., Lim, D., Brahim, A., Wong, A., Wood, A., Senthilselvan, A., et al. (2005). Sexually inappropriate behaviour in demented elderly people. *Postgraduate Medical Journal, 81,* 463–466.

American Cancer Society (ACS). (2012). *Cancer facts and figures, 2012.* Atlanta, GA: Author.

American Geriatrics Society Beers Criteria Update Expert Panel. (2012). American Geriatrics Society updated Beers Criteria for potentially inappropriate medication use in older adults. *Journal of the American Geriatrics Society, 60*(4), 616–631.

American Psychological Association. (2012). Guidelines for psychological practice with lesbian, gay, and bisexual clients. *American Psychologist, 67*(1), 10–42.

Annon, J. (1974). *The behavioral treatment of sexual problems: Volume I, Brief therapy.* Honolulu, HI: Enabling Systems.

Arias, E. (2011). United States life tables, 2007. *National Vital Statistics Reports, 59*(9). Hyattsville, MD: National Center for Health Statistics.

Assad, L. A. D. (2000). Urinary incontinence in older men. *Topics in Geriatric Rehabilitation, 16*(1), 33–53.

Averett, P., Yoon, I., & Jenkins, C. L. (2011). Older lesbians: Experiences of aging, discrimination, and resilience. *Journal of Women and Aging, 23,* 216–232.

Beers, M. H., & Berkow, R. (2000). *The Merck manual of geriatrics* (3rd ed.). Whitehouse Station, NJ: Merck Research Laboratories.

Bellino, F. (2007). Female reproductive aging and menopause. In P. S. Timiras (Ed.), *Physiological basis of aging and geriatrics* (4th ed., pp. 160–184). New York, NY: Informa Healthcare.

Beutel, M. E., Stobel-Richter, Y., & Brahler, E. (2008). Sexual desire and sexual activity of

men and women across their lifespans: Results from a representative German community survey. *BJU International, 101*(1), 76–82.

Bickley, L. S., & Szilagyi, P. G. (2007). *Bates' guide to physical examination and history taking* (9th ed.). Philadelphia, PA: Lippincott Williams & Wilkins.

Binstock, R. H. (1999). Older persons and health care costs. In R. N. Butler, L. K. Grossman, & M. R. Oberlink (Eds.), *Life in an older America* (pp. 75–96). New York, NY: Century Foundation Press.

Blieszner, R., & deVries, B. (2001). Perspectives on intimacy. *Generations, 25*(2), 7–8.

Bradway, C. (2005). Women's narratives of long-term urinary incontinence. *Urologic Nursing, 25,* 337–344.

Brazier, A. M., & Palmer, M. H. (1995). Collecting clean-catch urine in the nursing home: Obtaining the uncontaminated specimen. *Geriatric Nursing, 16,* 217–224.

Brotman, S., Ryan, B., Collins, S., Chamberland, L., Cormier, R., Julien, D., et al. (2007). Coming out to care: Caregivers of gay and lesbian seniors in Canada. *Gerontologist, 47,* 490–503.

Brown, A. D. G., & Cooper, T. K. (1998). Gynecologic orders in the elderly—Sexuality and aging. In R. Tallis, H. Fillit, & J. C. Brocklehurst (Eds.), *Brocklehurst's textbook of geriatric medicine and gerontology* (5th ed., pp. 987–997). Edinburgh, Scotland: Churchill Livingstone.

Bushman, W. (2009). Etiology, epidemiology, and natural history. *Urologic Clinics of North America, 36*(4), 403–415.

Butler, R. N., & Lewis, M. I. (2003). Sexuality and aging. In W. R. Hazzard, J. P. Blass, J. B. Halter, J. G. Ouslander, & M. E. Tinetti (Eds.), *Principles of geriatric medicine and gerontology* (5th ed., pp. 1277–1282). New York, NY: McGraw-Hill.

Carbone, D. J., & Seftel, A. D. (2002). Erectile dysfunction: Diagnosis and treatment in older men. *Geriatrics, 57*(9), 18–24.

Centers for Disease Control and Prevention. (2007). *HIV/AIDS surveillance report 2005* (vol. 17, rev. ed.). Atlanta, GA: Author.

Chen, P., Hu, P., Xie, D., Qin, Y., Wang, F., & Wang, H. (2010). Meta-analysis of calcium, vitamin D, and the prevention of breast cancer. *Breast Cancer Research and Treatment, 121,* 469–477.

Chorba, T., Tao, G., & Irwin, K. I. (2007). Sexually transmitted diseases. In M. S. Litwin & C. S. Saigal (Eds.), *Urologic diseases in America* (NIH Publication No. 07–5512, pp. 648–695). Washington, DC: U.S. Government Printing Office.

Chow, R. D. (2001). Benign prostatic hyperplasia: Patient evaluation and relief of obstructive symptoms. *Geriatrics, 56*(3), 33–38.

Comfort, A. (Ed.). (1974). *The joy of sex: A cordon bleu guide to lovemaking.* New York, NY: Fireside Books.

Cooperman, N. A., Arnsten, J. H., & Klein, R. S. (2007). Current sexual activity and risky sexual behavior in older men with or at risk for HIV infection. *AIDS Education and Prevention, 19,* 321–333.

Cronenwett, L., Sherwood, G., Barnsteiner, J., Disch, J., Johnson, J., Mitchell, P., Sullivan, D., & Warren, J. (2007). Quality and safety education for nurses, *Nursing Outlook, 55*(3) 122–131.

Daniluk, J. C. (1998). *Women's sexuality across the life span: Challenging myths, creating meanings.* New York, NY: Guilford Press.

Dellapasqua, S., Colleoni, M., Castiglione, M., & Goldhirsch, A. (2007). New criteria for selecting elderly patients for breast cancer adjuvant treatment studies. *The Oncologist, 12,* 952–959.

Dharmarajan, T. S., Yoo, J., Russell, R. O., & Norkus, E. P. (2012). Chronic kidney disease staging in nursing home and community older adults: Does the choice of Cockcroft-Gault, Modification of Diet in Renal Disease Study, or the Chronic Kidney Disease Epidemiology Collaboration Initiative equations matter? *Journal of the American Medical Directors Association, 13*(2), 151–155.

Duffy, L. M. (1998). Lovers, loners, and lifers: Sexuality and the older adult. *Geriatrics, 53*(Suppl. 1), S66–S69.

Emlet, C. A. (2006). "You're awfully old to have this disease": Experiences of stigma and ageism in adults 50 years and older living with HIV/AIDS. *The Gerontologist, 46,* 871–790.

Eriksson, I., Gustafson, Y., Fagerström, L., & Olofsson, B. (2010). Prevalence and factors associated with urinary tract infections (UTIs) in very old women. *Archives of Gerontology and Geriatrics, 50*(2), 132–135.

Esposito, C., Plati, A., Mazzullo, T., Fasoli, G., De Mauri, A., Grosjean, D., et al. (2007). Renal function and functional reserve in healthy elderly individuals. *Journal of Nephrology, 20,* 617–625.

Etzioni, R., Berry, K., Legler, J. M., & Shaw, P. (2002). PSA testing in black and white men: An analysis of Medicare claims from 1991–1998. *Urology, 59,* 251–255.

Focus on effects of commonly used drugs on sexual function. (2000). *Focus on Geriatric Care and Rehabilitation, 12*(10), 12.

Gandhi, S., & Verma, S. (2011). Early breast cancer and the older woman. *The Oncologist, 16,* 479–485.

Gill, J., Malyuk, R., Djurdjev, O., & Levin, A. (2007). Use of GFR equations to adjust drug doses in an elderly multi-ethnic group—A cautionary tale. *Nephrology Dialysis Transplantation, 22,* 2894–2899.

Griebling, T. L. (2007a). Urinary tract infection in men. In M. S. Litwin & C. S. Saigal (Eds.), *Urologic diseases in America* (NIH Publication No. 07–5512, pp. 620–645). Washington, DC: U.S. Government Printing Office.

Griebling, T. L. (2007b). Urinary tract infection in women. In M. S. Litwin & C. S. Saigal (Eds.), *Urologic diseases in America* (NIH Publication No. 07–5512, pp. 587–619). Washington, DC: US Government Printing Office.

Griffiths, D. J., Tadic, S. D., Schaefer, W., & Resnick, N. M. (2009). Cerebral control of the lower urinary tract: How age-related changes might predispose to urge incontinence. *Neuroimaging, 47,* 981–986.

Gupta, K., Hooten, T. M., Roberts, P. L., & Stamm, W. E. (2007). Short-course nitrofurantoin for the treatment of acute uncomplicated cystitis in women. *Archives of Internal Medicine, 167,* 2207–2212.

Haber, D. (2009). Gay aging. *Gerontology and Geriatric Education,* 267–280.

Hartford Institute for Geriatric Nursing. (2001). *Incorporating essential gerontologic content into baccalaureate nursing education and staff development* (3rd ed.). New York, NY: Author.

Hartford Institute for Geriatric Nursing. (2007). Urinary incontinence assessment in older adults: Part I, Transient urinary incontinence. In *Best nursing practices in care of older adults.* New York, NY: New York University. Retrieved from http://consultgerirn.org/uploads/File/trythis/try_this_11_1.pdf

Heath, H. (2011). Older people in care homes: Sexuality and intimate relationships. *Nursing Older People, 23*(6), 14–20.

Hennessey, B. T., Suh, G. K., & Markman, M. (2011). Ovarian cancer. In H. M. Kantarjian, R. A. Wolff, & C. A. Koller (Eds.). *The M. D. Anderson manual of clinical oncology* (2nd ed.). Retrieved from http://www.accessmedicine.com/content.aspx?aID=8308785

Hillman, J. (2007). Knowledge and attitudes about HIV/AIDS among community-living older women: Re-examining issues of age and gender. *Journal of Women and Aging, 19*(3/4), 53–64.

Hoffman, R. M. (2011). Screening for prostate cancer. *New England Journal of Medicine, 365,* 2013–2019.

Howlader, N., Noone, A. M., Krapcho, M., Neyman, N., Aminou, R., Waldron, W., Altekruse, S. F., Kosary, C. L., Ruhl, J., Tatalovich, Z., Cho, H., Mariotto, A., Eisner, M. P., Lewis, D. R., Chen, H. S., Feuer, E. J., Cronin, K. A., & Edwards, B. K. (Eds.). (2011). *SEER cancer statistics review, 1975–2008.* Bethesda, MD: National Cancer Institute.

Hu, T. W., Wagner, T. H., Bentkover, J. D., Leblanc, K., Zhou, S. Z., & Hunt, T. (2004). Costs of urinary incontinence and overactive bladder in the United States: A comparative study. *Urology, 63*(3), 461–465.

Jarvis, C. (2004). *Physical examination and health assessment* (4th ed.). Philadelphia, PA: Saunders.

Jassal, S. V., Trpeski, L., Zhu, N., Fenton, S., & Hemmelgarn, B. (2007). Changes in survival among elderly patients initiating dialysis from 1990 to 1999. *Canadian Medical Association Journal, 177*(9), 1033–1038.

Jassal, V., Fillit, H., & Oreopoulos, D. G. (1998). Diseases of the aging kidney. In R. Tallis, H. Fillit, & J. C. Brocklehurst (Eds.), *Brocklehurst's textbook of geriatric medicine and gerontology* (5th ed., pp. 949–971). Edinburgh, Scotland: Churchill Livingstone.

Johnson, B. K. (1996). Older adults and sexuality: A multidimensional perspective. *Journal of Gerontological Nursing, 22*(2), 6–15.

Johnson, T. M., & Ouslander, J. G. (2009). Incontinence. In J. B. Halter et al. (Eds.), *Hazzard's geriatric medicine and gerontology* (6th ed., pp. 717–728). New York, NY: McGraw-Hill.

Kane, R. L., Ouslander, J. G., & Abrass, I. B. (2004). *Essentials of clinical geriatrics* (5th ed.). New York, NY: McGraw-Hill.

Keilman, L. J. (2005). Urinary incontinence: Basic evaluation and management in the primary care office. *Primary Care: Clinics in Office Practice, 32,* 699–722.

Kim, H., Suzuki, T., Yoshida, Y., & Yoshida, H. (2007). Effectiveness of multidimensional exercises for the treatment of stress urinary incontinence in elderly community-dwelling Japanese women: A randomized, controlled, crossover trial. *Journal of the American Geriatrics Society, 55,* 1932–1939.

Lekan-Rutledge, D., & Colling, J. (2003). Urinary incontinence in the frail elderly. *American Journal of Nursing, 103*(Suppl. 3), 36–46.

Lichtenberg, P. A. (1997). Clinical perspectives on sexual issues in nursing

homes. *Topics in Geriatric Rehabilitation, 12*(4), 1–10.

Light, S. A., & Holroyd, S. (2006). The use of medroxyprogesterone acetate for the treatment of sexually inappropriate behaviour in patients with dementia. *Journal of Psychiatry and Neuroscience, 31*(2), 132–143.

Lin, K., Croswell, J. M., Koenig, H., Lam, C., & Maltz, A. (2011). *Prostate-specific antigen-based screening for prostate cancer: An evidence update for the U.S. Preventive Services Task Force* (Evidence Synthesis No. 90, AHRQ Publication No. 12-05160-EF-1). Rockville, MD: Agency for Healthcare Research and Quality.

Lindau, S. T. (2009). Sexuality, sexual function, and the aging woman. In J. B. Halter et al. (Eds.), *Hazzard's geriatric medicine and gerontology* (6th ed., pp. 567–581). New York, NY: McGraw-Hill.

Lindau, S. T., Schumm, L. P., Laumann, E. O., Levinson, W., O'Muircheartaigh, C. A., & Waite, L. J. (2007). A study of sexuality and health among older adults in the United States. *New England Journal of Medicine, 357,* 762–774.

Loue, S. (2005). Intimacy and institutionalized cognitive impaired elderly. *Case Management Journals, 6*(4), 185–190.

Manson, J. E., Hsia, J., Johnson, K. C., Rossouw, J. E., Assaf, A. R., Lasser, N. L., et al. (2003). Estrogen plus progesterone and the risk of coronary heart disease. *New England Journal of Medicine, 349,* 523–534.

McCance, K. L., & Huether, S. E. (2010). *Pathophysiology: The biological basis for disease in adults and children* (6th ed.). Philadelphia, PA: Elsevier.

McCue, J. D. (1999). Treatment of urinary tract infections in long-term care facilities: Advice, guidelines, and algorithms. *Clinical Geriatrics, 7*(8), 11–17.

McKnight, K. K., Wellons, M. F., Sites, C. K., Roth, D. L., Szychowski, J. M., Halanych, J. H., Cushman, M., & Safford, M. M. (2011). Racial and regional differences in age at menopause in the United States: Findings from the REasons for Geographical and Racial Differences in Stroke (REGARDS) study. *American Journal of Obstetrics and Gynecology, 205,* 353.e1–353.e8.

McVary, K. T., Roehrborn, C. G., Avins, A. L., Barry, M. J., Bruskewitz, R. C., Donnell, R. F. et al., (2011). Update on AUA guideline on the management of benign prostatic hyperplasia. *Journal of Urology, 185,* 1793–1803.

Meadows, E. (2000). Physical therapy for older adults with urinary incontinence. *Topics in Geriatric Rehabilitation, 16,* 22–32.

Monga, T. N., Monga, U., Tan, G., & Grabois, M. (1999). Coital positions and sexual functioning in patients with chronic pain. *Sexuality and Disability, 17,* 287–297.

Munster, P. N., & Hudis, C. A. (1999). Systemic therapy for breast cancer in the elderly. *Clinical Geriatrics, 7*(7), 70–80.

Nabi, G., Cody, J. D., Ellis, G., Hay-Smith, J., & Herbison, P. G. (2006). Anticholinergic drugs versus placebo for overactive bladder syndrome in adults. *Cochrane Database of Systematic Reviews, 4.*

NANDA International. (2012). *NANDA International nursing diagnoses: Definitions and classification, 2012–2014.* Philadelphia, PA: Wiley-Blackwell.

National Cancer Institute. (2003). *Physician data query.* Bethesda, MD: Author. Retrieved from http://www.cancer.gov/cancerinfo/pdq

National Center for Health Statistics (NCHS). (1999). *Health, United States, 1999 with health and aging chartbook.* Hyattsville, MD: Author.

National Institute of Diabetes and Digestive and Kidney Diseases. (2001). *Kidney and urologic diseases statistics for the United States* (NIH Publication No. 02-3895). Washington, DC: U.S. Department of Health and Human Services.

National Kidney and Urologic Diseases Information Clearinghouse (NKUDIC). (2007a). *Urinary incontinence in women.* Retrieved from http://kidney.niddk.nih.gov/kudiseases/pubs/uiwomen

National Kidney and Urologic Diseases Information Clearinghouse (NKUDIC). (2007b). *Urinary retention.* Retrieved from http://kidney.niddk.nih.gov/kudiseases/pubs/UrinaryRetention/index.htm

Nay, R. (1992). Sexuality and aged women in nursing homes. *Geriatric Nursing, 13*(6), 312–314.

Neville, S., & Henrickson, M. (2010). "Lavender retirement": A questionnaire survey of lesbian, gay, and bisexual people's accommodation plans for old age. *International Journal of Nursing Practice, 16,* 586–594.

Nicolle, L. E. (2009). Urinary tract infections. In J. B. Halter et al. (Eds.), *Hazzard's geriatric medicine and gerontology* (6th ed., pp. 1547–1558). New York, NY: McGraw-Hill.

Palacios, S., Henderson, V. W., Siseles, N., Tan., D., & Villaseca, P. (2010). Age of menopause and impact of climacteric symptoms by geographical region. *Climacteric, 13,* 419–428.

Pfisterer, M. H., Johnson, T. M., Jenetzky, E., Hauer, K., & Oster, P. (2007). Geriatric patients' preferences for treatment of urinary incontinence: A study of hospitalized, cognitively competent adults aged 80 and older. *Journal of the American Geriatrics Society, 55,* 2016–2022.

Pienta, K. J. (2009). Prostate cancer. In J. B. Halter et al. (Eds.), *Hazzard's geriatric medicine and gerontology* (6th ed., pp. 1149–1155). New York, NY: McGraw-Hill.

Pope, M. (1997). Sexual issues for older lesbians and gays. *Topics in Geriatric Rehabilitation, 12*(4), 53–60.

Schlanger, L., Bailey, J. L., & Sands, J. M. (2009). Renal disease. In J. B. Halter et al. (Eds.), *Hazzard's geriatric medicine and*

gerontology (6th ed., pp. 1017–1033). New York, NY: McGraw-Hill.

Sitruk-Ware, R. (2007). New hormonal therapies and regimens in the postmenopause: Routes of administration and timing of initiation. *Climacteric, 10,* 358–370.

Smith, L. J., Mulhall, J. P., Deveci, S., Monaghan, N., & Reid, M. C. (2007). Sex after seventy: A pilot study of sexual function in older persons. *Journal of Sexual Medicine, 4,* 1247–1253.

Song, H. J., & Bae, J. M. (2007). Prevalence of urinary incontinence and lower urinary tract symptoms for community-dwelling elderly 85 years of age and older. *Journal of Wound, Ostomy and Continence nursing, 34,* 535–541.

Stenzelius, K., Westergren, A., Mattiasson, A., & Hallberg, I. R. (2006). Older women and men with urinary symptoms. *Archives of Gerontology and Geriatrics, 43,* 249–265.

Stern, M. F. (1997). Erectile dysfunction in older men. *Topics in Geriatric Rehabilitation, 12*(4), 40–52.

Strandberg, T. E., Ylikorkala, O., & Tikkanen, M. J. (2003). Differing effects of oral and transdermal hormone replacement therapy on cardiovascular risk factors in healthy postmenopausal women. *American Journal of Cardiology, 92*(2), 212–214.

Sturdee, D. W., & Pines, A. (2011). Updated IMS recommendations on postmenopausal hormone therapy and preventive strategies for midlife health. *Climacteric, 14,* 302–320.

Talley, K. M. C., Wyman, J. F., & Shamliyan, T. A. (2011). State of the science: Conservative interventions for urinary incontinence in frail community-dwelling older adults. *Nursing Outlook, 59*(4), 215–220.

Taylor, H. S., & Manson, J. T. (2011). Update in hormone therapy in menopause. *Journal of Clinical Endocrinology and Metabolism, 96,* 255–264.

Tenover, J. L. (2009). Sexuality, sexual function, androgen therapy, and the aging male. In J. B. Halter et al. (Eds.), *Hazzard's geriatric medicine and gerontology* (6th ed., pp. 595–606). New York, NY: McGraw-Hill.

Timiras, M. L., & Leary, J. (2007). The kidney, lower urinary tract, body fluids, and the prostate. In P. S. Timiras (Ed.), *Physiological basis of aging and geriatrics* (4th ed., pp. 297–313). New York, NY: Informa Healthcare.

Timiras, M. L., & Luxenberg, J. S. (2007). Pharmacology and drug management in the elderly. In P. S. Timiras (Ed.), *Physiological basis of aging and geriatrics* (4th ed., pp. 355–361). New York, NY: Informa Healthcare.

Ünlü, H., Sardan, Y. C., & Ülker, S. (2007). Comparison of sampling methods for urine cultures. *Journal of Nursing Scholarship, 39*(4), 325–329.

U.S. Preventive Services Task Force. (2012). Screening for cervical cancer. Retrieved from

http://www.uspreventiveservicestaskforce.org/uspstf11/cervcancer/cervcancerrs.htm#clinical

U.S. Renal Data System. (2007). *USRDS 2007 annual data report: Atlas of end-stage renal disease in the United States.* Bethesda, MD: National Institutes of Health, National Institute of Diabetes and Digestive and Kidney Diseases.

Veldhuis, J. D., Keenan, D. M., Iranmanesh, A., Takahashi, P. Y., & Nehra, A. (2007). The ensemble male hypothalamo-pituitary-gonadal axis. In P. S. Timiras (Ed.), *Physiological basis of aging and geriatrics* (4th ed., pp. 185–203). New York, NY: Informa Healthcare.

Watters, Y., & Boyd, T. V. (2009). Sexuality in later life: Opportunity for reflections for the healthcare provider. *Sexual and Relationship Therapy, 24*(3-4), 307–315.

Wei, J. T., Calhoun, E., & Jacobsen, S. J. (2007). Benign prostatic hyperplasia. In M. S. Litwin & C. S. Saigal (Eds.), *Urologic diseases in America* (NIH Publication No. 07–5512, pp. 44–69). Washington, DC: U.S. Government Printing Office.

Wessels, H., Joyce, G. F., Wise, M., & Wilt, T. J. (2007). Erectile dysfunction and Peyronie's disease. In M. S. Litwin & C. S. Saigal (Eds.), *Urologic diseases in America* (NIH Publication No. 07–5512, pp. 482–528). Washington, DC: U.S. Government Printing Office.

Whitlock, E. P., Vesco, K., Eder, M., Lin, J. S., Senger, C. A., & Burda, B. U. (2011). Liquid-based cytology and human papillomavirus testing to screen for cervical cancer: A systematic review for the U.S Preventive Services Task Force. *Annals of Internal Medicine, 155,* 687–697.

Wiggins, J., & Patel, S. R. (2009). Changes in renal function. In J. B. Halter et al. (Eds.), *Hazzard's geriatric medicine and gerontology* (6th ed., pp. 1009–1015). New York, NY: McGraw-Hill.

Wildiers, H., Kunkler, I., Biganzoli, L., Fracheboud, J., Vlastos, G., Bernard-Marty, C., et al. (2007). Management of breast cancer in elderly individuals: Recommendations of the International Society of Geriatric Oncology. *Lancet Oncology, 8,* 1101–1115.

Woodford, H. J., & George, J. (2009). Diagnosis and management of urinary tract infections in hospitalized older people. *Journal of the American Geriatrics Society, 57,* 107–114.

Wound, Ostomy, and Continence Nursing Certification Board. (2008). *Support certification.* Retrieved from http://www.wocncb.org/administrators

Wyman, J. F. (2003). Treatment of urinary incontinence in men and older women. *American Journal of Nursing, 103*(Suppl. 3), 26–35.

Wyman, J. F., Burgio, K. L., & Newman, D. K. (2009). Practical aspects of lifestyle modifications and behavioural interventions in the treatment of overactive bladder and urge urinary incontinence. *International Journal of Clinical Practice, 63*(8), 1177–1191.

The Musculoskeletal System

Rita Olivieri, RN, PhD Associate Professor, Retired
WILLIAM F. CONNELL SCHOOL OF NURSING AT BOSTON COLLEGE

KEY TERMS

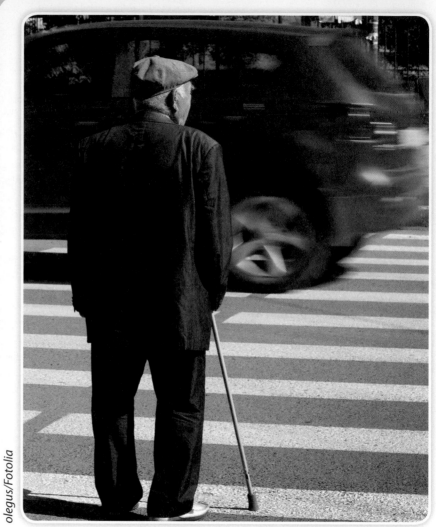

olegus/Fotolia

LEARNING OUTCOMES

On completion of this chapter, the reader will be able to:

1. Explain normal changes in the musculoskeletal system associated with aging.
2. Identify risk factors for the older person related to common musculoskeletal problems.
3. Formulate nursing diagnoses of older adults related to common musculoskeletal problems.
4. Compare the pharmacological management and nursing responsibilities related to the older person with common musculoskeletal problems, including osteoporosis, osteomalacia, Paget's disease, osteoarthritis, rheumatoid arthritis, gout, pseudogout, and hip fractures.
5. Discuss the nonpharmacological management of the older person with common musculoskeletal problems, including osteoporosis, osteomalacia, Paget's disease, osteoarthritis, rheumatoid arthritis, gout, pseudogout, and hip fractures.
6. Implement the nursing management principles related to the nursing care of older patients with arthritis.

The Normal Musculoskeletal System and Joints

The musculoskeletal system consists of the body's skeleton, muscles, ligaments, bursae, and joints. The skeleton provides form and support for the body. Bones provide protection for delicate body parts and are an important source of minerals as well as blood cells. The skeletal muscles provide movement of various body parts. All components of the system work together to produce the normal movement and actions that allow individuals to function independently in daily life.

Normal changes of aging often bring about complaints of musculoskeletal pain and various joint limitations, and aging appears to predispose an individual to the development of diseases such as osteoporosis and arthritis. The older person often suffers from these and other musculoskeletal chronic conditions that limit mobility and impair the ability to perform self-care activities such as bathing, dressing, and cooking resulting in a loss of independence. The older person may then be forced to give up an independent lifestyle and become increasingly dependent on others for assistance.

Skeletal System: Structure and Function

The adult body has 206 bones, which are divided into two major categories: the axial skeleton and the appendicular skeleton. Bones are also classified by shape, such as long bones (e.g., upper and lower extremities), short bones (e.g., tarsals, carpals), flat bones (e.g., ribs, cranium), and irregular bones (ear, vertebrae). The term *long* refers to the fact that the bone is longer than it is wide. For example, the bones of the fingers are considered long bones even though they are small. A typical long bone structure has a hard, compact diaphysis (or shaft) fused with the cancellous epiphysis at each end. The outer covering of the bone, the periosteum, is made up of fibrous connective tissue and is rich with blood vessels and nerves.

The two types of bones in the body based on texture are compact bone and cancellous bone. Both types of bone tissue have the same elements but are organized differently. **Compact bone** is solid and strong. At a microscopic level, compact bones are organized into structural units called haversian systems. These consist of concentric layers of crystallized matrix surrounding a central canal that contains blood vessels and nerves. **Cancellous bone,** which appears spongy, but is actually very strong, is less complex than compact bone and lacks the haversian systems. Together the two types of bones produce a skeleton that is light in weight but strong. A typical long bone structure has a hard, compact diaphysis (or shaft) fused with the cancellous epiphysis at each end. The outer covering of the bone, the periosteum, is made up of fibrous connective tissue and is rich with blood vessels and nerves.

Bones are composed of three types of cells and a bony matrix. The three types of cells are osteoblasts, osteocytes, and osteoclasts. Osteoblasts are bone-forming cells that lay down new bone. Osteocytes are mature bone cells that maintain bone. Osteoclasts are bone cells that reabsorb bone during repair and growth. The matrix consists of organic and inorganic substances. The organic substances, protein and fibers (especially collagen), are secreted by the osteoblasts and give tensile strength to the bone. The inorganic components of the matrix, calcium salts, account for the hardness that allows bone to resist compression.

Bone formation is an ongoing process and involves both the lengthening and thickening of the bone. The increase in diameter is called appositional growth. The rate of bone formation is determined by several factors including the amount of stress put on the bone, dietary intake, hormonal levels, and the activities of the bone-forming cells called the **osteoblasts.** Osteoblasts in the periosteum form compact bone around the external surface of the bone. At the same time osteoclasts break down bone on the internal bone surface. Working together these two processes allow the diameter of the bone to increase, while at the same time limiting the weight and size of the overall bone.

Bone tissue is very active with as much as 0.5 g of calcium entering or leaving the human body per day. When blood calcium levels drop below normal, calcium is released from the bones so that there will be an adequate supply for the metabolic needs of the body. When calcium levels become increased, the excess calcium is stored in the bone matrix.

The functions of the skeletal system include hematopoiesis, bone remodeling and repair, and homeostasis. Bone is the site for hematopoietic tissues, which manufacture blood cells. In adults, the most active site of hematopoiesis is the red marrow cavities found within the cancellous bone spaces of the skull, vertebrae, ribs, sternum, and shoulder.

Throughout life, new bone is continually deposited and reabsorbed in response to hormonal, dietary, and mechanical stimuli. Together, these processes are called *bone remodeling* or *renewing,* which is one of the major mechanisms for maintaining calcium balance in the body. An adequate diet during the early years of life is essential for maximal bone growth. Likewise calcium deficiency during teenage years will result in bones that are less dense later in life. Up to 90% of the calcium present in bones is deposited by the age of 18 in girls and age 20 in boys (National Institute of Arthritis and Musculoskeletal and Skin Diseases [NIAMS], 2012a).

Joints: Structure and Function

Joints, the area where two bones are attached, provide stability and mobility to the skeleton. A joint may be (1) freely movable, called a diarthrodial joint; (2) immobile, a synarthrosis joint; or (3) only slightly movable, an amphiarthrosis joint. Diarthrodial joints are the most complex, and allow various positions depending on the type of joint. The two ends of the bone are not directly connected but come together in a fibrous joint (articular) capsule that provides support. The joint capsule has two layers, an outer layer and a delicate inner layer called the synovial membrane. The synovial fluid, secreted by the synovial membrane, fills the joint cavity and provides lubrication and nourishment. Synovial joints have articulating surfaces covered by hyaline cartilage and a closed sac filled with fluid. The function of hyaline cartilage is to reduce friction in the joint and redistribute the forces of weight bearing. Bursae function as cushions in areas of potential friction. One example is the prepatellar bursa of the knee, which lies between the patella and the skin. It helps muscles and tendons glide smoothly over bone. Synovial joints include hinge, ball-and-socket, and pivot joints. Figure 18-1 ▶▶▶ illustrates the structure of a synovial joint.

Synarthrodial or fibrous joints are immovable and are found between the bones of the cranium, the bones of the lower arm (radius and ulna), and the bones of the lower leg (tibia and fibula). The amphiarthroses joints allow only slight movement. They are cartilaginous by construction and are found in the rib cage, vertebrae, and pubic bone.

Ligaments are fibrous connections between two bones that provide the joint with stability during movement. Ligaments both allow and limit joint motion. Commonly injured ligaments are the medial, collateral, anterior, and posterior cruciate ligaments of the knee. Tendons are collagen fibers that attach muscle to bone. These specialized tissues are surrounded by synovial-like tissue. Ligaments and tendons protect the limbs from various sudden movements or changes in speed.

Muscles: Structure and Function

Walking and running is the result of the coordinated action of the joints, bones, and skeletal muscles. Skeletal muscles are the largest organs of the body and account for 50% of lean body mass in a healthy young person. The more than 600 muscles in the body vary in size and shape. Their lengths range from 2 to 60 cm, and each muscle's shape is related to its function. Muscle consists of a three-layer framework composed of connective tissue covered by fascia. The fascia provides support and protection for the muscle, connects muscle to bony prominences, and is the structure that houses the blood, lymph, and nerve supply. The skeletal muscles have an abundant supply of blood vessels and nerves (Figure 18-2 ▶▶▶). This is important for their primary function, which is to contract. Each muscle fiber is covered by endomysium. A bundle of these fibers is called perimysium. Many bundles wrapped together form a muscle.

Skeletal muscles usually originate at one point of attachment to a tendon and terminate at the end of an adjoining bone (National Cancer Institute, 2012). A pair of skeletal muscles work together so that flexing of one muscle is balanced by the extension of the opposite pair. These opposite muscles can cause the opening and closing of such joints as the knee and elbow. Flexor muscles cause the closing of the joint and extensor muscles cause the opening of the joint.

Function of Skeletal Muscles

The motor unit is the functional unit of the neuromuscular system. A motor unit consists of muscle fibers innervated by a single motor nerve, its axon, and an anterior horn cell. When the motor unit receives an electrical impulse, it contracts as a whole. The number of motor units per muscle varies greatly.

Muscle contraction occurs on the molecular level and leads to the actual observed muscle movement. A contraction occurs when an electrical charge moves along a nerve and across the neuromuscular junction to the muscles. Neurotransmitters, such as acetylcholine, permit neurologic impulses to be transmitted to the muscle. Nerve fibers may supply more than 100 individual skeletal muscle cells.

Body movements like raising a hand or flexing the leg are voluntary (skeletal) muscle movements. Other movements are unconscious and happen without awareness or

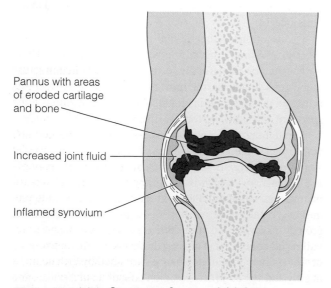

Pannus with areas of eroded cartilage and bone

Increased joint fluid

Inflamed synovium

Figure 18-1 ▶▶▶ Structure of a synovial joint.

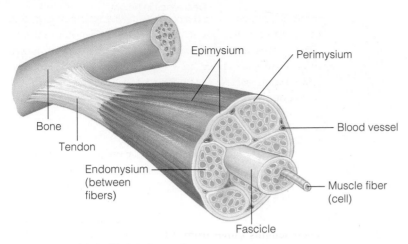

Epimysium

Perimysium

Bone

Tendon

Blood vessel

Endomysium
(between
fibers)

Muscle fiber
(cell)

Fascicle

Figure 18-2 ▶▶▶ Skeletal muscle.

conscious effort. Skeletal muscles are part of the somatic nervous system: involuntary muscles are controlled by the autonomic nervous system. Involuntary (smooth) muscles are those that line the stomach, and internal organs and blood vessels. Cardiac muscle is a third category; it is neither skeletal nor smooth muscle.

Isotonic contractions, such as those that allow the person to pick up an object, produce movement. Isometric contractions do not produce actual movement, but increase the tension within the muscle.

The number of muscle cells in the body does not change after birth. However, the size of the muscle cell will be determined by the work of the muscle. When the work of the muscle is demanding, the muscle will increase in diameter (hypertrophy). With lack of use, the muscle will shrink (atrophy).

The most important function of muscles is contractility. Most of the movement in the body is the result of muscle contraction. Functions of muscle contractions include movement, posture, joint stability, and heat production.

Normal Changes of Aging

Significant alterations in human structure, function, biochemistry, and genetic patterns are responsible for the changes in the muscles, tendons, bones, and joints of the older person. These changes contribute to the appearance of aging in many older adults such as decreased height, stooped shoulders, and rigid movements. Figure 18-3 ▶▶▶ illustrates the normal changes of aging in the musculoskeletal system.

Skeleton

The bone loss of normal aging has been described in two distinct phases: type I, or menopausal bone loss; and type II,

senescent bone loss. Menopausal bone loss is a rapid phase of bone loss that affects women in the first 5 to 10 years after menopause. Senescent bone loss is a slower phase that affects both sexes after midlife. These two phases are distinct in their clinical features, but in women there is eventual overlap, which leads to increased difficulty in differentiating the two phases. Other conditions may also contribute to skeletal deterioration in the older person and may alter the clinical symptoms.

In the older person, bones become stiff, weaker, and more brittle. Changes in appearance are evident after the fifth decade, and changes in height are the most obvious. At about 50 years of age, the long bones of the arms and legs appear disproportionate in size due to the shrinking stature. An average loss of height is 1 cm every 10 years after age 40. Height loss is even greater after 70 years old (National Library of Medicine [NLM], 2010a). This change in height is due to various processes that result in shortening of the vertebral column. Thinning of the vertebral disks occurs more commonly in midlife; in later years, there is a decrease in the height of individual vertebrae. As the older person enters the eighth and ninth decades, there is a more rapid decrease in vertebral height due to osteoporotic collapse of the vertebrae. The result is a shortening of the trunk and the appearance of long extremities. Additional postural changes are kyphosis and a backward tilt of the head to make eye contact. The result is a forward bent, or "jutting out" posture, with the hips and knees assuming a flex position.

Muscles

There is a great deal of variation in muscle function in the older person. Muscle function remains trainable well into advanced age, and the regenerative function of muscle tissue remains normal in the older person.

Maintaining muscle function is vital to maintaining functional independence. Muscle tone and tension decrease steadily after the fourth decade of life. **Sarcopenia** is a syndrome that involves a generalized loss of skeletal muscle mass, strength, and function that occurs in a progressive manner as a result of the aging process (Burton & Sumukadas, 2010). Some muscles decrease in size, resulting in weakness. The shape of muscles becomes more prominent and feels more distinct. Muscle strength declines slowly, but by 50 years of age a decline in stamina is often noticed. By 80 years of age, the maximum muscle strength

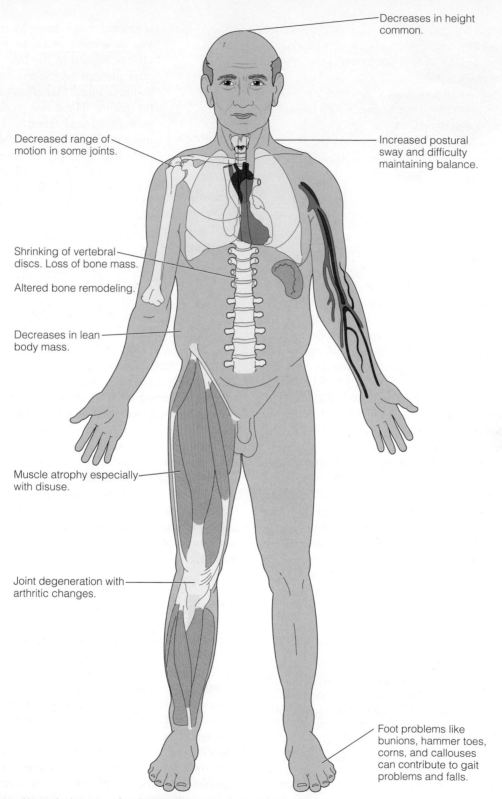

Decreases in height common.

Decreased range of motion in some joints.

Increased postural sway and difficulty maintaining balance.

Shrinking of vertebral discs. Loss of bone mass.

Altered bone remodeling.

Decreases in lean body mass.

Muscle atrophy especially with disuse.

Joint degeneration with arthritic changes.

Foot problems like bunions, hammer toes, corns, and callouses can contribute to gait problems and falls.

Figure 18-3 ▶▶▶ Normal changes of aging in the musculoskeletal system.

that the individual had in the mid-20s has decreased 65% to 85%. Epidemiologic studies estimate the prevalence of sarcopenia to be as high as 50% in people ages 80 years and older (Burton & Sumukadas, 2010). The faster contracting type II muscle fibers atrophy more than the slower contracting type I muscles. Type I fibers maintain posture and perform repetitive-type exercise; for the most part, they maintain this function in the older person.

The lower extremity muscles tend to atrophy earlier than those of the upper extremity. Routine daily activities most likely keep the upper extremities functioning on a regular basis. By comparison, walking may be limited to a small living area and for short periods of time. Despite age-related changes in muscle strength, the older adult can usually perform functional activities of daily living and demonstrate adequate muscle function when climbing stairs, walking a straight line, and rising from a sitting or squatting position.

Joints, Ligaments, Tendons, and Cartilage

Hyaline cartilage, which lines the joints, erodes and tears with advancing age, allowing bones to come in direct contact with one another. Knee cartilage is subjected to a great deal of wear and tear, and the result is a thinning as one ages. Thin, damaged cartilage and diminished lubricating fluid result in discomfort and slowness of joint movement.

Ligaments, tendons, and joint capsules lose elasticity and become less flexible. There is a decrease in the range of motion of the joints due to changes in ligaments and muscles. Nonarticular cartilage, as found in the ears and nose, grows throughout life, which may cause the nose to look large in relation to the face. The amount of collagen in cartilage does not change greatly but the collagen becomes stiffer, making the cartilage less able to handle mechanical stress.

Common Musculoskeletal Illnesses

Osteoporosis, osteomalacia, and Paget's disease are metabolic bone diseases. Osteoarthritis, rheumatoid arthritis, gout, and pseudogout are joint diseases (arthropathies). The two major categories of arthropathies are inflammatory and noninflammatory joint diseases. Noninflammatory joint diseases (osteoarthritis) are distinguished from inflammatory joint diseases (rheumatoid arthritis, gout, and pseudogout) by the (1) lack of synovial inflammation, (2) absence of systemic manifestations, and (3) normal synovial fluid (NLM, 2010b).

Osteoporosis

Osteoporosis is the most common metabolic disease, affecting 50% of women during their lifetime. In the United States 40 million people either have osteoporosis or are at risk for osteoporosis due to low bone mass (NIAMS, 2012a). Major risk factors for osteoporosis are increased age, female sex, White or Asian race, positive family history of osteoporosis, and thin body habitus. Most often, osteoporosis is a disease of White women. However, it is predicted that in the next 20 years, older men and also minorities will be affected in greater numbers because of changing demographics (Browder-Lazenby, 2011). Physical inactivity and a sedentary lifestyle as well as impaired neuromuscular function (e.g., reduced muscle strength, impaired gait and balance) are risk factors for developing fragility factors (International Osteoporosis Foundation [IOF], 2011). Additional risk factors include low calcium intake, prolonged immobility, excessive alcohol and caffeine intake, stress, cigarette smoking, and the long-term use of corticosteroids, anticonvulsants, or thyroid hormones (IOF, 2011).

Pathophysiology

Osteoporosis is characterized by low bone mass and deterioration of bone tissue leading to compromised bone strength that increases the risk for fractures. The bone strength reflects the integration of bone density and quality. Bone density is defined as grams of mineral per area or volume. Bone quality is explained as the architecture, turnover, and damage accumulation and mineralization.

At present, bone strength cannot be directly measured. Bone mineral density (BMD) is a replacement measure that accounts for 70% of a bone's strength. Bone loss in the older person is considered normal when the BMD is within 1 standard deviation (SD) of the young adult mean. Bone density between 1 and 2.5 SD below the young adult mean is termed osteopenic. Osteoporosis is defined as bone density 2.5 SD below the young adult mean (Jacobs-Kosmin, 2012). The three factors most likely to contribute to decreased bone mass in the older person are (1) failure to reach peak bone mass in early adulthood, (2) increased bone resorption, and (3) decreased bone formation.

Osteopenia and osteoporosis result in high mortality and morbidity. Estimated health costs are over $14 billion annually. Reduced BMD is highly predictive of spinal and hip fractures in women and men. One in three women over age 50 will experience osteoporotic fractures, as will one in five men (IOF, 2011). The greatest majority are fractures of the vertebrae, with about 700,000 individuals suffering from this injury each year. Hip and wrist fractures make up about one fifth of the total. One in five patients dies

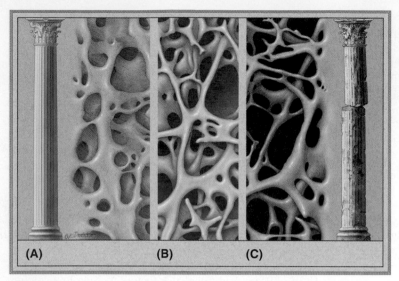

Figure 18-4 ▶▶▶ Normal bone compared to osteoporotic bone.
A. Normal bone. B. Osteopenia. C. Osteoporosis.

Source: John M. Daugherty/Photo Researchers, Inc.

within 1 year of a hip fracture, and only 40% regain their prefracture mobility and independence level (IOF, 2011). Figure 18-4 ▶▶▶ illustrates normal and osteoporotic bone structure.

Classification of Osteoporosis

Causes of both primary and secondary osteoporosis may include hyperparathyroidism, malignancy, immobilization, gastrointestinal disease, renal disease, or drugs that cause bone loss. Specific causes of secondary osteoporosis that commonly affect older adults are vitamin D deficiencies and the use of glucocorticoid drugs.

Menopausal Bone Loss

Before menopause, sex hormones (estrogen in women and testosterone in men) protect the body from bone loss. After menopause in women (or after castration in men), an over-production of interleukin-6 results in an increased loss of bone mass of up to 10-fold. The loss of bone matrix (resorption) occurs more rapidly than bone growth (deposition), resulting in the loss of bone density or osteoporosis. By age 70, susceptible women have lost an average of 50% of their peripheral **cortical bone** (dense solid bone) mass from the shafts of the long bones. Vertebral and Colles' fractures are the result of menopausal bone loss. As people age into their 70s and 80s, osteoporosis is a common disease (Jacob-Kosmin, 2012).

In **senescent bone loss** there is a decrease in the actual amount of bone formed during remodeling. This occurs in both sexes and is due to the aging process. Osteoblast formation, bone mineral density, and the rate of bone formation continuously decrease, leading to a decrease in bone wall thickness—especially in trabecular (cancellous) bone. Trabecular bone mass is found in the vertebrae, pelvis, and shafts of long bones. Vertebral and hip fractures may be the results of senescent bone loss.

Trajectory of Bone Loss for Women

In most cases, women in their third decade have lower peak bone mass than men. Women generally have thinner bones, so they have less in the "bone bank." Women who have children may lose additional bone mass with lactation. In the fifth decade during perimenopause, rapid withdrawal from the bone bank leaves the woman's bones even more depleted. The longer life span for women further extends the risk for osteoporosis (see Box 18-1 for gender differences in bone loss). Signs and symptoms of osteoporosis are usually absent. Osteoporosis is a silent disease; the first sign is often a fracture (IOF, 2011).

BOX 18-1 ▶ **Gender Differences in Bone Loss**

It is generally accepted that women have a greater risk of decreased bone density and possible osteoporosis. Several factors contribute to this risk:

1. Factors during the adolescent years:
   a. Women accumulate less bone mass than men and have smaller, narrower bones with thinner cortices.
   b. Men have more bone mass growth and have bigger and stronger bones.
2. Factors related to loss of sex hormones:
   a. Abrupt loss of estrogen after menopause causes rapid loss in bone.
   b. Men have a slower decline of testosterone. Although bone mass is lost, it is at a slower rate.
3. Factors related to reproduction:
   a. Women may also lose bone mass during the reproductive years, especially with prolonged lactation.
4. Factors related to longevity:
   a. Women live longer than men and thus have an increased risk for senescent bone loss.

Source: Data from IOF (2011) and Institute for Clinical Systems Improvement (2011).

Osteomalacia

Osteomalacia is a metabolic disease in which there is inadequate mineralization of newly formed bone matrix, usually resulting from vitamin D deficiency. Rickets, which is similar to osteomalacia, occurs in the growing bones of children. Although osteomalacia and rickets are not common in the United States, they are endemic in Asia. In the United States, these diseases are seen in older adults, premature infants, those who adhere to strict macrobiotic vegetarian diets, and women who have had multiple pregnancies and have breast-fed their children.

Pathophysiological Mechanisms

The most common causes of osteomalacia are vitamin D deficiency, abnormal metabolism of vitamin D, and phosphate depletion. In osteomalacia, the volume of bone remains normal, but new bone replacement consists of soft bony tissue rather than rigid bone. This soft bony tissue, known as *osteoid bone,* continues to be produced, in excess of mineralization, and results in deformities of the long bones, spine, pelvis, and skull. Osteomalacia may be due to primary vitamin D deficiency from a lack of exposure to the ultraviolet radiation of the sun, or to poor dietary intake. In the United States, primary vitamin D deficiency is rare because synthetic vitamin D is added to dairy and bread products. However, older adults are at risk for osteomalacia because of the inability to get outdoors, limited dietary intake of milk, as well as aging skin that is less able to produce vitamin D. In addition, many other pathological conditions in the older person may result in osteomalacia (Browder-Lazenby, 2011).

Clinical Manifestations

Osteomalacia causes varying degrees of bone pain and tenderness, which may be generalized or localized to the hips, pelvis, legs, ribs, or vertebrae. Bones are fragile, and fractures occur with minor injuries, making it difficult to differentiate from osteoporosis (NLM, 2012c). Vertebral collapse is common, resulting in changes in posture and height. Deformities (gibbus deformity, leg bowing) occur occasionally in the severely affected older person. In severe osteomalacia, muscle weakness and easy fatigability may cause an unsteady gait. The muscle weakness is caused by lack of vitamin D to the muscle cells, as well as low calcium and phosphorus levels.

Vitamin D Metabolism

Vitamin D is actually a group of vitamins that are essential for the metabolism of calcium and phosphorus. Each step in the process of vitamin D metabolism must be accomplished for the active form of the vitamin to be produced. Interference with any step may result in the insufficient bone mineralization that leads to osteomalacia.

The following are steps in the process of vitamin D metabolism and some of the pathological conditions that may cause a deficit at each step (Ignatavicius & Workman, 2010):

Step 1. Normal process.

Vitamin D_3 (cholecalciferol) is manufactured by skin (from sun or certain food such as salmon, tuna, and mackerel). *Vitamin D deficit occurs if there is* inadequate intake or inadequate exposure to sun or impairment of absorption in small bowel (postgastrectomy, small-bowel resection, or Crohn's disease).

Step 2. Normal process.

Vitamin D_3 (cholecalciferol) is then carried to the liver and partly converted to calcidiol (25-hydroxy D_3). *Vitamin D deficit occurs if there is* severe liver disease and if certain drugs are taken, such as phenytoin, barbiturates, or carbamazepine.

Step 3. Normal process.

Calcidiol (25-hydroxy D_3) is then carried to the kidney and converted to calcitriol (1, 25-dihydroxy D_3). The amount produced is regulated by parathyroid hormone and plasma phosphate levels. *Vitamin D deficit occurs if there is* severe renal disease.

Step 4. Normal process.

Calcitriol (1, 25-dihydroxy D_3) is the active hormonal form that stimulates intestinal absorption of calcium and phosphorus, resulting in mineralization of the bone.

> ***Practice Pearl*** ▶▶▶ Muslim women often cover their entire body when out in public. This may prevent them from obtaining adequate vitamin D through exposure to sunlight and may increase the risk of osteomalacia. The older Muslim woman can be taught to expose hands and face (15% of the body) in a private area such as a backyard, for about 15 minutes a day to absorb adequate vitamin D.

Paget's Disease

Paget's disease, or **osteitis deformans,** is a chronic, localized bone disorder of unknown etiology in which normal bone is removed and replaced with abnormal bone. Paget's lesions may involve one or more locations of the skeleton, but are most common in the pelvis (68%), vertebrae (49%), skull (44%), and femur (55%) in more men than women who are usually over 70 years of age (Browder-Lazenby, 2011). Following osteoporosis, it is the second most common bone remodeling disease, affecting between 1 million and 3 million Americans. Paget's disease may be asymptomatic, and the diagnosis is often made by abnormal X-ray findings for an unrelated problem.

Pathophysiology

Paget's disease begins with the accelerated activity of abnormally large osteoclasts, which resorb bone at specific sites. The resulting bone formation is too rapid, leading to new bone structure that is inferior to normal bone. The pagetic bone is less compact, more vascular, and especially prone to structural deformities, weakness, and pathological fractures. Although the etiology of Paget's disease is unknown, viral particles, genetics, and hereditary factors have all been implicated (NIAMS, 2012b).

Clinical Manifestations

The clinical manifestations of Paget's disease are determined by the affected bone sites. Bone pain, the most frequently reported symptom, may be described as deep and aching, and may be accompanied by muscle spasms. Pain may occur at the site of the pagetic lesion, or at the osteoarthritic joints (hips and knees) that result from the disease. Pain, as well as the inherent mechanical deformities of the long bones, may result in bowing of the femur or tibia (NLM, 2012d). Mobility impairments, gait changes, and stress fractures are also common lower extremity complications. Bony growths in the spine may cause kyphosis, cord compression, and paralysis.

When Paget's disease affects the skull, it may cause enlargement and disfigurement of the cranium, resulting in complications of the central nervous system such as mental deterioration and dementia. The older person may also experience headaches, tinnitus, and vertigo. Thickened bony growths on the interior of the skull may impinge cranial nerves, causing hearing loss and visual changes. Jaw and teeth deformities may result in dental problems such as malocclusion.

Paget's disease can also cause several different kinds of pain depending on areas of the body affected. The older person may complain of pain in joints, bone, muscle, or the nervous system due to damage or pressure caused by the disease (NIAMS, 2011c).

Joint Disorders: Noninflammatory and Inflammatory Categories

There are many joint diseases (arthropathies). The two major categories are inflammatory joint disease and noninflammatory joint disease. As mentioned previously, noninflammatory joint diseases (osteoarthritis) are distinguished from inflammatory joint diseases (rheumatoid arthritis, gout, and pseudogout) by the (1) lack of synovial inflammation, (2) absence of systemic manifestations, and (3) normal synovial fluid (Browder-Lazenby, 2011).

Noninflammatory Joint Disease: Osteoarthritis

Osteoarthritis is the most common form of arthritis in the United States. Osteoarthritis (OA) affects more than 50% of people over the age of 65 and is the leading cause of disability for this age group (Lozada, Diamond, & Agnew, 2011). OA is a chronic disease that is a daily presence in the lives of over 20 million older adults. Women are affected more than men. The severity of the disease may vary greatly from being an insignificant problem to causing a major life disruption. Nodal disease at middle age is frequently associated with the development of knee OA in the 60s and 70s (Lozada et al., 2011). Osteoarthritis is a significant predictor of whether older adults will be functionally limited in their self-care abilities. Recent studies have determined that aging alone does not cause this disease. Associated factors include obesity, overuse of a joint, trauma, and a cold climate.

Primary or idiopathic osteoarthritis has no single, clear cause. It is likely a group of similar disorders that involve various complex biomedical, biochemical, and cellular processes. The typical changes can occur in several joints but have various causes. Secondary arthritis has an underlying condition such as trauma, bone disease, or inflammatory joint disease.

Pathophysiology Osteoarthritis is characterized by the progressive erosion of the joint articular cartilage with the formation of new bone in the joint space. Figure 18-5 ▶▶▶ illustrates the hands of an older person diagnosed with osteoarthritis. The joints most commonly involved in OA are joints of the hands, the weight-bearing joints of the knee and hip, and the central joints of the cervical and lumbar spine. The process involves low-grade inflammation, articular cartilage, calcifications, genetic alterations, and metabolic disorders (Browder-Lazenby, 2011). Other components of the degenerative process include growth factors, enzymes, and cytokines.

Normal joint cartilage covers the joint and bone ends and provides a cushioning structure to reduce the mechanical force of the joint. In OA, the cartilage thins and erodes. The underlying bone (subchondral bone) is no longer

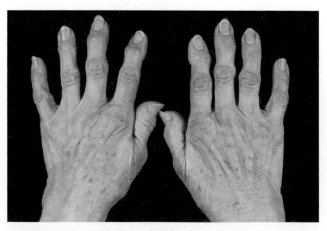

Figure 18-5 ▶▶▶ Osteoarthritis of the hands.
Source: Copyright 2012 Lee Samsami—Custom Medical Stock Photo. All rights reserved.

protected, particularly in areas of increased stress. Without the cartilage performing as a buffer, the subchondral bone becomes irritated, which leads to degeneration of the joint. As cartilage deteriorates, subchondral bone cells hypertrophy and eventually cause bony spurs (osteophytes). These bony spurs grow and enlarge, and often change the contour of the joint. Small pieces may break off (joint mice) and irritate the synovial membrane, causing a joint effusion and further limitation of movement.

Clinical Manifestations By age 40, about 90% of all people have X-ray evidence of primary osteoarthritis in their weight-bearing joints. However, only 40% of people with severe OA (as determined by X-ray) have pain. Generalized or systemic symptoms, such as fever and malaise, are not characteristic of OA. The most common symptoms are early morning stiffness and joint pain. Morning stiffness in the joints usually resolves in about 30 minutes. Pain usually occurs during activity and is relieved by rest. As the disease progresses, the pain may be present at rest and interrupt sleep patterns. The source of pain is often not known, but needs to be identified to provide treatment (NLM, 2012b).

> **Practice Pearl** ▶▶▶ The damaged articular cartilage, the distinct feature of OA, is not the direct source of the pain because cartilage lacks nerve endings. Rather, the articular cartilage and surrounding structures cause pain indirectly. Examples of etiologies of pain include stretching of the joint capsule, muscle spasm in the surrounding area, and the release of inflammatory cells into the synovial fluid (Lozada et al., 2011).

Joint involvement is usually asymmetrical at first, and patients may complain of the bony appearance of their joints (see Table 18-1 for specific joints and characteristics). Pain is not

TABLE 18-1 Osteoarthritis: Specific Sites, Joints, and Characteristics

Site	Joint	Features
Hand		
Women mainly in their 40s	Distal interphalangeal joint Proximal interphalangeal joint First carpometacarpal joint (thumb base)	Distal joint more common (flexion and lateral deviation have genetic component). Bony enlargement, malalignment (chronic). Can result in erosion, deformity, ankylosis.
Knee		
Women more than men in their 50s, 60s, and 70s	Medial, lateral, and patellofemoral compartment	Most often affected weight-bearing joint. Strong association with obesity. Crepitus on range of motion (chronic periarticular muscle atrophy). Limited range of motion (chronic). Bowed leg deformity—varus.
Spine		
	Lumbar area (facet joints) Cervical spondylosis	Pain referred to thigh—may mimic sciatic. Stiffness—muscle spasm. Spinal stenosis (chronic or severe).
Hip		
Men and women equally in their 40s, 50s, and 60s		Pain mainly at front of groin. Also at lateral thigh, buttocks, and radiating to knee. Characteristic limp (antalgic gait). Decreased range of motion, especially on internal rotation. Extremely disabling.
Foot		
	Big toe	Can result in pain with walking or prolonged standing, limiting mobility.

usually associated with inflammatory symptoms (as with rheumatoid arthritis). Joints affected may have crepitus (a grating sound on movement), deficits in range of motion, and muscle weakness. Osteoarthritis of the hands may show new bone growth with the appearance of Heberden's nodes (distal interphalangeal joint) and Bouchard's nodes (proximal interphalangeal joint). Pain can be elicited on both active and passive motion. The joint damage, chronic pain, and muscle weakness of OA result in impaired balance and decreased activity.

Inflammatory Joint Diseases

The three most common inflammatory joint diseases affecting the older person are rheumatoid arthritis, gout, and pseudogout. Redness, tenderness, and severe swelling around the circumference of the joints characterize inflammatory disease. Unlike osteoarthritis, inflammatory diseases are responsive to pharmacological intervention, which can improve the quality of life for the older person.

Rheumatoid Arthritis Rheumatoid arthritis (RA) is the

most prevalent inflammatory arthritis of any age group. It is quite common in older adults, and the incidence increases up to age 80. Women are affected more than men by a 3-to-1 ratio and tend to have more severe articular disease symptoms. The course of the disease varies greatly. For some patients, it may be a mild, remitting disease; for others, it brings severe disability, joint deformity, and even premature death.

Pathophysiology Rheumatoid arthritis is a chronic syndrome, characterized by symmetrical inflammation of the peripheral joints, with pain, swelling, significant morning stiffness, as well as general symptoms of fatigue and malaise. The cause of RA is unknown, but is most likely due to a variety of unknown environmental factors (infectious agents, chemical exposures) that trigger an autoimmune response to an unidentified antigen. Genetic predisposition is a major factor in both the susceptibility and the severity of RA.

In RA, the long-term intense exposure to the offending antigen (unknown virus or bacteria) causes normal antibodies (IgG and IgM) to convert to autoantibodies. These transformed antibodies (rheumatoid factors) can then perpetuate the inflammatory response indefinitely. Rheumatoid factors are commonly (not always) present in the synovial fluid and blood of the person with RA. The initial pathological changes appear in the synovial tissue and result in mild cell proliferation. Over time, complex immune and inflammatory processes form a neoplasm-like mass in the synovium, known as a *pannus* (Browder-Lazenby, 2011).

The pannus is made up of granulation tissue. It erodes joint, soft tissue, cartilage, and bone, and may cause the development of bone spurs and osteophytes. The end result of pannus formation is the development of scar tissue that shortens tendons and joints, resulting in subluxation and

contractures (loss of joint space, or juxta-articular bone erosion). The pannus formation causes the joint damage and is the focus of treatment for RA.

Clinical Manifestations The course of RA may be slow and insidious, or it may present with an acute process affecting several joints (polyarticular). RA causes tenderness and limitation of movement. The older person may experience the first symptoms of RA after the age of 65. This is known as *de novo* development of RA. Clinical manifestations include disabling morning stiffness and marked pain in the joints, chiefly in the upper extremities. The morning stiffness of RA lasts more than an hour and may also occur after a period of rest. On assessment, the joints will have severe redness, swelling, and warmth of the soft tissue. These symptoms cause severe pain on movement, limitation of movement, and a disrupted sleep pattern (NIAMS, 2011c). In the early stage of the disease, the older person may have symptoms that are severely disabling, but deformities are not present.

Rheumatoid arthritis commonly occurs in joints of the hands (proximal interphalangeal, metacarpophalangeal, wrist), elbows, shoulders, knees, ankle, and feet (metatarsophalangeal). Less frequently, joints of the shoulder, hip, and sternoclavicular are involved. Although RA is characterized by joint symptoms, it is a systemic inflammatory disease. Most patients with RA experience nonspecific systemic symptoms such as fatigue, malaise, weight loss, and fever, which often occur several weeks or months before the typical joint symptoms. Figure 18-6 ▶▶▶ illustrates the hands of an older person diagnosed with rheumatoid arthritis.

> **Practice Pearl** ▶▶▶ The stiffness of RA is caused by the inflammatory process in the synovium, which mechanically prevents the joint movement. The timing of the stiffness—lasting an hour—is especially characteristic of RA, and differentiates it from OA (stiffness due to OA lasts only a few minutes).

The second category of RA in older adults occurs in those who have been diagnosed with the disease before 65 years of age. Over time, rheumatoid arthritis becomes a symmetrical additive disease of the joints. The physical stresses and inflammatory changes of the disease result in the characteristic joint deformities. Within 2 years of the establishment of the disease, more than 10% of RA patients will develop deformities of the hands (Johnsson & Eberhardt, 2009). After 10 years, most RA patients will experience these changes. As described previously, these deformities are caused by the development of a pannus (long-term, severe proliferation of the synovial intimal layer).

Subcutaneous nodules also occur with advanced disease in more than one fourth of RA patients. They are located

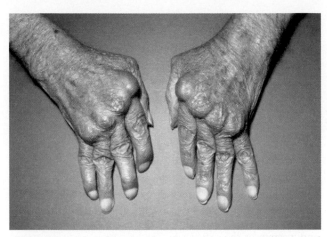

Figure 18-6 ▶▶▶ The hands of an older person diagnosed with rheumatoid arthritis.

Source: James Stevenson/Photo Researchers, Inc.

on pressure areas such as the elbows or sacrum, and are not attached to bone or underlying skin. Many older people who have had the disease for many years have multiple deformities due to progressive disease involvement. They may also have had various forms of drug treatment. In addition, these patients may have undergone one or more joint replacement surgeries.

Systemic and Nonarticular Manifestations In addition to joint symptoms, patients with severe and advanced RA have systemic and nonjoint manifestations of the disease. Although the disease is more common in women, these extra-articular manifestations are more common in men, especially pleural involvement, vasculitis, and pericarditis. It is often difficult to determine if these conditions are caused by the RA itself or by side effects of the drug used for treatment of the disease.

Systemic manifestations of RA include the following:

- Cutaneous manifestations: rheumatoid nodules, Sjögren's syndrome
- Ocular manifestations: episcleritis and scleritis

- Pulmonary involvement: pleurisy with effusion
- Cardiac: pericarditis and myocarditis
- Renal involvement
- Felty's syndrome (neutropenia and splenomegaly)
- Vasculitis

Multiple deformities of advanced RA are often present. These deformities are described in Table 18-2.

Gout Gouty arthritis is the most common form of inflammatory joint disease in men over 25 years of age. The peak onset of gout in men is between 40 and 50 years of age. Gout in women usually occurs after menopause. In general, gout occurs in 8.4 per 1,000 adults, with the prevalence increasing with age. For people between 65 and 74 years of age, the prevalence increases significantly to 16 per 1,000 for older women, and 24 per 1,000 for older men (Zhu, Pandya, & Choi, 2011). Gout is thought to be both misdiagnosed and underdiagnosed and consequently under- and overtreated.

Pathophysiology The pathophysiology of gout is closely linked to purine metabolism and kidney function. Uric acid is a by-product of purine, which is ingested or synthesized from ingested foods. Patients with gout have a genetic abnormality of purine metabolism that results in either an overproduction, or an underexcretion, of uric acid. For example, some patients with gout have an abnormally high rate of purine synthesis as well as an excess production of uric acid. For these patients, reducing intake of purine foods does not affect the level of uric acid production.

Serum urate levels greater than 7 mg/dL are associated with an increased risk of gout, with the risk increasing as the duration and level of urate increases. Hyperuricemia has recently been cited as an independent risk factor for cardiovascular disease (Hardy, 2011). Hyperuricemia is due to an underexcretion or overproduction of urate, or both. In most cases of gout, underexcretion of urate is considered the most common metabolic abnormality. The main predisposing factors for gout include family history, high purine diet, and obesity. Although genetics play a major role, drugs such as alcohol and acetylsalicylic acid (ASA) also result in low urate renal clearance.

TABLE 18-2	Deformities of Chronic Advanced Rheumatoid Arthritis	
Site	**Deformity**	**Description**
Hands	Swan neck deformity	Flexion of the distal interphalangeal and metacarpophalangeal joints, hyperextension of the proximal interphalangeal joint
	Boutonniere deformity	Avulsion of extensor hood of the proximal interphalangeal joint
	Ulnar deformity	Ulnar deviation of the fingers at the metacarpophalangeal joint
Feet	Hallux valgus	Displaced toes, lateral angulation

This may be a considerable problem for the older person who is frequently taking these drugs and may have decreased renal function, thus increasing the risk for hyperuricemia.

Clinical Manifestations   **Gout** results from the deposit of urate crystals in a peripheral joint where they initiate pain, inflammation, and destruction. Acute pain, warmth, and swelling in the metatarsophalangeal joint of the big toe are typically the first signs of gouty arthritis. A mild attack may last just a few hours, whereas a severe attack may last several weeks. Over time, the attacks continue and may affect other joints, including the knee, wrist, ankle, elbow joints of the hand or feet, or bursa. General malaise, fever, and chills accompany these painful joint symptoms. Pain and tenderness are often so severe that the older person cannot tolerate the weight of a sheet or blanket, or even move the affected joint. The diffuse periarticular erythema that is often present with an attack of gout may be mistaken for cellulitis. The white blood cell count (WBC) and erythrocyte sedimentation rate (ESR) may be elevated as well. The definitive finding for a diagnosis of gout is urate crystals in the aspiration fluid in a joint or tophus (Browder-Lazenby, 2011).

> **Practice Pearl** ▶▶▶ Although hyperuricemia is a common feature of gout, it is not obligatory. Serum urate concentrations may be normal during an acute attack. Most people with hyperuricemia do not develop gout.

Chronic gout, also known as tophaceous gout, can begin as early as 3 years or as late as 40 years after the initial acute attack. The person with chronic gout will have persistent complaints of aching joints, soreness, and morning stiffness, most commonly in the hands and feet. Urate crystal deposits (tophi) occur in cartilage, synovial membranes, tendons, and soft tissue. The development of tophi is directly related to the duration and severity of hyperuricemia. These white subcutaneous nodules, or tophi, vary in size and appear as irregular lumps or swellings of the joints. Tophi continue to grow and may eventually lead to severe limitation of movement and markedly deformed hands and feet.

> **Practice Pearl** ▶▶▶ In the older person, acute attacks of gout are less common. Instead, gout presents insidiously with symptoms of chronic arthritis and associated subcutaneous tophi deposits on the toes, fingers, and elbows.

Pseudogout   Pseudogout, or calcium pyrophosphate deposition disease, is a form of arthritis. It is caused by the formation of calcium pyrophosphate-dihydrate crystals in large joints. Pseudogout was so named because of the painfully similar goutlike nature of the acute attacks of joint pain that characterize the disease (see the earlier section on gout). This disease occurs in people 60 years of age or older, and women are affected more often than men. The knee is the most common joint affected. Other joints that may be affected include the shoulder, hip, and elbow.

Over time, pseudogout results in calcification of hyaline and fibrous cartilage (chondrocalcinosis). It may affect several joints at the same time and result in painful asymmetrical inflammatory polyarthritis. The mechanism of this disease is not fully understood. The tendency to develop pseudogout and chondrocalcinosis seems to run in families, although the exact genetic link is not clear. In some cases, the disease is associated with a history of hypothyroidism, hyperparathyroidism, and acromegaly.

Tendonitis and Bursitis   Tendonitis and bursitis are two of the most common and least understood causes of musculoskeletal pain. Many older adults who complain of acute pain in a joint area have soft tissue injuries and not the more serious, debilitating articular diseases. Both of these conditions are usually caused by repetitive injury due to age, sports, or occupational injuries. Bursitis is an irritation of subcutaneous tissue and inflammation of the underlying bursae. Bursitis also develops at pressure points such as the site of bunions. Acute bursitis is characterized by a deep aching pain on movement of any structure adjacent to the bursae. Tendonitis refers to inflammation of the tendon sheath (tenosynovitis). The course of soft tissue rheumatism, such as tendonitis and bursitis, is benign and responds to therapeutic regimens. The pain, however, is significant and will often temporarily decrease mobility.

Falls and the Older Person

Falls are a major health problem for the older person, with serious implications for medical as well as financial outcomes. Most falls occur in the home during normal routines. In the United States, falls are the leading cause of accidental death in people over 65 years of age (National Center for Injury Prevention and Control [NCIPC], 2011). The rate of death due to falls rises with increasing age. The statistics related to falls point out the seriousness of this problem and the need for ongoing prevention as part of the overall care of the older person. The NCIPC (2011) publishes a variety of statistics on this important topic. Information regarding falls and hip fractures in the older person includes the following:

- Each year, more than a third of people over age 65 sustain a serious fall.
- Among older adults, falls are the most common cause of injury-related deaths.
- In 2008, more than 19,700 older adults died from unintentional fall injuries.

- Among older adults, the majority of fractures are caused by falls.
- Osteoporotic fractures of the hip, spine, and forearm are the most common fall-related injuries.
- As a person ages, he or she is more likely to sustain a hip fracture. A person age 85 or older is 10 to 15 times more likely to sustain a hip fracture than a 65-year-old person.
- Of all fall-related fractures, hip fractures cause the greatest number of deaths. They also result in enormous quality of life changes and numerous health problems due to immobility.
- After sustaining a hip fracture, about one quarter of older people remain in an institution for at least a year. Many are never able to return to their homes.
- Treatment of injuries and complications associated with these falls costs the United States $20.2 billion annually (NCIPC, 2011).

An important part of nursing care of the older person is to maintain safety and prevent falls and fall-related deaths. The *Healthy People 2020* website contains the nation's goals and objectives for improved health for the years 2010 to 2020. One objective for the older adults states: "Prevent an increase in the rate of fall-related deaths" (Injury and Violence Prevention–23.2) (U.S. Department of Health and Human Services [USDHHS], 2010). The baseline data cited by *Healthy People 2020* is that 45.3 deaths per 100,000 population ages 65 years or older were caused by falls. The target for this goal is to maintain the baseline rate. A variety of government resources will focus on achieving the *Healthy People 2020* goals (USDHHS, 2010).

Prevention of falls in the clinical setting is one of the key goals of gerontological nursing practice. The goals are to recognize older adults at risk for falling; to identify and correct fall risk factors; to improve balance, gait, mobility, and functional independence using a structured interdisciplinary approach; to reduce or eliminate environmental factors that contribute to fall risk; and to evaluate outcomes with revision of the plan as needed. See the Best Practices feature.

Hip Fracture

Hip fractures are a serious problem for the older person. In the United States in 2007 hip fractures resulted in approximately 281,000 hospital admissions among people over age 65 (NCIPC, 2011). More than 95% of hip fractures among older adults are caused by falls. Hip fractures include those in the upper third of the femur, and may be intracapsular or extracapsular. Intracapsular fractures are those located within the joint capsule and are further categorized as femoral neck and subcapital fractures. Extracapsular fractures include intertrochanteric (in the trochanter) and subtrochanteric (below the trochanter).

Intracapsular fractures frequently impair the blood to the femoral head. A displaced femoral neck fracture can completely disrupt the blood supply to the femoral head, which may result in avascular necrosis and nonunion of the fracture. Extracapsular fractures cause acute blood loss from the vascular cancellous bone surfaces, but rarely cause avascular necrosis.

Most fractures in older adults result from low-energy trauma, and often occur in the home. Older adults with displaced fractures usually have a history of a fall and are unable to bear weight. Assessment findings usually reveal the older person lying with the injured leg shortened and externally rotated. The force of gravity and pull of the leg muscles cause this classic position. The extreme pain of the fracture prevents any movement, and the older person often cannot even crawl to reach a phone to call for help. Most hip fractures occur in women by falling sideways onto the hip.

Nursing Diagnoses

The following nursing diagnoses can be applied to many of the common musculoskeletal illnesses of older adults:

- *Mobility: Physical, Impaired* related to stiffness, pain, joint contractures, and decreased muscle strength
- *Pain, Acute* related to progression of inflammation
- *Pain, Chronic* related to joint abnormalities
- *Fatigue* related to pain and systemic inflammation
- *Body Image, Disturbed* related to chronic illness, joint deformities, impaired mobility
- *Coping, Ineffective* related to personal vulnerability in a situational crisis

NANDA-I © 2012.

The most common nursing diagnosis for the older person with musculoskeletal problems is *Mobility: Physical, Impaired* or a state where there exists a limitation of the ability for independent physical movement. The major defining characteristics include the inability to purposefully move within the physical environment, and limited range of motion. Minor defining characteristics are decreased muscle strength, less control, inability to sit unsupported, and impaired coordination. For a diagnosis to be accurate, the North American Nursing Diagnosis Association (NANDA) suggests the patient should have most of the major or critical defining characteristics. Examples of related factors for impaired mobility include decreased strength and endurance, external devices such as casts, and acute or chronic pain.

Older people who have chronic musculoskeletal illnesses, such as arthritis, will experience both acute and chronic pain. They often accept pain or a negative or unpleasant sensation as normal part of the aging process. As a result, pain is neither recognized nor well managed for this age group. Older people should be encouraged to express all their symptoms, including pain, so that they can be managed.

Chronic pain is defined as pain that is persistent for more than a 6-month period. The major defining characteristic of pain is the patient's report of pain. A rating scale of 0 to 10 should be used to identify the current pain level and to determine the goal for an acceptable pain level. Objective assessments of pain are variable and cannot be used in place of self-report. Some of the related factors for pain include actual or potential tissue damage, muscle spasm, and inflammation.

Diagnostic Tests and Values for Musculoskeletal Problems

Some of the laboratory and radiological tests that can assist in the diagnosis and evaluation of musculoskeletal problems in the older adult include the following:

- Bone mineral density test
- Bone and joint radiography
- Computerized tomography and magnetic resonance imaging
- Bone and joint scanning
- Blood serum tests
- Synovial fluid analysis

Bone Mineral Density Test

Dual-energy X-ray absorptiometry (DEXA) is a common method used to measure bone mineral density. DEXA of the proximal femur is the best way to predict hip fracture risk and is the gold standard for fracture prediction. Other sites tested include spine, wrist, or total body. Bone mineral density is measured by having the patient lie on a table. An arm of the machine passes over the body part that is being tested. The machine does not contact the patient, and radiation exposure is minimal. The test is considered expensive. The results of the DEXA test are expressed in mathematical terms and compare the patient's bone density reading to those of younger women in their thirties (T score) and women of the same age (Z score). The T scores are important because that provides a comparison to a time in life when bone density is considered to be the greatest and the patient will have an idea about present levels of bone density compared to these peak readings. Standard deviations are calculated with the T scores and scores of +1 to −1 indicate normal bone densities, while scores of −1 to −2.5 indicate osteopenia and scores above −2.5 indicate osteoporosis (Storck, 2011).

Despite the many benefits of DEXA bone density tests, the current densitometry systems have many pitfalls (Brown, 2011):

1. Older adults often have bone changes due to arthritis or disk disease in the lumbar spine, which complicates the measurement of BMD.

2. The cutoffs to determine diagnosis (−1 SD, etc.) are arbitrary and must be considered in light of other factors.
3. The site of the measurement changes the relative risk. A 1 SD below the mean of the young adult (measured in the femoral neck) increases the relative risk for hip fracture 2.7 times. If the BMD is measured at other body sites, the risk is considered to be increased between 1.5 and 2 times.
   a. BMD results vary with technique and the patient's position.
   b. Current criteria are based on postmenopausal Caucasian women and do not reflect sexual or cultural diversity.

Bone and Joint Radiography

The routine X-ray is the basic imaging technique for diagnosis and staging of all rheumatic diseases and for diagnosing fractures. X-rays detect musculoskeletal structure, integrity, texture, or density problems. X-rays also allow evaluation of disease progression and treatment efficacy. The routine X-ray is not sensitive enough to diagnosis BMD because change is not detected until 30% of bone mass is lost.

Computerized Tomography and Magnetic Resonance Imaging

Computerized tomography (CT) produces a computer reconstruction that allows detection of images in a small area of tissue. This allows more detailed and precise diagnosis. CT scan is obtained with an X-ray machine that rotates 180 degrees around the patient's body or head (Dugdale, 2010). Inflammation and degeneration that are not visible on a routine X-ray can be seen and diagnosed on a CT scan. CT also shows occult fractures and articular damage that are difficult to image on X-ray.

Magnetic resonance imaging (MRI) uses a large magnet and radio waves to produce an energy field that can be transferred to a visual image. It produces a more detailed image than CT without the use of radiation or a contrast medium. These factors give MRI advantages over CT.

However, MRI is more expensive than CT (by at least one third) and requires special facilities. MRI cannot show calcification or bone mineralization, and images of bone structure are not as useful as X-ray or CT. During an MRI, the patient hears noises that range from soft to thunderous. Earplugs may be used if desired. MRI can detect soft tissue changes such as synovitis, edema, and bone bruises that occur in traumatic injuries.

Bone Scan

A bone scan detects skeletal trauma and disease by determining the degree to which the matrix of the bone "takes up" a bone-seeking radioactive isotope. A bone scan may reveal the reason for an elevated alkaline phosphatase (ALP) level. It may help to diagnose a stress fracture in

Best Practices   Nursing Standard of Practice Protocol: Fall Prevention

The Hartford Institute for Geriatric Nursing (2008) recommends that the nurse consider the following risk factors when assessing fall risk in the older person:

- Cognitive impairment (dementia, impaired judgment, impulsive behavior)
- Medications (benzodiazepines, psychotropics, opioids)
- Impaired mobility, gait, or balance (cerebrovascular accident, osteoarthritis, peripheral neuropathies)
- Fall history (the occurrence of at least one previous fall)
- Acute or chronic illness
- Environmental factors (e.g., wet floor, loose and dangling wires, improper footwear, improper lighting, clutter)
- Sensory deficits (impaired vision, hearing, touch)
- Alcohol use (ataxia)
- Postural hypotension (may be iatrogenic related to pharmacological treatment of hypertension)
- Depression (inattention to environment)
- Use of assistive devices (improper use and maintenance of canes, walkers, raised toilet seats)
- Frailty or deconditioning (loss of endurance and lean muscle mass).

The nurse is urged to develop a restraint-free attitude regarding falls in the older adult. The professional responsibility is to assess the older person and develop an individualized nursing care plan to minimize risk for falls and injury.

A falls prevention program is essential to the provision of holistic care for older adults. Since normal and pathological changes, which are common in aging, contribute to falls, assessment of the risk factors for falls is necessary. Recommendations for fall prevention are abundant throughout the literature, and many tools exist to identify individuals at highest risk for injurious falls. The Hendrich II Fall Risk Model (Hendrich, Bender, & Nyhuis, 2003) presented here assesses patient factors that contribute to falls such as male gender, cognitive impairment, altered elimination, depression, including ability to rise from a chair, and use of high-risk medications such as benzodiazepines and antiepileptics. To administer the tool, the nurse circles the score that corresponds with the risk factor listed on the left-hand side of the instrument. The tool should be administered on admission to a long-term care facility or the first time an older patient is seen in an outpatient clinic. The assessment should be done again at specified intervals (yearly) and when warranted by changes in health status such as after an acute care hospitalization, the addition of a new medical diagnosis, or a significant change in the patient's condition. Scores of 5 and higher indicate high risk, and preventive fall measures should be implemented.

Instructions: Circle the score that corresponds with the risk factor listed on the left-hand side of the instrument. The tool should be administered on admission to the facility or agency and again at specified intervals and when warranted by changes in health status.

Older nursing home residents at risk for falls should have an appropriate safety plan, including resident and environmental interventions to prevent falls and serious injuries. The following illustrates appropriate interventions to prevent falls in long-term care facilities and delineates the roles and responsibilities of the members of the interdisciplinary team in fall prevention activities.

Resident and Environmental Interventions to Prevent Falls

Fall prevention interventions require a systemic and facility-wide approach to be effective. All care providers must commit to learning about safety principles, using standardized assessment instruments to assess fall risk, and committing to improve safety. The facility must provide a strong and clear message emphasizing the safety improvement goals and eliminating punitive reporting systems. Interdisciplinary team training should be provided that emphasizes the responsibilities of each team member on the multidisciplinary team. For instance, the maintenance and housekeeping departments must commit to provision of quick cleanup of spills and repairs of safety hazards. The nursing department should ensure that all older patients are wearing appropriate footwear with nonskid soles. Physicians should commit to the elimination of all unnecessary medications to decrease the risk of polypharmacy and medication interactions. Nursing administrators and family members can schedule visits with podiatry, ophthalmology, and audiology to ensure that toe nails are trimmed, glasses prescriptions are current, and hearing aids are maintained in good working order (Baker, Gustafson, Beaubien, et al., 2005).

(continued)

Best Practices **Nursing Standard of Practice Protocol: Fall Prevention (*continued*)**

HENDRICH II FALL RISK MODEL

RISK FACTOR	RISK POINTS	SCORE
Confusion/Disorientation/Impulsivity	4	
Symptomatic Depression	2	
Altered Elimination	1	
Dizziness/Vertigo	1	
Gender (Male)	1	
Any Administered Antiepileptics (anticonvulsants): (Carbamazepine, Divalproex Sodium, Ethotoin, Ethosuximide, Felbamate, Fosphenytoin, Gabapentin, Lamotrigine, Mephenytoin, Methsuximide, Phenobarbital, Phenytoin, Primidone, Topiramate, Trimethadi-one, Valproic Acid)[1]	2	
Any Administered Benzodiazepines:[2] (Alprazolam, Chloridiazepoxide, Clonazepam, Clorazepate Dipotassium, Diazepam, Flurazepam, Halazepam[3], Lorazepam, Midazolam, Oxazepam, Temazepam, Triazolam)	1	
Get-Up-and-Go Test: "Rising from a Chair" If unable to assess, monitor for change in activity level, assess other risk factors, document both on patient chart with date and time.		
Ability to rise in a single movement—No loss of balance with steps	0	
Pushes up, successful in one attempt	1	
Multiple attempts but successful	3	
Unable to rise without assistance during test If unable to assess, document this on the patient chart with the date and time.	4	
(A Score of 5 or Greater = High Risk)	**TOTAL SCORE**	

On-going Medication Review Updates:

1 Levetiracetam (Keppra) was not assessed during the original research conducted to create the Hendrich Fall Risk Model. As an antiepileptic, levetiracetam does have a side effect of somnolence and dizziness which contributes to its fall risk and should be scored (effective June 2010).

2 The study did not inculde the effect of benzodiazepine-like drugs since they were not on the market at the time. Hewever, due to their similarity in drug structure, mechanism of action and drug effects, they should also be scored (effective January 2010).

3 Halazepam was included in the study but is no longer availble in the United States (effective June 2010).

the older person who continues to experience pain after a skeletal X-ray has negative findings (Dugdale, 2010).

Blood Serum Tests

Several blood tests are important in diagnosing and treating musculoskeletal disorders:

- Electrolytes: calcium level
- Serum uric acid (SUA)
- Joint tests: rheumatoid factor (RF)
- Acute-phase reactants: C-reactive protein
- Bone and muscle enzymes: ALP
- CRP and ESR

Interpretation of these laboratory tests is guided by reviewing the following guidelines: electrolytes (serum calcium and phosphorus) are decreased in the older person. The normal range of serum calcium for an older adult is 8.8 to 10.2 mg/dL. The normal range of phosphorus for a person older than 60 years is 2.3 to 3.7 mg/dL. Serum calcium and phosphorus or phosphate have an inverse relationship in a normal healthy state. Calcium is increased in Paget's disease, bone fractures, and immobility; it is decreased in osteoporosis and osteomalacia. Phosphorus is increased in bone fractures in the healing state and decreased in osteomalacia.

Serum Uric Acid The value of SUA levels in the diagnosis of acute gout is not conclusive. A diagnosis of gout is not established unless SUA is found in tissue or synovial fluid. In general, the higher the level of SUA, the more likely the person is to have an attack of gout.

> **Practice Pearl** ▶▶▶ There are several limitations in the application of SUA levels. Elevated levels of SUA may occur in people who do not develop gout, and levels can be normal at the time of an acute attack. However, once the diagnosis of gout is made, the SUA levels can be helpful in monitoring medication levels.

Rheumatoid Factor Rheumatoid factor is an antibody (IgM, IgG) that binds to the Fc fragment of immunoglobulin G. In the early stages of the disease, the RF is negative. However, 70% to 80% of patients with RA will become RF positive (Lab Tests Online, 2011b). A high RF (positive RF high titers > = 1:320) is a predictor of an increase in the severity of symptoms such as greater disability and extra-articular disease. RF is also elevated in patients with liver disease, lung disease, and other conditions. Rheumatoid factor is not diagnostic for RA, but it can confirm the diagnosis. RF does not change rapidly, so once the titer is high, the test is not repeated (NLM, 2012e).

Acute-Phase Reactants: C-Reactive Protein and Erythrocyte Sedimentation Rate Acute-phase reactants are proteins that increase serum concentration in response to acute and chronic inflammation. C-reactive protein (CRP) and erythrocyte sedimentation rate (ESR) are common acute-phase reactants. CRP is used for determining if an inflammatory process is present, such as a bacterial infection or rheumatic disease. The CRP level increases and goes back to normal quicker than the ESR. ESR is the most common measurement of acute-phase proteins in rheumatic disease. Sedimentation of red cells is directly related to the acute-phase proteins. This test can be done in the office in 1 hour (NLM, 2012a).

Alkaline phosphatase (ALP) or SAP (serum alkaline phosphatase) is an enzyme associated with bone activity. Normal values for men are 45 to 115 units/L, and for women 30 to 100 units/L. Normal values tend to vary from laboratory to laboratory. Values tend to increase after the age of 50. ALP studies identify increases in osteoblastic activity and inflammatory conditions. A person with Paget's disease will have a pronounced elevation of ALP (at least 2× normal to up to 5× normal). Two isoenzymes—ALP_1 (liver origin) and ALP_2 (bone origin)—will help to determine if the source of the elevation is bone disease (NIAMS, 2011a; Paget Foundation, 2011a).

Synovial Fluid Analysis

Synovial fluid analysis involves evaluation of fluids drawn from a joint with a sterile needle. Synovial fluid is normally a viscous, straw-colored substance that is found in small amounts in a normal joint to provide lubrication and prevent friction during joint movement. The fluid is initially analyzed for color and clarity. Additional routine analysis may include evaluation of white blood cells, red blood cells, neutrophils, protein, glucose crystals, tests for rheumatoid factor (RF), uric acid for gout, and bacteria to establish the presence of infection. In RA, during active joint inflammation synovial fluid is turbid, yellow, and sterile and has reduced viscosity as well as 10,000 to 50,000 WBC/μL (Berman & Paget, 2009).

For many diseases that involve joint swelling, the aspiration and examination of synovial fluid is an important test to aid in the diagnosis. Based on visual inspection of the synovial fluid, it is classified into four groups (I = clear, II = translucent, III = opaque, IV = bloody), and the appearance, volume, and cellular contents are analyzed. These four groups are on a continuum. Group I fluids are noninflammatory, have a low WBC (<1,000/μL), and are associated with osteoarthritis. Group II fluids are inflammatory, have a moderate WBC (2,000 to 20,000/μL), and are associated with diseases such as rheumatoid arthritis. Group III fluids are purulent, have a high WBC (over 100,000/μL), and are infectious. Group IV fluids contain bloody fluid from a traumatic event.

Synovial fluid in groups II to IV should be cultured to determine if an infection is present in the joint. In addition, synovial fluids can be examined for monosodium urate crystals (gout) and calcium pyrophosphate-dihydrate crystals. Monosodium urate crystals are considered to be mandatory for establishing the diagnosis of gout and acute arthritis. Monosodium urate crystals are rod or needle shaped and can be seen with a light microscope (Berman & Paget, 2009).

Common Diagnostic Findings for Musculoskeletal Illnesses

A variety of tests (urine, blood, synovial fluid) and procedures may be done to diagnose and monitor the treatment of any musculoskeletal problem. Some of the common diagnostic findings are presented in Table 18-3.

Pharmacology and Nursing Implications

The physiological changes of aging and resulting altered drug metabolism frequently cause serious side effects as well as drug toxicities. The older person often has more than one clinical problem and may be taking over-the-counter drugs as well. A complete history and physical as

TABLE 18-3	Common Diagnostic Findings for Musculoskeletal Illnesses
Condition	**Diagnostic Findings**
Osteoporosis	• Decrease in bone mineral density (DEXA). • A bone mineral density of −1 SD below the mean (−1 SD) = osteopenia. Bone mineral density of −2.5 SD below the mean (−2.5 SD) = severe osteoporosis (National Osteoporosis Foundation [NOF], 2010). • Low bone mass and a U.S.-adapted World Health Organization algorithm: 10-year probability of a hip fracture > 3%.
Osteomalacia	• Serum alkaline phosphatase (ALP) elevated. • X-ray studies are similar to osteoporosis. However, the classic finding of Looser's lines due to stress fractures or pseudofractures that have not healed would confirm the diagnosis.
Paget's Disease	• ALP elevated. • Serum calcium levels (Ca) low or normal. • X-rays, bone scan, or CT scans will indicate areas of increased bone resorption. • Depending on the stage of the disease, the bone mass may be enlarged and deformities may be present. • A bone biopsy may be done to confirm findings.
Osteoarthritis	• The X-ray will show joint space narrowing, spur formation, and bony sclerosis. • Conventional X-rays do not show cartilage changes and therefore are not helpful for early OA. X-ray pathology may be present without corresponding clinical symptoms. • Synovial fluid—group I. • White blood cell count (WBC) and erythrocyte sedimentation rate (ESR) normal.
Rheumatoid Arthritis	• The X-ray will show symmetrical disease, soft tissue swelling, and loss of articular cartilage. In late disease, there is joint space narrowing and joint osteoporosis. • Synovial fluid—group II. • WBC and ESR elevated in 80% of cases. • Positive C-reactive protein during acute phase. • Rheumatoid factor (RF) elevated in 50% of cases. • High RF (> 1:80) is more specific to RA.
Gout	• Definitive finding is urate crystals in the synovial fluid of an affected joint. • WBC elevated. • ESR elevated. • Serum urate elevated (nonspecific).
Pseudogout	• Definitive finding is calcium pyrophosphate dihydrate crystals in the synovial fluid of an affected joint. • WBC elevated. • ESR elevated. • Serum uric acid elevated.
Fractures	• X-ray will show fracture, trauma, etc. • Hematocrit test determines blood loss from fractures. • ALP can be measured to show fracture healing.

well as baseline tests should be done to determine baseline function. It is important to determine all the medications and doses the older person takes. Medication should be added to the regimen in the most safe and effective manner. Drug dosage should be based on age and renal function. Blood work should be routinely monitored for signs of toxicity. Nonsteroidal anti-inflammatory drugs (NSAIDs) are of particular concern because of their serious renal and gastric side effects. These medications are taken frequently by the older person, sometimes in inappropriate doses.

Osteoporosis

Bisphosphonates, estrogen agonists/antagonists (formerly known as selective estrogen receptor modulators [SERMs]), and calcitonin are antiresorptive drugs prescribed for the treatment and prevention of osteoporosis in both men and women. Antiresorptive therapy preserves or increases bone density and decreases the rate of bone resorption.

Bisphosphonates—alendronate (Fosamax) and risedronate (Actonel)—are potent drugs that inhibit osteoclastic activity and have decreased the incidence of vertebral and nonvertebral fractures in postmenopausal women. Both of these drugs have been approved for the prevention of postmenopausal osteoporosis in women and for the treatment of osteoporosis in men and postmenopausal women (see Box 18-2 for drug dosages). Alendronate is now available as a generic preparation in the United States. Alendronate reduces the incidence of spine and hip fractures by about 50% over a 3-year period in patients with a prior vertebral fracture. The incidence is slightly less for those without a prior vertebral fracture (NOF, 2010).

Ibandronate (Boniva) offers the advantage of once-a-month dosing, instead of a weekly regimen and can be given IV every 3 months for treatment of severe osteoporosis. In a study by Bryan (2006), although Boniva increased bone density in the lumbar spine and the hip, it reduced the incidence of vertebral fractures only in the lumbar spine with hip fracture rates comparable to those taking only placebo. Many people who take these drugs experience adverse gastrointestinal symptoms, such as esophageal irritation, heartburn, and difficulty swallowing. Refer to a pharmacology text for complete information. Calcium should not be taken at the same time as bisphosphonates because this will interfere with the absorption of the drug.

Drug Alert ▶▶▶ On September 1, 2011, the U.S. Food and Drug Administration (FDA) issued an update to the drug label for zoledronic acid (Reclast) regarding the risk of kidney failure. Cases of acute renal failure requiring dialysis or having a fatal outcome have been reported to the FDA. Reclast is contraindicated in patients with evidence of acute renal failure.

Reclast is a drug that has been used to treat Paget's disease and has recently been approved for the treatment of osteoporosis. This drug is administered once yearly by IV and has been shown to increase bone strength and reduce fractures in the hips, spine, wrists, arms, legs, and ribs. Side effects include hypocalcemia, headache, dizziness, peripheral edema, musculoskeletal pain, and possibly osteonecrosis of the jaw.

Drug Alert ▶▶▶ The nurse is responsible for teaching the older person the specific instructions for taking Fosamax and Actonel. The older person must (1) take either drug on an empty stomach, first thing in the morning with 8 oz of water; (2) remain upright for 30 minutes; and (3) not eat or drink anything else for 30 minutes. Older adults taking oral Boniva must remain upright for 60 minutes.

BOX 18-2 **Common Pharmacological Interventions for Prevention and Treatment of Osteoporosis**

Bisphosphonates

Alendronate (Fosamax)
  Osteoporosis prevention: 5 mg daily or 35 mg weekly po
  Osteoporosis treatment: 10 mg daily or 70 mg weekly po
Ibandronate (Boniva)
  Osteoporosis prevention/treatment: 2.5 mg once daily or 150 mg monthly po
  Osteoporosis treatment: 3 mg IV once every 3 months

Estrogen Agonists/Antagonists

Raloxifene (Evista)
  Prevention: 60 mg daily po
Calcitonin (Miacalcin)
  Treatment: intranasally. One spray daily delivers 200 International Units.

Source: FDA, 2011; NOF, 2010.

Estrogen agonists/antagonists (formerly called SERMs) have been developed to provide the benefits of estrogens without the disadvantages. Raloxifene has been approved by the FDA for the prevention and treatment of osteoporosis in postmenopausal women. Raloxifene, brand name Evista, is a less effective antiresorptive drug than bisphosphonates, but it does reduce bone loss and decrease vertebral fracture risk (NOF, 2010). However, raloxifene has been associated with increased risk of venous thrombosis, hot flashes, and strokes, so it should be used with caution.

Calcitonin is generally considered to be a safe but less effective treatment for osteoporosis. It has been found to decrease spinal fractures by up to 33%. It may be given intranasally or subcutaneously. It is approved for women who are at least 5 years postmenopausal (NOF, 2010). Common pharmacological interventions for the prevention and treatment of osteoporosis are summarized in Box 18-2.

For many years, hormone replacement therapy (HRT) (e.g., Prempro) has been taken by postmenopausal women to reduce the risk of fractures and treat the symptoms of menopause. Many women believed that they gained extra benefits such as a reduction of cardiac events, cognitive changes, and mortality. However, many of those assumptions have been challenged. In 2000, the FDA withdrew its approval of estrogen replacement for the treatment of osteoporosis. More recent research results continue to raise concerns. Several additional reports from a long-term study conducted by the Women's Health Initiative and funded by the National Institutes of Health have greatly increased the concerns of women taking these drugs. Results from this study have demonstrated that postmenopausal women taking estrogen plus progesterone have an increased risk of heart attack, stroke, breast cancer, and blood clots (FDA, 2011). When HRT use is considered solely for prevention of osteoporosis, the FDA recommends that approved non-estrogen treatments should be carefully considered.

> ***Drug Alert*** ▶▶▶ Osteonecrosis of the jaw (ONJ) has been rarely reported with oral bisphosphonate use. In 2005, the FDA decided that a statement about ONJ would be included in the safety information provided in the package inserts of bisphosphonate products (FDA, 2008).

Paget's Disease

The many deformities, symptoms, and joint changes that occur in advanced Paget's disease are frequently irreversible. The FDA-approved treatment for Paget's disease includes two types of drugs: bisphosphonates and calcitonin (Paget Foundation, 2011a). The goal of this treatment is to relieve bone pain and prevent progression of the deformities of this disease. The therapies of choice are the most potent bisphosphonates: alendronate (Fosamax) and risedronate (Actonel). Common dosage examples include the following:

- Alendronate (Fosamax) given 40 mg daily for 6 months may produce a prolonged remission.
- Calcitonin (Miacalcin) by injection 50 to 100 units daily or 3 times a week for 6 months. A repeat course can be given after a short rest period (Paget Foundation, 2011a).

Osteonecrosis of the Jaw

In the past 10 years reports began appearing that a small percentage of patients taking biphosphates have been diagnosed with osteonecrosis of the jaw (ONJ). This is a rare condition that results in damage to jaw and cell death to the bone. The older person should be encouraged to maintain good dental hygiene before starting to take this drug.

Refer to the Paget Foundation website (www.paget.org) for information and additional references on the treatment of Paget's disease. For some older adults, mild bone pain can be managed with acetylsalicylic acid or NSAIDs. Adequate pain relief should be encouraged.

Osteomalacia

The goal of the pharmacological treatment of osteomalacia is to remineralize the bone. The treatment of osteomalacia will depend on the cause. Vitamin D replacement is given in doses of 50,000 to 100,000 units/day for 1 to 2 weeks and followed by a daily dose of 400 to 800 units/day. The older person should be monitored for serum and urine calcium levels. Other forms of vitamin D such as calcidiol and calcitriol are given for the specific cause of vitamin D deficiency. All older adults with osteomalacia need to have adequate calcium intake (1,000 to 1,500 mg/day).

Osteoarthritis

At present, there is no therapy that will slow or halt the progression of OA. Current therapy is directed at relief of pain and minimizing functional disability. Agents for pain relief for OA include topical agents, systemic oral agents, adjuvant agents, and intra-articular agents.

Capsaicin is a topical analgesic agent that is available as a nonprescription drug. It has been shown to be of value for OA. Capsaicin is believed to prevent the reaccumulation of substance P (a neurotransmitter) in peripheral sensory neurons. It is applied 2 to 4 times daily to the affected area, and may cause heat or burning. It has been found to be most effective for the hands and knees. Pain relief may require 4 to 6 weeks of applications. Acetaminophen (Tylenol) is one of the safest drugs available and is usually the first-line pharmacological therapy for OA (NIAMS, 2011c). Acetaminophen can be given up to 4 g/day with minimal toxicity. Higher doses may cause liver damage. This drug has a ceiling effect, which means that increasing the dose does not increase the analgesic benefit. Acetaminophen can be used alone or as an adjunct to NSAIDs.

NSAIDs are a large group of drugs that are the most common treatment for pain and inflammation of OA. Pain of OA is intermittent; therefore, medications can be too. With most traditional NSAIDs, analgesia can be obtained at smaller doses than anti-inflammatory effects. COX-2 inhibitors, a new category of anti-inflammatory drugs, are considered safer for the gastrointestinal tract but have other side effects such as renal impairment (see Chapter 9 ⊂⊃ for further information).

Intra-articular corticosteroids may be of value when synovial inflammation is present. Synovial effusion is removed prior to injections. Injection should be limited to four per year in any one joint. Few published trials support their benefit in OA.

Intra-articular hyaluronic acid is a substance considered a normal component of the joint and supports lubrication and nutrition of the joints. In general, hyaluronan derivatives have been found to decrease pain for longer periods than other intra-articular therapies. Intra-articular hyaluronic acid is administered in a series of 3 to 5 injections in the knee, on a weekly basis. It has been approved for use of OA of the knee, and studies on other joints are under way. There is conflicting evidence of the efficacy of hyaluronan derivatives. In October 2007 the Agency for Healthcare Research and Quality (AHRQ) announced the result of a systematic review of three treatments for osteoarthritis of the knee: (1) intra-articular viscosupplementation; (2) oral glucosamine, chondroitin, or a combination; and (3) arthroscopic lavage or debridement. The best available evidence does not clearly demonstrate clinical benefit. The AHRQ suggested an increase in rigorous random controlled trials as well as investigation of new approaches to prevention and treatment.

Rheumatoid Arthritis

Pharmacological therapies for RA include prednisone, NSAIDs, and disease-modifying antirheumatic drugs (DMARDs). Historically, treatment for the older person with RA started with corticosteroids and NSAIDs. The treatment regimen has evolved to now include DMARDs and then even fewer to biologic DMARDs. Recently, a more aggressive approach is advocated for people with RA to prevent joint deformity and decrease disease activity. It is currently recommended that DMARDs be prescribed within 3 months of a diagnosis of RA (Centers for Disease Control and Prevention [CDC], 2011b).

> *Practice Pearl* ▶▶▶ In relation to RA, the CDC reports that radiologic erosion is typically fastest in the first year of the disease. This highlights the importance of the older person seeking medical evaluation, diagnosis, and intervention as soon as possible (CDC, 2011b).

Corticosteroids such as prednisone are potent anti-inflammatory drugs used in the treatment of rheumatic diseases such as RA. They decrease inflammation rapidly and improve fatigue, pain, and joint swelling. The usual dose required for suppression of synovitis in the older person is low (2.5 to 7.5 mg per day) so toxicity is minimal. Low doses of prednisone take up to 10 years to produce osteoporosis, making it a good alternative for older adults who cannot tolerate other drugs. The long-term adverse effects of steroids (osteoporosis, cataracts, hypertension, and increased risk of infection) must be discussed with the patient and weighed against the functional and therapeutic benefits.

NSAIDs are another common drug category used for RA. However, the high doses required to relieve the inflammation in the older adult patient often cause toxic side effects such as gastrointestinal bleeding, gastrointestinal perforation, and renal failure. The COX-2 inhibitors are considered safer for the gastrointestinal tract, but have other damaging side effects such as renal impairment. Drugs in the category include celecoxib (Celebrex) and rofecoxib

(Vioxx). Vioxx was withdrawn from the market in 2004 because of studies showing an increased incidence of myocardial infarction related to its use in older people. Users of Celebrex are urged to take the lowest dose possible, use the drug for only short periods of time, and investigate the use of alternative drugs.

> *Practice Pearl* ▶▶▶ Treatment of acute RA that offers quick relief and return of function is particularly important for the older person to prevent immobility and loss of independence. The complications of immobility, such as pressure ulcers, occur more often in the older person. When these complications develop, return to the previous level of health, function, and independence is unlikely.

Disease-Modifying Antirheumatic Drugs (DMARDs)

For the older person who has been on low-dose steroids for several months, and whose symptoms have not subsided, the next pharmacological treatment offered may be the DMARDs (Box 18-3). These drugs may offer some pain relief, but the older person may not show improvement for weeks or months. However, most of these agents have been shown to slow the rate of joint erosion and dysfunction. Several studies have shown a benefit to the patient when the drug is offered

---

BOX 18-3 | **Examples of Disease-Modifying Antirheumatic Drugs (DMARDs)**

Immunosuppressive agents
Methotrexate
Antimalarial (hydroxychloroquine)
Sulfasalazine
Gold compounds (aurothioglucose)
Cytotoxic agents (azathioprine, cyclophosphamide, and cyclosporine)

Examples of Biologic Response Modifiers Approved for Arthritis

Etanercept (Enbrel) and infliximab (Remicade) reduce inflammation via tumor necrosis factor (TNF) blocking.
Anakinra (Kineret) works by blocking a cytokine called interleukin-1.
Rituximab (Rituxan) stops activation of a type of WBC called B cells.
Abatacept (Orencia) blocks a chemical that triggers an increase in T cells (NIAMS, 2009).

Source: National Institute of Arthritis and Musculoskeletal and Skin Disease (NIAMS), National Institute of Health, Department of Health and Human Services. (2009). Handout on health: Rheumatoid arthritis. Retrieved from http://www.niams.nih.gov/Health_Info/Rheumatic_Disease/default.asp.

early in the disease process (Majithia, Peel, & Geraci, 2009). The disease symptoms may return when treatment ends.

DMARDs include broad-spectrum immunosuppressive agents as well as newer biological agents. All of these drugs suppress lymphocyte destruction of the synovial membrane, and each has specific toxic effects that must be monitored. The typical first choice is often methotrexate (MTX). The long-term safety of the newer biological agents has not been proven. In addition, these agents require parenteral administration and have many contraindications for use such as a history of cancer or chronic infections, which are often present in older people (NIAMS, 2009).

Acute Gout and Chronic Gout

Pharmacological options for the treatment of acute gout include NSAIDs, oral colchicine loading, intra-articular steroid injections, and systemic steroids (Hardy, 2011). Prompt treatment in the older person is indicated to improve symptoms and ensure a better quality of life. The pharmacological options for the treatment of pseudogout include NSAIDs or a short course of oral corticosteroids (Box 18-4). If a large joint is involved, intra-articular corticosteroids may be effective.

Treatment for chronic gout includes colchicine, allopurinol, probenecid, and sulfinpyrazone (Box 18-5). Colchicine (0.5 mg qid) is used to decrease inflammation. Colchicine may be given long term to reduce repeated

---

BOX 18-4 | **Suggested Pharmacological Options for an Acute Gout Attack**

The drugs are given in the following situations:

1. NSAIDs for 2 to 7 days (should resolve the symptoms). If underlying pathology of renal, cardiac, or hepatic disease exists, NSAIDs are contraindicated.

2. If it is within 48 hours of the acute attack, introduction of the NSAID colchicine (marketed as Colcrys) can be given (normal renal function must be present). In the past, a dose of colchicine 0.6 mg given hourly to a 6-dose maximum was prescribed. This dosing schedule is no longer used because of the unacceptable GI toxicity. A reduced dose of 0.6 mg bid to qid is just as effective and less likely to cause adverse reactions (Hardy, 2011).

3. If symptoms are monoarticular, and the older person cannot tolerate other treatments, a long-acting steroid is injected (depomethylprednisolone) into the affected joint.

4. If the attack involves several joints, a course of oral steroids with a loading dose of 30 mg po initially, with a tapering of the dose over 2 weeks, is indicated (NIAMS, 2010).

BOX 18-5 | **Dose Ranges for Chronic Gout Medications**

Probenecid (500 to 2,000 mg/day)
Sulfinpyrazone (100 to 800 mg/day)
Allopurinol (100 mg daily bid up to 600 mg/day if needed)

---

attacks of gout. The maximum dose should be lowered for older adult patients. Colchicine is particularly useful in older adults who are intolerant of NSAIDs or who are receiving anticoagulants. It is used less often today because of its liver, renal, and bone marrow toxicity. If serum urate levels remain high and colchicine is not effective, other agents may be indicated.

Drugs such as probenecid, sulfinpyrazone, and allopurinol prevent long-term complications by lowering serum uric acid blood level (see Box 18-5 for dose ranges). Probenecid and sulfinpyrazone are uricosuric agents that work by increasing the excretion of uric acid. Allopurinol is a uric acid synthesis inhibitor, which means it lowers formation of uric acid. It is more versatile than uricosurics because it may be given at all levels of renal function. The goal of therapy with these agents is to decrease serum urate levels to 6.0 mg/dL or less (Hardy, 2011).

Bursitis

The treatment of bursitis will depend on the cause of the problem. If infection is present (usually gram-positive staphylococcus or streptococcus, group A), antibiotics can be given orally. If microcrystalline disease and infection are absent, aspiration of fluid and injection of the bursal sac with corticosteroid are usually successful. For milder cases, resting the joint during acute phases of pain, physical therapy, use of braces or splints, and oral use of NSAIDs are also effective.

Nonpharmacological Treatment of Musculoskeletal Problems

Lifestyle changes such as an increase in exercise, weight loss, and eating a healthy diet are important for all older adults. They are especially indicated for those with musculoskeletal problems to prevent disuse caused by immobility. Older adults should see their primary care provider, nurse, or other health professional for instructions or limitations related to fitness before beginning or changing normal routines. See specifics on exercise and rest later in the chapter.

HEALTHY AGING TIPS

Musculoskeletal Improvement

At home: walk on toes around the house, and stand on one foot at a time for as long as possible.

These activities will decrease risk for falling by improving balance.

Exercise routinely: find activities you like and find a partner to do them with.

Having a schedule with a friend improves your chances of keeping fit.

Implement healthy eating habits.

Weight loss decreases risk of osteoarthritis.

Osteoporosis

Nonpharmacological treatment of osteoporosis for the older person focuses on assessment of risk factors and education to promote positive behaviors related to healthy bones. Nonmodifiable risk factors for osteoporosis are increased age, female sex, White or Asian race, positive family history of osteoporosis, thin body habitus, and the long-term use of corticosteroids, anticonvulsants, or thyroid hormones. Modifiable risk factors include low calcium intake, prolonged immobility, excessive alcohol intake, and cigarette smoking. Prevention programs should be aimed at older adults with risk factors and those with osteoporosis as determined by bone density test results of 2 SD below the young adult mean. However, all older people will benefit from positive lifestyle changes for osteoporosis such as diet, exercise, and other risk modifications.

Assessment and Prevention of Risk Factors

The National Osteoporosis Foundation recommendations include the following:

1. All women should be educated on the risk factors for osteoporosis. One half of all White women will experience an osteoporotic fracture during their lifetime.
2. Any woman who has had a fracture should have a BMD test to determine osteoporosis diagnosis.
3. Any woman under age 65 who has any risk factors for osteoporosis should have a BMD test, and all women over age 65 should have a BMD test (NIAMS, 2011c).

Preventive activities are also important for older men. Many risk factors (with the exception of estrogen) are the same for men. Most men have bigger bones than women so they have increased protection. The following lifestyle modification activities to prevent or treat osteoporosis may be suggested by the nurse:

■ **Promote a diet with adequate calcium and vitamin D.** Calcium intake tends to decrease in older people, sometimes due to lactose intolerance. In addition, decreased absorption of calcium from the gastrointestinal tract and changes in vitamin D metabolism contribute to the decrease in calcium absorption of the older person. All older adults should obtain an adequate intake of dietary calcium and vitamin D. Calcium supplements may slow the rate of bone loss. Calcium intake of at least 1,500 mg/day is recommended. Calcium citrate is better absorbed than calcium carbonate and requires fewer pills. Patients should be instructed to take calcium with food to minimize side effects and enhance absorption. Vitamin D is necessary for calcium absorption into the bloodstream. The vitamin D requirement is 800 to 1,000 International Units/day for adults age 50 and over. Many supplement options are available (NOF, 2010).

■ **Encourage weight-bearing exercise.** Like muscle, bone is a living tissue that responds to exercise by becoming stronger. The older person should participate in weight-bearing exercise to improve muscle strength, mobility, and agility, and to reduce the risks of falls. Regular resistance and high-impact exercise are likely the most beneficial types of physical activity. Weight-bearing exercise such as dancing, walking, and stair climbing may slow bone loss that occurs in older adults because of disuse. The older person should exercise for 30 minutes, three times a week.

■ **Reduce or eliminate smoking.** Cigarette smokers tend to be thinner and experience more fractures. Smoking depletes the body of ascorbic acid and exposes it to toxins that damage bone and interfere with calcium absorption. Tobacco use is associated with decreased bone mass and an increased risk of hip fracture in men and women.

■ **Reduce or eliminate consumption of beverages containing alcohol, caffeine, and phosphorus.** Alcohol abuse is responsible for decreased bone mass and increased fractures. In addition, older adults with chronic alcoholism frequently use aluminum-containing antacids to treat gastrointestinal symptoms, which leads to calcium loss. The combination of alcohol and aluminum-containing antacids contributes to osteoporosis development. The general guideline for alcohol consumption is no more than one drink per day.

The older adult can reduce the risk of fractures and falls by implementing the personal and home safety guidelines listed in Box 18-6.

Osteomalacia

Nonpharmacological treatments of osteomalacia that may be suggested to the older patient include:

■ **Space activities to conserve energy.** By spacing tasks, the older person can partake in more activities, such as self-care, and work-related, social, or recreational pursuits.

BOX 18-6 ▶ **Fall Prevention Advice for Older Adults**

General Advice

- Have your vision and hearing checked regularly.
- Talk to your doctor or nurse about side effects of medications.
- Keep your intake of alcoholic beverages to a minimum.
- Wear rubber-soled shoes that fit well and support your feet.
- Avoid walking on icy sidewalks.
- Avoid slippery floor surfaces.
- Wear thin nonslip shoes at all times. Avoid the use of sneakers or slippers with deep treads.
- Wear hip protectors.
- Keep temperature at a comfortable level.

Home Safety Advice

- Clean house and remove clutter.
- Clean spills immediately.
- Keep lighting adequate and switches easy to reach.
- Have handrails installed where needed.
- Remove scatter rugs and mats.
- Ensure that bathtub and bathroom areas have nonskid mats.
- Secure all electrical cords.
- Use a cordless phone if possible.
- Find a safe stable place to balance while getting dressed such as a chair or leaning against the bed.

Source: Adapted from NIAMS, 2011c; NOF, 2010.

- **Monitor safety measures for the home.** Safety devices such as grab bars and ambulatory aids such as canes should be used to prevent falls and fractures. The fatigue experienced by the patient makes safety and protection an added concern to prevent falls and trauma.
- **Evaluate home hazards.** The risk of falls and fractures makes home safety important. Common home hazards such as scatter rugs, poor lighting, and furniture placement should be evaluated and proper steps taken to ensure safety.

Paget's Disease

Suggestions for nonpharmacological treatment of Paget's disease include:

- **Vitamin D and calcium.** Current evidence suggests that a high percentage of older people have inadequate intake and levels of vitamin D. In general, older people should be instructed to take adequate amounts of calcium and vitamin D and receive adequate sunshine. Older adults with Paget's disease should discuss the use of calcium and vitamin D if they have a history of kidney stones (see the instructions given earlier for osteoporosis).
- **Increase exercise.** Preventing fractures is very important for Paget's disease. The older person should avoid undue stress on affected bones and take proper measures to avoid falls. Exercise is important to maintain joint mobility and overall skeletal health. Weight gain should also be avoided (Paget Foundation, 2011b).

National Public Health Agenda for Osteoarthritis 2010

In 2010 the CDC and the Arthritis Foundation initiated a major effort to form a collaborative with over 75 other organizations to put a focus on osteoarthritis in order to achieve three major goals:

1. Ensure the availability of evidence-based interventions for those at risk for OA.
2. Establish support, communication, and strategies for OA prevention and management.
3. Initiate research to understand the burden of OA, risk factors, and interventions. (Arthritis Foundation, 2010).

This national effort brings much needed focus on this disease and the pain and suffering it causes. Osteoarthritis is the most common form of joint disease. It affects over 27 million Americans and places daily limits on their quality of life. Affecting mainly hands, hips, and knees, it causes weakness and pain, often leads to joint replacement, and has high socioeconomic costs.

The Arthritis Foundation and CDC have prepared many documents and reports on this agenda that are important for nurses to review and share with the public and patients (see www.arthritis.org/osteoarthritis-agenda.php).

Osteoarthritis

For the older person with OA, early treatment can significantly affect outcomes and improve the overall quality of life. Older patients should also be offered a variety of cognitive-behavioral modalities (relaxation, imagery) to help them cope with the adjustment to chronic illness. (See Chapter 9 ⫘ for cognitive-behavioral methods of pain management.) Nonpharmacological strategies are applicable to most types of arthritis. Each strategy must be individualized to the older person's needs. Nonpharmacological treatment of OA includes:

- Education about the disease.
- Weight reduction to decrease stress on joints.

- Exercise to relieve pain and stiffness (and many other benefits).
- General and specific rest as needed to control symptoms.
- The use of canes, crutches, and walkers to protect joints.
- The use of assistive technology to help with functional ability.
- Surgical intervention for joint replacement (hips and knees).

Prevention and Treatment

Older adults living with osteoarthritis may need to consider the following factors to prevent progression of their disease and to treat debilitating symptoms. Weight loss may be indicated for those who are overweight or obese, regular exercise may enhance joint health, and rest may ease pain and relieve fatigue for painful joints.

Weight Loss The most important risk factor for OA that can be modified is obesity. Reducing weight can improve quality of life and reduce healthcare costs associated with OA. Karlson et al. (2003) studied 568 participants from the ongoing Nurses' Health Study who received a hip replacement to treat OA. The researchers examined the following risk factors for (NIAMS, 2012c): body mass index (estimates body fat), use of hormone replacement therapy after menopause, age, alcohol consumption, physical inactivity, and cigarette smoking. Of all the risk factors, body mass index and age were associated with needing hip replacement. There was double the risk for a hip replacement for those with a high body mass index compared to participants with a low body mass index. The risk from obesity seems to begin early in life and to be established by age 18. This is one of the first long-term prospective studies to show an association between a modifiable risk factor and OA. The CDC (2011a) recently reported that obesity rates are 54% higher among adults with arthritis compared to those without the condition. A loss of just 11 pounds can decrease the occurrence (incidence) of new knee osteoarthritis, and losing just 5% of body weight (12 pounds in a 250-pound person) can reduce pain and disability (CDC, 2011a).

> ***Practice Pearl*** ▶▶▶ To prevent OA, the obese older person should lose weight. An obese person is five times more likely to have OA of the knees and twice as likely to have OA of the hips. Encourage the older adult to take control of arthritis. Be active and adopt good eating habits to lose weight.

Exercise to Relieve Pain and Stiffness Many older adults with OA (and other joint diseases) believe that exercise will cause a flare-up of their arthritis and lead to more pain. As a result, many are afraid to partake in activities that they previously enjoyed. Contrary to that misconception, exercise is an important part of treatment for the older

> **BOX 18-7** **Exercise Guidelines for Older Adults with Arthritis**
>
> 1. Stretch all muscle groups (prevent overstretching) 10 minutes daily.
> 2. Active range of motion daily for all joints.
> 3. Isometric exercises. Keep intensity low. Extremely forceful muscle contractions can cause intra-articular pressure and promote damage.
> 4. Isotonic exercises. Move the joint in an arc. Start gently and progress to weights. Attempts should be made to do full range of motion.
> 5. Resistive exercises twice a week. Increase weights gradually.
> 6. Aerobic exercises (aquatic, walking) are usually well tolerated by older adults with mild to moderate lower extremity OA. For some older adults with moderate to severe OA, walking as an aerobic exercise may not be well tolerated. Alternative exercises such as swimming, biking, and water walking can be offered. Aerobics and strength training improve strength, exercise capacity, gait, functional performance, and balance.

person with arthritis. In fact, joints are dependent on the surrounding muscles for strength, joint protection, and weight bearing. If the muscles are not used, atrophy may result and lead to weakness, falls, and mobility limitations (see exercise guidelines in Box 18-7).

Rest as Needed to Control Symptoms Rest is also an important part of an overall plan for the older person with arthritis. Teaching the older person about rest must include both general rest and rest for the specific joints involved. General rest includes adequate sleep at night and rest periods to ensure overall health and to prevent the excessive fatigue that often occurs with inflammatory conditions. Rest should occur at specific times with proper positioning and should be limited to prevent disuse that occurs with prolonged immobility. Frequent, short rest periods are better than long ones to prevent stiffness.

> ***Practice Pearl*** ▶▶▶ The correct balance between rest and exercise is extremely important for the patient with musculoskeletal problems such as OA and RA. Exercises such as swimming, stationary bicycling, and walking can be safely done with symptomatic (subacute or chronic) joints and not cause further aggravation of symptoms.

Specific rest relates to rest of joints that are painful or inflamed. This would include inflammatory arthritis (RA and gout) and osteoarthritis. This type of rest gives affected joints time to recover and prevents additional pain and injury, while maintaining overall physical activity and preserving function.

> ## BOX 18-8 ▸ Specific Methods to Rest a Painful Joint
>
> The following methods can be used during painful periods or when a joint is inflamed.
>
> **Modify Activities to Control Joint Loading**
>
> - Avoid stairs and climbing if knees or hip joints are painful.
> - Reduce time standing.
> - Alternate weight-bearing and non-weight-bearing exercises.
> - Choose low-impact activities (swimming).
> - Avoid carrying loads more than 10% of body weight.
>
> **Provide Biomechanical Support to Reduce Motion**
>
> - Shoe modification to reduce metatarsal extension.
> - Functional splints (usually of wrists, fingers, and thumbs).
> - Resting splints for nighttime use.
>
> **Provide Rest for Joint Repetitive Movement**
>
> - Keyboarding, sewing, playing musical instruments, and sitting are examples of repetitive movements.
> - A regular schedule of rest breaks from these activities should be implemented.

Source: Westby & Minor, 2006.

The older person should rest an acutely painful or inflamed joint by limiting particular activities and using assistive devices. It is important not to overstretch damaged tissues. During inflammation, tensile strength of the tissue is reduced by up to 50%; thus, overstretching and tearing can more easily occur. However, daily performance of range-of-motion exercises of the remaining joints should continue because strong muscles support the damaged joint. It is important to rest painful joints to prevent overuse, provide support, and maintain function (Box 18-8). Resting the joint should result in decreased pain, swelling, and fatigue.

Additional nonpharmacological strategies to enhance comfort for those with musculoskeletal problems such as OA and RA include:

- **Apply heat to painful joints.** Applying heat to a painful joint will decrease pain and improve flexibility. Hot packs can be applied for about 20 minutes to elevate skin temperature and then removed. Patients sometimes find hot showers and tub baths to be soothing. Moist heat is more effective than dry heat because it penetrates deeper.
- **Use cold applications to reduce pain and swelling.** Cold is applied to the skin with ice packs or cold packs, usually for 10 to 30 minutes depending on the intensity of the cold source and depth of the tissue. Mild cold can be used for swelling. According to Jacewicz (2009) cold application may be analgesic. Care should be taken not to frost the skin.
- **Use canes, crutches, and walkers to protect joints.** These devices are important for joint rest and safety, especially during times of acute joint pain and inflammation. The nurse should teach the patient the correct use of the device or consult with a physical therapist or occupational therapist for patient follow-up.
- **Use assistive technology.** Assistive devices are items that are used to maintain, increase, or improve function. They may be bought commercially or custom-made for the patient. It may be as simple as a kitchen grip, an enlarged pen, a specialized motor scooter, or a dressing aid such as a sock holder. Assistive devices are available for general daily living, home management, school, and work activities. Compliance with their use increases if the patient has been adequately taught. Specific guidelines are available for environmental accessibility. The Job Accommodation Network (a service of the U.S. Department of Labor's Office of Disability Employment) is a helpful resource for working with a patient in need of environmental modifications.

Rheumatoid Arthritis

The older person with RA generally has been living with the disease for many years. It is necessary for the patient and close family members to understand the disease, symptoms that it may cause, and special care it may require (see the following Teaching Guidelines section). General nonpharmacological treatment for RA is focused on reducing joint stress, maintaining joint function, promoting independence, and managing fatigue. Strength training can reverse muscle wasting. If a joint is inflamed, or if there is an exacerbation of the disease, high levels of activity are discouraged. Range of motion (ROM) of the joints, however, should be maintained to prevent contractures and muscle atrophy. In general, rest can reduce joint stress. Once the acute inflammation subsides, muscle strengthening should continue to prevent atrophy around inflamed joints.

For the older person with RA, fatigue is a common problem. The chronic inflammatory response, muscle atrophy, disrupted sleep patterns, and pain all play a role in causing fatigue. Long rest periods should be scheduled in the morning and afternoon. Total body rest is important to prevent the development of fatigue. Splinting, canes, and walking aids are also useful to protect joints and reduce stress. Special devices are available for the home such as grab bars, cups, and utensils.

A review of literature for thermotherapy for treating RA found that there were no significant effects for hot packs and ice packs applications and faradic baths on objective measures of RA disease such as joint swelling, pain medication need, and hand function compared to the control group. However, positive effects were found for paraffin wax baths alone for arthritic (RA) hands on measures such as stiffness and ROM compared to the control group (no treatment) after 4 weeks of treatment (Welch et al., 2001).

Teaching Guidelines

Education to prevent inappropriate treatment of RA includes:

- Contacting the local Arthritis Foundation for materials and references
- Visiting government websites to obtain accurate and up-to-date information
- Talking to healthcare providers regarding advertisements for RA treatments

Exercise and positioning to prevent contractures, muscle weakness, and atrophy include:

- Doing full ROM exercises daily
- Participating in an exercise program
- Staying active
- Avoiding positions of deformity

Steps to reduce joint stress during times of inflammation include:

- Resting the painful joint
- Losing weight
- Splinting specific joints (e.g., fingers, hands, wrist)
- Using larger stronger joints when possible

Rest periods to prevent fatigue should include:

- Planned rest periods in the morning and afternoon
- Whole body rest to reduce inflammatory response

Functional limitations can be minimized by:

- Using assistive devices to enhance self-care abilities
- Modifying the environment to ensure social activities
- Finding tools that allow leisure activities

Box 18-9 summarizes nonpharmacological interventions useful for older patients diagnosed with gout and pseudogout.

Nonpharmacological treatment for bursitis includes moving the affected area as much as possible to the point of pain. Limited movements of the shoulder area could cause long-term problems with range of motion such as "frozen

---

> **BOX 18-9** **Treatment for Gout and Pseudogout**
>
> - Rest the joint during an acute gout attack.
> - Increase fluid intake to 3 L/day to promote renal function and prevent stones.
> - Apply cold to relieve pain.
> - Avoid heat application (if inflammation present).
> - Avoid foods high in purine (shellfish and organ meats).
> - Avoid alcoholic beverages.
> - Prevent obesity to reduce urate production (for gout only).

shoulder." Exercises should be reinforced with the older person to prevent disuse.

Falls and Fall-Related Injuries

Approximately 30% of older adults not in hospitals or care facilities fall each year. Because many older people lose bone density as they grow older, the risk of fractures from falls is a major concern. Falls and fall-induced injuries are increasing at a tremendous rate. Vigorous prevention measures are needed to control the increasing numbers of injuries to the aging population (see Box 18-6). Changes in vision, balance, or judgment; cardiovascular problems; medications; urinary incontinence; and other physical conditions such as diabetes and malnutrition can contribute to an increased risk of falling (American Academy of Orthopedic Surgeons [AAOS], 2011a). Many of the so-called safety measures that have been used in the past such as restraints and side rails have not been found to be effective and may even cause injury. Assessment of functional mobility, such as gait, balance, and position changes, provides valuable clues regarding a person's risk for future falls.

The Osteoporosis and Related Bone Diseases National Resource Center (NIH, 2011a) has presented the Fracture Triangle as a way of analyzing the three causes/factors related to falls (Figure 18-7 ▶▶▶). The triangle sides represent:

1. **The *fall* itself.** Factors that caused the fall include tripping, loosing footing, reflexes and reaction time, balancing on chairs, and so forth.
2. **The *force* and **direction of the fall.** Factors to look at include the distance the person fell, how the fall was broken, and how the person landed.
3. **The *fragility* of the bones that take the impact.** Bones that were once strong are now fragile and this increases the risk for fractures.

If one of the three factors is modified, the chances of breaking a bone can be greatly reduced. This is the goal of the

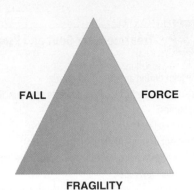

Figure 18-7 ►►► The Fracture Triangle.

triangle. For example, if home safety is maintained by, for example, removing clutter and scatter rugs, the fall could be avoided. Many strategies to support prevention in relation to the Fracture Triangle are discussed, for example, outdoor and indoor safety tips, balancing exercises, and decreasing bone fragility. See the Osteoporosis and Related Bone Diseases National Resource Center reference (NIH, 2011a) for additional guidelines.

Balance exercises are one way for older adults to increase confidence in their balance and take an active part in preventing falls and fractures. Teach the older person the following everyday, easy-to-do exercises:

1. Holding on to the sink, or back of a chair, stand on one foot at a time. Start with 1 minute and increase the time. Try closing your eyes and then try to do it without holding on.
2. Holding onto the sink, practice standing on your toes. Then rock back on your heels. Count to 10 for each position.
3. Holding on to the chair, make a big circle with your hips. Then make the circle in the opposite direction. Do each 5 times.

> **Practice Pearl** ►►► A simple assessment of routine mobility tasks can provide clinical information to determine fall risk. The older person is observed while doing the following activities: (1) getting up from a chair, (2) turning while walking, (3) raising the foot completely off the floor, and (4) sitting down. Difficulty with any of these activities often points to an increased risk for falls. The nurse should develop an individualized plan to increase muscle strength and prevent falls.

Difficulty with any one of the activities points to an increased risk for falls. The more difficulties the older person has, the greater the risk for falls. Many functional and performance assessment tools are available that will provide quantitative data (a score) on an older person's limitation

in mobility and risk for falls. Many exercise options are available to help the older person to regain and maintain muscle strength and improve general fitness. The CDC has developed a compendium of effective research-based community interventions from around the world to prevent falls in the older adult population (CDC, 2011a; NCIPC, 2011).

The older person should also be taught how to get up from a fall and how to get help. One method is to turn over on the stomach and crawl to the phone. Another is to scoot on the bottom or side to reach a phone. The person may be able to crawl to a stairway and climb up until able to stand. If the injury does not allow movement, the person should cover up with anything handy and try to stay warm. The older person should have an emergency plan such as a bell or a phone near the floor or carry a cordless or wireless phone to increase safety. Daily calls to the older person to check on his or her safety will also give a feeling of reassurance to a concerned family member or caregiver.

Treatment of Hip Fractures

Trained emergency staff should take the older person with a hip fracture to a hospital that offers 24-hour surgical care. Fractures must be immobilized immediately to prevent further damage. Surgery is the treatment of choice and should be performed as soon as possible. Older people will benefit from the increased mobility and pain relief that is experienced after surgery. In general, the more invasive the surgical procedure, the more risk involved for the older person. For some older people with acute or chronic disease, the risk of surgery may be too great, and medical management may be the preferred course. For example, a person with severe osteoporosis who has been bedridden may not benefit from surgical interventions. The following are examples of fracture types and common surgical procedures.

Fracture Types

There are two types of fractures: nondisplaced subcapital and femoral neck fractures and displaced fractures of subcapital and femoral neck.

1. **Nondisplaced subcapital and femoral neck fractures.** The surgical procedure includes internal fixation with multiple pins.
2. **Displaced fractures of subcapital and femoral neck.** The surgical procedure includes open reduction internal fixation (ORIF), with any of the following: intermedullary rod, pins, prosthesis, or a fixed sliding plate such as a compression screw.
   a. ORIF is the surgical preference for active older adults who are able to use crutches with partial weight bearing.

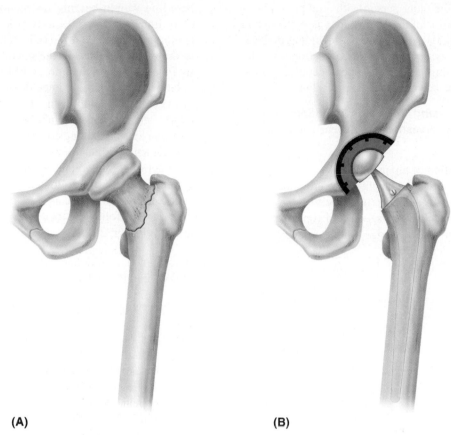

(A)   **(B)**

Figure 18-8 ►►► A hip fracture (A) and repair (B) with Moore's prosthesis in an older person.

b. Moore's prosthesis (hemiarthroscopy, replacement of the femoral head with a smooth metal sphere) is preferred for the less active older person. This treatment option allows full weight bearing and return to active function. Figure 18-8 ►►► illustrates the repair of a hip fracture using Moore's prosthesis.

c. Total hip replacement is done only when severe arthritis is present.

The type of injury, the overall condition of the person, and any preexisting orthopedic conditions will determine the type of surgical procedure.

Joint Replacement Surgery

Total joint replacement or arthroplasty involves removing the damaged part of the joint and replacing it with a prosthetic device made of metal or polyethylene. Joint replacements are indicated when pain, decreased range of motion, and increased disability interfere with daily function. The most common reason for a joint replacement is osteoarthritis, but other conditions such as RA, avascular necrosis, injury, and bone tumors may also require joint replacement.

The goals of joint replacement surgery are to decrease pain and increase joint function. Total joint replacement is becoming very common. In 2006, 542,000 total knee replacements and 231,000 total hip replacements were performed. As a nurse in acute care you will most likely give care to many older adults who have had these surgical procedures. Excellent nursing care, including knowledge of the procedures and specific assessment and critical thinking skills for the joint replacement patient, will help the older person to have the best possible outcome and return to function and activities with increased mobility and reduced pain.

In a total hip replacement, surgeons replace the head of the femur (the ball) and the acetabulum (the socket) with new parts that allow a natural gliding motion of the joint. The surgeon may use a cemented or uncemented prosthetic device. In the uncemented device, the person's own bone grows in the pores and holds the device in place. Cemented procedures were developed about 40 years ago, and have proven effective to reduce pain and increase function. They are used more frequently than cementless devices for people over 75 years old and for people with osteoporosis (NIAMS, 2012a).

Nursing care of the older person with total hip replacement or internal fixation of the hip includes assessment and prevention for common complications, including dislocation of the device, avascular necrosis, infection, and delayed healing. Nursing care for the postoperative patient would depend on the specific surgical procedure.

Postoperative Nursing Interventions Some major nursing care goals/interventions to prevent complications are as follows:

1. Prevent dislocation of hip prosthesis:
   a. Older person must be taught not to cross legs or sit on a low seat for at least 6 to 8 weeks.
   b. The nurse must place the affected (operative) hip in abduction with a wedge, splint or two pillows between the legs.
   c. Nurse supports leg in abduction when patient is turned.
   d. Position of the hip must not exceed 45 to 60 degrees.
   e. Patient will need teaching and reinforcement of these principles as well as follow-up care.
   f. See the AAOS website (www.orthoinfo.aaos.org) for further information regarding patient self-care at home.
2. Observe and record wound drainage and amount. Watch for excessive bleeding. Report immediately.
3. Provide nursing measures to prevent thromboembolism (see below).
4. Monitor vitals signs and assess for signs of infection of the operative site as well as other complications (pneumonia, urinary tract infection).

Total Knee Replacement

Total knee replacements (TKR) began about 50 years ago but did a poor job of mimicking the natural movement of the knee. In the past 15 years technology has improved and the prosthetic devices have better design and fit. Candidates for TKR usually range from 50 to 80 years of age.

About 90% of patients seem to experience a rapid decrease in pain, feel better overall, and have improved joint function after TKR (NIAMS, 2011b).

Postoperative Nursing Interventions Some major nursing care goals/interventions to prevent complications are as follows:

1. Provide adequate pain management. The nurse will need a strong background in pain assessment and reassessment and knowledge of both pharmacological and nonpharmacological modalities to manage the pain adequately for the patient.
2. Ensure safe and early mobilization and therapy. Safe early ambulation both for the patient and caregiver is

based on weight-bearing instructions, the ability of other limb, and overall safety risk (Parker, 2011). A continuous passive motion (CPM) machine is applied to the operative knee in the operating room to gently flex and extend the knee. CPM machines help the older person to increase knee flexion postoperatively.

3. Prevent thromboembolism. Deep vein thrombosis (DVT) and pulmonary embolism (PE) are the most common life-threatening complications after total joint replacement. Without prevention, up to 60% of patients undergoing a joint replacement would have a DVT within 1 to 2 weeks following surgery. The Centers for Medicare and Medicaid Services named DVT as a "never event" following total joint replacement surgery in 2008 (Parker, 2011).

Clinical practice guidelines (AAOS, 2011b) for prevention of DVT and PE include:

1. Mechanical prophylaxis: Use of intermittent compression stockings immediately postop, and constant use even when out of bed. Early ambulation and foot exercises, including plantar and dorsiflexion of foot.
2. Chemical prophylaxis: This will depend on physician preference and patient risk for PE. American Academy of Orthopedic Surgeons (2011b) guidelines include prescribing ASA, low-molecular-weight heparin, synthetic pentasaccharides, or warfarin.
3. Patients having a TKR will often have a Foley catheter inserted in the operating room because of the long duration of the surgery. This increases the patient's risk of developing the most common nosocomial infection: a catheter-acquired urinary tract infection (CAUTI). The Foley catheter should be removed as soon as possible and no longer than 24 hours after surgery to prevent infection (see elimination chapter).
4. Patient will need teaching and follow-up for self-care at home in relation to exercise, pain and prevention of complications. See "Total Knee Replacement Exercise Guide" (AAOS, 2011c).

QSEN Recommendations Related to the Musculoskeletal System

The Quality and Safety Education for Nurses (QSEN) project addresses the challenge of preparing future nurses with the knowledge, skills, and attitudes (KSAs) to continuously improve the quality and safety of the healthcare systems in which they work (Cronenwett et al., 2007). See the QSEN table for tips on meeting QSEN standards.

Patient and Family Teaching

Gerontological nurses require skills and knowledge related to teaching patients and families about the key concepts of gerontology and gerontological nursing. The guidelines in the following feature will assist the nurse to assume the role of teacher and coach.

Meeting QSEN Standards: The Musculoskeletal System

	KNOWLEDGE	SKILLS	ATTITUDES
Patient-Centered Care	Teach older person techniques that will help him or her to prevent further injury.	Review need to make home a safe place by removing scatter rugs and wearing nonskid shoes.	Show your understanding of the changes the older person is experiencing by listening and reinforcing positive behavior.
	Teach the family so that they can support and reinforce the plan of care.	Assess the older adult's awareness and need for change.	Give encouragement to patient and family.
Teamwork and Collaboration	As a team, review all acute care older patients for risks of falls. Incorporate entire team and share views.	Form a group to evaluate research on falls and fall prevention and share results of findings.	Write a short article about your group to show appreciation and get recognition.
	Be aware that the team approach may take time and patience.	Develop goals for the team that are short term.	Be open to others' ideas and discussion even if not in agreement.
Evidence-Based Practice	Know rheumatoid arthritis research related to drugs and patient responses and side effects.	Be familiar with NIH and other important websites to keep current about new FDA announcements.	Give encouragement to RA patients, show interest in their progress or areas that need attention.
Quality Improvement	Document patient functional ability and pain. Keep consistent records to determine trajectory.	Cultivate skills in data management. Review current practice guidelines at government websites.	Value the use of data and outcomes as a key component of QI efforts.
Safety	Provide older adults with current information on drugs and best way to adhere to medication plan for the best results.	Teach the older adult the side effects of drugs, both long and short term. Help them balance the pros and cons of their medication regimen.	Relate the importance of safety and prevention and be responsive to questions.
Informatics	Provide input into the formation and maintenance of patient databases needed for gathering QSEN data and providing patient care.	Utilize the electronic health record.	Protect patient confidentiality according to HIPAA standards.

Patient–Family Teaching Guidelines

The following are guidelines that the nurse may find useful when instructing older adults and their families about mobility problems.

MOBILITY PROBLEMS

1 I have osteoarthritis and chronic pain. What should I do to control my pain?

The pain of osteoarthritis should be managed with a variety of modalities. Pain initially occurs with increased activity and may be relieved by rest. As time goes on, the pain may take longer to subside and the pain may occur at rest as well. It is important that pain be managed effectively early in the disease in order to prevent inactivity that leads to muscle weakness and joint instability. Try Tylenol, topical rubs, hot and cold packs, and regular moderate exercise.

RATIONALE:

Pain levels should be adequately controlled so the older person can move about and stay active. If pain increases and limits activity, the older person may get discouraged and decide not to partake in activities because of fear of pain.

2 Why is it important to exercise?

To maintain or regain an active lifestyle, you need to maintain muscle strength, coordination, balance, flexibility, and endurance. Exercise can do all of that for you plus benefit your heart and keep off excess weight that can further stress your joints.

RATIONALE:

Many older people have very little exercise beyond the minimum required to carry out normal routines. The stereotype of the frail older person quickly becomes a reality as the older person faces the challenges of the aging process. The older person should begin with low-impact exercise and increase it gradually. Walking, dancing, and swimming are all examples of aerobic activities. A warm-up and cool-down period should be included. There are numerous ways to take part in exercise, including local programs at the YMCA, local senior citizens groups, and walking groups at the mall. Each older person should determine the type of exercise he or she prefers and will continue to do.

3 What exercise can I do to keep myself moving?

Key exercises and activities that will help you to maintain functional performance include walking, pool or water aerobics, yoga or stretching exercises, dancing, golfing, fishing, or anything that is enjoyable and gets you moving.

RATIONALE:

The quadriceps muscle groups are needed when rising from a chair, stair climbing, and walking. Weakness of these muscles may prevent older adults from maintaining independence in many functional activities and cause them to be homebound

or need assistance with activities of daily living. It is vital for the older person to maintain these activities on a regular basis as part of an exercise program.

4 What are some precautions I should take when I exercise?

Dress appropriately, wear proper footwear, and check with your doctor if you have chest pain, irregular heartbeat, shortness of breath, hernia, foot or ankle sores that do not heal, hot or red joints with pain, and certain eye conditions like bleeding in the retina or detached retina. If you have any of these conditions, it does not mean you cannot exercise, but modifications and precautions might be needed. See an expert who can help you get going.

RATIONALE:

Older people with chronic conditions should begin an exercise regimen slowly and seek advice from professionals familiar with their special needs, including cardiologists, physical therapists, sports medicine practitioners, and fitness instructors.

5 How do I know if exercise is helping me?

Begin by seeing how far you can walk in 5 minutes. (Use a watch and record your distance in feet or blocks.) Then time yourself as you walk up a flight of stairs (at least 10 steps). After 1 month of exercising, repeat these tests and compare your times. If you are on the right track, it should be taking less time. Keep a diary and bring it with you the next time you see your healthcare provider.

RATIONALE:

The nurse can discuss the patient's pain and activity diary and determine if the goals were achieved. If the patient is in the home or the primary care setting, the nurse can evaluate the older person's functional abilities and focus on areas of concern such as hips and knees. If the older person met the goal, the nurse and patient can determine if the exercise goal can be increased to include a longer time period or increase in intensity of activities. Praise is given for achievement.

If the goal has not been met, the nurse and patient need to evaluate the data and revise the care plan to reflect the abilities of the older person. Compassion and understanding are important so that the older person does not get discouraged. If the patient is having an episode of acute joint pain, range of motion should continue on all noninvolved joints. Stiffness, muscle weakness, and atrophy can occur quickly if the person becomes immobile. Prescribed pain medication, as well as nonpharmacological pain management techniques, should be implemented to allow the patient to remain as active as possible during the acute pain.

CARE PLAN A Patient With a Hip Fracture

Case Study

Mrs. Jerome is a patient in the orthopedic department of a large hospital. She is an 82-year-old widow who has lived alone for the past 5 years since her husband died. Her daughter found her on the floor of her home where she had fallen. Mrs. Jerome was admitted to the emergency department, where X-rays revealed a hip fracture due to severe osteoporosis. She is 4 days postoperative after an ORIF of the left femur. She is stable surgically and has been medicated for pain with Percocet, 1 tablet. The night nurse reports that Mrs. Jerome has been crying at times during the night. When the nurse tried to talk to her, Mrs. Jerome denies any problems and states she is fine.

Applying the Nursing Process

Assessment

The registered nurse completes the nursing assessment and discusses Mrs. Jerome's history, which includes hypertension, high cholesterol, and asthma. The physical examination shows blood pressure 160/90, pulse 88, respirations 28, and temperature 98°F. The nurse notes a large hip dressing, which is dry and intact. The patient has pain of 3 on a 0-to-10 scale. Mrs. Jerome states that she "has been living in her home alone and managing normal daily activities until this terrible thing happened." She enjoys cooking for herself, her daughter, and other family members when they visit. Her daughter, Rose, does her errands and takes her to the doctor. Mrs. Jerome does not go out alone. She gave up smoking many years ago and adheres to her diet to lower her cholesterol. She is on medications for asthma and hypertension. Mrs. Jerome starts to cry when she talks about her sister who recently passed away. She states, "My sister went to a nursing home after a fall and was never able to return to her own home again." Her daughter, Rose, has spoken with the nurse and doctor and does not feel that her mother would be safe living alone at home anymore. Rose is very upset about the situation. However, she does not wish to talk to her mother about this at the present time.

Diagnosis

The current nursing diagnoses for Mrs. Jerome include the following:

- *Mobility: Physical, Impaired* related to tissue trauma secondary to fracture
- *Anxiety* related to anticipated postoperative dependence and living situation
- *Pain, Acute* related to surgical procedure
- *Trauma, Risk for Falls* related to weakness
- *Fatigue* related to surgery

NANDA-I © 2012.

Expected Outcomes

Expected outcomes for the plan specify that Mrs. Jerome will:

- Demonstrate knowledge related to self-care after surgical procedure for a fractured hip.
- Verbalize fears to help cope with change due to injury and hospitalization.
- Report that the pain is tolerable (such as less than 3 on a 0-to-10 scale).
- Collaborate with the nurse and healthcare team to reach the goal of returning home with functional independence.

(continued)

CARE PLAN   A Patient With a Hip Fracture *(continued)*

Planning and Implementation

The following nursing interventions may be appropriate for Mrs. Jerome:

- Allow patient to complete self-care as much as possible to gain confidence in her abilities.
- Begin to explore the patient's problem-solving strategies to determine how she has resolved past changes or problems.
- Assess support systems that are available for the patient after hospitalization.
- Identify a plan to reduce the risk of falls in the future.
- Reinforce all exercises, ambulation, and transfer techniques that will achieve maximum physical mobility within restrictions of the surgery.

Evaluation

The nurse hopes to resolve this patient situation. The nurse will consider the plan a success based on the following:

- Mrs. Jerome will learn the major concepts of self-care after hip fracture.
- She will report minimal pain and will have adequate pain control.
- Mrs. Jerome will progress in her muscle strength and maintain functional ability as much as possible to prevent disuse.
- She and her daughter will discuss the short-term and long-term options and develop a plan based on Mrs. Jerome's progress and her overall health.

Ethical Dilemma

The primary ethical dilemma in this situation is the conflict between the moral obligation of the nurse to be honest with the patient (veracity) and the daughter's wish for the nurse not to disclose to the patient that she does not believe her mother should return home. The patient is interested in doing all she has to do to get better and return home. Her daughter has been visiting and giving encouragement to her mother but has not been honest about her true feelings about the discharge plan.

The nurse has an obligation to be honest with the patient. The nurse also has an obligation to do good, based on the principle of beneficence, and to respect the patient's autonomy.

The patient has the right to make decisions for herself and should be part of the discussions that affect her future.

The nurse plans to ask the daughter to speak openly with her mother. The nurse also plans to set up a meeting with the entire healthcare team so that the daughter can appreciate the true potential and progress that Mrs. Jerome can make. The risks and benefits of Mrs. Jerome returning to her home will also be discussed. The nurse hopes to help the daughter and mother make the decision together. The patient has the right to make the decision, but the daughter's help will be needed to support the patient in the home as she has been doing for the past 5 years.

Critical Thinking and the Nursing Process

1. What factors should the nurse consider when caring for older patients with osteoporosis?
2. What safety measures should the nurse and the older patient plan for in the home environment to prevent falls?
3. What type of exercise program are you comfortable suggesting to your older patients with mobility problems?

- Evaluate your responses in Appendix B.

Chapter Highlights

- The older person loses approximately 1 cm of height every ten years after age 40.

- By age 75, older adults lose about one half of the skeletal muscle mass they had at 30 years of age.

- The older person can usually perform the functional activities of daily living and demonstrate adequate muscle function.

- Older adults experience a decrease in range of motion of joints due to loss of elasticity in ligaments, tendons, and joint capsules.

- Diagnostic tests for musculoskeletal problems include bone mineral density, synovial fluid analysis, X-rays, CT, MRI, and blood tests including calcium level, rheumatoid factor, C-reactive protein, erythrocyte sedimentation rate, and serum uric acid.

- Osteoporosis is characterized by low bone mass and deterioration of bone tissue leading to a decrease in bone strength that increases the risk for fractures.

- The major risk factors for osteoporosis are increased age, female sex, White or Asian race, thin body, and positive family history of the disease.

- Treatment for osteoporosis includes increasing calcium in the diet and drug therapy with antiresorptive agents such as Fosamax.

- The older person with osteoporosis should exercise daily with a combination of weight-bearing exercise such as walking and strength training and balance training.

- Osteomalacia is a metabolic disorder caused by vitamin D deficiency that results in deformities of long bones. Muscle weakness and severe pain in the hip may cause gait problems.

- Paget's disease is a chronic disease of unknown etiology. It causes pain, physical deformity, motor impairments, and mental status changes that significantly affect the older person's quality of life.

- Gout is a metabolic disease caused by urate crystal deposits in joints, leading to local pain and inflammation in the joints. It primarily affects joints in the feet, often the big toe.

- Osteoarthritis is a chronic degenerative joint disease of the weight-bearing joints that is characterized by thinning and eroding of cartilage. Systemic symptoms such as fever are not present. Obesity is a major modifiable risk factor. Acetaminophen (Tylenol) is often used to relieve the pain.

- Rheumatoid arthritis is a chronic syndrome that is characterized by symmetrical inflammation of peripheral joints. It causes pain, swelling, and morning stiffness lasting up to an hour. RA may cause chronic deformities and systemic nonjoint symptoms including renal, lung, and vascular involvement. Anti-inflammatory treatment should be started early to prevent deformities.

- Total hip replacement and total knee replacement are common surgical procedures. Projections are that over a million of these procedures will be done yearly. These procedures have been successful in reducing or eliminating pain for many older adults suffering with osteoarthritis and/or rheumatoid arthritis.

- Education is the key to success in adapting to chronic diseases. A program of exercise and rest is an important part of preventing and reversing many of the disabilities that accompany joint diseases.

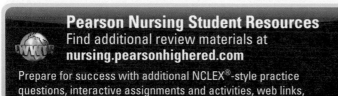

References

Agency for Healthcare Research and Quality (AHRQ). (2007). *Osteoarthritis of the knee.* Retrieved from http://www.ahrq.gov/clinic/tp/oakneetp.htm

American Academy of Orthopedic Surgeons (AAOS). (2011a). *Can in-hospital falls really be prevented?* Retrieved from http:www.orthoinfor.org/topic

American Academy of Orthopedic Surgeons (AAOS). (2011b). *New clinical treatment guideline recommendations to reduce blood clots after hip and knee replacement.* Retrieved from http://www.aaos.org/guidelines

American Academy of Orthopedic Surgeons (AAOS). (2011c). *Total knee replacement exercise guide.* Retrieved from http://www.orthoinfo.org/topic

Arthritis Foundation. (2010). *A national public health agenda for osteoarthritis.* Retrieved from http: www.arthritis.org / osteoarthritis-agenda.php

Baker, D., Gustafson, S., Beaubien, J., Salas, E., & Barach, P. (2005). Medical teamwork and patient safety: The evidence-based relation. Literature Review, *AHRQ. Publication No. 05-0053.* Rockville, Md: Agency for Healthcare Research and Quality. Retrieved from http://www.ahrq.gov/qual/medteam/

Berman, J., & Paget, S. (2009). Evaluation of the patient with joint disorders. *Merck Manual Professional.* Retrieved from http://www.merckmanuals.com/professional/musculoskeletal_and_connective_tissue_disorders/approach_to_the_ patient_with_joint_disease/evaluation_of_the_patient_with_joint_disorders.html

Browder-Lazenby, R. (2011). *Handbook of pathophysiology* (4th ed.). Philadelphia, PA: Lippincott Williams & Wilkins.

Brown, S. (2011). Bone density testing bias. *Better Bones Blog.* Retrieved from www.betterbones.com/blog/post/Bone-density-testing-biased-thin-small-women-take-note.asp

Bryan, R. (2006). Osteoporosis treatment: Boniva. *Advance for nurses.* Retrieved from http://nursing.advanceweb.com/Article/Osteoporosis-Treatment-Boniva.aspx

Burton, L., & Sumukadas, D. (2010). Optimal management of sarcopenia. *Clinical Intervention Aging, 5,* 217–228. Retrieved from www.ncbi.nlm.nih.gov/pmc/articles/PMC2938029

Centers for Disease Control and Prevention (CDC). (2011a). *Arthritis basics FAQ.* Retrieved from http://www.cdc.gov/arthritis/basics/faqs.htm#17

Centers for Disease Control and Prevention (CDC). (2011b). *Rheumatoid arthritis.* National Center for Chronic Disease and Prevention and Health Promotion. Division of Adult and Community Health. Retrieved from http://www.cdc.gov/arthritis/basics/rheumatoid

Cronenwett, L., Sherwood, G., Barnsteiner, J., Disch, J., Johnson, J., Mitchell, P., Sullivan, D., & Warren, J. (2007). Quality and safety education for nurses, *Nursing Outlook, 55*(3) 122–131.

Dugdale, D. (2010). CT scan. *Medline Plus.* Retrieved from http://www.nlm.nih.gov/medlineplus/ency/article/003330.htm

Hardy, E. (2011). Gout diagnosis and management: What NP's need to know. *Nurse Practitioner, 36*(6), 14–19.

Hartford Institute for Geriatric Nursing. (2008). *Falls: Nursing standard of practice protocols.* Retrieved from http://consultgerirn.org/topics/falls/want_to_know_more

Hendrich, A., Bender, P., & Nyhuis, A. (2003). Validation of the Hendrich II Fall Risk Model: A large concurrent case study of hospitalized patients. *Applied Nursing Research, 16*(1), 9–21.

Ignatavicius, D., & Workman, L. (2010). *Adult health nursing* (5th ed.). St. Louis, MO: Elsevier Saunders.

Institute for Clinical Systems Improvement. (2011). *Diagnosis and treatment of osteoporosis.* Retrieved from http://www.icsi.org/osteoporosis/diagnosis_and_treatment_of_osteoporosis__

International Osteoporosis Foundation (IOF). (2011). *Facts and statistics.* Retrieved from http://www.iofbonehealth.org/facts-and-statistics.html#factsheet

Jacewicz, M. (2009). Musculoskeletal and connective tissue disorders. *Merck Manual Professional.* Retrieved from http:www.merckmanuals.com/professional/musculoskeletal_and_connective_tissue_disorders/symptoms_of_joint_disorders/monarticular_joint_pain.html

Jacobs-Kosmin, D. (2012). Osteoporosis. *Medscape Reference.* Retrieved from http://emedicine.medscape.com/article/330598-overview

Johnsson, P., & Eberhardt, K. (2009). Hand deformities are important signs of disease severity in early rheumatoid arthritis. *Rheumatology (Oxford), 48*(11), 1398–1401.

Karlson, E., Mandl, L., Aweh, G., Sangha, O., Liang, M., & Grodstein, F. (2003). Total hip replacement due to osteoarthritis: The importance of age, obesity, and other modifiable risk factors. *American Journal of Medicine, 114*(2), 93–98.

Lab Tests Online. (2011a). *ALP.* Retrieved from http://labtestsonline.org/understanding/analytes/rheumatoid/tab/test

Lab Tests Online. (2011b). *Rheumatoid factor.* Retrieved from http://labtestsonline.org/understanding/analytes/rheumatoid/tab/test

Lozada, C., Diamond, H., & Agnew, S. (2011, October 11). Osteoarthritis treatment and management. *Medscape Reference.* Retrieved from http://emedicine.medscape.com/article/330487-treatment#showall

Majithia, V., Peel, C., & Geraci, S. (2009). Rheumatoid arthritis in elderly patients. *Geriatrics, 9*(64), 9. Retrieved from http://www.geri.com

National Cancer Institute, National Institutes of Health. (2012). *SEER training modules: Muscular system.* Retrieved from http://training.seer.cancer.gov/anatomy/muscular/

National Center for Injury Prevention and Control (NCIPC), Centers for Disease Control and Prevention. (2011). Older adult falls—Preventing falls among older adults. *Home and Recreation Safety—Injury Center.* Retrieved from http://www.cdc.gov/ncipc/factsheets/adulthipfx.htm

National Institute of Arthritis and Musculoskeletal and Skin Disease (NIAMS), National Institutes of Health. (2009). *Handout on health: Rheumatoid arthritis.* Retrieved from http://www.niams.nih.gov/Health_Info/Rheumatic_Disease/default.asp

National Institute of Arthritis and Musculoskeletal and Skin Diseases (NIAMS), National Institutes of Health. (2010). *Topics: Questions and answers about gout.* Retrieved from http://www.niams.nih.gov/hi/topics/gout/gout.htm

National Institute of Arthritis and Musculoskeletal and Skin Diseases (NIAMS), National Institutes of Health. (2011a). *Health topics: Questions and answers about arthritis and rheumatic diseases.* Retrieved from http://www.niams.nih.gov/Health_Info/Arthritis/arthritis_rheumatic_qa.as

National Institute of Arthritis and Musculoskeletal and Skin Diseases (NIAMS), National Institutes of Health. (2011b). *Knee problems: Questions and answers about knee problems.* Retrieved from htttp://www.niams.nih.gov/Health_Info/Knee_Problems/default.asp

National Institute of Arthritis and Musculoskeletal and Skin Diseases (NIAMS), National Institutes of Health. (2011c). *Osteoporosis: Handout on health.* Retrieved from http://www.niams.nih.gov/Health_Info/Bone/Osteoporosis/osteoporosis_hoh.asp#7pubnumber 07-5158

National Institute of Arthritis and Musculoskeletal and Skin Diseases (NIAMS), National Institutes of Health. (2012a). *Topic: Osteoporosis.* Retrieved from http://www.niams.nih.gov/health_info/bone/osteoporosis/bone_mass.asp

National Institute of Arthritis and Musculoskeletal and Skin Diseases (NIAMS), National Institutes of Health. (2012b). *Topic: Paget's disease of the bone*. Retrieved from http://www.niams.nih.gov/health_info/bone/pagets/diagnosis/_mass.asp

National Institute of Arthritis and Musculoskeletal and Skin Diseases (NIAMS), National Institutes of Health. (2012c). *Topics: Questions and answers about hip replacement*. Retrieved from http://www.niams.nih.gov/hi/topics/hip/hiprepqa.htm

NANDA International. (2012). *NANDA International nursing diagnoses: Definitions and classification, 2012–2014*. Philadelphia, PA: Wiley-Blackwell.

National Institutes of Health (NIH). (2011a). *Preventing falls and related fractures*. Osteoporosis and Related Bone Diseases National Resource Center. Retrieved from http://www.bones.nih.gov

National Library of Medicine (NLM). (2010a). Aging changes in the bones. *PubMed Health*. Retrieved from http://www.ncbi.nlm.nih.gov/pubmedhealth/PMH0004420

National Library of Medicine (NLM). (2010b). Osteoarthritis. *PubMed Health*. Retrieved from http://www.ncbi.nlm.nih.gov/pubmedhealth/PMH0001460/

National Library of Medicine (NLM). (2012a). ESR. *MedlinePlus*. Retrieved from http://www.nlm.nih.gov/medlineplus/ency/article/003638.htm

National Library of Medicine (NLM). (2012b). Osteoarthritis. *PubMed Health*. Retrieved from http://www.ncbi.nlm.nih.gov/pubmedhealth/PMH0001460

National Library of Medicine (NLM). (2012c). Osteomalacia. *PubMed Health*. Retrieved from http://www.nlm.nih.gov/medlineplus/ency/article/000376.htm

National Library of Medicine (NLM). (2012d). Paget's disease. *PubMed Health*. Retrieved from http://www.nlm.nih.gov/medlineplus/ency/article/000414.htm

National Library of Medicine (NLM). (2012e). *Rheumatoid factor*. Retrieved from http://www.nlm.nih.gov/medlineplus/ency/article/003548.htm

National Osteoporosis Foundation (NOF). (2010). *Clinician guide to prevention and treatment of osteoporosis*. Retrieved from http://www.nof.org/clinguide

Paget Foundation. (2011a). *A physician's guide to Paget's disease of the bone*. Retrieved from http://www.paget.org

Paget Foundation. (2011b). *Questions and answers about Paget's disease of the bone: General information about Paget's disease*. Retrieved from http://www.paget.org

Parker, R. (2011). Evidence-based practice: Caring for a patient undergoing a total knee arthroplasty. *Orthopedic Nursing, 30*(1), 4–8.

Storck, S. (2011). Bone mineral density test. *PubMed Health*. Retrieved from http://www.ncbi.nlm.nih.gov/pubmedhealth/PMH0004464

U.S. Department of Health and Human Services (USDHHS). (2010). *Healthy People 2020: Summary of objectives*. Retrieved from http://www.healthypeople.gov/2020/topicsobjectives2020/pdfs/EducationalPrograms.pdf

U.S. Food and Drug Administration (FDA), Center for Drug Evaluation and Research. (2008). *Highlights of prescribing information, Zometa*. Retrieved from http://www.fda.gov/cder/foil/label/2008/021223s016lbl.pdf

U.S. Food and Drug Administration (FDA), Center for Drug Evaluation and Research. (2011). Retrieved from http://www.fda.gov/Safety/MedWatch/SafetyInformation/SafetyAlertsforHumanMedicalProducts/ucm270464.htm

Welch, V., Brosseau, L., Casimiro, L., Judd, M., & Shea, B. (2001). Thermotherapy of treating rheumatoid arthritis. (2011). *Cochrane Database of Systemic Reviews,* Issue 2. Art. No.: CD002826. doi:10.1002/14651858.CD002826.

Westby, M., & Minor, M. (2006). Exercise and physical activity. In S. Bartlett (Ed.), *Clinical care in the rheumatic diseases* (3rd ed.). Atlanta, GA: American College of Rheumatology.

Zhu, Y., Pandya, B. J., & Choi, H. K. (2011), Prevalence of gout and hyperuricemia in the US general population: The National Health and Nutrition Examination Survey 2007–2008. *Arthritis & Rheumatism, 63,* 3136–3141. doi:10.1002/art.30520

The Endocrine System

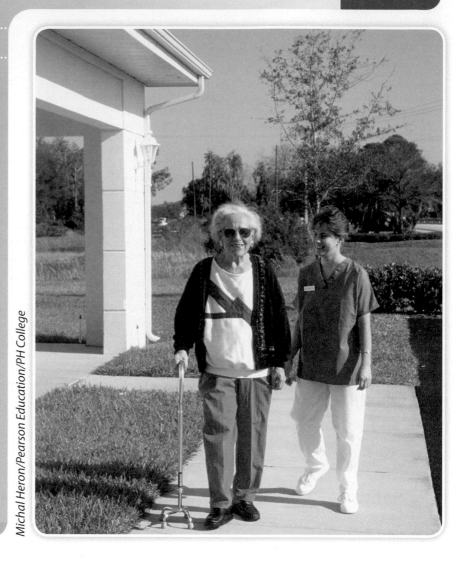

Michal Heron/Pearson Education/PH College

LEARNING OUTCOMES

On completion of this chapter, the reader will be able to:

1. Describe age-related changes that affect endocrine function.
2. Recognize the impact of age-related changes on endocrine function.
3. Identify risk factors to health for the older person with an endocrine problem.
4. Understand unique presentations of diabetes and thyroid problems in the older person.

5. Apply appropriate nursing interventions directed toward assisting older adults with endocrine problems to develop self-care abilities.
6. Identify and implement appropriate nursing interventions to care for the older person with endocrine problems.

The endocrine glands control the body's metabolic processes. The endocrine and metabolic control systems offer many of the greatest opportunities for preventing the disabilities associated with aging (Solomon, 2003). Endocrine glands respond to specific signals by synthesizing and releasing hormones into the circulation. The hormones affect cells with appropriate receptors and trigger specific cellular responses and activities. Most hormones operate via a feedback system that maintains an optimal internal environment or homeostasis within the body (Huether & McCance, 2012). Two major endocrine problems of importance to gerontological nursing are diabetes mellitus and thyroid disease. Thyroid disease is common, often undiagnosed, and easily treated in people of all ages. Early detection prevents unnecessary disability and loss of function. Diabetes mellitus (DM) is a chronic disease characterized by high levels of blood glucose resulting from problems with insulin production, insulin action, or both. DM can lead to serious complications such as heart disease, blindness, kidney failure, nontraumatic amputations, and premature death and disability. Regulation of blood glucose levels may minimize the devastating vascular and neurologic complications that often occur (American Geriatrics Society for Health in Aging, 2012). Knowledge of endocrine function and metabolism and an understanding of normal changes associated with aging is crucial for gerontological nurses in order to interpret signs and symptoms of illness and advise older adults on health promotion activities (Figure 19-1 ▶▶▶).

The hypothalamus, located in the brain, produces hormones that control the structures in the endocrine system. The pituitary gland, also located in the brain, reaches its maximum size in middle age and then gradually becomes smaller. The pituitary has two major functions: storing hormones produced by the hypothalamus and production of hormones that affect the ovaries, testes, breasts, and thyroid gland.

The thyroid gland is located in the neck and produces hormones that help control metabolism. Thyroid function is significantly altered with aging, and the thyroid gradually loses function and undergoes atrophy. The gland becomes more nodular, especially in areas with low iodine levels in the food and water. Fortunately, only about 2% of thyroid nodules are cancerous, and the presence of hypothyroidism and thyroid nodules rises dramatically with age (Solomon, 2003). Additionally, thyroid antibody levels rise with age, making it difficult to discern at what levels these antibodies indicate thyroiditis. Basic metabolic rate gradually declines, beginning around age 20. Less thyroid hormone may be produced, but because there is less body mass (because of loss of muscle and bone tissue), thyroid function tests usually show results within the normal range. Although the prevalence of hyperthyroidism is similar for younger and older people, the presentation of hyperthyroidism is often less dramatic in older adults, making it difficult to detect.

The parathyroids are four tiny glands located around the thyroid. Parathyroid hormone affects calcium and phosphate levels, which, in turn, affects bone strength. Changes in the level of parathyroid hormones may contribute to development of osteoporosis (see Chapter 18 ⬅ for further details). Insulin is produced by the pancreas. The average fasting glucose blood level rises 6 to 14 mg/dL for each 10 years after age 50. This is because the cells in the body become less sensitive to the effects of insulin, probably because of a loss in the number of insulin receptor sites in the cell wall. The adrenal glands are located just above the kidneys and these glands produce the hormones aldosterone (to regulate fluid and electrolyte balance) and cortisol (the "stress response" hormone). Aldosterone secretion decreases with age, which can contribute to light-headedness and a drop in blood pressure with sudden position changes (orthostatic hypotension). Cortisol secretion decreases with aging, but the blood level stays about the same.

The ovaries and testes produce the sex hormones that control secondary sex characteristics, such as breasts and facial hair. With aging, men experience a slightly decreased level of testosterone and women have decreased levels of estrogen after menopause (see Chapter 17 ⬅ for further details) (MedlinePlus, 2012).

Diabetes Mellitus

Diabetes mellitus (DM) is highly prevalent and its incidence is increasing in persons over age 65, particularly in racial and ethnic minorities (Centers for Disease Control and Prevention [CDC], 2011a). DM is a major cause of heart disease and stroke and is currently the seventh leading cause of death in the United States. Overall, the risk of death in people with diabetes is about twice as high as the risk of death in people without diabetes. DM is classified as type 1 (the result of insufficient insulin production) and type 2 (the result of insulin resistance). Type 1 DM is most often an autoimmune disease that develops when the body's immune system destroys pancreatic **beta cells** (specialized cells in the pancreas that make insulin), but also may be the result of pancreatic destruction secondary to a viral infection such as mumps, rubella, measles, influenza, and encephalitis (Huether & McCance, 2012). Beta cells are the only cells in the body that make the hormone insulin that regulates **blood glucose** (the main sugar that the body produces from ingested nutrients used by the cells of the body for energy). People with type 1 DM must take insulin every day either by injection, pump, or inhalation. Type 1 DM accounts for

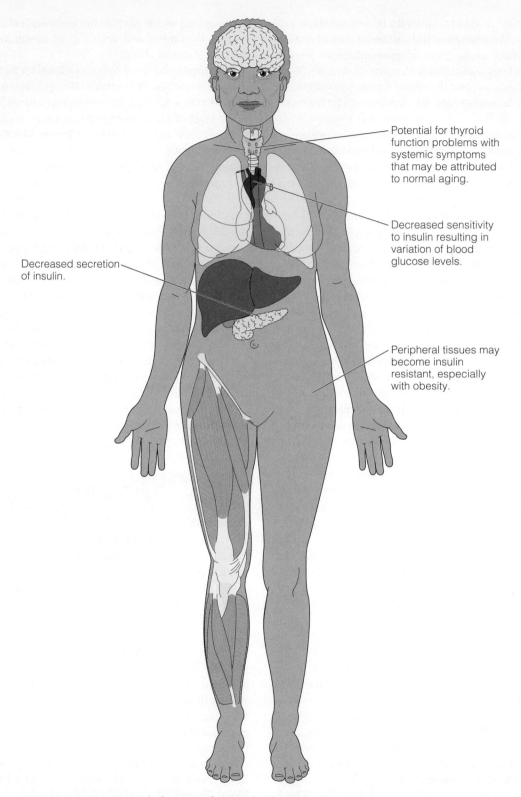

Potential for thyroid function problems with systemic symptoms that may be attributed to normal aging.

Decreased sensitivity to insulin resulting in variation of blood glucose levels.

Decreased secretion of insulin.

Peripheral tissues may become insulin resistant, especially with obesity.

Figure 19-1 ▶▶▶ Normal changes of aging in the endocrine system.

5% to 10% of all diagnosed cases of DM and usually affects children and young adults, although it may be diagnosed at any age (CDC, 2011a). Type 2 DM usually begins as insulin resistance because cells cannot use insulin properly. The need for insulin rises and the beta cells in the pancreas lose their ability to produce enough insulin over time. Type 2 DM accounts for 90% to 95% of cases of DM and is associated with older age, obesity, family history, physical inactivity, and racial/ethnic characteristics. Increasingly, type 2 DM is being diagnosed in adolescents and children and may be related to the obesity epidemic occurring in the United States (Figure 19-2 ▶▶▶) (CDC, 2011b).

In 2011, at least 18.8 million Americans were diagnosed with DM and 7.0 million were undiagnosed with DM accounting for approximately 8.3% of the population (CDC, 2011a). These two figures total about 25.6 million Americans with DM. Of these Americans, 10.9 million are over the age of 65 (CDC, 2011a). Between 1980 and 2000, the prevalence of diagnosed DM increased in all age groups. As Figure 19-3 ▶▶▶ illustrates, in 2010 the prevalence of diagnosed and undiagnosed DM among people over age 65 was about 26.9% (10.9 million people) compared to less than 11.3% in the 21- to 64-year-old age group. National estimates of diabetes by racial and ethnic groups reveal that minorities are disproportionately burdened with diagnosed and undiagnosed DM. Compared to non-Hispanic White

adults, the risk of diagnosed diabetes was 18% higher among Hispanics, and 77% higher among non-Hispanic Blacks. Among Hispanics compared to non-Hispanic White adults, the risk of diagnosed diabetes was about the same for Cubans and for Central and South Americans, 87% higher for Mexican Americans, and 94% higher for Puerto Ricans (CDC, 2011a).

Older adults often bear the greatest burden of diabetes. The statistics in Box 19-1 indicate the need to improve the quality of health care provided to older people with DM.

Complications of Diabetes Mellitus

DM affects people of all ages; however, the disease is particularly serious in the older person because of the many complications that can develop. Poor glycemic control may synergistically interact with normal changes of aging and other coexisting diseases to accelerate diabetes complications including the development of **retinopathy** (damage to the retina), **nephropathy** (kidney damage), and **neuropathy** (nerve damage resulting in sensory impairment) (Diabetes Guidelines Work Group, 2007). The prevalence and incidence of DM increases dramatically with age, and recognition of abnormal glucose metabolism in older adults and the development of age-appropriate preventive and therapeutic strategies assume major clinical importance (CDC, 2011b). Optimizing glucose control and

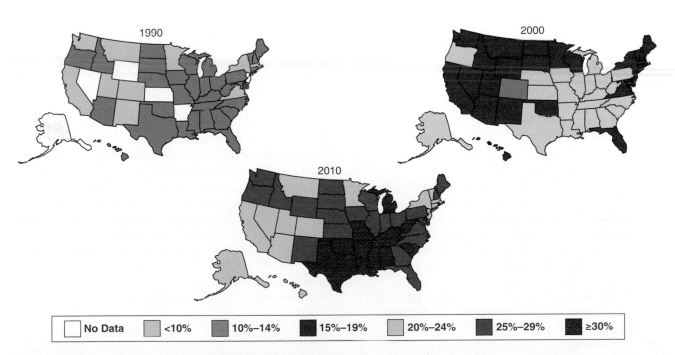

Figure 19-2 ▶▶▶ Obesity trends in the United States, 1990–2010.

Source: Centers for Disease Control and Prevention. (2011). *Obesity trends among U.S. adults between 1985 and 2010.* Retrieved from http://www.cdc.gov/obesity/downloads/obesity_trends_2010.ppt#531,5,Slide; Centers for Disease Control and Prevention. (2011). *Obesity trends.* Retrieved from http://www.cdc.gov/obesity/data/trends.html.

Diagnosed and undiagnosed diabetes among people aged 20 years or older, United States, 2010

Group	Number or percentage who have diabetes
Age ≥20 Years	25.6 million or 11.3% of all people in this age group
Age ≥65 Years	10.9 million or 26.9% of all people in this age group
Men	13.0 million or 11.8% of all men aged 20 years or older
Women	12.6 million or 10.8% of all women aged 20 years or older
Non-Hispanic Whites	15.7 million or 10.2% of all non-Hispanic Whites aged 20 years of older
Non-Hispanic Blacks	4.9 million or 18.7% of all non-Hispanic Blacks aged 20 years or older

Figure 19-3 ▶▶▶ U.S. diabetes prevalence in people age 20 years or older, 2010.

Source: Centers for Disease Control and Prevention. National diabetes fact sheet: National estimates and general information on diabetes and prediabetes in the United States 2011, Atlanta, GA: U.S. Department of Health and Human Services, Centers for Disease Control and Prevention, 2011.

decreasing risk factors for microvascular, macrovascular, and neurologic complications can improve the quality and quantity of life for patients of all ages. Complications that can develop due to inadequate glycemic control include the following:

- Eye disease leading to loss of vision or even blindness (macular degeneration)
- Kidney failure
- Heart disease or coronary artery disease and atherosclerosis
- Peripheral neuropathies
- Periodontal disease
- Neurogenic bladder
- Stroke
- Poor wound healing
- Amputations

The diagnosis of DM can shorten the average life span up to 15 years. Additionally, DM leads to higher death rates from other illnesses such as pneumonia, influenza, and heart disease. Care of persons with DM in the United States in 2007 was estimated to cost more than $174 billion annually, including direct and indirect costs such as disability, lost work productivity, and premature death (CDC, 2011a). Medical care for people with diabetes is more than two times higher than the cost of medical care for people without diabetes. The number of persons diagnosed with DM is expected to increase as a result of the rising number of older adults, along with the complication rates resulting from the diagnosis.

Pathophysiology of DM

DM can be caused by defective insulin secretion or use, resulting in abnormally high levels of blood glucose and damage or destruction to many organs in the body, including

---

BOX 19-1

Older Adults and the Burden of Diabetes

- About two in three people with DM die from heart disease or stroke. The risk for heart disease and stroke is two to four times higher in people with DM.
- DM is the leading cause of new cases of blindness among adults ages 20 to 74 years.
- The cost of direct care of older adults with DM exceeded $116 billion in 2007. The majority of these costs were paid by Medicare and Medicaid and by copayments and deductibles assumed by older adults themselves.
- DM is the leading cause of kidney failure, accounting for 44% of new cases in 2008. In 2008 in the United States, close to 202,290 people with end-stage kidney disease due to diabetes were living on chronic dialysis or with a kidney transplant.
- DM causes more than 60% of nontraumatic lower limb amputations each year. In 2006, about 65,700 nontraumatic lower limb amputations were performed in people with DM.
- DM is the seventh leading cause of death for persons ages 65 and older and a major contributor to heart disease, the leading cause of death for this age group.
- The death rates from all causes are higher among older adults with DM than among those without DM.

Source: CDC (2011a); National Diabetes Education Program (2007).

the eyes, kidneys, blood vessels, and nervous system. The nurse plays a key role in monitoring blood glucose levels, organizing and participating in screening activities, and providing ongoing assessment for early signs of complications in older patients with DM. Older patients with DM have higher rates of premature death, functional disability, and coexisting illnesses such as hypertension, coronary heart disease, and stroke than other older adults. With proper foot care, many of the lower limb amputations could be prevented. Older adults with DM are also at greater risk for depression, cognitive impairment, urinary incontinence, falls, and persistent pain (CDC, 2011a). Therefore, older people require attention and emphasis not only in the area of blood glucose control, but also in the area of identification and treatment of DM-related comorbidities.

It has been recommended that the terms *insulin-dependent diabetes mellitus* and *non–insulin-dependent diabetes mellitus* be replaced with the terms *type 1 diabetes mellitus* and *type 2 diabetes mellitus,* using Arabic numerals rather than Roman numerals (American Diabetes Association [ADA], 2011). This recommendation was made to improve communication between healthcare providers and patients, to reduce confusion and chance of error resulting from the use of Roman numerals, and to eliminate the artificial designation that occurs from the linkage with the use or nonuse of insulin, because both types of DM may be treated using insulin therapy.

Type 1 DM develops due to B-cell destruction and results in a lack or underproduction of insulin in the body. Type 1 DM can be the result of (1) autoimmune disease in which cell-mediated destruction of the B cells in the pancreas occurs, or (2) idiopathic DM that occurs for no apparent reason. Regardless of cause, patients with type 1 DM are insulin dependent and at risk for ketoacidosis.

Type 2 DM, the most prevalent form of diabetes in all age groups, results from a combination of insulin resistance and an insulin secretory defect. The insulin secretion is insufficient to compensate for the insulin resistance, which occurs in response to decreased insulin effectiveness in stimulating glucose uptake by skeletal muscle and failure to inhibit hepatic glucose production. The body attempts to compensate for rising blood glucose levels by producing more insulin. In some cases, this is adequate and the person does not develop DM. In others, genetic influences may play a role, and heightened insulin production results in hyperinsulinemia. This leads to further insulin resistance, characterized by visceral/abdominal obesity, hypertension, hyperlipidemia, and coronary artery disease along with slightly higher blood glucose levels. This condition has been termed **prediabetes.** Autoimmune destruction of B cells does not occur, ketoacidosis seldom occurs spontaneously, and insulin treatment is often not needed for survival; however, prediabetics have an increased risk of developing type 2 diabetes, heart disease, and stroke. Studies have shown that people with prediabetes who lose weight and increase their physical exercise can prevent or delay type 2 diabetes and in some cases return their blood glucose levels to normal. In 2008, 50% of older adults in the United States were considered prediabetic and the percentages were similar for non-Hispanic Whites, non-Hispanic Blacks, and Mexican Americans (CDC, 2011a).

Risk Factors for Development of Diabetes Mellitus

Patients with type 2 DM are often overweight and have higher percentages of body fat. In some patients, weight may be normal, but the waist-to-hip ratio is increased (greater than 1) as a result of upper body obesity. These patients may go undiagnosed for years because the hyperglycemia develops gradually. Blood glucose levels will decrease and may return to normal when the patient loses weight. A recent study demonstrated that lifestyle modification may delay or prevent the development of type 2 DM in high-risk individuals. In a study following nearly 200,000 older adults of both sexes for a period of 11 years, researchers found that when participants incorporated five lifestyle factors (not smoking, regular physical activity, moderate alcohol intake, healthy diet, and normal body weight) there was a strong reduction in the risk of developing type 2 DM (Reis et al., 2011).

Risk factors for the development of type 2 DM include:

- Age over 45 (the risk of DM increases with age).
- Overweight (body mass index greater than 25) and having a waist-to-hip ratio approaching 1.
- A waist circumference > 94 cm (37 in.) for men and > 80 cm (32 in.) for women represents an increased risk; > 102 cm (40 in.) in men and > 88 cm (35 in.) for women represents a substantially increased risk.
- African American, Hispanic or Latino American, Asian American or Pacific Islander, or Native American ethnicity.
- Parents or siblings with DM.
- Impaired glucose tolerance or impaired fasting glucose levels on laboratory examination.
- History of vascular disease.
- Medication use that may predispose to DM (steroids, atypical antipsychotics, protease inhibitors).
- Blood pressure above 140/90.
- Low levels of good cholesterol (less than 35 for men and less than 40 for women) and high levels of triglycerides (above 250 mg/dL).
- Sedentary lifestyle and exercise less than three times per week.

CDC, 2011a; Diabetes Guidelines Work Group, 2007.

Because older people at risk for development of type 2 DM are at greater risk of cardiovascular disease and other health problems, appropriate screening is indicated. Because one third of people with DM remain undiagnosed, finding and treating DM early may improve health outcomes. Because the early symptoms of DM are often vague and vary from person to person, obtaining measurements of fasting plasma glucose periodically as part of routine health screening in older people at high risk for DM is highly recommended. Early detection and treatment of the disease has great benefit and can delay or prevent the development of secondary complications.

> **Practice Pearl** ▶▶▶ Your patient is at risk for diabetes if he or she reports being tired or hungry, losing weight, urinating frequently, or having blurry vision, slow-healing cuts, and numb or tingling feet. A referral to the primary healthcare provider for a fasting blood glucose test is indicated.

Diagnostic Criteria

When an older person is identified as high risk for diabetes and presents with the symptoms of DM such as polyuria, polydipsia, unexplained weight loss plus a random plasma glucose concentration of >200 mg/dL, appropriate testing includes a fasting plasma glucose (FPG) level (preferred), a 2-hour oral glucose tolerance test (OGTT), and a HbA_{1c}. The FPG is performed by obtaining a blood sample and measuring the person's blood glucose after an overnight fast (8 to 12 hours). The 2-hour OGTT is performed after the overnight fast by measuring the person's blood glucose immediately before and 2 hours after drinking a 75-g glucose solution. The HbA_{1c} level is often obtained at an office or clinic visit without fasting. Generally, a fasting plasma glucose (FPG) of >126 mg/dL (confirmed on two separate occasions), a HbA_{1c} of >6.5%, a random plasma glucose (RPG) of >200 mg/dL and oral glucose tolerance test (OGTT) two-hour readings yielding a plasma glucose of >200 mg/dL is considered diagnostic for diabetes. Prediabetes can be diagnosed with the following laboratory values: HbA_{1c} of 5.7–6.4%, FPG of >100 and <126 mg/dL, and two-hour OGTT readings of >140 mg/dL but <200 mg/dL. Laboratory values are considered within normal limits with the following readings: HbA_{1c} of <5.7%, FPG <100 mg/dL and OGTT readings after two

hours of <140 mg/dL (Diabetes Guidelines Work Group, 2007; National Diabetes Information Clearing House, 2012; Nichols, 2009).

The nurse should inform older adults and their families regarding the need to prepare carefully for the FPG and the 2-hour OGTT and explain how the ingestion of food can raise the blood glucose levels and result in a false-positive diagnosis of DM. People with prediabetes or impaired glucose tolerance are at higher risk of developing DM. Older patients who have fasting blood glucose levels of 100 to 125 mg/dL and 2-hour OGTT levels of 140 to 199 mg/dL or HbA_{1c} levels of 5.7% to 6.4% meet the criteria for diagnosis of prediabetes (ADA, 2011). Use of glucocorticoids, some diuretics, peritoneal dialysis, infection, or an acute event such as myocardial infarction can also elevate blood glucose levels. Elevated blood glucose levels obtained from older adults in these circumstances are not considered diagnostic of DM.

> **Practice Pearl** ▶▶▶ The presence of hyperglycemia does not meet the diagnostic criteria for DM and is referred to as impaired fasting glucose (IFG) or impaired glucose tolerance (IGT). Modest weight loss (5% to 10% of body weight) and increased physical activity (about 150 minutes/week) can delay or prevent the progression to diagnosis with type 2 DM. Lifestyle modification can be more effective than treatment with medication.

Source: Diabetes Guidelines Work Group (2007).

> **Drug Alert** ▶▶▶ Use of glucocorticoids or diuretics can greatly and suddenly increase blood glucose levels both in older patients with DM and in those without DM.

Follow screening with a history, physical examination, and comprehensive geriatric assessment including nutritional status, functional capabilities, and psychosocial issues. Some symptoms of DM in the older person include anorexia, incontinence, falls, pain intolerance, and cognitive or behavioral changes (Green, Bierman, Foody et al., 2009). Older patients with DM may complain of symptoms of hyperglycemia (usually above 200 mg/dL), including polydipsia (excessive thirst), weight loss, polyuria (excessive urination), polyphagia (excessive hunger), blurred vision, fatigue, nausea, and fungal and bacterial infections

(Reuben et al., 2012). Older women may complain of perineal itching due to vaginal candidiasis. Additionally, older women with DM may experience frequent urinary tract infections. However, these signs may not be present at all in many older adults and the diagnosis of DM may be made based almost entirely on results of blood glucose testing.

> **Practice Pearl** ▶▶▶ Cranberry juice may be helpful in prevention of urinary tract infections. It is thought to prevent bacteria from adhering to the lining of the bladder. The optimal dosage remains unclear; however, no adverse effects have been reported with intake of less than 3 L/day (Gutierrez, 2008).

Once DM has been diagnosed, the physician will determine whether the patient has the type 1 or type 2 form. The majority of older people have type 2 DM with gradual onset of symptoms and obesity. The patient with type 1 DM is typically younger than 40, is lean, exhibits a rapid onset of symptoms, and may have ketonuria. However, type 1 DM can occur at any age and in persons who are obese. The onset symptoms of hyperglycemia in the older adult with type 1 DM may occur more slowly and without the presence of **ketones** (a waste product of fat breakdown indicating the body is unable to metabolize blood glucose for energy), making an accurate diagnosis difficult.

Table 19-1 presents the typical history and onset of symptoms common to type 1 and type 2 DM.

The initial physical examination includes blood pressure measurement (including orthostatic changes), weight, dilated retinal examination by an ophthalmologist or eye specialist, cardiovascular examination for evidence of cardiac or peripheral vascular disease, complete skin inspection, and neurologic examination to rule out any peripheral or autonomic neuropathy (Medical Examination.org, 2008). Funduscopic examination may reveal the presence of microaneurysms, hemorrhages, exudates, or increased intraocular pressure indicative of glaucoma. Assess peripheral pulses, capillary filling, and warmth of extremities to indicate the presence of macrovascular pathology. Mental status, deep tendon reflexes, and ability to detect peripheral sensation are key components of

TABLE 19-1	**Typical History of Symptom Onset in Type 1 and Type 2 Diabetes Mellitus**
Type 1	**Type 2**
Sudden onset, severe symptoms	Gradual onset, less severe symptoms
Polyuria, polyphagia, polydipsia	Atypical presentation: weight loss, depression, gastrointestinal problems, incontinence
Weight loss with normal or increased appetite	Gradual weight loss, decreased appetite
Orthostatic hypotension (secondary to dehydration)	Normal blood pressure with orthostatic changes, hyperlipidemia
Blurred vision	Attributes vision changes to aging
Fatigue/weakness	Attributes fatigue/weakness to aging
Nausea/vomiting	Decreased appetite may make presentation more vague
Vaginal itching	Recurrent vaginitis, urinary tract infection, fungal skin infections
Ketones in urine	Protein in urine
Dry, flaky skin	Slow-healing skin ulcerations
Sensation usually intact	Paresthesias

the neurologic examination. A visual foot examination (without shoes and socks) is recommended for every older person with DM initially and at every subsequent clinical visit to the healthcare provider. The nurse should counsel older adults to discontinue smoking, and refer those ready to undertake smoking cessation to ongoing support groups and counseling centers. The nurse should counsel older adults with diabetes who are overweight regarding weight loss.

The following laboratory tests are recommended:

- Thyroid evaluation (thyroid-stimulating hormone and palpation of the thyroid)
- Urinalysis to test for albuminuria, serum creatinine for renal function
- Electrocardiogram if older person has not had one within 10 years
- Electrocardiogram for those diagnosed with DM more than 10 years ago
- Fasting blood glucose and lipid profile to assess cardiovascular risk
- **Glycosylated hemoglobin (HbA_{1c})**

Diabetes Guidelines Work Group, 2007.

The HbA_{1c} is not specific for diagnosing diabetes; however, elevated HbA_{1c} levels confirm the degree of estimated blood glucose control during the past 3 months. The HbA_{1c} test measures how much glucose attaches to the hemoglobin in the red cells. Because the average life of a red cell is about 4 months, the test summarizes how high the glucose levels have been during the life of the cell. Table 19-2 illustrates the relationship between the HbA_{1c} level and average blood sugar readings. The ideal HbA_{1c} goal is less than 7%. Levels of 8% or greater indicate the need to adjust the treatment plan (Diabetes Guidelines Work Group, 2007). The formula for converting A_{1c} levels to average glucose levels is:

$$28.7 \times HbA_{1c} - 46.7 = \text{average blood sugar reading}$$

> **Practice Pearl** ▶▶▶ The HbA_{1c} measurement serves as an excellent marker of disease control and an indicator of risk level for the development of complications.

An in-depth foot examination includes the presence of protective sensation, vascular status, skin integrity, and foot structure. Approximately 15% of all older adults with DM will develop a foot or leg ulcer during the course of their disease. More than 60% of nontraumatic lower limb amputations occur in people with diabetes. In 2004, about 71,000 nontraumatic lower limb amputations were performed in

TABLE 19-2	The Relationship Between the HbA_{1c} Level and Average Blood Sugar Readings
HbA_{1c} Level	**Blood Glucose Test Average**
12	300
11	270
10	240
9	210
8	180
7	150
6	120
5	80

Source: Diabetes Pro (2012); National Institute of Diabetes and Digestive and Kidney Diseases (2008).

people with diabetes (NIDDKD, 2008). Older adults with DM have sensory, motor, and autonomic neuropathies; lower extremity peripheral vascular disease; impaired host defenses against infection; and delayed wound healing. When a diabetic ulcer occurs, ischemia, neuropathy, and infection delay healing and raise the risk of complications.

A monofilament or a tuning fork can be used to assess for the presence of protective sensation that can alert the older person to the development of a blister or foot ulcer. It is recommended that a visual examination of the diabetic foot be conducted at each healthcare encounter and a more in-depth inspection be done annually. Saving the diabetic foot and preventing amputation requires the following:

- Identification of feet at risk
- Prevention of foot ulcers
- Early treatment of foot ulcers
- Prevention of recurrence of foot ulcers

Dunphy, Winland-Brown, Porter et al., 2011.

The older person can be classified as high or low risk depending on the outcome of the foot examination. The nurse should follow the foot status of high-risk older adults closely, teach preventive self-care of the feet, and refer for therapeutic shoes and footwear. A small mirror placed on or near the floor (like those in a shoe store) can assist older adults to monitor and inspect their own feet. After sitting in a chair, shoes and socks are removed

The sensory testing device used to complete a foot examination is a 10-gram (5.07 Semmes-Weinstein) nylon filament mounted on a holder that has been standardized to deliver a 10-gram force when properly applied. Research has shown that a person who can feel the 10-gram filament in the selected sites is at reduced risk for developing ulcers.

- ■ The sensory examination should be done in a quiet and relaxed setting. The patient must not watch while the examiner applies the filament.
- ■ Test the monofilament on the patient's hand so he or she knows what to anticipate.
- ■ The five sites to be tested are indicated on the screening form.
- ■ Apply the monofilament perpendicular to the skin's surface (see diagram A below).
- ■ Apply sufficient force to cause the filament to bend or buckle (see diagram B below).
- ■ The total duration of the approach, skin contact, and departure of the filament should be approximately 1½ seconds.
- ■ Apply the filament along the perimeter and *not on* an ulcer site, callus, scar, or necrotic tissue. Do not allow the filament to slide across the skin or make repetitive contact at the test site.
- ■ Press the filament to the skin such that it buckles at one of two times as you say "time one" or "time two." Have patients identify at which time they were touched. Randomize the sequence of applying the filament throughout the examination.

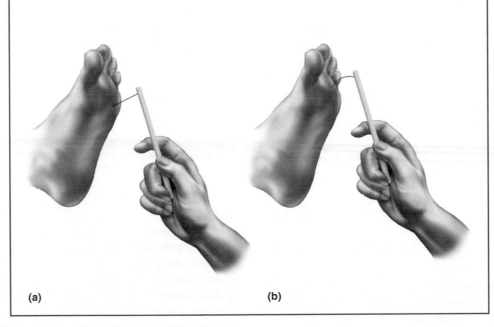

(a)   (b)

Figure 19-4 ▶▶▶ Foot inspection and monofilament use for sensory foot examination.

Source: National Diabetes Education Program (2011).

and the feet are raised in front of the mirror to inspect the heels, toes, and dorsal aspects. The nurse should educate older adults with DM to not attempt to cut their own toenails because of the risk of cutting their skin. Rather, they should see the podiatrist on a regular basis for toenail care and cutting. Figure 19-4 ▶▶▶ illustrates the procedure for foot inspection and monofilament use for sensory foot examination.

Practice Pearl ▶▶▶ Podiatry services including routine foot care, trimming of toenails, and in some cases, purchase of therapeutic shoes are covered by Medicare in older adults who have been diagnosed with DM. The nurse should make sure the diagnosis of DM is carefully noted on the problem list to ensure this important service is covered (Medical Learning Network, 2007).

Use a nylon filament to test an older person's foot for sensation. Older adults who can sense that their foot is being touched with the monofilament have protective sensation. Additional nursing assessments include using a 128-cps tuning fork to assess vibratory sensation in the feet and checking peripheral pulses including the dorsalis pedis, posterior tibial, popliteal, and femoral pulses. Loss of vibration and diminished pulses may indicate early findings of neuropathy and circulatory impairment. When protective sensation is lost and the skin is broken, whether by an ulcer or a blister, bacteria and fungi can enter the skin. The older person with neuropathy may not feel the infection until it is well established. Peripheral vascular disease makes healing less likely (NIDDKD, 2005).

Practice Pearl ▶▶▶ Foot care in the older person with DM includes hygiene and protection. It is important to lubricate dry areas with lotion, carefully dry moist areas (between toes), and care for the nails. Urge older adults with DM to not cut their own toenails, see the podiatrist regularly, and use an emery board to keep nails short and smooth between visits.

In addition to the history and physical examination, nursing assessment of older adults with DM includes the following components:

- Nutritional assessment
- Medication review
- Functional assessment
- Psychosocial assessment
- Gait and balance evaluation

Complications of DM can develop at an accelerated rate in older adults because of poor glycemic control. The principal goals of therapy are to enhance quality of life, decrease chance of complications, improve self-care through education, and maintain or improve general health status (Dunphy et al., 2011). The approach the nurse selects should be individualized and take into account life expectancy, coexisting illness, functional capability, level of independence, disease trajectory, and economic and social considerations.

Therapeutic Management

The goals of management of DM in the older person include achieving normal or near-normal blood glucose levels through self-management techniques, including self-monitoring of blood glucose levels; recognition, treatment, and prevention of hypoglycemia; prevention, early detection, and treatment of chronic complications; nutrition therapy; regular physical activity; and provision of continuing education (Diabetes Guidelines Work Group, 2007).

HEALTHY AGING TIPS TO AVOID DIABETES MELLITUS

1. Eat more nutritious food with fewer calories.
2. Achieve and maintain a healthy weight. Stay active by engaging in regular physical exercise. Don't smoke.
3. Limit your intake of sugar, fat, salt, caffeine, alcohol, and soft drinks.
4. Eat regular, balanced meals that include the four food groups (grain products, vegetables and fruit, milk products, meat and alternatives).
5. Keep cholesterol to a minimum and maintain a normal blood pressure.

The goals must reflect the fact that older adults with DM have varying degrees of frailty, differences in underlying chronic conditions, varying degrees of DM-related comorbidity, and highly variable life expectancies. In general, the more functional the older person and the longer the life expectancy, the more aggressively the DM will be treated by the healthcare provider to decrease the probability of DM-related complications. If an older person is close to death from cancer or other chronic illness, they often become anorexic with increased risk of hypoglycemic episodes. Therefore, the multiple insulin injections and frequent (four to six times per day) blood glucose monitoring may not be justified and the standard of care changes from tight glycemic control to maintenance of comfort and enhancement of quality of life (Ferrell & Coyle, 2010). Likewise, any older person with frequent and severe hypoglycemia will require less intensive glycemic goals (Diabetes Guidelines Work Group, 2007). Hypoglycemic events in the older person are associated with cardiovascular events, stroke, impaired cognition, and falls (American College of Physicians, 2007). Older adults are more likely to have neurologic symptoms related to hypoglycemia such as dizziness, weakness, and mental status changes as opposed to the tremor, palpitations, and sweating typically seen in middle-aged or younger adults. As a result, hypoglycemic episodes in the older person may be undiagnosed or diagnosed as a primary neurologic event (American College of Physicians, 2007). A less aggressive approach may be indicated because the dangers of hypoglycemia may be more serious and significant than the worry of hyperglycemia complications.

> **Practice Pearl** ▶▶▶ Special considerations are needed when establishing goals of glycemic control for frail older adults. Consult the geriatric interdisciplinary team for input into the discussion.

For highly functional older adults with good vision, manual dexterity, and cognitive function, a more aggressive management plan can be implemented with support from the primary healthcare provider, the nurse, and the family. Aggressive glycemic control decreases microvascular complications of DM, but also increases the risk of hypoglycemic episodes. Older people who live alone, those with cognitive or physical deficits, or those with serious underlying chronic illnesses are more likely to suffer serious consequences from hypoglycemic episodes, including falls, disorientation, metabolic problems, and dehydration.

The goals of therapy for the highly functional older person include the following:

	Normal	Goal
Preprandial plasma glucose	<100 mg/dL	80–120 mg/dL
Bedtime plasma glucose	<110 mg/dL	100–140 mg/dL
Peak postprandial (2-hour) plasma glucose	<120 mg/dL	<180 mg/dL
AIC	<6%	<7%

Source: Reuben et al. (2012). *Geriatrics at your fingertips.* 14th ed. New York: The American Geriatrics Society.

The goals of therapy for the older person with advanced microvascular complications (neuropathy or retinopathy), cognitive deficits, serious associated cardiovascular problems, frailty, high risk for hypoglycemia, polypharmacy, or drug interactions or those diagnosed with underlying serious illness are more conservative and set the target for the HbA_{1c} at under 8%. Intensive control of DM to a HbA_{1c} level of under 6.5% reduces the likelihood of nephropathy but does not improve macrovascular events such as stroke and heart attack, causes more hypoglycemia, and may increase overall mortality (Reuben et al., 2012).

Figure 19-5 ▶▶▶ illustrates a glucometer used to test blood sugar. Equipment and techniques vary. Visit the American Diabetes Association website for a full description of

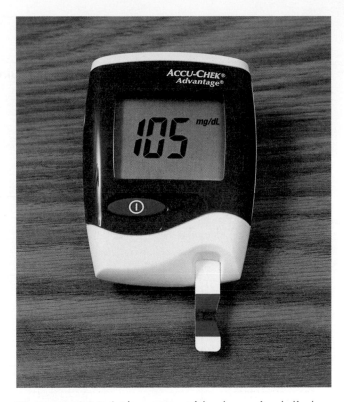

Figure 19-5 ▶▶▶ A glucometer with a large visual display.
Source: Michal Heron/Pearson Education/PH College.

glucometers that function in high- and low-temperature environments, have backlighting and a large display area for people with visual impairments, have an audio capability for the blind, or have large amounts of memory for storing results. Well-cared-for glucometers can last for years and should maintain their accuracy when used with in-date test strips. If doubt about accuracy exists, ask the patient to bring his or her glucometer to the laboratory for the next scheduled fasting blood sugar and perform simultaneous testing with the glucometer at the time of the blood draw to check for accuracy when the laboratory test results are returned.

Teach older adults to perform blood glucose testing and to keep track of their readings using a daily log. This log will provide feedback to the older person and guide day-to-day choices regarding exercise, food, and medication. The finger or forearm is pricked with a lancet, and a drop of blood is placed on a test strip and read by the machine. The normal readings and treatment goals (70 to 140 mg/dL) should be clearly written in the log book for easy referral. Newer glucometers have large digital readouts, making them easier for older adults to read. The sample daily diabetes record shown in Figure 19-6 ▶▶▶ illustrates the kind of information to be recorded and shared with the healthcare provider.

Daily Diabetes Record

Week Starting _____

	Other Blood Glucose	Breakfast Blood Glucose	Medicine	Lunch Blood Glucose	Medicine	Dinner Blood Glucose	Medicine	Bedtime Blood Glucose	Medicine	Notes: (Special events, sick days, exercise)
Monday										
Tuesday										
Wednesday										
Thursday										
Friday										
Saturday										
Sunday										

Figure 19-6 ▶▶▶ Sample daily diabetes record.
Source: NIDDK (2004).

Controlling DM in the older person requires intervention in several areas: weight management, appropriate use of medications, aggressive management of comorbid conditions, and prevention of complications. There is an increased obesity and lipid abnormality risk independent of glycemic control in type 2 DM. The low-density lipoprotein (LDL) goal for older adults is less than 100 mg/dL. A second goal is to raise high-density lipoprotein (HDL) to greater than 45 mg/dL in men and greater than 55 mg/dL in women. Control of hypertension reduces the progression rate of diabetic nephropathy, cardiovascular disease, and cerebrovascular disease. A desired blood pressure reading is below 130/80. Monitor postural blood pressure readings in older adults to prevent falls and dizziness during and immediately after changes in position (Dunphy et al., 2011).

> **Practice Pearl** ▶▶▶ For younger and healthier older adults with BMI > 35 who have type 2 DM and who cannot lose weight with healthy eating and increased activity, consider recommending a consultation for bariatric surgery (Reuben et al., 2012).

Weight Management

The nutrition goals for the older person with DM include maintenance of near-normal blood glucose levels, achievement of optimal serum lipid levels, provision of adequate caloric intake to attain or maintain normal weight, prevention and treatment of complications, and improvement of overall health through optimal nutrition (McPhee & Papadakis, 2011). For older adults with obesity and DM, weight loss is encouraged. Insulin sensitivity increases when older adults who are obese begin to lose weight. When insulin sensitivity is improved, medication doses may be lowered and blood glucose levels are more responsive to medications. A registered dietitian can provide advice on meal planning that is consistent with the cultural, social, and energy requirements of the older person. The recommendations should also address associated risk factors such as elevated lipids, protein and calcium requirements, and sodium restrictions. Ideally, the older person with DM should attempt to keep blood glucose levels stable throughout the day by eating smaller portions of carbohydrates and fats at mealtime and scheduling snacks during peak times of insulin or oral hypoglycemic medication action. The federal government's MyPlate food guide is a good starting point for educating the older person regarding healthy eating (see Chapter 5 ▭ for more information on nutrition and diabetes).

The nurse should teach older adults with diabetes to eat at regular times and not skip meals, and to take snacks at the same time each day. The nurse should encourage them to eat a variety of foods to keep the meal plan interesting and to meet nutritional needs. Once the older person becomes skilled at choosing healthy foods that are consistent with nutritional needs and blood glucose control, nutritional status and overall health often improve. A sample daily menu for the older person with DM is shown in Figure 19-7 ▶▶▶.

Additional nutritional guidelines for older adults with DM include:

- **Eat less fat.** Avoid fried foods and trans fat. Choose baked, broiled, grilled, or steamed foods to reduce fat. Eat two or more servings of fish per week. Limit dietary cholesterol to less than 200 mg/day. Choose reduced-fat dairy products. Limit fat to less than 30% of total calories, saturated fat to less than 7% of calories, and monounsaturated fat to between 10% and 15% of calories.
- **Eat less sugar.** Read the labels on jars, cans, and food packages before buying them. If one of the first four ingredients is dextrose, sucrose, corn sweeteners, honey, molasses, or sugar, try to find a less-sweetened substitute. Try to avoid highly sweetened cereal, cakes, pastries, and candy.
- **Eat less salt.** Taste food before salting it. Use additional spices when cooking food. Cut down on processed foods and salty snacks. Try to consume no more than 3 g of sodium daily. For persons with hypertension, the goal is 2 g or less.
- **Eat foods with higher fiber.** High-fiber foods improve glycemic control and decrease hyperinsulinemia. Because foods high in fiber take longer to be digested and absorbed, postprandial hyperglycemia is decreased and medications can work more effectively. Try to consume 20 to 35 g dietary fiber from soluble and insoluble fiber sources daily including cereal, whole-grain products, fruits, and vegetables.
- **Avoid or reduce alcohol.** Alcohol can cause problems for people with DM. In addition to adding empty calories, it can interact with diabetic medications. An occasional drink can be incorporated into meal plans with the guidance of a dietitian. It is recommended that older adults with DM consume no more than two drinks per day for men and no more than one drink per day for women (one alcoholic beverage is 12 oz of beer, 5 oz of wine, or 1.5 oz of distilled spirits). Alcohol must be consumed with food to prevent hypoglycemia, and calories from alcohol must be calculated as part of the total caloric intake and are best substituted for fat calories (Diabetes Guidelines Work Group, 2007).
- **Limit protein intake to about 20% of daily energy intake.** Include meat, fish, eggs, cheese, milk, and soy. High-protein diets for weight loss are not recommended (ADA, 2008).

Physical exercise slows the progression of DM, improves weight control, and maintains overall function. Older patients should set a goal of achieving and maintaining a normal body mass index (BMI) of 18.5 to 24.9 kg/m^2. Regular physical activity is encouraged for all older people with DM

Meal	Food Example
Breakfast	
3 carbohydrate servings	1/2 grapefruit
0–1 meat servings	1/2 cup cooked oatmeal
0–1 fat servings	1 cup low-fat milk
Lunch	
3–4 carbohydrate servings	1 cup chicken noodle soup
2–3 meat servings	1 oz sliced chicken or turkey
0–1 fat servings	1 slice whole wheat bread
	1 serving of fresh fruit
Afternoon Snack	
1 carbohydrate serving	1 low-fat granola bar or 1 cup cereal with
0–1 fat servings	low-fat milk
Evening Meal	
3–4 carbohydrate servings	1 slice whole wheat bread with 1 pat of margarine
3–4 meat servings	1 cup vegetable of choice
1–2 fat servings	3–4 oz lean meat or fish
	1/2 cup low-fat cottage cheese or yogurt
	1 serving of fresh fruit
Evening Snack	
2 carbohydrate servings	1 cup low-fat milk
1 fat serving	1 serving low-calorie cookie (ginger snap)

Figure 19-7 ▶▶▶ A sample daily menu for the older patient with DM.

Source: Adapted from Blair, E. (1999). Diabetes in the Older Adult. Advance for NPs and PAs. Retrieved from http://nurse-practitioners-and-physician-assistants.advanceweb.com/Article/Diabetes-in-the-Older-Adult.aspx.

and should be begun slowly and built up gradually. Regular exercise can reduce cardiovascular risk factors, decrease risk of falls, improve functional capacity, and improve blood glucose control. Sedentary older adults should avoid strenuous exercise because of the risk of injury, retinal detachment, or vitreous hemorrhage but resistance training and moderate activity are recommended. After initial medical evaluation, the current recommendation is for 150 minutes of moderate intensity activity per week such as brisk walking. For functional older adults, additional exercise to improve flexibility and strength training is encouraged (American Association of Clinical Endocrinologists [AACE], 2011a; Diabetes Guidelines Work Group, 2007). Because of marked improvement in glycemic control in people who are morbidly obese, bariatric surgery should be considered in those older adults with BMIs of >35 kg/m^2 who have tried and failed numerous weight loss attempts and are able to tolerate anesthesia and surgical intervention (ADA, 2008).

Older adults taking insulin who engage in strenuous physical exercise may suffer from hypoglycemia, primarily because absorption from the injection site increases and metabolism also increases. Older adults taking insulin should check their blood glucose levels before exercising and eat additional carbohydrates if their glucose levels are below 100 mg/dL prior to exercise. Monitoring blood glucose before and after exercise helps to identify necessary changes in insulin or food intake. The goal is to adjust the insulin and food regimen to allow safe participation in exercise; an individualized exercise plan is needed based on the older patient's unique metabolic requirements. To avoid hypoglycemia, the older person may have carbohydrate foods available during and after exercise. The older person should avoid exercise if fasting glucose levels are poorly controlled because of the risks of hypo- and hyperglycemia.

Older adults with DM are advised to obtain a detailed medical evaluation before beginning an exercise program, including medical history, physical examination, diagnostic studies, and screening for heart disease (AACE, 2011a). The healthcare provider may obtain a graded exercise test or radionuclide stress test to assess cardiac function. Recommended exercises include walking, swimming, bicycling, rowing, chair exercises, arm exercises, and other non–weight-bearing exercises. Strenuous exercise such as prolonged walking, treadmill use, jogging, or step exercise should be avoided in those older adults with significant peripheral neuropathies (AACE, 2011a).

Walking or swimming three times a week for 30 minutes is a good way to keep or become more active. An older person who has not been physically active is urged to begin gradually. If there is doubt about strength and endurance, advice from the physical therapist and primary healthcare provider is helpful. The nurse should urge the older person to begin a form of exercise that is acceptable and safe. If walking is chosen, a safe place to walk and good footwear are essential. When older people walk outside during the winter months in northern climates, they risk falling on ice or snow. Additional hazards include uneven sidewalks, cold weather, and criminal activity. Some older adults engage in mall walking. Usually malls are warm, well lit, and have security personnel, so they are ideal places for older people to engage in physical activity. As they grow in strength, older adults are encouraged to add a minute or two of activity to their daily exercise. Older people who are already active are encouraged to maintain and even increase their activity levels. If they experience pain, shortness of breath, or dizziness, they should stop and wait until the feeling subsides. The nurse should refer older adults with recurrent symptoms of exercise intolerance such as shortness of breath, chest pain, and excessive fatigue for evaluation by the healthcare provider because underlying undiagnosed heart disease may be responsible for these symptoms.

Gerontological nurses may encourage older adults to begin walking by teaching them and their families the benefits of regular activity. Education enables people with DM to participate more actively in their treatment and prevention of complications. The nurse should present diabetes education simply and in a straightforward manner. As time progresses, the instruction defines and addresses the individual needs of the older person and his or her family. For example, the nurse may educate the older person regarding the benefits of walking.

Walking is one of the easiest ways to be active. It can be done almost anywhere and anytime. The older person can purchase a good pair of walking shoes and then may enjoy the following benefits:

- Increased energy
- Reduced stress
- Improved sleep
- Toned muscles
- Controlled appetite
- Increased number of calories burned daily
- Prevention of complications of diabetes

Diabetes Guidelines Work Group, 2007.

The nurse should integrate the walking program into the older person's schedule in a way that will work best. Recommendations by the nurse may include the following actions:

- Choose a safe place to walk and find a partner or exercise group at about the same fitness level to walk with.
- Wear shoes with thick, flexible soles to cushion each step and absorb shock. (Figure 19-8 ▶▶▶ illustrates

---

Improper or poorly fitting shoes are major contributors to diabetes foot ulcerations. Counsel patients about appropriate footwear. All patients with diabetes need to pay special attention to the fit and style of their shoes and should avoid pointed-toe shoes or high heels. Properly fitted athletic or walking shoes are recommended for daily wear. If off-the-shelf shoes are used, make sure that there is room to accommodate any deformities.

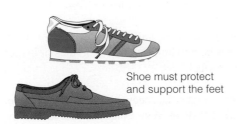
Shoe must protect and support the feet

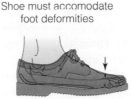
Shoe must accommodate foot deformities

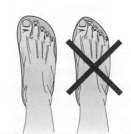
Shoe shape must match foot shape

High-risk patients may require therapeutic shoes, depth-inlay shoes, custom-molded inserts (orthoses), or custom-molded shoes, depending on the degree of foot deformity and history of ulceration.

Figure 19-8 ▶▶▶ Guidelines for footwear assessment.
Source: NDEP (2011).

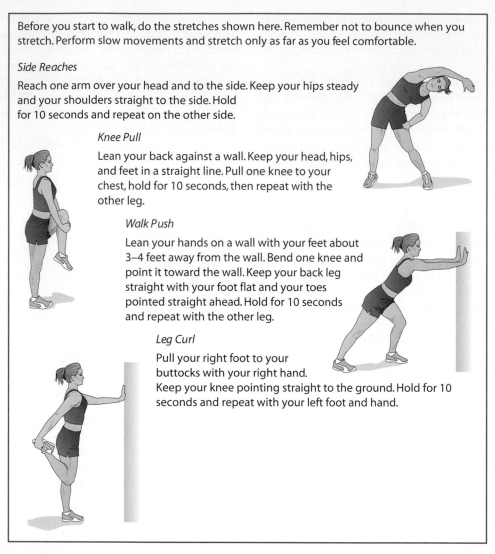

Before you start to walk, do the stretches shown here. Remember not to bounce when you stretch. Perform slow movements and stretch only as far as you feel comfortable.

Side Reaches

Reach one arm over your head and to the side. Keep your hips steady and your shoulders straight to the side. Hold for 10 seconds and repeat on the other side.

Knee Pull

Lean your back against a wall. Keep your head, hips, and feet in a straight line. Pull one knee to your chest, hold for 10 seconds, then repeat with the other leg.

Walk Push

Lean your hands on a wall with your feet about 3–4 feet away from the wall. Bend one knee and point it toward the wall. Keep your back leg straight with your foot flat and your toes pointed straight ahead. Hold for 10 seconds and repeat with the other leg.

Leg Curl

Pull your right foot to your buttocks with your right hand. Keep your knee pointing straight to the ground. Hold for 10 seconds and repeat with your left foot and hand.

Figure 19-9 ▶▶▶ Warm-up exercises to prepare the older person with diabetes for walking.

Source: NDEP (2011).

factors to be considered when an older person with DM is being fitted for shoes.)

- Wear clothes that are dry and comfortable. Dress in layers so that a jacket or coat can be removed to prevent overheating.
- Think of the walk in three parts. Walk slowly for 5 minutes, and subsequently increase the speed for 5 minutes. Slow the pace at the end of the walk for 15 minutes to cool down.
- Try to walk at least three to five times per week. Add 2 to 3 minutes per week to the walk.
- Start slowly to avoid stiff muscles and joints. Work up gradually and increase distance and pace slowly. Engage in warm-up exercises. Figure 19-9 ▶▶▶ illustrates

warm-up exercises, and Figure 19-10 ▶▶▶ gives guidelines for how to build up to 30 minutes of brisk walking 5 days a week.

Bariatric surgery has been increasingly recommended for those with a BMI of more than 35 (morbid obesity). Older adults who are morbidly obese and also have DM are at risk for many health complications including cardiovascular disease, mobility problems, depression, lipid disorders, and worsening DM. Bariatric surgery is not without risk; however, DM and hypertension improve rapidly as weight loss progresses. Because of the risks of surgery and anesthesia, bariatric surgery is the intervention of last resort, while

first step	A sample walking program			
	Warm Up Time	Fast Walk Time	Cool Down Time	Total time
	Week 1			
	Walk slowly 5 min.	Walk briskly 5 min.	Walk slowly 5 min.	15 min.
	Week 2			
	Walk slowly 5 min.	Walk briskly 8 min.	Walk slowly 5 min.	18 min.
	Week 3			
	Walk slowly 5 min.	Walk briskly 11 min.	Walk slowly 5 min.	21 min.
	Week 4			
	Walk slowly 5 min.	Walk briskly 14 min.	Walk slowly 5 min.	24 min.
	Week 5			
	Walk slowly 5 min.	Walk briskly 17 min.	Walk slowly 5 min.	27 min.
	Week 6			
	Walk slowly 5 min.	Walk briskly 20 min.	Walk slowly 5 min.	30 min.
	Week 7			
	Walk slowly 5 min.	Walk briskly 23 min.	Walk slowly 5 min.	33 min.
	Week 8			
	Walk slowly 5 min.	Walk briskly 26 min.	Walk slowly 5 min.	36 min.
	Week 9 & Beyond			
	Walk slowly 5 min.	Walk briskly 30 min.	Walk slowly 5 min.	40 min.

Walking right is very important.

Walk with your chin up and your shoulder held slightly back.
Walk so that the heel of your foot touches the ground first. Roll your weight forward.
Walk with your toes pointed forward.
Swing your arms as you walk.

If you walk less than three times per week, increase the fast walk time more slowly.

Figure 19-10 ▶▶▶ A sample walking program.
Source: NDEP (2011).

lifestyle modifications such as consuming a healthy diet and engaging in regular exercise remain the interventions of choice.

The nurse can help the older person to set realistic goals and not to be discouraged if progress proceeds more slowly than anticipated. Beginning a regular activity program involves a major lifestyle modification. Most older adults will need ongoing support and encouragement before they finally incorporate this healthy habit into their lifestyle.

Medications Used to Control DM

Pharmacologic therapy is recommended for older adults who have been unable to achieve optimal blood glucose control after 6 months of intensive lifestyle modification (exercise and improved diet); have symptomatic hyperglycemia; are ketotic; and/or have concurrent illness, medications, or surgery that worsen glycemic control (Diabetes Guidelines Work Group, 2007). Oral hypoglycemic drugs are used for type 2 DM only. Single or combination drugs can result in good glycemic control and have been used successfully for years. However, newer drugs have emerged during the past 10 years. Each medication addresses a different glycemic problem, and they can be used as monotherapy or in combination with other drugs.

Oral antidiabetic drugs include the following:

■ Sulfonylureas, meglitinide analogs, d-phenylalanine derivatives, GLP-1 receptor agonists, and DPP-4 inhibitors (to stimulate insulin release from the pancreatic B cells)

- Biguanides (primary action is on the liver, reducing hepatic glucose production)
- Thiazolidinediones, alpha-glucosidase inhibitors (to sensitize peripheral tissues to insulin and slow digestion, delaying absorption of carbohydrates)

The oldest class of oral hypoglycemic drugs is the sulfonylureas, and these drugs have been improved during the past 20 years to increase their effectiveness. These second-generation sulfonylureas stimulate the beta cells in the pancreas to secrete insulin. They are effective drugs that depend on the presence of functioning pancreatic beta cells, but sometimes can stimulate the release of too much insulin, resulting in hypoglycemia, hunger, and weight gain. Approximately 60% to 70% of older adults with type 2 DM respond to sulfonylurea therapy resulting in a fasting blood sugar (FBS) of 60 to 70 mg/dL and lowered HbA_{1c} level by 1% to 2% (Reuben et al., 2012). Hypoglycemia can be especially dangerous in the older adult and occurs most often with long-acting sulfonylureas (glyburide). Sulfonylurea-induced hypoglycemia can be severe and last or recur for days after treatment is stopped. All older adults treated with sulfonylureas who develop hypoglycemia should be closely monitored for 2 to 3 days and have their doses of medication carefully evaluated. The extended-release formulations offer the advantage of simplifying dosing to once a day. Because they contain sulfa, these drugs are contraindicated in older adults who are allergic to sulfa.

Metformin is a biguanide introduced in 1994 that improves insulin sensitivity and achieves potent antihyperglycemic properties by enhancing glucose uptake and use by the muscles (McPhee & Papadakis, 2011). Additional benefits include mild weight loss and favorable changes in lipid profiles for older adults with high lipid levels (decreasing LDL and triglycerides) and as such metformin is a first-line therapy. Gastrointestinal side effects are common during initial dosing but are usually mild and resolve spontaneously. Metformin should not be used by older adults over age 80 or those with renal insufficiency (serum creatinine above 1.4 in women and above 1.5 in men) (Reuben et al., 2012). Metformin reduces FBS by 50 to 70 mg/dL and HbA_{1c} levels by 1% to 2%. Additionally, metformin does not cause weight gain. In contrast with oral antihyperglycemics, these drugs rarely cause hypoglycemia and may be safer for older adults. Metformin therapy should be temporarily stopped on the day patients are scheduled to receive radiocontrast agents and for 2 days afterward to prevent lactic acidosis and acute renal failure (McPhee & Papadakis, 2011).

Alpha-glucosidase inhibitors decrease postprandial hyperglycemia by slowing digestion and delaying intestinal absorption of carbohydrates. These drugs are helpful in older adults who exhibit baseline blood glucose levels in the normal range but become hyperglycemic immediately after eating a meal. Alpha-glucosidase inhibitors reduce FBS levels by 35 to 40 mg/dL and HbA_{1c} levels by 0.5% to 1% (Reuben et al., 2012). Alpha-glucosidase inhibitors do not cause insulin secretion or hypoglycemia when administered as monotherapy. The major side effects of these drugs are gastrointestinal and include flatulence, bloating, and diarrhea as a result of undigested carbohydrate reaching the lower bowel, so many older adults wish to discontinue taking these medications (McPhee & Papadakis, 2011). Sometimes starting at a low dose and slowly titrating up to the therapeutic dose will minimize adverse effects.

Thiazolidinediones were introduced in 1997 with troglitazone (Rezulin). This drug was withdrawn in 2000 after it was associated with several deaths and liver failure resulting from hepatotoxicity. Since then, new thiazolidinediones have been approved (Actos and Avandia) and both of these medications have been combined with metformin for a combination drug; however, safety concerns and troublesome side effects continue to emerge that potentially limit their use. These drugs enhance insulin sensitivity through activation of intracellular receptors and also suppress hepatic glucose production. Absolute contraindications include active liver disease (alanine aminotransferase [ALT] more than 2.5 times the upper limit of normal) and congestive heart failure (New York Heart Association [NYHA] Class III or IV) (Reuben et al., 2012). Regular monitoring of liver function tests is recommended at baseline and every 2 months for the first year and periodically thereafter. An additional side effect is weight gain. Recently, Avandia has been linked with a significant increase in the risk of angina and/or myocardial infarction and an increased risk of death from all cardiovascular causes (McPhee & Papadakis, 2011). This may be related to the increased cholesterol readings associated with this drug. Additionally, increases in fluid retention may be related to increases in heart failure, prompting the FDA to request manufacturers place a "black box" warning. However, at this time older adults are urged to continue taking this medication and it has not been withdrawn from the market. These drugs reduce FBS levels by 25 to 50 mg/dL and decrease HbA_{1c} levels by 0.5% to 1.5% (Reuben et al., 2012).

Another class of oral hypoglycemics is the meglitinides. Drugs in this class are insulin secretagogues and act by stimulating insulin release in response to a meal. Although they are considered rapid-onset drugs, their duration of action is short and they must be taken with each meal for maximum effect. These drugs offer flexibility for older adults who do not eat regularly scheduled meals and are appropriate for older adults with high postprandial glucose levels. These drugs should not be taken without food (Reuben et al., 2012). The meglitinides lower FBS levels by 65 to 76 mg/dL and reduce HbA_{1c} by 1.0% to 2%.

The final class of drugs includes injectable and oral drugs in the DPP-4 category. These drugs stimulate insulin release from the pancreas by binding to a membrane receptor and may be used alone or in combination with other drugs. Because this class of drug is new and many are still in development, long-term outcome data are not available in clinical trials with older adults. Side effects include nausea, hypoglycemia, weight gain, acute pancreatitis, headache, pharyngitis, and upper respiratory and urinary tract infections (McPhee & Papadakis, 2011). HbA_{1c} levels are lowered from 0.4% to 1%.

Some older adults take combination drugs such as glyburide-metformin (Glucovance), glipizide-metformin (Metaglip), and repaglinide-metformin (PrandiMet). These drugs simplify the dosing requirements and may be less expensive than taking each of the combined drugs individually. They combine drugs with different mechanisms of action to achieve better basal glucose levels and prevent postprandial peaks. However, the use of combination drugs incurs more risk in the older person. If an adverse effect occurs, it may not be clear which drug in the combination is responsible. Further, drug combinations limit the clinician's ability to optimally adjust the dosage of each individual drug and for that reason are not recommended (McPhee & Papadakis, 2011). Extra caution and monitoring are needed to prevent hypoglycemia and ensure success with combination medications. Table 19-3 illustrates the commonly used medications and their starting and maximum doses.

Drug Alert ▶▶▶ Metformin is associated with lactic acidosis and acute renal failure when intravenous iodinated contrast material is given for radiologic studies. It is recommended that metformin be withheld for 48 hours prior to testing and be restarted after the procedure once kidney function has been evaluated and found to be within normal limits (Reuben et al., 2012).

Insulin

Insulin is used alone in type 1 DM and may be used alone or in combination with oral hypoglycemic medications in type 2 DM whose hyperglycemia does not respond to diet therapy either alone or combined with other hypoglycemic drugs (McPhee & Papadakis, 2011). Although most older adults with type 2 DM will not need insulin, it may be used in any older person whose diabetes cannot

be adequately controlled with oral agents alone. Insulin is injected with special insulin syringes. The 0.5-mL syringes are preferred by older adults who inject doses of 50 units or less, because these syringes facilitate the accurate measurement of smaller insulin doses. A multiple-dose insulin injection device (e.g., Novolin Pen) uses a cartridge containing several days' dosage. The accuracy and ease of use of the insulin pen is ideal for some older adults. Insulin should be refrigerated but never frozen. Most insulin is stable at room temperature and will safely last about a month, but it should not be stored near a heat source or transported in an overheated car or trunk (ADA, 2012). If extra bottles of insulin are stored in the refrigerator, take the bottle out ahead of time and allow it to come to room temperature to avoid painful injections with cold insulin. For older adults with visual difficulties, magnifying glasses can be helpful, or the medication can be drawn up by the visiting nurse or a family member. Use prefilled syringes within a week.

As with oral hypoglycemics, the insulin regimen mimics normal physiology with control of both basal and postprandial glucose levels. Long-acting insulin controls blood glucose levels and uses glucose as a fuel long after the meal has been digested (basal insulin). Short-acting insulin satisfies the need for insulin after meals or ingestion of food and is usually injected around mealtime. Newer insulins are made from recombinant DNA and do not require extraction from the pancreas of animals. Animal insulins are no longer available in the United States (McPhee & Papadakis, 2011). Lispro (Humalog), aspart (NovoLog), and glulisine (Apidra) are rapid-acting insulins with onset of action within 15 to 30 minutes. They are usually injected several times daily immediately prior to eating a meal. Longer-acting insulins such as glargine (Lantus) are designed to release insulin evenly throughout the day and control basal glucose levels. Lantus cannot be mixed with other insulins because of its acidic pH. Older adults who take Lantus experience less overnight hypoglycemia compared to those using NPH (McPhee & Papadakis, 2011).

Drug Alert ▶▶▶ Lipodystrophy occurs as a result of insulin impurity or poor injection technique. Rotate insulin injection sites and avoid injecting insulin directly into one of these fatty thickenings, as absorption can be delayed.

Mixtures of insulin preparations with different onsets and durations of action are often given in a single injection to simplify the dosing and better control blood glucose levels. These insulin combinations are more suitable for older

TABLE 19-3 **Oral Hypoglycemic Medications**

Class	Generic Name Strength	Trade Name®	Usual Dosage	Comments Regular testing of blood glucose and A_{1c} is recommended to assess medication effect.
Biguanides	metformin 500, 850, 1000 metformin extended-release (ER) 500, 750 mg	Glucophage Glucophage XR	500–2550 mg 1500–2000 mg q pm	Decreases hepatic glucose production and increases insulin sensitivity. When used as monotherapy, does not cause hypoglycemia. Take with food to lessen gastrointestinal (GI) side effects. Do not use with impaired renal or hepatic function. Hold for iodinated contrast study. Start at 500 mg bid or 850 mg daily, increase 500 mg weekly or 850 mg every 2 weeks. Max 2550 mg/day; however, most studies show little benefit over 2000 mg/day. Start dose low and titrate slowly to minimize GI effects. The ER formulation may be given once daily. Do not crush. Monitor serum creatinine (SCr) level at baseline and at least yearly, more often if indicated. Discontinue if age greater than 80 or SCr is > 1.5 in males and 1.4 in females. Hold if dehydrated or septic; increases risk of lactic acidosis. Potential for vitamin B_{12} deficiency.
Second-generation sulfonylureas (First-generation sulfonylureas are no longer used due to their adverse effect profiles.)	glipizide 5, 10 mg	Glucotrol	2.5–40 mg daily to bid	Stimulates pancreatic islet beta-cell insulin release. Start at 5 mg daily or 2.5 mg daily if an older adult. The ER formulation may allow for once daily dosing. For non-ER form, divide doses > 15 mg/day. Max 40 mg daily. Do not cut or crush the ER form.
	glipizide ER 2.5, 5, 10 mg	Glucotrol XL	5–20 mg daily	
	glyburide 1.25, 2.5, 5 mg	Micronase DiaBeta	1.25–20 mg daily	Start at 2.5 to 5 mg daily or 1.25 mg daily if at risk for hypoglycemia. Max 20 mg daily. Take with breakfast or first meal.
Caution in older patients.	glyburide (micronized) 1.5, 3, 4.5, 6 mg	Glynase PresTab	1.5–12 mg daily	No advantage over the nonmicronized products. Start at 1.5–3 mg daily or 0.75 mg daily if at risk for hypoglycemia. Take with breakfast or first meal.
	glimepiride 1, 2, 4 mg	Amaryl	1–4 mg daily	Dosage once daily with first main meal. Start at 1–2 mg po daily. Titrate by 1–2 mg every 1–2 weeks. Max 8 mg daily. Take with first main meal.
Alpha-glucosidase inhibitors	Acarbose 25, 50, 100	Precose	50–100 mg q8h, just before a meal	GI side effects common. Monitor liver function tests (LFTs). Avoid if creatinine (CR) > 2.
	Miglitol 25, 50, 100	Glyset	25–100 q9h with first bite of meal	Same as Acarbose but no need to monitor LFTs.
Thiazolidinediones	Pioglitazone 15, 30, 45	Actos	15–30 mg daily with max 45 as monotherapy; 30 mg daily max in combination therapy.	Avoid if NYHA Class III or IV cardiac status. Monitor cardiac function. Check LFTs at start and q2mo during first year. DC if serum ALT levels >2.5 times upper limit of normal; may increase risk of fractures in women.
	Rosiglitazone 2, 4, 8	Avandia	Restricted access. Can be used only if glucose cannot be controlled with other medications.	Check LFTs at start and q2mo during first year. DC if serum ALT levels > 2.5 times upper limit of normal; may increase risk of fractures in women.

TABLE 19-3	Oral Hypoglycemic Medications (*continued*)			
Class	**Generic Name Strength**	**Trade Name**®	**Usual Dosage**	**Comments** *Regular testing of blood glucose and A_{1c} is recommended to assess medication effect.*
DPP-4 enzyme inhibitors	Sitagliptin 25, 50, 100	Januvia	100 mg daily as monotherapy or with metformin or a thiazolidinedione; 50 mg daily for decreased renal function.	
	Saxagliptin 2.5, 5	Onglyza	5 mg; 2.5 mg if decreased renal function.	
Meglitinides	Nateglinide 60, 120	Starlix	Take 30 minutes before a meal.	Caution in decreased hepatic and renal function.
	Repaglinide 0.5, 1, 2	Prandin	Take 30 minutes before a meal.	Adjust dose gradually. Potential for many drug interactions. Caution in hepatic and renal function.

Source: Diabetes Guidelines Work Group (2007); Nurse Practitioners' Prescribing Reference (2012); Reuben et al. (2012).

adults with type 2 DM because those with type 1 DM are totally reliant on insulin and would lose the ability to make individual dose adjustments based on food consumption and metabolic demands imposed by exercise.

Table 19-4 lists the available insulins and duration of action. Caution and careful monitoring are indicated during the initial dosing period. The major determinant of the onset and duration of action is the rate of insulin absorption from the injection site, and this can vary widely among older adults (UpToDate, 2012).

Inhaled insulin (Exubera) was FDA-approved for monotherapy or in combination with oral hypoglycemics in older adults with type 2 DM and as an adjunct to injected insulin for those with type 1 DM. However, due to lack of demand and consumer interest, it was withdrawn from the market in 2007.

Hypoglycemia as a Complication of Insulin Treatment

Hypoglycemia can be caused by too high a dose of insulin, missing a meal or eating a smaller meal, unplanned exercise, or the onset of illness that alters metabolic need. Older adults need to recognize the symptoms of hypoglycemia, including feeling nervous, shaky, sweaty, or excessively fatigued. However, in older adults these classic signs and symptoms may be absent or greatly diminished. These warning signs may be mild at first, but may progress rapidly to confusion, loss of consciousness, slurred speech, or having seizures as blood levels continue to drop.

Older adults are advised to test their blood glucose levels if they experience these symptoms, and if glucose levels are less than 60 to 70 mg/dL, treatment is needed immediately. Those who are unable to test their glucose levels are advised to initiate treatment anyway. The usual treatment recommendation is to eat 10 to 15 g of carbohydrates right away. Table 19-5 lists examples of food or liquids with this amount of carbohydrate.

After ingesting 15 to 30 g of carbohydrate, the older person is advised to wait 15 minutes and test the blood glucose level again. More carbohydrates may need to be ingested. This process is repeated until the blood glucose is above 70 mg/dL or the signs of hypoglycemia have resolved. Older adults must be cautioned that eating the foods on this list will keep the blood glucose level up for only about 15 to 30 minutes. If the next meal or snack is a long way off, then eating something more substantial like crackers with peanut butter or a slice of cheese or meat is advised. In the in-patient setting, glucagon 0.5 to 1 mg subcutaneous or intramuscular or 25 to 50 g of D50 intravenous may be administered if the patient is unconscious or cannot swallow (Reuben et al., 2012). All older adults with DM are advised to carry a card that identifies them as having diabetes and to wear a medical bracelet or necklace. Family members, caregivers, and close friends should be taught to administer glucagon with an easy-to-use injection device as part of an emergency kit. Glucagon is available by prescription and is a powerful antihypoglycemic. The usual dose is 1 mg (International Unit) given subcutaneously, intramuscularly, or

TABLE 19-4	Available Insulins and Duration of Action			
Insulin Type	**Onset**	**Peak**	**Duration**	**Comments** *Regular testing of blood glucose and A_{1c} is recommended to assess medication effect.*
Very short-acting insulin lispro Humalog® (Lilly)	20 minutes	30–90 minutes	3–4 hours	Insulins lispro, aspart, and glulisine are very short-acting products. Both lispro and aspart are available mixed with intermediate-acting preparations as fixed-ratio combinations that provide the benefit of rapid and intermediate action.
Very short-acting insulin aspart NovoLog® (Novo Nordisk)	30 minutes	60–180 minutes	5–8 hours	
Very short-acting insulin glulisine Apidra® (Sanofi-Aventis)	10–20 minutes	30–90 minutes	3–4 hours	Humalog mix 75/25 is a mixture of 75% insulin lispro protamine suspension and 25% insulin lispro. NovoLog 70/30 is a mixture of 70% insulin aspart protamine and 30% insulin aspart.
Short-acting regular insulin Humulin R (Lilly), Novolin R (Novo Nordisk)	30 minutes–1 hour	2–3 hours	5–8 hours	NPH and regular insulins are also available as fixed-ratio combinations of 50/50 and 70/30.
Intermediate-acting NPH insulin Humulin N (Lilly), Novolin N (Novo Nordisk)	1–1.5 hours	4–12 hours	24 hours	NPH and regular insulins are also available as fixed-ratio combinations of 50/50 and 70/30.
Long-acting insulin glargine Lantus® (Sanofi-Aventis) approved in pediatric population > 6 years of age Insulin detemir Levemir® (Novo Nordisk) approved in pediatric population ≥ 6 years	1–2 hours	No pronounced peak	24 hours	Once daily subcutaneous administration at a consistent time in patients who require basal (long-acting) insulin for the control of hyperglycemia. Neither should be diluted nor mixed with any other insulin or solution, and is not intended for intravenous administration.

Source: Diabetes Guidelines Work Group (2007); McPhee & Papadakis (2011); Nurse Practitioners' Prescribing Reference (2012); Reuben et al., (2012).

TABLE 19-5	Food and Liquids Providing 10 to 15 g of Carbohydrates for Low Blood Glucose Levels
Food Item	**Amount**
Glucose gel (amount equal to 15 grams of carbohydrate)	1 serving
Fruit juice	1/2 cup (4 oz)
Soda pop (not diet)	1/2 cup (4 oz)
Hard candy	5 to 6 pieces
Sugar or honey	1 tablespoon
Glucose tablets	3 to 4

Source: National Diabetes Information Clearing House (2008).

intravenously. If no one is available to help and the symptoms do not subside, the nurse should instruct the older person to call for emergency assistance and hospital evaluation. It is unsafe for the older person to drive themselves to the hospital, as confusion or loss of consciousness from low glucose levels may occur.

Morning Hyperglycemia

The dawn phenomenon refers to the normal tendency of blood glucose levels to rise in the early morning before breakfast. This normal phenomenon is exaggerated in older adults with type 1 and type 2 diabetes. The liver may produce increased glucose as a result of a midnight surge of growth hormone. In some older adults, nocturnal hypoglycemia may be followed by a marked increase in fasting blood glucose with an increase in plasma ketones (Somogyi phenomenon) (McPhee & Papadakis, 2011).

Injection Site Reactions

At the injection site, local fat hypertrophy, atrophy, or allergic reactions can occur. Pain and burning at the injection site may last for a few hours, followed by redness, itching, and induration. These reactions may disappear on their own as the body becomes desensitized to the insulin. Rotate injection sites routinely to prevent fat hypertrophy or atrophy.

Effect of Acute Illness

If an older person with DM experiences an acute illness such as pneumonia or urinary tract infection, hyperglycemia can be the result. However, if the older person has lost his or her appetite or is vomiting, continuing to take the same dose of oral hypoglycemics or insulin can result in hypoglycemia. If the older person is hospitalized or in a long-term care facility, the nurses will routinely check blood glucose levels and "cover" the older person with a sliding scale of insulin until the acute illness resolves and the blood glucose levels stabilize. Current practice standards recommend scheduled basal and prandial insulin doses with correction doses with rapid-acting analog (aspart, glulisine, or lispro) as preferred over sliding-scale insulin regimens. If the patient is critically ill, target blood glucose levels should be 140 to 180 mg/dL and if not critically ill, fasting blood glucose levels should be <140 mg/dL and random levels <180 mg/dL (Reuben et al., 2012). The physician may request that hypoglycemic drugs be withheld or the dosage decreased during an acute condition associated with decreased food intake or persistent nausea and vomiting. The effects of surgical procedures, stress, and trauma can markedly increase blood glucose levels. The nurse and other members of the healthcare team will attempt to regulate medications and oral intake to prevent dangerous variations in blood glucose levels.

Instruct older adults and their families to call their healthcare provider if any of the following conditions occur:

- Inability to keep food or liquids down or eat normally for over 6 hours
- Severe diarrhea
- Unintentional weight loss of 5 lb
- Oral temperature over 101°F
- A blood glucose level lower than 60 mg/dL or over 300 mg/dL
- Presence of large amounts of ketones in the urine
- Difficulty breathing
- Sudden onset of sleepiness or inability to think clearly

Diabetes Guidelines Work Group, 2007.

Nonketotic Hyperglycemic-Hyperosmolar Coma

Nonketotic hyperglycemic-hyperosmolar coma (NKHHC) is a complication of type 2 DM that has a high mortality rate (McPhee & Papadakis, 2011). It usually develops after a period of symptomatic hyperglycemia during which fluid intake is inadequate to prevent extreme dehydration from osmotic diuresis. Symptoms of hyperglycemia include dry mouth, extreme thirst, excessive urination, fatigue, blurred vision, weight loss, nausea, abdominal pain, and vomiting. NKHHC can occur in some older adults with undiagnosed or untreated type 2 DM when they receive drugs that impair glucose tolerance such as glucocorticoids or drugs that increase fluid loss such as diuretics. Older adults with severe dementia may also be at risk because the decreased thirst and hunger drive may prevent them from eating and drinking adequate amounts of fluid and nutritious foods.

NKHHC may begin as mild confusion and progress to coma or seizures. Laboratory studies reveal hyperglycemia (above 500 mg/dL), hyperosmolarity, and metabolic acidosis. Serum sodium and potassium levels are usually normal, but blood urea nitrogen (BUN) and serum creatinine levels are increased. Because the average fluid deficit is usually significant, acute circulatory collapse is common. Widespread thrombosis is a frequent finding on autopsy and may lead to disseminated intravascular coagulation (DIC) (McPhee & Papadakis, 2011). Treatment must begin immediately and intravenous fluids are needed to expand the intravascular volume, stabilize blood pressure, and improve circulation and urine flow. Insulin treatment is not always necessary, because adequate hydration may decrease blood glucose levels.

Difficulties in Caring for Older Adults With DM

Six geriatric syndromes were selected by the California Healthcare Foundation and the American Geriatrics Society Panel on Improving Care for Elders with Diabetes based on literature reviews and expert opinions (2003). These syndromes represent areas where gerontological nurses can intervene and collaborate with other healthcare professionals to improve the quality of care provided to older adults with DM. They include:

1. **Polypharmacy.** Older adults with DM may require several medications to manage their overall health problems, including elevated blood glucose levels, hypertension, hyperlipidemia, and other associated conditions. Perform a careful and accurate drug assessment at each visit and document whether the

person is taking the medications as ordered. Provide older adults and their families with information describing the expected benefits, risks, and potential side effects of each medication.

2. **Depression.** Older adults with DM are at an increased risk for depression that may be undetected and untreated. Screen for depression using a standardized instrument (for example, the Geriatric Depression Scale) at baseline and periodically thereafter. Note symptoms of depression on the chart, and refer to the primary care provider for drug therapy or counseling as needed. Note progress toward symptom relief in the chart.

3. **Cognitive impairment.** Older adults with DM are at increased risk for cognitive impairment. Subtle or unrecognized cognitive impairment may interfere with the older person's ability to manage this complicated disease. Therefore, screening for cognitive impairment on the initial visit using a standardized assessment instrument (Mini-Mental State Examination) is necessary and should be repeated periodically thereafter. The healthcare team will investigate any increased difficulty with self-care or failure of self-management. Consult with caregivers (with the older adults' permission) and involve them with the ongoing education and management plan to provide care to the older person with DM and a cognitive impairment.

4. **Urinary incontinence.** Older women with DM are at increased risk of urinary incontinence. Assess for urinary incontinence initially and periodically thereafter. Older age and disease-associated conditions that can contribute to urinary incontinence include polyuria, neurogenic bladder, atrophic vaginitis, urinary tract infection, and vaginal candidiasis.

5. **Injurious falls.** Falls in older people are associated with higher rates of morbidity, mortality, and functional decline. Older adults with DM are at increased risk for injurious falls because of higher rates of frailty and functional disability, visual impairment, peripheral neuropathy, hypoglycemia, and polypharmacy. Screen for fall risk initially and periodically thereafter. Once risk factors have been identified, they can be addressed by the healthcare team to prevent or reduce the risk of injurious falls.

6. **Pain.** Older adults with DM are at risk for neuropathic pain, which often goes untreated. Screen older adults for persistent pain initially and periodically thereafter. Older adults with persistent pain should be monitored, treated, and provided with appropriate therapy with results of treatment noted in the older person's healthcare record.

General Health Promotion

Coordinated care is essential in the management of the older person with DM. Treatment emphasizes dietary modification, exercise, weight reduction, and appropriate use of medication as described in this chapter. At each visit, the older person's progress is evaluated by the nurse who identifies and reviews problems. The nurse revises and reassesses the plan on an ongoing basis.

The nurse should teach older adults with DM and their families self-management skills including self-monitoring for signs of hypoglycemia, blood glucose monitoring skills and medication adjustment, nutrition management, and development and maintenance of a physical activity plan. The nurse should administer the influenza vaccine to older adults with DM every fall. The pneumococcal vaccine is recommended at age 65. Revaccination is suggested if the older person is over the age of 65 and the initial vaccine was given over 5 years ago and the older person was under 65 years at that time.

The nurse should counsel older adults with DM regarding smoking cessation, psychosocial adjustment and depression, sexuality and erectile dysfunction, urinary incontinence, falls, presence of pain or neuropathy, and foot and skin assessment. Referral to a certified diabetes educator may be indicated for additional education and self-management skills consistent with the National Standards for Diabetes Patient Education Programs. The nurse should schedule podiatry and dental consultations as needed. An annual comprehensive dilated eye and visual examination by an ophthalmologist is recommended so that microvascular complications can be detected and treated early to prevent vision loss.

At each visit, the older person is weighed and the blood pressure is recorded. The feet and skin are carefully examined. Any irritation, ulceration, deformity, or loss of sensation is carefully noted and referred for treatment. It is recommended that laboratory tests be obtained as indicated in Table 19-6.

Hope for the Future

Continuous subcutaneous insulin infusion pumps are being used more widely. These small devices (about the size of a beeper) can be programmed to deliver an individualized basal dose of insulin and can be bolused by the older person before a meal to control the postprandial glucose levels. A small tube connects to a subcutaneous catheter usually placed in the abdomen. Older adults wearing the pumps must be motivated to perform frequent self-monitoring of blood glucose levels and be able to calculate the need for the insulin bolus depending on the size and content of their meal. Usually four to six fingersticks to test blood glucose are needed daily to ensure appropriate dosing and prevent

TABLE 19-6	**Massachusetts Guidelines for Adult Diabetes Care**	
	Diabetes Care Summary	
Frequency	**Test/Care**	**Comments**
Every Visit	Weight/BMI	BMI: Goal: <25 kg/m^2
	Blood Pressure	Goal: $<130/80$ for most patients
		Higher or lower systolic BP targets based on response to therapy and patient characteristics
	A_{1c}	Every 6 months if at goal with stable glycemia
		Every 3 months if not meeting goals or change in therapy
		Target $<7\%$ for most patients
	Foot Exam	Visual exam without shoes and socks
	Self-management	Check self-monitoring log book, diet, physical activity, and medications
		Review self-management goals
		Refer for Diabetes Self-Management Education if indicated
	Nutrition Plan	Ongoing
	Physical Activity Plan	Ongoing
	Tobacco Use	Ongoing: Ask, Advise, Refer
		MA Smokers' Helpline: 1-800-QUIT-NOW (1-800-784-8669)
		www.makesmokinghistory.org
	Preconception/ Pregnancy	Discuss need for tight glucose control 3-6 months preconception
		Consider early referral to OB/GYN
	Psychosocial Assessment	Assess for depression or other mood disorder
	Sexuality/Impotence/ Erectile Dysfunction	Discuss diagnostic evaluation and therapeutic options
Annually	Flu Vaccine	Every fall
	Microalbumin	Initial urinalysis at diagnosis; annual microalbumin thereafter.
		If abnormal, recheck x2 in a 3-month period, then treat if 2 out of 3 collections show elevated levels
	Dilated Eye Exam	Type 1 DM: initial exam after 3–5 years disease duration
		Type 2 DM: initial exam shortly after diagnosis
		A qualified eye care professional may recommend less frequent exams; more frequent examinations will be required if retinopathy is progressing
	Fasting Lipid Profile	Targets: • LDL (goal <100; <70 if overt CVD) • HDL (men: goal >40; women: goal >50) • Triglycerides (goal <150) Fasting Lipid Profile every 2 years if values fall in lower risk levels
	Creatinine/GFR	To estimate glomerular filtration rate (GFR) and stage level of chronic kidney disease
	Comprehensive Lower Extremity Exam	Comprehensive lower extremity evaluation (LEE) every 3–6 months if patient has high-risk foot conditions
	MNT Referral	Initially and ongoing as needed
	DSME Referral	Initially and ongoing as needed
	Dental Exam	(2 $\times$ year)
At Least Once	Pneumonia Vaccine	Also revaccination $\times$ 1 if >65 and first vaccine >5 years ago and patient <65 at the time of first vaccine
	EKG	If >40 years and/or DM >10 years

Source: These recommendations are based on the *Massachusetts Guidelines for Adult Diabetes Care* and are not intended to replace the clinical judgment of health care providers. Please refer to the *Guidelines* for more extensive review of recommendations and supporting evidence: http://www.maclearinghouse.com/CatalogDiabetes.htm

hypo- or hyperglycemia. Newer models allow the catheter to be disconnected for bathing.

An insulin pump without a catheter has been developed in which the insulin reservoir and infusion set are integrated into a pod. The pod is placed on the skin and can administer subcutaneous basal and bolus insulin based on wireless instructions from a personal digital assistant. These devices are appropriate for motivated older adults who are well educated about their DM. Additionally, these devices are expensive and some of the cost may not be covered by Medicare. Transplantation of islet cells from one human pancreas to another is also being tested. Although insulin independence is achieved immediately after transplantation, most subjects experienced a marked decline in insulin production over a period of 2 years (McPhee & Papadakis, 2011). Additionally pancreas transplantation at the time of kidney transplantation is becoming more widely accepted. Solitary pancreas transplantation in the absence of need for kidney transplantation should be considered only in those patients with frequent life-threatening hypoglycemia who have failed all other methods of treatment.

Despite the possibilities for improving future treatment, nurses should work with older adults to prevent DM from developing through rigorous lifestyle modification including diet, exercise, weight loss, and reducing cardiac risk factors. After diagnosis, these same lifestyle modifications will improve the effect of medications, delay or perhaps prevent secondary complications, preserve strength and function, and improve the quality of life for the older person.

Thyroid Disorders

The prevalence of thyroid disease rises with age. The rate of **hypothyroidism** (the metabolic state resulting from inadequate amounts of thyroid hormone) is much higher in women than in men of all ages, and is higher in older adults living in institutions than in older community-residing persons (Lowrence, 2009). Hypothyroidism is common, affecting approximately 1% of the general population and about 5% of older adults (McPhee & Papadakis, 2011). The prevalence of **hyperthyroidism** (the metabolic state resulting from excessive amounts of thyroid hormone) in older people is similar to the rates in the general population. Approximately 5% to 10% of persons over age 65 have hypothyroidism, and 0.2% to 2% have hyperthyroidism. When the thyroid is functioning well, the nurse will observe an older person who is functioning well metabolically. When thyroid dysfunction is present, and insufficient or excessive amounts of thyroid hormone are produced, the nurse may see dramatic effects in the cardiovascular system, hematologic system, and central nervous system. Because thyroid dysfunction often occurs gradually, the signs and symptoms may be imperceptible to the older person and family and may be attributed to normal changes of aging.

Hypothyroidism is characterized by a generalized reduction in metabolic function that most often manifests as a slowing of physical and mental activity. The complaints may vary from asymptomatic, mild, moderate, or severe, and depend on a variety of factors such as the person's age, general health status, cognitive abilities, and rate at which the disease develops (AACE, 2011b). Because older adults may not complain of classic symptoms of thyroid disease, their complaints may be attributed to other causes. The necessary testing is often not done, leaving the condition undiagnosed for long periods of time. This can result in expensive and unnecessary testing, inappropriate use of healthcare resources, and prolonged suffering for the older person (AACE, 2011b). Undiagnosed thyroid disease can have a profound effect on the body, making early and accurate diagnosis and treatment a necessity.

Normal Anatomy and Physiology

The thyroid is an endocrine gland that produces thyroxine (T_4) and triiodothyronine (T_3), two hormones that play a key role in regulating the body's energy levels and metabolic function. Normally, thyrotropin-releasing hormone (TRH) is produced by the hypothalamus, stimulating the anterior pituitary gland to produce thyroid-stimulating hormone (TSH). This in turn stimulates the thyroid to produce T_4 and T_3. Additionally, TSH increases carbohydrate, protein, and lipid metabolism and stimulates cell proliferation, thus affecting many systems of the body (Huether & McCance, 2012). High levels of T_4 and T_3 provide negative feedback to the pituitary gland and hypothalamus, decreasing the production of TSH and TRH. If free T_4 and T_3 levels are low, feedback to the pituitary gland and hypothalamus stimulates increased production of TRH and TSH, which stimulates the thyroid to produce more hormone. More than 99% of T_4 and T_3 is bound to thyroxine-binding globulin (TBG) and albumin, leaving only a small amount free to influence metabolic effect. Figure 19-11 ►►► illustrates the physiology of the normally functioning thyroid gland.

Practice Pearl ►►► Deficient amounts of thyroid hormones stimulate TSH secretion, whereas excess levels inhibit TSH secretion. Therefore, an older person with hypothyroidism will have an elevated TSH, and an older person with hyperthyroidism will have an abnormally low TSH level.

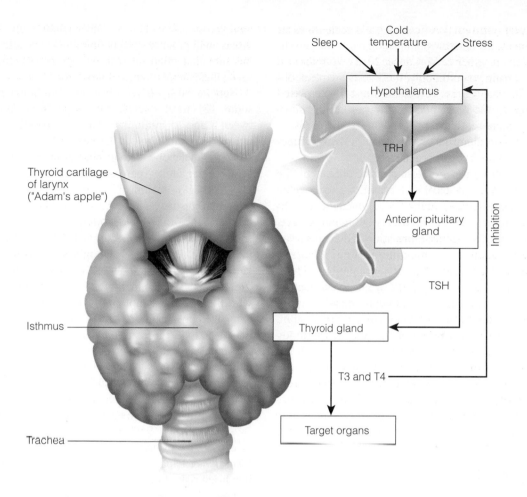

Figure 19-11 ▶▶▶ Physiological function of the thyroid gland.

Both T_3 and T_4 rely on an adequate supply of iodine from the diet that is taken up by the gland from the circulating blood. T_4 comprises the main hormone produced by the thyroid (about 80%); T_3 is formed from T_4 and is the active form of hormone, but much less is produced (20%). Once T_4 and T_3 are released into the circulation, they are bound by plasma proteins including TBG and albumin. T_3 and T_4 are inactive when bound to circulating proteins, and only the free fraction is able to bind to specific thyroid hormone receptors in peripheral tissue and stimulate biological activity. The bound hormones form a circulating reservoir of T_3 and T_4 that is available to the body to use as needed for regulating metabolic activity.

Thyroid Function Testing

Thyroid function tests help to diagnose and detect the presence of thyroid disease. With laboratory testing, thyroid disease is detectable at early stages, before significant loss of function occurs in the older person. The American Thyroid Association recommends initially checking free T_4 and TSH levels to test thyroid function. Serum TSH level remains the best test of thyroid function because TSH is central to the negative-feedback system, small changes in serum thyroid function cause major changes in TSH secretion, and the most advanced measurement methods can detect both elevation and lowering of TSH levels and are capable of reliably measuring values below 0.1 milliunits/L (McPhee & Papadakis, 2011). Total serum T_4 levels, measured by radioimmunoassay, have high sensitivity, with elevated readings exhibited in approximately 90% of older adults with hyperthyroid disease and decreased T_4 levels in 85% of persons with hypothyroid disease. Interpretation of T_3 levels can be more misleading because diminished peripheral conversion of T_4 to T_3 contributes to low serum T_3 levels. Therefore, T_3 levels are low in only 50% of hypothyroid patients.

The presence of nutritional deficiencies and acute illnesses such as cirrhosis, uremia, or malnutrition can slow peripheral conversion (Huether & McCance, 2012). With thyroid disorders occurring so commonly, these tests are often obtained in the clinical setting. Test results must be interpreted in relationship to the older person's overall health status, presence of diagnosed illnesses, and medications taken. Table 19-7 lists common laboratory tests of thyroid function and interpretation of abnormal findings.

Additional thyroid function tests may be ordered by the primary healthcare provider or endocrinologist to make an accurate diagnosis in older adults with atypical or complicated presentation of thyroid disease. Although expensive, these tests can yield valuable information and are reserved for those older adults with multiple systemic illnesses, multiple medications, and atypical presentations. These tests include T_3-resin uptake (T3RU), an assessment of binding in both thyroxine and triiodothyronine; thyroglobulin levels (Tg), a measure of circulating thyroglobulin, a useful marker for thyroid cancer; thyroid autoantibody levels, which are elevated in 95% of older adults with autoimmune thyroiditis (Hashimoto's thyroiditis); iodine 131 uptake, useful in differentiating a hyperfunctioning thyroid **(Graves' disease)** from a nonfunctioning gland (subacute thyroiditis); and radioactive iodine scan or sonogram, which provides a functional picture of the thyroid and is useful in the evaluation of thyroid nodules.

Hypothyroidism

Hypothyroidism is relatively common and can be caused by dysfunction of the thyroid gland (primary), pituitary (secondary), or hypothalamus (tertiary). The most common cause of primary hypothyroidism is **Hashimoto's thyroiditis,** an autoimmune disease with subtle onset and minimal symptoms while the thyroid gland undergoes progressive inflammatory destruction. Hypothyroidism may also be caused by factors that negatively affect the synthesis of thyroid hormones such as iodine deficiency or excess and inherited defects in thyroid hormone biosynthesis (Huether & McCance, 2012). The cause of Hashimoto's disease is unknown, but it is accompanied by elevated levels of antithyroglobulin or antimicrosomal antibodies. Older adults with Hashimoto's disease will progress to hypothyroidism because the chronic inflammation will result in scarred, nonproductive glandular tissue that cannot produce thyroid hormone.

Subclinical hypothyroidism is a condition in which the serum TSH level is between the upper limits of normal (between 5 and 15 milliunits/L) and the free T_4 is within the normal range, but below the mean of the **euthyroid** standard (the metabolic state of normal thyroid function) used for the older adult. Approximately 17% of persons over the age of 60 with subclinical hypothyroidism progress to overt hypothyroidism over a 1-year period (McPhee & Papadakis, 2011). Many of these older adults have no clinical signs or symptoms of hypothyroidism and usually careful monitoring of laboratory values and ongoing assessment for debilitating signs and symptoms of hypothyroidism is indicated. Treatment of subclinical hypothyroidism in older patients with no signs or symptoms of hypothyroidism is controversial (Reuben et al., 2012). The serum TSH measurement may need to be repeated in older adults with concurrent illnesses because it may be subnormal during the illness and elevated during the recovery phase in response to the body's metabolic demands. Evaluation of thyroid function in the critically ill patient is not recommended unless thyroid dysfunction is strongly suspected (Reuben et al., 2012).

In more than 95% of older adults, hypothyroidism is caused by primary dysfunction of the thyroid gland (McPhee & Papadakis, 2011). Factors associated with the increased risk of developing hypothyroidism include older age; female gender; a history or diagnosis of thyroid disease including goiter, thyroid nodules, thyroiditis, hyperthyroidism, treatment of head or neck cancer with external radiation or iodine 131; family history of thyroid disease; diagnosis of nonthyroid autoimmune disease; and certain medications (Esherick, 2010; Reuben et al., 2012; McPhee & Papadakis, 2011). Medications associated with hypothyroidism include lithium, amiodarone, sulfonylureas, salicylates, furosemide, phenytoin, rifampin, and radioactive contrast dyes (Gutierrez, 2008; Reuben et al., 2012).

Older adults with goiter or enlarged thyroid glands detected through physical examination are euthyroid with the

TABLE 19-7	Common Laboratory Tests of Thyroid Function		
	Normal Value	**Value in Hypothyroidism**	**Value in Hyperthyroidism**
TSH	0.32–5.0 milliunits/mL	↑Usually >10–20	↓Usually low (<0.30) or undetectable
Free T$_4$	4.5–12 mcg/dL	↓Decreased	↑ Increased
Free T$_3$	75–200 ng/dL	Normal	↑ Increased

goiter representing a proliferation of thyroid tissue in response to inadequate serum levels of T_3. Older adults with goiter will often undergo thyroid function tests, antithyroid antibody tests, and thyroid scans to rule out Graves' disease, nodular goiter, hypothyroidism, or some other thyroid dysfunction (Esherick, 2010).

Signs and Symptoms of Hypothyroidism

Thyroid hormone deficiency results in a reduction in the metabolic rate. The onset of symptoms is usually gradual, and older adults can present with a wide range of symptoms. The typical older person diagnosed with hypothyroidism is a female over the age of 50; however, the condition can occur in either sex at any time (Gutierrez, 2008). It is easy to attribute symptoms like constipation, fatigue, depression, and decreased hearing to aging when hypothyroidism may be responsible.

See Box 19-2 for typical symptoms of hypothyroidism.

Hypothyroidism can cause a variety of symptoms associated with all of the major body systems. Neurologic symptoms include headache, vertigo or tinnitus, relaxation of the deep tendon reflexes, psychiatric disorders, cognitive deficits, and visual disturbances. Sensory disorders include numbness, tingling, and paresthesias. The primary care provider will most likely evaluate thyroid function in all older adults with symptoms of depression before treatment is begun. Cardiovascular effects of hypothyroidism can mimic heart failure with cardiac enlargement and decreased contractility of cardiac muscle. Pulse rate and stroke volume are diminished. These changes may be difficult to detect, especially if the older person is being treated with a beta-blocker for hypertension. Musculoskeletal changes attributed to hypothyroidism include generalized muscle fatigue, cramps, myalgias, joint effusions, and pseudogout. Osteoporosis may be aggravated by hypothyroidism because the growth of new bone can be inhibited. Gastrointestinal effects of hypothyroidism include constipation and gaseous distention as a result of prolonged gastric emptying and intestinal transit. Achlorhydria and pernicious anemia occur more frequently in older adults with hypothyroidism. The manifestations of hypothyroidism are diverse and numerous. Thyroid hormone is important for normal metabolic functioning, cardiac function, regulation of the gastrointestinal tract, respiration, renal function, red blood cell production, and regulation of total body water (Huether & McCance, 2012).

The evaluation of thyroid function in chronically ill older adults may be confusing. Many illnesses, medications, and treatments can affect thyroid function tests, and these abnormal values do not reflect abnormal thyroid function. This syndrome has been named *euthyroid sick syndrome* and can result from illness, hospitalization, and starvation as the body attempts to decrease metabolic rates and compensates by decreasing TSH levels with corresponding low free T_4 levels. The chronically ill or hospitalized older person with abnormal thyroid function tests should be evaluated by a clinical endocrinologist (AACE, 2011b).

Older adults with hypothyroidism have fewer symptoms than younger persons (Esherick, 2010). Most often, the older person will present with chronic, nonspecific complaints. The older person may fall, exhibit poor coping patterns, experience declining mental function, exhibit new-onset incontinence, and become less mobile. Physical findings are often difficult to interpret. Complications of hypothyroidism include hypertension and hyperlipidemia. Untreated hypothyroidism may lead to myxedema coma, a life-threatening emergency. In myxedema, mental confusion progresses to stupor and coma and is accompanied by hyponatremia, hypoglycemia, or hypercapnia. Treatment of myxedema coma involves hospitalization in the intensive care unit with the older person receiving large intravenous doses of thyroid hormones supplemented by intravenous adrenal corticosteroids. Additional interventions are needed to treat hyponatremia, hypoglycemia, and respiratory failure, if present (McPhee & Papadakis, 2011).

Diagnosis

Hypothyroidism is diagnosed by precise measurement of serum TSH and T_4 levels. In primary hypothyroidism, the TSH is elevated and free serum T_4 levels are below normal.

BOX 19-2   **Symptoms of Hypothyroidism**

- Fatigue
- Increased need for sleep
- Muscle aches
- Delayed relaxation of deep tendon reflexes
- Dry skin
- Bradycardia
- Increased cholesterol levels (elevations in LDL)
- Ataxia and balance difficulties
- Hearing loss
- Depression
- Cold intolerance
- Hair loss
- Voice changes
- Hypothermia
- Periorbital swelling
- Decreased appetite and weight loss

Source: Esherick, 2010; Reuben et al., 2012.

The free serum T_3 level has little value because it is normal in about one third of older adults with hypothyroidism and because low T_3 levels are associated with acute illness and inadequate caloric intake (Reuben et al., 2012). An older person with chronic thyroiditis may have an atrophic, normal, or enlarged thyroid gland, but thyroid autoantibodies are positive in 95% of these older adults, making high titers a valuable diagnostic tool. Thyroid nodules or sudden enlargement of the thyroid requires a thyroid scan or ultrasound (AACE, 2011b).

The thyroid is examined first with a visual inspection of the neck to identify any enlargements or irregularities. The nurse observes the neck using tangential lighting and stands a foot or two away to identify any shadows. Asking the older person to swallow will accentuate any irregularities during movement. The nurse begins to palpate the thyroid by placing fingers on the trachea at either side of the larynx and moving them gently up and down. The older person is asked to swallow to assess symmetry during movement. The nurse palpates underneath the muscles on either side of the trachea to ensure that the entire gland has been examined, and places a finger gently over the larynx to palpate the isthmus, the part of the thyroid that crosses over the larynx and forms the center of the butterfly-shaped gland. The thyroid will feel soft and spongy without nodules or irregularities. Giving the older person a sip or two of water may make it easier to swallow.

A comprehensive health assessment and history may suggest the development of hypothyroidism. However, because the symptoms are vague and many older adults experience few symptoms, laboratory assessment of thyroid function is required to confirm the diagnosis.

Treatment and Nursing Management

The goals of therapy are to relieve symptoms and to provide sufficient thyroid hormone to decrease raised serum TSH levels to the normal range. The treatment of hypothyroidism will be tailored to meet the needs of the older person. Long-standing untreated hypothyroidism is a risk factor for coronary artery disease. The older person with heart disease may need cardiac stress testing and complete cardiovascular risk assessment before treatment is begun. Thyroid hormone replacement should be started cautiously because in some older adults, an increase in levels of thyroid hormones can increase myocardial oxygen demand and result in myocardial infarction, angina, and cardiac arrhythmia (Nurse Practitioners' Prescribing Reference, 2012). If cardiac symptoms develop or worsen, stop the therapy pending evaluation of the symptoms.

The treatment of choice is T_4 replacement with levothyroxine sodium. The average dose for persons over 65 years of age is 25 to 50 mcg/day by mouth. If the older person has coronary artery disease, the initial dose should be started very cautiously and increased slowly to prevent the occurrence of cardiac arrhythmias or angina. The patient's dose should be increased gradually (25 mcg) over 4-week intervals and the serum TSH level should be monitored to assess the effectiveness of treatment. If the TSH levels are below normal, decrease the dose of levothyroxine. If the TSH levels are above normal, then increase the dose slowly until the TSH is normal. Close monitoring of blood levels, overall function, cardiac status, and cognitive function is indicated during the initial period. After the TSH has stabilized in the normal range, assess thyroid function every 6 to 12 months by an appropriate health assessment and laboratory testing (Esherick, 2010). Overly suppressed TSH levels indicate that the older person is at increased risk for osteoporosis; however, T_4 replacement with carefully monitored TSH levels has not been associated with decreased bone density (AACE, 2011b).

Several brands and generic preparations of levothyroxine sodium are now available. Although no one preparation appears distinctly superior to another, many older adults experience a change in thyroid status when switching brands; therefore, it is best to maintain older adults on the same preparation they have been taking during the initial titration period. Because the half-life of levothyroxine is 1 week, dose adjustments will not be immediately apparent. If it is necessary to change from one brand to another, a dose adjustment may be needed. Reevaluation of thyroid status is indicated because some preparations are more bioavailable than others (Esherick, 2010). Since levothyroxine has a narrow therapeutic range, small differences in absorption can produce subclinical or clinical hypothyroidism (AACE, 2011b). The two most popular brand names are Synthroid and Levoxyl, with Levoxyl's retail price being about 30% to 50% less than that of Synthroid (Epocrates.com, 2012).

Oral levothyroxine should be taken on an empty stomach at the same time every day. The nurse should advise the patient to avoid, or urge discontinuation of, drugs that can decrease the absorption of levothyroxine and cause harmful drug interactions. Drugs that interfere with levothyroxine absorption include aluminum hydroxide, calcium preparations, cholestyramine, colestipol, iron preparations, and sucralfate (AACE, 2011b). Other drugs such as anticonvulsants and antitubercular agents (rifampin) may accelerate levothyroxine metabolism, necessitating a higher replacement dose (AACE, 2011b). The nurse should carefully monitor the older person's medications on an ongoing basis to prevent harmful drug interactions.

> **Drug Alert ▶▶▶** Thyroid replacement hormones increase the metabolic rate in the body, including the cardiac system. It is important to start at a low dose (25 mcg daily), monitor response, and check a serum TSH level periodically to prevent cardiovascular collapse.

The American Thyroid Association recommends screening every 5 years by measuring serum TSH for all men and women over age 35. For those with risk factors for thyroid disease, check the serum TSH level more often and as indicated by the presence of new or unexplained symptoms of decreased metabolism. Screening for thyroid function should be performed in populations that have a high incidence of thyroid dysfunction because of disease state, drug therapy, or other predisposing factor, and when early intervention is crucial to prevent irreversible pathology once the diagnosis of hypothyroidism is made (AACE, 2011b). The TSH assay is the screening method of choice for identifying hypothyroidism.

Hyperthyroidism

Hyperthyroidism, or thyrotoxicosis, is the result of excess thyroid hormone with metabolic overstimulation of body function. The prevalence of hyperthyroidism in the older person is similar to that of the general population (about 2%) (McPhee & Papadakis, 2011). Hyperthyroidism in the older person is often due to Graves' disease or toxic goiter, an autoimmune disorder associated with the production of immunoglobulins that attach to and stimulate the TSH receptor, leading to sustained thyroid overactivity (Esherick, 2010). Older people are prone to the development of toxic nodular goiters, abnormal growths within the thyroid gland that can secrete excessive amounts of TSH. Additionally, hyperthyroidism may be medication induced as a result of taking amiodarone, a cardiac drug containing iodine that deposits in tissue and delivers iodine to the general circulation over long periods. Hyperthyroidism may also result from overtreatment with levothyroxine. Less common causes include pituitary tumors, pituitary resistance to thyroid hormones, and malignancies such as thyroid cancer (Reuben et al., 2012). Regardless of the cause, hyperthyroidism is the result of high levels of thyroid hormones, especially T_3 and to a lesser extent T_4 as the peripheral tissue will convert excess T_4 to T_3 (Huether & McCance, 2012).

Signs and Symptoms

Hyperthyroidism in the older person is even more difficult to assess than hypothyroidism because older adults exhibit fewer and different signs and symptoms than do younger adults. Only about 25% of hyperthyroid patients over the age of 65 exhibit classic symptoms (Esherick, 2010). The severity of signs and symptoms relates to duration of the illness, magnitude of the hormone excess, and age of the person (AACE, 2011b). Common clinical features of hyperthyroidism in the older person may include the following:

- Cardiac arrhythmias and tachycardia
- Tremor
- Weight loss and appetite changes
- Sleep disturbances
- Changes in vision, photophobia, diplopia, eye irritation
- Fatigue and muscle weakness

In the older person, the most common presentation of hyperthyroidism is tachycardia, weight loss, fatigue, and weakness or apathy. Decreased appetite is common. Because of decreases in baseline heart rate with age, tachycardia is interpreted as a resting heart rate greater than 90 beats per minute. Most often, the thyroid is not enlarged or easily palpated. Some of the classic symptoms of hyperthyroidism commonly exhibited in younger persons are rather uncommon in the older person, including feelings of nervousness and anxiety, hyperactive deep tendon reflexes, heat intolerance with excessive sweating, diarrhea or frequent bowel movements, and enlarged thyroid (Esherick, 2010).

Cardiac symptoms are experienced by 27% of older adults with hyperthyroidism. New onset atrial fibrillation, heart failure, and angina are common presentations. Because cardiac disease is common in the older person, underlying hyperthyroidism may not be suspected. Gastrointestinal symptoms may be confused with malignancy or other bowel disease. Other commonly overlooked symptoms of hyperthyroidism in the older person include depression (called apathetic thyroidism), myopathy, and osteoporosis (AACE, 2011b).

Thyroid storm is a rare, life-threatening situation that can occur when a physical illness is superimposed on an older person with hyperthyroidism. Report extreme tachycardia, fever, nausea, vomiting, heart failure, and changes in mental status or level of consciousness in an older person with hyperthyroidism to the physician. Emergency treatment will be required. Treatment includes large doses of propylthiouracil (PTU) and intravenous propranolol to slow the heartbeat to 90 to 110 beats per minute. Intravenous glucocorticoid and oral ipodate sodium are also given to decrease inflammation and lower serum T_3 levels (Reuben et al., 2012).

Diagnosis

The nurse should obtain a comprehensive health history and physical assessment with emphasis on weight and blood pressure, pulse rate and rhythm, thyroid palpation, neuromuscular examination, eye examination, vision assessment, and cardiovascular assessment. The TSH is the best screening test for hyperthyroidism, and subnormal or undetectable values are considered to be diagnostic (Esherick, 2010). Serum T_4, T_3, and thyroglobulin levels are, on average, lower in older adults with hyperthyroidism than in younger persons, but are not considered diagnostic of the disease. Ultrasound and radioisotope scans are needed when nodules are detected by palpation. Fine-needle aspiration may be done to rule out malignancies. Thyroid cancer is rare over the age of 60 and should be suspected when masses are painless and rapidly growing, the gland is hard and fixed, lymph nodes are palpable, and hoarseness or vocal cord paralysis is present, indicating laryngeal nerve involvement.

Treatment and Nursing Management

The prognosis for hyperthyroidism is excellent with treatment, usually leading to euthyroid or hypothyroidism with supplementation of levothyroxine (Reuben et al., 2012). The treatment of choice for most older adults is ingestion of radioactive sodium iodide (^{131}I). It is easy to administer and avoids the option of surgery with all the complications related to anesthesia and hospitalization. No consensus exists on the appropriate dose of ^{131}I for hyperthyroidism. One option is to administer a low dose and monitor for return to euthyroid state; another option is to administer a single large dose intended to produce hypothyroidism and treat with levothyroxine to achieve normal thyroid function. The large-dose option may provide the older person with more years of well-being because the relief of hyperthyroidism is faster and more reliable (AACE, 2011b).

Drugs other than ^{131}I may be used to treat hyperthyroidism under the following circumstances: (1) ^{131}I is refused by the older person; (2) to control symptoms before the administration of ^{131}I; or (3) to deplete the thyroid gland of stored hormone in order to prevent hyperthyroidism or "dumping" of hormone into the blood after treatment with ^{131}I (Esherick, 2010). These drugs are designed to block thyroid hormone production. The remission rates are variable, but relapses are frequent (AACE, 2011b). PTU is given initially at 150 to 300 mg/day in divided doses every 8 hours. Based on signs and symptoms and serum hormone levels that are monitored every 2 months, the dose of PTU may be decreased to 100 to 150 mg/daily. Methimazole can be given as a single daily dose, usually starting at 15 to 40 mg/day. The dose is monitored and changed every 1 to 2 months as needed based on symptoms. Side effects of PTU and methimazole are dose related and include skin rash, nausea, hepatitis, and arthritis. The most serious side effect is granulocytopenia. Warn older adults to stop taking the medications and to seek medical attention when a sore throat or generalized infection occurs.

Propranolol and other beta-blockers can help to manage symptoms of hyperthyroidism, including atrial fibrillation. Although it protects the heart from the effects of excessive thyroid hormone, it can cause adverse effects such as hypotension, heart failure, and bronchospasm. It will conceal the symptoms of thyrotoxicosis, but does not affect thyroxine levels or readings on thyroid function tests.

When hyperthyroidism is due to subacute thyroiditis, Hashimoto's disease, or radiation damage, the only effective treatment is to administer beta-blockers and closely observe the older person's function and cardiac status for complications. Antithyroid drugs are ineffective because they do not decrease the uncontrolled output of hormone from the damaged thyroid follicles (McPhee & Papadakis, 2011).

Another therapeutic option for hyperthyroidism is surgery to remove a significant portion of the thyroid gland. This procedure is usually a last option for older adults and reserved for those with suspicious nodules, those allergic or intolerant of antithyroid drugs, and those with symptoms so severe that they cannot wait for ^{131}I to become effective (McPhee & Papadakis, 2011).

Nursing Diagnoses Associated with Endocrine Problems

Nursing diagnoses associated with older adults with endocrine problems are diverse and depend on the older person's severity of illness and success of treatment. For older adults with type 2 DM and obesity, *Nutrition, Imbalanced: More Than Body Requirements* is appropriate. All older adults with DM may also be diagnosed with *Infection, Risk for*. Because DM requires many lifestyle modifications and therapeutic interventions, the effect of therapeutic regimen (family, community, and individual) should be assessed and ineffective patterns noted. The nurse should assess noncompliance to any aspect of diet, exercise, medication, or other self-care strategy.

Older adults with thyroid problems may be noted to have *Sleep Deprivation, Fatigue, Activity Intolerance, Risk for, Thermoregulation, Ineffective* and *Body Temperature: Imbalanced, Risk for*. Because of the many signs and symptoms manifested by the older person with endocrine problems, focus on principles of disease management, health promotion, safety, and patient and family coping.

COMPLEMENTARY AND ALTERNATIVE THERAPIES

Bladderwrack is a kelp-like tablet or powder that is sometimes used to achieve weight loss related to thyroid dysfunction and as a treatment for hypothyroidism because it contains high concentrations of iodine. Prolonged ingestion of bladderwrack reduces iron absorption and can lead to anemia. It can potentiate the effect of warfarin and cause excessive bleeding and interact with lithium to enhance thyroid activity. Additionally, it contains high amounts of sodium and can negate the effects of diuretics or lead to the formation of congestive heart failure (Gutierrez, 2008). Older adults are urged to check with their physician before using bladderwrack.

QSEN Recommendations Related to the Endocrine System

The Quality and Safety Education for Nurses (QSEN) project addresses the challenge of preparing future nurses with the knowledge, skills, and attitudes (KSAs) to continuously improve the quality and safety of the healthcare systems in which they work (Cronenwett et al., 2007). See the QSEN table for tips on meeting QSEN standards.

Patient and Family Teaching

Gerontological nurses require skills and knowledge related to teaching patients and families about the key concepts of gerontology and gerontological nursing. The guidelines in the following feature will assist the nurse to assume the role of teacher and coach.

Meeting QSEN Standards: The Endocrine System

	KNOWLEDGE	SKILLS	ATTITUDES
Patient-Centered Care	Involvement of patient and family in plan of care is crucial.	Family assessment and adult learning principles. Be able to individualize the plan of care.	Appreciate uniqueness of each patient/family.
	Examine barriers that may keep patients from being active in formulating their plan of care.	Evaluate for depression, vision/hearing, cognitive status, functional ability, knowledge deficits.	Provide patient-centered care to improve successful nursing outcomes.
Teamwork and Collaboration	Recognize scope of practice for interdisciplinary team members including endocrinologist, dietitian, social worker, occupational therapist, and others as needed.	Use leadership skills to coordinate team and share knowledge.	Value the contribution of each member of the team to improve outcomes.
	Be aware of organizational problems that can inhibit effective team functioning.	System assessment skills.	Be open to input from team members on effective means to improve communication and collaboration.
Evidence-Based Practice	Describe effective interventions to decrease CV and endocrine risk factors and improve overall health and function.	Access current evidence-based protocols to guide interventions.	Possess confidence in necessary skills to evaluate and incorporate nursing interventions from the literature.

(continued)

Meeting QSEN Standards: The Endocrine System *(continued)*

	KNOWLEDGE	SKILLS	ATTITUDES
Quality Improvement	Recognize the importance of measuring patient outcomes to improve comprehensive nursing care.	Skills in data management, technology, and U.S. government and DM and thyroid websites describing current incidence and prevalence of endocrine disease.	Value the use of data and outcomes as a key component of QI efforts.
Safety	Describe common errors and risks related to hypo- and hyperglycemia and patient/family characteristics that increase the likelihood of such errors occurring.	Use appropriate strategies to provide written information to compensate for memory loss (if present).	Appreciate the impact of cognitive, sensory, and functional deficits on the occurrence of adverse drug reactions.
Informatics	Provide input into the formation and maintenance of patient databases needed for gathering QSEN data and providing patient care.	Utilize the electronic health record.	Protect patient confidentiality according to HIPAA standards.

Patient–Family Teaching Guidelines

The following are guidelines that the nurse may find useful when instructing older adults and their families about diabetes mellitus.

DIABETES MELLITUS

Focus the education of the older person and his or her family on disease management principles, lifestyle modification, and promotion of health and safety. The goal is to assist older adults to acquire and maintain the knowledge, skills, and behaviors needed to successfully manage their disease.

Without comprehension of the relationship between home blood glucose readings, meal planning, and physical activity, older adults with diabetes will be hindered in their ability to achieve optimal blood glucose control and are at higher risk for long-term complications.

1 I have diabetes. What can I do to stay healthy?

General goals of health maintenance for older adults with diabetes include:

- Achieving and maintaining near-normal blood glucose levels by balancing food intake and medication with physical activity

- Achieving optimal serum lipid levels

- Providing adequate calories for attaining and maintaining reasonable weight

- Preventing and treating the acute and long-term complications of diabetes (damage to the eyes, kidneys, nerves, and heart)

- Improving overall health through optimum nutrition

Patient–Family Teaching Guidelines *(continued)*

RATIONALE:

Older people with DM are at increased risk for morbidity and mortality related to microvascular and macrovascular complications. Education regarding prevention of complications is crucial.

2 **I have just been diagnosed with diabetes. What are the most important things for me to know?**

Important things to know include:

a. The relationship of food and meals to blood glucose levels, medication, and activity including action, side effects, timing, and interactions of all medications:
   - Recognition, causes, treatment, and prevention of hypo- and hyperglycemia
   - Benefits of control
   - Importance of lifestyle modification
   - Use of glucagon if appropriate
   - Use of blood glucose meter and establishment of blood glucose target with guidelines for reporting high or low levels
   - Disposal of lancets and other contaminated materials

b. Basic food and meal plan guidelines—referral to a dietitian if necessary

c. Consistent times each day for meals and snacks

d. Recognition, prevention, and treatment of hypoglycemia

e. Sick day management

f. Self-monitoring of blood glucose

g. Complication prevention and recognition:
   - Self-foot care and podiatry consultation
   - Need for yearly eye examination
   - Impact of lipids and need for yearly lipid evaluation
   - Need for blood pressure control and establishment of regular monitoring schedule
   - Identification of symptoms; treatment and methods for preventing kidney disease, peripheral vascular disease, cardiovascular disease, periodontal disease, and peripheral neuropathy
   - Need for pneumococcal vaccine and annual flu immunization

RATIONALE:

Older adults and their families can become overwhelmed when they realize that managing this disease will affect every aspect of their lives and daily activities. Making a list and providing one or two key points of information on each of the items listed earlier will assist older adults and their families in the management of diabetes and prevention of diabetic complications.

3 **What are some things I will need to know over time?**

As you and your family become more familiar with the management of DM and blood glucose levels, additional content beyond basic meal planning is needed. As you make changes in your weight, exercise regimen, medications, and functional status, we will schedule follow-up sessions and focus on increasing your knowledge, skills, and flexibility to improve the quality of your life. Additional content may include:

- Sources of essential nutrients and their effect on blood glucose and lipid levels
- Label reading and grocery shopping guidelines
- Dining out and restaurant guidelines
- Modifying fat intake
- Use of sugar-containing foods, and dietetic foods and sweeteners
- Alcohol guidelines
- When to modify blood glucose testing schedules for glucose patterning and increased control
- Adjusting mealtimes
- Adjusting food for exercise
- Special occasions and holidays
- Travel and schedule changes
- Vitamin and mineral supplementation

RATIONALE:

As older adults become more sophisticated in the management of diabetes, they will be ready to adapt the basic principles to accommodate a more flexible lifestyle. This information will be helpful for the older person who has mastered the basics.

Patient–Family Teaching Guidelines

The following are guidelines that the nurse may find useful when instructing older adults and their families about thyroid conditions.

THYROID CONDITIONS

Education of the older person and his or her family should focus on disease management principles, lifestyle modification, and promotion of health and safety. The goal is to assist older adults to acquire and maintain the knowledge, skills, and behaviors needed to successfully manage their disease.

1 **I have just been diagnosed with a thyroid problem. What should I know about my thyroid?**

People live long and healthy lives with thyroid problems. The essential knowledge for you to understand about your thyroid disorder includes:

- Understanding the relationship between the thyroid hormones and the body's metabolic rate
- Correctly identifying the body's reaction to excess or deficient thyroid hormone levels (signs and symptoms of hypo- or hypermetabolic state)
- Preventing or delaying complications resulting from hypo- or hyperthyroidism
- Participating in the plan of care and improving your disease management skills

RATIONALE:

Older people with thyroid problems are at risk for the development of fatigue or anxiety, sleep disorders, changes in their weight, and other vague symptoms that may be falsely attributed to normal changes of aging. Education regarding prevention of complications is crucial.

2 **What are some things I need to know right away?**

Some basic information that you need to begin to manage your thyroid problem includes:

- The importance of taking thyroid medication daily and avoiding other drugs that are known to interact with thyroid medications
- Awareness of the signs and symptoms of thyroid disease such as appetite changes, fatigue, cardiovascular symptoms, changes in bowel movements, weight changes, and mood changes
- Need for careful ongoing monitoring of TSH by the healthcare provider and the importance of keeping appointments
- Need to tell all healthcare providers about the diagnosis and treatment of hypo- or hyperthyroidism
- Importance of not changing brand of levothyroxine without careful monitoring of thyroid function

RATIONALE:

As with diabetes, the older person may be overwhelmed at the amount of information needed to manage this newly diagnosed disease. Making a list of important items and listing one or two key points under each item may ease the older person's and family's anxiety. Make sure the older person knows that you are available to answer any questions that might arise in the future.

CARE PLAN   A Patient With Chest Pain Related to Hyperthyroidism

Case Study

Mrs. Jones is an 82-year-old woman who presents in the emergency department with complaints of fatigue, palpitations, and intermittent chest pain. She is highly functional and lives alone with the support of her daughter who lives close by and visits regularly. She denies nausea or vomiting. Physical examination reveals that her lungs are clear, blood pressure is 150/96, and pulse is 96 and irregular. Mrs. Jones's skin is clammy and she has trouble lying still for the electrocardiogram because she feels the need to move about. Her pulse oximetry is 99% on room air. Laboratory values reveal a TSH of 0.1 and a T_4 of 19. The electrocardiogram reveals atrial fibrillation.

Mrs. Jones has a regular care provider but has not seen her physician for about 6 months. She states she has never had any problems with her heart before.

Applying the Nursing Process

Assessment

Mrs. Jones is in need of emergency evaluation and stabilization of her cardiac status. New-onset atrial fibrillation, elevated pulse rate and blood pressure, and abnormal laboratory values need immediate attention. Intermittent chest pain and atrial fibrillation could indicate a myocardial infarction in progress.

Diagnosis

Appropriate nursing diagnoses for Mrs. Jones may include the following:

- *Tissue Perfusion: Cardiac, Risk for Decreased and Cardiac Output, Decreased*
- *Fatigue* and *Activity Intolerance* based on her cardiac status
- *Fear* and *Anxiety* related to her altered metabolic and cardiac status
- *Pain, Acute*

NANDA-I © 2012.

Expected Outcomes

The expected outcomes for Mrs. Jones may include the following:

- Mrs. Jones's vital signs and cardiac rhythm will gradually return to normal.
- She will report no further chest pain.
- She will report decreased levels of anxiety.
- She will begin to establish a therapeutic relationship with the nurse.

Planning and Implementation

The main issue is to decrease Mrs. Jones's heart rate and stabilize her cardiac status. An intravenous line should be established and a cardiologist consulted. Laboratory values reveal the older person is in a metabolic hyperthyroid state because her TSH is low. Her increased metabolic drive has triggered increases in systolic blood pressure, increased heart rate, and myocardial irritability. She is at risk for embolic stroke because of her atrial fibrillation. Her cardiac situation should improve spontaneously once the atrial refractory period is lengthened. The cardiologist may use a beta-blocker to slow the heart rate.

Mrs. Jones will need reassurance and a calm approach. She may wish her daughter to be called in for additional support. Deliver instructions in a reassuring manner with appropriate use of calming touch.

(continued)

CARE PLAN **A Patient With Chest Pain Related to Hyperthyroidism** (continued)

Evaluation

The nurse hopes to work with the emergency department team to stabilize Mrs. Jones's medical condition and rule out myocardial infarction. Once stabilized, Mrs. Jones can be admitted to the hospital. The nurse will consider the plan a success based on the following criteria:

■ Mrs. Jones will demonstrate knowledge of her condition and medications.

■ Mrs. Jones and her family will identify safe living arrangements and a plan for rehabilitation if needed after hospital discharge.

■ Mrs. Jones will institute advance directives by establishing a living will or naming a healthcare proxy.

■ A family meeting will be held to discuss Mrs. Jones's overall health and future.

Ethical Dilemma

Change the previous scenario slightly to reflect that Mrs. Jones has been taking levothyroxine for many years because she was diagnosed with hypothyroidism years ago. Lately, she reports she has been having trouble remembering things and often takes her medicine three or four times a day because "if one pill is good, then three or four are probably better." When informed of this, Mrs. Jones's daughter replies in anger, "OK. That's it. You're going to a nursing home. I'd rather have you safe than dead." Mrs. Jones is devastated and begins to cry uncontrollably.

Mrs. Jones's autonomy is in conflict with her daughter's beneficence or need to do good for her mother. Try to diffuse the emotionally charged situation by urging both Mrs. Jones and her daughter not to say anything in anger or make any immediate decisions. With team involvement and appropriate safeguards, there may be a way to offer Mrs. Jones more support with her medication management and home safety while satisfying her daughter's concerns regarding her mother's safety. A social worker referral and early discharge planning with identification of additional resources is needed.

Critical Thinking and the Nursing Process

1. What strategies can a gerontological nurse use to educate older people about the need for lifestyle modification when they are unaware that they are at risk for type 2 DM?

2. Examine your own nutrition and exercise habits. Do you have risk factors for development of type 2 DM? Are you setting a good example for your patients?

3. How can you increase your colleagues' level of suspicion regarding symptoms relating to hypo- and hyperthyroidism when the signs and symptoms are vague and atypical in the older person?

4. Imagine that you have been diagnosed with type 1 DM and have to be reliant on insulin injections for the rest of your life. What thoughts go through your head? What fears do you have? What kinds of support would make you feel better? What interventions would empower you to manage your life?

5. Discuss with a colleague the importance of genetics and lifestyle in the development of type 2 DM. Try to reach some agreement on which of these factors is most crucial to the development of type 2 DM in the older person.

■ Evaluate your responses in Appendix B. ⊂⊃

Chapter Highlights

- The endocrine glands control the body's metabolic processes. The endocrine and metabolic control systems offer many of the greatest opportunities for preventing the disabilities associated with aging.

- Two major endocrine problems of importance to gerontological nursing are diabetes mellitus and thyroid disease.

- Thyroid disease is common, often undiagnosed, and easily treated in people of all ages. Early detection prevents unnecessary disability and loss of function.

- Diabetes mellitus is common, and normalization of blood glucose levels may minimize the devastating vascular and neurologic complications that often occur.

- Knowledge of endocrine function and metabolism is crucial for gerontological nurses to interpret signs and symptoms of illness and advise older adults on health promotion activities.

- Type 1 DM develops due to B-cell destruction and results in a lack of or underproduction of insulin in the body. Older adults with type 1 DM are insulin dependent and at risk for ketoacidosis.

- Type 2 DM, the most prevalent form of diabetes in all age groups, results from a combination of insulin resistance and an insulin secretory defect.

- The prevalence of thyroid disease rises with age. Hypothyroidism is much higher in women than in men of all ages, and is higher in older adults living in institutions than in community-residing older adults.

- Symptoms of hyperthyroidism and hypothyroidism are vague and can be debilitating, affecting many body systems. Detection and treatment of thyroid problems can improve quality and length of life.

Pearson Nursing Student Resources
Find additional review materials at
nursing.pearsonhighered.com

Prepare for success with additional NCLEX®-style practice questions, interactive assignments and activities, web links, animations and videos, and more!

References

American Association of Clinical Endocrinologists (AACE). (2011a). *AACE diabetes care plan guidelines*. Retrieved from https://www.aace.com/sites/default/files/DMGuidelinesCCP.pdf.

American Association of Clinical Endocrinologists (AACE). (2011b). ATA/AACE guidelines: Hyperthyroidism and other causes of thyrotoxicosis: Management guidelines of the American Thyroid Association and the American Association of Clinical Endocrinologists. *Thyroid Guidelines Task Force*. Retrieved from https://www.aace.com/sites/default/files/HyperGuidelines2011.pdf

American College of Physicians. (2007). *Diabetes in elderly patients*. Retrieved from http://diabetes.acponline.org/custom_resources/ACP_DiabetesCareGuide-CH14.pdf?dbp

American Diabetes Association (ADA). (2008). *Nutrition recommendations and interventions for diabetes*. Retrieved from http://care.diabetesjournals.org/content/31/Supplement_1/S61.full

American Diabetes Association (ADA). (2011). *Standards of medical care in diabetes*. Retrieved from http://professional.diabetes.org/content/CPR/2011/ADA%20Standards%20of%20Medical%20Care%202011.ppt#256,1,Slide1

American Diabetes Association (ADA). (2012). *Insulin storage and syringe safety*. Retrieved from http://www.diabetes.org/living-with-diabetes/treatment-and-care/medication/insulin/insulin-storage-and-syringe.html

American Geriatrics Society for Health in Aging. (2012). *Diabetes*. Retrieved from

http://www.healthinaging.org/agingintheknow/chapters_ch_trial.asp?ch=29#Consequences of Diabetes

California Healthcare Foundation & American Geriatrics Society Panel on Improving Care for Elders with Diabetes. (2003). *Guidelines for improving the care of older persons with diabetes mellitus. Journal of the American Geriatrics Society, 51*(5), S5265–S5280.

Centers for Disease Control and Prevention (CDC). (2011a). *National diabetes fact sheet*. Retrieved from http://www.cdc.gov/diabetes/pubs/pdf/ndfs_2011.pdf

Centers for Disease Control and Prevention (CDC). (2011b). *Obesity trends among US adults* . Retrieved from http://www.cdc.gov/obesity/downloads/obesity_trends_2010.ppt#531,5,Slide

Cronenwett, L., Sherwood, G., Barnsteiner, J., Disch, J., Johnson, J., Mitchell, P., Sullivan, D., & Warren, J. 2007. Quality and safety education for nurses, *Nursing Outlook, 55*(3) 122–131.

Diabetes Guidelines Work Group. (2007). *Massachusetts guidelines for adult diabetes care*. Boston: Massachusetts Department of Public Health, Massachusetts Health Promotion Clearinghouse.

Diabetes Pro. (2012). *Estimated average glucose*. Retrieved from http://professional .diabetes.org/GlucoseCalculator.aspx

Dunphy, L., Winland-Brown, J., Porter, B., & Thomas, D. (2011). *Primary Care* (3rd ed.). Philadelphia, PA: F. A. Davis.

Epocrates.com. (2012). Thyroid function testing. *Drug and formulary reference*. Retrieved from https://online.epocrates .com/u/29111121/Thyroid+function+testing/ Summary/Overview

Esherick, J. (2010). *Tarascon primary care pocketbook*. Sudbury, MA: Jones and Bartlett.

Ferrell, B., & Coyle, N. (2010). *Palliative nursing* (3rd ed.). Oxford, UK: Oxford University Press.

Green, M., Bierman, J., Foody, J., Robertson, R., & Martin, G. (2009). *Primary care mentor*. Philadelphia, PA: F. A. Davis.

Gutierrez, K. (2008). *Pharmacotherapeutics: Clinical reasoning in primary care*. St. Louis, MO: Saunders.

Huether, S., & McCance, K. (2012). *Understanding pathophysiology* (5th ed.). St. Louis, MO: Mosby.

Lowrence, J. (2009). How many Americans suffer thyroid disorders? *General Medicine@ Suite 101*. Retrieved from http://jim-lowrance

.suite101.com/how-many-americans-suffer-thyroid-disorders-a135894

McPhee, S., & Papadakis, M. (2011). *Current medical diagnosis and treatment*. New York, NY: McGraw-Hill Medical.

Medical Examination.org. (2008). *Diabetes examination*. Retrieved from http://www.medical-examination.org/ diabetes-medical-examination

Medical Learning Network. (2007). *Overview of Medicare podiatry services*. Retrieved from http://www.cms.hhs.gov/MLNProducts/ downloads/MedicarePodiatryServicesSE_ FactSheet.pdf

MedlinePlus. (2012). *Aging changes in hormone production*. Retrieved from http:// www.nlm.nih.gov/medlineplus/ency/ article/004000.htm

NANDA International. (2012). *NANDA International nursing diagnoses: Definitions and classification, 2012–2014*. Philadelphia, PA: Wiley-Blackwell.

National Diabetes Education Program. (NDEP). (2011). Four steps to control your diabetes for life. Retrieved from http://www .ndep.nih.gov/diabetes/control/4steps.htm

National Diabetes Education Program. (2007). *Diabetes: The numbers*. Retrieved from http://ndep.nih.gov/resources/presentations/ diabetesthenumber0107

National Institute of Diabetes and Digestive and Kidney Diseases (NIDDK). National Diabetes Information Clearinghouse (2005). National Diabetes Statistics. Retrieved from http://diabetes.NIDDK.NIH.gov/dm/pubs/ statistics/

National Diabetes Information Clearing House. (2012). *Diagnosis of diabetes and

prediabetes, publication 12-4642*. National Institutes of Diabetes and Digestive and Kidney Diseases, National Institutes of Health. Retrieved from http://diabetes.niddk .nih.gov/dm/publs/diagnosis/#3.

National Diabetes Information Clearinghouse. (2008). *Hypoglycemia*. Retrieved from http://diabetes.niddk.nih.gov/dm/pubs/ hypoglycemia

National Institute of Diabetes and Digestive and Kidney Diseases (NIDDKD). (2008). *National diabetes statistics*. Retrieved from http://www.diabetes.NIDDK.NIH.gov/dm/ pubs/statistics

Nichols, G. (2009). International expert committee urges clinicians to use A1c Assay in the diagnosis of diabetes. *Diabetes Care, 32*: 1327–1334.

Nurse Practitioners' Prescribing Reference. (2012). *Winter 2011–2012, 18*(4). New York, NY: Prescribing Reference LLC.

Reis, J., Loria, C., Sorlie, P., Park, Y., Hollenbeck, A., & Schatzkin, A. (2011). Lifestyle factors and risk of new-onset diabetes. *Annals of Internal Medicine, 155*(5), 292–299.

Reuben, D., Herr, K., Pacala, J., Pollock, B., Potter, J., & Semla, T. (2012). *Geriatrics at your fingertips* (14th ed.). New York, NY: American Geriatrics Society.

Solomon, D. (2003). Metabolic and thyroid disorders. In M. Beers & R. Berkow (Eds.), *Merck manual of geriatrics*. Rahway, NJ: Merck.

UpToDate. (2012). Patient information: Diabetes mellitus type 1: Insulin treatment. Retrieved from http://www.uptodate.com/ contents/patient-information-diabetes-mellitus-type-1-insulin-treatment

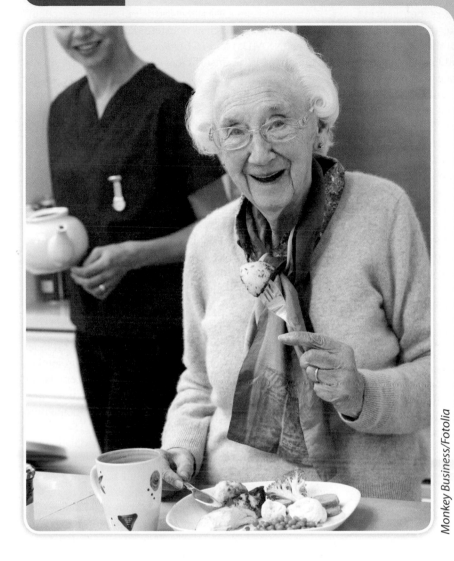

Monkey Business/Fotolia

LEARNING OUTCOMES

On completion of this chapter, the reader will be able to:

1. Describe age-related changes that affect gastrointestinal function.
2. Recognize the impact of age-related changes on gastrointestinal function.
3. Identify risk factors to health for the older person with gastrointestinal problems.
4. Interpret unique presentations of gastrointestinal problems in the older person.
5. Define appropriate nursing interventions directed toward assisting the older adult with gastrointestinal problems to develop self-care abilities.
6. Formulate and implement appropriate nursing interventions to care for the older person with gastrointestinal problems.

The gastrointestinal (GI) tract is responsible for four major functions relating to food ingestion: digestion, absorption, secretion, and motility. The GI tract begins at the mouth and ends at the rectum and includes the accessory organs of digestion, the liver, gallbladder, and pancreas. Throughout life, the GI tract is constantly remodeling with the endothelial lining shedding and regenerating every 24 to 48 hours. Ingested food, partially degraded by chewing in the mouth, enters the stomach where it is churned and mixed with acid, mucus, enzymes, and other secretions, beginning the process of digestion. After the food passes from the stomach to the small intestine, the liver and pancreas secrete enzymes to further break it down into protein, fat, and carbohydrates for easy absorption and metabolic use. These substances pass through the walls of the small intestine into the blood vessels and lymphatic system where they are transported to the liver for processing and storage. The peristaltic movements of the intestine are regulated by hormones and by the autonomic nervous system. The autonomic innervation is controlled by centers in the brain and local stimuli mediated by networks of nerve fibers within the walls of the GI tract (Huether & McCance, 2012).

Unabsorbed food continues into the large intestine, and fluid is absorbed and transported to the kidneys for elimination as urine. Under normal circumstances, the colon absorbs approximately 1 to 2 L of water per day. Solid waste and fiber are transported to the rectum and held for elimination. When the rectum is distended with stool, a signal is sent to relax the anal sphincter and triggers the urge to defecate. Normal bowel continence is dependent on the individual's ability to recognize rectal distention and to delay defecation. Figure 20-1 ▶▶▶ illustrates the normal configuration of the GI tract.

NORMAL CHANGES OF AGING

Figure 20-2 ▶▶▶ illustrates the normal changes of aging related to the gastrointestinal tract. Biological changes in GI function that occur in older adults result from the physical, mental, and psychological changes of aging and other factors associated with aging, such as immobility, impaired fluid balance, neuromuscular disorders, endocrine and metabolic problems, and the effects of medications. Age-related changes in the gastrointestinal system begin before age 50 and continue gradually throughout life (Huether & McCance, 2012). These changes include:

- Changes in the mouth, including potential for loss of teeth, periodontal disease, decline in sense of taste and smell, and decreases in salivary secretion

- Decreased esophageal motility
- Diminished gastric motility with increased stomach-emptying time
- Diminished capacity of the gastric mucosa to resist damage from factors such as nonsteroidal anti-inflammatory drugs (NSAIDs) and *Helicobacter pylori*
- Achlorhydria or insufficient hydrochloric acid in the stomach
- Decreased production of intrinsic factor leading to increased risk of developing pernicious anemia
- Decreased intestinal absorption, motility, and blood flow
- Decreased pancreas size with duct hyperplasia and lobular fibrosis
- Increased incidence of cholelithiasis (gallstones) and decreased production of bile acid synthesis
- Decreased liver size and blood flow
- Decreased thirst and hunger drive due to cognitive changes or psychological conditions such as depression
- Increased medication use and possible adverse drug reactions

Huether & McCance, 2012; Shaheen, 2006.

Medications with great potential to affect the GI tract include the anticholinergics (antidepressants, neuroleptics, antihistamines, antiparkinsonian agents), antihypertensives (calcium channel blockers, ACE inhibitors, diuretics), iron and calcium supplements, antiemetics, aluminum-containing antacids, opioids, and laxatives (Gutierrez, 2008). See Chapter 6 ▭ for further information relating to medication use and the GI tract.

Older adults with diseases of the GI tract and visceral organs are much more likely than younger adults to present atypically. For instance, older adults with peptic ulcer disease exhibit impaired visceral pain perception and take longer to recognize and report pain. This often leads to delayed diagnosis, a longer hospital stay, and a higher probability of mortality due to perforation (Gray-Miceli, 2012). Additionally, older people will also exhibit changes in GI function as the result of other illnesses (diabetes, neurologic illness, vascular disorders).

Common GI Disorders

Because of the large functional reserve capacity of most of the GI tract, aging alone has very little impact on GI function. However, aging is associated with an increased prevalence of many GI disorders, and these should be evaluated carefully and not attributed to normal aging.

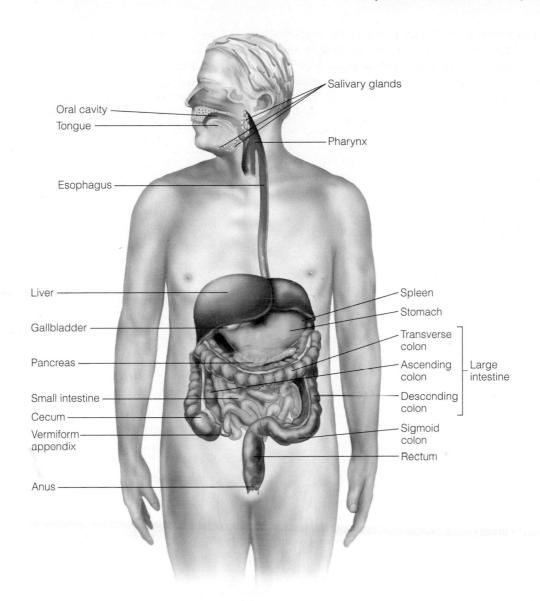

Figure 20-1 ►►► Normal configuration of the GI tract.

Esophageal Disorders

In healthy older adults, aging has only minor effects on esophageal motor and sensory function. Upper esophageal sphincter pressure and the amplitude of peristalsis decrease slightly with age, but these changes do not significantly affect function. Older adults with significant esophageal disorders usually have underlying systemic diseases, including vascular or neurologic problems. Gastroesophageal reflux appears to be more common in older than in younger people, possibly because of weakening of the lower esophageal sphincter and increased incidence of **hiatal hernia.** A hiatal hernia occurs when the stomach protrudes into the chest cavity through the opening in the diaphragm that usually only allows the esophagus to pass through. By age 60, 60% of people have developed hiatal hernia to some degree (eMedicineHealth, 2008). Many drugs can cause injury to the esophagus, including NSAIDs, potassium chloride, tetracycline, quinidine, alendronate, ferrous sulfate, and theophylline (Castell, 2012). Older people are at risk for esophageal injury as a result of taking these drugs. They should be advised to swallow these medications in an upright position, drink at least 8 oz of water when taking any medication, and remain in an upright position for 30 minutes to prevent reflux into the esophagus.

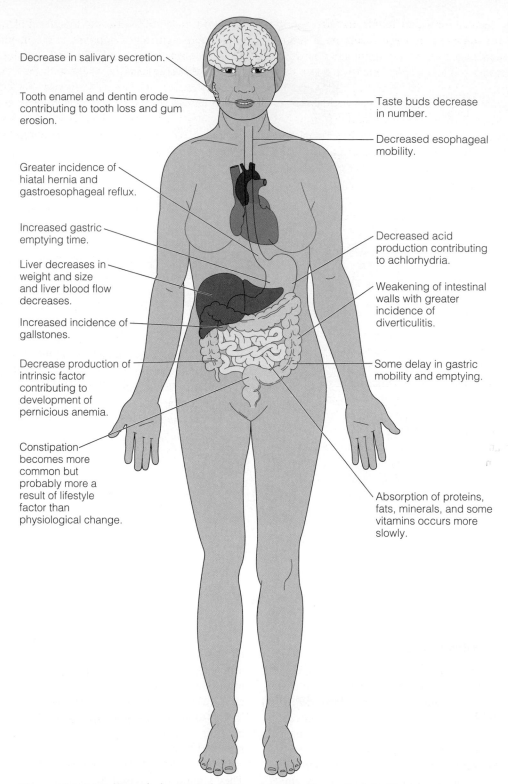

Decrease in salivary secretion.

Tooth enamel and dentin erode contributing to tooth loss and gum erosion.

Taste buds decrease in number.

Decreased esophageal mobility.

Greater incidence of hiatal hernia and gastroesophageal reflux.

Increased gastric emptying time.

Decreased acid production contributing to achlorhydria.

Liver decreases in weight and size and liver blood flow decreases.

Weakening of intestinal walls with greater incidence of diverticulitis.

Increased incidence of gallstones.

Decrease production of intrinsic factor contributing to development of pernicious anemia.

Some delay in gastric mobility and emptying.

Constipation becomes more common but probably more a result of lifestyle factor than physiological change.

Absorption of proteins, fats, minerals, and some vitamins occurs more slowly.

Figure 20-2 ▶▶▶ Normal changes of aging related to the gastrointestinal tract.

Aggravating factors for hiatal hernia include obesity, smoking, and consumption of large meals on a routine basis. Hiatal hernias are often asymptomatic; however, common symptoms might include belching, chest pain, difficultly swallowing, or heartburn, especially when lying down. If the symptoms are not severe, symptoms of hiatal hernia can be managed with lifestyle modification including weight loss, avoiding consumption of large meals, sitting upright for at least 1 hour after eating, and using blocks to elevate the head of the bed at night to prevent food from refluxing above the diaphragm. Antacids may also be used to decrease stomach acidity. If testing is needed, a barium swallow may be performed to visualize the anatomy of the esophagus, diaphragm, and stomach. In extreme cases such as strangulation or entrapment of the hernia or repeated episodes of aspiration pneumonia, surgical repair may be indicated.

Dysphagia

Dysphagia is the most common esophageal disorder in older people (WcbMD, 2012). Dysphagia is defined as difficulty in any part of the process involved with swallowing solid foods or liquids. Whether acute or chronic, the condition affects oral intake and is usually indicative of some other disease process. The act of swallowing involves approximately 50 muscles and requires intact oropharyngeal anatomy and unimpaired nerve conduction, permitting coordination between the respiratory and digestive systems. From start to finish, a single swallow takes about 20 seconds (Dahlin, 2004; WebMD, 2012).

An estimated 60% of institutionalized older adults have identifiable signs and symptoms of dysphagia. This is especially common in older adults with neurologic problems. A high incidence of older adults with Parkinson's disease (52% to 82%), Alzheimer's disease (84%), and stroke (30%) admitted to the hospital had signs and symptoms of dysphagia with risk for aspiration and development of pneumonia (Rofes et al., 2011). The normal swallow consists of three stages:

1. **Oral stage.** Food is prepared for transfer from the mouth to the oropharynx. Older adults need to be able to chew, have the desire to eat, and be able to see or smell the food. The food is mixed with saliva and forms a bolus for swallowing. When the bolus is pushed to the back of the mouth, the soft palate is raised, and coordinated muscular movements occur in the pharynx and larynx to move the bolus downward.
2. **Pharyngeal stage.** The bolus is propelled into the esophagus, and the larynx moves upward under the base of the tongue to prevent food from entering. The epiglottis lowers to protect the airway. This phase takes about a second in the normal swallow.
3. **Esophageal stage.** The bolus is propelled toward the stomach by peristalsis. This phase can take 8 to 20 seconds depending on the consistency of the food, the strength of the peristaltic movements, and the older person's position and anatomy.

Figure 20-3 ▶▶▶ illustrates the anatomy of the oral cavity and the esophagus.

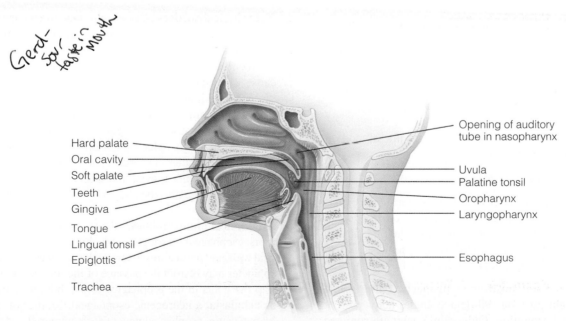

Figure 20-3 ▶▶▶ Anatomy of the oral cavity and the esophagus.

Any of the phases of normal swallowing may be disrupted in older adults with dysphagia. For instance, an older person may have poor tongue control and thus experience delay in initiating the swallow reflex. The bolus of food may be poorly prepared for swallowing, and the food may collect in the pharynx and spill over into the trachea. Poor dentition and poor-fitting dentures may contribute to chewing problems. Psychotropic drugs may cause excessive lethargy or oversedation. Lack of saliva, a common side effect of anticholinergic medications, may make food excessively dry and difficult to swallow. Most often, older adults will experience more than one probable cause for dysphagia, although diagnosis with a neurologic disorder (e.g., dementia, stroke) may be a common underlying theme (Dahlin, 2004; Rofes et al., 2011).

Older Adults at Risk for Dysphagia

Signs and symptoms observable in older adults at risk include the following:

- Reports from the older person or his or her family that swallowing food or medications is difficult
- Difficulty controlling food or saliva in the mouth (drooling, dribbling)
- Facial droop, open mouth
- Dementia, frailty, confusion, extreme lethargy, decreased level of consciousness
- Inability to sit in an upright position and maintain trunk position for a reasonable length of time
- Choking or coughing while eating or drinking
- Increased nasal or oral congestion or secretion after a meal
- Weak voice, cough, and tongue movements
- Slurred speech
- Change in voice during meal (wet, gurgling, or hoarse voice)
- Recurrent upper respiratory infections or pneumonia
- Retention or pocketing of food in mouth
- Oral thrush
- Refusal to open mouth or accept a large bite of food
- Unexplained weight loss

Dahlin, 2004; Reuben et al., 2011.

Early detection of dysphagia is vital because its complications can be life threatening. Aspiration of food or fluid into the respiratory tract can cause choking, airway obstruction, hypoxia, and aspiration pneumonia. Risk factors associated with dysphagia include the following:

- **Older adults not positioned properly.** Eating while in an upright position (90-degree angle) helps prevent choking and aspiration. Older adults who are confined to bed should not be fed in the semireclined position.

- **Older adults fed inappropriate food and liquid.** Thin food and liquids such as tea, juice, water, and clear broth are difficult for older people with dysphagia to swallow. Thin liquids quickly drain into the esophagus before the swallow reflex is triggered. Thickened liquids slow the swallow process, give the older person time to prepare for the swallow, and help prevent aspiration and dehydration.

- **Older adults fed quickly with large bites of food.** Older adults with dysphagia must be fed slowly and given small bites of food to minimize the risk of choking and aspiration. Busy and overburdened staff may feel time pressure to feed the older person due to the demands of other duties resulting in aspiration and choking as a result.

- **Older adults labeled as "difficult" or "uncooperative."** Some older adults are labeled as "combative" or "resistive" to the person feeding them and are noted to turn their heads and constantly push away the spoon. These older adults may be protecting themselves from choking because they need extra time to swallow the food remaining in their mouths. The older person may be at risk for use of additional medications (psychotropic, antianxiety, or sedatives) resulting in increased drowsiness and sedation, further exacerbating swallowing problems. Weight loss may be the inevitable result.

Rofes et al., 2011.

Because dysphagia is associated with underlying illness or disorders, the older person with multiple comorbidities is considered to be at risk for aspiration. Causes of dysphagia include:

1. **Neurologic disorders.** Any disease that affects neuromuscular function, including movement or sensation, may cause dysphagia. Stroke, especially in the midbrain or the anterior cortical areas, is the most common cause of dysphagia in the older person. Parkinson's disease, multiple sclerosis, brain tumors, and central nervous system degenerative diseases (Alzheimer's disease) may cause dysphagia by inhibiting movements of the tongue, pharynx, or upper esophagus.

2. **Muscular disorders.** Disorders such as muscular dystrophy, myasthenia gravis, and extreme frailty at the end of life may cause dysphagia by inhibiting muscular function.

3. **Anatomical abnormalities.** Abnormalities such as tumors, esophageal scarring, outpouchings of the esophageal wall, and premature closure of the upper esophageal sphincter may restrict the passage of the food bolus and trap the bolus in the esophagus. In a condition known as **achalasia,** a neurogenic esophageal disorder of unknown cause, esophageal peristalsis is impaired and the lower esophageal sphincter fails to relax, trapping food

in the esophagus. Zenker's diverticulum is an outpouching of the posterior pharyngeal wall immediately above the upper esophageal sphincter. Esophageal strictures or localized narrowing of the esophagus can develop in people with long-standing **gastroesophageal reflux disease (GERD)** due to acid reflux into the unprotected esophagus causing erosion and scarring. Strictures can also result from swallowing caustic agents (bleach, lye) and certain drugs such as doxycycline, tetracycline, benzodiazepines, clindamycin, NSAIDs, and alendronate (Huether & McCance, 2012; Rofes et al., 2011).

> **Drug Alert** ▶▶▶ Older adults should be advised to swallow their medication with a full 8 oz of water and remain upright for 30 minutes to decrease the risk of reflux and formation of esophageal erosion, stricture, and scarring.

Nursing Assessment

Often, the gerontological nurse is aware that the older person has a swallowing disorder based on the signs and symptoms previously presented. In other cases, the nurse must carefully observe the older person at rest and during the process of eating and drinking. Speech and occupational therapists can assist the nurse and provide valuable professional opinions during the assessment process. The following questions should be included in a dysphagia assessment:

- Have you ever choked while eating or drinking? If so, how recently? Does choking occur frequently?
- Does your mouth feel dry? Do you have enough saliva to chew your food easily?
- Do you have problems with drooling or controlling saliva?
- Does food ever fall out or get stuck in your mouth?
- Do you ever spit up food after a meal?
- Do you feel the need to clear your throat frequently?
- Do you have problems sitting upright during mealtime?

If the answer to any of these questions is positive, the gerontological nurse should notify the primary care provider and request a formal swallowing evaluation by the speech pathologist. A bedside evaluation may be carried out with the older person drinking a variety of liquids (thin to thickened) and being observed for swallowing functionality. In some cases, videofluoroscopic radiographic evaluation of the swallowing process is conducted. The older person drinks a chalklike radiopaque solution, and the movement of the oropharyngeal structures is evaluated. A report is issued that notes any anatomical abnormalities, abnormal movements, or esophageal scarring or strictures. This information helps the interdisciplinary team determine how best to meet the older person's nutrition needs and prevent aspiration.

> **Practice Pearl** ▶▶▶ The chalk mixture used in swallow studies is constipating, and the nurse should carefully monitor bowel function after the procedure to prevent fecal impaction.

All older adults at risk for aspiration should have a notation made on the nursing care plan to inform all involved with the older person's care regarding this risk and appropriate interventions to facilitate safe eating and drinking. Nurses and others caring for the older person should follow the guidelines listed in Box 20-1.

BOX 20-1 ▶ Guidelines to Avoid Risk of Aspiration

- Minimize distractions during eating and provide a pleasant and calm environment during mealtime.
- Use consistent feeding techniques with notations as to the older person's likes, dislikes, eating and drinking habits, and consumption patterns.
- Properly position and support posture during mealtime. Positioning techniques include use of a chair at a table, raising the head of the bed to a 90-degree angle, and use of pillows to support an upright position.
- Maintain the upright position for at least 1 hour after eating.
- Ensure the older person has swallowed one bite before giving another. Do not try to rush. The older person may become resistive.
- Monitor the older person's respirations. A change in breathing pattern or rate can signal the onset of aspiration.
- Provide oral hygiene before and after the meal. A clean, fresh, odor-free mouth will stimulate the older person's appetite. Ensure dentures are in place and in good repair.
- Plan meals at times when the older person is rested and alert. Present meals to people with dementia according to routine.
- Offer food and liquid consistencies according to the speech pathologist's and dietitian's recommendations. Do not overly thicken liquids. The older person will resist "chewing" juice or liquids (rightly so).
- Keep conversation to a minimum and focus attention on the task at hand. For instance, "Now here's a bite of vegetables. Chew them slowly and let me know when you are ready to swallow." Assess mental status to ensure the older person can understand instructions and follow instructions.
- Instruct all people who assist the older person with feeding in the appropriate techniques. Nurses' assistants should sit comfortably at the same level as the older person.
- Never engage in forceful feeding techniques. Everyone has times when they are not hungry and do not feel like eating. Forcing an older person to eat may set the stage for a power struggle at the next meal.

Source: Amella & Lawrence, 2007; Reuben et al., 2011.

Ongoing monitoring of weight, functional status, and the older person's satisfaction during mealtime should be carefully recorded in the older person's record. Weigh older adults weekly if weight fluctuates and then monthly to monitor weight on an ongoing basis. Periodic swallowing evaluation is recommended every 6 months, after a significant change in the older person's condition, or with the onset or return of signs and symptoms of dysphagia. If the older person is unable to tolerate oral feeding, the alternatives may include administration of total parenteral nutrition or placement of a gastric tube for administration of liquid nourishment. Total parenteral nutrition is discussed in detail in Chapter 5 ⬜. Nasogastric tubes (tubes placed through the nose and down the throat into the stomach) should be avoided because they increase the risk of aspiration by keeping the esophagus open, interfere with swallow recovery, and may be uncomfortable for the older person. The head of the bed should be elevated at least 30 degrees during continuous feeding of liquid nourishment through a gastric tube and for 1 hour after intermittent feeding to prevent regurgitation and aspiration (Dahlin, 2004).

Nursing Diagnoses

Nursing diagnoses related to dysphagia include the following:

- *Swallowing, Impaired*
- *Self-Care Deficit: Feeding*
- *Fluid Volume: Imbalanced or Deficient, Risk for*
- *Airway Clearance, Ineffective*
- *Aspiration, Risk for*
- *Dentition, Impaired* (if appropriate)

NANDA-I © 2012.

Related factors identified by the North American Nursing Diagnosis Association include the following:

- Neuromuscular impairment
- Decreased strength or excursion of muscles involved in mastication
- Perceptual impairment
- Mechanical obstruction (edema, tracheostomy tube, tumor)
- Fatigue
- Limited awareness
- Reddened, irritated oropharyngeal cavity

Nursing Management Principles

Nurse-sensitive outcomes that would indicate use of appropriate nursing interventions include improvement in the older person's weight, skin turgor, food and fluid intake, and laboratory values including hemoglobin, hematocrit, and serum albumin levels. Additionally, patients and their families should express satisfaction with the dysphagia prevention plan and no new aspiration events should occur. The well-nourished patient will enjoy improved function and possess appropriate levels of energy.

Gastroesophageal Reflux Disease

Gastroesophageal reflux disease (GERD) involves reflux of gastric contents into the esophagus. Many people occasionally experience heartburn, but for some, it is a frequent and continual problem. Heartburn is often thought to be a trivial problem but in reality it is a serious health issue capable of causing permanent damage. In the United States, symptoms of GERD occur at least once a month in about 25% of adults, amounting to about 60 million people (Slowik, 2012). GERD occurs more frequently in men than in women. According to the National Institute of Diabetes and Digestive and Kidney Diseases, GERD results in 18.3 million ambulatory care visits, 3.1 million hospitalizations, and 64.6 million prescriptions each year in the United States (Everhart, 2009). GERD is a common diagnosis in all age groups, but most diagnoses are found in the over-65 age group. Older adults are more at risk for GERD complications because of prolonged esophageal acid exposure over a period of years. Additionally, the higher frequency of hiatal hernia, decreased saliva volume, and use of drugs that reduce lower esophageal sphincter tone may contribute to the development and progression of GERD in older adults (Huether & McCance, 2012). Hiatal hernias, or diaphragmatic hernias that allow a small portion of the stomach to slide into the chest, are so common in older people that they are sometimes classified as a normal change of aging and are often asymptomatic.

Those with thyroid disease, diabetes, scleroderma, or connective tissue disorders may develop esophageal motility problems and heighten their risk for GERD. In the majority of older adults with GERD, the cause of the problem is not overproduction of acid, but length and frequency of esophageal acid exposure (McPhee & Papadakis, 2011). In healthy people, the contractile motions in the esophagus move substances quickly out of the esophagus into the stomach, and these clearance mechanisms limit the amount of time that the esophageal tissues are exposed to reflux. The longer the reflux is in contact with the unprotected esophageal lining, the greater the opportunity for esophageal injury, erosion, and scarring.

The symptoms of GERD include heartburn (sensation of burning in the substernal or sternal area), indigestion, belching, hiccups, and regurgitation of gastric contents into the mouth (sour mouth). The heartburn will typically worsen with lying flat or bending over. Chest pain can be so severe and persistent that it is sometimes confused with cardiac pain or angina. The older person may seek emergency evaluation because he or she fears the onset of a heart attack. Erosive esophagitis occurs when the caustic gastric contents remain in contact with the esophageal mucosa and begin to cause damage to the esophageal lining. Chronic laryngeal irritation can cause voice hoarseness, wheezing, bronchitis, asthma, and aspiration pneumonia. Symptoms may be worsened by eating large meals, using certain medications, eating foods and drinking beverages high in fat or caffeine, using tobacco and alcohol, reclining after eating, and obesity (Reuben et al., 2011). Drugs that may worsen reflux symptoms include those listed in Box 20-2.

In addition to physical consequences, GERD is associated with psychosocial consequences. Some older adults may be fearful of eating out or attending social events because stress and certain foods may trigger symptoms. Because the symptoms of GERD may be heightened when the older person is lying flat, sleep is often disrupted. Complications from untreated GERD include esophagitis, bleeding, scarring, and stricture formation. Barrett's esophagus occurs in about 10% to 15% of older adults with GERD and results when chronic acid exposure causes the cells lining the esophagus to become inflamed, with cellular changes considered to be precancerous for development

of adenocarcinoma. Hemorrhage can occur from deep erosions and ulcerations, resulting in anemia, black tarry stools, or vomiting of bright red blood.

Nursing Assessment

The older person's report of symptoms, past medical history, medications, and dietary and sleep habits are the most useful sources of information to diagnose GERD. The nurse should question the older person about characteristics of the symptoms, onset, duration, frequency, aggravating and alleviating factors, and prior methods of treatment and symptom control. These questions may include:

- When did your symptoms begin?
- How long does the pain last?
- Have you had heartburn before?
- What do you usually eat at a meal? How long does it usually take you to eat a meal?
- Do you drink coffee, alcohol, or caffeinated beverages? Do you smoke?
- Have you experienced unintentional weight loss?
- Does the pain go to your neck, jaw, back, or arm?
- What medications—herbals, vitamins, and dietary supplements—are you taking?
- Do you vomit red blood or something that looks like coffee grounds?
- Do you have black stools or red blood in your stool?
- What else (if anything) goes along with your heartburn, such as nausea or abdominal pain?

Adapted from Dunphy et al., 2011; Reuben et al., 2011.

Generally, pain resulting from GERD can be distinguished from cardiac pain because esophageal pain worsens after a large meal, worsens after lying down, often is accompanied by belching and regurgitation, and is relieved by antacids. Referral to the primary care provider for a thorough cardiac evaluation is necessary to rule out cardiac disease and will confirm the chest discomfort as GERD. Older adults with atypical pain, unexplained weight loss, or iron deficiency anemia should be referred to a gastroenterologist for diagnostic testing. Upper endoscopy with biopsy is the best way to document the type and extent of tissue damage in GERD, for ruling out serious pathology and other possible causes of reflux, and for detecting complications such as scarring and stricture (McPhee & Papadakis, 2011). Upper endoscopy enables the physician to look inside the esophagus, stomach, and duodenum by passing a small tube down the throat. Acid perfusion tests are usually not necessary and require the placement of an esophageal probe above the esophageal sphincter to collect esophageal contents. Patients considering antireflux

---

BOX 20-2 ▶ **Drugs That May Worsen Reflux Symptoms**

Alendronate	Nitrates
Anticholinergics	Nonsteroidal anti-inflammatory agents
Benzodiazepines	Oral antineoplastic agents
Beta-blockers	Phentolamine
Bisphosphonates	Potassium supplements
Caffeine and alcohol	Progesterone
Calcium channel blockers	Prostaglandins
Codeine and opioid narcotics	Quinidine
Dopamine	Sedatives and hypnotics
Estrogen	Tetracycline
Glucagon	Theophylline
Nicotine	

Source: Dunphy, Winland-Brown, Porter et al., 2011; Gillson, 2011.

surgery may benefit from esophageal reflux pH monitoring. Most often, the older person's diagnosis is based on signs and symptoms and improvement of symptoms with treatment.

> *Practice Pearl* ▶▶▶ "Red flags" or signs and symptoms that require immediate evaluation and referral include heartburn accompanied by weight loss, lack of response to treatment, black or bloody stools, unexplained anemia, swallowing problems, choking while eating, hoarse voice, and radiation of pain to the neck, arm, jaw, or back accompanied by diaphoresis or shortness of breath (Dunphy et al., 2011). These problems could indicate the presence of a malignancy or serious heart condition.

Treatment Goals

The goal of treatment is to control symptoms and heal esophageal mucosal injury. Many healthcare providers recommend lifestyle changes first to avoid the use of medications, or they may recommend lifestyle changes along with the prescription of medications to maximize the treatment effects. Lifestyle modifications include those listed in Box 20-3.

BOX 20-3 ▶ **Lifestyle Modifications to Control Symptoms of GERD**

- Elevate the head of the bed 6 to 10 inches on wooden blocks.
- Reduce portion sizes so the stomach is not overfilled. Cut back on late-night eating.
- Avoid foods that increase reflux such as chocolate, cola, certain spices, onions, garlic, tomatoes, raw onions, vinegar, and citrus fruits.
- Drink 6 to 8 oz of water with all medications.
- If you are taking medications daily (prescription or over-the-counter), ask your healthcare provider if they can be contributing to your symptoms of GERD.
- Stop drugs that promote reflux (if possible).
- Avoid tight-fitting clothes and girdles.
- Decrease fat, alcohol, and caffeine intake.
- Avoid supine position immediately after eating. Stay upright for 1 to 3 hours after a meal.
- Avoid lying on right side when reclining, because this position encourages reflux.
- Avoid vigorous exercise within 1 hour after meals.
- Lose weight if indicated.
- Stop smoking.

Medications Used to Manage GERD

Over-the-counter antacids buffer the gastric pH and are widely available and useful for treating episodic heartburn. The cost is reasonable, but side effects may include diarrhea, constipation, altered mineral metabolism, and acid–base disturbances. Magnesium-containing antacids (milk of magnesia) can cause diarrhea and should be used with caution in older adults with renal dysfunction, including chronic or acute renal failure, because of the potential for hypermagnesemia and related toxicity. Aluminum-containing antacids (Maalox, Mylanta) can cause constipation, osteomalacia, hypophosphatemia, and related toxicity (Nurse Practitioners' Prescribing Reference, 2012).

Histamine$_2$ receptor agonists (Zantac, Pepcid) decrease acid production by inhibiting histamine stimulation of the parietal cells. They are now available over the counter at lower strength than the prescription medication. These medications are potent inhibitors of gastric acid secretion and are generally well tolerated in older people with a low incidence of side effects. Risk factors for side effects include advanced age, hepatic or renal impairment, and diagnoses of additional medical conditions. Cimetidine (Tagamet), a drug available without prescription, has the greatest chance for adverse effects, including erectile dysfunction, gynecomastia, confusion, agitation, anxiety, and depression, and should be used with caution. Further, cimetidine inhibits the cytochrome P-450 oxidase system, increasing the probability of interactions with other medications. See Chapter 6 ▭ for further information related to the P-450 oxidase system and the potential for drug interactions. More general side effects of histamine blockers include headache, diarrhea, and constipation. Clinically significant interaction between H$_2$-blockers and other medications may occur because of an alteration in absorption, metabolism, or excretion of these drugs due to inhibition of gastric acid production.

> *Practice Pearl* ▶▶▶ Older adults taking H$_2$-blockers may not absorb enteric-coated medications because they lack the gastric acid necessary to dissolve the protective coating. The nurse should obtain a complete medication history (including over-the-counter medications) before the dosage of any medication is altered.

Proton pump inhibitors (PPIs) (Nexium, Prilosec, Protonix) suppress acid secretion by inhibiting the hydrogen/potassium adenosinetriphosphatase pump at the parietal cell. The effect is dose related. In the older person, the acid-reducing effect of the medication and the duration of action and bioavailability are increased. However, these drugs are usually well tolerated in the older person, with healing and rate of adverse reactions similar to those in younger people. Common side effects of proton pump inhibitors include atrophic **gastritis,** headache, diarrhea and constipation, dizziness, rash, cough, backache, and abdominal pain (Nurse Practitioners' Prescribing Reference, 2012; Reuben et al., 2011). The danger of long-term acid suppression with a PPI has been debated. The major concern is that use of PPIs results in an overproduction of gastrin, which is associated with cell hyperplasia and liver adenomas and carcinoma in animals. Studies in humans note a relationship between nutritional deficiencies and increased risk of infectious processes (Ali, Roberts, & Tierney, 2009). Additionally, PPIs inhibit the biotransformation of oral anticoagulants, diazepam, theophylline, and phenytoin, leading to elevated serum levels of these drugs. Pantoprazole (Protonix) is less likely to have significant drug interactions compared with the other PPIs (Gutierrez, 2008).

Other medications besides acid-suppression agents can help control the symptoms of GERD, including promotility agents (Reglan) that enhance esophageal clearance and gastric emptying. However, these drugs are considered second-line treatments because of the prevalence of adverse effects, including abdominal cramping, diarrhea, gynecomastia, galactorrhea, fatigue, drowsiness, and movement disorders (tremor, rigidity, and tardive dyskinesia).

The mucosal protectant agent sucralfate (Carafate) aids in mucosal healing by reducing direct tissue exposure to acid. Sucralfate works locally by forming an adherent complex that coats the ulcer site and protects it from further injury from acid, pepsin, and bile salts. It is minimally absorbed, but bowel function should be carefully monitored because it may cause constipation. Sucralfate should be used with caution in older adults with renal impairment because of the potential for aluminum absorption and associated toxicity. Further, sucralfate can reduce the absorption of other drugs, including quinolone antibiotics, phenytoin, and warfarin (Nurse Practitioners' Prescribing Reference, 2012). Older adults taking these drugs should have drug levels carefully monitored if sucralfate is added to the medication regimen.

Misoprostol (Cytotec), a combination drug that has an antisecretory and mucosal protective effect, is a synthetic prostaglandin E analogue. It is indicated only for prophylactic treatment in older adults taking NSAIDs (U.S. National Library of Medicine, 2010). It has been shown to prevent NSAID-induced damage to the gastric mucosa but does not protect against duodenal ulcers. The major side effects are diarrhea (13% to 40% of older adults) and abdominal pain (7% to 20%). The severity of these side effects is sometimes improved with dose reduction. Older adults should be instructed to report the onset of diarrhea or abdominal pain immediately to prevent dehydration and associated secondary problems. Table 20-1 lists medications used to manage GERD.

To minimize adverse effects, medications are usually begun at a low dose and then "stepped up" until symptoms resolve. If symptoms persist after 6 to 8 weeks of treatment, the older person should return to the primary care provider for further evaluation. The underlying problem may be more serious than initially determined, and further testing may be needed. If the older person's symptoms are controlled, therapy at the initial dose is usually continued for about 8 weeks to allow complete healing. However, some older adults will relapse and require long-term maintenance therapy to prevent future recurrences and return of symptoms. Maintenance therapy should consist of the least costly, most convenient, and most effective (desired effect achieved without troubling side effects) drug for the older person (Dunphy et al., 2011).

> **Practice Pearl** ▶▶▶ Most antacids impede the absorption of certain drugs by binding to them to form insoluble compounds. These drugs include antibiotics (tetracycline and quinolones), oral thyroid replacement hormones, digoxin, captopril, and acetaminophen. If these drugs are needed, they should be scheduled to be taken several hours after ingestion of the antacid (Gutierrez, 2008).

Older adults with GERD and with Barrett's esophagus require aggressive treatment with PPIs and regular endoscopic examination. Surgery may be required if esophageal erosion does not reverse with treatment. The surgery of choice is Nissen fundoplication and involves closing any hiatal hernia and restoring an antireflux barrier by creating a pressure gradient in the distal esophagus. The surgery is usually 85% successful. The most common side effect is dysphagia and inability to belch or vomit. Increasingly, Nissen fundoplication is being performed laparoscopically as an alternative to major surgery. Use of NSAIDs increases the risk of recurrence and GI complications two to six times, depending on the dose and half-life of the drug, the dosing frequency, and duration of use. Older adults should be discouraged from taking these drugs following healing and resolution of their symptoms (McPhee & Papadakis, 2011).

Nursing Diagnoses

Nursing diagnoses related to GERD include the following:

- *Swallowing, Impaired*
- *Skin Integrity, Impaired*
- *Social Interaction, Impaired* (if appropriate)
- *Sleep Pattern Disturbance* (if appropriate)
- *Pain, Acute* or *Chronic*

NANDA-I © 2012.

TABLE 20-1	Medication Management of Gastroesophageal Reflux Disease		
Drug	**Initial Dose**	**Maximum Dose**	**Formulation**
Antacids (neutralize acids)			
Tums, Rolaids, Mylanta	1–2 tbs or tablets PRN between meals and bedtime		Chewable, liquid
Histamine Blockers (suppress acid production)			
Cimetidine (Tagamet)	400–800 mg bid	2 × initial dose	Tablets, liquid
Famotidine (Pepcid)	20 mg bid × 6 wks	2 × initial dose	Tablets
Nizatidine (Axid)	150 mg bid	2 × initial dose	Tablets
Ranitidine (Zantac)	150 mg bid	2 × initial dose	Tablets, liquid
Proton Pump Inhibitors			
Esomeprazole (Nexium)	20 mg daily × 4 wks		Delayed-release tablets
Lansoprazole (Prevacid)	15 mg daily × 8 wks	60 mg	Delayed-release tablets
Omeprazole (Prilosec)	20 mg daily × 4–8 wks		Tablets
Pantoprazole (Protonix)	40 mg daily × 8 wks		Enteric-coated tablets
Mucosal Protective Agents			
Sucralfate (Carafate)	1 g q6h, 1h ac and hs	4 g/day	Oral suspension
Antisecretory/Mucosal Protective Agent			
Misoprostol (Cytotec)	100–200 mcg po/qid	800 mcg/day	Tablets
Prokinetic Agents (speeds stomach emptying)			
Metoclopramide	5 mg q6h, ac and hs	15 mg qid	Tablets, sugar-free syrup, injection syrup

Source: Data from Nurse Practitioners' Prescribing Reference (2012); Reuben et al. (2011).

Nursing Management Principles

Nurse-sensitive outcomes that would indicate use of appropriate nursing interventions for patients with GERD include positive relief of signs and symptoms, no significant side effects of medications, sustained progress on lifestyle modification plan, and adequate nutrition as measured by weight and nutritional markers.

Gastric Disorders

Gastric disorders occurring in the older person will exhibit different signs and symptoms, complications, and treatment options (Gray-Miceli, 2012). Symptoms may be more vague and less specific than those of younger adults, are more likely to be attributed to changes of aging, and may be diagnosed and treated in the more severe stage of the disease progression. Common gastric disorders include gastritis, ulcers, hiatal hernias, and stomach tumors.

Gastritis

Gastritis, or inflammation of the gastric mucosa, is classified by the severity of the mucosal inflammation, the site of involvement, and the inflammatory cell type. Erosive (hemorrhagic) gastritis may be caused by ingestion of substances that irritate the gastric mucosa such as NSAIDs, alcohol, radiation therapy, gastric trauma, or ischemia as a result of arterial insufficiency or circulatory problems. Diagnosis is based on endoscopic appearance of the stomach lining, and biopsy is usually not necessary to confirm the diagnosis. Antral gland gastritis (type B) is the most common form of gastritis and is associated with *H. pylori* and duodenal ulcers. Fundic gland gastritis (type A) is associated with diffuse severe mucosal atrophy and the presence of pernicious anemia. Treatment of gastritis is directed at the underlying cause, including reducing factors contributing to the inflammatory process, acid neutralization and suppression (with antacids, H₂-blockers, PPIs), protection of the gastric mucosa (sucralfate), and antibiotic therapy to eradicate *H. pylori* (Dunphy et al., 2011). Older adults with severe gastritis may be diagnosed with anemia and require transfusion, careful ongoing monitoring of hemoglobin and hematocrit levels, and periodic evaluation of stool for occult blood testing.

Peptic and Duodenal Ulcer Disease

In the United States, about 4.5 million adults have peptic ulcer disease. The specific incidence in older people is unknown, but hospitalization, morbidity, and mortality rates from peptic ulcer disease are higher for older adults than the general population (Anand, 2012). Most duodenal ulcers occur in patients between the ages of 30 and 55, but gastric ulcers are more prevalent between ages 55 and 70 (Dunphy et al., 2011). **Peptic ulcer disease** is defined as an excoriated area of the gastric mucosa (peptic ulcer) or first few centimeters of the duodenum (duodenal ulcer) that penetrates through to the muscularis mucosae. Duodenal ulcers are more common than gastric ulcers. Bleeding from duodenal ulcers occurs more frequently in older adults. Chronic or slow upper gastrointestinal bleeding may present with anemia, melena (black, tarry stools), or a positive fecal occult blood test. Pain from a peptic ulcer may occur when food is in the stomach or shortly after eating, whereas pain from a duodenal ulcer occurs when the stomach is empty and may awaken the older person in the middle of the night. Upper gastrointestinal endoscopy is required to definitively evaluate and diagnose the cause of the pain.

H. pylori is an important factor in the development of ulcers, and the prevalence of *H. pylori* infections increases with age. *H. pylori* gastritis is implicated in 90% to 95% of both duodenal and gastric ulcers that are not associated with NSAIDs (Dunphy et al., 2011). In the United States, about 70% to 90% of older adults with gastric ulcers and 90% to 100% of older adults with duodenal ulcers are infected with *H. pylori*. Although nearly all older adults with *H. pylori* will develop gastritis, only 15% develop a peptic ulcer. Eradication of *H. pylori* is associated with more rapid ulcer healing and a decrease in recurrence rates

(Dunphy et al., 2011). A serology blood test can detect the presence of *H. pylori* as can direct analysis of cells biopsied during esophagogastroduodenoscopy (EGD), which is much more expensive and invasive. An *H. pylori* breath test can also detect the presence of this bacterium, but this test is less reliable because false negatives and true negatives are difficult to distinguish.

The first signs of peptic ulcer disease may be serious gastrointestinal bleeding episodes requiring emergency evaluation, treatment, and transfusion. NSAID use increases the incidence of peptic ulcer disease, especially early in treatment (during the first 3 months). Higher doses of NSAIDs, history of peptic ulcer disease, and concurrent use of anticoagulants (warfarin, aspirin) predispose older adults to larger ulcers. Approximately 50% of these older adults do not experience abdominal pain and the first sign of the ulcer may be a massive GI bleed. Defensive factors to protect the stomach lining, such as the production of a mucous-bicarbonate barrier, are overwhelmed by the production of acid-induced aggressive factors, resulting in the penetration of the mucous barrier and allowing tissue injury. The strength of the mucous barrier is dependent on the production of prostaglandin, and older adults have decreased prostaglandin concentrations in the stomach and duodenum (McPhee & Papadakis, 2011). These factors contribute to the development of peptic and duodenal ulcers in older people and are a key reason why the use of NSAIDs in older people often results in GI side effects and problems.

> **Practice Pearl ▶▶▶** Taking an NSAID with food helps to protect the stomach only slightly from local irritation but damage to the stomach lining is more likely to result from decreased prostaglandin production, which will occur at the same rate whether the medication is taken with or without food.

Zollinger-Ellison syndrome is characterized by gastric hypersecretion and peptic ulceration caused by a gastrin-producing tumor (gastrinoma) of the pancreas or duodenal wall. The continuous high-gastrin output stimulates the parietal cells to produce acid. The onset of Zollinger-Ellison syndrome is usually between the ages of 30 and 50, and 7% of the older adults developing this syndrome are over the age of 60 (Roy, 2012). Peptic ulcer occurs in 90% of older adults with Zollinger-Ellison syndrome with persistent symptoms that progress and do not respond to drug treatment. For these older adults, referral to a gastroenterologist for additional testing and assessment of gastrin levels is indicated. Treatment may include tumor removal and surgical resection for older adults without surgical risk or treatment with omeprazole (Prilosec).

Signs and Symptoms In older people, the classic signs and symptoms of peptic ulcer disease are rare. The classic sign of abdominal pain occurs in only 35% to 50% of older adults. When pain is present, it is often vague and diffuse throughout the abdomen. Often the presenting sign is blood loss and iron deficiency anemia.

Dyspepsia (indigestion with bloating, early satiety, abdominal distention, anorexia, vomiting, dysphagia, belching, or nausea) is a common symptom but often is not vigorously investigated and is attributed to normal changes of aging. These symptoms most often are the result of lifestyle such as ingestion of excess alcohol or may be related to use of medications such as NSAIDs, erythromycin, or theophylline. However, they may signal the onset of serious organic disease such as gastric cancer. Older adults with persistent symptoms of dyspepsia associated with anorexia and weight loss should be referred to a gastroenterologist for further assessment and treatment.

Nursing Diagnosis The older person's report of symptoms, past medical history, use of medications, and dietary habits are the most useful sources of information to diagnose peptic ulcer disease. The nurse should question the older person about characteristics of the symptoms, onset, duration, frequency, aggravating and alleviating factors, and prior methods of treatment and symptom control. A history of iron deficiency anemia or occurrence of new-onset anemia should be aggressively investigated by the healthcare provider. Generally, pain resulting from peptic ulcer disease is described as dyspepsia localized in the epigastric area, occurring hours after a meal (on an empty stomach), and relieved by food or antacids. Abdominal pain that awakens the older person at night can be a symptom of peptic ulcer disease. Referral to a gastroenterologist for an upper endoscopy or X-ray is the best method to diagnose ulcer disease. Upper endoscopy is the most sensitive and specific test for assessing abnormalities in the upper GI tract. Biopsies can be taken, if needed, during the procedure. Gastric ulcers are often difficult to distinguish from stomach cancer, and biopsy is required to eliminate the possibility of malignancy. For those who are very frail or who have cognitive impairments, symptomatic treatment with antiulcer medications may be tried to assess if troublesome symptoms can be reduced and quality of life improved without invasive testing or treatment. Avoidance of all medications associated with gastric ulcers is indicated.

The morbidity and mortality rates from peptic ulcer disease have increased significantly in older adults. These trends are thought to be related to the increased use of NSAIDs among older adults. It was hoped that the introduction of cyclooxygenase (COX-2) inhibitors (celecoxib) would decrease this trend; however, recent evidence indicates that the use of these pain-relieving medications may be associated with increased risk of stroke and heart attack and casts doubt on the continued utility of these medications. In 2004 and 2005, rofecoxib (Vioxx) and valdecoxib (Bextra) were withdrawn from the market and as of this writing only celecoxib (Celebrex) is available in the United States. Older patients taking Celebrex require careful monitoring and supervision.

Treatment Goals Older adults should discontinue the use of all NSAIDs, alcohol, tobacco, and caffeine. Alcohol stimulates acid secretion, and tobacco and caffeine delay healing. Eating small frequent meals and avoiding offending foods is helpful to relieve symptoms. The goal of treatment is to promote healing of the gastric mucosa through the use of lifestyle modification and medications that neutralize acid, inhibit gastric acid secretion, improve gastric mucosal defense mechanisms, and eradicate the presence of *H. pylori*.

Medications used to treat peptic ulcers are similar to those used in the treatment of GERD. Refer to Table 20-1 on page 566, which illustrates these agents by category. In older adults with documented *H. pylori* infection, the use of antisecretory drugs combined with an antibiotic results in more rapid duodenal ulcer healing. Eradication of *H. pylori* has proven difficult due to antibiotic resistance. In the United States, up to 50% of strains are resistant to metronidazole and 13% are resistant to clarithromycin. It is recommended to include amoxicillin in first-line therapy for most patients and reserve metronidazole for penicillin-allergic patients (McPhee & Papadakis, 2011). Recurrence of duodenal ulcers can be as high as 80% within 1 year if eradication of *H. pylori* is not part of treatment and less than 5% when *H. pylori* is eradicated. Among the factors that can contribute to ulcer formation after eradication of *H. pylori* are NSAID use, smoking, and continued acid hypersecretion (Dunphy et al., 2011). The classic treatment involves triple therapy over a period of 10 to 14 days of a PPI plus clarithromycin 500 mg q12h plus amoxicillin 1000 mg q12h. For those with a penicillin allergy, Metronidazole 500 mg q12h can be substituted (Reuben et al., 2011). These protocols achieve eradication rates of >75% after 10 to 14 days but eradication rates are declining due to antibiotic resistance. Monotherapy (use of only one antibiotic) is not recommended because of its limited effectiveness and potential for stimulating antimicrobial resistance. Surgery is recommended for older adults with ulcers without comorbidities who do not respond to treatment or who are at high risk for serious complications (perforation, hemorrhage) (McPhee & Papadakis, 2011).

Nursing Diagnoses Nursing diagnoses related to peptic ulcer disease include the following:

- *Nutrition, Imbalanced: Less than Body Requirements*
- *Infection, Risk for*
- *Tissue Integrity, Impaired*
- *Sleep Pattern: Disturbed* (if appropriate)
- *Fatigue* (if appropriate)
- *Activity Intolerance, Risk for* (if appropriate)
- *Pain, Acute* or *Chronic*

NANDA-I © 2012.

Nursing Management Principles Nurse-sensitive outcomes that would indicate use of appropriate nursing interventions include:

- Positive relief of signs and symptoms
- No significant side effects of medications
- Sustained progress on lifestyle modification plan
- Adequate nutrition as measured by weight and nutritional markers
- Resolution of ulcer disease as evidenced by tissue healing and stable hemoglobin and hematocrit levels

Gastric Volvulus

Gastric volvulus, or a turning, twisting, or telescoping of the stomach into or onto itself, occurs more commonly in older adults than in younger adults because of relaxation of the ligaments supporting the stomach. A complete twist can lead to strangulation of the blood supply and tissue death and is considered a surgical emergency. Symptoms include acute pain localized to the abdomen or chest, shock and hypotension, abdominal distention, an inability to vomit, and dyspnea. Emergency evaluation is needed and treatment is always surgical. The mortality rate is as high as 60%.

Lower Gastrointestinal Tract Disorders

The lower GI tract is composed of the colon and the rectum. The function of the lower GI tract is affected by metabolic or endocrine disorders, lifestyle and environmental factors, neurologic disorders or injury, and many medications. Many older people experience problems or dysfunction of the lower GI tract.

Anatomy and Physiology

The main functions of the colon and rectum are the storage and passing of feces. Fecal storage is enhanced by the ability of the colon to stretch and adapt to the amount of fecal matter contained within. Rhythmic colonic contractions and peristaltic waves, known as mass movements, regulate the progression of stool and allow water to be absorbed, thus decreasing stool

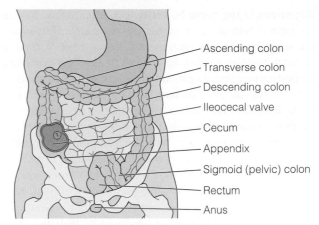

Figure 20-4 ▶▶▶ The lower digestive tract.

Source: National Digestive Disease Information Clearinghouse. (2003). *Your digestive system and how it works.* Retrieved from http://www.digestive.NIDDK.NIH.gov.

volume. Normally, the colon absorbs approximately 1 to 2 L of water each day. The colon has both intrinsic and extrinsic innervations. The intrinsic nervous system regulates motility in response to immediate factors such as distention and intraluminal irritants. The extrinsic nervous system originates from the autonomic nervous system and regulates colonic motility (Huether & McCance, 2012). Bowel continence and controlled defecation are dependent on the older person's ability to sense fullness and accurately identify contents in the rectum and to coordinate function of the internal and external anal sphincters. The anal canal is 3 to 5 cm long and is formed by circular muscles known as the internal and external anal sphincters. The internal sphincter is smooth muscle and under autonomic control, while the external sphincter is under voluntary control. Figure 20-4 ▶▶▶ illustrates the anatomy of the lower GI tract.

NORMAL CHANGES OF AGING

Colonic motility and transit in healthy older adults are similar to those in younger people; however, aging is associated with diminished anal sphincter tone and strength (Bharucha, 2007). The structural weakening of colonic muscle may contribute to the development of **diverticula,** or saclike mucosal projections through the muscle wall. Colonic diverticular disease is rare in developing nations but common in the United States, accounting for approximately 130,000 hospitalizations each year. The risk of having diverticular disease increases with age with 30% at age 60 and 50% of those at age 80 having this diagnosis (McPhee & Papadakis, 2011; Nguyen, Sam, & Anon, 2011). Older adults with the presence of diverticula are diagnosed with **diverticulosis.** Several factors can alter colonic function and lead to alterations in the lower bowel function, including diagnosis with a metabolic or endocrine disorder, lifestyle and environmental factors such as insufficient fiber or fluid in the diet, neurologic disorders or injury, mobility problems, cognitive impairment or mood disorders, and many medications. These factors may make the older person more susceptible to fecal incontinence, constipation, or diarrhea.

In the healthy older adult, the large intestine does not experience major changes with regard to colonic motility. Although 50% of nursing home residents suffer from fecal incontinence, this is commonly caused by chronic constipation, fecal impaction, laxative use, and mobility or neurologic disorders. There is, however, a slight decrease in the older person's ability to recognize rectal wall distention and this may play a role in the pathogenesis of constipation (Bharucha, 2007). Dementia, depression, medications, chronic pain, and lack of mobility may further compound the problem and contribute to the development of fecal incontinence over time.

Common Lower Gastrointestinal Disorders

The major lower gastrointestinal disorders in older adults are constipation, diarrhea, abdominal pain, rectal bleeding, and fecal incontinence. Lower GI disorders that occur more commonly in the older person than in younger people include diverticular disease, colonic ischemia, antibiotic-associated diarrhea and colitis, and fecal incontinence. Additionally, inflammatory bowel diseases occur in all age groups, and new onset is common in the older person (Bharucha, 2007).

Diverticular Disease or Diverticulosis

Diverticula can potentially trap feces, become inflamed and infected, and rupture. Usually diverticula are found in the sigmoid and descending colon where blood vessels penetrate to the submucosa (Bharucha, 2007). Lifestyle-related factors include inadequate intake of dietary fiber and a diet high in refined carbohydrates. A low-fiber diet increases the density of the stool with increases in intraluminal pressure, forcing the saclike projections of the colon wall through the muscular layers of the colon. Additional aggravating factors include physical inactivity, constipation, obesity, smoking, and treatment with NSAIDs.

Bleeding may occur from rupture of the penetrating arteriole contained within the mucosal diverticula and is usually painless. Although 10% to 20% of older adults continue to bleed chronically, bleeding usually stops spontaneously unless the older person is taking medications that increase clotting times such as anticoagulants. Usually, diverticula are asymptomatic and occur commonly in the older person. Older adults with diverticulosis or diverticula without inflammation should be urged to increase dietary fiber to prevent complications such as diverticulitis (Huether & McCance, 2012).

Diverticulitis is an infection or inflammation occurring in the diverticula. Diverticulitis develops in 15% to 25% of older adults with diverticulosis, and the probability of infection increases with the length of time from diagnosis. Diverticulitis is caused when normal bowel flora (aerobic and anaerobic gram-negative bacilli) overgrow and flourish in the diverticular pouch when stool becomes entrapped. With inflammation, the diverticular opening becomes obstructed and a pouch forms, trapping the infection. Symptoms of diverticulitis may include fever, leukocytosis, left lower quadrant pain, or abdominal tenderness, but the very old or frail older person may exhibit none of these classic symptoms and suffer more severe negative outcomes (obstruction and abscess) because of their immunocompromised status and inability to mount an effective immune response (Nguyen et al., 2011).

Nursing Assessment The gerontological nurse should perform a careful abdominal examination on the older person with complaints of abdominal pain or discomfort. Diverticulosis is usually asymptomatic; however, the older person may experience mild abdominal pain in the lower left quadrant, cramping, and bloating. Occasional constipation or diarrhea may also be symptomatic of diverticulosis. Diverticulitis usually presents more dramatically with symptoms of abdominal pain (severe at times), cramping (usually on the left side), fever, nausea or vomiting, and disturbed bowel habits such as constipation, diarrhea, and watery stools with flatus.

Examination of the abdomen for abnormal peristaltic waves and auscultation of bowel sounds should always precede palpation because palpation may stimulate or alter peristaltic movement. Hyperactive bowel sounds, rebound tenderness, or the presence of an abdominal mass may indicate a bowel obstruction or perforation and require immediate referral and medical attention. The older person or caregiver should be questioned as to the time and nature of the last normal bowel movement. Diarrhea and fecal oozing may accompany bowel obstruction and complicate recognition of the problem. Some older adults and caregivers may confuse rectal oozing with diarrhea and administer antidiarrheal medications, further compounding the problem. Rectal bleeding is usually not present.

Most often, a gastroenterologist will obtain an abdominal computerized tomography (CT) scan or ultrasound to assess colonic wall thickness and extraluminal structures for suspected diverticulitis. The CT scan has high diagnostic accuracy, but pelvic ultrasonography or barium enema may also be considered (McPhee & Papadakis, 2011). Invasive studies such as barium enema and colonoscopy should be delayed until the inflammation and infection resolve with treatment because of the increased risk of bowel perforation. Surgery may be recommended for some older adults who fail to respond to medical therapy within 72 hours, for those with repeated attacks of diverticulitis, and for the immunocompromised older person (including those on chemotherapy, chronic steroid users, and those with diabetes mellitus). Emergency surgery is required for generalized peritonitis, persistent bowel obstruction, and uncontrollable GI bleeding, however with appropriate management, fewer than 10% of older adults admitted to the hospital with acute diverticulitis will require surgery (Jacobs, 2007).

> **Practice Pearl ▶▶▶** When palpating the abdomen of an older person with abdominal discomfort or pain, always begin with very light palpation and warm hands in an area as remote from the area of pain as possible. Deep palpation or cold hands can trigger intense pain, causing the older person to become uncooperative and resist further examination attempts.

Treatment

The goal of treatment is to eliminate the bacterial infection that is the source of pain and inflammation. Mild infections may be treated with oral antibiotics on an outpatient basis, whereas severe infections may require hospitalization with intravenous antibiotics. Drugs of choice include one of the following: metronidazole (Flagyl) and a quinolone (Cipro) (orally or by intravenous regimen); amoxicillin-clavulanate orally; or a beta-lactam with a beta-lactamase inhibitor via intravenous delivery (Jacobs, 2007). Sometimes a liquid diet progressing to a low-fiber diet may be suggested to allow the colon to rest and heal (Dunphy et al., 2011).

To prevent recurrence of diverticulitis and manage diverticular disease, the nurse may suggest the following interventions:

- Eat more fiber and drink plenty of fluids (try to drink eight full glasses of water per day). This will decrease intraluminal pressure and soften the consistency of the stool.
- Do not ignore the urge to have a bowel movement. Holding stool in the colon and rectum longer will encourage further water absorption, causing stool to become drier, more compact, and more difficult to pass. Older adults who regularly resist the urge to have a bowel movement will, over time, become unaware of the need and may suffer from chronic constipation.
- Exercise regularly (e.g., walking, swimming) to aid digestion and increase colonic peristalsis.
- Avoid foods that precipitate painful attacks. Some foods with seeds, such as popcorn, sesame seeds, and poppy

seeds, can become trapped in the diverticula and trigger an infection and inflammatory response.

Irritable Bowel Disease

Irritable bowel disease (IBS) is defined as chronic (more than 3 months) abdominal pain, bloating, or discomfort that occurs in association with altered bowel function including constipation and diarrhea. Other symptoms include pain relief with defecation, lumpy or loose stool, straining at stool or incomplete evacuation, and passage of mucus. The symptoms may be continuous or intermittent. Approximately 66% of people with irritable bowel disease are women (McPhee & Papadakis, 2011). Approximately 10% to 20% of older people have symptoms consistent with the diagnosis (Ehrenpreis, 2005). IBS is considered a functional disease, meaning no structural or biochemical pathophysiology can be linked to the diagnosis.

Because several other bowel diseases present with symptoms similar to those of IBS, careful monitoring is required. Older patients with a family history of colon cancer or inflammatory bowel disease should seek evaluation by a gastroenterologist. Danger signs or "red flags" requiring immediate evaluation include new-onset diagnosis of anemia, persistent fever, weight loss, and chronic diarrhea (Ehrenpreis, 2005).

Treatment

Treatment includes avoidance of fatty foods and caffeine and avoidance of foods causing bloating and diarrhea (corn syrup, wheat-based products, brussel sprouts, cabbage). A high-fiber diet may be of little value and may increase gas and distention (McPhee & Papadakis, 2011). Drug therapy is reserved for older patients with severe symptoms not responsive to conservative measures. Antispasmodic agents, antidiarrheal agents, anticonstipation agents, and the probiotic *Bifidobacterium infantis* have been demonstrated to have a therapeutic effect in clinical trials (McPhee & Papadakis, 2011). Counseling, relaxation techniques, and hypnotherapy also have been effective in some older patients.

Inflammatory Bowel Disease

Inflammatory bowel disease includes **ulcerative colitis** and **Crohn's disease.** The age of onset for these diseases occurs at two points in life: first in the 20s and then again between the ages of 50 and 80. The reason for the differences in the age of occurrence and the causes of these diseases are unknown (Dunphy et al., 2011).

Ulcerative Colitis Ulcerative colitis is a chronic inflammatory process that affects the superficial layers of the wall of the colon in a continuous distribution. Pathological changes to the epithelial lining of the colon include inflammatory changes such as widespread ulceration, epithelial necrosis, depletion of goblet cells, and leukocyte infiltration. The disease can occur at any age but usually occurs between ages 10 and 40. Risk factors include Caucasian race, family history, and Jewish descent (Huether & McCance, 2012).

The major signs and symptoms of ulcerative colitis include bloody diarrhea, left lower quadrant abdominal pain, and weight loss. Systemic manifestations may also occur and include uveitis and arthralgia. Diagnosis is made by referral to a gastroenterologist for sigmoidoscopy, colonoscopy, and rectal mucosa biopsy. Stool samples may be obtained and cultured or examined for toxins indicating the presence of pathogens such as *Salmonella, Shigella,* and **Clostridium difficile** in older adults with recent history of antibiotic use. Although part of the normal bowel flora, *C. difficile* diarrhea can occur when antibiotics allow overgrowth of the *C. difficile* bacterium. *C. difficile* produces a toxin that is irritating to the lining of the bowel and results in inflammation and a frothy diarrhea.

Toxic megacolon may occur in the older person as a result of chronic ulcerative colitis. Symptoms of toxic megacolon include abdominal distention, fever, colonic dilatation, and rapid deterioration. The risk of developing colorectal cancer increases substantially in older adults with ulcerative colitis. Frequent colonoscopy with biopsy to detect mucosal dysplasia (premalignant lesions in ulcerative colitis) is recommended along with monitoring symptoms and laboratory data.

Crohn's Disease Crohn's disease is a chronic inflammatory process that usually affects the terminal ileum or colon and is characterized by inflammation, linear ulcerations, and granulomas. The inflammatory process affects all layers of the bowel and can often result in scarring and fibrosis. Unlike ulcerative colitis, Crohn's disease exhibits "skip areas" or areas where normal bowel exists between areas of inflammation (McPhee & Papadakis, 2011).

Signs and symptoms of Crohn's disease in the older person are similar to those in younger people but may be less dramatic and include diarrhea, fever, abdominal pain, and weight loss. The diagnosis is confirmed by barium enema or colonoscopy when visualization of the colon reveals discontinuous or skip areas of ulceration and inflammation followed by areas of healthy bowel. Abdominal CT scans are being used more often nowadays to diagnose Crohn's disease because they are noninvasive and identify abnormalities of the colon wall more easily. A complete blood count may confirm leukocytosis or elevated white cell count and a sedimentation rate should also be checked as it is often elevated as a result of the inflammatory process. If the disease is of long-standing duration or severe, the older person may exhibit signs of systemic illness such as hypoalbuminemia or anemia due to chronic blood loss and malabsorption syndromes. Treatment is based on the extent, severity, distribution, and complications. Drug therapy includes all the drugs used for ulcerative colitis. In some older adults, antibiotics are used to supplement treatment (Huether & McCance, 2012). Unlike ulcerative colitis, Crohn's disease is not cured by surgery. For older adults who are candidates for surgery, complications of Crohn's disease such as abscesses and fistulas may be treated by colectomy or ileostomy to prevent peritonitis.

Treatment Treatment is based on the extent and severity of the disease. For older adults with severe ulcerative colitis or toxic megacolon, hospitalization for administration of intravenous corticosteroids may be necessary. For older adults with moderate disease, oral corticosteroids are used to decrease inflammation. Prednisone 40 to 60 mg per day may be given initially and then tapered to 20 mg every morning as symptoms resolve. To avoid adverse effects from long-term corticosteroid use, the dose of prednisone should be tapered by 5 mg per week as long as symptoms do not recur. Long-term corticosteroid use may cause or induce hyperglycemia in older adults with diabetes, induce steroid psychosis or acute delirium, accelerate osteoporosis, and worsen heart failure and hypertension. Corticosteroid retention enemas may be used for older adults with left-sided disease; however, approximately 60% of rectal corticosteroid may be absorbed and systemic effects may occur (Nurse Practitioners' Prescribing Reference, 2012).

Sulfasalazine, olsalazine, or mesalamine (5-ASA drugs) are often given with oral corticosteroids; however, adverse effects occur in up to 30% of older adults. Adverse effects are dose related and include nausea, anorexia, diarrhea, headache, and rash. Treatment should be maintained indefinitely for older adults who can tolerate these drugs. The usual maintenance dose of sulfasalazine is 1 g po bid (Nurse Practitioners' Prescribing Reference, 2012).

Surgery may be necessary for functional older adults with acute disease, when drug therapy fails, and when multiple precancerous lesions are detected. The most common surgical procedure is subtotal colectomy and ileostomy.

> **Drug Alert** ▶▶▶ The use of NSAIDs may activate inactive inflammatory bowel disease. Their use should be avoided in older adults with a history of inflammatory bowel disease unless absolutely necessary.

Benign and Malignant Tumors

Benign colorectal tumors and polyps are present in 30% of people over the age of 50 (McPhee & Papadakis, 2011).

Polyps take 9 yrs to become cancerous [handwritten annotation]

Most benign tumors are polyps. Polyps are classified as hyperplastic (nonneoplastic), adenomatous (neoplastic), or submucosal (lipomas). Adenomatous polyps are thought to be the precursors of malignant adenocarcinomas, which comprise more than 95% of all malignant tumors of the colon (Dunphy et al., 2011). Predisposing factors include age, diet, family history, and prior diagnosis of polyps. Most polyps are asymptomatic, but occasionally rectal bleeding can occur. Diagnosis is usually confirmed by sigmoidoscopy, colonoscopy, or barium enema. During colonoscopy, polyps can be removed for biopsy.

Malignant tumors or colorectal cancer accounts for 9% of all cancer deaths in the United States and becomes more common after the age of 65; the median age for diagnosis is 71 years of age (Dunphy et al., 2011). Predisposing factors include family history, inflammatory bowel disease, and history of colorectal tumors. In early stages, colorectal cancer is asymptomatic and diagnosis is most often made by barium enema or endoscopy. Later stage tumors may be accompanied by change in bowel habits, abdominal pain, abdominal mass, onset of anemia, rectal bleeding, and weight loss. Carcinoembryonic antigen (CEA) levels may be elevated in older adults with cancer of the colon as well as those with benign conditions. Therefore, CEA levels cannot be considered a diagnostic tool but it may be used to follow the effectiveness of treatment and management of those diagnosed with colon cancer (Dunphy et al., 2011). As with most cancers, early diagnosis and treatment of colorectal cancer improves outcomes and survival rates.

Surgical resection of the primary tumor is needed to prevent perforation, bleeding, and obstruction of the bowel. Segmental resection, subtotal colectomy, or colostomy may be performed, depending on the stage and extent of the disease and the older person's underlying health status. About 25% of older adults with colorectal cancer develop hepatic metastases, and adjuvant chemotherapy is frequently used as a treatment in these older adults. Radiation therapy can ease the pain of recurrent rectal cancer, and laser therapy has been used to reduce inoperable rectal tumors and prevent obstruction (Dunphy et al., 2011). For end-stage older adults with bowel obstruction, nasogastric tubes can be used to relieve distention and prevent the vomiting of fecal material. The overall survival rate for patients with colorectal cancer is about 55% and is attributed to more emphasis on early detection and screening.

Annual fecal occult blood testing increases detection of colorectal tumors in the early and curable stage and improves long-term survival. Sigmoidoscopy and colonoscopy have been established as cost-effective screening tools. Initial screening should begin at age 50 and be repeated every 10 years until age 75 (Reuben et al., 2011). If polyps are identified, the procedures should be repeated every 3 to 5 years (Dunphy et al., 2011).

Antibiotic-Associated Colitis and Diarrhea

Diarrhea that occurs during or shortly after the administration of antibiotics is often caused by a cytotoxin produced by *C. difficile.* This cytotoxin produces inflammation in the bowel and epithelial necrosis resulting in diarrhea and pseudomembranous colitis (diarrhea caused by *C. difficile*). These conditions are more common in older people receiving treatment in hospitals or residing in nursing homes and may indicate underlying frailty and the presence of acute and chronic illnesses. The organism can also be spread on the hands of staff providing care to the older person. Nosocomial transmission and environmental contamination with the organism are common. Risk factors for the acquisition of *C. difficile* include recent surgery, spending time in the intensive care unit, nasogastric or gastric intubation, taking a proton pump inhibitor (PPI) and extended hospital stays. Although most antibiotics are associated with the development of *C. difficile* infection, cephalosporins, extended-spectrum penicillins (ampicillin), and clindamycin are implicated most often as are several antineoplastic agents including cyclophosphamide, doxorubicin, fluorouracil, and methotrexate (Reuben et al., 2011).

antibiotics have wiped out normal flora [handwritten annotation]

> **Practice Pearl ▶▶▶** Careful hand washing done on a regular basis is the best way to stop the spread of nosocomial infections like *C. difficile.* Wearing rings and having long fingernails increases the chances of transmitting bacteria even with careful hand washing. It is easier and safer to prevent an infection than to cure one.

The signs and symptoms of *C. difficile* infection range from mild diarrhea to severe colitis often associated with pseudomembranes that adhere to necrotic colonic tissue. Typically, the older person passes watery nonbloody or bloody diarrhea, complains of lower abdominal pain and cramping, and exhibits a low-grade fever. The stool may contain fecal leukocytes. Older patients may become symptomatic a few days to 10 weeks after taking an offending drug (Reuben et al., 2011). In severe cases and in those who are not treated, dehydration, hypotension, and colonic perforation may occur. The stools have a characteristic odor that many nurses over time recognize as associated with this infection.

Diagnosis is confirmed by stool analysis and examination by enzyme-linked immunoassay or stool culture.

Often, several stool samples are necessary to diagnose the condition and at least two negative fecal examinations are needed to exclude the diagnosis (Reuben et al., 2011). Flexible sigmoidoscopy can confirm the presence of gray pseudomembranous tissue but should be performed only as a last resort on the most seriously ill older adults because of the invasive nature of the procedure and the risk of perforation. Usually, barium enemas and abdominal CT scans are not useful.

Treatment includes metronidazole 500 mg po qid for 10 to 14 days. Refractory cases are treated with vancomycin 125 mg po q6h for 10 to 14 days. Metronidazole is about as effective as vancomycin in mild to moderate cases and much less expensive, making it the drug of choice under these circumstances. Fever usually resolves within 24 hours, and diarrhea decreases over 4 to 5 days. Antidiarrheal drugs should not be used because they expose the colonic tissue to the toxin for longer periods of time and place the older person at risk for developing necrotic tissue and pseudomembranes. Aggressive nursing interventions to prevent dehydration should be implemented, including frequently assessing pulse and blood pressure, assessing postural blood pressure if the older person is ambulatory, establishing a schedule to offer the older person oral fluids (water, juice, and the beverage of choice) every 15 to 30 minutes, monitoring urinary output and skin turgor, and notifying the primary care provider of imminent dehydration so that intravenous fluids may be initiated if necessary. If the older person is receiving diuretics, these drugs should be held until the diarrhea subsides, because they may exacerbate dehydration.

Relapse rates average 20% to 25% after successful treatment with metronidazole or vancomycin. Older adults who relapse are likely to continue with higher relapse rates over time. Relapses can be treated successfully with another course of metronidazole or vancomycin. Older adults who are prone to relapse should avoid the offending antibiotic if possible. *Lactobacillus acidophilus* 500 mg qid or eating yogurt with active acidophilus cultures may be helpful to recolonize the bowel with normal flora and prevent overgrowth by *C. difficile*, but probiotic products containing *Lactobacillus casei*, *Streptococcus thermophilus*, and *L. bulgaricus* are not recommended to prevent primary infections (Reuben et al., 2011).

Constipation

Constipation is a common problem in older people and affects up to 20% of those residing in the community and 50% to 75% of nursing home residents. The number of people reporting constipation increases with age. Constipation means different things to different people, and many older adults feel that a daily bowel movement is necessary for good health. Approximately 30% of older people in the community report taking laxatives, and 24% report chronic constipation (Tariq, 2007). However, constipation is not defined by the absence of daily stool passage, but rather as infrequent defecation (fewer than two to three bowel movements per week), a hardened or reduced caliber of stool (pencil stools), a sensation of incomplete evacuation, or the need to strain at bowel movements (Reuben et al., 2011). Usually three bowel movements a week or less is considered indicative of constipation. Factors contributing to constipation include dehydration, side effects of medication, depression, insufficient fiber intake, cognitive impairment, and immobility. Presence of physical illness can also predispose an older person to constipation, including metabolic and endocrine disorders (diabetes, hypothyroidism, chronic renal failure), muscular dystrophy, neurologic disorders (spinal cord injury, multiple sclerosis, Parkinson's disease, cerebrovascular accident, Alzheimer's disease), and recent abdominal surgery (Reuben et al., 2011). Obstructive disorders are also associated with constipation and include **rectal prolapse,** or protrusion of part of the rectum through the anus, presence of a tumor, and megacolon resulting from chronic constipation and storage of large amounts of feces in the colon over time. Surgical adhesions and hernias sometimes inhibit transport of stool, causing constipation and obstruction. Constipation can lead to abdominal discomfort, loss of appetite, and nausea and vomiting.

Drug Alert ▶▶▶ Drugs known to cause constipation include all of those with anticholinergic side effects (antidepressants, neuroleptics, antihistamines, antiparkinsonian agents), some antihypertensive agents (calcium channel blockers, beta-blockers, ACE inhibitors, diuretics), iron supplements, muscle relaxants, calcium supplements, aluminum-containing antacids, benzodiazepines, antiarrhythmics, and opiates. The nurse should carefully monitor bowel function in older adults taking these medications.

Because hard stool is difficult to expel, the major complication of constipation is fecal impaction, which can result in intestinal obstruction, colonic ulceration, overflow incontinence with leakage of stool around the obstructing feces, and paradoxical diarrhea (Tariq, 2007). Urinary incontinence, urinary tract infection, and urinary retention are also associated with fecal impaction. Excessive straining to pass stool is associated with syncope, transient ischemic attacks, hemorrhoids, anal **fissures,** and rectal prolapse. Over time, older adults with chronic constipation and straining at stool will dread having a bowel movement and may ignore the need to defecate, further compounding the problem.

Nursing Assessment When assessing an older person with constipation, the gerontological nurse should carefully evaluate the complaint. It is important to understand the older person's beliefs about bowel habits and frequency of bowel movements. The older person should be questioned as to the basis of the complaint of constipation, such as frequency of bowel movement (fewer than three per week), consistency of stool (hard or difficult to pass), presence of excessive straining, or feeling of fullness in the rectum after completing a bowel movement. The presence of bright red blood on the stool or toilet tissue may indicate bleeding from internal or external hemorrhoids or perhaps a more serious underlying condition such as a rectal fissure or tumor. This information should be reported to the primary healthcare provider for further investigation and diagnosis.

A careful review of the older person's medications, medical conditions, level of exercise, fluid and fiber, and psychological status (somatization, anxiety, and depression) is indicated. The nursing assessment should also include an abdominal examination with auscultation of bowel sounds and palpation to detect the presence of large amounts of stool in the colon. The rectum may be examined digitally for the presence of hard, impacted stool in the rectal vault. The primary healthcare provider may, when appropriate, seek further diagnostic testing such as barium enema, colonoscopy, or X-ray of the abdomen.

A multidisciplinary approach is needed for management of constipation in older adults, with the primary care provider assessing predisposing and underlying diseases and side effects of medication, and the nurse addressing nutrition and hydration issues, monitoring bowel function, and administering laxatives as needed. Nursing management of constipation involves education of older adults so that they understand the importance of fluid and fiber intake, exercise, and avoidance of medications that can cause constipation. Older people should be aware that changes in bowel function occur naturally with change in routine such as travel, hospitalization, illness, stress, taking pain medication, or other transitory conditions.

Constipation is often relieved by adequate hydration, increased mobility, fiber supplementation (20 to 35 g/day), and use of laxatives. One nursing study reported that laxatives can sometimes be discontinued for an older person with bran intake that reached 25 g daily (Howard, West, & Ossip-Klein, 2000). A classic nursing study formulated a bran mixture that significantly reduces laxative use for older adults and includes 3 cups unsweetened applesauce,

2 cups coarse wheat bran, and 1-1/2 cups unsweetened prune juice. Administering 4 tablespoons per day (2 before breakfast and 2 before supper) will stimulate natural bowel movements and decrease dependence on laxatives (Smith & Newman, 1989). Fiber should be consumed as wheat or oat bran, fruits, vegetables, or nuts. When fiber intake is increased, excessive gas may be initially present but this annoying problem usually resolves as the body becomes accustomed to the change. It is recommended to increase fiber intake slowly with 5 g daily, adding small increments until the desired results are achieved with good tolerance and minimal gas and bloating. Contraindications to use of the fiber mixture include bowel obstruction, severe dysphagia, dietary restriction to low-fiber diet, and limited fluid intake. Lack of sufficient fluid intake with increased fiber diets or use of fiber supplements is associated with impaction, bowel obstruction, and large amounts of dry stool accumulating in the colon. The older person should be instructed in techniques of bowel training and counseled not to delay the urge to have a bowel movement and to take advantage of the natural defecation reflex that usually occurs about 30 minutes after a meal.

Laxatives

When lifestyle modification has failed, the primary care provider may prescribe a laxative. These agents can be divided into several categories based on pharmacological action. Refer to Table 20-2 which illustrates these agents by category.

Bulk laxatives contain soluble and insoluble fibers that absorb water (in states of adequate hydration) into the intestinal tract and increase stool mass. The increased mass will stimulate colonic peristalsis. Bulk laxatives are contraindicated in the presence of intestinal obstruction or when peristaltic activity is compromised (paralytic ileus). Stool softeners should be limited to older adults who complain of straining at stool, painful defecation with the presence of hemorrhoids, or anal fissures. Stool softeners are sometimes used to facilitate bowel movements and prevent constipation in high-risk older adults (postoperative abdominal surgery). Osmotic laxatives draw water into the colon by osmotic pressure. If the osmotic laxative is metabolized by bacteria in the colon, production of gases may lead to flatulence, abdominal bloating, or cramping. Magnesium-containing products should not be used in older adults with chronic renal failure, and sodium agents should be avoided in the presence of congestive heart failure and hypernatremia (Nurse Practitioners' Prescribing Reference, 2012). Laxatives containing senna increase peristalsis and secretion of water into the bowel. These agents tend to be more harsh than other agents and can sometimes cause

TABLE 20-2   Laxatives by Category

Type	Action	Examples
Bulk laxatives	Increase stool bulk and urge to defecate with adequate fluid intake	Metamucil, Citrucel, FiberCon
Stool softeners	Surfactant wetting agent	Colace, Surfak
Lubricants	Lubricate stool surface	Mineral oil
Saline	Hypertonic increase in stool water content	Milk of Magnesia, Fleet Phospho-Soda
Stimulants	Increase colonic peristalsis	Dulcolax, Ex-Lax, senna, Senokot
Osmotic agents	Hypertonic increase in stool water content	Sorbitol, lactulose
Enemas and suppositories	Local rectal stimulants	Fleet enemas, glycerine suppositories

Source: Data from Nurse Practitioners' Prescribing Reference (2012); Reuben et al. (2011).

unpleasant cramping. Suppositories and enemas are usually reserved for those older adults who have not responded to the other laxatives because they are invasive and sometimes uncomfortable for the older person; therefore, they should be used as a last resort. Enemas are the treatment of choice if colonic fecal impaction is suspected. Plain tap water, saline, or sodium phosphate enemas are recommended. Soap-suds enemas produce mucosal damage and cramping and should be avoided. Because rectal volumes increase with age, the enema should be administered slowly to prevent cramping and should generally contain about 150 to 300 milliliters or 5 to 10 fluid ounces of solution. After the initial blockage has been passed or removed manually, a second enema may be needed to remove additional stool that has moved into the proximal colon. Because this procedure is uncomfortable and unpleasant, fecal impaction should be avoided by paying close attention to the older person's bowel function.

For drug-induced constipation, the best action is to seek advice from the primary care provider as to whether the offending medication may be discontinued. Some

drugs (such as verapamil) cause more constipation than others, and the primary care provider may wish to substitute a less constipating antihypertensive agent if the older person experiences problems with constipation. However, when the medication cannot be discontinued (for example, opioids for pain), a careful bowel management plan is needed to prevent constipation and fecal impaction. Opioids inhibit gastric emptying time and decrease peristaltic movements. About 50% of older people taking opioids report symptoms of constipation. Correcting constipation associated with opioid use requires a senna or osmotic laxative to overcome the strong opioid effect. Stool softeners and bulking agents alone are inadequate because of the opioid-related constipation resulting from slowed gut motility. A prophylactic bowel regimen should be initiated whenever an older person is started on an opioid pain medication to prevent fecal impaction (Dunphy et al., 2011). Fecal impactions high in the rectum or in the sigmoid can lead to nausea and vomiting, anorexia, pain, obstruction, perforation, and fecal peritonitis.

HEALTHY AGING TIPS

Maintaining Bowel Health

1. Increase fiber in your diet by eating more fresh fruits and vegetables and more whole-grain cereal and bread. Dried fruit such as apricots, prunes, and figs are especially high in fiber.

2. Drink plenty of liquids (1 to 2 quarts/day) unless you have heart or kidney problems.

3. Consider adding small amounts of unprocessed bran to baked goods, cereal, and fruit. Start slowly with fiber to avoid cramping and gas to allow your body to adapt over time.

4. Stay active. Walking, dancing, and swimming are great forms of exercise.

5. Don't expect to have a bowel movement each and every day. Every person has a different pattern of elimination.

6. Avoid laxatives and enemas as a cure for constipation. If you use harsh laxatives and enemas on a regular basis, your body may forget how to work on its own.

Diarrhea

Diarrhea is defined as abnormally loose stool accompanied by a change in frequency or volume (Reuben et al., 2011). As with constipation, diarrhea is a subjective symptom and careful nursing assessment is required. The nurse should assess for the presence of urgency, cramping, bloating, incontinence, pain on defecation, and blood in the stool. A history of gastric tube feeding or recent antibiotic use may suggest the presence of *C. difficile*.

The incidence of diarrhea in the older person is unknown, but older people may be more susceptible to diarrhea because of hypochlorhydria or achlorhydria when taking gastric acid-suppressing drugs, increased use of antibiotics, and decreased mucosal immune function (Reuben et al., 2011). The likelihood of morbidity and mortality increases with persistent diarrhea. In nursing homes, outbreaks of *Escherichia coli* infections have been documented with three times the morbidity and mortality occurring in younger people. The higher mortality rate (16% to 35%) occurs mostly because the older person is more susceptible to the harmful effects of fluid loss, dehydration, and hypovolemia.

Diarrhea of less than 2 weeks' duration is considered acute; diarrhea occurring longer than 4 weeks is defined as chronic. Most diarrhea in the older person is acute and self-limited. Causes include infection (viral, bacterial, or parasitic), medications and drug changes, and food intolerances. Acute bloody diarrhea needs immediate medical evaluation. Causes include ischemia, diverticulitis, or inflammatory bowel disease. Viruses responsible for infectious diarrhea include the Norwalk virus and rotavirus. Both viruses are spread by the fecal–oral route and have caused epidemic diarrhea in nursing homes. Toxic diarrhea can result from food poisoning (*Salmonella, Staphylococcus aureus, E. coli*) or ingestion of contaminated food. Careful hand washing and food preparation in sanitary conditions are required to prevent infectious diarrhea in the older person.

Chronic diarrhea may occur as a result of tumors, surgery, and medications. Almost all drugs can cause diarrhea. Commonly associated drugs include NSAIDs, magnesium-containing antacids, antiarrhythmics, beta-blockers, quinidine, colchicine, and digoxin (Reuben et al., 2011). If the pattern of diarrhea suggests lactose intolerance (diarrhea after ingestion of dairy products), a trial lactose-free diet or treatment with lactase can be tried and bowel function carefully monitored. Older adults who are immunosuppressed, such as those receiving chemotherapy or those diagnosed with HIV/AIDS (10% of people with HIV/AIDS are older people), may experience chronic diarrhea secondary to bowel infections caused by giardiasis, microsporidiosis, and *Mycobacterium avium-intracellulare* (McPhee & Papadakis, 2011).

Nursing Assessment Assessment should focus on quantifying the nature of the stool, frequency of passage, and presence of associated symptoms. Overflow diarrhea and oozing can occur as a result of fecal impaction, and the date of the last normal bowel movement should be carefully identified. Older adults at risk for dehydration will require aggressive fluid replacement, including frequent offerings of oral fluids, consultation with the primary healthcare provider to temporarily hold diuretics, and perhaps administration of intravenous fluids. Hospitalization may be required for complete evaluation and treatment. Nursing assessment includes a careful examination of the abdomen, including visual examination for bloating or excessive peristaltic movements, auscultation of bowel sounds, palpation to identify masses or rebound tenderness, and digital rectal examination to determine presence of impacted stool. Older adults with recent antibiotic use, those who have experienced recent foreign travel, and those who may have been exposed to food poisoning should have stool collected for culture and analysis. A plain abdominal X-ray (kidneys, ureter, bladder) may indicate the presence of an intestinal obstruction or fecal impaction.

If toxin-producing and infectious diarrhea are not suspected, antidiarrheal agents can be administered. However, administration of these drugs in the presence of toxins and infectious agents can lead to colon damage and systemic adverse effects by allowing the toxic substance to remain in the bowel for longer periods of time and thus to be absorbed into the general circulation. Soluble fiber (Metamucil) adds bulk to the stool and is sometimes helpful to slow bowel movements in people requiring bulk. Kaopectate, Pepto-Bismol, and Imodium A-D can be administered after each loose stool in divided doses. Lomotil should be avoided because of significant atropine-like side effects (Nurse Practitioners' Prescribing Reference, 2012).

Fecal Incontinence

Fecal incontinence is embarrassing and can cause an older person to severely limit social activity. Approximately 2% of the community-residing older adults and 54% of institutionalized older adults suffer from fecal incontinence (Reuben et al., 2011). Continence requires adequate sensation and ability to discriminate between feces and flatus, coordination of internal and external anal sphincters, and adequate pelvic floor muscles to retain stool in the rectum. Sometimes mobility problems, severe depression, or cognitive impairment may inhibit the older person's motivation and ability to remain continent. Immobilized and functionally impaired older adults may be unable to suppress the urge to defecate and suffer fecal incontinence while waiting for assistance to use the bedpan or toilet. A regular toileting program, administration of a high-fiber diet, elimination of medications associated with diarrhea, and treatment of infections are appropriate interventions for older adults with fecal incontinence.

Hemorrhoids and Rectal Bleeding

Hemorrhoids are a common cause of bright red rectal bleeding. **Hemorrhoids** are varicose veins of the anorectal junction and are classified as internal or external with external hemorrhoids protruding through the anus. Although hemorrhoids have been commonly thought to develop as a result of straining and constipation, hemorrhoids may actually develop because of sliding of the lining of the anal canal (McPhee & Papadakis, 2011). A thrombosed external hemorrhoid is a localized clot that forms in the vein of an external hemorrhoid or arises from a ruptured blood vessel. Thrombosed hemorrhoids appear bluish in color and may be painful.

Hemorrhoids tend to be asymptomatic in the early stages but may bleed over time. Bleeding is usually scant and involves bright red blood on toilet tissue but may be more severe with blood dripping into the toilet after bowel movement. External hemorrhoids may be easily seen, but internal hemorrhoids require visualization by sigmoidoscopy or colonoscopy because they cannot be reliably felt with a digital examination. Any rectal bleeding should be referred to a gastroenterologist for an accurate diagnosis and followed up with endoscopic examination to rule out malignancy.

Treatment of hemorrhoids depends on size. Grade 1 hemorrhoids are those that do not prolapse. Grade 2 hemorrhoids reduce spontaneously after prolapse. Grade 3 hemorrhoids prolapse and require manual reduction, and grade 4 hemorrhoids are nonreducible. Grade 1 and 2 hemorrhoids may be treated with rubber banding, high-fiber diet, and bulking agents such as psyllium. Rubber band ligation is contraindicated in patients who are anticoagulated, and antiplatelet drugs (including aspirin) should be discontinued 5 to 7 days before and after banding (Reuben et al., 2011). Heavy lifting and straining at stool should be avoided, because those actions can worsen prolapse. Sitz baths and suppositories with benzocaine can relieve symptoms. Sclerotherapy, cryosurgery, and laser therapy may also be effective options for some older adults. Hemorrhoidectomy should be reserved for those older adults with persistent symptoms who have not been helped by nonsurgical techniques (Dunphy et al., 2011).

Rectal prolapse or passage of the rectum through the anus is common in older adults, affecting women more than men (Tariq, 2007). The main symptom is protrusion of the rectum with the passage of stool or upon standing. Continued rectal prolapse can lead to fecal incontinence, and surgical repair may be necessary. Conservative therapy includes instruction on avoiding heavy lifting and prolonged standing and prevention of constipation and straining at stool.

Liver and Biliary Disorders

With aging, the liver is more susceptible to the effects of drugs and other toxins. An older person with liver disease may present with vague and ambiguous symptoms, including fatigue, weight loss, anorexia, and malaise. The older person with viral hepatitis may complain of nausea, fatigue, and loose stools. Acute hepatitis A is much less common in the older person than in younger people; since introduction of the hepatitis A vaccine, the rate of hepatitis A has declined by over 76% with a corresponding decline in the mortality rate of 32% (McPhee & Papadakis, 2011). Acute hepatitis B and C are also less common in the older person than the younger person. The incidence of hepatitis B has decreased by over 75% since the 1980s. Groups at risk include healthcare providers and patients at hemodialysis centers and those working at blood banks, but the greatest number of cases results from heterosexual transmission (McPhee & Papadakis, 2011). If an older person is infected with the hepatitis virus, the likelihood the disease will become chronic is heightened and poorer clearance of the virus results from treatment. Older adults who have abnormal liver function tests, who have a history of intravenous drug use, who have recently traveled in underdeveloped countries, or who engage in unsafe sexual practices should consult a gastroenterologist for further evaluation and treatment.

Hepatic cysts are common in the older person and are usually benign. If a cyst enlarges and causes discomfort, excision or draining may be necessary. Hemangioma, a common benign liver tumor, is found in about 5% of older adults. Benign tumors and cysts are usually asymptomatic and are often found when a CT scan or ultrasound is done for another reason. Liver function tests are usually normal. Typically no treatment is required; however, for older adults with complaints of abdominal discomfort, the cysts may be aspirated under local anesthesia as needed for comfort.

Metastatic carcinoma is the most common form of liver cancer, and many cancers metastasize to the liver. In the United States, the incidence of liver cancer is highest in people over 65 years of age, higher in men and in Asians and Pacific Islanders (New York State Department of Health, 2011). Primary liver cancer or hepatocellular cancer rates are higher in parts of the world where the incidence of viral hepatitis is higher. In most cases, the tumor develops in cirrhosis resulting from hepatitis B or C infection. The 5-year probability of an older person with cirrhosis developing hepatocellular carcinoma is about 20%. Other predisposing factors include excessive alcohol and tobacco use. Because the liver functions as a filter in the body, other types of cancer such as breast and colon cancer, frequently metastasize to the liver.

Only 20% of older adults with hepatocellular cancer will have symptoms at the time of diagnosis. These symptoms usually include jaundice, variceal bleeding, ascites, right upper quadrant abdominal pain, weight loss, or an enlarged liver. Liver function tests are usually abnormal with increased serum bilirubin levels, elevated serum alkaline phosphatase, and decreased serum albumin concentrations. Definitive diagnosis follows after abdominal ultrasound, CT scan, MRI with contrast enhancement, and liver biopsy (Dunphy et al., 2011).

Treatment is determined by the tumor stage and the older person's functional status. Small tumors (less than 2 cm) may be treated with percutaneous hepatic injection with ethanol under ultrasound control. This minimally invasive technique may be used in older patients who are not candidates for resection or liver transplant. This treatment often results in complete tumor necrosis. Other options include tumor embolization, chemotherapy, and immunotherapy (McPhee & Papadakis, 2011). Many of these treatments are experimental, and the effect on the older person's survival has not been clearly established. Surgical resection is usually restricted to highly functional older adults with solitary tumors that have not metastasized. Liver transplantation may be curative for nonmetastasized tumors, but most centers will not perform liver transplantation in adults over age 65, especially if they have coexisting medical conditions. Regardless of treatment, the gerontological nurse should provide holistic care including careful attention to pain and symptom control, nutritional issues, skin care, emotional support for the older person and family, and issues relating to death and dying.

In the United States, cancer of the bile ducts accounts for 3% of all cancer deaths (McPhee & Papadakis, 2011). Bile duct cancer, usually adenocarcinoma, is more common in men. The diagnosis is more prevalent in people 50 to 70 years of age. Adenocarcinoma also accounts for 80% of all gallbladder cancers (more common in women), and gallstones are present in 85% of cases. Symptoms include intermittent vague pain in the upper right quadrant. Later in the progression of the disease, jaundice and weight loss are common. Abdominal ultrasound and CT provide definitive diagnosis.

The prognosis for cure for cancer of the gallbladder is poor with only 5% of older adults experiencing 5-year survival. Radical cholecystectomy is the treatment of choice for nonmetastasized tumors of the gallbladder. Radiation therapy and chemotherapy are ineffective. Whipple operation (radical resection of the bile duct and pancreatoduodenectomy) provides some promising benefit for bile duct cancer with 5-year survival rates of about 20% to 30%, but older adults over the age of 70 have a high surgical risk (McPhee & Papadakis, 2011). As previously mentioned, the gerontological nurse should address issues of symptom palliation and death and dying.

Gallstones

The incidence of gallstones rises with age. In the United States, the prevalence of gallstones is 5.5% in men and 8.6% in women, higher in those over the age of 60, and higher in Mexican Americans and African Americans (McPhee & Papadakis, 2011). Typical symptoms include right upper quadrant pain, gas, distention, and nausea and vomiting. Acute cholecystitis, a complication of gallstones, is characterized by increased local tenderness, fever, and increased white blood count. If a gallstone migrates into the common bile duct, blockage and pancreatitis can result with increases in serum amylase levels (Dunphy et al., 2011). Surgery should be performed within 2 or 3 days from the onset of symptoms of acute cholecystitis, especially after several acute attacks.

Ultrasound visualizes gallstones in 95% of cases, and abdominal CT scans will diagnose biliary problems. Treatment includes laparoscopic cholecystectomy, stone dissolution by chenodeoxycholic acid, and extracorporeal shock wave lithotripsy (McPhee & Papadakis, 2011). Many older adults decide to avoid aggressive treatment for gallstones and instead manage their symptoms by avoiding high-fat and other foods that cause them pain or distress.

Pancreatitis

Acute pancreatitis occurs more frequently and is more severe in older adults than in younger people. Factors that increase risk include gallstone, medications, alcohol abuse, and cancer. Drugs increasing the risk of pancreatitis include estrogen, furosemide, ACE inhibitors, and mesalamine. Diagnosed hyperlipidemia and hypercalcemia also increase the risk. Typical presenting symptoms are epigastric pain, nausea, and vomiting. Serum amylase, lipase, bilirubin, and alkaline phosphatase levels may be elevated. Abdominal ultrasonography or CT scanning should be done to confirm the diagnosis.

Treatment for acute pancreatitis includes nasogastric suction, pain management, hyperalimentation, and fluid replacement. In 90% of older adults, acute pancreatitis is self-limiting and conservative measures are sufficient.

Chronic pancreatitis results in weight loss, diarrhea, diabetes, and presence of persistent pain. Diagnosis is based on symptoms and specialized testing. All older adults with chronic pancreatitis must refrain from drinking alcohol. Surgical treatment may be necessary when conservative measures fail.

Pancreatic cancer accounts for 5% of all cancer deaths in the United States and risk factors include age, tobacco and alcohol use, obesity, chronic pancreatitis, history of abdominal radiation, and family history of the disease (McPhee & Papadakis, 2011). Painless jaundice, pruritus, and weight loss are common presenting symptoms. The prognosis of pancreatic cancer is poor with 5-year survival rates ranging from 2% to 5% (McPhee & Papadakis, 2011).

Endoscopic Gastrointestinal Procedures

Upper or lower gastrointestinal endoscopic procedures can be done to view body cavities with fiberoptic tubing. Conventional X-rays cannot identify color changes, bleeding, or vascular malformations. Endoscopy allows biopsy of abnormalities, allows stent placement, and helps surgeons determine if surgery is needed.

Esophagogastroduodenoscopy visualizes the upper gastrointestinal tract. Inspection of the esophagus to the duodenum is indicated for evaluation of the esophageal and gastric areas and provides information on upper GI bleeding. Therapeutic indications include dilating esophageal strictures, vaporizing gastric and esophageal neoplasms, endoscopic injection therapy or thermal coagulation of upper GI bleeding, sclerotherapy for esophageal varices, and removal of polyps. Older adults are at risk of complications due to lowered oxygen intake during the passage of the tube. Using a small-caliber endoscopic tube and administering additional oxygen during the procedure may help these older adults (Waye, 2004).

Before endoscopy, food and drink may be restricted to allow the stomach to empty, and a strong laxative is taken to clean the bowel for colonoscopy preparation. Consequences of the vigorous bowel preparation may include dehydration, fatigue resulting from frequent trips to the bathroom, and changes in blood glucose levels secondary to dietary restrictions. Because transient bacteremia may occur during endoscopy, older adults at high risk for infection (those with valvular heart disease or artificial heart valves) should receive antibiotics (usually ampicillin or gentamicin) before the procedure (Waye, 2004).

Most endoscopies are performed while the older person is consciously sedated. Usually, benzodiazepines are given for relaxation. Midazolam is given for conscious sedation. Aggressive cleansing protocols are difficult for some older adults to tolerate. Harsh cathartics can result in dehydration in an older person, and adequate fluid intake must be maintained during preparation for the procedure.

A sigmoidoscopy permits inspection of the rectum and distal sigmoid colon, and most of the descending colon. The flexible sigmoidoscope (about 60 cm in length) may be used to evaluate the left side of the colon where two thirds of neoplasms appear (Waye, 2004). Polyps are usually not removed during examination with the flexible sigmoidoscope. Sedation is not required, and one or two phosphate enemas cleanse the bowel adequately. The older person usually lies on the left side during the procedure.

Colonoscopy allows visual examination of the entire colon. Colonoscopy is indicated for routine testing or when anemia is present, positive fecal occult blood testing is noted, or polyps are suspected. Screening in asymptomatic older people should begin at age 50 and continue every 10 years. No data indicate at what age screening should be stopped, but some geriatricians recommend screening of highly functional older adults until the age of 85 (Waye, 2004). Colonoscopy allows the removal of colonic polyps and evaluation of bleeding sites with electrocautery treatment. Strictures may be dilated and stents may be placed in strictures resulting from malignant growths to prevent bowel obstruction. Contraindications to colonoscopy include fulminant colitis, acute diverticulitis, perforated bowel, and recent myocardial infarctions (Waye, 2004).

The colon must be cleansed to allow complete visualization during a colonoscopy. Typical preparation is 1 or 2 days of a liquid diet and administration of a cathartic the night before the procedure. Even the smallest amount of feces in the colon can hide important details and compromise the examination. Two doses of sodium phosphate should be administered. Older adults with cardiovascular or renal instability should be carefully monitored. The nurse should consult with the gastroenterologist who is to perform the procedure and the primary care provider regarding the administration of regularly scheduled medications. Usually the procedure focuses on identifying and removing elevated mushroom-like polyps that were thought to be more dangerous than flat polyps. However, recent studies have revealed that flat or sunken polyps that are similar in color to healthy bowel tissue are more difficult to visualize and may be more dangerous (Soetikno et al., 2008). The bowel must be meticulously cleaned of stool in order to identify these flat or sunken lesions, thus reinforcing the necessity of an aggressive bowel cleansing regimen.

Complications from colonoscopy when performed by a skilled clinician are minimal. Colonoscopy is a relatively safe procedure and reliable results are valuable for accurate diagnosis. Risk of colonic perforation and excessive bleeding is low. Complications from sedative use include arrhythmias, aspiration, and, rarely, cardiac arrest (Waye, 2004). Older adults should be instructed to bring a friend or relative to the procedure because they will be unable to drive for at least 24 hours after the administration of the sedation. The older person will usually receive a smaller dose of the sedating drug but still may be lethargic and sleepy for 24 hours.

Nursing Diagnoses

Nursing diagnoses for problems associated with the gastrointestinal tract include the following:

- *Nutrition Imbalanced: Less Than Body Requirements* for those with anorexia
- *Infection, Risk for* for those undergoing endoscopic examination and needing antibiotic prophylaxis
- *Constipation* and *Constipation, Perceived*
- *Diarrhea*
- *Bowel Incontinence*
- *Constipation, Risk for*
- *Tissue Perfusion, Peripheral: Ineffective*
- *Aspiration, Risk for*
- *Mucous Membrane: Oral, Impaired*
- *Social Isolation* (if appropriate)
- *Noncompliance* (if appropriate)
- *Health Maintenance, Ineffective*
- *Self-Care Deficit: Toileting*
- *Pain, Acute* or *Chronic*
- *Nausea*

NANDA-I © 2012.

The nurse should educate older adults and their families regarding the causes, prevention, and treatment of gastrointestinal diseases.

COMPLEMENTARY AND ALTERNATIVE THERAPIES

Milk thistle (a member of the daisy family) is used for its hepatoprotective characteristics and to treat cirrhosis, chronic hepatitis, fatty infiltration caused by alcohol and other toxins, and gallbladder disorders (National Center for Complementary and Alternative Medicine [NCCAM], 2010). There is some evidence that it protects and promotes the growth of liver cells. Some studies report a therapeutic effect and others are inconclusive, so further study is needed. Usually, side effects are few and generally mild including headache, nausea, vomiting, diarrhea, flatulence, skin rashes, erectile dysfunction, hypoglycemia, conjunctivitis, malaise, and insomnia (NCCAM, 2010).

Acidophilus capsules contain active cultures that can be used to treat a variety of gastrointestinal problems including irritable bowel syndrome, diarrhea, flatulence, and bad breath, and as an adjunct to antibiotic therapy to prevent antibiotic-associated diarrhea caused by overgrowth of *C. difficile* (NCCAM, 2011). These capsules contain probiotic microorganisms that confer benefit to the host and flood the bowel with friendly bacteria, thus preventing the overgrowth of pathogens. In addition, some foods are considered to be probiotic, including yogurt with live cultures, miso, tempeh, fermented and unfermented milk, and some juices and soy beverages. NCCAM (2011) reports there is encouraging evidence that probiotics can be useful in certain cases including for the treatment of diarrhea and irritable bowel syndrome. The amount of active cultures in acidophilus products varies and ideally there should be no less than 1 billion organisms per capsule (Gutierrez, 2008). Side effects are mild and include flatulence.

QSEN Recommendations Related to the Gastrointestinal System

The Quality and Safety Education for Nurses (QSEN) project addresses the challenge of preparing future nurses with the knowledge, skills, and attitudes (KSAs) to continuously improve the quality and safety of the healthcare systems in which they work (Cronenwett et al., 2007). See the QSEN table for tips on meeting QSEN standards.

Patient and Family Teaching

Gerontological nurses require skills and knowledge related to teaching patients and families about the key concepts of gerontology and gerontological nursing. The guidelines in the following feature will assist the nurse to assume the role of teacher and coach.

Meeting QSEN Standards: The Gastrointestinal System

	KNOWLEDGE	SKILLS	ATTITUDES
Patient-Centered Care	Involvement of patient and family in plan of care is crucial.	Family assessment and adult learning principles	Appreciate uniqueness of each patient/family.
	Examine barriers that may keep patients from being active in formulating their plan of care.	Evaluate for depression, vision/hearing, function, tobacco/alcohol use, and dietary preferences.	Provide patient-centered care to improve successful nursing outcomes.
Teamwork and Collaboration	Recognize scope of practice for interdisciplinary team members.	Use leadership skills to coordinate team and share knowledge.	Value the contribution of each member of the team to improve outcomes.
	Be aware of organizational problems that can inhibit effective team function.	System assessment skills	Be open to input from team members on effective means to improve communication and collaboration.
Evidence-Based Practice	Describe effective interventions to decrease gastrointestinal risk factors and improve overall health and functioning.	Access current evidence-based screening and health promotion protocols to guide interventions.	Possess confidence in necessary skills to evaluate and incorporate nursing interventions from the literature.
	Be aware of drug side effects impacting on GI function.	Conduct complete medication reviews yearly and after each hospitalization.	Advocate for medication changes and use of nonpharmacologic interventions as needed.
Quality Improvement	Recognize the importance of measuring patient outcomes to improve gastrointestinal system care.	Skills in data management, technology, and U.S. government and ALA websites describing current incidence and prevalence of GI disease	Value the use of data and outcomes as a key component of QI efforts.
Safety	Describe common medication and treatment errors and health system characteristics that increase the likelihood of such errors occurring.	Use appropriate strategies to deliver patient/family education and provide written information to compensate for functional deficits (if present).	Appreciate the impact of frailty and cognitive loss on the occurrence of adverse drug reactions.
	Recognize the factors that increase the risk of nosocomial infections.	Avoid the use of unnecessary antibiotics and unsafe food handling and storage methods that increase the risk of *C. difficile* infection.	Institute infection control practices to decrease the incidence of food contamination and other infections.

Meeting QSEN Standards: The Gastrointestinal System *(continued)*

	KNOWLEDGE	SKILLS	ATTITUDES
Informatics	Provide input into the formation and maintenance of patient databases needed for gathering QSEN data and providing patient care.	Utilize the electronic health record.	Protect patient confidentiality according to HIPAA standards.

Patient–Family Teaching Guidelines

The following are guidelines that the nurse may find useful when instructing older adults and their families about gastrointestinal problems.

GASTROINTESTINAL DISEASE

1 How can I prevent gastrointestinal disease?

Many people experience heartburn, constipation, diarrhea, and other problems with the gastrointestinal tract as they get older. Some problems are common and will go away on their own such as occasional constipation or diarrhea. Other problems are more serious and require further investigation such as blood in the stool and change in normal elimination patterns. Some suggestions for general health of the gastrointestinal tract include the following:

- Know your family history. Do you have a blood relative with polyps in the colon, colon cancer, Crohn's disease, or diverticulitis? If so, you may be more at risk than others without a family history.
- Eat a balanced diet that is high in fiber and low in fat and processed carbohydrates.
- Maintain a normal weight.
- Stop smoking or using tobacco products.
- Decrease the size of portions at mealtime and avoid lying down for 2 to 3 hours after eating.
- Ask your healthcare provider to provide you with occult blood stool testing cards every year, and begin having colonoscopies at age 50 and periodically thereafter.
- Take medications with 8 oz of water and sit upright for 20 minutes after taking them.
- Limit the use of nonsteroidal anti-inflammatory agents such as ibuprofen because they can interfere with the protective covering in the stomach and cause ulcers.

RATIONALE:

Many of the problems that develop in the gastrointestinal tract are preventable with healthy lifestyle choices and early

disease prevention. Older adults should be encouraged to preserve GI function by making healthy lifestyle choices.

2 If I already have gastrointestinal disease is there anything I can do to stop it?

Yes. Take medications prescribed by your healthcare provider and begin lifestyle changes immediately. Also carry out all suggestions previously discussed. If your doctor prescribes medication for you, take it exactly as directed. Report any worsening of your condition or new symptoms to your doctor or nurse. Avoid straining at stool and heavy lifting if you have hemorrhoids. Drink plenty of fluids and try to get daily exercise. With treatment and lifestyle changes, most gastrointestinal problems can be successfully treated.

RATIONALE:

Most older adults who already have diseases or problems of the GI tract will have improvement in symptoms by following treatment suggestions and making healthy lifestyle choices. It is important to stress to older adults and families that it is never too late to work toward good health.

3 Is there anything else I should do to make the most of living with gastrointestinal disease?

Yes. Exercise to keep your muscles fit and strong, eat a healthy diet, control your weight, and see your healthcare provider on a regular basis. Screening tests, no matter how unpleasant, save lives. Your healthcare provider can give you specific instructions that will help you to lead a long and healthy life.

RATIONALE:

Following general health promotion principles and engaging in periodic screening are good ideas for everyone.

CARE PLAN A Patient With GERD

Case Study

Mrs. Stein is an overweight 67-year-old woman who is complaining of heartburn that she has had on and off for over a year. She has seen the commercial on television warning people that they could have serious problems with erosive esophagitis if they do not take an expensive prescription drug to ease the symptoms.

Specifically, she says the pain is worse when lying flat after a big meal. The symptoms include nausea at times, and the burning is worse when she has her evening glass of wine. Other medications include ibuprofen 200 mg three times a day for arthritis and one of the bisphosphonates (Fosamax) for osteoporosis.

Applying the Nursing Process

Assessment

The gerontological nurse should carefully question Mrs. Stein regarding the nature of her symptoms. How consistently are they occurring? Has she noticed a pattern with certain foods? Have the symptoms become worse since taking the ibuprofen and bisphosphonate? What is her pattern of alcohol use? Does she drink alcoholic beverages in addition to her evening glass of wine? What has she done to make it better? Has she had any weight loss or gain? Does she see her healthcare provider regularly? Does she have any other diagnosed illnesses? A complete nursing assessment is indicated.

Diagnosis

The current nursing diagnoses for Mrs. Stein include the following:

- *Pain, Chronic*
- *Nausea (occasional)*

Expected Outcomes

The expected outcomes for the plan of care specify that Mrs. Stein will:

- Become aware of the harmful effects of alcohol, ibuprofen, and Fosamax on esophageal function.
- Use weight loss techniques to begin gradual weight reduction.
- Develop a therapeutic relationship with the nurse to begin a variety of lifestyle modifications that will improve her GI symptoms and health status in general.
- Agree to see a gastroenterologist for further diagnosis of her GI symptoms.

Planning and Implementation

The following nursing interventions may be appropriate for Mrs. Stein:

- She should be weighed to establish a baseline weight. If previous weights are documented, the baseline weight can be compared with previous readings. Over 2 or 3 lb of unintentional weight loss could be significant even in an overweight older person. A careful review of her eating habits and preferences will assist the nurse in this area.
- Mrs. Stein may be advised to discontinue use of ibuprofen, because chronic heartburn can result in damage to the lining of the esophagus, including inflammation, ulcers, bleeding, and scarring. Further risks include formation of peptic erosion or ulcer with slow blood loss. The pain will be dulled by the pain-relieving qualities of the medication.
- Mrs. Stein should be carefully questioned as to how she takes her Fosamax. It should be taken on an empty stomach with a full 8 oz glass of water. Additionally, she must sit upright or stand for 30 minutes to prevent esophageal reflux and erosion.

Because Mrs. Stein's pain has persisted for about a year and she has risk factors for gastroesophageal reflux disease and peptic ulcer formation, with Mrs. Stein's permission, the nurse should contact the primary care provider and report the change in condition and the information

A Patient With GERD *(continued)*

gathered in the nursing assessment. Mrs. Stein and her family should schedule an appointment with the health-care provider for further evaluation. If the nurse has access to screening cards for fecal occult blood testing, Mrs. Stein should gather the specimens at home and bring them with her for analysis at the next appointment. This will provide valuable information at the time of the visit.

Evaluation

The nurse hopes to work with Mrs. Stein over time to provide support and improve overall health and function. The nurse will consider the plan a success based on the following criteria:

- Mrs. Stein will agree to meet with a social worker to assess caregiver strain, the situation in the home, and the need for supportive services (see ethical dilemma below).

In the meantime, Mrs. Stein should be instructed to:

- Avoid foods that seem to make her situation worse (such as wine).
- Decrease the size of portions at mealtime.
- Avoid lying down for 2 to 3 hours after eating.
- Elevate the head when resting or sleeping.
- Take an antacid for symptom relief.

- A family meeting will be held to discuss Mrs. Stein's overall health.
- She will begin to decrease her alcohol consumption at bedtime and report improvement in GI symptoms.
- She will begin a gradual weight reduction program to decrease her GI symptoms and enjoy a general improvement in overall health status.

Ethical Dilemma

On the way out the door, Mrs. Stein tells the nurse that her 80-year-old husband is ill with dementia and she is exhausted caring for him. He is incontinent and often soils himself. She has to constantly clean him and is unsure how long she can keep providing his care without assistance. When the nurse offers to have Elder Services come to the home and do an assessment for assignment of home services, Mrs. Stein refuses. She states, "I can't have strangers in my home right now. It's a mess and I'm too exhausted to clean." How should the nurse respond?

The issue here is the conflict between Mrs. Stein's autonomy (the right to determine her husband's care and control entry into her home) and beneficence (what is in Mrs. Stein's and her husband's best interest). Clearly, further information and involvement of the healthcare team are needed. On the surface, it seems to make sense to allow

Mrs. Stein more time to organize her life and seek treatment for herself. However, her husband's dementia may be progressive and irreversible and therefore the likelihood of improvement may not be realistic. Should something happen to Mrs. Stein, who would care for her husband? Is there a family member who can help? Why has Mrs. Stein not gotten help thus far? Would she be willing to meet with the social worker and explore these issues further?

The nursing code of ethics supports the older person's right to self-determination and believes that nurses will and must play a primary role in implementing this right. The nurse should identify and mobilize mechanisms in place within Mr. and Mrs. Stein's support network and community. Mrs. Stein is trying to act responsibly but, by not accepting help, she may be denying her husband and herself of much needed physical and psychosocial support services.

Critical Thinking and the Nursing Process

1. What reaction have you observed when a physician or nurse recommends that an older person undergo a colonoscopy as a health maintenance measure?
2. When working with older adults experiencing GI problems, what barriers to lifestyle modification suggestions can you anticipate?

3. What is the perception of society in general regarding older adults and bowel function? Discuss this with your classmates to see if you can understand why some older people are "bowel obsessed" and overly concerned about bowel function.

- Evaluate your responses in Appendix B.

Chapter Highlights

- The gastrointestinal tract performs four major functions: digestion, absorption, secretion, and motility.

- Gastrointestinal problems are common in older adults and range from mild, self-limiting problems to serious problems requiring immediate attention and intervention.

- Comorbid illness and polypharmacy can contribute to gastrointestinal problems and exacerbate normal changes of aging. Frail older adults and those residing in nursing homes may be most at risk for adverse events and experience worse outcomes as a result of adverse events.

- Changes in bowel habits, swallowing disorders, unintentional weight loss, melena, rectal bleeding, and abdominal pain are all examples of significant abnormalities in the GI system that require careful investigation and should not be attributed to normal aging.

- The risk of colorectal cancer and peptic ulcer disease secondary to NSAID use rises rapidly with age.

- Dysphagia is the most common esophageal disorder of the older person and is estimated to occur in up to 50% of institutionalized older adults. Swallowing difficulties can be successfully assessed and risk of aspiration pneumonia minimized by the gerontological nurse.

- Gastroesophageal reflux disease can cause chest pain, exacerbate asthma and insomnia, and negatively affect quality of life. An integrated approach involving lifestyle modification, pharmacological therapy, and referral to specialists if needed can greatly improve the older person's comfort level, ability to eat, and overall quality of life.

- Constipation and diarrhea are common motility disorders that result in malnutrition, social isolation, and fluid and electrolyte imbalances. Medications are often implicated as causative factors of motility disorders.

- Diverticulosis increases with age. Complications include bleeding, diverticulitis, and perforation. Inflammatory bowel disease may present for the first time after the age of 65.

- The rate and incidence of GI malignancies rises with age, and the presenting symptoms may be more vague in the older person than in the younger adult. Most GI malignancies are more successfully treated with early detection.

- Beginning at age 50, yearly occult blood testing and colonoscopy every 10 years are recommended. While the colonoscopy itself is relatively safe, the preparation and bowel cleansing routine can be difficult. Older people with respiratory and cardiac problems may need additional supervision and monitoring of fluid and electrolyte status.

Pearson Nursing Student Resources
Find additional review materials at
nursing.pearsonhighered.com

Prepare for success with additional NCLEX®-style practice questions, interactive assignments and activities, web links, animations and videos, and more!

References

Ali, T., Roberts, D., & Tierney, W. (2009). Long term safety concerns with proton pump inhibitors. *American Journal of Medicine, 122*(10), 896–903.

Amella, E., & Lawrence, J. (2007). Eating and feeding issues in older adults with dementia: Part II: Interventions. *Try this: Best practices in nursing care for older adults with dementia* (No. D11.2). Hartford Institute of Geriatric Nursing. Retrieved from http://

consultgerirn.org/uploads/File/trythis/try_this_d11_2.pdf

Anand, B. (2012). Peptic ulcer disease. *Medscape Reference*. Retrieved from http://emedicine.medscape.com/article/181753-overview#a0101

Bharucha, A. (2007). Approach to the patient with lower GI complaints. *Merck manual for professionals*. Retrieved from http://

www.merckmanuals.com/professional/gastrointestinal_disorders/approach_to_the_patient_with_lower_gi_complaints/introduction.html

Castell, D. (2012). Medication induced esophagitis. *UpToDate*. Retrieved from http://www.uptodate.com/contents/medication-induced-esophagitis

Cronenwett, L., Sherwood, G., Barnsteiner, J., Disch, J., Johnson, J., Mitchell, P., Sullivan, D., & Warren, J. (2007). Quality and safety education for nurses, *Nursing Outlook, 55*(3) 122–131.

Dahlin, C. (2004). Oral complications at the end of life. *American Journal of Nursing, 104*(7), 40–47.

Dunphy, L., Winland-Brown, J., Porter, B., & Thomas, D. (2011). *Primary care: The art and science of advanced practice nursing* (3rd ed.). Philadelphia, PA: F. A. Davis.

Ehrenpreis, E. (2005). Irritable bowel syndrome. *Geriatrics*. Retrieved from http://geriatrics.modernmedicine .com/geriatrics/data/articlestandard// geriatrics/032005/142662/article.pdf

eMedicineHealth. (2008). *Hiatal hernia*. Retrieved from http://www.emedicinehealth .com/hiatal_hernia/article_em.htm

Everhart, J. (2009). Gastroesophageal reflux disease. In *The burden of digestive disease in the United States*. National Institute of Diabetes and Digestive and Kidney Diseases. Retrieved from http://www2.niddk .nih.gov/NR/rdonlyres/E1D07DDD-712A-4445-8F71-3C08C31698A6/0/BurdenDD_ ch14_Jan2009.pdf.

Gillson, S. (2011). Medications that may cause heartburn. *About.com: Heartburn/ GERD*. Retrieved from http://heartburn.about .com/od/whatcausesheartburn/a/Medications-That-May-Cause-Heartburn.htm

Gray-Miceli, D. (2012). *Assessment and management of atypical presentation of illness in older adults*. American Association of Colleges of Nursing & Hartford Institute of Geriatric Nursing. Retrieved from http:// consultgerirn.org/uploads/File/aprncenter/ slidelibrary/APRN-SlideLib_AtypicalPres .ppt#441,2,Adult-Gerontology APRN Slide Library

Gutierrez, K. (2008). *Pharmacotherapeutics: Clinical reasoning in primary care* (2nd ed.). St. Louis, MO: Saunders.

Howard, L., West, D., & Ossip-Klein, D. (2000). Chronic constipation management

for institutionalized older adults. *Geriatric Nursing, 21*(2), 78–82.

Huether, S., & McCance, K. (2012). *Understanding pathophysiology* (5th ed.). St. Louis, MO: Mosby.

Jacobs, D. (2007). Diverticulitis. *New England Journal of Medicine, 357*(20), 2057–2066.

McPhee, S., & Papadakis, M. (2011). *Current medical diagnosis and treatment*. New York, NY: McGraw-Hill Medical.

National Center for Complementary and Alternative Medicine (NCCAM). (2010). *Herbs at a glance: Milk thistle*. Retrieved from http://nccam.nih.gov/health/milkthistle/ ataglance.htm

National Center for Complementary and Alternative Medicine (NCCAM). (2011). *Oral probiotics: An introduction*. Retrieved from http://nccam.nih.gov/health/probiotics/ introduction.htm

National Digestive Disease Information Clearinghouse. (2003). *Your digestive system and how it works*. Retrieved from http://www .digestive.niddk.nih.gov

New York State Department of Health. (2011). *About liver cancer*. Retrieved from http:// www.health.ny.gov/statistics/cancer/registry/ abouts/liver.htm

Nguyen, G., Sam, J., & Anon, N. (2011). Epidemiological trends and geographic variation in hospital admissions for diverticulitis in the United States. *World Journal of Gastroenterology*. Retrieved from http://www.wjgnet.com/1007-9327/pdf/v17/ i12/1600.pdf

Nurse Practitioners' Prescribing Reference. (2012). *Winter 2011–2012, 18*(4). New York, NY: Prescribing Reference LLC.

Reuben, D., Herr, K., Pacala, J., Potter, J., Pollock, B., & Semla, T. (2011). *Gastrointestinal diseases: Geriatrics at your fingertips*. New York, NY: American Geriatrics Society.

Rofes, L., Arreola, V., Almirall, J., Cabre, M., Campins, L., Garcia-Peris, G., Speyer, R., & Clave, P. (2011). Diagnosis and management of

oropharyngeal dysphagia and its nutritional and respiratory complications in the elderly. *Gastroenterology Research and Practice*. Retrieved from http://www.hindawi.com/ journals/grp/2011/818979

Roy, P. (2012). Zollinger-Ellison syndrome. *Medscape Reference*. Retrieved from http://emedicine.medscape.com/ article/183555-overview#a0199

Shaheen, N. (2006). Effects of aging on the digestive system. *Merck manual home health handbook*. Retrieved from http://www .merckmanuals.com/home/digestive_disorders/ biology_of_the_digestive_system/effects_of_ aging_on_the_digestive_system.html

Slowik, G. (2012). What is GERD? *EhealthMD*. Retrieved from http://ehealthmd .com/content/what-gerd

Smith, D., & Newman, D. (1989). The bran solution. *Contemporary Long Term Care, 12*, 66.

Soetikno, R., Kaltenbach, T., Rouse, R., Park, W., Maheshwari, A., Sato, T., et al. (2008). Prevalence of nonpolypoid (flat and depressed) colorectal neoplasms in asymptomatic and symptomatic adults. *Journal of the American Medical Association, 299*(9), 1027–1035.

Tariq, S. (2007). Constipation in long-term care. *Journal of the American Medical Directors Association, 8*, 209–218.

U.S. National Library of Medicine. (2010, September 1). *Misoprostol*. Retrieved from http://www.ncbi.nlm.nih.gov/pubmedhealth/ PMH0000886

Waye, J. (2004). Endoscopic gastrointestinal procedures. In M. Beers & R. Berkow (Eds.), *Merck manual of geriatrics*. Retrieved from http://www.merck.com

WebMD. (2012). *Difficulty swallowing (dysphagia)—Overview*. Retrieved from http:// www.webmd.com/digestive-disorders/tc/ difficulty-swallowing-dysphagia-overview

The Hematologic System

KEY TERMS

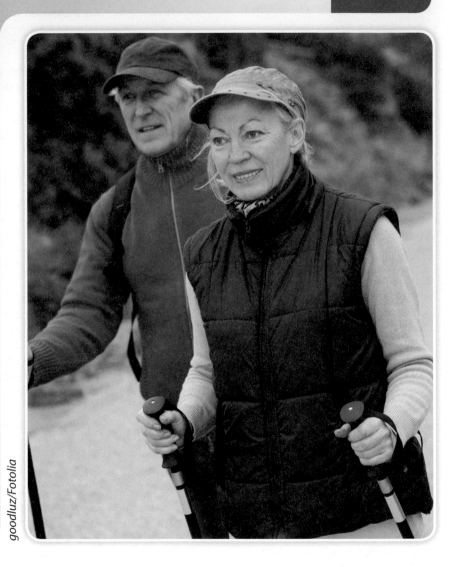

goodluz/Fotolia

LEARNING OUTCOMES

On completion of this chapter, the reader will be able to:

1. Describe age-related changes that affect hematologic function.
2. Recognize the impact of age-related changes on hematologic function.
3. Identify risk factors to health for the older person with hematologic problems.
4. Interpret the unique presentation of hematologic problems in the older person.

5. Devise appropriate nursing interventions directed toward assisting the older person with hematologic problems to develop self-care abilities.
6. Identify and prioritize appropriate nursing interventions to care for the older person with hematologic problems.

The hematologic system is responsible for many functions in the body and serves as a medium of exchange between the outside environment and the body's internal environment. The main function of the circulating blood is to carry oxygen and nutrients to and remove carbon dioxide and waste products from the internal organs and peripheral tissue. **Oxyhemoglobin** (oxygen bound to hemoglobin) is normally about 100% when measured in arterial blood but decreases to about 60% in venous return, which indicates that body cells are aggressive oxygen consumers (Holcomb, 2005). Additionally, blood transports other substances such as hormones, proteins, solutes, water, and medications to sites where they are needed. Blood contributes to homeostasis along with the renal and respiratory systems and helps to maintain the acid–base balance. Blood carries various ions, oxygen, and carbon dioxide to the renal and respiratory systems, thus participating in acid–base balance. This contribution helps to maintain a constant internal body environment. Blood consists of red blood cells, white blood cells, **platelets,** and **plasma.** Plasma accounts for about 55% of the blood, and blood volume accounts for 7% of total body weight (National Heart, Lung, and Blood Institute [NHLBI], 2007). Blood volume in healthy, hydrated adults is about 5.5 L (6 quarts). Older adults with diseases associated with blood and blood-forming organs may experience health problems that range from minor disruptions in functional ability to major life-threatening problems.

Erythrocytes, or red blood cells (RBCs), have a life span of about 120 days. They are flexible, concave disks that arise from stem cells in the **bone marrow.** Erythrocytes contain **hemoglobin,** a protein that binds with oxygen to form oxyhemoglobin. Old RBCs are destroyed in the spleen, liver, bone marrow, and lymph nodes by **phagocytes** that save and reuse key materials from the destroyed RBCs, including proteins and iron. The number of circulating RBCs remains fairly stable under normal conditions, but chronic and acute illness, blood loss, toxic substances, and nutritional deficiencies can decrease the number of circulating cells and result in **anemia.** Anemia occurs whenever the hemoglobin content of the blood is insufficient to satisfy body demands (Huether & McCance, 2011). Erythropoiesis, or the production of RBCs, is regulated by erythropoietin, a hormone secreted by the kidneys that stimulates the cells in the bone marrow. Erythropoietin is released by the kidneys in response to hypoxia and stimulates the bone marrow to produce RBCs. This process usually takes about 5 days to reach a maximum and will result in the release of a higher percentage of reticulocytes or immature RBCs into the circulation.

> **Practice Pearl** ▸▸▸ Anemia is a sign and symptom of disease—not a disease itself. When an older person is diagnosed with anemia, the underlying condition should be diagnosed before the anemia is corrected.

Normally, about 4,000 to 10,000 **leukocytes,** or white blood cells (WBCs), are present in a microliter of adult blood. The function of WBCs is to protect the body and form a defense against invading microorganisms. The WBCs include granulocytes (65%), lymphocytes (30%), and monocytes (5%). The granulocytes are composed mostly of neutrophils (40% to 60%), eosinophils (4%), and basophils (1%). Granulocytes and monocytes (immature macrophages) are produced in the bone marrow, and lymphocytes are produced in the lymph nodes, spleen, and thymus. The function of the granulocytes and monocytes is to engage in phagocytosis and help the body to fight off infections by surrounding and dissolving invading microorganisms. When stimulated by an antigen (a foreign protein or allergen), some lymphocytes are transformed into plasma cells to release antibodies. Antibodies are carried by the bloodstream to the site of infection and will bind with foreign proteins to destroy or neutralize their biological functions (Huether & McCance, 2011).

Platelets begin as small cell fragments residing in bone marrow. When mature, they enter the circulation as platelets. Platelets are essential for blood coagulation and they help to control bleeding by forming the foundation for a clot. The spleen holds about one third of the platelets in reserve for use in the body. A platelet lives approximately 10 days, after which it dies and is removed by macrophages (Huether & McCance, 2011).

Humans have four major types of blood groups: O, A, B, and AB. These groups differ by the nature of the antigens (A and B) present on the RBCs. People with blood type A have A antigens present, those with type B have B antigens, those who are type AB have both antigens, and those who are type O have neither antigen. ABO antibodies develop in the serum of people whose RBCs lack the corresponding antigen. These antibodies are called anti-A and anti-B. People with blood type A have anti-B antibodies, and people with blood type B have anti-A antibodies. Because plasma of people with blood types A, B, and AB has no antibodies to group O red blood cells, people with group O blood have traditionally been called universal donors. Conversely, people with AB blood have been called universal recipients, because their plasma has no antibodies to antigens in the other three groups. A third antigen on the red blood cell is D. People who are Rh positive have the D antigen, and those who are Rh negative do not have this antigen. The presence of these antigens and antibodies may cause ABO and Rh incompatibilities unless the appropriate blood type is administered during transfusions. Currently, because of a better understanding of complex immune reactions, blood type O is no longer considered the universal donor and all transfusions undergo typing and crossmatching (MayoClinic.com, 2008). An acute hemolytic transfusion reaction can occur when an ABO incompatibility results. This is because an antigen–antibody reaction will occur between the blood of the recipient and the blood of the donor who has a different antigen.

NORMAL CHANGES OF AGING

Most of the changes of aging in the hematologic system are the result of the bone marrow's reduced capacity to produce RBCs quickly when disease or blood loss has occurred. However, without major blood loss or the diagnosis of a serious illness, the bone marrow changes of aging are not clinically significant. Figure 21-1 ▶▶▶ illustrates the normal changes of aging in the hematologic system.

At about age 70, the amount of bone marrow in the long bones (where most RBCs are formed) begins to decline steadily. Additional changes of aging in the hematologic system include the following:

- The number of stem cells in the marrow is decreased.
- The administration of erythropoietin to stimulate use of iron to form RBCs is less effective in older adults than in younger people.
- Lymphocyte function, especially cellular immunity, appears to decrease with age.
- Platelet adhesiveness increases with age.
- Average hemoglobin and **hematocrit** values decrease slightly with age but remain within normal limits.

Many functions of the hematologic system remain constant in healthy older adults, including RBC life span, total blood volume, RBC volume, total lymphocyte and granulocyte counts, and platelet structure and function (Huether & McCance, 2011; NHLBI, 2007; Reuben et al., 2011).

Common Disorders

With aging, several common disorders can occur in the hematologic system. The most common of these disorders is anemia, a condition often falsely attributed to normal aging.

Anemia

Anemia, or insufficient hemoglobin content to meet the body's needs, is defined as a decrease in the number of circulating RBCs (and thus hemoglobin) resulting from blood loss, impaired production of RBCs, or increased RBC destruction. Anemia is common in older adults. Although old age alone does not increase the chances of developing anemia, many chronic illnesses that occur with aging can contribute to the diagnosis of anemia. Chronic disorders such as kidney disease, chronic infections or inflammation, and endocrine disorders, as well as nutritional deficiencies, medication use, and blood loss from surgery or trauma, are associated with various types of anemia (Dunphy, Winland-Brown, Porter, et al., 2011). It is estimated that more than 3 million Americans over the age of 65 are anemic, occurring in about 10% of the older adult population. African Americans are three times more likely than Caucasians to be diagnosed with anemia (Vanassa & Berliner, 2010). As many as one third of hospitalized patients have anemia related to serious diagnoses such as kidney disease, cancer, diabetes, HIV/AIDS, and other serious illnesses (NHLBI, 2007).

Although anemia is common in older people, it is never normal and it requires complete and thorough investigation. Some anemias are simply markers of chronic illness and nutritional deficiencies, whereas others indicate serious underlying illness such as malignant neoplasms. All anemias result in a loss of oxygen-carrying capacity of the blood and produce generalized tissue hypoxia. The body tries to compensate by raising the heart and respiratory rates, shunting blood to vital organs away from the skin, and increasing blood viscosity to supply oxygen to hypoxic tissues. The physiological results may include skin pallor, chronic fatigue, dyspnea on exertion, and bone and joint pain as well as the potential for clot-related disorders, such as stroke (Dunphy et al., 2011).

The presentation of anemia depends on the underlying pathophysiology that caused the disease. Anemias are usually classified by measuring the size of the RBCs and computing the **mean corpuscular volume (MCV).** The resulting groups include **microcytic** (smaller RBCs), **macrocytic** (larger RBCs), and **normocytic** (RBCs of normal size). Additional classifications include hypochromic (abnormally low hemoglobin concentration), hyperchromic (abnormally high hemoglobin concentration), or normochromic (normal hemoglobin concentration). However, some anemias fall into more than one category, and sometimes an older person may be diagnosed with more than one type or a mixed anemia.

Symptoms of anemia are similar for older and younger people; however, older adults, especially those with chronic illness and mobility problems, may not experience symptoms until their disease has become more severe because they are not physically active and are less likely to notice the troubling signs and symptoms accompanying

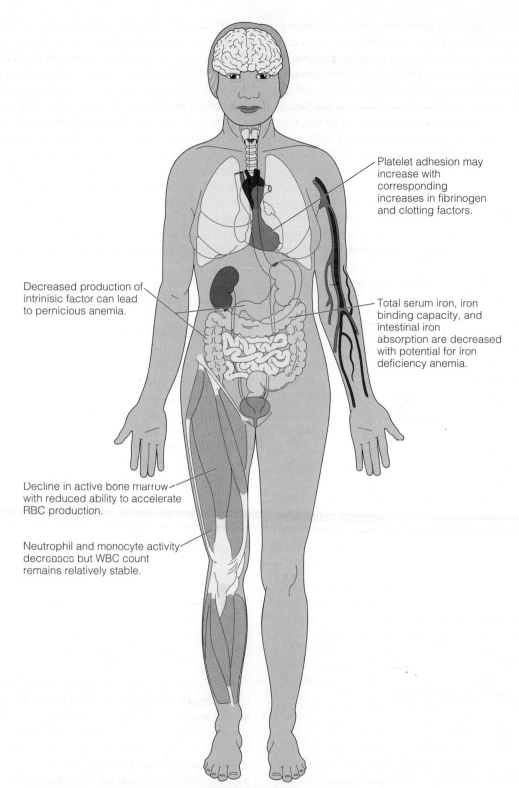

Platelet adhesion may increase with corresponding increases in fibrinogen and clotting factors.

Decreased production of intrinisic factor can lead to pernicious anemia.

Total serum iron, iron binding capacity, and intestinal iron absorption are decreased with potential for iron deficiency anemia.

Decline in active bone marrow with reduced ability to accelerate RBC production.

Neutrophil and monocyte activity decreases but WBC count remains relatively stable.

Figure 21-1 ▶▶▶ Normal changes of aging in the hematologic system.

anemia. Anemia in the older person is associated with negative health outcomes and increased mortality (St. Louis University, 2006). Symptoms include fatigue, shortness of breath, worsening angina, developing or worsening of peripheral edema, falls, increased hospitalizations, and decreased quality of life. Dizziness and mental status changes such as confusion, depression, agitation, and apathy may also occur as symptoms of anemia, especially in the frail older adult who is less likely to be physically active and to exhibit the more common musculoskeletal and cardiac signs of aging. Pallor, usually less obvious in the older person and people of color, may be noticed in the oral mucosa and conjunctiva (Dunphy et al., 2011). Severe anemia may result in tachycardia, palpitations, systolic murmurs, and angina with ischemic changes evident on electrocardiogram. Despite the abundance of medical clues, anemia is often underdiagnosed and undertreated in older adults (St. Louis University, 2006).

> **Practice Pearl** ▶▶▶ In the United States, the most common type of anemia is iron deficiency anemia followed by the anemia of chronic disease (American Society of Hematology, 2010).

The diagnosis of anemia increases with age. In community-residing older adults over age 65, the rate is between 11%; after age 85, the rate increases to 20% (Vanassa & Berliner, 2010). In nursing home residents (average age over 80 years of age) the rate of anemia is found to be around 50% (Anemia.org, 2010). Chronic kidney failure results in a twofold increase in the chance of being diagnosed with anemia. For each 0.6 g/dL fall in hemoglobin, there is approximately a 30% increased risk of the older person developing left ventricular hypertrophy (an independent risk factor for myocardial infarction and stroke) (St. Louis University, 2006).

> **Practice Pearl** ▶▶▶ Judicious blood testing in hospitalized patients would minimize anemia resulting from blood loss for laboratory testing, especially in intensive care patients and others subjected to frequent blood draws (Salisbury et al., 2011).

Evaluation of the older person with suspected anemia should begin with laboratory tests including measurement of hemoglobin, hematocrit, RBC count and indices, reticulocyte count, WBC count and differential, and platelet count. Older men are considered anemic with a hemoglobin concentration below 14 g/dL and older women below 12 g/dL; however, all older adults regardless of their gender should be evaluated when their hemoglobin falls

below 13. Additionally, older adults whose hemoglobin falls more than 1 g/dL in 1 year should be evaluated (Reuben et al., 2011). Hemoglobin concentrations will be artificially higher in a dehydrated older person and in those who smoke cigarettes or live at high altitudes. Hemoglobin concentrations will be artificially lower in an overhydrated older person such as those with heart failure.

A hematocrit level of greater than 47 for men and postmenopausal women is considered within normal limits (National Kidney Foundation, 2011). A hematocrit of less than 41% in men and 37% in women is diagnostic of anemia (McPhee & Papadakis, 2011). It is important to remember that hematocrit levels are greatly influenced by hydration status with dehydrated older adults exhibiting artificially high hematocrit levels and overhydrated people exhibiting artificially low levels.

Important laboratory tests to determine anemia and their normal values are listed in Table 21-1.

Microcytic Anemias

Anemias are classified as microcytic if the MCV is less than 80 fl. In older people, microcytic anemias can result from iron deficiency and thalassemia minor (a result of inadequate globin synthesis). Anemia of chronic disease can be microcytic but is more commonly normocytic, especially early in the disease process (Dugdale, 2010). Iron deficiency anemia is characterized by small, pale (hypochromic) RBCs and eventual depletion of iron stores. The body cannot synthesize hemoglobin without iron, and gradually the number of RBCs decreases. Serum ferritin levels usually accurately reflect bone marrow iron stores; however, these may remain normal early in the process before iron stores are depleted. The reticulocyte count is usually decreased. Serum ferritin levels of less than 10 mcg/L are highly diagnostic of iron deficiency (Gersten, 2010).

> **Practice Pearl** ▶▶▶ Serum ferritin concentrations can be falsely elevated in older adults with liver damage and certain cancers (Gersten, 2010).

Iron deficiency can occur as the result of acute blood loss (from surgery or trauma) or chronic blood loss (from gastrointestinal bleeding, hemorrhoids, or cancer). It may also result from inadequate dietary intake of iron or malabsorption of iron. In menstruating women, blood loss is the most common cause of iron deficiency; however, in men or postmenopausal women, the first site to consider for possible blood loss is the gastrointestinal tract. Black stools or melena might indicate upper GI bleeding, whereas the presence of red blood in the stool or on toilet tissue is indicative of lower GI or rectal bleeding. Excessive blood

TABLE 21-1	Laboratory Tests to Determine Anemia	
Test	**Purpose**	**Normal Geriatric Value**
Transferrin	Regulates iron absorption and transport. *Increased* in iron deficiency anemia due to hemorrhage, thalassemia, early B$_{12}$ and folate deficiency, and acute hepatitis. *Decreased* in anemia of chronic disease, hypothyroidism, hemorrhage, and protein deficiency. Transferrin levels are usually normal in the anemia of chronic disease, hemorrhage, and hypothyroidism.	240–480 mg/dL
Serum iron	Transferrin-bound iron. Used in combination with transferrin test and TIBC. Serum iron levels vary throughout the day and are higher in the morning. Serum iron levels are decreased in iron deficiency due to blood loss, malnutrition, and chronic inflammation and increased in B$_{12}$ and folate deficiency, liver disease, and lead toxicity.	Men: 60–180 mcg/dL Women: 50–165 mcg/dL
Total iron-binding capacity (TIBC)	Reflects the transferrin content of the serum. When the body is deficient in iron (iron deficiency anemia), the TIBC is increased; the TIBC is decreased in the presence of chronic inflammation. The TIBC is usually normal in the presence of B$_{12}$ and folate deficiency.	250–450 mg/dL
Serum ferritin	An iron compound found in the intestinal mucosa, spleen, and liver. Contains >20% iron and is essential for **hematopoiesis,** the production and differentiation of red blood cells occurring in the bone marrow. Indicates adequacy of iron stores. *Increased* in iron overload, acute hepatitis, metastatic cancer, and chronic inflammatory disorders. *Decreased* in iron deficiency anemia. Serum ferritin levels greater than 100 mg/mL exclude iron deficiency anemia and levels less than 18 mg/mL usually confirm the diagnosis of iron deficiency anemia. Serum ferritin is usually normal in the presence of anemia of chronic disease.	Men: 18–270 ng/mL Women: 18–160 ng/mL
Mean corpuscular volume (MCV)	Index for classifying anemias on size of the red cell. Indicates whether the RBC is normocytic, microcytic, or macrocytic. *Decreased* in iron deficiency anemia, lead poisoning, and thalassemia. *Increased* with B$_{12}$ and folic acid deficiency, alcoholism, and hemolytic anemia. *Normal* in anemia of chronic disease, renal disease hypothyroidism, and early hemorrhage.	Men: 80–100 fl Women: 76–96 fl
Mean corpuscular hemoglobin concentration (MCHC)	A measure of the average hemoglobin concentration in the RBCs. *Decreased* in iron deficiency anemia and thalassemia. *Increased* in vitamin B$_{12}$ and folic acid deficiency and chronic inflammation.	27–36 g/dL
Reticulocyte count	Reticulocytes are immature cells in the RBC cycle and last 1–2 days in the circulation before the RBC matures. *Increased* in hemolytic anemia, leukemia, sickle cell anemia, and after acute hemorrhage. *Decreased* in iron deficiency and aplastic anemia, untreated pernicious anemia, anemia of chronic disease, and bone marrow disease.	Men: 0.5–1.5% of total RBCs Women: 0.5–2.5% of total RBCs

Source: Dunphy et al. (2011); Reuben et al. (2011); St. Louis University (2006).

donation and frequent phlebotomies (older adults who are on warfarin or hospitalized) are causes that are often overlooked (Salisbury et al., 2011).

Once the cause of the iron deficiency has been identified, oral iron therapy is the preferred treatment. Stool should be tested for occult blood, and additional gastrointestinal testing (colonoscopy or barium studies) may be necessary. Iron therapy should never be recommended for an older person with iron deficiency anemia without identifying the reason for occult blood loss. Correcting the symptom without knowing the underlying cause of the problem can mask the symptoms of serious disease like cancer.

The usual treatment is ferrous sulfate 325 mg daily. To minimize gastrointestinal distress, ferrous sulfate should be taken with meals. Enteric-coated and sustained-release formulations should be avoided, because they are poorly absorbed. A single daily dose of ferrous sulfate reduces the risk of constipation and gastric irritation. Increasing the dose only minimally increases iron absorption; however, the nurse should carefully monitor the older person taking iron supplements and report new onset of constipation and symptoms of gastrointestinal distress. Ferrous gluconate causes less gastrointestinal distress. Therapeutic response is monitored by measuring a reticulocyte count after 1 to 2 weeks of therapy and remeasuring the serum hemoglobin, hematocrit, and ferritin levels in about 2 months. It may take up to a year to fully replenish iron stores in the marrow (Reuben et al., 2011).

Thalassemia is an inherited disorder of hemoglobin synthesis in which parts of the hemoglobin molecular chain are missing or defective. As a result, the RBC is fragile, hypochromic, and microcytic (60 to 75 fL). Thalassemia occurs mostly in people of Mediterranean (Greek or Italian) descent, but may be found in people of Southeast Asia and China descent (McPhee & Papadakis, 2011). The disease is usually diagnosed in infancy or childhood, and most undiagnosed adults will have the disease in a milder form that may go unnoticed until late in life. The diagnosis is made by a hematologist using serum electrophoresis. Iron replacement is not indicated and may result in iron overload. Patients with thalassemia should be identified so that they are not subjected to repeated evaluation for iron deficiency. There is no treatment but it is recommended that a folate supplement be taken and oxidative drugs such as sulfonamides be avoided. Older patients with severe thalassemia may require periodic transfusions (McPhee & Papadakis, 2011).

Additional microcytic, hypochromic anemias include those caused by lead poisoning, aluminum toxicity, and parasitic infections (Gersten, 2010). Referral to a hematologist is indicated in these complex situations.

Normocytic Anemia

The most common types of normocytic anemia in the older person are anemia of chronic disease, hemolytic anemia, and aplastic anemia. In this form of anemia, the red blood cells are normal size and contain normal amounts of hemoglobin, but there are too few RBCs to carry the amount of oxygen needed by the cells. Anemia in which the MCV is 80 to 100 fL is considered normocytic because the RBCs are of normal size. Normocytic anemia is usually caused by concurrent chronic illness (heart, respiratory, or renal disease, or malignancy), and anemia of chronic disease is the most common type of normocytic anemia.

Anemia of chronic disease is usually associated with malnutrition or conditions such as chronic infection or inflammation, renal insufficiency, chronic liver disease, endocrine disorders, malnutrition, and cancer. These diseases influence RBC production in the following manner:

- **Chronic infection and inflammation.** After 4 to 8 weeks of illness, anemia may result from slightly decreased erythropoietin production, decreased RBC survival, and impaired transport of iron to the bone marrow. The reticulocyte count is low, serum iron is normal or slightly reduced, and serum ferritin is normal or elevated. When the underlying disease is treated and the infection or inflammation resolves, the anemia disappears.

- **Renal insufficiency.** This anemia results from decreased erythropoiesis and decreased RBC survival. Serum iron stores are normal. In hemodialysis patients, injections of erythropoietin may reverse the anemia. In nondialysis patients, erythropoietin is not as effective because erythropoietic inhibitors can accumulate. Erythropoietin is given intravenously to hemodialysis patients and subcutaneously to nondialysis patients with renal failure in an attempt to produce more prolonged bone marrow stimulation. The Hct should be carefully monitored as Hct measurements greater than 60% to 65% may develop, placing the patient at risk for stroke or myocardial infarction (Dunphy et al., 2011).

- **Chronic liver disease.** Normocytic anemia results from decreased RBC production and survival. Large quantities of alcohol are toxic to the bone marrow and the liver as well as other organs of the body. The result is decreased serum iron levels and total iron-binding capacity. Treatment is aimed at stopping the progression of, or correcting, the underlying liver disease.

- **Malnutrition.** When essential nutrients such as folic acid and vitamin C are missing, RBC production decreases, resulting in a normocytic anemia. Nutritional deficiencies can also result from malabsorption disorders or heightened need for nutrients when nutritional intake is adequate.

- **Malignancies.** Cancer in the later stages is nearly always accompanied by anemia of chronic disease. Chemotherapy can suppress bone marrow function and contribute to decreased appetite, nausea and vomiting, and nutritional deficiencies leading to inadequate caloric, protein, and vitamin intake. Erythropoietin injected subcutaneously is sometimes used to treat anemia and fatigue in older patients with nonmyeloid cancers.

Erythropoietin-like agents can increase hemoglobin levels in older adults with chronic kidney disease, those with cancer and receiving cancer therapy, and in those with anemia of chronic disease. Erythropoietin administration has been shown to correct anemia and reduce transfusion needs. Ferritin levels must be monitored and corrected, if deficient, in order to maximize treatment effects (St. Louis University, 2006). Erythropoietin can be administered monthly and the hemoglobin level should not be increased more than 1 g/dL per month. Medicare will stop reimbursement when hemoglobin levels rise above 13 g/dL for three consecutive billing cycles (Centers for Medicare & Medicaid Services, 2007). These drugs are usually well tolerated in the recommended dosage; however, side effects may include alopecia, nausea, vomiting, diarrhea, fever, and fatigue (Nurse Practitioners' Prescribing Reference, 2012). High dosages may also be associated with increased risk of adverse cardiovascular events, increased tumor growth, and death in older adults with cancers of the breast, head and neck, lung, and cervix (U.S. Food and Drug Administration [FDA], 2007). The FDA has recommended that physicians target hemoglobin ranges in the range of 10 to 12 g/dL to minimize the occurrence of these adverse events.

Diseases associated with anemia of chronic disease include but are not limited to:

- Acute infections—bacterial, fungal, or viral
- Chronic infections—osteomyelitis, infective endocarditis, chronic urinary tract infection, tuberculosis, or chronic fungal disease
- Inflammatory disorders—rheumatoid disease, systemic lupus erythematosus, burns, severe trauma, and acute and chronic hepatitis
- Malignancy—carcinoma, myeloma, lymphoma, and leukemia
- Radiation and chemotherapy
- Vitamin deficiency (folate) and other forms of malnutrition
- Chronic renal failure

Huether & McCance, 2011; McPhee & Papadakis, 2011.

Hemolytic anemia is also a normocytic anemia that can occur at any age, but it becomes more common with aging. When the **hemolysis** or premature destruction of RBCs increases, the body compensates by increasing production of immature RBCs in the bone marrow, resulting in increased numbers of circulating reticulocytes in the blood. If the RBC life span is reduced to less than 40 days, the older person has a hemolytic disorder that may be manifested by an increased production of RBCs and/or an increased destruction of RBCs (Reuben et al., 2011). The causes of increased RBC destruction may be associated with increased autoimmune antibodies; inherited enzyme deficits (G6PD deficiency); infections such as syphilis, leukemia, Hodgkin's disease, and non-Hodgkin's lymphoma; trauma; mechanical factors (prosthetic heart valves); burns; exposure to toxic chemicals and venoms; and drugs (Huether & McCance, 2011).

Drugs capable of causing hemolytic anemia include ibuprofen, L-dopa, penicillin, drugs classified as cephalosporins, tetracycline, acetaminophen, aspirin,

erythromycin, hydralazine, hydrochlorothiazide, insulin, isoniazid, methadone, phenacetin, procainamide, quinidine, rifampin, streptomycin, sulfonamides, nitrofurantoin, and triamterene (Dugdale, 2010; Nurse Practitioners' Prescribing Reference, 2012). Increased destruction of RBCs results in increased levels of unconjugated bilirubin. The indirect Coombs' test is used to detect antibodies on the RBC. Drug-related hemolysis usually stops quickly when the drug is withdrawn (Dugdale, 2010).

All hemolytic anemias require folic acid treatment because this vitamin is used up with increased bone marrow production of RBCs. Folic acid is absorbed from the intestine and is found in green leafy vegetables, fruits, cereals, and meats. Deficiencies are often found in chronically undernourished people. When the cause of the hemolytic anemia cannot be found, prednisone is sometimes used to treat idiopathic autoimmune hemolysis. More commonly, the offending drug can be identified. Drug-induced hemolysis is usually treated by simply discontinuing the responsible drug or replacing it with another drug, if needed.

Although aplastic anemia is not very common and is usually a disease of adolescents and young adults, it can occur in old age. The cause of aplastic anemia is unknown in the majority of cases, but this anemia may sometimes develop as a result of damage to the cells in the bone marrow by radiation or chemical substances (benzene, arsenic, chloramphenicol, and chemotherapeutic agents). The overall mortality rate is greater than 50%. In this disorder, the reticulocyte count is low, and bone marrow function is suppressed and hypoplastic. It does not produce adequate numbers of RBCs. Treatment involves discontinuation of all medications and administration of ongoing blood transfusions. Bone marrow transplantation is usually not effective in older adults (McPhee & Papadakis, 2011).

Macrocytic Anemias

Anemias are classified as macrocytic if the MCV is greater than 100 fL. The most common cause of macrocytic anemia in the older person is B_{12} or folate deficiency. Additional causes include liver disease, alcoholism, and thyroid disorders (McPhee & Papadakis, 2011). Vitamin B_{12} deficiencies can occur when the amount of the vitamin in the diet is inadequate or when sufficient amounts are not absorbed from the gastrointestinal tract. Failure to absorb vitamin B_{12} from the gastrointestinal tract is called pernicious anemia and results from a lack of intrinsic factor. About 12% of older people have low serum vitamin B_{12} levels (<300 pg/mL). Vitamin B_{12}–related neurologic damage, such as neuropathies, paresthesias, and cognitive impairment, may occur before the anemia is discovered. Additional causes of macrocytic anemia include hypothyroidism, chronic liver disease, and drugs such as chemotherapeutic agents and anticonvulsants (Huether & McCance, 2011). The signs and symptoms of B_{12} deficiency may take years to develop and are often subtle. Mental status may be affected, and cognitive impairment, depression, mania, and other psychiatric syndromes may develop. Neurologic findings will include peripheral neuropathies, numbness and tingling in the extremities, and ataxia and difficulty walking and maintaining balance. Unfortunately, correcting the B_{12} deficiency does not usually reverse or improve mental status but may halt the progression of the symptoms. Laboratory tests used to detect low levels of B_{12} may not be abnormal until the older person becomes overtly anemic. In addition to a large MCV, leukopenia and thrombocytopenia may occur.

Pernicious anemia results when an older person lacks the needed intrinsic factor to absorb vitamin B_{12}. Because only about 1% of older adults lack intrinsic factor, a more common cause of low serum vitamin B_{12} results from the inability to split vitamin B_{12} from proteins in food. This inability may be the result of a deficiency of hydrochloric acid or pancreatic enzymes. Other causes of B_{12} deficiency include gastrectomy, small bowel disease, *Helicobacter pylori* infection, prolonged use of antacids, intestinal bacterial overgrowth, cachexia, and adherence to a strict vegetarian diet (McPhee & Papadakis, 2011).

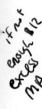

The diagnosis of vitamin B_{12} deficiency has traditionally been based on low serum vitamin B_{12} levels, usually less than 150 pg/mL; however, some older adults become symptomatic at levels between 150 and 300 pg/mL. Common B_{12} deficiency symptoms include cognitive impairment and neurologic deficits such as paresthesias. Measurements of metabolites such as methylmalonic acid and homocysteine have been shown to be more sensitive in the diagnosis of vitamin B_{12} deficiency than measurement of serum B_{12} levels alone. Regardless of the test results, successful treatment can still be achieved with oral replacement therapy (Reuben et al., 2011).

> **Drug Alert** ▶▶▶ The widespread use of gastric acid–blocking agents may contribute to the eventual development of vitamin B_{12} deficiency because these medications neutralize the acidic environment that is needed to break down and release vitamin B_{12} bound to the ingested food. When caring for an older person on long-term acid suppression therapy, methylmalonic acid and homocysteine levels should be monitored periodically.

For those with pernicious anemia, treatment usually consists of lifelong B_{12} replacement. Because most clinicians are generally unaware that oral vitamin B_{12} therapy is effective, the traditional treatment for B_{12} deficiency has

been intramuscular injections. The usual intramuscular dose is 1,000 mcg/day for the first week, then 1,000 mcg/week for 4 weeks, and then 1,000 mcg/month for life. Although the daily requirement of vitamin B_{12} is approximately 2 mcg, the initial oral replacement dosage consists of a single daily dose of 1,000 to 2,000 mcg. This high dose is required because of the variable absorption of oral vitamin B_{12} in smaller doses. The oral replacement should be taken on an empty stomach. It has been shown to be safe, cost effective, and well tolerated by older adults (Reuben et al., 2011). Approximately 1 month of treatment is needed to correct the anemia. Treatment with folic acid alone may improve the anemia, but it will not prevent further decline or improve existing neurologic changes associated with the B_{12} deficiency. Folic acid supplementation may mask an occult vitamin B_{12} deficiency and further exacerbate or initiate neurologic disease.

Folic acid deficiency produces laboratory results similar to those found with B_{12} deficiency. Serum folate levels will measure below 3 ng/mL, and B_{12} levels are normal in early folate deficiencies. Folate deficiency is not common in the healthy older person but may be found in older people with malabsorption syndromes, poor nutrition, alcoholism, and underlying malignancies. Foods high in folate include liver, orange juice, cereals, whole grains, beans, nuts, and dark green leafy vegetables like spinach. Chronic use of certain drugs such as triamterene, trimethoprim, anticonvulsants, and nitrofurantoin can also cause folic acid deficiency by blocking folic acid metabolism. It usually takes about 6 months to deplete the folic acid from body storage. Laboratory testing usually reveals a macrocytic RBC and low serum folate levels (<2 ng/mL) or low RBC folate levels (<100 ng/mL). However, RBC folate levels are a more stable marker and more clinically reliable. Treatment consists of folic acid 1 mg/day by mouth (Reuben et al., 2011).

> **Drug Alert** ▶▶▶ In older adults with macrocytic anemia due to a B_{12} deficiency, treatment with folic acid alone may correct the anemia but will not prevent or reverse neurologic damage resulting from B_{12} deficiency.

Sickle Cell Anemia

Sickle cell anemia is an inherited disease found mostly in people of West African descent in which the RBCs are crescent shaped. As a result, the RBCs tend to clump together and form small clots, causing vaso-occlusive crises and cellular death due to lack of oxygen. These clots give rise to recurrent painful hypoxic episodes called sickle cell crises. Crises can be triggered by stress, illness, infection, temperature changes, and other unknown reasons. Crises can occur infrequently or six or more times per year. Complications include stroke, cardiomegaly, pulmonary hypertension, renal failure, blindness, skin ulcerations, and chronic joint pain (Dunphy et al., 2011).

Symptoms of sickle cell disease begin within the first year of life. Approximately 1 out of every 400 to 500 African Americans has sickle cell disease, and about 8–10% carries the trait or carries the gene that can cause the disease if he or she has a child with another carrier. In the past, death from organ failure occurred between the ages of 20 and 40 years in most people with sickle cell disease. Now with better management, older adults are living into their 50s and 60s. People with sickle cell disease should avoid infection, consume a balanced diet, avoid dehydration and stress, and take folic acid supplementation of 1 mg/day by mouth as infection, poor nutrition, lack of fluids, and high stress levels can precipitate a sickle cell crisis (Dunphy et al., 2011).

Transfusions

Many older people gradually adjust to being anemic by conserving energy and adopting sedentary lifestyles. Some care providers attribute lack of energy to aging and, hence, fail to diagnose anemia. Therefore, severe anemias may be present for long periods of time and avoid detection. Severe anemia can lead to myocardial infarction, falls, confusion, and other serious complications. When quick reversal of anemia is indicated, a transfusion may be needed. There is no agreement among clinicians on when a transfusion is needed, but when the older person's hemoglobin is below 7 to 8 g/dL and he or she is experiencing symptoms such as shortness of breath or chest pain, a blood transfusion may be indicated (Artz, 2011). Transfusions carry the risk of infection, fluid overload, and transfusion reactions. Older adults receiving two units of packed red cells may be at risk for fluid overload if they have cardiac dysfunction; however, for severe anemia transfusion may be warranted.

Practice Pearl ▶▶▶ Members of the Jehovah's Witness religious denomination reject the use of blood transfusions and blood products. Blood-sparing strategies should be used with these older adults including use of hemostatic agents in wound healing, blood salvage techniques, decreased use of phlebotomy associated with diagnostic testing, and use of hemoglobin substitutes, erythropoietin, and less restrictive blood transfusion triggers (Tinmouth, McIntyre, & Fowler, 2008).

Older adults are subject to fluid overload and are at risk for acute heart failure. Therefore, the physician may request transfusion with packed red blood cells (most of the plasma removed) to reduce the volume to be transfused. By administering packed red blood cells, anemia can be improved when volume replacement is not required. Signs of fluid overload include elevated systolic blood pressure, jugular venous distention, crackles, dyspnea, tachycardia, peripheral edema, cyanosis, and headache. Early detection and physician notification allow more time for the implementation of appropriate treatments including discontinuation of further intravenous fluids and administration of diuretics.

Transfusions for older people should be given slowly over a 2- to 4-hour period. If several units of packed cells are to be infused, often a diuretic (20 mg furosemide) is given orally or intravenously between units to prevent fluid overload and congestive heart failure. Older people may have more fragile veins, and venous access may be more difficult. Therefore, older people are at increased risk for infiltration. The IV site should be carefully secured and frequently observed for signs of infiltration including bruising, swelling, and accumulation of fluid into the soft tissue surrounding the site. The gerontological nurse should carefully monitor the older person's vital signs and urinary output during the transfusion process.

As with all transfusions, the older person's blood type must match the donor's. To prevent transfusion errors and potentially fatal hemolytic reactions, the blood will be tested by type and crossmatch each time the older person requires a transfusion. The hemolytic reaction that can occur when an older person receives an incompatible blood transfusion is life threatening, and every precaution must be taken both in the laboratory and at the bedside to ensure that the older person and the blood type are correctly identified and matched. Hemolytic reactions can progress to oliguria, renal failure, and disseminated intravascular clotting with uncontrolled hemorrhage.

Chronic Myeloproliferative Disorders

Chronic myeloproliferative disorders are characterized by abnormal proliferation of one or more hematopoietic processes and become more common with age. These classic disorders include primary thrombocythemia, polycythemia vera, and myelofibrosis.

Thrombocythemia is characterized by an increased number of circulating platelets in the blood. Older adults with thrombocythemia are more likely to exhibit uncontrolled bleeding with hemorrhage or develop clot formation. The average age of diagnosis is 60 years, and it is more common in women. Symptoms are absent or vague and may include headache, visual disturbances, and burning pain and erythema of the hands and feet. Accurate

iliac crest site @ bedside   *routine bloodwork*

diagnosis requires bone marrow aspiration. Usually, the treatment includes administration of hydroxyurea to suppress platelet formation, and the goal is to keep the platelet count below 400,000/μL. Older adults with thrombocythemia are at significantly increased risk of thrombosis, and careful monitoring of platelet levels and symptoms is indicated (Dunphy et al., 2011).

Polycythemia vera is a chronic stem cell disorder characterized by an increase in hemoglobin concentration and uncontrolled production of mature RBCs. Approximately 90% of people with this disease are diagnosed after age 60. The condition is relatively rare but is most common in Caucasian men of European Jewish ancestry (Huether & McCance, 2011). Symptoms of the disease are absent initially but later progress to findings common in hypervolemia, including headache, dizziness, hypertension, visual disturbances, weight loss, and night sweats. Itching after bathing is a common complaint. Complications include thrombosis (20% of cases) and transformation to acute leukemia after 10 to 20 years of disease progression. Phlebotomy significantly decreases the risk of thrombosis. About 500 mL of blood may be removed daily until the hematocrit is below 45% in men and 42% in women. Hydroxyurea can decrease the risk of thrombosis and can supplement phlebotomy in older adults. Gentle bathing, use of soft towels, and starch baths may decrease postbathing pruritus.

Myelofibrosis is a chronic disease characterized by bone marrow fibrosis (scarring of the bone marrow), splenomegaly, and teardrop-shaped RBCs. It is usually diagnosed at about age 60. The cause is unknown, and the liver and spleen become enlarged as the disease progresses. Symptoms include weight loss, pallor, abdominal distention, fatigue, low-grade fever, and night sweats. The diagnosis is made by examination of a peripheral blood smear and bone marrow biopsy. Survival time after diagnosis is about 3 to 5 years. There is no specific treatment, but blood transfusions can eliminate symptoms of anemia, and administration of erythropoietin may stimulate RBC production. In younger people, allogeneic bone marrow transplantation may be effective, but this intervention is usually not indicated in the older person. For seriously ill older adults, palliative care with attention to pain and symptom control is indicated. Splenectomy can improve symptoms and may be indicated in some older adults (Tefferi, 2004).

can die from acute bleed/infection

Hematologic Malignancies

Hematologic malignancies arise when immature lymphoid and myeloid cells are overproduced with associated bone marrow failure. Large numbers of immature WBCs accumulate in the bone marrow, liver, spleen, lymph nodes, and central nervous system and eventually cause failure. Acute leukemia is primarily a disease of children and older adults (Dunphy et al., 2011). The incidence of acute leukemia is slightly more common in men than in women over the age of 50. In most cases, the cause of acute leukemia is unknown. Predisposing factors include exposure to chemical agents such as benzene, genetic factors, viruses, immune disorders, certain antineoplastic drugs, and radiation exposure (Huether & McCance, 2011). An increased incidence of leukemia has been noted in the atomic bomb survivors of Hiroshima and Nagasaki, radiologists, and older adults receiving radiation therapy. Careful monitoring of radiation exposure is mandatory for all healthcare workers caring for older adults receiving radiation treatments or diagnosis by X-ray.

Acute leukemia presents dramatically in children with high fevers, but in the older person the onset is more insidious with weakness, pallor, and acute confusion. Often the liver, spleen, and lymph nodes are enlarged. The WBC count may or may not be elevated. Diagnosis is confirmed by bone marrow aspiration. The prognosis is poor without treatment. Advanced age, bleeding, and concurrently diagnosed chronic illness are indicators of poor prognosis. Treatment consists of a combination of drugs designed to inhibit WBC production, including vincristine, prednisone, anthracycline, and asparaginase. Most older adults experience relapse within 1 year. Because of the risks, bone marrow transplantation is rarely used for older adults over age 65.

Infections are a major cause of morbidity and mortality. The lack of mature WBCs to fight infection compromises the ability to fight disease. Acute leukemia in older adults is most often fatal within 1 to 2 years. The risks and benefits of aggressive chemotherapy must be discussed with the older person and the family so they can make an informed decision about treatment choices. Palliative care with emphasis on pain and symptom control and hospice care (when and if appropriate) will enhance the quality of life of the older person diagnosed with acute leukemia.

Chronic leukemia usually progresses more slowly than acute leukemia. Chronic lymphoid leukemia (CLL) is primarily a disease of older adults and accounts for 25% to 40% of all leukemias. CLL is characterized by a proliferation and accumulation of small, abnormal mature lymphocytes in the bone marrow, peripheral blood, and body tissues. These cells are usually unable to produce adequate antibodies to maintain normal immune function. Men are affected twice as often as women and the majority are over the age of 60. The cause of CLL is unknown, but there is a predisposition in some families, and the Epstein-Barr virus has also been suggested as a possible cause (Tsimberidou, Keating, Bueso-Ramos, et al., 2006). Common symptoms include fatigue, malaise, rapid worsening of coronary artery disease, and decreased exercise tolerance. Enlarged lymph nodes occur in the cervical, axillary, and supraclavicular areas. The spleen may also be enlarged as the disease progresses.

As with acute leukemia, infections and fever are frequent complications of CLL. The diagnosis of CLL requires repeated measurement of sustained lymphocytosis and examination of the bone marrow. The 5-year survival rate is about 50%, and 25% to 30% of older adults with CLL live 10 years or more. Older adults with CLL have a heightened risk of developing a second malignancy. Although CLL is very responsive to chemotherapy and radiation, early treatment has not been shown to increase survival; therefore, treatment should not be started until the older person manifests symptoms of weight loss, night sweats, fever, or enlarged lymph nodes. Oral alkylating agents combined with prednisone provide effective treatment (Stannard, 2011). As the disease progresses, older adults will increasingly require nutritional support, pain control, skin care, and emotional support from the gerontological nurse.

Multiple myeloma is a malignancy that results from the overproduction and accumulation of immature plasma cells in the bone marrow, lymph nodes, spleen, and kidneys. Multiple myeloma is a disease of aging and the median age at diagnosis is 65 (McPhee & Papadakis, 2011).

Bone pain in the lower back or ribs is the most common early symptom of multiple myeloma. Additional symptoms include bone fractures, pallor, weakness, fatigue, dyspnea, and palpitations. Bruising and excessive bleeding from trauma are common. Renal disease occurs in about 50% of older adults, including urinary tract infections, calcium or uric acid calculi, and dehydration. Most older adults have a normocytic anemia and osteolytic bone lesions or osteoporosis, monoclonal proteins (*Bence Jones protein*) in blood serum, and increased plasma cells in the bone marrow. Treatment involves administration of steroids, immunomodulatory biologic agents, and radiation therapy for localized tumors and to relieve back pain from osteolytic lesions.

Autologous transplantation with peripheral blood stem cells is being used for people up to age 76, depending on functional status. All older adults should be urged to stay as active as possible to counteract bone demineralization and the deconditioning common with prolonged bed rest. All infections, fevers, and night sweats should be reported to the healthcare provider and treated aggressively and promptly. Fluid intake should be 2 to 3 L/day to increase urinary output and increase the excretion of calcium, uric acid, and other metabolites. There is no cure for multiple myeloma. The disease is progressive and the prognosis has improved in the past decade, with death occurring 4 to 6 years from diagnosis (McPhee & Papadakis, 2011). Palliative care with the emphasis on pain management and

symptom control, referral to hospice (if and when appropriate), and emotional support will be needed by the older person and family.

Lymphomas

A malignant lymphoma is a neoplastic tumor affecting the lymphoid tissue. The disease is diagnosed by the presence of excess lymphocytes and progressive enlargement of the lymph nodes. The major types of lymphoma are Hodgkin's disease and non-Hodgkin's lymphoma. These diseases have differences in origin, patterns of spread, and clinical presentation.

Hodgkin's Disease

Hodgkin's disease occurs most often in people between the ages of 15 and 35 or over age 50. The disease usually presents as one or more painlessly enlarged lymph nodes. Other symptoms include persistent fever, night sweats, fatigue, weight loss, malaise, pruritus, and anemia (Huether & McCance, 2011). The diagnosis is made by lymph node biopsy. Additional testing includes computerized tomography (CT) scans, magnetic resonance imaging (MRI), splenectomy, and liver biopsy. Treatment of the disease depends on the stage, but older people usually receive chemotherapeutic drugs and or radiation therapy for 6 to 8 months. The 5-year survival rate for adults is 88% (Huether & McCance, 2011).

Non-Hodgkin's Lymphoma

Malignant disorders that originate from lymphoid tissue but are not diagnosed as Hodgkin's disease are classified as non-Hodgkin's lymphoma. Non-Hodgkin's lymphoma can begin with one node and spread throughout the lymphatic system and then metastasize to bones, the central nervous system, and the gastrointestinal tract. Because of the more systemic nature of non-Hodgkin's lymphoma, the prognosis is generally poorer than the prognosis of an older person with Hodgkin's lymphoma. The risk of acquiring the disease increases with age. The cause is unknown, but those with impaired immune system abnormalities or those taking phenytoin are more at risk.

In non-Hodgkin's lymphoma, the normal lymphoid tissue is replaced by malignant cells leading to infection and immunodeficiency. Tumors can also form in the spleen, liver, and gastrointestinal tract. Symptoms include cervical or inguinal lymph node enlargement. Diagnosis is made by lymph node biopsy, bone marrow aspiration, blood testing, and chest X-ray. Chemotherapy is used to treat intermediate and high-grade lymphomas but does not prolong survival time in early disease. Aggressive chemotherapy in older adults with comorbidities can be extremely difficult, resulting in disability and inability to engage in self-care. Older adults with early disease are closely monitored for progressive problems, and radiation can be used to treat enlarged lymph nodes. The gerontological nurse should provide ongoing pain control, symptom management, nutritional guidance, and counseling during the treatment and recuperative phases of the illness.

Both lymphomas may be curable with radiation and intensive chemotherapy; however, aggressive treatment in the older person with comorbidities is often difficult and may not be tolerated. Older people living alone may need assistance with activities of daily living, nutrition, and pain and symptom control during the required 6 or more months of aggressive treatment.

Nursing Assessment

The nursing assessment of an older person with hematologic problems includes a complete review of the older person's past medical history and current health status. When taking the history of the older person with anemia, the nurse should focus not on the anemia, but rather on discovering the functional implications of the condition. The complaints of an older person with anemia or a blood disorder may be vague and often confused with normal changes of aging or symptoms of chronic disease. Any complaints of fatigue, shortness of breath, loss of appetite, weight loss, mental status changes, bruising, and activity intolerance should be carefully investigated. The nurse can play a key role in advising the older person to seek treatment and report symptoms to the healthcare provider. Anemia and other blood disorders can be caused by nutritional problems, blood loss, chronic illness, medications, or a variety of other factors that may respond to treatment.

The nurse can begin by gathering the following information:

- Diagnosis of any concurrent chronic or progressive illness such as cancer or heart or kidney disease
- Medication listing, including over-the-counter and herbal remedies
- History of surgery or trauma
- Baseline level of function, activity level, and documentation of change of status
- Lifestyle factors that can be related to the older person's status, including smoking, alcohol use, depression, obesity, poor nutrition, and sedentary lifestyle
- Family history and diagnosed blood disorders in first-degree relatives
- Occupational exposures during the older person's work career to chemicals or pollutants and current hobbies

Because anemia is a sign of disease and not an actual disease itself, further investigation and careful assessment of the person with vague symptoms of fatigue, activity intolerance, and weakness should always be carried out. The skin should be examined for pallor, bruising, and poor turgor. The axillary, cervical, and inguinal areas should be checked for lymphadenopathy. Carefully note the presence of purpura, ecchymoses, and petechiae. Older adults with pernicious anemia may experience paresthesias. The liver and spleen should be palpated for enlargement. The presence of rashes, urticaria, and itching should be noted. Balance and endurance should be observed and documented. Although there is no single recommended test of endurance, the nurse can observe the older person walking in a protected environment for several minutes and then assess for the presence of increased heart and respiratory rate, irregular respiratory or cardiac rate, weakness, and decreased pulse oximetry after exercise. A complete dietary assessment for reduced intake of iron-containing foods and an assessment of occult bleeding from the gastrointestinal tract are essential. Because depression can contribute to and be a result of chronic illness, the older person should be carefully screened for depression (see Chapter 7 ⊂⊃ for further information).

Referral to a healthcare provider for a complete health assessment is indicated for older adults who might be experiencing anemia. A complete physical examination, electrocardiogram, test of thyroid function (because chronic hypothyroidism may be related to anemia), and complete blood count with differential are indicated (Dunphy et al., 2011). Older adults with a decreased WBC count should be protected from infection and placed in reverse isolation if necessary until their WBC count returns to normal.

Nursing diagnoses as defined by the North American Nursing Diagnosis Association that may be associated with an older person experiencing anemia or other hematologic problems include, but are not limited to, the following:

- *Activity Intolerance*
- *Falls, Risk for*
- *Poisoning, Risk for*
- *Infection, Risk for*
- *Nutrition, Imbalanced: Less Than Body Requirements*
- *Skin Integrity, Impaired*
- *Breathing Pattern, Ineffective*
- *Anxiety*
- *Hopelessness*

NANDA-I © 2012.

Some nursing interventions that may be appropriate for the older person with hematologic problems are as follows:

- Provide support and teaching for the older person and family.
- Protect the skin from dryness, cracking, and injury.

- Provide teaching and administration of medications to relieve nausea and vomiting.
- Encourage recreational and diversional activities consistent with the older person's general functional ability.
- Advise and provide referrals regarding nutritional intake.
- Assess and treat pain with appropriate pharmacological and nonpharmacological techniques.
- Treat associated symptoms, including constipation, diarrhea, and dry mouth.
- Involve the multidisciplinary team to address physical, social, psychological, and spiritual needs.

Nurse-sensitive outcomes include lessened symptom severity, increased effectiveness of cardiac pump, improved vital signs, improved ambulation and endurance, improved nutritional status, discontinuation of toxic medication, improved quality of life and overall functional ability, and improved depressive symptoms. If serious underlying disease is found during the investigation of the older person with anemia or other hematologic problems, the nurse can provide support during aggressive therapy and palliative care, with hospice referral if appropriate.

Hypercoagulability and Anticoagulation

Deep vein thrombosis (DVT) and pulmonary embolism can lead to myocardial infarction and stroke, and the incidence increases with age. Hospitalized older patients are more at risk due to impaired mobility, surgical interventions, and orthopedic procedures. The older person is more at risk because of three components:

1. Abnormalities in the vessel walls caused by trauma, atherosclerosis, or intravenous medication administration
2. Abnormalities within the circulating blood and hypercoagulability seen with coagulation disorders, some cancers, and hormone (estrogen) use
3. Stasis of blood flow secondary to immobility, heart failure, or age-related changes

Huether & McCance, 2011; McPhee & Papadakis, 2011.

The major danger associated with DVT is that a portion of the thrombus will embolize to the lungs, causing pulmonary embolism (Huether & McCance, 2011). It is estimated that each year, DVT affects 2 million Americans, with 300,000 dying from pulmonary embolism and complications (Fox & Bertaglio, 2011). The mortality rate for older people with deep vein thrombosis is 21%, and 39% for pulmonary embolism in the year following the occurrence (Wick, 2006). Aggressive therapy is needed to treat DVT because it is a potentially life-threatening situation.

Anticoagulation and bed rest are critical to prevent movement of clots to the lungs, heart, or brain where they can block vital circulation.

Risk factors for venous thromboembolism include recent major surgery, traumatic injury, age over 70 years, immobility, obesity, and diagnosis of inflammatory disease. While rare in youth, the incidence of deep vein thrombosis doubles for each decade of life after age 40 (Wick, 2006).

The clinical manifestations of DVT include edema, skin discoloration, and pain. The hallmark of DVT is the rapid onset of unilateral leg swelling with pitting edema. The diagnosis is made with Doppler ultrasonography, plethysmography, or venogram.

> **Practice Pearl** ▶▶▶ In older adults with heart failure and dependency edema, both legs will be swollen. Edema from a single DVT is unilateral.

Preventive approaches are individualized to minimize the risk factors that can predispose to DVT. Specific conditions warranting prevention include these:

- **Orthopedic procedures.** Examples include total hip replacement, traumatic hip fracture, and total knee replacement. For total hip replacement, the incidence of DVT without prophylaxis is 25%; for traumatic hip fracture, about 50%; and for total knee replacement, as high as 60%.
- **Atrial fibrillation.** Older adults with atrial fibrillation can form thrombi within the atria that can enter the general circulation and cause stroke. Transesophageal echocardiography identifies older adults at risk for thromboembolism.
- **Acute myocardial infarction.** The risk of DVT in older adults who are post–myocardial infarction approaches 20%. Older adults with heart failure, recurrent angina, or ventricular arrhythmias are most at risk.
- **Ischemic stroke.** In older adults with stroke and paralyzed lower extremities, the incidence of DVT is 40%.

WebMD, 2012.

The following nursing interventions are designed to prevent DVT formation:

- Identify older adults at risk, including those with a history of DVT, clotting disorders, heart failure, orthopedic surgery, and other risk factors.
- Get older adults up and walking as soon as possible after surgery or injury.
- Change the position of bed-bound older adults at least every 2 hours to prevent circulatory compromise.
- Urge older adults at risk for DVT to wear fitted support stockings, avoid sedentary lifestyle, maintain adequate

hydration, elevate legs during periods of rest, and perform meticulous skin care to keep skin clean and intact.

- Urge the use of intermittent pneumatic compression boots postoperatively until older adults are ambulatory.
- Administer anticoagulants as prescribed.

Many anticoagulants are available and each has distinct uses. In general, drugs given intravenously, such as heparin or the fibrinolytic agents, are used short term for hospitalized patients. Oral drugs, such as warfarin and antiplatelet drugs, are used long term for outpatients. Low-molecular-weight heparins, administered subcutaneously, are used in both settings (WebMD, 2012). Drugs are given for prevention and treatment of thrombotic conditions.

HEALTHY AGING TIP

How to Avoid Deep Vein Thrombosis

Use these tips to help your patients stay healthy and avoid DVTs:

1. Stay well hydrated.
2. Avoid prolonged sitting and bed rest.
3. When flying on an airplane, get up and walk every half hour; don't cross your legs; keep your feet on the floor and flex your feet and legs often to keep the blood moving.
4. If you are on blood thinning medications, keep on a regular schedule and try not to skip or miss any doses.
5. Avoid wearing tight clothing and short, tight stockings.
6. Consider wearing support hose or compression stockings during travel.

Laboratory tests to monitor efficacy and to determine the dosage of medications are usually done every 3 to 4 days of therapy. They include the prothrombin time (PT) and the partial thromboplastin time (PTT). The PT, a measure of the time required for a firm fibrin clot to form after reagents have been added to the blood sample, is the standard measure of efficacy. It is commonly reported in an international normalized ratio (INR) because the World Health Organization urged the adoption of a standardized reagent so that all laboratories would report standardized results. Warfarin will prolong the INR. The higher the INR, the longer it takes the blood to clot. Guidelines suggest various target INR measurements and duration of therapy. The PTT is used to evaluate the time required for a firm fibrin clot to form after phospholipid reagents have been added to the specimen. Heparin will prolong the PTT.

Anticoagulant Medications

Heparin is the most widely used anticoagulant. It accelerates the inhibitory interaction between hemostatic proteins and clotting factors. Unfractionated heparin is used in older adults to prevent and to treat venous or arterial thromboembolism.

Low-molecular-weight heparin therapy is prophylactic therapy for DVT in older adults who have the following:

- Most general and orthopedic surgery
- Acute myocardial infarction and heart failure
- Ischemic stroke with lower extremity paralysis
- Cancer patients on bed rest

High-dose heparin therapy (intravenous administration) is indicated in the following older adults:

- Those with DVT, pulmonary embolism, or unstable angina
- Those who have had hip fracture surgery or total hip or knee replacement
- Those with spinal cord injury

Reuben et al., 2011; WebMD, 2012.

The most common adverse effect of heparin is hemorrhage. Other adverse effects include thrombocytopenia, alopecia, and skin necrosis. The risk of bleeding increases with increased dosage. Other risk factors include older age, low body weight, recent trauma or surgery, and performance of invasive procedures with concurrent use of aspirin. Mild bleeding can be handled by reducing the dose; severe bleeding requires discontinuation of the heparin and possibly treatment with reversal agents (Reuben et al., 2011).

Excessively high INRs (3.5 and over) should be reported immediately to the healthcare provider or anticoagulation clinic so that dosage adjustment and possible action to reduce the INR reading can be accomplished. For INRs between 3.5 and 5, the usual recommendation is to omit the next dose and lower the maintenance dose. For INRs between 5 and 9, the recommendation may be to omit the next several doses and restart at a lower dose. Some healthcare providers recommend administration of vitamin K 1.0 to 2.5 mg by mouth. For INRs over 9 with or without bleeding, the warfarin would probably be discontinued and vitamin K given orally or intravenously until the INR returns to normal levels.

Low-molecular-weight heparins are used for DVT prophylaxis and in the treatment of DVT with acute coronary syndromes such as unstable angina and myocardial infarction. Low-molecular-weight heparins can be given intravenously or subcutaneously. Because of the predictable bioavailability, dose-independent clearance rates, and a more stable anticoagulant response, these drugs have been increasingly used in the clinical setting and monitoring of the PTT is not required (Dunphy et al., 2011). However, as a precaution, older adults receiving low-molecular-weight heparins should be carefully monitored for signs of excessive bleeding.

Warfarin is frequently used for anticoagulation in the prevention or treatment of DVT. It is rapidly absorbed from the gastrointestinal tract, reaches maximal serum concentration in about 90 minutes, and takes up to 7 days to reach stable serum levels on fixed doses (Reuben et al., 2011). Warfarin interacts with many substances, and older adults taking the medication should be instructed to report any changes in their medication regimen to their healthcare providers so that INRs can be monitored and warfarin dosage adjusted in response. Table 21-2 lists substances that affect warfarin response.

Hepatic clearance of warfarin declines with age. The older person is more likely than a younger person to experience bleeding complications, so the drug is usually started at lower doses. Frequent monitoring is required to safely titrate dosage during the induction period. Risk factors for anticoagulant-related bleeding include increased age, history of gastrointestinal bleeding, history of stroke, diabetes mellitus, anemia (hematocrit < 30%), and creatinine greater than 1.5 mg/dL. Older adults with three or more of these risk factors have a 50% chance of developing abnormal bleeding within 1 year (Wick, 2006). Table 21-3 lists anticoagulation indications for conditions with target INRs.

Contraindications to warfarin therapy include older adults with bleeding disorders, those who fall frequently and are at risk for intracranial bleeding, and those who are not compliant with dosage adjustments and laboratory testing. Some surgeons will request that warfarin be held for four doses prior to surgery to decrease the risk of intraoperative bleeding.

Protamine sulfate is indicated in the treatment of heparin overdosage. Protamine sulfate should be administered by very slow intravenous injection over a 10-minute period in doses not to exceed 50 mg. All serious or significant bleeding requires emergency treatment and evaluation for an older person taking any anticoagulant. Signs of bleeding may occur as blood in the urine or stool, vomiting of blood, nosebleeds, blood in the sputum, bleeding gums, bruising out of proportion to or in the absence of injury, fatigue, severe headache, and loss of vision or weakness on one side of the body. All older adults taking warfarin should be instructed to take the medication as ordered, regularly monitor INR levels, check for interactions before starting any new medications, recognize dietary sources of vitamin K and ingest stable amounts, and recognize the signs of bleeding and the need to seek treatment (Patel, 2011).

TABLE 21-2 Substances That Affect Warfarin Response

These agents **increase** the INR in conjunction with warfarin.	Alcohol (binge) Allopurinol Amiodarone Antibiotics Acetaminophen Aspirin Corticosteroids Isoniazid Omeprazole	Phenytoin Propoxyphene Selective serotonin reuptake inhibitors Tamoxifen Vitamin E Herbals (ginkgo, bladderwrack, capsaicin, garlic) Flu vaccine
These agents **decrease** the INR in conjunction with warfarin.	Alcohol (moderate) Barbiturates Carbamazepine Cholestyramine Cyclosporine	Estrogen Rifampin Sucralfate Vitamin K Herbals (coenzyme Q-10, St. John's wort)

Source: Nurse Practitioners' Prescribing Reference (2012); Reuben et al. (2011); Wick (2006).

TABLE 21-3 Indications for Anticoagulation With Target International Normalized Ratios

Condition	Target INR	Duration of Therapy
Orthopedic surgery	2.0–3.0	11–35 days postoperatively or until older person is fully ambulatory
Deep vein thrombosis	2.0–3.0	At least 3 months
Pulmonary embolism	2.0–3.0	At least 6 months
Atrial fibrillation	2.0–3.0	Indefinitely for chronic atrial fibrillation and at least 3 weeks before and 4 weeks after cardioversion
Mechanical heart valve	2.0–3.0	Indefinitely
Mechanical heart valve with atrial fibrillation	2.5–3.5	Indefinitely
Acute myocardial infarction	2.0–3.0	1–3 months

Source: Nurse Practitioners' Prescribing Reference (2012); Reuben et al. (2011).

Platelet Antagonists

Platelets participate in the thrombotic process by adhering to abnormal surfaces, aggregating to form a plug, and triggering the coagulation cascade. Aspirin irreversibly inhibits platelet aggregation by blocking enzymes in the clotting process and impairing prostaglandin metabolism. Aspirin is used for primary and secondary prevention of myocardial infarction and stroke and is used with other antiplatelet agents (clopidogrel or ticlopidine) after the placement of intracoronary stents (Reuben et al., 2011).

Ticlopidine is a potent inhibitor of platelet aggregation by impairing platelet adhesion and inhibiting platelet release action. Ticlopidine has been used in the treatment of transient ischemic attacks, strokes where aspirin was already being taken, unstable angina, and cardiac stent placement. Side effects include two serious conditions: neutropenia and thrombocytopenic purpura. Clopidogrel reduces the risk of myocardial infarction and recurrent myocardial infarction among older adults with atherosclerotic vascular disease. It has a more favorable side effect profile than ticlopidine, and the longer half-life requires only once-a-day dosing (Nurse Practitioners' Prescribing Reference, 2012).

Dabigatran (Pradaxa) has recently been introduced and is indicated for patients at risk of stroke and embolism diagnosed with nonvalvular atrial fibrillation. Dabigatran is a direct thrombin inhibitor and routine laboratory testing is not recommended. Coagulation tests in patients on dabigatran should be interpreted with caution and peak effect generally occurs within 2 to 4 hours after administration (University of Utah Healthcare, 2011).

Nursing Assessment

Older adults at risk for hypercoagulability and DVT formation include those with atherosclerosis, circulating blood abnormalities, and slowing of blood flow. Immobility and orthopedic surgery greatly increase the risk of DVT formation, and the older person should be assisted to ambulate as soon as possible after surgery. Postoperative nursing care involves use of compression stockings, intermittent pneumatic compression boots, early and consistent ambulation of older adults, maintenance of adequate hydration, and careful administration of anticoagulants. Postoperative and chronic pain should be carefully assessed and treated to prevent the hazards of immobility.

Practice Pearl ▶▶▶ The older person who says "It only hurts when I move, so I don't need any pain medication" is at risk for immobility and DVT formation.

Older adults receiving anticoagulation medications require careful and ongoing nursing assessment of frank or occult bleeding and laboratory examination of clotting times. Older adults taking warfarin should report any bleeding or medication changes immediately to the healthcare provider.

The following nursing diagnoses as defined by NANDA may be associated with an older person experiencing potential hypercoagulability:

- *Activity Intolerance*
- *Falls, Risk for*
- *Injury, Risk for*
- *Poisoning, Risk for*
- *Infection, Risk for*
- *Health Behaviors, Risk-Prone* (inability to recognize signs and symptoms of bleeding)
- *Noncompliance* related to laboratory monitoring procedures

NANDA-I © 2012.

Nurse-sensitive outcomes may include the following: lessening of symptom severity, increased effectiveness of cardiac pump, improvement of vital signs, improvement of ambulation and endurance, improvement of mobility, discontinuation of toxic medication, and adherence to monitoring and laboratory requirements.

Many older adults with anemia lack sufficient energy to carry out their daily activities and suffer from functional impairment, including cognitive and mood impairment. The gerontological nurse may find that many older adults and their families lack knowledge regarding the significance, assessment, and treatment of anemia in later life. The patient–family teaching guidelines at the end of the chapter will assist the nurse in the education of older adults and their families regarding anemia.

COMPLEMENTARY AND ALTERNATIVE THERAPIES

Herbal remedies for anemia include the following:

- Dong quai—an herb rich in vitamins and minerals
- Spirulina (blue-green algae)—a source of complete protein containing all essential amino acids
- Quinoa—a grain that contains essential vitamins and amino acids
- Gentian—an herb popular in England that can be brewed into a tea
- An assortment of other herbs including dandelion, alfalfa, grape skins, parsley, watercress, red raspberries, and goldenseal

Holisticonline.com, 2008; University of Maryland Medical Center, 2011.

No scientific evidence of effectiveness has been shown for any of these remedies. Because iron replacement in large amounts can be toxic, older adults are urged to refrain from taking large doses of iron for extended periods of time. Dandelion may be a platelet inhibitor useful to prevent clotting because of its high vitamin A content. Likewise, capsaicin may inhibit platelet aggregation with a more pronounced effect in Asians. Coenzyme Q-10 may counteract coagulation by serving as a vitamin K antagonist (Wick, 2006).

QSEN Recommendations Related to the Hematologic System

The Quality and Safety Education for Nurses (QSEN) project addresses the challenge of preparing future nurses with the knowledge, skills, and attitudes (KSAs) to continuously improve the quality and safety of the healthcare systems in which they work (Cronenwett et al., 2007). See the QSEN table for tips on meeting QSEN standards.

Meeting QSEN Standards: The Hematologic System

	KNOWLEDGE	SKILLS	ATTITUDES
Patient-Centered Care	Recognize and treat anemia and hypercoagulation.	Recommend and monitor laboratory testing results and report abnormal levels to the health care provider.	Recognize the value and importance of ongoing laboratory monitoring to lessen the probability of adverse outcomes in the patient diagnosed with anemia and hypercoagulation.
	Involve patient and family in plan of care.	Family assessment and adult learning principles.	Appreciate uniqueness of each patient/family.
	Examine barriers that may keep patients from being active in formulating their plan of care.	Evaluate for depression, vision/hearing, function, tobacco/alcohol use, and dietary preferences.	Provide patient-centered care to improve successful nursing outcomes.
Teamwork and Collaboration	Recognize scope of practice for interdisciplinary team members.	Use leadership skills to coordinate team and share knowledge.	Value the contribution of each member of the team to improve outcomes.
	Be aware of organizational problems that can inhibit effective team functioning.	System assessment skills.	Be open to input from team members on effective means to improve communication and collaboration.
Evidence-Based Practice	Describe effective interventions to decrease hematologic risk factors and improve overall health and functioning.	Access current evidence-based screening and health promotion protocols to guide interventions.	Possess confidence in necessary skills to evaluate and incorporate nursing interventions from the literature.
	Be aware of drug side effects impacting on bleeding and clotting dysfunction.	Conduct complete medication reviews yearly and after each hospitalization.	Advocate for medication changes and use of nonpharmacologic interventions as needed.
Quality Improvement	Recognize the importance of measuring patient outcomes to improve care of the patient with hematologic system problems.	Skills in data management, technology, and U.S. government NHLBI websites describing current incidence and prevalence of hematologic disease.	Value the use of data and outcomes as a key component of QI efforts to prevent hospitalization from excessive bleeding, stroke/myocardial infarction, and anemia.

(continued)

Meeting QSEN Standards : The Hematologic System   *(continued)*

	KNOWLEDGE	SKILLS	ATTITUDES
Safety	Describe common medication, laboratory and treatment errors, and health system characteristics that increase the likelihood of such errors.	Use appropriate strategies to deliver patient/family education and provide written information to compensate for functional deficits (if present).	Appreciate the impact of frailty and cognitive loss on the occurrence of adverse drug reactions.
	Recognize the factors that increase the risk of nosocomial infections in those with decreased WBC counts.	Isolate patients at risk for acquiring secondary infections in the acute care setting.	Institute infection control practices.
Informatics	Provide input into the formation and maintenance of patient databases needed for gathering QSEN data and providing patient care.	Utilize the electronic health record.	Protect patient confidentiality according to HIPAA standards.

Patient–Family Teaching Guidelines

The following are guidelines that the nurse may find useful when instructing older adults and their families about anemia, the most common hematologic problem experienced by older people.

THE OLDER PATIENT WITH ANEMIA

1 How do I know if I have anemia?

There is no one main symptom of anemia. Often, the symptoms are vague and may be noticed as fatigue, lack of energy, shortness of breath on physical exertion, pale skin color, memory problems, and worsening of other problems like heart or lung conditions.

RATIONALE:

Often, the symptoms of anemia develop gradually and are attributed to normal changes of aging. The nurse can help the older person and his or her family to examine current function and make a comparison to previous functional ability to identify changes over time.

2 What are the most common causes of anemia?

Anemia is caused by either an underproduction of red blood cells or excessive loss or destruction of red blood cells. Iron deficiency is common in older people who have had blood loss due to injury or surgery. Unexplained blood loss should be investigated to make sure there is no hidden bleeding in the stomach or intestinal tract. Some medications can cause red blood cells to be broken down and destroyed, causing anemia. Sometimes red blood cells are not formed quickly enough to replace the ones that live a natural life span. The bone marrow slows production because of chronic illness in the heart, lungs, or kidneys. Sometimes a nutritional deficiency is responsible. Whatever the cause, it is important to pinpoint the kind of anemia and treat the cause.

RATIONALE:

Most people attribute anemia to iron deficiency or nutritional problems; however, the causes of anemia in the older person are diverse and varied. It is often necessary to think beyond the obvious and simple causes of anemia.

3 What kinds of tests is my healthcare provider likely to order to diagnose anemia?

The most basic test is a complete blood count with differential. This test gives a measure of the number of circulating red blood cells and the types and numbers of other cells, including white blood cells and platelets. Sometimes, iron studies are performed and vitamin B_{12} and folate levels examined, depending on the

Patient–Family Teaching Guidelines *(continued)*

kind of anemia suspected. If the physician suspects bleeding in the stomach or intestine, an endoscopy or examination of the stomach or colon with a small tube and camera may be performed. Because anemia is not a disease itself but a symptom of some other condition, a careful search for the cause is indicated.

RATIONALE:

Older adults and their families should be instructed that finding the cause of the anemia is as important as treating the anemia and a variety of tests may be ordered to pinpoint the cause of the problem. To treat anemia in the older person without knowing the cause is inappropriate and may mask the symptoms of serious underlying diseases or health problems.

4 **How often should I ask my healthcare provider to check my blood for the presence of anemia?**

Healthy older people should be checked for anemia every year. A complete blood count may be ordered and stool checked for occult bleeding. Those with chronic conditions, recent injury or trauma, or symptoms should be checked more frequently.

RATIONALE:

Regular health maintenance and disease detection in the healthy older person is indicated yearly to diagnose and treat

diseases early and improve chances of success. Healthy older adults and those with chronic conditions should be urged to have blood testing, fecal occult stool testing, and colonoscopy/ sigmoidoscopy on a regular basis.*

5 **What can I do to prevent anemia?**

Eat a balanced diet, keep active, avoid taking unnecessary medications, and report any fatigue or loss of energy to your healthcare provider. Taking a once-a-day multivitamin can help. There is no need to take iron pills unless you are instructed to do so by your healthcare provider. Be sure to report any gastrointestinal distress, black stools, or red blood in the stool to your healthcare provider immediately.

RATIONALE:

General good health, regular exercise, and avoidance of medications will help promote overall health, including hematologic health, at all ages and stages of life. A multivitamin will help to ensure adequate vitamin intake when an occasional meal is skipped. Usually, iron replacement is not necessary in an older person who has not had recent surgery or trauma. Taking iron unnecessarily can cause gastrointestinal problems and constipation.

CARE PLAN A Patient With a Bleeding Disorder

Case Study

Mr. Thayer is a 78-year-old man who has been diagnosed with chronic atrial fibrillation. He is receiving warfarin therapy for anticoagulation to prevent pulmonary embolism from his decreased cardiac output. His INR goal is 2.5 to 3.0. He is usually quite responsible with his warfarin regimen and monitoring requirements. He recently has not been feeling well and calls the clinic office to report he has a nosebleed that he cannot stop.

Applying the Nursing Process

Assessment

The nurse should conduct a brief focused history of the bleeding event over the phone. An older person's assessment of bleeding is often subjective and influenced by anxiety, so it would be helpful to accurately assess how long the bleeding has occurred and the approximate quantity of blood. The nurse may ask, "Is it gushing? Is it trickling? Is it soaking a handkerchief? Is it soaking a towel?" Large amounts of blood and uncontrolled bleeding need immediate attention and may constitute a medical emergency. Smaller amounts of blood may be controlled with ice packs to the nose, pressure on the external nose, and sitting upright to avoid swallowing blood.

(continued)

CARE PLAN   **A Patient With a Bleeding Disorder** *(continued)*

Upon further questioning, Mr. Thayer reports he has been taking an antibiotic that was prescribed when he went to the local hospital emergency department because he had a bad cold. The nurse knows that many antibiotics can interact with warfarin and cause the INR to be elevated. An elevated INR means that the older person is at risk for uncontrolled bleeding. Additionally, Mr. Thayer may have taken other medications such as aspirin or cold and flu preparations that can interact with warfarin.

Diagnosis

The current nursing diagnoses for Mr. Thayer include the following:

- *Anxiety* related to uncontrolled nasal bleeding
- *Bleeding, Risk for* related to lack of current INR laboratory testing
- *Airway Clearance, Ineffective* related to nosebleed
- *Tissue Perfusion: Peripheral, Ineffective* related to uncontrolled nosebleed secondary to insufficient clotting factors
- *Activity Intolerance* due to hypovolemia and possible anemia as the result of excessive bleeding
- *Falls, Risk for*
- *Poisoning, Risk for* related to drug reactions between warfarin and many other medications
- *Infection, Risk for*
- *Breathing Pattern, Ineffective*

NANDA-I © 2012.

Expected Outcomes

The expected outcomes for the plan of care specify that Mr. Thayer will:

- Become aware of the harmful effects of drug interactions on clotting time.
- Administer emergency measures including applying ice to the nasal area, applying gentle pressure to the upper nose, and sitting in an upright position.
- Call his healthcare provider who is responsible for his anticoagulation regimen and report changes in the medication regimen when he begins taking an antibiotic or any other new medication (his healthcare provider could have altered his warfarin dose and requested extra INR monitoring during the period he was taking the antibiotic).
- Seek immediate medical help and attention for his nosebleed if it is assessed to be of a serious nature.
- Agree to establish a therapeutic relationship with the nurse and develop a mutually acceptable plan to work toward these outcomes.

Planning and Implementation

Some nursing interventions that may be appropriate for Mr. Thayer include the following:

- Provide support and teaching for the older person and family.
- Urge him to contact his healthcare provider for an INR reading as soon as possible.
- Teach Mr. Thayer about any dose adjustment in warfarin that may be required as a result of his INR reading.
- Involve the multidisciplinary team to address physical, social, psychological, and spiritual needs.

Evaluation

The nurse hopes to work with Mr. Thayer over time and formulate a mutually agreeable plan to achieve the identified outcomes. The nurse will consider the plan a success based on the following criteria:

- Mr. Thayer will become more compliant and responsive to his warfarin regimen and dose adjustments based on regularly scheduled INR readings.
- A family meeting will be held to discuss Mr. Thayer's overall health and psychosocial function.
- Mr. Thayer will verbalize an understanding of the many possible drug interactions between warfarin and other medications and report all changes in his medication regimen to his healthcare provider.

CARE PLAN   A Patient With a Bleeding Disorder *(continued)*

Ethical Dilemma

Mr. Thayer admits he does not always adhere to his medication regimen. Lately he and his wife have been arguing, and he reports: "I just don't care if I live anymore." It is not a cognitive or financial problem, but perhaps represents depression due to marital stress. The nurse suggests further evaluation with a geriatric social worker, but he refuses.

The nurse realizes that Mr. Thayer sounds as if he is truly depressed. Assuming he has no suicidal ideation or plan to harm himself or his wife, the principle of autonomy must be honored. However, the nurse realizes that depressed older adults often lack the will and energy to engage in behaviors that will improve depressive symptoms.

The nurse should stress to Mr. Thayer that failure to take his medication can result in serious adverse health events such as stroke. His depression may be transient, but a devastating stroke will adversely impair his function and self-care for the rest of his life. Perhaps Mr. and Mrs. Thayer would agree to a joint session with the social worker, or Mr. Thayer might engage in a short-term trial of an antidepressant. The nurse could attempt to set some short-term goals with Mr. Thayer and encourage him to identify some actions to reach those goals. Support, encouragement, and ongoing monitoring of this older person's depression and medication regimen will be required.

Critical Thinking and the Nursing Process

1. What physical, emotional, and environmental factors make Mr. Thayer more at risk for stroke?
2. The INR obtained on Mr. Thayer was 5.4. What safety measures should the nurse implement while this older person has an elevated INR?
3. What nutritional modifications should be made, if any?
4. What additional support is needed from members of the interdisciplinary healthcare team?

- Evaluate your responses in Appendix B.

Chapter Highlights

- The hematologic system is responsible for many functions, including the transport of oxygen and nutrients to, and the removal of carbon dioxide and waste products from, the peripheral tissue.
- Disturbances to the hematologic system are common in the older person, and often the symptoms are vague and attributed to normal aging.
- Anemia or a decrease in the number of red blood cells can be the result of nutritional problems, drug toxicity, chronic illness, and metabolic disorders. Because anemia is a sign, not a diagnosis, further evaluation of the older person with anemia is always indicated.
- White blood cell production can be affected by disorders of the bone marrow, lymph nodes, spleen, and thymus. When lymphocyte formation is impaired, the older person will have problems with humoral and cell-mediated immunity and will be unable to mount an effective immune response.
- Platelet adhesiveness increases with age. Older adults are at risk for the development of deep vein thrombosis and pulmonary embolism, especially after suffering a traumatic injury, in the presence of atherosclerosis, or with changes within the blood clotting factors. With proper administration, monitoring, and support, anticoagulation therapy can be a lifesaving intervention for older people.
- Many functions of the hematologic system remain constant in healthy older adults, including RBC life span, total blood volume, RBC volume, total lymphocyte and granulocyte counts, and platelet structure and function. Average hemoglobin and hematocrit values decrease slightly with age, but remain within normal limits.

Pearson Nursing Student Resources
Find additional review materials at
nursing.pearsonhighered.com
Prepare for success with additional NCLEX®-style practice
questions, interactive assignments and activities, web links,
animations and videos, and more!

References

American Society of Hematology. (2010). *Anemia*. Retrieved from http://www .hematology.org/Patients/Blood-Disorders/ Anemia/5225.aspx

Anemia.org. (2010). *Anemia*. Retrieved from http://www.anemia.org/patients/feature- articles/content.php?contentid=490& sectionid=15

Artz, A. (2011). Anemia in elderly persons. *Medscape Reference*. Retrieved from http://emedicine.medscape.com/ article/1339998-overview#a30

Centers for Medicare and Medicaid Services. (2007). *Monitoring of erythropoietin stimulating agents for beneficiaries with end stage renal disease*. Retrieved from https:// www.cms.gov/medicare-coverage-database/ details/medicare-coverage-document-details .aspx?MCDId=11&McdName=Monitoring+ of+Erythropoietin+Stimulating+Agents+for+ Beneficiaries+with+End+Stage+Renal+ Disease&mcdtypename=CMS+Solicitation+of +Public+Comments&MCDIndexType=4&bc= AgAEAAAAAAAA&

Cronenwett, L., Sherwood, G., Barnsteiner, J., Disch, J., Johnson, J., Mitchell, P., Sullivan, D., & Warren, J. (2007). Quality and safety education for nurses, *Nursing Outlook, 55*(3) 122–131.

Dugdale, D. (2010). RBC indices. *MedlinePlus*. Retrieved from http://www.nlm .nih.gov/medlineplus/ency/article/003648.htm

Dunphy, L., Winland-Brown, J., Porter, B., & Thomas, D. (2011). *Primary care: The art and science of advanced practice nursing*. Philadelphia, PA: F. A. Davis.

Fox, J., & Bertaglio, K. (2011). Emergency physician performed ultrasound for DVT evaluation. *Thrombosis*, Article ID 938709,1155/2011/938709.

Gersten, T. (2010). Ferritin. *MedlinePlus*. Retrieved from http://www.nlm.nih.gov/ medlineplus/ency/article/003490.htm

Holcomb, S. (2005). Recognizing and managing anemia. *The Nurse Practitioner, 30*(12), 16–31.

Holisticonline.com. (2008). *Conventional, holistic and integrative treatments for anemia*. Retrieved from http://www.holisticonline.com/ Remedies/anemia.htm

Huether, S., & McCance, K. (2011). *Understanding pathophysiology* (5th ed.). St. Louis, MO: Elsevier Mosby.

MayoClinic.com. (2008). *Universal blood donor type: Is there such a thing?* Retrieved from http://www.mayoclinic.com/health/ universal-blood-donor-type/HQ00949

McPhee, S., & Papadakis, M. (2011). *Current medical diagnosis and treatment*. New York, NY: McGraw-Hill Medical.

National Heart, Lung, and Blood Institute (NHLBI). (2007). *Anemia*. Retrieved from http://www.nhlbi.nih.gov/health/dci/Diseases/ anemia/anemia_whatis.html

National Kidney Foundation. (2011). *Guidelines for anemia of chronic disease*. Retrieved from http://www.kidney.org/professionals/kdoqi/ guidelines_updates/doqiupan_i.html

Nurse Practitioners' Prescribing Reference. (2012). New York: Prescribing Reference LLC.

Patel, K. (2011). Deep vein thrombosis. *Medscape*. Retrieved from http://emedicine .medscape.com/article/1911303-medication#3

Reuben, D., Herr, K., Pacala, J., Pollock, B., Potter, J., & Semla, T. (2011). *Geriatrics at your fingertips* (13th ed.). New York, NY: American Geriatrics Society.

Salisbury, A., Reid, K., Alexander, K., Masoudi, F., Lai, S., Chan, P., Bach, R., Wang, T., Spertus, J., & Kosiborod, M. (2011). Diagnostic blood loss from phlebotomy and hospital-acquired anemia during acute myocardial infarction. *Archives of Internal Medicine, 171*, 1646–1653.

St. Louis University, Division of Geriatric Medicine. (2006). Anemia in older persons. *Aging Successfully, XVI*(2), 1–23.

Stannard, L. (2011). List of cancer drugs. *Livestrong*. Retrieved from http://www .livestrong.com/article/26716-list-cancer- drugs

Tefferi, A. (2004). Chronic myeloid disorders. In M. Beers & R. Berkow (Eds.), *Merck manual of geriatrics*. Retrieved from http:// www.merck.com

Tinmouth, A., McIntyre, L., & Fowler, R. (2008). Blood conservation strategies to reduce the need of blood transfusion in critically ill patients. *Canadian Medical Association Journal, 178*(1), 49–57.

Tsimberidou, A. M., Keating, M. J., Bueso- Ramos, C. E., & Kurzrock, R. (2006). Epstein-Barr virus in patients with chronic lymphocytic leukemia: A pilot study. *Leukemia and Lymphoma, 47*(5), 827–836.

University of Maryland Medical Center. (2011). *Anemia*. Retrieved from http:// www.umm.edu/altmed/articles/ anemia-000009.htm

University of Utah Healthcare. (2011). *Dabigatran (Pradaxa) laboratory monitoring overview*. Retrieved from http://healthcare .utah.edu/thrombosis/newagents/TS.Dabi_lab .monitor.pdf

U.S. Food and Drug Administration (FDA). (2007). *Procrit/Epogen label: Increased mortality, serious cardiovascular events*. Retrieved from http://www.fda.gov/cder/foi/ label/2007/103234s5158lbl.pdf

Vanassa, G., & Berliner, N. (2010). Anemia in elderly patients: An emerging problem in the 21st century. In *American Society of Hematology education program book*. Retrieved from http://asheducationbook .hematologylibrary.org/content/2010/1/271.full

WebMD. (2012). *Deep vein thrombosis health center*. Retrieved from http:// www.webmd.com/dvt/news/20091204/ post-op-blood-clot-risk-high

Wick, J. (2006). Beyond the basics: Special issues in venous thromboembolism prevention. *Annals of Long-Term Care, 14*(1), 17–22.

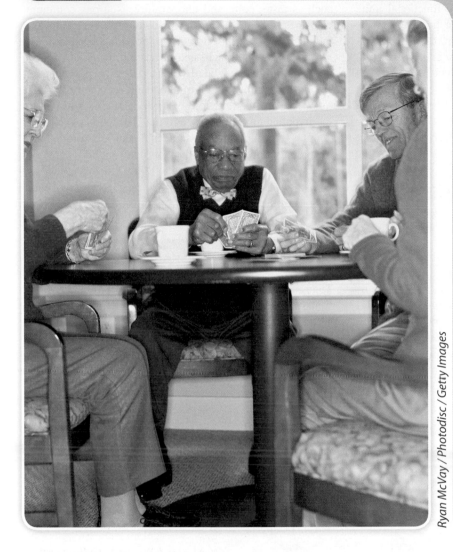

Ryan McVay / Photodisc / Getty Images

LEARNING OUTCOMES

On completion of this chapter, the reader will be able to:

1. Describe the components of the neurologic system.
2. Identify progressive dementias.
3. Recognize the stages of Alzheimer's disease and implications for nursing care.
4. Apply a contextual model to direct behavioral and pharmacological interventions for behavioral symptoms of Alzheimer's disease.
5. Discuss Parkinson's disease in terms of diagnosis, treatment strategies, and nursing interventions.
6. Recognize symptoms of brain attack/stroke in older adults.
7. Develop nursing interventions for older patients with brain attack/stroke.
8. Formulate nursing interventions for older patients with seizures.
9. Categorize the difference between epilepsy and seizures and nursing implications.
10. Differentiate seizure classifications.

Our neurologic system defines who we are. When brain function ceases, life itself is determined to have ceased. The neurologic system consists of two systems: the central and peripheral. The functional units are the sensory and motor neurons. The human nervous system controls consciousness, cognition, ethics, and behavior. Each mature brain has 100 billion neurons, several miles of axons and dendrites, and more than 10^{15} synapses. The functional health of older adults is dependent on a healthy functioning neurologic system. From cognitive ability to pain sensation, the neurologic system is the key. The functions of all other body systems rely on the intact function of the neurologic system.

The Central Nervous System

The central nervous system includes the cerebral cortex, basal ganglia, diencephalon, cerebellum, brain stem, and spinal cord. The brain is divided into right and left halves and is further divided into four lobes: frontal, temporal, parietal, and occipital. The function of the frontal lobes includes language (Broca's area), motor function, judgment, problem solving, impulse control, reasoning, memory, and **executive function** (ability to plan and think abstractly). The temporal lobes are responsible for language (Wernicke's area), memory, hearing, perception, and recognition. The occipital lobes process visual information and the parietal lobes integrate sensory information such as taste, pain, and temperature. Neurons communicate messages through neurotransmitters, chemicals that include acetylcholine, dopamine, norepinephrine, and serotonin. Two amino acid neurotransmitters, glutamate and gamma-aminobutyric acid (GABA), are less well understood. Neurotransmitters influence memory and cognition, mood, and motor function. Neurotransmitters also control the hypothalamic-pituitary-adrenal (HPA) axis, which integrates the endocrine, immune, and nervous systems. This neuroendocrine system is the link between the neurologic system and the endocrine system that maintains homeostasis in the body. See Figure 22-1 ▶▶▶ for an illustration of the regions of the brain and their function.

The Peripheral Nervous System

The peripheral nervous system consists of the cranial nerves, spinal nerves, the somatic and autonomic nervous system, and the reflex arc. The somatic nervous system is the link between the brain through the spinal cord to the muscles and sensory receptors. It is responsible for movement and receiving messages. The autonomic nervous system maintains

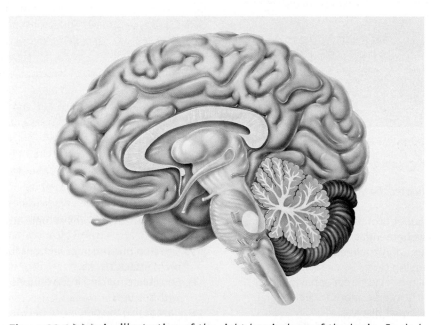

Figure 22-1 ▶▶▶ An illustration of the right hemisphere of the brain. In dark brown, the cerebellum. In beige, from bottom to top, the medulla oblongata and the pons. Just above it and slightly lighter, the corpus callosum.

Source: BSIP/Photo Researchers, Inc.

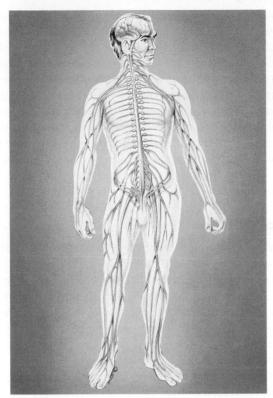

Figure 22-2 ▶▶▶ An illustration of the central and peripheral nervous systems. The brain (at top) and spinal cord constitute the central nervous system (CNS). The CNS integrates all nervous activities. Nerves outside of the CNS are part of the peripheral nervous system. This nerve anatomy allows the human body to respond to outside stimuli, and to move, feel, and make intelligent choices.

Source: Paul Singh-Roy/Photo Researchers, Inc.

homeostasis within the body and is divided into the parasympathetic and sympathetic nervous system. It controls heart rate, size of the blood vessels, blood pressure, contraction and relaxation of smooth muscle in various organs, visual accommodation, pupillary size, and secretions from exocrine and endocrine glands (Huether & McCance, 2011). The anatomy of the central nervous system allows the human to maintain homeostasis, move, feel, and interact with the environment. Figure 22-2 ▶▶▶ depicts the peripheral nervous system.

NORMAL CHANGES OF AGING

It is difficult to determine what constitutes normal changes of aging. The variability among adults increases as does the incidence of chronic disease. Not only is there variability

among adults, but even among organ systems in an adult and among different cell populations within an organ system. The challenge of caring for older adults is not to treat normal aging changes as disease. It is just as important not to delay treatment for disease by attributing it to normal aging. A common myth regarding the aging adult is that cognitive decline is inevitable. Memory, attention, and executive function do experience changes with aging, but the ability to learn new material and meet the cognitive demands of independent living remains intact without the presence of neurologic disease.

Central Nervous System

The brain decreases in size and weight with aging. The healthy human brain is made up of tens of billions of neurons acting as information messengers. It is estimated that one neuron may have synaptic connections to as many as 7,000 other neurons. The function and survival of neurons depends on key biological processes and with aging there is neuronal death and changes in the synapse between neurons. These changes are especially pronounced in neurodegenerative diseases such as Alzheimer's disease (a progressive and irreversible disease causing dementia) or Parkinson's disease (a progressive disease causing rigidity, tremor, and slowness of movement). Like the vessels in the rest of the body, vessels in the central nervous system (CNS) may be affected by atherosclerosis and are vulnerable to clots or rupture, which result in stroke. The brain consumes up to 20% of the energy used by the human body, more than any other organ, and has one of the richest blood supplies to keep it adequately perfused (U.S. Department of Health & Human Services, 2010). Decreased arterial perfusion to the brain may result in age-related changes in cognition.

The level of most neurotransmitters decreases with aging and the chemicals' receptors decline in number. The less understood amino neurotransmitters have recently drawn increased attention. The effect of aging on levels of glutamate and GABA is unknown, but there does seem to be a decline in their receptors with aging (Huether & McCance, 2011). New medications for Alzheimer's are directed at the amino neurotransmitters, clearing away or reducing damage caused by abnormal accumulations of tau and amyloid proteins, and other therapeutic targets.

Neuroendocrine changes also occur with aging. The change in regulation of glucocorticoids is especially important. There is a mean increase in glucocorticoids with aging, which in effect puts the body in a chronic stress condition. This increase in glucocorticoids may influence the development of depression and the development of type 2 diabetes mellitus, a common disease of older adults (Mattson, 2004; Sam & Frohman, 2008).

[handwritten top margin: slowed responses + movements / intermittent hand tremors / –impairment of coordination]

Peripheral Nervous System

The spinal cord is not spared in aging. Cells of the spinal cord decline in number and narrowing of the interior of vertebral bodies puts pressure on the spinal cord. Peripheral nerves decline from years of wear and tear. With aging bilateral loss of vibratory sense in the feet is almost universal, but it should not advance to the knees. Achilles reflex may be absent in older adults, but quadriceps reflex should be preserved in the absence of disease. Cranial nerve 1, the olfactory nerve, is the most exposed cranial nerve and also susceptible to decreased sensation. Smell is important in the sense of taste, and changes in smell and taste can affect appetite in older adults. The effects on the autonomic nervous system affect both the sympathetic and parasympathetic pathways. There is a slower response to the drop in blood pressure that occurs with position change, putting older adults at a greater risk for orthostatic hypotension. Thermoregulation is also affected and explains the reason that older adults are the victims of hyper- and hypothermia at a disproportionate rate.

From the perspective of directing nursing care, the neurologic conditions of the central nervous system fall into the categories of memory, movement, seizure disorders, and stroke. The conditions of the peripheral nervous system fall into the categories of motor, sensory, and autonomic disorders. Understanding the clusters of symptoms surrounding the neurologic disorders in general and in specific neurologic diseases and their impact on older adults is important when planning and providing nursing care. Figure 22-3 ▶▶▶ provides an overview of normal changes of aging in the neurologic system.

Conditions of the Central Nervous System

Mental status includes more than just cognitive ability; level of consciousness, appearance and behavior, speech and language, mood (depression or anxiety) and affect, perception and thought content, and insight and judgment all are factors in mental health status. Substance use is also an important factor to assess when someone has questionable function or behavior. Memory loss is not a normal part of growing older. When older people have difficulties with their memory or changes in their behavior, they need to be carefully assessed to determine if there is a treatable cause. Distinguishing between the "three D's"—**depression** (a mood disorder characterized by sadness), **dementia** (a progressive cognitive impairment), and **delirium** (potentially reversible acute confusional state)—is one of the

most important lessons that gerontological nurses must learn. Although these three syndromes have unique distinguishing features, they also may not be exclusive. It is possible for an older person with delirium to have an undiagnosed dementia or an older person with dementia to develop an acute delirium. Depression can occur along with either of the other conditions and it is conceivable that all three could be present at the same time. Knowing the baseline mental status of the older person is an important step in sorting out the issues if there are problems with cognition. Family members are a good resource to help define the baseline level of the older person's cognition.

Depression

Depression is covered more fully in Chapter 7 ⊂⊃. One clue that an older person may be suffering from depression rather than dementia is the apathy that is common in depression. For example, when the nurse is performing a mental status exam, an older person with depression may just not care to answer or feel that it is just too much trouble to answer. The older person with dementia may try hard to do their best or even confabulate. The Geriatric Depression Scale is an excellent tool for screening older people for the presence of depressive symptoms. In its short form there are only 15 questions and the test is highly valid and reliable. Depression is a very common comorbidity often accompanying dementia and the diagnosis is made more difficult because the older person with Alzheimer's may be less able to express those feelings that guide the diagnosis, including sadness, hopelessness, and guilt, than the cognitively intact older person. The incidence of depressive mood may be as high as 40%, while 10% to 20% meet the _Diagnostic and Statistical Manual of Psychiatric Disorders, Text Revision,_ 4th ed. (DSM-IV-TR) (APA, 2012) criteria for major depressive disorder. With treatment, there is often an improvement in function and behavior (Alzheimer's Association, 2012).

Delirium

[handwritten: causes: dementia, older age, fever, acute infection, previous delirium episodes, visual or hearing impairment, dehydration, chronic illness, multiple med problems, treatment w/ multiple drugs, alcohol or withdrawal drugs]

Delirium is an acute disorder of cognition that affects functional independence. Older adults do not develop dementia overnight, so any sudden change in mental status needs to be aggressively evaluated. The American Psychiatric Association (APA, 2012) recognizes two forms of delirium including hyperactive and hypoactive presentations. Delirium must be ruled out because cognitive impairment caused by delirium may be reversible. The development of delirium may indicate decreased reserve capacity of the brain and signal an increased risk for dementia (Fong, Tulebaev, & Inouye, 2009). To rate delirium and distinguish delirium from other types of cognitive impairment, the Hartford Institute for Geriatric Nursing _Try This_ assessment series

[handwritten bottom margin left: loss of independence]

[handwritten bottom margin right: cumulative loss: loss of spouse, driving, home]

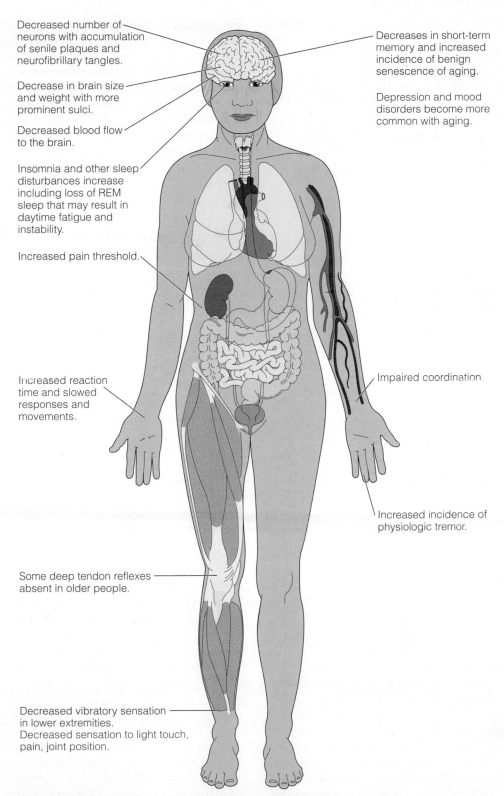

Decreased number of neurons with accumulation of senile plaques and neurofibrillary tangles.

Decrease in brain size and weight with more prominent sulci.

Decreased blood flow to the brain.

Insomnia and other sleep disturbances increase including loss of REM sleep that may result in daytime fatigue and instability.

Increased pain threshold.

Increased reaction time and slowed responses and movements.

Some deep tendon reflexes absent in older people.

Decreased vibratory sensation in lower extremities.
Decreased sensation to light touch, pain, joint position.

Decreases in short-term memory and increased incidence of benign senescence of aging.

Depression and mood disorders become more common with aging.

Impaired coordination.

Increased incidence of physiologic tremor.

Figure 22-3 ▶▶▶ Normal changes of aging in the neurologic system.

-help them manage meds

recommends use of the Confusion Assessment Method (CAM) (Inouye et al., 1990). The CAM includes two parts: Part 1 is an assessment instrument that screens for overall cognitive impairment; Part 2 includes only those four features that distinguish delirium. The tool can be administered in less than 5 minutes. It closely correlates with DSM-IV criteria for delirium. Visit the Hartford Institute of Geriatric Nursing website for further information on the use and scoring of the CAM-ICU. Please refer to the Best Practices feature below noting the signs and symptoms of delirium in the older adult.

Dementia

Dementia is a syndrome whose signs and symptoms may be the result of several acquired, progressive, life-limiting disorders that erase memory and the person's usual way of being in the world. The person with dementia has both a chronic illness and a terminal illness, first losing the ability to independently perform activities of daily living and finally becoming completely dependent in all aspects of self-care. Because the disease can affect different areas of the brain and different

hint *greatest risk factor is older age*

Best Practices Signs and Symptoms of Delirium in the Older Adult

Please note that not all of these signs and symptoms need be present in order to confirm the diagnosis of delirium and the intensity of symptoms may fluctuate and vary during any given time period.

1. **Reduced Level of Consciousness**—Observe the patient. Does he/she fall asleep during the interview or routine patient care?

2. **Disorientation**—Check orientation to time, place and person. Disorientation is common in acutely ill older adults, but often reorientation efforts in those without delirium to current circumstances are successful. An older adult with delirium is often unable to be reoriented.

3. **Short Term Memory Impairment**—Sudden onset loss of recent memory is common in delirium. Ask the older adult about his/her care earlier in the day. Patients who forget family visits, bathing or showering, or eating breakfast may have memory impairment.

4. **Agitation**—The patient may not be able to tolerate an IV line or indwelling urinary catheter. He/she may attempt to pull out these and other medical devices or otherwise refuse needed care. Agitated patients are at risk for receiving sedative/hypnotic medications that have the potential to further increase orientation, memory and level of consciousness.

Best Practices Signs and Symptoms of Delirium in the Older Adult (*continued*)

5. **Attention Impairment**—The patient may not be able to maintain attention or complete a task. Ask the patient to spell a word backwards or subtract 7 from 100. These patients are unable to cooperate with rehabilitation efforts or follow instructions regarding medication regimens.

6. **Perceptual Disturbance**—Delirious patients may experience visual or auditory hallucinations. A photograph of a person on the wall may be perceived to be a long-lost relative who is speaking or a bedside curtain may appear to be crawling with insects. These hallucinations may be troubling and upsetting to the patient, family and healthcare providers.

7. **Delusions**—A persistent false thought may be present and difficult to dispel in the older adult with delirium. He/she may think that a loved one long dead is alive and the nursing staff is not allowing the presence of this loved one at the bedside. These delusions are often related to disorientation and memory impairment and can fluctuate widely during the course of the day.

8. **Sleep-wake Cycle Disturbance**—Older patients with delirium will often sleep soundly during the day and experience significant nighttime awakenings. Daytime sleeping removes the patient from enjoying family visits, participating in needed rehabilitation activities, eating routine meals and escalates the risk of further time and place disorientation.

levels of the cortex, there is no uniform course and no predictability. The diagnostic criteria for dementia are defined in the DSM-IV-TR (APA, 2012). The syndrome must include the presence of cognitive or behavioral symptoms that:

1. Interfere with the ability to function at work or at usual activities and
2. Represent a decline from previous levels of functioning and performance and
3. Are not explainable by delirium or major psychiatric disorders.
4. Cognitive impairment is present and diagnosed through a combination of history supplied by the patient and/or caregiver; objective cognitive assessment including bedside mental status examination or neuropsychological testing. Neuropsychological testing should be done when the history and bedside examination cannot provide a confident diagnosis.
5. The cognitive or behavioral impairment involves a minimum of two of the following domains:
   a. Impaired ability to acquire and remember new information—symptoms include repetitive questions or conversations, misplacing personal belongings, forgetting events or appointments, getting lost on a familiar route.
   b. Impaired reasoning and handling of complex tasks, poor judgment—symptoms include poor understanding of safety risks, inability to manage

interaction between genetic & environmental factors

finances, poor decision-making ability, inability to plan complex or sequential activities.

c. Impaired visuospatial abilities—symptoms include inability to recognize faces or common objects or to find objects in direct view despite good acuity, inability to operate simple implements, or orient clothing to the body.

d. Impaired language functions (speaking, reading, writing)—symptoms include difficulty thinking of common words while speaking, hesitations; speech, spelling, and writing errors.

e. Changes in personality, behavior, or comportment—symptoms include uncharacteristic mood fluctuations such as agitation, impaired motivation, initiative, apathy, loss of drive, social withdrawal, decreased interest in previous activities, loss of empathy, compulsive or obsessive behaviors, socially unacceptable behaviors.

McKhann et al., 2011.

The greatest risk factor for developing dementia is older age. Currently, more than 5 million Americans suffer with Alzheimer's disease with the highest prevalence in the oldest age groups (Davis, Hendrix, & Superville, 2011). With the increasing age of the population in the United States and the oldest old being the fastest growing segment of the population, the prospects for increasing prevalence of this disease in the future is daunting. In the year 2050 one American will be diagnosed with Alzheimer's disease (AD) every 33 seconds with the number of Americans afflicted expected to more than triple to 16 million persons.

Types of Dementia

– multiple concussion pts ↑↑ @ risk

Multiple diseases can result in dementia, but the most common causes can be divided into four major dementia groupings:

1. Alzheimer's disease (AD) is the most common cause of dementia, being responsible for nearly 80% of the dementia diagnoses (Davis et al., 2011). AD has an insidious onset and although the exact cause is unknown, it may have a genetic, lifestyle, and environmental component. It presents clinically with language, memory, and visual spatial disturbances.

2. Vascular dementia (VaD) is the second most common form and usually presents more abruptly. It progresses with stepwise deterioration, executive dysfunction, and gait changes. It is thought to be caused by cardiovascular factors.

3. Lewy body dementia includes Parkinson's disease with dementia (PDD) and dementia with Lewy bodies (DLB). This dementia has a special pathology with the presence of round structures, or Lewy bodies, and neuritis found in the brain. Clinical symptoms include visual hallucinations, **delusions** (fixed beliefs held despite evidence to the contrary) and extrapyramidal symptoms such as tremor, rigidity, and postural instability.

4. The frontotemporal lobe dementia group includes Pick's disease. This dementia presents with personality changes and atrophy of the frontotemporal lobe of the brain.

Dementia can also be a mixture of AD with DLB or with VaD. Normal pressure hydrocephalus is a rare cause of dementia and is distinguished by an accompanying gait disorder and new-onset urinary incontinence. Surgical intervention and placement of a shunt to drain fluid from the brain may successfully treat the disorder (Factora & Luciano, 2008).

Early detection and diagnosis of memory loss is essential in order to slow the progression of memory loss and allow the older person and his or her family time to plan for the future.

Alzheimer's disease is progressive and is characterized by slow, progressive cognitive and functional decline. When detected, appropriate treatments can slow the decline and cognitive function may be extended. To identify and treat older adults with dementia earlier in their disease trajectory, in 2011 a workgroup formed by the National Institute on Aging and the Alzheimer's Association set guidelines and criteria for the clinical diagnosis and staging of AD. This group established three stages of AD: (1) preclinical, (2) mild cognitive impairment due to AD, and (3) dementia due to AD (McKhann et al., 2011).

Preclinical Stage of AD

The preclinical stage occurs before memory loss and functional impairment have occurred. During this stage changes in biomarkers such as beta-amyloid proteins are thought to occur, but there are no reliable diagnostic testing criteria associated with this stage and the use of the preclinical diagnosis is currently not recommended until further research has been conducted. Some persons in the preclinical phase will progress to AD with an annual conversion rate of 6% to 15% (Reuben et al., 2011).

Alzheimer's Disease

Alzheimer's disease (AD) is named after Dr. Alois Alzheimer who in 1906 first described the disease in a 55-year-old woman. AD presents with an insidious onset and decline in multiple cognitive abilities. Early in the disease, older people have difficulty remembering names and recent events and later they demonstrate symptoms that include impaired judgment, disorientation, confusion, behavior changes, and trouble speaking, swallowing, and walking.

Neuropathological criteria for AD include the presence of two abnormal structures: neuritic plaques and neurofibrillary tangles. The plaques and tangles each contain a specific protein that may play a role in pathogenesis of AD. Beta-amyloid protein is present in the plaques, and the tau protein is found in the tangles. AD disrupts the three processes that keep neurons healthy: (1) communication, (2) metabolism, and (3) repair. As a result, nerve cells are destroyed or die, causing memory failure, personality changes, problems carrying out activities of daily living, and other deficits. Although the definitive diagnosis is provided only after histopathological confirmation at autopsy, the clinical diagnosis can be made from history, physical examination, and neuropsychological testing with almost 90% accuracy (Ala, Mattson, & Frey, 2003). Figure 22-4 ▶▶▶ illustrates the underlying pathology in the formation of these plaques and tangles.

The majority of cases of AD result from complex interactions between genetic and environmental factors, with advanced age being the single greatest factor. From ages 65 to 74, the risk is about 2%, rising to 19% at age 75 and 42% at age 85. Higher risk is also associated with having a parent or sibling with AD and increases as the number of family members with the disease increases (Alzheimer's Association, 2012). Higher education has been correlated with later onset of dementia, as are more and more varied activities and greater social networks. Medical risks for AD include a history of head trauma, diabetes mellitus, frailty, high cholesterol levels, cigarette smoking, lack of physical activity, obesity, low levels of vitamin D, high levels of stress, and clinical depression (National Institute on Aging, 2012). Genetic causes are responsible for fewer than 5% of the cases of AD. Adult children of a parent with AD are often concerned about their own risk of developing the disease and may seek genetic testing. While age is the biggest risk factor for developing the disorder, having one or both parents with the disorder comes second. Researchers have found that children who had a parent with late-onset Alzheimer's were more likely than those without an Alzheimer's parent to show Alzheimer's-associated changes in two biomarkers and on brain scans although they did not have symptoms of the disease themselves (Mosconi et al., 2010). Alzheimer's disease is more common in people whose mothers had the disease than in those whose fathers had it indicating a possible "maternal effect." Older adults whose mothers had late-onset Alzheimer's exhibited Alzheimer's-like brain shrinkage patterns more often than those whose fathers had the disease (Honea, Swerdlow, Vidoni, et al., 2010). As more is understood about the human genome, the interest in genetic testing and risk factors for identifying, treating, and preventing AD will continue to grow.

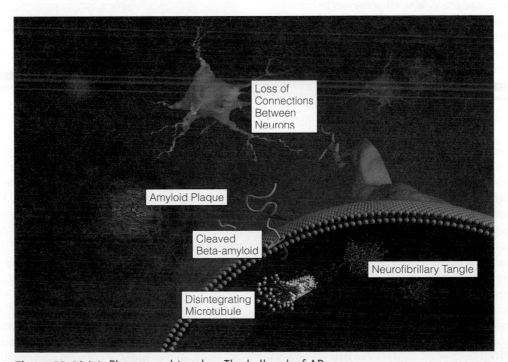

Figure 22-4 ▶▶▶ Plaques and tangles: The hallmark of AD.

Source: National Institutes of Health. (2006). *Plaques and tangles: The hallmark of AD.* Alzheimer's Disease Education and Referral Center. Retrieved from http://www.nia.nih.gov/NR/rdonlyres/F562167C-D864-4C02-8636-E01AD2C66312/2401/tangles_big1.jpg

Vascular Dementia

Vascular dementia, the second most common cause of dementia, is characterized by a cerebrovascular abnormality. Diagnostic criteria for vascular dementia are an abrupt onset of dementia, focal neurologic findings (abnormal reflexes or nerve functions), low-density areas (indicating vascular changes in the white matter), or presence of multiple strokes in computerized tomography (CT) or magnetic resonance imaging (MRI) scans. Other criteria include fluctuation of impairment, unchanged personality, emotional lability, and a temporal relation between a stroke and development of dementia. Control of those factors that affect vascular health has the potential to decrease the risk and improve the course of this cause of dementia. That includes controlling blood pressure, lipids, blood sugar, weight, nutrition, and any factors that cause vascular disease.

Lewy Body Dementia

Parkinsonism is a group of symptoms and signs in which there are variable combinations of tremor, rigidity, bradykinesia, and a disturbance in gait and posture. In **Parkinson's disease (PD),** Lewy bodies are present in the substantia nigra located in the midbrain, the basal ganglia, brain stem, spinal cord, and sympathetic ganglia. Lewy bodies are a complex protein aggregate. Not all older adults with Parkinson's disease develop dementia and dementia develops later in the disease process. Estimates of the prevalence of Parkinson's disease with dementia (PDD) vary greatly. A review of several studies found an average prevalence of 40%, but this is a cross-sectional prevalence and does not help determine an individual's risk of developing dementia. Like dementia of the Alzheimer's type, the risk of PDD increases with increasing age, with almost all persons developing dementia by 8 years after diagnosis (Gross, Siderowf, & Hurtig, 2007).

Dementia with Lewy bodies (DLB) has some similarities to PDD with the earliest symptoms being parkinsonism, but the onset of dementia is usually within 1 year of the motor symptoms. DLB may be confused with delirium because of the presence of wide swings in alertness and attention and other symptoms such as visual hallucinations which may take the form of seeing shapes, colors, or people who aren't present (Mayo Clinic, 2010). When compared to AD, DLB has early prominent frontal/executive dysfunction along with visuospatial deficits, while language is relatively preserved, although speech may be affected (Gross et al., 2007). The disease progression is often more rapid than that of AD. Autopsy confirmation reveals the presence of Lewy bodies in the brain tissue. Treatment includes use of cholinesterase inhibitors and Parkinson's disease medications to improve cognitive and motor functioning. Antipsychotics should be avoided because approximately one third of persons diagnosed with DLB have a dangerous sensitivity to these drugs and may suffer irreversible Parkinson's like symptoms and worsening of confusion (Mayo Clinic, 2010).

Frontotemporal Dementia

Frontotemporal dementia, which includes **Pick's disease,** is diagnosed on the basis of personality changes and the presence of frontal brain area atrophy in neuroimaging studies (CT scan or MRI). Less common in older adults, onset usually occurs in the mid-50s. Personality changes observed in frontotemporal dementia are similar to changes induced by damage to frontal lobes from other causes (injury, stroke) and include behavioral disinhibition, loss of social or personal awareness, or disengagement with apathy. Decline in memory occurs later in the disease process. Atrophy of the brain's frontal and temporal lobes and proliferation of nonneuronal glial cells in these areas characterize pathological findings in frontotemporal dementia. Pick's disease is characterized by two specific neuropathological findings on autopsy: (1) Pick's bodies inside nerve cells and (2) ballooned nerve cells.

Stages of Dementia

Dementia is generally described as occurring in three stages. This staging of dementia is based on the staging of AD, but may be applied to other causes of dementia as well. Six domains are evaluated to determine the older person's classification: memory, orientation, judgment and problem solving, community affairs, home and hobbies, and personal care. The stages are generally classified as stage 1, early–mild; stage 2, middle–moderate; and stage 3, late–severe. Preclinical cognitive impairment would precede stage 1, and sometimes a terminal stage is added as a classification after stage 3. Treatment options vary depending on the stage of the older person's dementia.

Dementia is a clinical diagnosis. At the present time, there are no laboratory tests or X-rays that can definitively diagnose the disease or the cause. When labs and X-rays are ordered during the diagnostic process, they are used to determine if there are other diseases that may respond to treatment. The standard workup for diagnosing dementia includes a complete physical examination, formal or informal neuropsychological tests, laboratory studies (B_{12} levels, thyroid function tests, complete blood count, and a basic metabolic panel), and imaging studies

(CT and/or MRI) to rule out subdural hematoma or brain tumor (Davis et al., 2011). The nurse is a very important partner in recognizing the symptoms of cognitive decline and in helping to determine the probable underlying cause. Complete geriatric assessment conducted by key members of the healthcare team will help to ensure the accuracy of the diagnosis. Key members of the team include the geriatrician, geriatric social worker, gerontological nurse, dietitian, and physical, occupational, and speech therapists as needed. Screening tools can be used to determine if observed concerns can be quantified. Once it has been established that cognitive decline is present, the DSM-TR-IV has classifications to help the provider clarify the cause (APA, 2012). Nurses who are aware of the differences in the types of dementia can contribute data to assist in the diagnostic process.

Pharmacological Therapies

There is no cure available at the present time for dementia; treatments are directed at improving function and slowing the progression of the disease. Available pharmacological therapies have been developed with the pathophysiology of Alzheimer's disease in mind because it is the most prevalent type of dementia and often a comorbidity with other causes of dementia. All of the neurotransmitters are affected by AD, but research has focused on the cholinergic system and blocking the enzyme that destroys acetylcholine to provide for increased availability of that neurotransmitter that is essential to memory. The first cholinesterase inhibitor was introduced in 1993, tacrine (Cognex), and is rarely used today because of the need for the four times daily dosing requirement and the potential for hepatotoxicity that requires careful monitoring of liver functions. Three other cholinesterase inhibitors are approved for treatment of mild and moderate dementia: donepezil (Aricept), rivastigmine (Exelon), and galantamine (Razadyne) (Davis et al., 2011). Donepezil has also been approved for use in moderate to severe dementia and rivastigmine is approved for use in Parkinson's disease with dementia. Donepezil has recently been released in a 23-mg tablet for those patients who have been treated with the 10-mg dose for more than 3 months, but the safety and efficacy of this larger dose had not been established at the time of this writing. These medications may also be used with patients with vascular dementia or dementia with Lewy bodies. These medications are not curative but can produce slight improvements in mental status testing scores although improvement in function is not often detected. Most importantly, cholinesterase inhibitors have not been convincingly shown to delay institutionalization (McPhee & Papadakis, 2011). The major side effects of these medications are gastrointestinal disturbances.

Review of the scientific data collected in studies using these medications question the impact of their effects and that when choosing a cholinesterase inhibitor the efficacy of the medications is roughly equivalent. Therefore, the choice of medication should be based on cost, patient tolerance, and convenience (Kennedy, 2006). Although each drug is chemically similar, each has unique characteristics that may result in an individual older person having a better tolerance or response to one over the other. The nurse needs to explore with the older person and family what they expect will be the result of treatment. Families may be happy with even subtle improvement that may not be measured using research instruments. Because each older person and family is unique, with varying expectations, values, and goals, the treatment of dementia often encompasses treating the older person along with the family as the unit of care.

Memantine (Namenda) was introduced in 2003 and was approved for use in moderate and severe AD. It is an *N*-methyl-D-aspartate (NMDA) antagonist, the only drug in its class. The drug modulates the activity of glutamate, an amino acid neurotransmitter. Memantine may be neuroprotective by blocking abnormal glutamate activity. Because memantine is not the same class of medication as the cholinesterase inhibitors, it can be added to those medications. In a study that examined the effect of donepezil and placebo versus donepezil and memantine, older people who had memantine added to their treatment did show improvement in function. However, long-term and meaningful functional outcomes have yet to be demonstrated (McPhee & Papadakis, 2011). Table 22-1 summarizes the drugs, dosing, and side effects of these medications.

COMPLEMENTARY AND ALTERNATIVE THERAPIES

Free radicals are produced when the body breaks down food. These negatively charged particles are the result of oxidation, a chemical reaction that transfers electrons to an oxidizing agent. Free radicals, in turn, can damage cells. Antioxidants can stop this destruction by being oxidized themselves. Vitamin E is an antioxidant and it is theorized that its use could help prevent or delay the development of AD. Early studies looked promising, but a recent Cochrane review found no evidence of the efficacy of vitamin E for people diagnosed with Alzheimer's disease or mild cognitive impairment (Mgekn, Quinn, & Tabet, 2008). Additional research is needed to further investigate the relationship between vitamin E and other antioxidants and dementia.

Ginkgo biloba is another antioxidant used for treatment of memory disorders. It is presumed to improve blood flow to the brain as well. Although many studies have been conducted using ginkgo biloba as prevention or treatment for

TABLE 22-1	Pharmacological Agents Used to Treat Cognitive Impairment		
Drug Name	**Dose**	**Precautions**	**Side Effects**
Aricept (donepezil)*	5–10 mg daily at bedtime	Abrupt withdrawal can cause cognitive decline; caution in cardiac conduction defects, seizure diagnosis, NSAID use, asthma	GI upset, bradycardia, syncope, seizures, urinary obstruction, AV block
Exelon (rivastigmine)*	1.5–6 mg bid; max: 12 mg daily	Take with food to avoid GI upset; titrate at 4-week intervals; caution in asthma, COPD, cardiac conduction defects, history of GI bleed, seizure diagnosis, NSAID use	GI upset (usually transient), seizures, urinary obstruction, hypotension, syncope, respiratory depression, paranoia, vomiting
Razadyne (galantamine) (previously named Reminyl)*	4–12 mg bid; max: 24 mg daily	Take with food to avoid GI upset; titrate at 4-week intervals; caution if NSAID use, seizure disorder, impaired liver function, asthma, COPD, cardiac conduction defects	GI upset (usually transient), arrhythmias, GI bleed, urinary obstruction, somnolence, tremor, abdominal pain, rhinitis
Namenda (memantine)+	5 mg daily. Increase 5 mg q week; max: 20 mg daily.	Reduce dose in renal impairment, use cautiously in those with seizure disorder	Dizziness, headache, hypertension, constipation, cough, pain, fatigue

*Indicates cholinesterase inhibitors.

+Indicates NMDA agonists.

Source: Nurse Practitioners' Prescribing Reference (2012); Reuben et al. (2011).

memory disorders, none meet the stringent requirements of the double-blind study considered necessary to support the claims and its use is not recommended. Side effects include bleeding, nausea, anxiety, gastrointestinal disturbance, and headache (Reuben et al., 2011).

Other medications, vitamins, and herbal remedies have been examined for use to prevent or slow the progression of AD. Because persons using nonsteroidal anti-inflammatory drugs (NSAIDs) for treating arthritis were found to have lower rates of AD, epidemiological studies were conducted and the results indicate that older adults with a certain genetic background (those possessing the APOE e4 allele) had a lower risk of developing AD regardless of age (Szekely, Breitner, & Fitzpatrick, 2008). In epidemiological studies, the drug group statins, when given to reduce cholesterol levels, did not reduce the risk of AD (McGuinness, 2009).

Nursing Considerations

Nurses are the crucial interface between the older person and the healthcare system. With increased knowledge of gerontology and the needs of older adults and their families, nurses will be better prepared to help them negotiate the challenges of dementia. As a chronic illness, dementia may require 20 years of home care, assisted living, or long-term institutional care with an array of community and acute care services to maintain independence, prevent excess disability, ensure safety, and manage medical complications. Even with the finest efforts of caregivers, the disease progresses

and creates dependency in activities of daily living and ultimately results in death if the care recipient has not died from another cause. Clinical baseline evaluations using reliable instruments are necessary to monitor treatment and evaluate progress. Mental status testing scores, ADL ratings, and other pertinent data should be noted in the chart and updated regularly in order to monitor clinical progress and the effectiveness of medical and nursing interventions. Figure 22-5 ▶▶▶ depicts the progressive decline observed in dementia.

The Hartford Institute for Geriatric Nursing suggests the use of the Mini-Cog to assess cognitive ability in the older adult (Doerflinger, 2007). This instrument can be easily done in the clinical setting and assesses a person's registration, recall, and executive function. The Mini-Cog takes about 3 minutes to administer, requires no special training, and is not influenced by the patient's education, culture, or language. See Chapter 3 ▭ for details on administering the test.

At the Time of Diagnosis

Early diagnosis provides the family and the older person with the opportunity to discuss treatment options and wishes while the older person still has decision-making capacity. The goals of treatment are directed toward cognitive symptom management, maintenance of functional status and easing stress in family caregivers. The nurse can work with the healthcare team to initiate discussions about advance directives and desired treatment modalities, selecting a healthcare proxy (power of attorney for health care), and

What do they want done w/ their care?

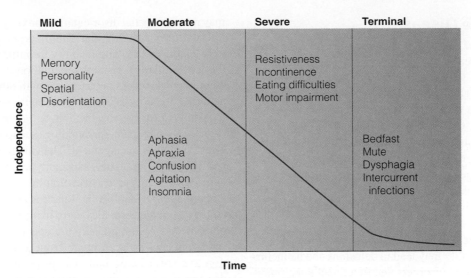

Figure 22-5 ▶▶▶ Progressive decline observed in AD.

Source: Volicer, L., Brandeis, G. H., & Hurley, A. C. (1998). Infections in advanced dementia. In L. Volicer & A. Hurley (Eds.), *Hospice care for patients with advanced progressive dementia* (pp. 29–47). New York, NY: Springer. Reproduced with the permission of Springer Publishing Company, LLC, New York, NY 10036.

informing the proxy about desired care to be provided when unable to make those decisions later in the disease. Referrals to the local Alzheimer's Association for support groups, services, and assistance locati can benefit both the older pers

In this stage, there is a nee tonomy. Caregivers need to a not driving, not leaving the p viding the least restrictive prot

Strategies used to prevent modified to provide a *safer* out infantilizing persons with To make the home safer and decrease the chances of falls, fires, burns, and getting lost, the caregiver (with another person such as the visiting nurse or occupational therapist) should tour the home to identify safety issues and develop a plan to rectify them. Areas of importance include placing door locks to prevent entry into hazardous areas, use of rug tape to prevent loose scatter rugs, decreasing the temperature of the water heater to 120 degrees to prevent scalding, and placing handrails in the bathroom to prevent falls.

Advance Directives and Establishing a Proxy

Early diagnosis allows for inclusion of the older person in making decisions and plans for the future. The older person's participation helps prevent the struggle families face to make decisions about care in the later stages if these issues were not discussed. Persons with dementia should be given an opportunity to establish advance directives. As early as

practicable, they should select a healthcare proxy to carry out their wishes. Educated decision making should be established and maintained throughout the progressive course, h the roles changing from the early stage when older pple can represent themselves, to later stages when their xy presents older adults' wishes. With a better under nding of the progression of the disease, families should encouraged to be realistic about the demands of caregiv and avoid making promises such as "I'll never put you a nursing home" that may not be realistic in the long run.

Preparing for a Progressive Decline

Progression of dementia does not occur uniformly in all individuals. Health teaching should be geared to the older person's current stage and the anticipated issues. As the disease progresses, the role of the caregiver becomes more active to compensate for the older person's cognitive losses and the development of behavioral symptoms. Families will need support from their professional caregivers as they make and live through some of the most difficult decisions of their lives—selecting life-prolonging treatments that may also increase discomfort, or choosing care that will provide comfort but may be seen as hastening death. Palliative care is an option for all older people with dementia because often aggressive medical care such as surgery and chemotherapy carries the burden of pain and troublesome symptoms like nausea, vomiting, and diarrhea. Nurses can help guide older adults and their families as they face some of these difficult end-of-life choices. See Chapter 11 for further discussion of palliative care.

Effect of the Disease

The appearance of behavioral symptoms is a common consequence of dementia and creates an imperative for nursing interventions to prevent, alleviate, or minimize these symptoms. Managing behavioral symptoms is as central to care of the person with dementia as pain management is to cancer. However, the various etiologies of the symptoms, their variability, and their appearance and disappearance at different times during the progressive stages of disease make their management complex. Figure 22-6 ▶▶▶ illustrates the relationship between behavioral symptoms and the social, caregiving, physical, and medical treatment environments.

Progressive dementia in combination with the person's underlying personality may lead to delusions and hallucinations as well as mood disorders and functional impairment. This may impose numerous challenges for caregivers, such as older adults' dependence for activities of daily living, inability to initiate meaningful activities, anxiety, and **spatial disorientation** (not knowing where one is in relation to the environment). These core and secondary symptoms often cause peripheral symptoms. Processes at each level influence the next level in a comprehensive way. Thus, delusions may result in spatial disorientation, anxiety, and dependence in activities of daily living. The mood disorder depression may lead to anxiety and inability to initiate meaningful activities. Similarly, spatial disorientation may lead to elopement, combativeness, interference with other residents, and agitation. Inability to initiate meaningful activities may lead to apathy, repetitive vocalization, agitation, and insomnia.

The four quadrants surrounding the model in Figure 22-6 direct symptom management. The caregiving environment and caregiving strategies, especially a nonpharmacological approach to management of symptoms (Volicer, Mahoney, & Brown, 1998), establish the tone for nursing care. The social environment provides caregiving in a milieu that recognizes and accommodates the special needs of persons with dementia and can range from a one-on-one interaction to a special care unit. The physical environment emphasizes the importance of environmental design, both as a treatment for dementia and support to help compensate for cognitive and functional deficits. Medical treatment ensures that physical problems, related or unrelated to dementia, are addressed.

The overall approach is first to focus on prevention. If known triggers result in problematic behaviors, the caregiver should remove those stimuli. Secondly, nurses should

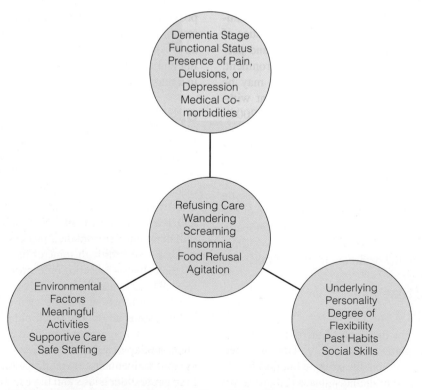

Figure 22-6 ▶▶▶ Context for evaluation of troublesome behaviors in dementia.

TABLE 22-2	Management Guidelines for Alzheimer's Disease	
Problem	**Goal**	**Treatment**
• Recent injury (e.g., unwitnessed fall) • Discomfort or pain (e.g., undertreated arthritis) • Physical complications (e.g., urinary tract infection) • Uncomfortable environment (e.g., too hot or too cold)	1. Eliminate physical and medical causes.	• Individualized care • Analgesic medication given liberally and possibly prophylactically before routine physical care • Adjust environmental conditions by providing more heat or cooling • Treat infections with antibiotics if needed
• Frustrating interaction • Chaotic environment • Overly complex task request • Nothing to occupy time • Patterns, e.g., time of day (fatigue), after a certain drug administration (untoward effect), before meals (hungry) • Events (e.g., change in physical or caregiving environment)	2. Remove immediate precipitants and eliminate, reduce, or compensate for "triggers."	• Never say "no" but instead offer options • Provide a calm environment with music/change of scenery • Avoid stress • Provide meaningful activities • Give rest breaks such as afternoon naps • Trial of drug "holiday" or discontinue drug • Ensure caregiver and environmental continuity
• Dementia • Mood disorders (depression) • Delusions or hallucinations • Functional impairment • Anxiety • Dependence in activities of daily living • Inability to initiate meaningful activities • Spatial disorientation	3. Treat core and/or primary or secondary symptoms that may be the cause of the behavior.	• Cholinesterase inhibitors • Correct amount of assistance (to preserve independence/prevent excess disability without overtaxing ability) • Implement nonpharmacological approaches and medications as needed • Personalize living space with family pictures and items from home to provide familiar environment

provide and suggest behavioral strategies (Table 22-2). When nonpharmacological strategies have been instituted and the older person still suffers from symptoms, pharmacological interventions should be added to the care plan (Table 22-3). Medications are given for the benefit of the older person and for no other reason.

Dementia causes older adults to act in ways that make them uncomfortable, is distressing to their caregivers, and would embarrass them if they had their normal faculties. Nurses and other caregivers need to assess symptoms and intervene to prevent troublesome behaviors or to minimize those that are inevitable, while providing opportunities for success and pleasure. Discussion of the 12 core, primary, and peripheral symptoms follows.

Functional Impairment

Functional impairment is a primary consequence of dementia and has both cognitive and physical components. The physical component may result from the underlying dementia, other comorbid conditions, or disuse. Improving

or supporting functional ability will have a positive effect on multiple behavioral consequences of dementia.

> *Practice Pearl* ▶▶▶ Provide verbal prompts one at a time to decrease the chances of the older person becoming confused. Even when verbal language is lost, nonverbal communication by way of tone of voice, smiling, and body language may be comforting. It is important to avoid any pressure to perform and to allow persons with dementia to continue with patterns that give a sense of security. Fatigue, nonroutine activities, alcohol, and a high-stimulus environment should be avoided because they increase functional impairment.

Apraxia, or inability to carry out learned and purposeful movements, interferes with the ability to follow a command such as "wash your face." However, older people with AD may be able to wash their face if handed a washcloth, or to continue an activity such as eating if

TABLE 22-3	Commonly Used Medications for Older Adults With Alzheimer's Disease		
Drug Class	Name	Dose Range (mg)/Frequency*	Comments
Selected Antidepressant Medications			
Selective serotonin reuptake inhibitors	Fluoxetine (Prozac)	10–60 mg/day	With older adults, any new medication should be initiated at a lower dose, and a longer time period should be allowed before increasing the dosage.
	Paroxetine (Paxil)	10–40 mg/day	
	Sertraline (Zoloft)	50–200 mg/day	
	Citalopram (Celexa)	20–30 mg/day	
	Escitalopram (Lexapro)	10–20 mg/day	Medications that are highly protein bound may be problematic and medications with anticholinergic properties should be avoided.
			Other considerations include onset of action and indications for treatment of both depression and generalized anxiety syndrome.
Other	Mirtazapine (Remeron)	15–45 mg/day	Mirtazapine may be useful in older adults who suffer from insomnia. As always, the dose will be decreased in older adults with renal impairment.
	Desvenlafaxine (Pristiq)	50–400 mg/day	
	Venlafaxine (Effexor)	75–225 mg/day	
	Duloxetine (Cymbalta)	40–60 mg/day	
Selected Drugs Used in Treatment of Delusions and Hallucinations			
Typical neuroleptics	Haloperidol (Haldol)	0.5–2 mg/day	Do not give a drug with a long half-life for an intermittent symptom of short duration.
Atypical neuroleptics	Risperidone (Risperdal)	0.25–1.5 mg/day	
	Olanzapine (Zyprexa)	2.5–10 mg/day	
	Quetiapine (Seroquel)	25–100 mg/bid-tid	
Selected Medications to Treat Anxiety			
Several Antidepressants Are Also Useful for Anxiety: Duloxetine (Cymbalta), Venlafaxine (Effexor XR), Escitalopram (Lexapro), and Paroxetine (Paxil)			
Benzodiazepines	Lorazepam (Ativan)	0.5–1 mg/bid-tid	Side effects are sedation, impaired motor coordination, akathisia, risk of falls, memory loss, respiratory or CNS depression, and paradoxical reaction. Must be tapered slowly.
	Alprazolam (Xanax)	0.25–0.5 mg/tid	
	Oxazepam (Serax)	10–20 mg/tid-qid	
	Clonazepam (Klonopin)	0.25–0.5 mg/bid	
Azapirone	Buspirone (BuSpar)	5–20 mg/tid	Side effects are headache, nausea, drowsiness, and light-headedness.

*bid = twice a day, tid = three times a day, qid = four times a day, qam = every morning, qhs = every evening

Note: All of these medications contain a black box warning for use in older adults and the risks and benefits of treatment need to be discussed with families.

someone helps them get started. **Agnosia** is the inability to recognize objects. Unlike **anomia,** or severe problems naming objects or finding words, agnosia causes functional impairment and predisposes to safety hazards, such as putting inedible things into the mouth or pouring water into a toaster. Persons with dementia may not recognize the bathroom or remember how to use the toilet. If the

functional consequences of agnosia and apraxia decrease self-care independence, the nurse should use multiple channels to overcome the deficit. Physical impairment may result from specific brain pathology. If the person has vascular dementia, the infarcts may have caused weakness of an extremity, exaggerated deep tendon reflexes, or gait abnormalities. Persons with diffuse Lewy body disease may exhibit parkinsonian symptoms that affect posture, balance, and gait. AD may result in abnormal reflexes, seizures, myoclonic jerks and rigidity, loss of the ability to walk, and loss of the ability to stand. The hazards of immobility, when combined with neuromotor deterioration, create a double jeopardy for the person with dementia.

Interventions for physical impairment should be targeted at maintaining the highest level of functional capacity for as long as possible and restoring capacity that may be remediable. Some nursing intervention guidelines to retard physical impairment and maintain functional ability include the following:

1. Prevent excess disability. To prevent immobility, provide assisted ambulation versus allowing the person to remain on bed rest. Encourage safe movement to the maximum degree possible in order to avoid problems related to immobility and dependency.
2. Treat other conditions that lead to physical decline. If pain interferes with walking, be sure pain relief is ordered and provided. Pain medications may need to be scheduled routinely rather than PRN to ensure they are administered to older people with limited ability to express their symptoms.
3. Identify and respond rapidly to acute changes in function. Be alert to symptoms suggesting an infection in order to make an early diagnosis.
4. Adapt care to accommodate neuromotor changes secondary to the progression of dementia. Compensate for changes in muscle tone and reflexes that affect posture, balance, range of motion, and ability to cooperate with care. Establish a preventive program to assess mobility, prevent falls, promote proper positioning, and implement environmental adaptations, such as redesigning furniture or introducing appropriate assistive devices (Trudeau, 1999).

> ***Practice Pearl*** ▶▶▶ An individualized assessment should be conducted to develop specific interventions to prevent excess disability, create a therapeutic environment, actualize functional potential, and promote dignity.

Mood Disorders

Depression may be a core consequence of AD and cause secondary and peripheral symptoms such as agitation and inability to initiate meaningful activities. Depression is difficult to diagnose since many of its clinical signs also result from other complications of dementia (e.g., insomnia and agitation), and many older people cannot respond to most standardized assessment instruments or express sadness.

Caregivers should be alert for changes in appetite, disinterest and **anhedonia** (loss of interest in activities that were once enjoyable), sleep abnormality, and fatigue.

Delusions and Hallucinations

Paranoid delusions are common psychotic symptoms in AD as first described by German neurologist Alois Alzheimer in 1906. Delusions and hallucinations may also be caused by delirium induced by drugs, electrolyte imbalance, hyperglycemia, urinary tract infection, seizure disorder, hypothyroidism, and Parkinson's disease. Delusions in AD may be due to (1) an intercurrent confusional state (delirium), (2) an interaction of dementia and personality, (3) a separate mental disorder that coexists with the dementia, or (4) a disinhibition of cortical functions resulting in "released" symptomatology.

The nursing role is to attempt to control the consequences of delusions and hallucinations. Nonpharmacological approaches such as reassurance and creating a calming environment targeted to presumed causes should be initiated and evaluated. If delusions and hallucinations are causing other behavioral problems, pharmacological treatment may be necessary (see Table 22-3). Careful nursing assessment is needed to document the frequency and severity of the problem, the response to medications and behavioral interventions, and the presence of side effects related to medication treatment. Very potent and effective neuroleptic medications for treatment of delusions and hallucinations are available, but they should be avoided unless absolutely necessary when quality of life is adversely affected. Extrapyramidal symptoms (EPS) are common with neuroleptics and, if present, cessation of the drug should be considered. Some of these symptoms include akathisia (restless feet and legs), Parkinson-like movements (tremors, rigidity, facial masking), dyskinesia (abnormal lip and mouth movement), and dystonic reactions (back arching, dysphagia, hoarse voice) (Davis et al., 2011).

> ***Practice Pearl*** ▶▶▶ Delusions and hallucinations should not be treated when they are pleasant and comforting, such as the "happy confabulator" who is mentally living in an earlier happy time of life with a long-dead spouse. Environmental interventions such as turning off the television set or covering a mirror may prevent distressing delusions and hallucinations when the older person fears another person in the room.

Dependence in Activities of Daily Living

Persons with AD will need varying degrees of assistance depending on their retained capacities and deficits. The goal is to preserve and promote functional independence. The nurse should determine the best time for activities of daily living and develop a preventive care plan to avoid potential problems. For maintaining continence as long as possible, a prompted voiding plan should be established. The nurse can devise a schedule where the older person is assisted to the bathroom to void every 2 hours in order to routinely empty the bladder and prevent episodes of incontinence. There are many ways to encourage independence. To assist with dressing, it is helpful to use garments that are easy to put on (jogging clothes, sneakers with Velcro closures), lay out the clothes in the order to be put on, provide a verbal prompt, and repeat if necessary. When assistance is needed, the nurse should provide what is necessary to prevent stressing the older person, but not so much as to cause excess disability.

> **Practice Pearl** ▶▶▶ Not all dependence in activities of daily living is attributable to dementia. Preventing avoidable decrements in capacity can be accomplished by knowledgeable caregivers. Since there may be other reasons for decreased ability to carry out daily activities, a complete assessment should be done. For example, new incontinence may be related to a urinary tract infection, which when treated may reverse the incontinence.

Inability to Initiate Meaningful Activities

Inability to initiate meaningful activities, although easy to overlook, affects persons with dementia and their caregivers. This inability has roots in functional impairment and depression, and its effects are far reaching. Lack of meaningful activity may result in apathy or agitation for the person with dementia, and frustration and burden for the caregiver. Involvement with meaningful activity is important for maintenance of functional abilities and social involvement—providing a feeling of success and accomplishment, improving mood, and reducing disruptive behaviors.

> **Practice Pearl** ▶▶▶ Since the person with dementia cannot initiate meaningful activities, caregivers must select appropriate activities that match the person's capacity and provide pleasure.

Anxiety

Anxiety may be a primary disorder or a symptom of depression. It may result from delusions, hallucinations, or functional impairment. Environmentally focused and behavioral interventions should be used before prescribing anxiolytics (see Table 22-3). The nurse should plan specific interventions to minimize stress level, enhance feelings of trust and safety, and promote stability by providing a daily routine with few variations. Diversional activities such as music therapy can be provided.

> **Practice Pearl** ▶▶▶ Anxiety is an unpleasant symptom. Caregivers must identify and treat anxiety before it channels the person's energy into defensive behaviors.

Spatial Disorientation

Even when persons with AD have no eyesight problem, space and location may be distorted, objects may be interpreted incorrectly, or directions may be misunderstood. Spatial disorientation may cause misunderstanding of the environment and lead to the development of fear, anxiety, suspicions, illusions, delusions, and safety problems such as getting lost. This can be especially distressing when the older person is placed in a new or unfamiliar environment, for instance, when they are hospitalized or newly admitted to a nursing home. Placing family photos or recognizable familiar items in a prominent spot can help orient the older person with spatial disorientation. In the early stage of dementia, the person may become confused when in an unfamiliar place. In the later stages, the person can become confused when in previously familiar places.

Two basic concepts, pop-up cues and environmental landmarks, can guide interventions. A pop-up (contrasting color should be used, such as a red wall in the bathroom) can help when a person does not use a white toilet in a white bathroom or will not sit on a blue chair in front of a blue wall. Landmarks capitalize on long-standing memory and use objects that are associated with the years the individual best remembers. Personal effects associated with specific rooms should be used as orientation devices.

> **Practice Pearl** ▶▶▶ Specific color-cued interventions should be targeted for individuals in their environment. The same furniture should be kept in the same place, and no changes should be made in room decorations except to simplify rooms and remove clutter.

Elopement

Caregivers are justifiably fearful that their care recipient will wander away and become lost, get injured, or die. Elopement is a potential problem in all settings. Community-dwelling older adults with dementia are more likely to wander if they have severe cognitive impairment, exhibit more than one challenging behavior, and spend long periods of time alone. Other risk factors include a darkened or unfamiliar environment, boredom, stress, tension, lack of control, lack of exercise, and nocturnal delirium.

In designing prevention strategies, the primary care provider should ask caregivers two questions: (1) Is the older person ever left alone? (2) Is the older person registered with the Alzheimer's Association Safe Return Program? Safe Return is a national program in cooperation with the MedicAlert Foundation that helps to find and return registered older people with AD and helps guide the family through elopement.

> **Practice Pearl** ▶▶▶ It is important to remove the precipitants of elopement such as unmet physical needs, boredom, easy exit, or reminders stimulating leaving. Safe walking activities provide exercise, offer social interaction, fill time, and use energy. Exits should be locked. The caregiver must not leave cues to leaving, such as car keys or coats, by the door.

Resistiveness to Care

Resistiveness to care is common during the middle to late stages of dementia and stresses both older adults and caregivers. If unmanaged, it is also a major reason for institutionalization and the use of psychotropic medications and restraints. Resistiveness to care occurs during interactions among care recipient, caregiver, and their environment. At times, simply responding with a relaxed and smiling manner may achieve calm and functional behavior. A time-out with a pleasant distraction should divert the older person's attention from the disturbing stimulus. For example, an older person with dementia who is refusing to take a medication might enjoy looking at family photos for a few minutes before the nurse attempts to give the medication again. Because the neurologic conditions are chronic, older adults and families manage the disorder for their entire lives. Nursing interventions can often be incorporated into activities of daily living. For example, the nurse may provide a hand massage with a warm washcloth to an older person who is resisting handwashing, thus stimulating circulation, providing range of motion, and cleansing the hands before eating.

> **Practice Pearl** ▶▶▶ There are no medications to directly prevent or treat resistiveness to care. Core consequences and secondary symptoms of AD that may lead to resistiveness can be managed by behavioral or pharmacological interventions (see Tables 22-2 and 22-3). Because resistiveness occurs intermittently for short periods, a medication with a long duration and poor side-effect profile should not be used.

Food Refusal

Specific issues related to food refusal occur during each of the progressive stages of dementia as a consequence of primary or secondary symptoms. In all stages, changes in environment and disruption of usual routines can be upsetting, so mealtime rituals and consistency are helpful. Mealtimes should be a focal point of the day, and other activities can be built around structured eating times. The primary caregiver should know the individual's current likes and dislikes, his or her level of physical activity and degree of independence, and how to make eating pleasant and nutritious to provide adequate calories, nutrition, and hydration. Nursing interventions to make mealtime pleasant include playing calming music, presenting food in an attractive place setting, placing real or artificial flowers, and making sure that unpleasant odors are eliminated. A nourishment plan should specify which foods will be provided and how they will be prepared, identify the best eating areas, and establish routines for the eating process.

In addition to the problems related to food refusal in dementia, normal changes with aging in the sense of taste can lead to decreased appetite and decreased food intake. Furthermore, older people with ill-fitting dentures or lack of natural teeth to properly chew food may refuse to eat because they anticipate the discomfort that will be associated with chewing. Sense of smell is also affected by aging and these losses result in the decreased flavor of food. See Table 22-4 for recommendations for preventing food refusal.

Because persons with dementia tend to lose weight later in the disease, caloric density should be maximized, unless they are above ideal weight. Use of finger foods (sandwiches) is one way to address misperception or inability to use a knife, fork, or spoon. In the terminal stage, when older people are bedfast, mute, dysphagic, and subject to infections, eating difficulties can become very problematic. Choking may appear in the severe-to-terminal stage and may be prevented or at least minimized by avoiding thin liquids, feeding the person in a sitting position or keeping the head of the bed at a 90-degree angle, and using foods in which the bolus has sufficient moisture content to help passage through the pharynx and facilitate swallowing.

> **Practice Pearl** ▶▶▶ If a person likes a food, the caregiver should serve it. The same meals and snacks can be served until the person cannot eat them or does not want to eat them. Some medications can be eliminated if they alter the taste of food, take away appetite, or interfere with the ability to use eating utensils.

Insomnia

Insomnia in older adults is discussed in Chapter 8 ⊂▭, but AD may present more difficulties with insomnia since it causes death of nerve cells in many areas of the brain,

TABLE 22-4	Suggestions for Encouraging Food Intake for Older Adults with Severe Cognitive Impairment
Observed Behavior	**Suggested Nursing Actions**
Older person seems distracted and uninterested in eating his/her meal.	1. Make eye contact and address the older person by name along with a gentle touch on the hand or shoulder. "Mr. Smith, good morning. Here is your delicious lunch." 2. Place the meal in the line of vision of the older person and unwrap or prepare the meal so that the sight and aroma are apparent. 3. Eliminate distractions if possible such as turning off the television or closing the door to the room if the hall is noisy. 4. Place a piece of finger food in the older person's hand and gently guide it to his/her mouth. A small piece of bread or a cracker might be appropriate. 5. Using a spoon place a small amount of sweet or soft food on the older person's lips. Hopefully the older person will lick it off and become aware of the meal.
Older person seems to not want to eat. He/she may turn head away, keep mouth closed, or hold food in his/her mouth without swallowing.	1. Maintain smile and pleasant, calm behavior. Do not attempt to "force feed" or push the spoon into the older person's mouth. 2. Gently stroke the older person's throat to stimulate swallowing. 3. Offer a sample of each food contained on the plate. If the older person seems to prefer one food over the other, continue to offer that food first before moving on to the other foods. 4. If all attempts to feed the older person fail, refrigerate the meal for later. The older person may become hungry and the meal can be reheated and enjoyed at a more appropriate time.
Older person pushes food away or becomes angry at feeding attempts.	1. Assess for comfort. Is the older person in pain or does he/she need other care? 2. If the older person continues to push food away after two feeding attempts, discontinue all attempts. Do not force the issue. Come back at a later time.

Source: National Institute on Aging, 2013. Caregiver Guide: Tips for Caregivers of People with Alzheimer's Disease. Retrieved from http://health.nih.gov/category/SeniorsHealth.

including the suprachiasmatic nucleus. Cell loss in the suprachiasmatic nucleus leads to abnormalities of circadian rhythms in persons with AD. Approximately 70% of persons with AD will experience sleep disruption during the course of their disease (Lee-Frye, 2010). Circadian rhythm disruption leads to changes of sleep, body temperature, melatonin secretion, and possibly other physiological functions. When sleep disturbance is linked with increased agitation and disorientation during the late afternoon and early evening hours, it is referred to as "sundowning." Sundowning may be related to exhaustion, loss of visual cues as darkness approaches, and inability to distinguish dreams from reality (Lee-Frye, 2010).

When persons with AD experience insomnia, several strategies may be used. Lifestyle changes should be explored to establish proper sleep hygiene. Activities inconsistent with maintaining high-quality sleep and daytime alertness should be avoided, such as irregular use of daytime naps, extended amount of time in bed, irregular sleep–wake schedules, or inactivity. It is important to avoid using products that interfere with sleep (caffeine, nicotine, and alcohol), scheduling exercise close to bedtime, engaging in exciting or emotionally upsetting activities close to bedtime, and having a poor sleep environment, such as an uncomfortable bed or a bedroom that is too bright, stuffy, hot, cold, or noisy.

Practice Pearl ▶▶▶ Insomnia places a burden on persons with AD and their caregivers—depriving family caregivers of their sleep and precipitating institutionalization of the person with AD dementia. In an institution, residents suffering from insomnia may disturb the sleep of other residents.

Drug Alert ▶▶▶ All persons with AD are choline deficient, and anticholinergic drugs have the potential to worsen the symptoms of AD. It is essential to be wary of over-the-counter sleeping medications that may contain an anticholinergic component or other drugs that may have anticholinergic properties.

The Beers list is an excellent resource for information about anticholinergic drugs (see Tables 6-6 and 6-7 in Chapter 6 ▭).

Apathy and Agitation

Apathy and agitation are likely to occur as dementia worsens and persons experience more functional and cognitive decline. Persons with dementia are unable to make sense of their environment, to filter the stimulation that comes their way, and to handle the stress of what is happening to them.

Engagement, the opposite of apathy, involves attention to and participation in the external environment such as involvement in a conversation or other meaningful activities. Persons with dementia need help to become active and interested in what is going on around them. It is common for persons with dementia to have bouts of apathy followed by agitation. By uncovering the causes, it is easier to treat agitation before it escalates into assaultive or even violent behavior.

Treatment and relief of agitation and apathy are central to promoting psychological well-being specific for persons with dementia. Worsening of dementia over time restricts the capacity to express emotions. As the ability to express emotions verbally declines, older adults with dementia resort to other, primarily nonverbal, means of communication such as reaching out to others.

Practice Pearl ▶▶▶ The right amount of stimulation will promote pleasure and prevent apathy without inciting agitation. The nurse should identify appropriate activities and help the older person become engaged with them and assess causes and management of overstimulation (too many visitors or television set).

Pharmacological Interventions

Pharmacotherapy is indicated only when nonpharmacological interventions do not prevent or alleviate challenging behaviors. Prevention or treatment of challenging behaviors is critical to older adults' overall well-being since behavioral dysregulation can be associated with functional impairment (Schultz, Ellingrod, Turvey et al., 2003). In all cases, medications are prescribed to promote the older person's comfort and for no other reason such as sedation. Two traditional principles of geriatric nursing—start low and go slow, and monitor treatment continuously—must be followed. Exactly which medication to select is dependent on the older person's clinical condition and the balance between the desired action and side-effect profile.

Practice Pearl ▶▶▶ Although it is always important to consider the older person first when developing nursing interventions for persons with a neurologic disorder, these conditions are family disorders because they affect the entire family. Families will be stressed and in crisis as a result of their loved one's dementia and symptoms.

Late-Stage Issues

There often comes a time when the family cannot manage home care any longer and must seek institutionalized long-term care. This difficult decision carries dual concerns: (1) finding an appropriate facility, and (2) managing the guilt of transferring care to another. Many assisted-living facilities have dementia special-care units. When the person's needs

overwhelm home or assisted-living care, a skilled nursing facility will be required. An ideal skilled nursing facility provides for basic safety needs, meets overall health needs, and promotes quality of life in daily living. Nursing home placement should be considered the best choice for the older person and his or her family, not the last choice. By discussing placement issues as early as possible in the placement process, hopefully crisis and emergency placement can be avoided, allowing adequate time to investigate all options. The nurse can help the family by suggesting questions to ask the nursing director (Table 22-5). Additionally, the federal government sponsors a website that compares the quality of nursing homes in a specific geographic area using the Five-Star Quality Ratings including health inspection results, nursing home staff data, quality measures, and fire safety inspection results. Families can enter their zip codes and find comparison results of nursing homes in their geographic area.

Practice Pearl ▶▶▶ Too much information can be overwhelming. The nurse should teach what the older person and family will need to know tomorrow, not next year.

Family caregivers must be supported in dealing with their guilt at "failing" the person with AD. The nurse can help by stating, "You have done such a fine job of caregiving. Look at the nursing home staff. It takes a team of nurses working three shifts a day, seven days a week to do what you have been doing." The nurse should reiterate that AD will continue to worsen and the older person will continue to decline. If nursing home placement or relocation to an assisted living facility is anticipated, time will be needed to prepare the older person and his or her family. Often bringing the older person with AD to view the facility and meet some of the staff will ease the transition. However, despite careful preparation and planning it often takes the older person with AD from 3 to 6 months to adjust to changes in living environment and functional decline may be inevitable and to be expected.

The family may confront four issues: (1) Should cardiopulmonary resuscitation (CPR) be attempted? (2) Will the person be transferred to an acute care facility? (3) Should a feeding tube be used? (4) How should life-threatening infections be managed?

Do Not Resuscitate For persons with late-stage dementia, CPR should not be offered (Robinson, 2002). If the person does not have an advance plan stipulating either CPR or do not resuscitate (DNR), the DNR decision should be discussed with the surrogate decision maker. DNR does not present an ethical dilemma, as clinicians recognize both the futility and adverse effects of CPR on long-term care older adults in general, and its use is low. Resuscitation for an unwitnessed cardiac arrest in this population has

TABLE 22-5	Helping Families Choose a Nursing Home
Issues	**Questions to Ask the Medical Director, Nursing Director, and Administrator**
Safe physical environment	Is the unit locked? Are there protected inside and outdoor wandering paths?
	How is elopement prevented? How are falls prevented? Are physical or chemical restraints ever used? What types of assistive devices are used?
Dementia health	How often does a physician or nurse practitioner routinely visit each resident? What memory-enhancing medications are typically used? What cognitively enhancing activities are used?
Overall health	What drugs and treatment are available for other medical conditions without being transferred from the unit? From the nursing home?
	How are chronic preexisting and other new problems assessed and managed?
	What is the procedure if acute care is needed? Where is end of life care provided? Is hospice available on the unit?
Knowledgeable and available staff	What kinds of staff training programs are there? How often are they provided?
	What percentage of staff attend? What percentage of nursing assistants are certified?
	What percentage of nursing assistants are certified in dementia care? What special consultants are available? How many hours of direct nursing care does each resident receive each 24 hours? How many full-time equivalent registered nurses are there per resident?
Quality-of-life issues	What programs are there to maintain physical functioning (toileting, feeding assistance, ambulation)? What is the pain management program? How much time in each 24-hour period do residents spend outside their bedrooms? What are the ongoing activities and daily events?
Support services	What types of family support groups are there and how frequently do they meet? What family education programs are provided?
Interdisciplinary team approach	How are individual resident's care plans developed, evaluated, revised, and shared with the family? How frequently does the team evaluate each resident's care plan? Is there a system to include family input?

Source: Adapted from Medicare.gov (2012). Nursing Home Checklist. Retrieved from http://www.medicare.gov/files/nursing-home-checklist.pdf.

a very low probability of restoring life (Robinson, 2002). Older people who survive and are discharged back to their long-term care unit are invariably in a much more advanced stage of dementia than they were before the arrest. A DNR order would spare the few older adults who survive the resuscitation event from living in an uncomfortable state for the remainder of their lives. If the definition of success is to restore older adults to their previous functional capacity, no matter how limited, there is no place for resuscitation attempts when older adults with AD have a cardiac or respiratory arrest.

Although healthcare workers may understand that CPR is futile in late-stage AD, the family may not. Education should be provided to families who make the ultimate decision about DNR for persons who do not have the capacity to do so for themselves. Older adults living in the community who have decided to be designated as DNR should place large and clear instructions on the refrigerator, notify neighbors, family and friends, and place a "No CPR" card in their wallet in case emergency care is needed.

Transfer to an Acute Care Site There are many reasons why older adults in general and persons with AD in particular are transferred from a long-term care facility to a hospital, and often these reasons are not centered around the older person's care. Hospital transfers are sometimes carried out because of an insufficient number of adequately trained nursing home staff to administer and monitor intravenous therapy, lack of diagnostic services, and pressure from staff and family. Additionally, nurses influence the decision to transfer dying residents because of insufficient knowledge of resident or family preferences, lack of technological and personnel resources in the nursing home, and concerns about liability (Bottrell, O'Sullivan, Robbins et al., 2001). Staffing in nursing homes may be less than ideal, and staffing problems may further contribute to hospitalization of older adults with AD. Some long-term care sites prefer not accept older adults with advanced AD. In this case, the older person may qualify for hospice, which is paid for by Medicare.

Once in the hospital, older adults with dementia are at risk for complications such as delirium, being tube-fed, relocation stress, and dying. Delirium or acute confusional state, superimposed on AD, was found in 50% older adults with documented dementia (Andrew et al., 2006). The problems of delirium during an acute phase of illness are well documented, but the long-term outcomes, or the results of an entire episode of delirium, are lacking. It is not known how the hospital-induced delirium episode affects an already frail individual's cognitive and physical functioning long term; however, it is known that older delirious patients often refuse care and are subject to highly sedating medications and physical restraints. Identification and treatment of delirium offers the opportunity to reverse the causes, thus lowering the risk of injury to the older patient. Refer to pages 616–617 for information on assessing delirium in the older adult.

When discussing the issue of transferring, healthcare providers have to help the family understand the differences between reversing an acute care problem in an otherwise healthy individual and extending the dying process in a person with AD. For instance, coronary bypass surgery might extend the life of a older person who has severe coronary disease. However, living on a long-term care unit without perceiving the stresses of the world and receiving care in a low-stimulus environment may be clinically advantageous. Cataract surgery may be advocated to allow older people the ability to connect visually with their environment. However, older people with AD will be at risk of removing an intraocular lens because, unless restrained, they would be likely to rub their eyes. A transfer to an acute care unit means that older people will be vulnerable to nosocomial infections and cared for by staff who may be experts in critical care but not in dementia care. According to Holzer and Warshaw (2002), "Traditional patterns of caring for older people in an acute care hospital in which the nursing staff bathes, toilets, feeds, and grooms these older people without ensuring that they can perform these tasks by themselves may contribute to a lack of independence. In addition, enforced bed rest, use of sedating drugs, indwelling bladder catheters, physical restraints, and medications that lead to acute confusional states contribute to the loss of independence of these older people" (p. 192). Many older patients who are incontinent of urine when discharged from the hospital were continent on admission. Older people with pneumonia were more likely to experience decline in their activities of daily living if hospitalized than comparable older people with similar severity of illness treated in the skilled nursing facility (Gillick, 2002). Almost one third of older adults hospitalized for acute medical or surgical illness decline in their ability to perform daily activities (Holzer & Warshaw, 2002). Thus, hospital-acquired decrements last beyond hospitalization.

On acute care units, there is an increased potential for the use of restraints, which can predispose older people to increased delirium and the complications of immobility. A vicious cycle of events leading to increased iatrogenesis can be set in motion. The issue of using restraints to deliver technology the older person cannot understand is complex. One could argue that the older person will forget being restrained and the long-term benefit outweighs the short-term requirement of being in restraints. However, because older people with AD appear to live in the present, the stress associated with being restrained is not outweighed by the ability to deliver technology. Older people with late-stage AD have a reduced life span, which needs to be considered when asking if the burden is outweighed by the benefit. All nurses, even those not working in specialized geriatric settings such as orthopedic or coronary care units, would benefit from increased education regarding dementia, palliative care, and provision of specialized acute care of the older adult with dementia.

Feeding Tube The "need" for feeding tubes may be avoided by promoting eating and preventing food refusal. Caregivers should sit and make eye contact, chat, and make eating an important and pleasurable component of long-term institutional care. More than one third of severely cognitively impaired nursing home residents in the United States have feeding tubes (Lee & Kolasa, 2011). Even though older people with AD may refuse food, turn away when food is offered, push the spoon or hand away, or spit out food, they can be successfully fed by hand.

Even older people with advanced AD can revert to natural feeding after tube feeding. An individualized care plan, based on the older person's target body weight and functional eating abilities, should be developed by an interdisciplinary team that includes a nurse, dietitian, and physician. Natural feeding can begin with the tube in place until the older person's eating is reestablished. Then the tube may be removed. Skillful hand feeding should continue, and a program of functional feeding using the older person's remaining skills should be initiated. To promote independence, the caregiver may place a hand over the older person's hand, take a large spoon, place a small amount of sweetened food such as applesauce on the tip of the spoon, move it to the older person's mouth, and follow the steps outlined earlier in Table 22-4. Placement of a nasogastric tube will contribute to the risk of aspiration pneumonia and elevating the head of the bed to a 30-degree angle for an hour after feeding will decrease this risk.

Permanent tube feeding is not recommended for persons with advanced AD, even those who choke on food and liquids. Tube feeding does not prevent aspiration, improve functioning or quality of life, increase comfort, or promote weight gain (Lee & Kolasa, 2011). One widely held misconception about tube feeding is that it is ordinary care like spoon feeding. However, tube feeding does not resemble eating or drinking in any way. Although some family members and healthcare workers may fear that the older person will "starve to death," older people with advanced AD do not feel the desire to eat or drink. Body functions are shutting down during the dying process, and food and liquids are no longer necessary. In fact, dehydration is beneficial during the dying process because it decreases the sensation of pain and prevents edema and excessive respiratory secretions. Dehydration also decreases the incidence of vomiting and diarrhea. The only consequence of dehydration that may lead to discomfort is dryness of the mouth, lips, or eyes, which can be prevented or alleviated by moisturizing spray, swabs or salve, or ice chips.

Treatment of Infections Infections are an inevitable consequence of advanced dementia because of several risk factors that cannot be avoided, such as changes in immune function, incontinence, decreased mobility, and aspiration. Because of the atypical presentation of pneumonia and infection in the older person, leukocytosis, fever, and cough may not be present. The presentation may instead be altered level of function, falls, increased confusion, or new-onset incontinence. Infections may be treated by the administration of oral antibiotics that are as effective as parenteral antibiotics and do not require restraints to prevent removal of an intravenous catheter. However, the effectiveness of antibiotic treatment is diminished in the terminal stage of dementia when infections become recurrent. Pneumonia is the most common cause of death in individuals with dementia, reflecting the limited effectiveness of antibiotic therapy in this patient population. Antibiotics are not necessary to maintain comfort of the older person during an infectious episode because comfort can be maintained by administration of analgesics and antipyretics.

In summary, successfully caring for the person with dementia requires the humane, empathetic, and skillful application of evidence-based interventions. "Good endings" are possible. Caregivers can provide the education, guidance, and support needed to appropriately care for AD patients, who may live for many years or more from the onset of symptoms (Hurley & Volicer, 2002).

Parkinson's Disease

Parkinson's disease (PD) is a chronic, progressive neurologic disorder in which idiopathic parkinsonism appears without other widespread neurologic symptoms, such as cognitive impairment. PD symptoms are caused by the loss of nerve cells in the pigmented substantia nigra pars compacta and the locus coeruleus in the midbrain. In PD, Lewy bodies are present in the basal ganglia, brain stem, spinal cord, and sympathetic ganglia. PD is considered an extrapyramidal syndrome because of the anatomical structures involved and the resulting symptoms of tremor, **chorea** (involuntary twitching of the limbs or facial muscles), and **dystonia** (involuntary muscle contractions forcing unusual or painful positions).

> **Practice Pearl** ▶▶▶ PD may progress to PD with dementia, and the nurse will be caring for an older person with two characteristic groups of neurologic symptoms, including movement and memory disorders.

Similar to Alzheimer's disease, PD is a disorder for which the risk increases dramatically with age. PD occurs at similar rates in all ethnic groups, is equally distributed in males and females, and has a prevalence of 1 to 2 per 1,000 persons in the general population, which increases to 2% of adults over age 65. The exact cause of PD is unknown, but it is hypothesized that exposure to environmental toxins or a genetic predisposition leads to PD. The disease can be induced in primates by chemical exposure leading to death of nigrostriatal neurons, depletion of dopamine in the basal ganglia, and parkinsonism. First-degree relatives of older people are twice as likely to develop PD as are controls. Currently, there is no exact diagnostic test for PD. It is considered a disease of exclusion, that is, the diagnosis is made when all other causes of chronic parkinsonism are ruled out.

The pathology of PD is related to the loss of the dopaminergic cells situated deep in the midbrain in the substantia nigra (the black substance so named because of the melanin seen in those neurons). With the depletion of dopamine, which inhibits neurotransmitters, an abnormal movement syndrome characterized by rigidity and tremor can occur. Neurotransmission that takes place at the nerve terminals produces dopamine, which is necessary to initiate movement. Thus, therapy directed to correct dopamine deficiency currently drives the pharmacological bases of treatment. Pharmacological intervention by administration of levodopa, the metabolic precursor of dopamine, provides symptomatic relief of symptoms, particularly bradykinesia.

Although the replacement hypothesis sounds like a straightforward solution, two factors complicate the issue. First, the active medication must pass into the brain through the blood–brain barrier. Because the enzyme dopa decarboxylase in the intestinal mucosa converts ingested levodopa to dopamine, most is lost before it even enters the general circulation. Thus, levodopa is combined with a peripheral dopa-carboxylase inhibitor. The combination of medication is available commercially as carbidopa-levodopa (Sinemet, Parcopa) in formulations of 1:10 and 1:4 ratios. A common starting dose is one half tablet of 25/100 mg carbidopa/levodopa three times daily and increased gradually to 25/250 mg up to three times daily to control symptoms as needed. To maximize absorption and facilitate crossing the blood–brain barrier, carbidopa-levodopa should be taken on an empty stomach. The nurse should incorporate timing of the administration of this medication into the older person's care plan. Both the older person and caregiver should be taught that this medication should be taken 1 hour before or 2 hours after a meal. Nursing interventions should be planned to minimize potential side effects of nausea and vomiting. The older person may experience postural hypotension. The nurse needs to teach strategies to prevent falling, such as sitting on the side of the bed before standing or holding onto a table when arising from a chair.

The second issue related to levodopa therapy is that the older person may at times appear to have developed a drug-induced tolerance. However, the older person's symptoms can vary widely despite constant levels of the drug in the peripheral circulation and in the brain. During the "off" time, the drug becomes ineffective and the older person may freeze up momentarily and lose mobility. During the "on" time, side effects such as involuntary and hyperactive movements and dystonia occur. The exact pathogenesis of this on–off phenomenon is unknown, but the older person and family need to be prepared for this possibility and request a change in dose or timing of the medication.

The anticholinergics are another class of medications used for symptomatic treatment of PD. These drugs are prescribed to relieve tremors. The nurse needs to be vigilant in managing the side effects of dry mouth, constipation, blurred vision, and urinary retention. Because PD is a movement disorder, a vision problem can further increase the risk of falling. In older men, urinary retention could complicate symptoms of an enlarged prostate. Another drug, amantadine, alone or in combination with an anticholinergic drug, may help by potentiating the release of endogenous dopamine. However, this benefit may be transitory. Another class of medications are dopamine agonists, which directly stimulate the dopamine receptors, such as Permax (Parkinson's Study Group, 2000). Dopamine agonists are often initiated in early PD before starting levodopa and are also used in combination with levodopa through the progressive course of PD. Thus, because of the on–off effects of levodopa, some older people are tried on other

medications at the onset of symptoms. Dopamine agonists such as pramipexole (Mirapex) and ropinirole (Requip) may be added to the drug regimen should the movement disorders become refractory to drug treatment (Nurse Practitioners' Prescribing Reference, 2012). Patients should be closely monitored for sleepiness, drowsiness, and dizziness.

Deep brain stimulation is replacing surgery to treat older people unresponsive to drug therapy. Gene therapy and stem and fetal cell implants hold promise for treatment in the future and research is ongoing (McPhee & Papadakis, 2011).

Nursing care should be directed to helping the older person manage parkinsonism—that is, to design individualized interventions to promote mobility, prevent falls, assess and treat dysphagia, and preserve independence for as long as possible. In the early stage, the older person may have mild symptoms on one side only, which are inconvenient but not disabling, and changes in posture, walking, and facial expression (masklike, as originally described by English physician James Parkinson). In the middle stages, older people often will have difficulty rising from bed or chair, tend to assume a flexed posture when standing, and have difficulty initiating walking. They lean forward increasingly to "get started." They may walk with small shuffling steps with no arm swing, have an unsteady gait especially on turning, and have difficulty in stopping. Some older people walk at an increased speed to counteract their abnormal center of gravity and to prevent themselves from falling. In the very late stage, the older person cannot stand or walk, becomes cachectic, and requires constant nursing care.

Nurses should assess fall risk (see Chapter 18 ▭ for fall risk assessment) using an agreed-on assessment measure such as the functional reach test (Behrman, Light, Flynn et al., 2002). Based on the older person's retained capacity, the nurse should develop a plan to include the older person and family. An interdisciplinary approach to care is important. The nurse should be part of a team that includes the physical and occupational therapists to help retain skills and promote independence in activities of daily living. Exercise is another way to preserve independence and protect against the hazards of immobility and deconditioning.

Stroke and TIA

A stroke is a rapidly developing loss of consciousness due to lack of blood circulating to the brain. Stroke is a leading cause of death and disability and the third leading cause of death in the United States (McPhee & Papadakis, 2011). The pathology typically is caused by hemorrhage into the brain, rupture of an artery, or an embolus or thrombus occluding an artery.

A transient ischemic attack (TIA) is a mini-stroke that causes no permanent or lasting damage. Survivors of a TIA have an increased risk of another stroke with the 90-day risk of stroke estimated to be as high as 10.5% and the greatest risk occurring in the first week after the TIA (American Stroke Association, 2006). Stroke and TIA have common underlying pathologies and both require immediate evaluation and treatment. If neurologic symptoms continue for greater than 24 hours, an older person will be diagnosed as having had a stroke; otherwise, neurologic deficits that resolve before 24 hours are classified as a TIA.

Control of risk factors can decrease the number of strokes each year. Risk factors include hypertension, diabetes mellitus, hypercholesterolemia and hyperlipidemia, cigarette smoking, excessive alcohol consumption, obesity, and lack of physical activity. Older people with these risk factors should work with their healthcare providers to reduce their risk factors by instituting lifestyle modification and pharmacological treatment. Older people with symptomatic atherosclerotic carotid stenosis >70% should be evaluated for carotid endarterectomy in order to reduce their risk of stroke. Older people with persistent and paroxysmal atrial fibrillation should receive anticoagulation with warfarin with a target INR in the 2.0 to 3.0 range. For older people who are a high fall risk or those with a history of gastrointestinal bleeding, aspirin 325 mg/day, ticlopidine (Ticlid), or clopidogrel (Plavix) may be indicated as an alternative treatment. Postmenopausal hormone therapy is not beneficial for prevention of heart disease and stroke and is not recommended for women who have a history of myocardial infarction, TIA, or stroke (American Stroke Association, 2006).

Immediate treatment of stroke is targeted to lifesaving techniques, prevention of extension of the stroke, and early treatment using a plasminogen activator if appropriate. Stroke is an emergency, is often called a *brain attack,* and the benefits of reducing further morbidity have to be balanced against the risks of increasing the possibility of intracerebral hemorrhage. An adequate airway needs to be established and maintained with ventilation and oxygenation provided as needed. The nurse assesses for neurologic status using the Glasgow Coma Scale (Ingersoll & Leyden, 1994), vital signs, papillary responses, respiratory patterns, and sensory and motor responses to verbal, tactile, and painful stimulation (Crosby & Parsons, 1989). An experienced team needs to make the decision about movement of the older person and transport depending on severity of the stroke and stability of the older person.

After an acute stroke, the older person is typically transferred to an emergency department. Usually, the National Institutes of Health (NIH) Stroke Scale (Figure 22-7 ▶▶▶) is used to gauge the degree of cerebral infarction by determining level of consciousness. Also used are performance and examination of tests of gaze, visual fields, facial palsy, motor strength, ataxia, sensation, language, dysarthria, and extinction or inattention (Brott et al., 1989). The NIH Stroke Scale is considered to be a valid and reliable clinical examination scale to determine stroke severity (Reuben et al., 2011).

If thrombolytic therapy is not contraindicated, then often recombinant tissue plasminogen activator (rt-PA) will be administered within 3 hours to treat the acute ischemic stroke although outcome data on the risk/benefit of IV thrombolysis in older adults are limited (Reuben et al., 2011). Contraindications to antithrombotic therapy include heparin use in the last 48 hours, blood pressure greater than 185/110 mmHg, and history of intracranial hemorrhage.

For those stroke survivors who are able to return home, the physical, cognitive, and emotional sequelae can place great burdens on the older person and family. Many of their post-discharge needs are responsive to nursing interventions. An examination of community-dwelling stroke survivors found that the most commonly reported interventions were directed toward ensuring continuity of care between the hospital and home, family care, and modifying risk factors (McBride, White, Sourial et al., 2004). Structured nursing interventions and provision of physical, occupational, and speech therapy during the rehabilitative period have resulted in better functional status, less depression, and higher self-perceived health, self-esteem, and dietary adherence (Nir, Zolotogorsky, & Sugarman, 2004). Nursing interventions include provision of skin care, attention to bowel and bladder continence, and ensuring safety and mobility. Post-stroke depression and mood swings are common in stroke survivors and careful monitoring of mood is indicated. Older patients with a hypercholesterolemia and a LDL of less than 70 should be discharged from the hospital on a statin drug (Reuben et al., 2011).

Although the prognosis is grave, many older people survive and rehabilitation becomes the cornerstone of nursing care. The major issues for older people who survive a stroke have to do with activity limitations across multiple domains (basic and instrumental activities of daily living), psychological distress, and communication difficulties. In contrast to AD, which worsens, stroke survivors' conditions often improve with rehabilitation. However, persons who experience a stroke associated with small vessel disease are at risk for both motor and cognitive impairment problems (Mok et al., 2004), thus underscoring the importance of preventing strokes by promoting good cardiovascular health.

Although the onset of stroke is precipitous, the risk factors have often developed over the years. Stroke prevention is best accomplished by adopting a prudent heart-healthy lifestyle. Prevention activities include maintaining normal blood pressure, not smoking, exercising, and maintaining normal weight. The nurse has an important role in prevention and health education. These interventions should begin in the formative years in elementary school.

HEALTHY AGING TIPS FOR STROKE PREVENTION

||||||||||||||||||||||||||||||||||||||||||||||||||||||||||||||||||||

To reduce stroke risk in your patients, urge them to:

▶ Stop smoking.

▶ Reduce blood pressure to at least 140/90 but 120/80 is more desirable.

▶ Reduce cholesterol and triglyceride levels.

▶ Seek anticoagulation treatment if they have atrial fibrillation.

▶ Follow a low-sodium (<2 to 3 g/day), high-potassium (>4.7 g/day) diet.

▶ Begin or maintain an exercise program (>30 minutes of moderate intensity daily).

▶ Lose weight if overweight (BMI < 25 kg/m^2).

National Institute on Aging, 2012; Reuben et al., 2011.

Patient Identification ——⁻————⁻————   Pt. Date of Birth ——/——/——

Hospital —————————— (————⁻————)   Date of Exam ——/——/——

Interval: [ ] Baseline [ ] 2 hours post treatment [ ] 24 hours post onset of symptoms ±20 minutes

[ ] 7–10 days [ ] 3 months [ ] Other ————————— (—— ——)

Time: —— : —— [ ] am [ ] pm   Person Administering Scale —————————

Administer stroke scale items in the order listed. Record performance in each category after each subscale exam. Do not go back and change scores. Follow directions provided for each exam technique. Scores should reflect what the patient does, not what the clinician thinks the patient can do. The clinician should record answers while administering the exam and work quickly. Except where indicated, the patient should not be coached (i.e., repeated requests to patient to make a special effort).

Instructions	Scale Definition	Score
1a. Level of Consciousness: The investigator must choose a response if a full evaluation is prevented by such obstacles as an endotracheal tube, language barrier, or orotracheal trauma/bandages. A 3 is scored only if the patient makes no movement (other than reflexive posturing) in response to noxious stimulation.	0 = **Alert;** keenly responsive. 1 = **Not alert;** but arousable by minor stimulation to obey, answer, or respond. 2 = **Not alert;** requires repeated stimulation to attend, or is obtunded and requires strong or painful stimulation to make movements (not stereotyped). 3 = Responds only with reflex motor or autonomic effects or totally unresponsive, flaccid, and flexic.	————
1b. LOC Questions: The patient is asked the month and his/her age. The answer must be correct—there is no partial credit for being close. Aphasic and stuporous patients who do not comprehend the questions will score. 2. Patients unable to speak because of endotracheal intubation, orotracheal trauma, severe dysarthria from any cause, language barrier, or any other problem not secondary to aphasia are given. It is important that only the initial answer be graded and that the examiner not "help" the patient with verbal or nonverbal	0 = **Answers** both questions correctly. 1 = **Answers** one question correctly. 2 = **Answers** neither question correctly.	————
1c. LOC Commands: The patient is asked to open and close the eyes and then to grip and release the non-paretic hand. Substitute another one-step command if the hands cannot be used. Credit is given if an unequivocal attempt is made but not completed due to weakness. If the patient does not respond to command, the task should be demonstrated to him or her (pantomime), and the result scored (i.e., follows none, one, or two commands). Patients with trauma, amputation, or other physical impediments should be given suitable one-step commands. Only the first attempt is scored.	0 = **Performs** both tasks correctly. 1 = **Performs** one task correctly. 2 = **Performs** neither task correctly.	————

Figure 22-7 ▶▶▶ NIH Stroke Scale.

Source: National Institutes of Health (2003); http://www.stroke-site.org/stroke_scales/stroke_scales.html. Pictures, words, and sentences used to score item 9 of the Stroke Rating Scale.

(continued)

Patient Identification ——⁻———⁻———   Pt. Date of Birth ——/——/——

Hospital ———————————— (————⁻————)   Date of Exam ——/——/——

Interval: [ ] Baseline [ ] 2 hours post treatment [ ] 24 hours post onset of symptoms ±20 minutes

[ ] 7–10 days [ ] 3 months [ ] Other ———————————— (—— ——)

Instructions	Scale Definition	Score
2. **Best Gaze.** Only horizontal eye movements will be tested. Voluntary or reflexive (oculocephalic) eye movements will be scored, but caloric testing is not done. If the patient has a conjugate deviation of the eyes that can be overcome by voluntary or reflexive activity, the score will be if a patient has an isolated peripheral nerve paresis (CN III, IV or VI), score a 1. Gaze is testable in all aphasic patients. Patients with ocular trauma, bandages, pre-existing blindness, or other disorder of visual acuity or fields should be tested with reflexive movements, and a choice made by the investigator. Establishing eye contact and then moving about the patient from side to side will occasionally clarify the presence of a partial gaze palsy.	0 = **Normal.** 1 = **Partial gaze palsy;** gaze is abnormal in one or both eyes, but forced deviation or total gaze paresis is not present. 2 = **Forced deviation,** or total gaze paresis not overcome by the oculocephalic maneuver.	_____
3. **Visual:** Visual fields (upper and lower quadrants) are tested by confrontation, using finger counting or visual threat, as appropriate. Patients may be encouraged, but if they look at the side of the moving fingers appropriately, this can be scored as normal. If there is unilateral blindness or enucleation, visual fields in the remaining eyes are scored. Score 1 only if a clear-cut asymmetry, including quadrantanopia, is found. If patient is blind from any cause, score 3. Double simultaneous stimulation is performed at this point. If there is extinction, patient receives a 1, and the results are used to respond to item 11.	0 = **No visual loss.** 1 = **Partial hemianopia.** 2 = **Complete hemianopia.** 3 = **Bilateral hemianopia** (blind including cortical blindness).	_____
4. **Facial Palsy:** Ask—or use pantomime to encourage—the patient to show teeth or raise eyebrows and close eyes. Score symmetry of grimace in response to noxious stimuli in the poorly responsive or non-comprehending patient. If facial trauma/bandages, orotracheal tube, tape, or other physical barriers obscure the face, these should be removed to the extent possible.	0 = **Normal** symmetrical movements. 1 = **Minor paralysis** (flattened nasolabial fold, asymmetry on smiling). 2 = **Partial paralysis** (total or near-total paralysis of lower face). 3 = **Complete paralysis** of one or both sides (absence of facial movement in the upper and lower face).	_____
5. **Motor Arm:** The limb is placed in the appropriate position: extend the arms (palms down) 90 degrees (if sitting) or 45 degrees (if supine). Drift is scored if the arm falls before 10 seconds.The aphasic patient is encouraged using urgency in the voice and pantomime, but not noxious stimulation. Each limb is tested in turn, beginning with the non-paretic arm. Only in the case of amputation or joint fusion at the shoulder, the examiner should record the score as untestable (UN), and clearly write the explanation for this choice.	0 = **No drift;** limb holds 90 (or 45) degrees for full 10 seconds. 1 = **Drift;** limb holds 90 (or 45) degrees, but drifts down before full 10 seconds; does not hit bed or other support. 2 = **Some effort against gravity;** limb cannot get to or maintain (if cued) 90 (or 45) degrees, drifts down to bed, but has some effort against gravity. 3 = **No effort against gravity;** limb falls. 4 = **No movement.** UN = **Amputation** or joint fusion, explain: _____ **5a. Left Arm** **5b. Right Arm**	_____ _____

Figure 22-7 ▶▶▶ (continued)

Patient Identification ——ˉ————ˉ———   Pt. Date of Birth ——/——/——

Hospital ———————————— (————ˉ—————)   Date of Exam ——/——/——

Interval: [ ] Baseline [ ] 2 hours post treatment [ ] 24 hours post onset of symptoms ±20 minutes

[ ] 7–10 days [ ] 3 months [ ] Other ——————————— (—— ——)

Instructions	Scale Definition	Score
6. Motor Leg: The limb is placed in the appropriate position: hold the leg at 30 degrees (always tested supine). Drift is scored if the leg falls before 5 seconds. The aphasic patient is encouraged using urgency in the voice and pantomime, but not noxious stimulation. Each limb is tested in turn, beginning with the non-paretic leg. Only in the case of amputation or joint fusion at the hip, the examiner should record the score as untestable (UN), and clearly write the explanation for this choice.	0 = **No drift;** leg holds 30-degree position for full 5 seconds. 1 = **Drift;** leg falls by the end of the 5-second period but does not hit bed. 2 = **Some effort against gravity;** leg falls to bed by 5 seconds, but has some effort against gravity. 3 = **No effort against gravity;** leg falls to bed immediately. 4 = **No movement.** UN = **Amputation** or joint fusion, explain: _____ **6a. Left Leg** **6b. Right Leg**	_____
7. Limb Ataxia: This item is aimed at finding evidence of a unilateral cerebellar lesion. Test with eyes open. In case of visual defect, ensure testing is done in intact visual field. The finger-nose-finger and heel-shin tests are performed on both sides, and ataxia is scored only if present out of proportion to weakness. Ataxia is absent in the patient who cannot understand or is paralyzed. Only in the case of amputation or joint fusion, the examiner should record the score as untestable (UN), and clearly write the explanation for this choice. In case of blindness, test by having the patient touch nose from extended arm position.	0 = **Absent.** 1 = **Present in one limb.** 2 = **Present in two limbs.** UN = **Amputation** or joint fusion, explain:	_____
8. Sensory: Sensation or grimace to pinprick when tested, or withdrawn from noxious stimulus in the obtunded or aphasic patient. Only sensory loss attributed to stroke is scored as abnormal and the examiner should test as many body areas (arms [not hands], legs, trunk, face) as needed to accurately check for hemisensory loss. A score of 2, "severe or total sensory loss," should only be given when a severe to total loss of sensation can be clearly demonstrated. Stuporous and aphasic patients will, therefore, probably score 1 or 0. The patient with brainstem stroke who has bilateral loss of sensation is scored 2. If the patient does not respond and is quadriplegic, score 2. Patients in a coma (item 1a = 3) are automatically given a 2 on this item.	0 = **Normal;** no sensory loss. 1 = **Mild-to-moderate sensory loss;** patient feels pinprick is less sharp or is dull on the affected side; or there is a loss of superficial pain with pinprick, but patient is aware of being touched. 2 = **Severe to total sensory loss;** patient is not aware of being touched in the face, arm, and leg.	_____

Figure 22-7 ▶▶▶ (continued)

(continued)

Patient Identification ——ˉ————ˉ————   Pt. Date of Birth ——/——/——

Hospital ———————————— (————ˉ—————)   Date of Exam ——/——/——

Interval: [ ] Baseline [ ] 2 hours post treatment [ ] 24 hours post onset of symptoms ±20 minutes

[ ] 7–10 days [ ] 3 months [ ] Other ———————————— (—— ——)

Instructions	Scale Definition	Score
9. Best Language: A great deal of information about comprehension will be obtained during the preceding sections of the examination. For this scale item, the patient is asked to describe what is happening in the attached picture, to name the items on the attached naming sheet, and to read from the attached list of sentences (see the following page). Comprehension is judged from responses here, as well as to all of the commands in the preceding general neurological exam. If visual loss interferes with the tests, ask the patient to identify objects placed in the hand, repeat, and produce speech. The intubated patient should be asked to write. The patient in a coma (item 1a = 3) will automatically score 3 on this item. The examiner must choose a score for the patient with stupor or limited cooperation, but a score of 3 should be used only if the patient is mute and follows no one-step commands	0 = **No aphasia;** normal. 1 = **Mild-to-moderate aphasia;** some obvious loss of fluency or facility of comprehension, without significant limitation on ideas expressed or form of expression. Reduction of speech and/or comprehension, however, makes conversation about provided materials difficult or impossible. For example, in conversation about provided materials, examiner can identify picture or naming card content from patient's response. 2 = **Severe aphasia;** all communication is through fragmentary expression; great need for inference, questioning, and guessing by the listener. Range of information that can be exchanged is limited; listener carries burden of communication. Examiner cannot identify materials provided from patient response. 3 = **Mute, global aphasia;** no usable speech or auditory comprehension.	_____
10. Dysarthria: If patient is thought to be normal, an adequate sample of speech must be obtained by asking patient to read or repeat words from the attached list. If the patient has severe aphasia, the clarity of articulation of spontaneous speech can be rated. Only if the patient is intubated or has other physical barriers to producing speech, the examiner should record the score as untestable (UN), and clearly write an explanation for this choice. Do not tell the patient why he or she is being tested.	0 = **Normal.** 1 = **Mild-to-moderate dysarthria;** patient slurs at least some words and, at worst, can be understood with some difficulty. 2 = **Severe dysarthria;** patient's speech is so slurred as to be unintelligible, in the absence of or out of proportion to any dysphasia, or is mute/anarthric. UN = **Intubated** or other physical barrier, explain:	_____
11. Extinction and inattention (formerly Neglect): Sufficient information to identify neglect may be obtained during the prior testing. If the patient has severe visual loss preventing visual double simultaneous stimulation, and the cutaneous stimuli are normal, the score is normal. If the patient has aphasia but does appear to attend to both sides, the score is normal. The presence of visual spatial neglect or anosognosia may also be taken as evidence of abnormality. Since the abnormality is scored only if present, the item is never untestable.	0 = **No abnormality.** 1 = **Visual, tactile, auditory, spatial, or personal inattention** or extinction to bilateral simultaneous stimulation in one of the sensory modalities. 2 = **Profound hemi-inattention or extinction to more than one modality;** does not recognize own hand or orients to only one side of space.	_____

Figure 22-7 ▶▶▶ (*continued*)

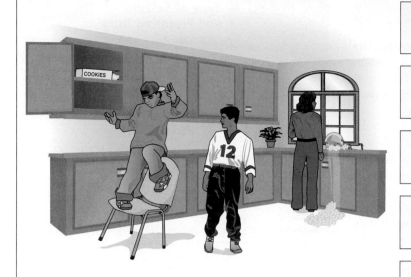

You know how.

Down to earth.

I got home from work.

Near the table in the dining room.

They heard him speak on the radio last night.

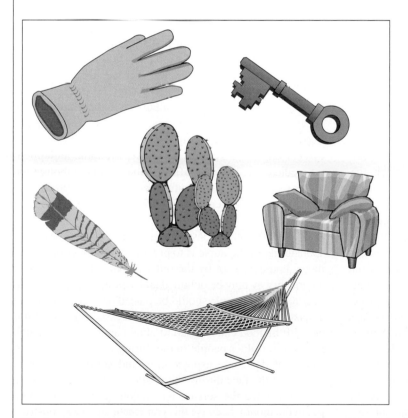

MAMA

TIP-TOP

FIFTY-FIFTY

THANKS

HUCKLEBERRY

BASEBALL PLAYER

Pictures, words, and sentences used to score item 9 of the Stroke Rating Scale.

Figure 22-7 ▶▶▶ (*continued*)

Seizures

Seizure is an abnormal, abrupt release of electrical activity in the brain. A seizure can cause a variety of symptoms (e.g., spasticity, flaccidity) based on the area of the brain affected. **Epilepsy** is defined as two or more unprovoked seizures. The incidence of epilepsy increases with advanced age; people over age 75 are twice as likely to develop new-onset epilepsy as all adult age groups under 65.

Seizures are classified as either generalized, partial (focal), or unclassified using the international classification of epileptic seizures (Commission on Classification and Terminology of the International League Against Epilepsy, 1981). There has been no significant change in this classification since 1981. Classification is based on the area of the brain from which the electrical activity originated, regardless of whether it then spreads to other areas. In generalized seizures, both hemispheres of the brain are involved. There are six types of generalized seizures, each with separate symptoms: (1) Tonic–clonic seizures (also called grand mal) have a duration of 2 to 5 minutes and begin with a period of rigidity and stiffening (extension) of the muscles and loss of consciousness. The second phase entails rhythmic jerking (flexion) of the extremities, but this may not always occur. (2) Absence seizures (petit mal) are common in children and involve brief loss of attention with no loss of consciousness, as if daydreaming. (3) Myoclonic seizures last only a few seconds and involve rhythmic jerking of the muscles. (4) A tonic seizure, like the first phase of the tonic–clonic seizure, entails rigidity. (5) Clonic seizure involves repetitive motor activity (e.g., lip smacking). (6) An atonic seizure is sudden loss of muscle tone (Cotton, Fuoto, & Shemansky, 2007).

Partial (focal) seizures occur in only one hemisphere of the brain and are either complex or simple. Complex partial seizures are 1 to 3 minutes in duration and involve loss of consciousness and automatisms. During a simple partial seizure, the older person remains conscious and often feels an aura (e.g., ringing in ears) before the seizure takes place. The older person may exhibit unilateral movements in a limb. Determining the type of seizure is important to be able to choose the appropriate medication. Table 22-6 lists the preferred antiseizure drug based on type of seizure.

Several nursing interventions are used when caring for an older person with a history of seizures. It is the nurse's responsibility to obtain an accurate patient history, including the age at onset of the initial seizure and frequency of attacks. In addition, the nurse should inquire about the dates and duration of the seizures as well as medication name, dosage, and frequency. It is important

TABLE 22-6	Type of Seizure and Preferred Drug
Type of Seizure	**Preferred Drug(s)**
Partial (focal)—simple	phenytoin (Dilantin), carbamazepine (Tegretol)
Partial (focal)—complex	phenytoin (Dilantin), carbamazepine (Tegretol)
Tonic–clonic	phenytoin (Dilantin), carbamazepine (Tegretol)
Absence	valproic acid (Depakene), clonazepam (Klonopin)
Myoclonic	valproic acid (Depakene), clonazepam (Klonopin)

for the nurse to be aware of the medication dose, because many older people are not initially given a high enough dose. The antiepileptic medications act differently in older adults. Older adults have an increased ratio of body fat to lean body mass so drugs such as phenytoin that are fat soluble may remain in the system longer. This is also the case for renally excreted drugs because of the decline in creatinine clearance that occurs with aging. Protein-bound drugs may have higher concentrations because of the decrease in albumin concentrations, and because most of the antiepileptic medications are metabolized by the liver, they may alter other medications in the cytochrome P450 system. All of the available antiepileptic medications have significant side effects, although the newer medications have an improved side-effect profile and have equivalent efficacy (Table 22-7) (Carlson, Macera, & Price, 2007).

If an older person has a seizure, the most important responsibility of the nurse is to prevent injury. Suction equipment should be kept by the older person's bedside so that an oral airway may be obtained and aspiration prevented. In addition, older people should be placed on their side during a seizure to prevent aspiration. If necessary, the head-tilt/chin-lift method can be used to obtain an airway. Although it is rare for older people to die during a seizure, the chief causes of death are asphyxiation and suffocation due to turning of the face during the postictal unconscious phase. However, once the seizure has begun, nothing should be put in the mouth, because this can create an airway obstruction and cause injury to the oral mucosa. Oxygen and intravenous access should always be made available. Oxygen is used if the older person experiences signs of hypoxia (change of skin color), and intravenous access is needed in

TABLE 22-7 Antiepileptic Medications and Their Side Effects

Commonly Used Antiepileptic Medications	Common Side Effects
phenytoin (Dilantin) gabapentin (Neurontin) lamotrigine (Lamictal) topiramate (Topamax) carbamazepine (Tegretol)	Dizziness, headache, gastrointestinal upset, blood dyscrasia, bone marrow suppression, tremor, somnolence, hepatic dysfunction, parkinsonian movements, weight gain, rash, nystagmus, hematologic abnormalities
levetiracetam (Keppra) valproic acid (Depakote) zonisamide (Zonegran) pregabalin (Lyrica)	Dizziness, drowsiness, irritability, weakness

case emergency medication must be administered. Side-rail pads are used to prevent injury to the older person. Another important nursing intervention is to carefully observe the seizure and document the progression of symptoms. Appropriate treatment is based on specific symptom progression.

A seizure that lasts more than 10 minutes or groups of seizures that occur in rapid succession and last a combined time of 30 minutes are status epilepticus, a neurologic emergency. In the event of status epilepticus, the physician should be notified, an airway should be established, and oxygen should be given. If an intravenous access is not already available, one should be started and the older person should receive 0.9% sodium chloride. The provider may prescribe medications to cease the motor movement (intravenous diazepam, lorazepam, or valproate) followed by an AED to prevent recurrence. Vital signs should be closely monitored during the entire event and vital signs are best obtained during the tonic or rest period between seizure movements. If the older person needs to be transported, only padded carts should be used because there is a great risk of a fall with the use of a wheelchair.

Patient family education is an important intervention of the nurse. Older people and families should be provided with audiovisual aids they may review at their own pace (e.g., handouts and videotapes). Identifying and avoiding precipitating factors associated with seizures should be taught, such as alcohol withdrawal, stress, and lack of sleep. It is important to emphasize taking medication correctly and the dangers of not adhering to the prescribed self-care regimen. The family should be taught what to do in the event of a seizure (lay the older person on his or her side, surround with soft objects, and do not place anything in the mouth) and how long to wait before taking the older person to the emergency department for treatment of possible status

epilepticus. For older people who suffer chronic seizures, falling is a great concern, because injury can often occur as a result of the fall. The older person should be taught to keep a seizure calendar (including date, time, duration, and specific descriptions) to assist with the treatment program. A discussion of medication adherence is important, because failure to take medications as prescribed can lead to subtherapeutic levels and trigger further seizures and status epilepticus.

Multiple Sclerosis

Multiple sclerosis (MS) is a central nervous system disease affecting the myelin sheath of the brain and spinal cord. Over time, messages cannot be transmitted smoothly, leading to muscle weakness, incoordination, visual problems, paresthesias, and memory and cognition disturbances. The exact cause of MS is unknown but it may be related to an autoimmune disorder. The disease is more common in women than men and usually begins between the ages of 20 and 40. For most people, the disease is mild but for others the symptoms progress rapidly and severely. Diagnosis is difficult, as the symptoms are vague and neurologic testing is required. The treatments include physical and occupational therapy, medications to control symptoms such as tremor (beta-blockers) and spasticity (Baclofen) and disease-modifying agents (Rebif Copaxone). Side effects of the disease-modifying agents are similar to those of the disease and include fatigue, weight gain, and tremor. Careful monitoring of the disease progression and treatment is required (National Multiple Sclerosis Society, 2008).

QSEN Recommendations Related to the Neurologic System

The Quality and Safety Education for Nurses (QSEN) project addresses the challenge of preparing future nurses with the knowledge, skills, and attitudes (KSAs) to continuously improve the quality and safety of the healthcare systems in which they work (Cronenwett et al., 2007).

See the QSEN table for tips on meeting QSEN standards.

Patient and Family Teaching

Gerontological nurses require skills and knowledge related to teaching patients and families about the key concepts of gerontology and gerontological nursing. The guidelines in the following feature will assist the nurse to assume the role of teacher and coach.

Meeting QSEN Standards: The Neurologic System

	KNOWLEDGE	SKILLS	ATTITUDES
Patient-Centered Care	Involvement of patient and family in plan of care is crucial.	Family assessment and adult learning principles.	Appreciate uniqueness of each patient/family and variability of coping and disease patterns and progression.
	Examine barriers that may keep patients from being active in formulating their plan of care.	Evaluate for depression, function, vision/hearing, cognitive status.	Provide patient-centered care to improve successful nursing outcomes.
Teamwork and Collaboration	Recognize scope of practice for interdisciplinary team members.	Use leadership skills to coordinate team and share knowledge.	Value the contribution of each member of the team to improve outcomes.
	Be aware of organizational problems that can inhibit effective team functioning. Utilize valid and reliable assessment instruments and share information during transfers/patient handoffs.	System assessment skills.	Be open to input from team members on effective means to improve communication and collaboration.
Evidence-Based Practice	Describe effective interventions to decrease neurologic risk factors and to improve the overall health and functioning of the neurologic system.	Access current evidence-based protocols to guide interventions.	Possess confidence in necessary skills to evaluate and incorporate nursing interventions from literature about the neurologic system.
Quality Improvement	Recognize the importance of measuring patient outcomes to improve patient-centered care.	Skills in data management, technology, and U.S. government and NIND websites describing current incidence and prevalence of neurologic disease.	Value the use of data and outcomes as a key component of QI efforts.
Safety	Describe common medication errors and patient/family characteristics that increase the likelihood of such errors occurring.	Use appropriate strategies to provide written information to compensate for memory loss (if present).	Appreciate the impact of cognitive loss on the occurrence of adverse drug reactions.
Informatics	Provide input into the formation and maintenance of patient databases needed for gathering QSEN data and providing patient care.	Utilize the electronic health record.	Protect patient confidentiality according to HIPAA standards.

Patient–Family Teaching Guidelines

The following are guidelines that the nurse may find useful when instructing older adults and their families about memory problems.

THE OLDER PATIENT WITH ALZHEIMER'S DISEASE

Many older patients and their families are fearful of memory loss and the possibility of developing AD. These patient–family teaching guidelines will assist the nurse in the education of older people and families regarding memory loss in later life.

1 **Sometimes I forget things. Should I be worried that I'm developing Alzheimer's disease?**

A lot of people forget things and experience memory lapses. Sometimes this is serious and sometimes it is not. Serious changes in memory accompanied by changes in personality, behavior, or the ability to care for oneself often accompany the diagnosis of dementia. Symptoms of dementia include asking the same question repeatedly; getting lost or disoriented in a familiar environment; being unable to follow directions; becoming disoriented to time and place; neglecting personal safety, hygiene, and nutrition; and being unable to manage personal affairs and finances. Alzheimer's disease is one of the many types of dementia.

RATIONALE:

Nurses can greatly assist older people and families to distinguish between benign senescence of aging (memory loss that does not affect a person or the ability to remain safe and independent) and the more serious memory loss of dementia. Supplying concrete examples of serious symptoms may help.

2 **What causes dementia or serious memory problems?**

Dementia has many causes, some of which are reversible by treatment and some of which are permanent and progressive. Some reversible conditions that may cause dementia include high fever, dehydration, vitamin deficiencies, poor nutrition, side effects of medications, thyroid conditions, head injuries, and undiagnosed serious illness like urinary tract infection or pneumonia. Sometimes older people who are depressed, bored, or worried can have memory problems. Seeing a doctor as soon as possible after the detection of memory problems can assist in the diagnosis and treatment of these reversible conditions.

RATIONALE:

Many older people and their families will try to cover up or hide memory problems because they are fearful. The nurse should reassure them that seeking medical attention can be beneficial, because some memory problems are correctable.

3 **How is the diagnosis of Alzheimer's disease confirmed?**

Your doctor will carry out a complete medical, neurologic, psychiatric, and social evaluation of your health status. Information will be gathered about your medical history, use of medications, diet, past medical problems, and general health and function. A family member should accompany you if you have problems relating specific information regarding your symptoms or past medical history. Tests of blood and urine will also be done. A CT scan may be done to examine the brain. It usually takes one or two visits to gather all of the information needed for an accurate diagnosis.

RATIONALE:

It is important to prepare the older person and the family for the intensive examinations and questioning that are needed to diagnose Alzheimer's disease. Because there are so many causes of memory problems in the older person, the diagnosis is carefully arrived at and other potential causes must be ruled out or eliminated.

4 **How is Alzheimer's disease treated?**

In the early and middle stages of Alzheimer's disease, drugs like donepezil (Aricept) and galantamine (Reminyl) are used to delay the worsening of the disease and the progression of symptoms. Medications are also used for behavioral problems like agitation, anxiety, depression, and sleep disorders. Careful use of drugs is important, and nurses will keep track of symptoms to make sure that they are improving as a result of medication administration. General health care such as diet, exercise, social activities, and memory aids such as calendars, lists of important phone numbers, and other notes about day-to-day activities can help improve the quality of life of older people with dementia.

RATIONALE:

At present, there is no cure for Alzheimer's disease but treatment is possible and can improve an older person's quality of life even in the face of this serious and debilitating illness.

5 **What can I do to prevent dementia?**

The research shows that people who remain active and engaged in life stimulate their bodies and brains to continue to function effectively. Develop hobbies and interests, enjoy your life, exercise to remain or become fit, eat a balanced diet, avoid smoking and heavy drinking, do not take unnecessary drugs, avoid stress and anxiety, and stay connected with at least

(continued)

Patient–Family Teaching Guidelines *(continued)*

one other person on a daily basis. Some physical and mental changes occur with age in healthy people; however, dementia is a disease and not a normal part of aging. Report any memory problems to your physician or nurse and seek an accurate diagnosis as soon as possible to identify reversible causes.

RATIONALE:

General health promotion activities will help to prevent disabling illness and comorbidities that can hasten or exacerbate the symptoms of memory loss or dementia. Minimizing threats to good health is always an appropriate intervention.

CARE PLAN | A Patient With a Neurologic Disorder

Case Study

Mr. Dalton is a 75-year-old man who has been admitted to the hospital. He fell in his home and suffered a fractured left hip and had an open reduction with internal fixation this morning. When Mr. Dalton first arrived, he was quiet and pleasant but now he is agitated, attempting to get out of bed, yelling, and throwing his sheets on the floor. The nurse attempts to reason with him and reassure him, but he is not responding.

Applying the Nursing Process

Assessment

The nurse suspects Mr. Dalton is delirious because his symptoms had an acute onset. Delirium poses a common and serious problem in older patients with hip fracture. Systematic determination of an older person's mental status is of major importance for early recognition and treatment of delirium. The nurse knows that delirium can be caused by any of the following factors:

- Infection
- Medications (antihistamines, anticholinergics, benzodiazepines)

- Anesthesia
- Electrolyte imbalance
- Pain
- Sleep disturbance
- Underlying dementia (diagnosed or undiagnosed)

A complete assessment of each of these factors using standardized assessment instruments is indicated while the older person is protected from injury.

Diagnosis

Nursing diagnoses that may be appropriate for Mr. Dalton include the following:

- *Confusion, Acute*
- *Fluid Volume: Imbalanced, Risk for*
- *Injury, Risk for* (due to falls)
- *Communication: Verbal, Impaired*

- *Mobility: Physical, Impaired*
- *Surgical Recovery, Delayed*
- *Pain, Acute*
- *Anxiety*
- *Fear*

NANDA-I © 2012.

Expected Outcomes

The expected outcomes for the plan of care specify that Mr. Dalton will:

- Be free from injury.

- Begin to exhibit resolution of his symptoms of delirium.
- Experience correction of the underlying mechanisms causing his delirium.

■ Receive consultation, assessment, and treatment from appropriate members of the interdisciplinary team, including physicians, nurses, physical therapists, dietitians, social workers, and others as appropriate to resolve and improve his delirium.

Planning and Implementation

The following nursing interventions may be appropriate for Mr. Dalton:

■ Establish a therapeutic relationship by being present and using gentle touch and a soft voice for communication.
■ Review all current medications.
■ Evaluate basic laboratory studies (complete blood count, serum electrolytes, and urinalysis).
■ Provide supportive and restorative care.
■ Treat behavioral symptoms.
■ Correct sensory deficits (place glasses and hearing aids if used by the older person).

■ In consultation with the physician, consider further testing as appropriate that may include chest radiology, blood culture, drug levels, serum B_{12}, thyroid function tests, pulse oximetry, electrocardiogram, brain imaging, lumbar puncture, or electroencephalogram.
■ Administer medications as ordered by the physician (haloperidol 0.5 to 2.0 mg or lorazepam 0.5 to 2.0 mg by mouth every 4 to 6 hours).
■ Reassure, educate, and involve family.
■ Maintain a quiet and peaceful environment to decrease noise stimuli to the extent possible.

Evaluation

The nurse will consider the plan a success based on the following criteria:

■ Mr. Dalton will return to normal cognitive and physical function.

■ He will be free from injury.
■ He will cooperate with a rehabilitation program and be discharged to home or a rehabilitation facility (as appropriate).

Ethical Dilemma

Mr. Dalton's daughter requests that he be restrained to prevent falls. She has seen older people with waist restraints and feels the use of this device will keep her father safe from injury. The nurse wishes to be responsive to the daughter's request, but professional standards indicate that restraints can worsen delirium and injure the older person. The ethical dilemma involves threats to the older person's and surrogate's autonomy versus nonmaleficence or the desire to do no harm. The nurse should educate and inform the daughter regarding the risks of entrapment and strangulation that accompany the use of restraints. Agitation and anxiety can be exacerbated as the older person fights to free himself from the restraints, and larger doses of medication may be needed to reduce symptoms. Physical restraints should be used cautiously (if at all) and only as a last resort. Additionally, a delirious physically restrained older person will need constant observation to prevent injury, entrapment, and strangulation.

Critical Thinking and the Nursing Process

1. How would you explain the diagnosis of Alzheimer's disease to a family?
2. What resources are available in your community or professional setting to assist older people and their families caring for a loved one with dementia?
3. Identify three major changes you would like to see implemented in your clinical agency that would facilitate the care of older people with dementia.

4. Caring for older people with cognitive impairments (dementia and delirium) can be stressful for nurses and other healthcare providers. What types of support services and resources in the clinical setting would assist you to provide the highest quality care to older people with cognitive impairments?

■ Evaluate your responses in Appendix B. ▭

Chapter Highlights

- The nursing care of patients with neurologic disorders often involves care of a person with both a memory and a movement disorder, thus ensuring patient safety while encouraging independence is a significant consideration.

- Secondary symptoms appear at various stages of illness and may resolve only because the person's condition has worsened and the individual no longer has the physical capacity to express the symptom (e.g., elopement because the person can no longer walk) or sign

(e.g., elevated temperature because the older person is too frail to mount a typical fever response).

- Some secondary symptoms cause more suffering than does the primary disorder.

- Neurologic disorders are very amenable to nursing interventions. While focusing on care rather than cure, nurses can attend to quality-of-life issues, prevent suffering, and promote positive coping.

Pearson Nursing Student Resources
Find additional review materials at
nursing.pearsonhighered.com

Prepare for success with additional NCLEX®-style practice questions, interactive assignments and activities, web links, animations and videos, and more!

References

Ala, T. A., Mattson, M. D., & Frey, W. H. (2003). The clinical diagnosis of Alzheimer's disease without the use of head imaging studies. A cliniconeuropathological study. *Journal of Alzheimer's Disease, 5*(6), 463–465.

Alzheimer's Association. (2012). *Depression and Alzheimer's.* Retrieved from http://www .alz.org/living_with_alzheimers_depression.asp

American Psychiatric Association (APA). (2012). Delirium, dementia, amnestic disorders, and other cognitive disorders. *Diagnostic and statistical manual of mental disorders, fourth edition, text revision.* Retrieved from http://www.psych.org/ MainMenu/Research/DSMIV/DSMIVTR/ DSMIVvsDSMIVTR/SummaryofText ChangesInDSMIVTR/DeliriumDementia AmnesticDisorderandOtherCognitive Disorders.aspx

American Stroke Association Healthcare Professionals Expert Panel. (2006). Guidelines for prevention of stroke in patients with ischemic stroke or transient ischemic attack. *Stroke, 37,* 577–617.

Andrew, M., Freter, S., & Rockwood, K. (2006). *Prevalance and outcomes of delirium in community and nonacute care settings in people without dementia: A report from the Canadian study of health and aging.* BMC Medicine, 4(15), 4-15.

Behrman, A. L., Light, K. E., Flynn, S. M., & Thigpen, M. T. (2002). Is the functional reach test useful for identifying falls risk among individuals with Parkinson's disease? *Archives of Physical Medicine & Rehabilitation, 83,* 538–542.

Bottrell, M. M., O'Sullivan, J. F., Robbins, M. A., Mitty, E. L., & Mezey, M. D. (2001). Transferring dying nursing home residents to the hospital: DON perspectives on the nurse's role in transfer decisions. *Geriatric Nursing, 22,* 313–317.

Brott, T., Adams, H. P., Olinger, C. P., Marler, J. R., Barsan, W. G., Biller, J., et al. (1989). Measurements of acute cerebral infarction: A clinical examination scale. *Stroke, 20,* 864–870.

Carlson, S. L., Macera, L., & Price, D. M. (2007). Treatments for seizure disorder in the elderly. *Counseling Points, 1*(2), 4–12.

Commission on Classification and Terminology of the International League Against Epilepsy. (1981). Proposal for revised clinical and electroencephalographic classification of epileptic seizures. *Epilepsia, 22*(4), 489–501.

Cotton, A. E., Fuoto, A., & Shemansky, C. (2007). Seizures in the elderly—A current overview. *Counseling Points, 1*(1), 4–12.

Cronenwett, L., Sherwood, G., Barnsteiner, J., Disch, J., Johnson, J., Mitchell, P., Sullivan, D., &

Warren, J. (2007). Quality and safety education for nurses. *Nursing Outlook, 55*(3), 122–131.

Crosby, L., & Parsons, L. C. (1989). Clinical neurologic assessment tool: Development and testing of an instrument to index neurologic status. *Heart and Lung, 18,* 121–129.

Davis, N., Hendrix, C., & Superville, J. (2011). Supportive approaches for Alzheimer disease. *The Nurse Practitioner, (36)*8, 22–29.

Doerflinger, D. M. C. (2007). Mental status testing of older adults: The Mini-Cog. *Try this: Best practices in nursing care to older adults* (No. 3). Hartford Institute for Geriatric Nursing. Retrieved from http://consultgerirn .org/uploads/File/trythis/try_this_3.pdf

Ely, E. W., Inouye, S. K., Bernard, G. R., Gordon, S., Francis, J., May, L., . . . Dittus, R. (2001). Delirium in mechanically ventilated patients: Validity and reliability of the confusion assessment method for the intensive care unit (CAM-ICU). *Journal of the American Medical Association, 286*(21), 2703–2710.

Factora, R., & Luciano, M. (2008). When to consider normal pressure hydrocephalus in the patient with gait disturbance. *Geriatrics, 63*(2), 32–37.

Fong, T., Tulebaev, S., & Inouye, S. (2009). Delirium in elderly adults: Diagnosis, prevention and treatment. *National Review of Neurology, 5*(10), 2010–2020.

Gillick, M. R. (2002). Do we need to create geriatric hospitals? *Journal of the American Geriatrics Society, 50,* 174–177.

Gross, R., Siderowf, A., & Hurtig, H. (2007). Cognitive impairment in Parkinson's disease and dementia with Lewy Bodies: A spectrum of disease. *Neurosignals, 16,* 24–34.

Holzer, C., & Warshaw, G. A. (2002). Perioperative care and hospital care. In R. J. Ham, P. D. Sloane, & G. A. Warshaw (Eds.), *Primary care geriatrics, A care-based approach* (4th ed., pp. 183–197). St. Louis, MO: Mosby.

Honea, R., Swerdlow, R., Vidoni, E., Goodwin, J., & Burns, J. (2010). Reduced gray matter volume in normal adults with a maternal family history of Alzheimer disease. *Neurology, 74*(2), 113–120.

Huether, S., & McCance, K. (2011). *Understanding pathophysiology.* St. Louis, MO: Mosby.

Hurley, A. C., Gauthier, M. A., Horvath, K. J., Harvey, R., Smith, S. J., Trudeau, S. A., et al. (2004). Promoting safer home environments for persons with Alzheimer's disease. *Journal of Gerontological Nursing, 30*(6), 43–51.

Hurley, A. C., & Volicer, L. (2002). Alzheimer's disease. It's okay, Mama, if you want to go, it's okay. *Journal of the American Medical Association, 288,* 2324–2332.

Ingersoll, G. L., & Leyden, D. B. (1994). The Glasgow Coma Scale for patients with head injuries. *Critical Care Nurse, 7*(5), 26–32.

Inouye, S., van Dyck, C., Alessi, C., Balkin, S., Siegal, A., & Horwitz, R. (1990). Clarifying confusion: The confusion assessment method. A new method for the detection of delirium. *Annals of Internal Medicine, 113*(12), 941–948.

Kennedy, G. J. (2006, April). Therapeutic approaches to combating Alzheimer's disease. *Alzheimer's Disease Early Intervention for Optimal Management* (a supplement to the *Clinical Advisor*), pp. 15–20.

Lee, T., & Kolasa, K. (2011). Feeding the person with late stage Alzheimer's disease. *Nutrition Today, 46*(2), 75–79.

Lee-Frye, B. (2010). Sleep disorders and Alzheimer's disease. *About.com.* Retrieved from http://alzheimers.about.com/lw/ Health-Medicine/Conditions-and-diseases/Sleep-Disorders-and-Alzheimers-Disease.htm

Mahoney E. K., Volicer, L., & Hurley, A. C. (2000a). Introduction. In E. K. Mahoney, L. Volicer, & A. C. Hurley (Eds.), *Management of challenging behaviors in dementia* (pp. 1–9). Baltimore, MD: Health Professions Press.

Mahoney, E. K., Volicer, L., & Hurley, A. C. (2000b). *Management of challenging behaviors in dementia.* Baltimore, MD: Health Professions Press.

Mattson, M. (2004). Infectious agents and age-related neurodegenerative disorders. *Aging Research Reviews, 3*(1), 105–120.

Mayo Clinic. (2010). *Lewy body dementia.* Retrieved from http://www.mayoclinic .com/health/lewy-body-dementia/DS00795/ DSECTION=treatments-and-drugs

McBride, K. L., White, C. L., Sourial, R., & Mayo, N. (2004). Postdischarge nursing interventions for stroke survivors and their families. *Journal of Advanced Nursing, 47,* 192–200.

McGuinness, B. (2009). Statins do not help reduce Alzheimer's disease. *Cochrane Review.* Retrieved from http://www.medicalnewstoday .com/releases/146041.php

McKhann, G., Knopman, D., Chertkow, H., Hyman, B., Clifford, R., Kawas, C., Klunk, W., Koroshetz, W., Manly, J., Mayeux, R., Mohs, R., Morris, J., Rossor, M., Schettens, P., Carrillo, M., Thies, B., Weintraub, S. & Phelps, C. (2011). The diagnosis of dementia due to Alzheimer's disease: Recommendations from the National Institute on Aging–Alzheimer's Association workgroups on diagnostic guidelines for Alzheimer's disease. *Alzheimer's and Dementia.* Retrieved from http://www.alzheimersanddementia.com/ article/S1552 5260(11)00101-4/fulltext

McPhee, S., & Papadakis, M. (2011). *Current medical diagnosis and treatment.* New York, NY: McGraw-Hill Medical.

Mgekn, I., Quinn, R., & Tabet, N. (2008). No evidence of the efficacy of vitamin E for people suffering from Alzheimer's disease and mild cognitive impairment. *Cochrane Summaries.* Retrieved from http://summaries.cochrane.org/CD002854/ no-evidence-of-the-efficacy-of-vitamin-e-for-people-suffering-from-alzheimers-disease-ad-and-mild-cognitive-impairment-mci

Mok, V. C., Wong, A., Lam, W. W., Fan, Y. H., Tang, W. K., Kwok, T., et al. (2004). Cognitive impairment and functional outcome after stroke associated with small vessel disease. *Journal of Neurology, Neurosurgery & Psychiatry, 75,* 560–566.

Mosconi, L., Glodzik, L., Mistur, R., McHugh, P., Rich, K., Javier, E., Williams, S., Pirraglia, El, DeSanti, S., Mehta, P., Zinkowski, R., Blennow, K., Pratico, D., & de Leon, M. (2010). Oxidative stress and amyloid-beta pathology in normal individuals with a maternal history of Alzheimer's. *Biological Psychiatry, 68*(10), 913–921.

National Institute on Aging. (2012). *2010 Alzheimer's disease progress report: A deeper understanding.* Retrieved from http://www.nia .nih.gov/alzheimers/publication/2010-alzheimers-disease-progress-report-deeper-understanding

National Institutes of Health. (2006). *Plaques and tangles: The hallmark of AD.* Alzheimer's Disease Education and Referral Center. Retrieved from http://www.nia.nih.gov/NR/

rdonlyres/F562167C-D864-4C02-8636-E01AD2C66312/2401/tangles_big1.jpg

National Multiple Sclerosis Society. (2008). *Medications used in MS.* Retrieved from http:// www.nationalmssociety.org/about-multiple-sclerosis/treatments/medications/index.aspx

Nir, Z., Zolotogorsky, Z., & Sugarman, H. (2004). Structured nursing intervention versus routine rehabilitation after stroke. *American Journal of Physical Medicine & Rehabilitation, 83,* 522–529.

Nurse Practitioners' Prescribing Reference. (2012). New York, NY: Haymarket Media.

Parkinson's Study Group. (2000). A randomized controlled trial comparing pramipexole with levodopa in early Parkinson's disease: Design and methods of the CALM-PD Study. *Clinical Neuropharmacology, 23,* 34–44.

Reuben, D., Herr, K., Pacala, J., Pollock, B., Potter, J., & Semla, T. (2011). *Geriatrics at your fingertips.* New York, NY: American Geriatrics Society.

Robinson, E. (2002). An ethical analysis of cardiopulmonary resuscitation for elders in acute care. *AACN Clinical Issues, 13*(1), 132–144.

Sam, S., & Frohman, L. A. (2008). Normal physiology of hypothalamic pituitary regulation. *Endocrinology and Metabolism Clinics, 37*(1), 1–22.

Schultz, S. K., Ellingrod, V. L., Turvey, C., Moser, D. J., & Arndt, S. (2003). The influence of cognitive impairment and behavioral dysregulation on daily functioning in the nursing home setting. *American Journal of Psychiatry, 160,* 582–584.

Szekely, C. A., Breitner, J. C. S., & Fitzpatrick, A. L. (2008). NSAID use and dementia risk in the cardiovascular health study. *Neurology, 70*(1), 17–24.

Trudeau, S. A. (1999). Prevention of physical limitations in advanced Alzheimer's disease. In L. Volicer & L. Bloom-Charette (Eds.), *Enhancing quality of life for persons with advanced Alzheimer's disease* (pp. 80–90). Philadelphia, PA: Taylor & Francis.

U.S. Department of Health & Human Services. (2010). *Progress report on Alzheimer's disease.* Retrieved from http://www.nia.nih.gov/alzheimers/ publication/2010-alzheimers-disease-progress-report-deeper-understanding

Volicer, L., Mahoney, E., & Brown, E. J. (1998). Nonpharmacological approaches to the management of the behavioral consequences of advanced dementia. In M. Kaplan & S. B. Hoffman (Eds.), *Behaviors in dementia: Best practices for successful management* (pp. 155–176). Baltimore, MD: Health Professions Press.

CHAPTER
23

The Immune System

Gail A. Harkness, DRPH, RN, FAAN
PROFESSOR EMERITUS, UNIVERSITY OF CONNECTICUT

KEY TERMS

antibody *652*

antigens *652*

autoimmunity *651*

cell-mediated immune response *652*

granulocytes *652*

histocompatibility antigens *652*

humoral immune response *652*

hypersensitivity *655*

immune deficiency *651*

immune dysregulation *651*

immunoenhancing drugs *668*

immunoglobulins *652*

immunosenescence *654*

lymphocytes *652*

macrophages *652*

memory *652*

monocytes *652*

primary immune response *653*

nosocomial infections *668*

secondary immune response *653*

self-recognition *651*

specificity *652*

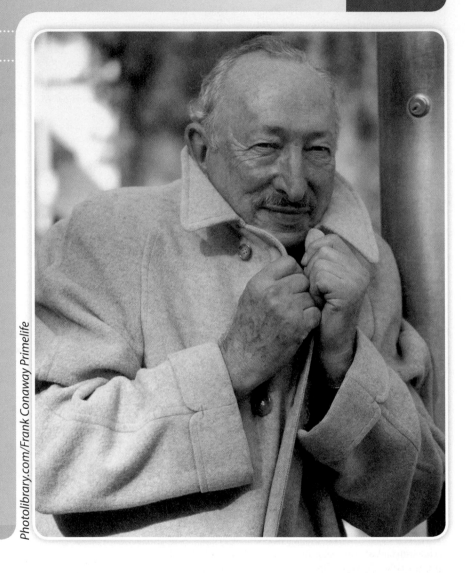

Photolibrary.com/Frank Conaway Primelife

LEARNING OUTCOMES

On completion of this chapter, the reader will be able to:

1. Define the role of the immune system in the maintenance of health.

2. Describe the three unique characteristics of the immune system.

3. Identify factors that affect proper immune system function.

4. Distinguish the similarities, differences, and interactions among the humoral immune response and the cellular immune response.

5. Associate the pathology that underlies illnesses associated with both excessive and deficient immune responses.

6. Outline the unique characteristics associated with HIV infection in the older person.

7. Relate the care of the patient with a rheumatoid disorder to the pathology involved.

8. Explain the physiological processes that increase the susceptibility of the older person to infections.

9. Identify nursing interventions that can be effective in improving immune status in the older person.

hree major biological defense mechanisms protect the human body from injurious chemicals, foreign bodies, microorganisms, and parasites. The first line of defense is the physical, anatomical, and biochemical barriers provided by our skin and the mucous membranes that line our digestive, respiratory, urinary, and reproductive tracts. Viruses, bacteria, fungi, parasites, chemicals, and foreign bodies must penetrate these barriers to harm the individual. The second line of defense is often called the "innate" immune system because it is present from birth in all animals. It includes mechanical clearance, such as sloughing of the skin, the actions of the respiratory cilia, mucous secretions, vomiting, defecation, and urination. These actions prevent substances from entering the body or assists in expelling them. The inflammatory response is also part of the second line of defense. It is evoked immediately at the site of entry when external barriers are breached. Fluids, cells, and body secretions attempt to isolate, neutralize, destroy, and remove the invaders by surrounding the affected area (see the Components of the Immune System section below). These first two lines of defense target all invaders, and therefore are nonspecific defense mechanisms (Huether & McCance, 2009; Sompayrac, 2012).

The third line of defense is the immune response or the "adaptive" immune system, a highly complicated, integrated system that is controlled by a complex communication mechanism. The immune system is briefly reviewed here. Anatomy and physiology or pathophysiology textbooks should be accessed for more detailed information.

The Immune System

Although the immune response occurs more slowly in the older adult than the middle-aged or young adult, it has the capability to confer long-term and, sometimes, permanent protection against living organisms such as bacteria, viruses, and parasites. It also protects the body from its own cancer cells. It is a diverse and complicated system made up of interrelated parts that function as a whole. The immune system includes the thymus gland, red bone marrow, spleen, lymph nodes, lymph vessels, lymphatic tissues, and skin. Cells belonging to the immune system are carried throughout the body by the blood and lymphatic fluids. Anything that is not a normal part of the body is identified, and the invader is blocked from entering the body, attacked, chemically neutralized, or destroyed, leaving the normal tissues of the body undisturbed.

Multiple factors affect the individual's immune system; some factors can be modified by healthcare interventions,

and some cannot. The internal characteristics of the individual include factors such as age, gender, and inherited genetic sequence. These factors are permanent characteristics and cannot be modified. However, other internal factors such as nutritional status and existence of underlying disease potentially can be modified through primary and secondary interventions. External factors also can have a substantial effect on a person's immune system. These include environmental pollutants, radiation, ultraviolet light, and drugs. If known, exposure to external factors can be modified by healthcare professionals. The intensity and effectiveness of any immune response depends on the combination of all characteristics of the individual's immune system, especially when a challenge to the immune system occurs. Occasionally, the immune system needs to be suppressed, such as after organ transplantation. Also, a person's immune system may overreact to a substance, and allergies or hypersensitivities result.

The Immune Theory of Aging

The immune theory is one of multiple theories of aging. It proposes that the normal process of aging in humans and animals is related to altered immunological processes in all body tissues that have developed over a lifetime. There are three major components of this theory: autoimmunity, immune deficiency, and immune dysregulation. **Autoimmunity,** a misdirected immune process that produces antibodies against the body itself, occurs as a person ages and the ability of the immune system to differentiate between invaders and normal tissues diminishes. As a result, immune cells begin to attack normal body tissues, causing conditions that are often associated with aging, such as arthritis in joints. Heredity is a major factor in autoimmunity, as are exposures to biological and environmental stressors.

It is believed that **immune deficiency** occurs with increasing age, resulting in more difficulty defending the body from foreign invaders. Also, the changes in the immune system may disrupt the regulation between the multiple components of the immune process; this is **immune dysregulation.** The result is progressive destruction of the body cells. The decline in immune response, the association of this decline with specific diseases such as cancer, and the increased production of substances that attack body tissues are arguments in favor of immune theories of aging.

Characteristics Unique to the Immune System

Three characteristics are unique to the immune system: self-recognition, specificity, and memory. In **self-recognition** (tolerance), the immune system differentiates between substances that are normal constituents of a person's body and those that are not. A wide range of substances that are identified as "non-self" and stimulate an immune response are called **antigens.** Antigens are large protein or polysaccharide molecules found on the surfaces of living cells such as viruses, bacteria, fungi, or parasites. They are also on environmental substances such as pollen and foods, and on drugs, vaccines, transfusions, and transplanted tissues. Some types of cancer cells have surface molecules that are identified as foreign, and these will also stimulate an immune response.

Self-antigens on body cells will not stimulate an immune reaction. These are found on the surface of almost every cell of the body. These self-antigens are called **histocompatibility antigens,** or human leukocyte antigens (HLAs). Each person has HLA proteins on his or her body cells that are different from those of all other people. Exceptions occur with genetically identical twins. With some abnormalities, however, the immune system will attack self-antigens and an autoimmune condition, such as rheumatoid arthritis, will occur.

Specificity means that the immune response reacts only to one antigen. Each time a new antigen is identified, a different immune response is stimulated. For example, an immune response against chickenpox will not confer immunity against any other disease. The immune response results in production of antigen-specific glycoprotein molecules called antibodies that attach to the antigen and render it harmless.

Memory means that the immune system has the capacity to develop long-lasting protection against specific invaders. A residual set of cells that are specific to each antigen remains in the body, to be stimulated when the antigen presents itself at a later time. Each successive time the antigen is encountered, a quicker and more intense reaction is stimulated by the immune system in the healthy older person.

Components of the Immune Response

White blood cells are associated with both inflammation and the immune response. The three primary types of white blood cells are granulocytes, monocytes, and lymphocytes. **Granulocytes** ingest and digest debris and foreign material throughout the body and release powerful chemicals such as histamine and heparin that assist in the inflammatory process. **Monocytes** become large phagocytic cells, or **macrophages,** when stimulated by chemicals released by the body, and play an important part

in inflammation by removing cellular debris in order to stimulate healing.

Lymphocytes are the primary cells concerned with the development of immunity. Of all white blood cells, only lymphocytes have the ability for self-recognition, specificity, and memory. They arise from undifferentiated stem cells in the bone marrow, liver, and spleen. To become mature cells that can elicit an immune response, lymphocytes must pass through lymphoid tissue in various parts of the body. In doing so, they are committed to one of two types of lymphocytes: B or T lymphocytes. Cells destined to become B lymphocytes (B cells) mature in the bone marrow and migrate to the lymphatic system. When mature B lymphocytes come in contact with antigens, they are stimulated to become mature plasma cells and secrete antibodies to counteract the antigen. This reaction is called the **humoral immune response.** Cells destined to become T lymphocytes (T cells) migrate through the thymus gland when the person is very young. When mature T lymphocytes come in contact with antigens, the lymphocyte attacks the antigen directly. This reaction is called the **cell-mediated immune response.**

Humoral Immune Response

The humoral immune response is initiated when an antigen binds with **antibody** receptors on the surface of the mature B cell. This triggers a sequence of events, including assistance from helper T cells, resulting in production of plasma cells that secrete antibodies (immunoglobulin molecules). These antibodies are specific to the antigen that initially bound to the B-cell surface receptors. Also, memory cells are produced that live for months or years and can react swiftly when the antigen once again presents itself.

There are five classes of **immunoglobulins:** IgG, IgA, IgM, IgD, and IgE (Table 23-1). The classes of immunoglobulins differ in antigenic properties, structure, and function. The antibodies function in a number of ways to enhance the removal of antigens from the body. These functions are precipitation, agglutination, neutralization, opsonization, and complement activation.

Antibodies and antigens bind together (agglutination) to form large insoluble complexes (immune complexes) that fall out of body fluids (precipitation) (Figure 23-1 ▶▶▶). Phagocytic cells, such as macrophages, can find these complexes easily and then engulf and destroy them. Antibodies also can inactivate an antigen (neutralization) by binding with it before it can interact with body cells. Some antibodies can coat the foreign antigen (opsonization) and

TABLE 23-1	Characteristics of Immunoglobulins
Class	**Characteristics**
IgG	Approximately 75% to 80% of total; four subclasses
	Present in serum, interstitial fluid, and amniotic fluid
	Crosses placenta; protects newborns
	Responsible for most of the antibody functions; activates complement
	Enhances phagocytosis
IgA	Approximately 15% of total; two subclasses
	Present in serum, tears, saliva, and body secretions from the pulmonary system, vagina, gastrointestinal tract, and other areas
	Prevents attachment and invasion of pathogens through mucosal membranes
	Passes to neonate through breast milk
IgM	Approximately 10% of total; largest immunoglobulin
	Present in serum; activates complement
	First antibody produced during the initial response to antigen
	Forms antibodies for ABO blood antigens
IgD	Less than 1% present in serum and umbilical cord
	Located on surfaces of developing B lymphocytes
	Action is relatively unknown
IgE	Less than 1% of circulating antibodies
	Present in serum and tissues
	Principal antibody in allergic reactions; combats parasitic infestations

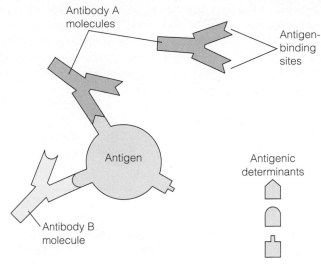

Figure 23-1 ►►► Antigen–antibody reaction.

make it more susceptible to phagocytosis. Many bacteria produce toxins that can harm the older person who may become septic as a result of systemic infection. Antibodies produced against these toxins function as antitoxins that neutralize the bacterial toxins. Antibodies also protect people against some viral infections by preventing the attachment and entrance of viral cells into body cells. Neutralized viral particles may agglutinate or be ingested and destroyed by phagocytes. However, many viruses do not circulate in the bloodstream where antibodies are plentiful. Instead, they enter cells and spread by cell-to-cell contact (Huether & McCance, 2009).

The antigen–antibody complexes also trigger the complement system, which consists of approximately 25 plasma proteins that normally circulate inactivated in the bloodstream. The plasma proteins work together to "complement" the action of antibodies in destroying bacteria. When an antibody locks into an antigen, a series of steps called the complement cascade is initiated. The result is dilatation of blood vessels and stimulation of the inflammatory response. Leukocytes are drawn to the antigen site, and the destruction of abnormal cells is increased.

The body has many weapons when mounting a primary immune response. Figure 23-2 ►►► illustrates various immune responses when a virus is threatening to invade the body's defenses.

Primary and Secondary Immune Responses

The characteristic of memory is involved in both primary and secondary immune responses (Figure 23-3 ►►►). The first exposure to the foreign antigen results from active infection or immunization, and a **primary immune response** begins. A latent period occurs initially, during which no antibodies can be detected.

With a second exposure, however, the **secondary immune response** is evoked. Due to presence of memory cells, there is a more rapid production of large amounts of antibodies than occurred in the primary immune response. IgG is the predominant type of antibody associated with the secondary immune response, although IgM is also produced. The production of these antibodies is immediate, and high levels may last for several years. The characteristics of the primary and secondary

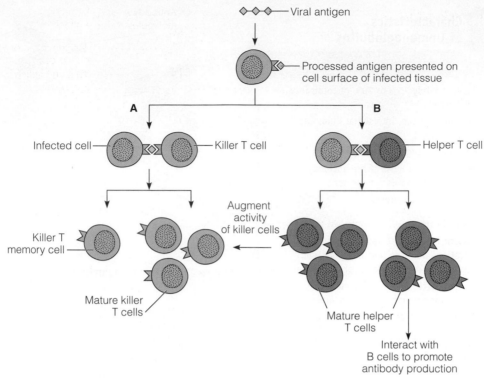

Figure 23-2 ▶▶▶ Various mechanisms of the primary immune response.

Source: National Institute of Allergy and Infectious Diseases (2007).

response allow clinicians to determine the individual's stage of an infectious disease by evaluating a series of antibody titers for a specific antigen such as those obtained in a hepatitis panel.

Cell-Mediated Immune Response

During the process of maturation in the thymus gland, T cells begin producing several types of new proteins that become attached to the surface of the T cell. The two major types of mature T cells are helper T (Th) cells and cytotoxic (Tc) cells. Helper (Th) cells have CD4 proteins on their surface. When presented with an antigen, helper T cells produce signaling substances such as interleukin, interferon, and tumor necrosis factor. These stimulate other T cells and B cells in such a way that inflammation and other body activities are promoted.

The humoral and cell-mediated immune responses are complex and interdependent. A highly regulated communication system with a series of positive and negative feedback systems regulates and coordinates the immune response so that normal body tissues are not injured. These regulatory functions can be affected by the aging process and the presence of chronic disease.

Normal Changes of Aging

Generally, aging is associated with physiological changes that cause stiffness or rigidity and decreased levels of functioning in many systems. As a result, it is difficult to differentiate age changes that occur simultaneously in organs throughout the body from specific changes in the immune system. Aging is the result of a lifetime of cumulative effects of environmental exposures, such as sunlight, radiation, pesticides, and other chemicals, as well as a lifetime of exposure to illness and stress.

One of the most important biological changes occurring during human aging is a progressive decrease in immune functioning, or **immunosenescence.** Since regulatory mechanisms also are diminished, the activation of the immune response is inefficient and poorly controlled. This increases risk for infectious, autoimmune, neoplastic, cardiovascular, and neurodegenerative diseases and other disorders.

Older individuals have more variation in the effectiveness of their immune system than younger people. However, data that compare the function of the immune

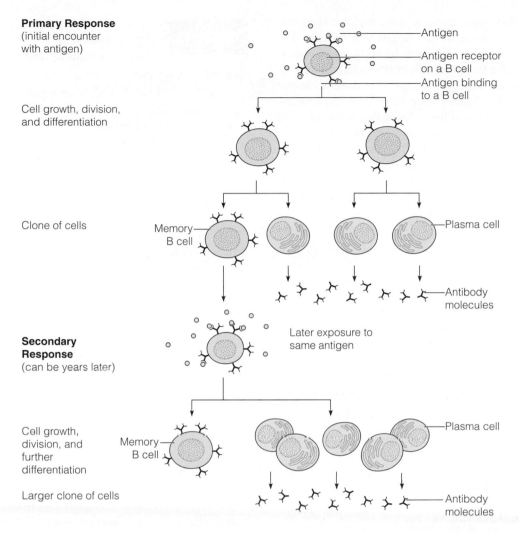

Primary Response
(initial encounter
with antigen)

Antigen

Antigen receptor
on a B cell

Antigen binding
to a B cell

Cell growth, division,
and differentiation

Clone of cells

Memory
B cell

Plasma cell

Antibody
molecules

**Secondary
Response**
(can be years later)

Later exposure to
same antigen

Cell growth,
division, and
further
differentiation

Memory
B cell

Plasma cell

Larger clone of cells

Antibody
molecules

Figure 23-3 ▶▶▶ Primary and secondary immune responses.

Source: National Institute of Allergy and Infectious Diseases (2007).

system between the young and old often conflict. Some older people show relatively little change, and others are severely compromised. There is a trend, however. As the age of a population increases, the proportion of people with declining humoral and cellular immune function increases (National Institute of Allergy and Infectious Diseases [NIAID] & National Cancer Institute [NCI], 2007). Within the individual, there is a decrease in the speed, strength, and duration of both the immune response and the regulation of immune activities.

A decreased ability to respond to antigenic stimulation by B lymphocytes is a common characteristic of the aging humoral immune system. Although the secondary immune response of the humoral (B-cell) immune system may be normal due to the presence of memory cells, the response to new antigens is decreased. More antigenic material may

be needed to prompt antibody production, and the production is slower. A lower peak antibody concentration may occur, and antibody levels decline faster as the person ages. As a result, risk of an insufficient humoral immune system response increases with the age at which antigens are first encountered.

Over time, the secondary immune response may also show changes. The number of B cells in the circulation decreases in some individuals. As a result, tissues are slower to repair and are more vulnerable to disease, especially infections. A decline in the production of IgE leads to a decrease in allergic or **hypersensitivity** reactions. An increase in antibody production that reacts against the person's own body cells also may occur, contributing to the development of autoimmune diseases such as rheumatoid arthritis. All changes in B cells develop slowly until the age of 60, when they begin to occur more rapidly. Therefore, in general, vaccinations should be given by the age of 60 to have the greatest effectiveness; however, exceptions to this rule exist. For example, vaccination with pneumococcal vaccine is recommended at age 65 with revaccination recommended after 5 years if the initial dose was administered before age 60, or if the individual was less than age 65 at the time of the first vaccination (Centers for Disease Control and Prevention [CDC], 2011).

There is consensus among investigators that normal aging, when no pathological conditions exist, is associated with diminished responses by the cell-mediated immune system, particularly with the T lymphocytes when the body is exposed to some antigens. T lymphocytes mature in the thymus, which begins to shrink after adolescence. By middle age, it is only about 15% of its maximum size. This is regarded as a key age-related factor in the gradual reduction in effectiveness of the immune system (National Library of Medicine [NLM], 2012). A decrease in T-cell proliferation leads to reductions in all the subsequent parts of the immune response. Cell secretions such as interleukin-2 decline. The ratio of helper T cells (CD4) and cytotoxic T cells (CD8) to other T cells is often reduced. There is a slower response to delayed hypersensitivity reactions, and regulation of the immune system is impaired. As a result, the incidence of infectious diseases, cancer, and autoimmune diseases increases. A summary of age-related changes in the immune system is found in Box 23-1. Figure 23-4 ▶▶▶ illustrates the structures of the immune system and normal changes associated with aging.

Factors Affecting Aging of the Immune System

Many factors directly or indirectly associated with aging can affect the immune system. These factors include stress, chronic illness, exercise, and dietary nutrients.

Stress

Stress initiates a physiological fight-or-flight response that evolved over time as a result of threats to one's physical well-being. However, people now rarely encounter the type of stress that predators or natural disasters evoked in our ancestors. Instead, psychological threats that come from worrying about bills, work, or relationships, or traumatic experiences from the distant past, trigger a chronic fight-or-flight response. The extent to which this type of stress has affected the immune system, and its relationship to disease susceptibility, remains under investigation.

Older people are at a higher risk for acute and chronic diseases in which the aging immune system may play a role. It is generally believed that the stress response, resulting

---

> ### BOX 23-1 ▶ Aging Influences on the Immune System
>
> - Overall decrease in:
>   - Speed and strength of the immune response.
>   - Neuroendocrine regulation of immune activities.
> - Decrease in humoral immunity:
>   - The B-cell response to new antigenic stimulation decreases.
>   - The number of B cells in the circulation decreases.
>   - The production of IgE declines.
>   - Antibody production against self increases, which contributes to development of autoimmune diseases.
>   - The humoral immunity decrease is slow until the age of 60, then occurs more rapidly.
> - Decrease in cellular immunity:
>   - The key factor in the gradual reduction in effectiveness of the immune system is diminished proliferative responses by T lymphocytes.
>   - Reductions in all the subsequent parts of the immune response occur.
>   - Cell secretions such as interleukin-2 decline.
>   - Helper T cells (CD4) and cytotoxic T cells (CD8) are often reduced in their ratio to other T cells.
>   - There is slower response to delayed hypersensitivity reactions.
> - Regulation of the immune system is impaired.

---

in sympathetic nervous system stimulation and hormonal changes, can suppress the immune system in older adults. In some illnesses, such as respiratory infections, a short-term change in immune function may be all that is required to increase susceptibility. However, since chronic diseases often take years to develop, it may also take many years of stress-induced alterations of the immune system to affect the progress and severity of chronic diseases such as cardiovascular disease or cancer.

The cumulative effect of stress over time most likely contributes to the physical aging of the immune system and associated effects on health. Individuals who characteristically react more strongly to stress may have greater stress-related effects over the course of their lives. Older people often have increased psychosocial stressors such as caring for an infirm spouse or partner. High levels of stress and social isolation have been reported among caregivers of dementia patients. The stress that accompanies this kind of caregiving has been equated to multiple and severe long-term stressors. However, every individual has a different exposure to the type, frequency, intensity, and duration of stressful events in everyday life. This is a major factor in the heterogeneity demonstrated in the variation of effectiveness of immune systems in older people.

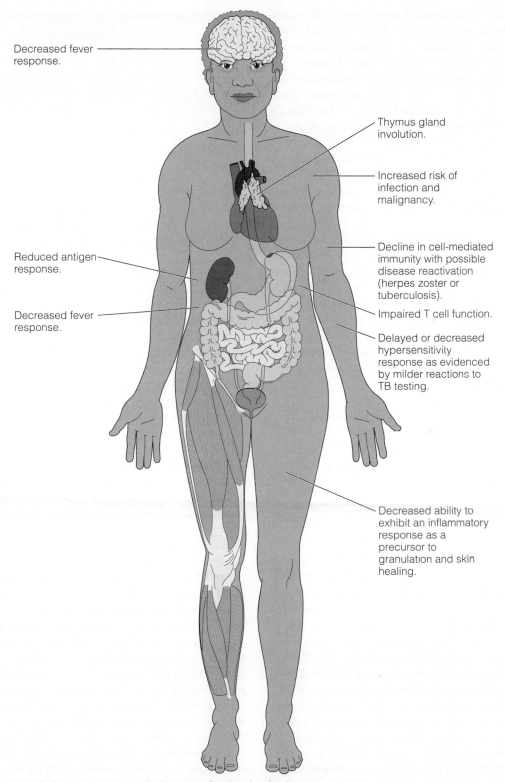

Decreased fever response.

Thymus gland involution.

Increased risk of infection and malignancy.

Reduced antigen response.

Decline in cell-mediated immunity with possible disease reactivation (herpes zoster or tuberculosis).

Impaired T cell function.

Decreased fever response.

Delayed or decreased hypersensitivity response as evidenced by milder reactions to TB testing.

Decreased ability to exhibit an inflammatory response as a precursor to granulation and skin healing.

Figure 23-4 ▶▶▶ Normal changes of aging in the immune system.

An increase in the amount of stress perceived by individuals is generally associated with poorer cellular immunity. However, this relationship is modified by the amount and type of coping used by the individual. Coping styles are likely to differ among individuals, even when faced with a similar stressful situation. Successful coping strategies deal with the perceived cause of the stress. This includes an increased awareness of the problem, obtaining and processing information about the problem, and carrying out a new series of actions to address the problem that leads to a peaceful resolution (Seaward, 2012). This process of active coping can have positive effects on immune function, particularly at high stress levels (Kemeny & Schedlowski, 2007).

Psychoneuroimmunology studies the interaction between psychological processes and the nervous and immune systems of the human body. There is now sufficient data to conclude that the immune system is modified by psychosocial stressors that can lead to actual health changes. Changes related to infectious disease and wound healing have provided the strongest evidence, but it is believed that diverse conditions and diseases could result from increased stress. Negative emotions over time may lead to immune dysregulation.

> **Practice Pearl** ▶▶▶ If older adults have assistance coping with stress-inducing events, such as death of a spouse, for a period of approximately 6 months after the event, resolution and stabilization of the immune system is likely to occur.

Chronic Illness

The central nervous system, the immune system, the endocrine system, and the psyche are interrelated. Aberrations in one system can adversely affect another system. Lymphocytes have receptors on their surface for many neuroendocrine hormones that consequently have regulatory effects on the lymphocytes. Mood, stress, depression, and mental illness influence the immune system. For example, patients with schizophrenia have increased presence of autoantibodies and decreased immune responses to antigens. Patients with systemic lupus erythematosus, an autoimmune disease, are associated with a psychosis that has symptoms similar to those seen in patients with schizophrenia (NLM, 2012). Several feedback systems between the central nervous and immune systems exist. For example, an antigen induces the production of interleukin-1, which increases levels of glucocorticoids. The glucocorticoids, in turn, inhibit the production of interleukin-1.

Improving the Immune Response

Lifestyle strategies, such as physical exercise and nutrition, improve the functions of immune cells, leading to increased longevity. However, there is still a lack of understanding about the processes by which this occurs.

Exercise

In healthy older adults, regular exercise of moderate intensity appears to boost the immune system. Exercise helps to offset diminished immune responses and chronic inflammation, and those who exercise are less likely to develop an infection than their sedentary counterparts. The age-related decline in the immune response may be prevented or slowed by exercise, and it is particularly effective in slowing the decline in cell-mediated immunity. Long-term, moderate physical activity appears to be associated with several benefits for the older adult. In addition to reduction in infectious disease risk, benefits include increased rates of vaccine efficacy, reduction of inappropriate inflammation such as within arteries, increased wound healing, and improvements in both physical and psychosocial aspects of daily living. Although long-term, moderate exercise appears to affect multiple components of the immune response, including both cellular and humoral immune responses, the underlying mechanisms remain to be identified (Friedrich, 2008; Senchina & Kohut, 2007). The type of exercise (aerobic or resistance), the amount of exercise, and the characteristics of the populations who will benefit the most from exercise, are still under study. Nevertheless, moderate physical activity performed on a regular basis does seem to decrease immunosenescence, and an increase in physical activity programs by the healthcare community can result in improved health for the older adult.

Tai chi is a popular, moderate Chinese exercise that has beneficial effects on the immune system as well as other body systems. Various studies in China have found that practicing tai chi has an impact on circulating levels of IgG and IgM. Yang et al. (2008) at the University of Illinois investigated whether 5 months of tai chi and qigong practice could improve the immune response to influenza vaccine in older adults when compared with controls who were not practicing tai chi. Subjects received influenza vaccine during the first week of intervention. Blood samples were then collected 3, 6, and 20 weeks after administration of the influenza vaccine and analyzed for signs of antibody response. The findings indicate a significant increase in the magnitude and duration of the antibody response to the influenza vaccine in the tai chi group compared to controls. Other studies have found beneficial effects of improved muscle strength and flexibility from practicing tai chi in balance control, prevention of falls, and in the treatment of chronic diseases such as rheumatoid arthritis, chronic heart failure, Parkinson's disease, and Alzheimer's disease.

> **Practice Pearl** ▶▶▶ Regular, moderate exercise, as appropriate for the individual older person, may reduce signs of aging and promote the health of the immune system. Urge active older adults to continue appropriate exercise and urge those who are inactive to consult with their primary healthcare provider for recommendations on how to begin an exercise program.

Nutrients and Herbal Remedies

Adequate intake of vitamins and trace elements is required for the immune system to function effectively. However, deficiencies of vitamins and trace elements are observed in almost one third of all older adults, inducing low immune responses and increasing susceptibility to infections. Vitamins A, C, D, E, B_6, folate, B_{12}, iron, copper, selenium, and zinc all contribute to the cellular immune response. Vitamins A and D play important roles in both the cellular and humoral antibody response (Wintergerst, Maggini, & Hornig, 2007). Studies suggest that supplements containing micronutrients that approximate the recommended dietary allowances improve delayed-type hypersensitivity and assist in preventing infections.

The prevalence of vitamin D deficiency is rising worldwide, but the condition remains undiagnosed and untreated in the vast majority of people. While current evidence overwhelmingly indicates that supplemental doses greater than 800 International Units per day have beneficial effects on the musculoskeletal system, evidence is also accumulating on the beneficial effects of vitamin D in improving the health of the immune system. Wimalawansa (2012) states that most older adults need vitamin D supplementation ranging from 600 to 2,000 International Units per day.

Zinc is a micronutrient that helps maintain many body homeostatic mechanisms, including the effectiveness of the immune system. Zinc is required for proper production of many enzymes and proteins in the body, and for cellular proliferation. However, mild zinc deficiency is prevalent in the older population, with intake below 50% of the recommended daily allowance on a given day. Zinc deficiency results in impaired immune response and, subsequently, degenerative diseases develop (Mocchegiani et al., 2012). Multiple studies have evaluated zinc supplementation and its effect on the immune system. Supplementation improved selected components of the cellular immune system and decreased respiratory infections. Zinc should be administered with caution, however. High doses of zinc can cause toxicity, copper deficiency, and immunosuppression.

Some older adults taking zinc supplements also take copper supplements to prevent copper deficiency.

A year's supply of micronutrients is relatively inexpensive. Since there is no evidence that the recommended daily allowances given for prolonged periods have any toxic or adverse consequences, many clinicians feel that supplements in modest amounts can be recommended for all older individuals. Ideally, the maximum physiological and health benefit will be obtained with the least risk of toxicity. The exact types and optimum amounts have not yet been determined (see Chapter 5 ▭).

Ginseng is thought by some to improve overall health and boost the immune system. The root of Asian ginseng contains chemicals that are thought to be responsible for the herb's medicinal properties. This herb when dried can be made into tablets, capsules, and extracts and also into teas and cream for external use. Side effects include headache, sleep disruption, and gastrointestinal disturbances. To date, the research on ginseng does not support the claim that it is an immune booster. Further study is needed to support these claims (National Center for Complementary and Alternative Medicine, 2012).

As part of the probiotic (for life) movement, some yogurt drinks have been developed and marketed to improve immune function. These drinks are supplemented with *L. casei immunitas* cultures and claim to strengthen the body's defense when consumed daily. There is no established body of scientific evidence to support this claim; however, dairy drinks that are low in calories and high in calcium and vitamins could benefit health in general.

> **Drug Alert** ▶▶▶ There is a need for caution if a patient is taking anticoagulants along with any vitamin and/or herbal supplements.

> **Practice Pearl** ▶▶▶ Many clinicians support the use of a daily multivitamin/mineral supplement for all older adults.

HEALTHY AGING TIPS

▶ Engage in regular, moderate, exercise 30 minutes a day, 5 days a week. Suggested activities include walking, gardening, swimming, and tai chi.

▶ Take a daily multivitamin/mineral supplement.

▶ Consider vitamin D supplementation, ranging from 600 to 2,000 International Units per day.

▶ Maintain a healthy weight.

▶ Report increased infections to your healthcare practitioner.

Excessive Immune Responses

Excessive responses of the immune system result from an increase in the normal activities of the immune system. Hypersensitivity and autoimmunity are types of excessive responses. Overreaction of the immune system is believed to result from interplay between environmental factors and the genetic makeup of the individual. For instance, type 1 diabetes is thought to be an autoimmune disease where misguided T cells attack the beta cells in the pancreas and eventually destroy their ability to produce insulin. Figure 23-5 ▶▶▶ illustrates the pathological process.

Hypersensitivity

Hypersensitivity is either an excessive response to antigen stimulation or a normal response that is inappropriate. It usually does not occur on the first exposure to the antigen when the primary immune response occurs (sensitization). Reexposure to the antigen and initiation of the secondary immune response can stimulate hypersensitive reactions in predisposed individuals. The four types of hypersensitivity are characterized by a specific humoral or cell-mediated response. Types I, II, and III are primarily reactions of the humoral immune system (B cells). Type IV hypersensitivity is a response of the cellular immune system (T cells). A complex interrelationship exists between some hypersensitivity reactions and several autoimmune diseases. Characteristics of the four types of hypersensitivity and the diseases associated with each type are found in Table 23-2.

Type I Hypersensitivity

Type I hypersensitivities are immediate and may be life threatening. Reactions normally occur within 15 to 30 minutes after exposure to an antigen (allergen). Manifestations vary in severity, but often include hives, localized swelling, tightening of the throat, shortness of breath, wheezing, tachycardia, and hypotension. Anaphylactic allergic reactions leading to shock can occur.

TABLE 23-2	Characteristics and Diseases Associated With Hypersensitivity	
Type	**Action**	**Diseases**
Type I	Immediate reaction: IgE-mediated local or systemic allergic response	Anaphylaxis; atrophic disorders
Type II	Cytotoxic reactions: IgG- and/or IgM-mediated destruction of cells	Drug and transfusion reactions
Type III	Immune complex reactions: IgM- or IgG-mediated formation of antigen–antibody complexes	Serum sickness or localized arthus reactions
Type IV	Cell-mediated reactions: mediated by sensitized T cells	Allergic contact dermatitis; delayed hypersensitivity reactions

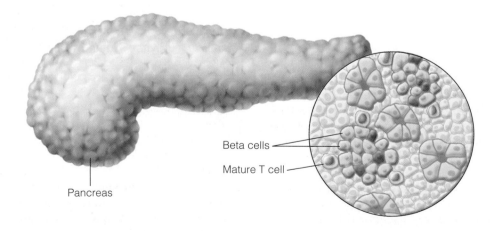

Beta cells

Mature T cell

Pancreas

Figure 23-5 ▶▶▶ The pathological process of misguided T cells attacking beta cells in the pancreas.

Source: National Institute of Allergy and Infectious Diseases (2007).

Asthma is a common hypersensitivity type I problem that is often underdiagnosed and suboptimally treated in the older person. The prevalence of asthma increases steadily with age; however, it is not identified well in older adults. The symptoms are often attributed to other diseases of the respiratory system such as congestive heart failure, chronic obstructive pulmonary disease, and other pulmonary disorders, especially chronic bronchitis. Patients with asthma are more likely to have had symptoms earlier in life. Older people also may have less awareness of symptoms. Asthma medications may aggravate coexisting medical conditions, and some drugs commonly used for the older person (aspirin and beta-blockers) may adversely influence asthma (Buttaro, Trybulski, Bailey et al., 2012). Interventions should be aimed at identifying allergens that precipitate attacks and reducing them in the home.

Type II Hypersensitivity

Type II hypersensitivities occur within minutes or hours of exposure. Examples of this type of reaction include transfusion reactions, drug reactions, myasthenia gravis, thyroiditis, and autoimmune hemolytic anemia. Autoimmune thyroiditis can result in both hyperthyroidism and hypothyroidism. Other than hypothyroidism, none of these conditions is a particularly prevalent disorder in the older person. Hypothyroidism does occur in women over 60 years of age, and often the symptoms are subtler than in younger people. As a result, thyroid-stimulating hormone (TSH) screening is recommended. If older adults require thyroid hormone replacement medications, a low dose should be given initially. After the dose has stabilized, periodic TSH measurements are required. Also, patients should be aware that supplementation is lifelong.

Type III Hypersensitivity

Type III hypersensitivity is characterized by a failure to remove antigen–antibody complexes from the circulation and tissues. The subsequent inflammatory reaction can lead to cell and tissue injury. The underlying cause may be a persistent low-grade infection by a viral or bacterial agent; chronic exposure to an environmental antigen from molds, plants, or animals; or an autoimmune process. For example, glomerulonephritis typically occurs about 10 to 14 days after an infection by a *Streptococcus* bacterial organism. The immune complex is deposited in the glomerular capillary wall of the kidney with resulting proteinuria, hematuria, hypertension, oliguria, and red cell casts in the urine. This may lead to acute or chronic renal failure.

Systemic lupus erythematosus (SLE) is another example of a type III hypersensitivity reaction caused by autoantibody production. Although 15% of the people with SLE develop it later in life after age 55, the prevalence of the disease is considered to be underreported. Late-onset SLE affects women eight times more often than men and is found primarily in Caucasians (Lupus Foundation of America, 2012). In SLE, antibodies are formed against nuclear DNA and RNA throughout the body. The resulting inflammatory response causes a cycle of cell damage and further formation of antigen–antibody immune complexes that are deposited in connective tissues. The signs and symptoms vary significantly since any organ of the body can be involved. Lesions of the skin, mucosal ulcerations, nephritis, restrictive pulmonary disease, retinal changes, neuritis, and gastrointestinal ulceration are but a few. Because symptoms of SLE in older people mimic other diseases, diagnosis may be delayed or missed. Progressive use of anti-inflammatory agents, systemic corticosteroids, and immunosuppressive drugs can decrease symptoms and increase the person's quality of life.

Rheumatoid arthritis is believed to be another example of type III hypersensitivity that affects the older person. About 1% of all adults have rheumatoid arthritis, and it is more frequent in women. Peak incidence is between the fourth and sixth decade of life. A number of theories exist to explain the etiology, all related to components of the immune system and the development of autoimmunity.

There does seem to be a genetic predisposition to rheumatoid arthritis. It is two to three times more common in women with a familial history. Pathological changes occur initially in the synovial tissue of joints. Antibodies form against the person's own IgG, and the resulting complex is identified as foreign. The inflammatory process, stimulated by infiltrating T cells, gradually destroys articular cartilage. Bone erosion occurs, causing swelling, pain, and loss of motion. The freely movable joints of the hands, wrists, ankles, and feet are the most commonly affected, in a symmetrical pattern. Characteristic ulnar deviations lead to swan neck deformities of the hands. The elbows, knees, and shoulders may also be involved. Eventually, proper functioning of the joints becomes impossible and crippling deformities occur.

Rheumatoid arthritis is a chronic, fluctuating, systemic disease, and widespread damage can occur. Fibrous materials everywhere in the body can be attacked. Along with specific joint pain, patients are chronically tired and may complain of generalized aching. Prolonged inactivity increases stiffness and swelling. As the disease progresses, activities such as climbing stairs and opening jars become difficult. A low-grade fever, weight loss, and depression are common. Cardiac, pulmonary, and ophthalmic manifestations may occur in later stages of the disease. Drug therapy often consists of a combination of nonsteroidal anti-inflammatory drugs (NSAIDs), antirheumatic drugs, low-dose chemotherapeutic agents (methotrexate), and glucocorticoids. A summary of the care of patients with rheumatic disorders is found in Box 23-2. A thorough discussion of rheumatoid arthritis can be found in Chapter 18 ⊂⊃ of this text.

BOX 23-2 **Nursing Diagnoses and Interventions for Rheumatic Disorders**

Nursing Diagnosis: *Pain, Chronic* related to inflammatory process and advancing disease process.
Outcome: Pain decreased below current level or relieved to a level that is acceptable to the older person. Incorporation of pain relief measures into daily life.
Interventions:
- Measure the level of pain on a pain scale; in those unable to report pain levels, observe for improvement in functional ability.
- Provide a variety of nonpharmacological comfort measures:
  - Heat or cold
  - Massage
  - Position change
  - Supportive equipment such as splints, positioning, and mobility aids
  - Relaxation techniques
  - Diversion activities
- Encourage verbalization.
- Administer anti-inflammatory analgesics and antirheumatic medications on an individualized plan.
- Encourage exercise routine while protecting joints.
- Teach pathophysiology of pain.

Nursing Diagnosis: *Activity Intolerance* or *Fatigue* related to disease process.
Outcome: Increased tolerance for daily activities.
Interventions:
- Assist in development of an activity/rest/sleep schedule.
- Explain the relationship of the disease to fatigue.
- Encourage use of energy-saving techniques.
- Encourage adequate nutrition.
- Encourage adherence to medication and treatment plans and evaluate effects.

Nursing Diagnosis: *Mobility: Physical, Impaired* caused by disease process or surgical intervention.
Outcome: Achieves and maintains optimal mobility.
Interventions:
- Encourage independence in mobility.
  - Assess need for physical or occupational therapy.
  - Develop a routine exercise program, including range-of-motion, strengthening, and endurance exercises along with rest periods.
  - Use appropriate ambulatory devices such as canes, walkers, braces, and splints.
  - Explain importance of supportive shoes.

- Assess environmental barriers.
- Refer to community health agency for assistance.

Nursing Diagnosis: *Self-Care Deficit* related to loss of motion and fatigue.
Outcome: Improve functional ability by decreasing dependence and moving toward optimal levels of function and self-care using necessary resources.
Interventions:
- Assist patient and family in identifying factors that interfere with self-care activities, and ways to ameliorate problems.
- Develop goals and a plan for meeting self-care needs.
  - Protect joints.
  - Conserve energy.
  - Simplify activities.
- Assess need for assistive devices and instruct on their safe use.

Nursing Diagnosis: *Body Image, Disturbed*
Outcome: Takes an active part in improving self-concept.
Interventions:
- Assess concerns about body image.
- Encourage expression of feelings about deformities with support and concern.
- Teach strategies for improving body image (how to dress, apply makeup, improve hygiene).
- Assist significant others to understand the impact of the limitations and solicit their help in identifying methods to promote a positive body image.
- Seek assessment from members of the multidisciplinary team such as physical and occupational therapists in order to gain access to assistive devices to improve mobility and function.

Nursing Diagnosis: *Skin Integrity, Impaired* related to altered peripheral perfusion.
Outcome: Skin remains intact.
Interventions:
- Assess skin color, pulses, capillary refill, sensation, and temperature.
- Discourage use of nicotine products.
- Avoid exposure to cold and protect extremities in cold environment.
  - Wear natural fiber clothing.
  - Use lanolin-based ointments.
- Monitor complaints of numbness and tingling.
- Encourage routine skin care.
- Promote adequate nutrition.

NANDA-I © 2012.

Type IV Hypersensitivity

Type IV hypersensitivity is also called delayed hypersensitivity. Tissue is damaged as a result of a delayed T-cell reaction to an antigen. The reaction normally occurs within 1 to 14 days after exposure, although it is often slower in older adults. Contact hypersensitivity such as dermatitis from a latex allergy, tuberculin reactions, and transplant rejections are examples. In people with multiple sclerosis, a variety of studies have documented abnormalities in both B cells and T cells.

Deficient Immune Responses

Deficient immune responses occur when there is a functional decrease in one or more components of the immune system. These are either primary or secondary immunodeficiency disorders.

Primary Immunodeficiency Disorders

Primary immunodeficiency disorders are either congenital or acquired, and are not attributed to other causes.

HIV/AIDS

Infection with the human immunodeficiency virus (HIV) and the resulting acquired immunodeficiency syndrome (AIDS) is the best example of a primary immunodeficiency disorder. The hallmark of this infection is a decrease in cellular (T-cell) immunity. Helper T (CD4) cells are primarily affected by the virus. These T cells mediate between the antigen presenting cells (macrophages) and other B and T cells. HIV is an example of an emerging infectious disease that jumped from animal to human, probably in the 1950s. It is a chronic disease spread primarily through sexual contact with an infected person. The widespread organ involvement associated with the infection has caused much human suffering and death. Extensive information regarding the pathophysiology, interventions, and outcomes associated with HIV infection can be found in pathophysiology and medical–surgical textbooks and in medical journals. Only the effects of HIV infection in the older person are described here.

People age 50 and older now represent almost one fourth of all people with HIV/AIDS in the United States. Because older people do not get tested for HIV/AIDS on a regular basis, there may be even more cases than currently known (CDC, 2012b). HIV infection in the older person is often underdiagnosed and underreported.

Many factors contribute to the increasing risk of infection in older people. In general, older Americans know less about HIV/AIDS and sexually transmitted infections (STIs) than younger age groups. Older people have been compared to teenagers in their knowledge of HIV. They have not known people who have suffered from HIV/AIDS, and so they have little knowledge, personal awareness, or interest in preventing the disease. Education and prevention messages have not been directed to older adults in the past. However, many senior centers now have AIDS awareness programs that provide information about HIV prevention and safe sex. Also, older people are less likely than younger people to talk about their sex lives or drug use with their physicians; conversely, many physicians do not ask older patients about sex or drug use. Finally, older people often mistake the symptoms of HIV/AIDS for the aches and pains of normal aging, so they are less likely to get tested (CDC, 2012b; National Institutes of Health [NIH], 2012b).

Survival rates for those infected with HIV have improved due to advances in diagnostic resources, antiviral treatment, and prophylaxis; those infected at a relatively young age are now becoming older adults. The entire senior population is increasing and so are their expectations regarding their sex lives. Male sexual function has been enhanced by medications such as sildenafil citrate (Viagra), and medications to enhance female sexual drive and response have been developed. The sexually permissive baby boomers are entering the ranks of the older population. Some older adults continue their risky sexual behaviors and pay little attention to preventive measures, believing that HIV infection is not an issue in their age group. These factors have not only contributed to an increased incidence of HIV/AIDS in older adults, but also to an increase in other STIs, often among people who live in over-55 communities.

Late diagnosis of HIV infection among older adults is a considerable problem. To address this, CDC recommends routine HIV screening for all people ages 13 to 64. People ages 64 and older should be counseled to receive HIV testing if they have risk factors for HIV infection. A number of HIV screening tests are available that can be performed in ambulatory settings. They are interpreted visually and give results rapidly, but require confirmation using other techniques if the test is positive. This type of routine testing will identify people who are unaware that they are HIV infective, and also remove the stigma of being tested. Since many symptoms of AIDS mimic those of normal aging, such as memory loss, fatigue, and weight loss, physicians can miss a diagnosis of HIV infection. Earlier diagnosis resulting in treatment and referral to other medical and social services improves a person's chance for living a longer and healthier life.

> **Practice Pearl** ▶▶▶ The CDC recommends routine HIV testing in all healthcare settings for people ages 13 to 64. People older than age 64 should receive HIV testing if they have risk factors for HIV infection such as engaging in unprotected sexual activity with multiple partners and intravenous drug use.

Antiretroviral therapy, which typically contains at least three antiretroviral medications, is used to treat older people with HIV infection. When compared to younger people,

older patients in one study had somewhat better virological responses and similar immunological responses to antiretroviral therapy. Older patients had fewer interruptions in the therapy and were able to tolerate and adhere to the therapy regimen relatively well. An older patient's failure to respond to antiretroviral therapy should be analyzed and not attributed to age alone. The prognosis for seniors diagnosed with HIV today is good. Although they live fewer years after diagnosis, they can still live long, productive lives. Care of the older patient with an HIV infection is presented in Box 23-3.

BOX 23-3 ▶ **Nursing Diagnoses and Interventions: The Older Patient With an HIV Infection**

Nursing Diagnosis: *Knowledge, Deficient* related to preventing transmission of HIV.
Outcome: Can describe preventive measures related to prevention of transmission of HIV infection through sexual activity.
Interventions:
- Instruct patient, family, and friends on preventing transmission of HIV.
- Avoid sexual contact with multiple partners.
- Use condoms if the partner's HIV status is uncertain.
- Avoid oral contact with genitals.
- Avoid sexual practices that can cause injury to tissue.
- Use water-based lubrication during intercourse.
- Avoid having sex with people at high risk.
- Do not use intravenous recreational drugs.

Nursing Diagnosis: *Infection, Risk for* due to immunodeficiency.
Outcome: Infections do not occur.
Interventions:
- Monitor for symptoms of new infection:
  - A body temperature of 37.8°C (100°F)
  - White blood cell count and differential
  - Classic symptoms may not be present in older adults
- Instruct patient, family, or caregiver in ways to prevent infection.
- Administer antimicrobial therapy as prescribed.
- Encourage adequate nutrition.
- Use strict aseptic techniques for any invasive procedure.

Nursing Diagnosis: *Infection, Risk for* related to CNS infection or other potential complications.
Outcome: Describe to the extent possible using verbal and nonverbal communication techniques.
Interventions:
- Assess mental status and sensory changes.
- Monitor for drug interactions, infections, nutrition and electrolyte imbalances, depression, and other associated conditions.
- Create an environment that will minimize disorienting stimuli.
- Orient to changes in the environment.

- Help obtain a power of attorney if necessary to handle legal and financial matters.
- Assess self-care deficits.

Nursing Diagnosis: *Self-Care Deficit* related to factors such as mental changes, neurologic impairment, and depression.
Outcome: Becomes independent in self-care using necessary resources.
Interventions:
- Assist patient and family in identifying factors that interfere with self-care activities, and ways to ameliorate problems.
- Encourage adherence to antiviral medications.
- Take steps to avoid medication errors due to memory loss.
- Develop goals and a plan for meeting self-care needs.
- Assess need for assistive devices and instruct on their safe use.

Nursing Diagnosis: *Poisoning, Risk for* from drug toxicity.
Outcome: Tolerates medication regimen.
Interventions:
- Encourage adherence to antiviral drug therapy.
- Explain dosage, route of administration, action, and side effects of all medications.
- Instruct when to discontinue drugs and call for assistance.
- Keep list of medications and time of administration.

Nursing Diagnosis: *Social Isolation* related to fear of AIDS, rejection by family, and withdrawal from social activities, and fear of infecting others.
Outcome: Contacts with people are maintained.
Interventions:
- Observe for behaviors that suggest isolation, such as hostility, depression, withdrawal, feelings of rejection, or loneliness.
- Encourage maintenance of important personal relationships.
- Encourage visitors and telephone calls.
- Encourage diversional activities such as reading, watching TV, or crafts.
- Educate patient, family, and friends about how HIV is transmitted.
- Refer to support groups and community resources.

NANDA-I © 2012.

Secondary Immunodeficiency Disorders

Secondary immunodeficiency disorders are a consequence of other disorders or treatment regimens. Many factors can lead to the development of secondary immunodeficiency disorders, including physical, nutritional, environmental, psychosocial, and pharmacological factors (Table 23-3). For example, an excessive neuroendocrine secretion of corticosteroids in response to stress can lead to increased susceptibility to infectious disease and cancer. Low levels of corticosteroids may enhance autoimmune diseases. People who have high levels of physical and psychosocial stress, limited social support, depression, and bereavement show decreased immune functioning. Older people are often exposed to these types of stressors.

The stress of surgery, including the effects of anesthesia, can decrease the number of both B and T cells, and the deficiency can last for up to 1 month. This is particularly true for removal of the spleen, a structure of the immune system. Diabetes mellitus, cirrhosis, severe trauma and burns, malignancies, and severe infections are associated with secondary immune deficiencies. Medications, such as the cancer pharmacotherapeutic drugs, also cause a state of general immunosuppression. Others, such as antibiotics, anticonvulsants, antihistamines, and steroids, affect various mechanisms of the immune system. X-rays can destroy the rapidly proliferating cells of the immune system. Malnutrition can lead to protein and other deficiencies that impair immune function. Many of these factors affect older adults, many of whom already have a decreased ability to reproduce new cells of the immune system.

Susceptibility to Infections

Infections are one of the most frequently encountered problems in the older population. Although specific relationships between an aging or compromised immune system and infection are not clear, the decline in responsiveness of the immune system to harmful foreign invaders leads to an increase in the incidence and severity of infections. Sometimes they are difficult to diagnose. The febrile response that signals infections may be blunted in the older person. Medications commonly taken may also decrease the normal fever response. The baseline body temperature in older people is approximately 1°F lower than the normal temperature in younger people. Therefore, a rise in body temperature may not be immediately evident. Any temperature of 37.8°C (100° F) when other symptoms are present may indicate an infection. Other classic signs and symptoms of infection, such as redness, swelling, and pain, may also be altered.

TABLE 23-3 Effects of Selected Medications and Therapy on the Immune System

Drug	Action on Immune System
Antibiotics in High Doses	Bone marrow suppression: aplastic anemia
chloramphenicol	Leukopenia
gentamicin sulfate	Agranulocytosis
streptomycin	Leukopenia, pancytopenia
penicillin	Agranulocytosis
Antithyroid Drugs	Agranulocytosis, leukopenia
Nonsteroidal anti-inflammatory drugs (NSAIDs) in high doses	Prostaglandin synthesis/release inhibited Agranulocytosis, leukopenia
Adrenal Corticosteroids	Immunosuppression
prednisone	
Cancer Chemotherapeutic Drugs	Immunosuppression
(Cytotoxic Drugs)	
Alkylating agents	Leukopenia, agranulocytosis
cyclosporine	Decreased T-cell function, leukopenia
Antimetabolites	Immunosuppression
fluorouracil	Leukopenia, eosinophilia
mercaptopurine	Leukopenia, pancytopenia
methotrexate	Leukopenia, aplastic bone marrow
Ionizing Radiation	Suppression of stem cell division; pancytopenia

Source: Adapted from Smeltzer, S. C., & Bare, B. B. (2010). *Brunner & Suddarth's textbook of medical-surgical nursing* (12th ed.). Philadelphia, PA: Lippincott.

Practice Pearl ▶▶▶ A body temperature of 37.8°C (100°F), combined with other symptoms, may often herald an infection in the older person; however, many older adults will not exhibit an elevated temperature, illustrating the body's inability to mount an effective immune response.

Pneumonia

Pneumonia is a common condition in immune-deficient people, and is the leading cause of death in people over 65 years of age. It is the most common hospital-associated infection, and it has the highest mortality rate. The combination of pneumonia and influenza causes the greatest number of deaths. *Streptococcus pneumoniae* (pneumococcus) remains the single most common cause of pneumonia in the older person, and the risk for acquiring this disease increases with age. It accounts for approximately 40% to 60% of the cases. Pneumococcal pneumonia may occur as a primary illness or as a complication of a chronic disease. *S. pneumoniae* is a common resident of the human upper respiratory tract, and has been isolated in up to 70% of healthy adults.

Clearance of foreign invaders by the action of mucus production and cilia is less effective in the older person. As part of the aging process, there is a loss of both alveolar ducts and the surrounding elastic tissue. Demineralization of bones in the chest and a decreased effectiveness of the respiratory musculature further predispose the older person to lower respiratory infections. Under these conditions, pneumonia can occur following aspiration of microorganisms into the lungs. A serious complication of pneumonia is the development of bacteremia in nearly one fourth of those infected.

The signs and symptoms of pneumonia in older people are likely to be atypical. Often, the classic signs of fever, productive cough, chest pain, and leukocytosis are muted, and the diagnosis may be missed. Instead, other symptoms such as general deterioration, lethargy, falls, changes in mental status and orientation, anorexia, gastrointestinal symptoms, and tachycardia may signal the onset. Older people who live alone are particularly at risk of advanced illness since no one may be present to notice early changes in their general function. Underlying conditions may also mask the symptoms of pneumonia. For example, purulent sputum or slight changes in respiratory symptoms may be the only sign of pneumonia in patients with chronic obstructive pulmonary disease. Chest X-rays may determine whether chronic congestive heart failure or other processes are involved.

To prevent serious complications, all people 65 years of age and older should receive pneumococcal vaccine. Antibody response is often lower in the older person and may decline after 5 to 10 years. Revaccination is occasionally recommended after 5 years, especially in those older adults who received the first dose of pneumococcal vaccine before the age of 60. Yearly influenza immunizations are also highly recommended for the older person. The only contraindication is an allergy to eggs. More than 90% of the deaths during previous U.S. influenza epidemics were attributed to pneumonia as a complication of influenza. The vaccine reduces influenza-related morbidity and mortality by 70% to 90% among vaccinated individuals (CDC, 2012d).

> **Practice Pearl** ▶▶▶ All people age 65 and over should receive an initial dose of pneumococcal vaccine at age 65, and a yearly influenza immunization. Pneumococcal vaccine immunization can be repeated after 5 years if the first dose of vaccine was received before age 60 (Reuben et al., 2010).

Urinary Tract Infection (UTI)

Urinary tract infections (UTIs) are one of the most common problems in older adults, especially in women. Fecal contamination of the urinary tract with *E. coli* is the usual cause. The prevalence of urinary bacteriuria increases with age. It is found in approximately 20% of women over the age of 70 years. It is important to differentiate between asymptomatic bacteriuria that generally is not treated, and symptomatic infection that can range from painful urination to severe systemic illness. Although less common, older men can also suffer from UTIs mostly as a result of benign prostatic hypertrophy causing urinary retention and bacterial growth. Bladder dysfunction, a hypertrophied prostate gland, the relaxation of pelvic musculature, and other coexisting illnesses increase the incidence of infection. Indwelling catheters will eventually become infected, so long-term catheterization should be avoided whenever possible.

Symptomatic infections usually include urinary frequency, urgency, and suprapubic or flank pain. Fever may or may not occur. As with other infections in the older person, the presenting symptoms may vary. Mental status may change, falls may occur, and a decline in activities of daily living may be noticed. Generalized observations such as these may signal a smoldering urinary tract infection. All older people who are symptomatic should be treated promptly. While a short course of oral antibiotic therapy is often an effective treatment, resistant strains of *E. coli* (methicillin-resistant) are increasing. Therefore, a mucosal vaccine for prevention of UTIs in high-risk groups is being investigated (Centers for Disease Control and Prevention (CDC), 2012f) .

Bacteremia

Microorganisms can be introduced into the bloodstream spontaneously, as a result of indwelling catheters, or from dental, gastrointestinal, genitourinary, or other procedures. Bacteremia may also be a complication of pneumonia, UTIs, infection of skin and soft tissues, and other infectious processes. The urinary tract is the most common source of bacteremia, followed by the respiratory tract. Perirectal abscesses are frequently missed and can be a source of infection. Once in the bloodstream, microorganisms are disseminated to other organs throughout the body. Endocarditis, especially in those with valvular heart abnormalities, is a serious complication. Therefore, patients with certain underlying heart conditions should receive prophylactic antibiotics before procedures that may introduce bacteria into the bloodstream, such as dental procedures. Increased age and associated illness contribute to a poorer prognosis, and mortality rates increase.

As with most infections in the older person, the clinical clues vary. Often, the older person becomes confused and agitated, with altered mental status. Decreased consciousness may occur. Fever, while usually present, may be low grade. Blood cultures confirm the diagnosis, and immediate antibiotic treatment is essential. Septic shock is a serious complication that develops in 25% to 40% of patients with significant bacteremia.

Tuberculosis

One third of the world's population is infected with tuberculosis. It is a chronic pulmonary and extrapulmonary infectious disease that is acquired through exposure to *Mycobacterium tuberculosis.* It spreads from person to person by airborne transmission. The number of cases of tuberculosis is highest in people over 65 years of age, with the exception of those who are infected with HIV. The majority of active cases occur through reactivation of a dormant infection in an older person who has not been effectively treated in the past. Older adults are also at increased risk of initial infection, particularly those who are chronically ill or debilitated and residing in nursing homes. A discussion of tuberculosis is found in Chapter 16 .

The TB Education and Training Network (TB ETN) was formed to bring TB professionals in the United States together to network, share resources, and build education and training skills. Membership is free and open to all people and includes representatives from TB programs, correctional facilities, hospitals, nursing homes, federal agencies, universities, the American Lung Association, regional training and medical consultation centers, and international organizations interested in TB education and training issues (CDC, 2012e).

Skin Infections

As the skin becomes thinner and less elastic with age, the older person becomes more susceptible to injury and breakdown of tissue. Peripheral neuropathy with decreased sensation and circulation may lead to abrasions, burns, and stasis ulcers. Reduced physical activity, malnutrition, dehydration, and other systemic illnesses are also predisposing factors. Immobilized people who are convalescing at home are at high risk for the development of pressure ulcers. Any interruption of skin integrity leads to infection, especially with organisms that are a part of the normal skin flora.

Erysipelas, a superficial cellulitis of the skin caused by group A streptococcus, usually affects the lower extremities or the face (Figure 23-6 ▶▶▶). Any illness that compromises skin integrity, such as diabetes mellitus or alcohol abuse, may increase the risk of this infection. The involved area is bright red and raised with well-defined borders. Skin infections such as this can predispose the individual to bacteremia and septic shock. Although antibiotic treatment is effective, the most important method of therapy is prevention. Necrotizing fasciitis, although uncommon, can cause extensive invasion of the subcutaneous tissues. Immediate surgical intervention and appropriate antibiotic treatment are required.

The reactivation of the herpes zoster (varicella) virus that has lingered in nerve tissue for years following chickenpox infection can lead to shingles. Shingles has been a common condition among those over 60 years of age. However, the Zoster vaccine is now available and recommended routinely for people in this age group. The expanded use of this vaccine should decrease the incidence

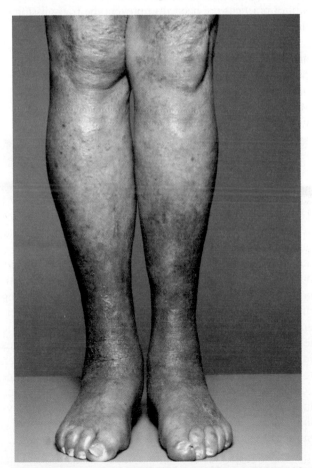

Figure 23-6 ▶▶▶ Erysipelas, a superficial cellulitis of the skin caused by group A streptococcus.
Source: NMSB/Custom Medical Stock.

of shingles. Vesicular lesions occur along spinal nerves, most frequently affecting T_3 to L_2 nerves and the fifth cranial nerve. Extreme discomfort may occur. Early treatment with acyclovir or other antiviral medications should begin within 72 hours after appearance of the rash. This treatment reduces acute pain and shortens the period of infectivity. Otherwise, treatment is largely supportive, with administration of analgesics and topical cleansing. Occasionally, chronic pain develops that will require longer term analgesics and possibly antidepressants.

Because of the overuse of antibiotics and increasing levels of frailty in older adults in nursing homes, hospitals, and outpatient clinics, healthcare-acquired (**nosocomial infections**) are increasing. A growing number of pathogenic organisms are resistant to one or more antimicrobial drugs, threatening older adults receiving care in a variety of settings. These pathogens include vancomycin-resistant enterococci (VRE), methicillin-resistant *Staphylococcus aureus* (MRSA), and *Clostridium difficile*–associated disease (CDAC) (CDC, 2012a). Careful hand washing and infection control practices are needed to prevent the transmission of the multidrug-resistant organisms to older patients.

> **Practice Pearl** ▶▶▶ The one-time Zoster vaccine is recommended routinely for people 60 years of age and older. People who have had shingles can receive the vaccine to help prevent future occurrences of the disease.

Trends in Immunology

Monoclonal Antibodies

The scientific community can now mass produce immune cell secretions, such as antibodies. The availability of these products has revolutionized the study of the immune system, and has not only had a significant impact on medicine, but on agriculture and industry as well. Monoclonal antibodies are identical antibodies made by multiple cloning of a single B cell. Due to antibody specificity for different antigens, monoclonal antibodies are used in diagnostic tests to identify invading pathogens and to identify changes in the body's proteins. Monoclonal antibodies can attach to cancer cells and block the chemicals that stimulate uncontrolled multiplication. They can also carry potent toxins into specific cells, altering or destroying the cell, but leaving nearby cells intact. Monoclonal antibodies are promising for the future treatment of a wide variety of diseases.

Genetic Engineering

Genetic engineering, recombinant DNA technology, genetic modification/manipulation, and gene splicing are all terms that are applied to the direct manipulation of an organism's genes. Segments of DNA from the cells of one organism are removed and then combined with genetic material from a second organism. This technique forms artificial DNA, combining DNA sequences that would not normally occur together.

Immunoenhancing drugs, produced by genetic engineering, are available that help boost both the number of white blood cells and red blood cells in the bloodstream. These drugs are used in patients who are receiving immunosuppressant chemotherapy drugs that target cancer cells but also can have an adverse affect on healthy cells. Pegfilgrastim (Neulasta) is a protein that stimulates the production of white blood cells (neutrophils) that are depleted during chemotherapy. This drug appears to be self-regulating in that it remains in the blood while the patient is deficient, and is cleared when the neutrophils increase and the drug is no longer needed. A single injection is administered per chemotherapy cycle. The resulting increase in white blood cells reduces risk of infection. Darbepoetin alfa (Aranesp), an erythropoiesis-stimulating protein designed to increase red blood cell production, is also produced through genetic engineering. Administered in single-dose subcutaneous injection, it stimulates the production of red blood cells, counteracting anemia associated with some types of chemotherapy and chronic renal failure, thereby decreasing the need for transfusions. Because these are powerful drugs, patients should be monitored closely for side effects. Over time, the healthcare community will see more of these types of drugs approved for use in a variety of conditions.

Nursing Assessment

Multiple factors underlie immune problems in the older person. Therefore, a health history and physical examination are essential. The key assessment areas include the following factors:

- Age
- Nutrition
- Recent infections
- Immunization status
- Allergies
- Disorders and diseases
  - Autoimmune disease
  - Neoplastic disease
  - Chronic illness
  - Surgery
- Pain
- Medications
- Blood transfusions
- Lifestyle, stress, and other factors

Nursing Interventions

Nursing interventions that can improve immune status in the older person include the following:

- Consider older people who are under substantial stress at high risk for conditions associated with a decreased immune status.
- Evaluate stress levels and biologic markers of stress such as hypertension, insomnia, and anxiety to identify older people at high risk.
- Assist people in identifying active, positive coping strategies, especially following stressful events.
- Educate the person, family, and friends about the effects of stress.
- Administer pneumococcal vaccine at age 65 or revaccinate after the age of 65 as recommended by the primary care provider.
- Stress the importance of obtaining yearly influenza immunizations.
- Encourage daily vitamin and mineral supplementation and discourage megadosing leading to possible toxicity.
- Encourage all older adults to develop an exercise plan appropriate for their physical status.

- Encourage community senior centers to offer education about HIV and STD prevention.
- Routinely screen for HIV infection in older people.
- Encourage older adults with a history of risky sexual behaviors to seek advice from healthcare professionals if symptoms of HIV such as fatigue or lymphadenopathy occur.

The nurse will often engage in teaching older patients and families about prevention of infectious diseases like influenza. Refer to the patient–family teaching guidelines feature below.

QSEN Recommendations Related to the Immune System

The Quality and Safety Education for Nurses (QSEN) project addresses the challenge of preparing future nurses with the knowledge, skills, and attitudes (KSAs) to continuously improve the quality and safety of the healthcare systems in which they work (Cronenwett et al., 2007). See the QSEN table for tips on meeting QSEN standards.

Meeting QSEN Standards: The Immune System

	KNOWLEDGE	SKILLS	ATTITUDES
Patient-Centered Care	Involvement of patient and family in the plan of care is crucial.	Family assessment and adult learning principles.	Appreciate uniqueness of each patient/family.
	Examine barriers that may keep patients from actively participating in their plan of care.	Evaluate for signs and symptoms related to dysfunction of the immune system.	Provide patient-centered care to improve successful outcomes.
Teamwork and Collaboration	Recognize scope of practice for interdisciplinary team members.	Use leadership skills to coordinate team and share knowledge.	Value the contribution of each member of the team to improve outcomes.
	Be aware of organizational problems that can inhibit effective team functioning.	System assessment skills.	Be open to input from team members on effective means to improve communication and collaboration.
Evidence-Based Practice	Describe effective interventions to treat immune disorders and to improve the overall health and functioning of the immune system.	Access current evidence-based protocols to guide interventions.	Possess confidence in necessary skills to evaluate and incorporate nursing interventions from literature about the immune system.

(continued)

Meeting QSEN Standards: The Immune System   *(continued)*

	KNOWLEDGE	SKILLS	ATTITUDES
Quality Improvement	Recognize the importance of measuring patient outcomes to evaluate interventions related to the immune system.	Skills in data management, technology, and U.S. government and AHA sites describing current incidence and prevalence of immune disorders.	Value the use of data and outcomes as a key component of QI efforts.
Safety	Realize the risk factors associated with immune system aging, hypersensitivity, and deficiency.	Assess safety risk factors associated with specific immune disorders and institute proper safeguards.	Appreciate the importance of moderate exercise and proper nutrition in preventing and modifying immune system dysfunction.
Informatics	Provide input into the formation and maintenance of patient databases needed for gathering QSEN data and providing patient care.	Utilize the electronic health record.	Protect patient confidentiality according to HIPAA standards.

Patient–Family Teaching Guidelines

The following are guidelines that the nurse may find useful when instructing older adults and their families about preventing the flu (adapted from CDC, 2012c; NIH, 2012a).

PREVENTION OF INFLUENZA

1 Can the flu be prevented?

A flu shot greatly reduces your chances of getting the flu. No vaccine is completely effective, but studies show that older people who get the flu shot are 70% less likely to be hospitalized and 85% less likely to die as a result of getting the flu.

The flu is highly contagious and spreads easily from person to person. It is caused by viruses that infect the nose, throat, and lungs. When you are out in crowded places like church, the grocery store, or the mall, try to avoid contact with people who are coughing and sneezing. Wash your hands often and do not put things found in public places in or near your mouth. The flu can be life threatening in an older person or a person with other chronic illness like diabetes or diseases of the kidneys, liver, heart, or lungs.

RATIONALE:

Administration of yearly influenza vaccine and avoiding contact with persons infected with the flu are effective preventive measures.

2 Who should get a flu shot?

In general, anyone who wants to reduce their chances of getting influenza can get vaccinated. The CDC recommends the following people receive flu shots, trivalent inactivated influenza vaccine (TIV), each year because these persons are categorized as high risk for serious illness and complications from the flu:

- People over the age of 50
- Residents of nursing homes and other long-term care facilities where older adults live in close contact
- People of any age with chronic health conditions such as asthma, diabetes, and kidney, liver, heart, or lung disease
- Healthcare workers in contact with people in high-risk groups
- Caregivers or people who live with someone in a high-risk group

Patient–Family Teaching Guidelines *(continued)*

RATIONALE:

Persons in these high-risk groups are at risk for life-threatening complications from the flu, including hospitalization, development of pneumonia and sepsis, and death. Healthcare workers are less likely to develop a serious case of the flu, but may inadvertently spread the flu virus from person to person by transmitting the virus carried in their noses and throats.

3 Will my insurance cover the cost of the shot?

The cost of the flu shot is covered by Medicare. Many private health insurance plans also pay for the flu shot. You can get a flu shot at your healthcare provider's office or you may receive it from your local health department or at flu shot clinics sponsored by some drug or department stores.

RATIONALE:

It makes sense for insurance companies and Medicare to cover the cost of flu shots, because they greatly reduce costs by preventing hospitalization, treatment of serious complications, and death.

4 When is the best time to get the flu shot?

In the United States, the flu season usually starts in December and ends in April. The best time to get the flu shot is between mid-September and mid-November. It takes about 1 to 2 weeks to develop immunity after you receive the flu shot.

RATIONALE:

Although the impact and start of the flu season vary from year to year, it is always best to plan ahead and make sure high-risk older patients are immunized by mid-November.

5 What about side effects of the flu shot?

The vaccine is made from killed flu viruses, so you cannot possibly get the flu. The vaccine is grown in eggs, so people who are severely allergic to eggs should not get the flu shot. Some people (fewer than one third who get the flu shot) report soreness, redness, or swelling in the arm where the flu shot was given. These side effects can last up to 2 days and usually are controlled with acetaminophen.

RATIONALE:

The danger of getting the flu is far greater than any risks from getting a flu shot. Reassurance and education can empower some older adults to request and receive the flu shot.

6 What are the symptoms of the flu?

Flu causes fever, chills, dry cough, sore throat, runny nose, headache, muscle aches, and fatigue. Usually, symptoms are worse than the symptoms of a cold or upper respiratory infection. If you get the flu, make sure to rest, drink plenty of fluids, and take acetaminophen to control aches and fever. Call your doctor or primary healthcare provider if:

- Your fever (usually over 100°F) lasts for more than a few days.
- You are diagnosed with heart, lung, liver, or kidney problems.
- You are taking drugs to fight off cancer or other drugs that weaken your body's immune response.
- You feel sick and do not seem to be getting better.
- You have a cough with phlegm.
- You, or someone caring for you, is worried about your condition.

RATIONALE:

If serious side effects or complications of the flu develop, early treatment improves the chance of success.

7 How is the flu treated?

Because the flu is caused by a virus, antibiotics (only effective against bacterial infections) are not an effective treatment. The four drugs approved to treat the flu include:

- Amantadine (Symmetrel)
- Rimantadine (Flumadine)
- Zanamivir (Relenza)
- Oseltamivir (Tamiflu)

These drugs must be taken within 48 hours of the onset of symptoms, so it is important to call your doctor or primary healthcare provider if you think you have the flu. These drugs shorten the duration of the illness and prevent complications like pneumonia. They are only available by prescription and are not right for everyone. Other drugs may be given to make you feel better, including cough medication and antibiotics, should you develop a bacterial pneumonia as a complication of the flu.

RATIONALE:

Early treatment with an antiviral medication can ease the symptoms and prevent complications in high-risk persons. High-risk patients should contact their doctor quickly if symptoms of the flu are detected during flu season.

CARE PLAN A Patient With Joint Pain From an Autoimmune Disease

Case Study

On the first home visit to Mrs. Ryan for a health assessment, the visiting nurse notes that the patient walks with difficulty and complains of pain in her knee joints. Mrs. Ryan is an 83-year-old woman who has enjoyed good health all her years. She has had rheumatoid arthritis for years and no other medical problems. She gets some pain relief from daily naproxen (Aleve) but does not ambulate much during the day, spending her time on the couch. She states, "I just don't like to move around much now. My darn knees hurt too much so I mostly sit here on my couch and rest." Family members shop for her and visit weekly, but the apartment seems dirty and disorganized and there is spoiled food in the refrigerator.

On examination, the nurse finds warm, swollen knees with little active range of motion (ROM). Passive ROM produces pain after 30 degrees flexion. Mrs. Ryan denies weight loss, but her clothing fits her loosely, indicating she may have recently lost a significant amount of weight. She also has a bruise on her left hip that she cannot explain. The rest of the examination is negative.

Applying the Nursing Process

Assessment

The nurse should assess whether Mrs. Ryan has seen her healthcare provider for evaluation of her rheumatoid arthritis recently. The presence of warm swollen knees, weight loss, and bruising (from a possible fall) might indicate an exacerbation of this chronic illness. A complete functional assessment, dietary history, medication assessment, and safety inventory in the home are needed.

Diagnosis

Current nursing diagnoses for Mrs. Ryan may include the following:

- *Pain, Chronic* in knee joints (related to progression of rheumatoid arthritis)
- *Mobility: Physical, Impaired*
- *Activity, Deficient Diversional*
- *Disuse Syndrome, Risk for* (related to immobility and pain on movement)
- *Walking, Impaired*
- *Falls, Risk for*
- *Nutrition, Imbalanced: Less Than Body Requirements*

- *Constipation, Risk for* (potentially as a result of immobility and dehydration)
- *Urinary Incontinence* (potentially as a result of pain on movement)
- *Fluid Volume: Deficient* (related to possible dehydration)
- *Social Isolation*
- *Loneliness, Risk for*
- *Caregiver Role Strain*
- *Failure to Thrive, Adult*

NANDA-I © 2012.

Planning and Implementation

Appropriate nursing interventions for Mrs. Ryan may include the following:

- Referral to members of the interdisciplinary team, including social worker, physical therapist, occupational therapist, nutritionist, and primary care provider.
- Consultation with primary care provider about pain evaluation and possible referral to a rheumatologist.
- Educate the patient and family regarding mobility issues and resulting problems related to immobility.

- Development of a home safety plan including improving fall risk and food safety measures.
- Gaining additional services for Mrs. Ryan to ease caregiver strain, including Meals-on-Wheels and homemaker services.
- Requesting a family meeting to clarify care issues, identify involved family members, and clarify end-of-life goals, values, and advance directives.

A Patient With Joint Pain From an Autoimmune Disease *(continued)*

Expected Outcomes

The expected outcomes for Mrs. Ryan may include the following:

- Mrs. Ryan's pain will be decreased with active and passive exercises, use of topical rubs, heating pads, and optimum doses of appropriate medications, including NSAIDs, methotrexate, sulfasalazine, corticosteroids, or other medications as recommended by the rheumatologist to prevent further joint destruction.

- Mrs. Ryan will maintain mobility, strengthen muscles, prevent deformity, and minimize the risk of falls and injury.
- Mrs. Ryan's home environment will be free of barriers to mobility, and she will begin appropriate use of mobility assistive devices, such as a cane or walker.
- Caregiver strain will be eased and family involvement improved.
- The healthcare team will arrange for ongoing support and evaluation of progress.

Evaluation

The nurse hopes to work with Mrs. Ryan over time to provide support and improve overall health and function. The nurse will consider the plan a success based on the following criteria:

- Mrs. Ryan will agree to meet with a social worker to assess caregiver strain, the situation in the home, and the need for supportive services.
- A family meeting will be held to discuss Mrs. Ryan's overall health.

- Mrs. Ryan will arrange an appointment with her primary healthcare provider for further assessment and evaluation of her rheumatoid arthritis.
- She will improve her nutrition and establish and maintain a normal healthy weight.
- She will not exhibit further unexplained bruising and will remove safety hazards from her home.
- Advance directives will be established with healthcare goals and appropriate levels of treatment specified.

Ethical Dilemma

The visiting nurse requested permission from Mrs. Ryan to contact her son and daughter-in-law who live in a nearby town and visit her on weekends. She granted permission, but warned: "My son and his wife are fed up with me. I'm afraid to be a burden on them. I'm afraid to ask them for anything because they might put me in a nursing home and I could never stand that." When the nurse reached Mrs. Ryan's son at work, he agreed to a family meeting but said, "I can't schedule a long meeting. I'm busy at work and Mom is requiring more and more help. I want her to be safe, but I can't do any more for her. Let's just pursue nursing home placement. Is this meeting really necessary?" The nurse responded that it was necessary and the meeting would last 1 hour or less. The ethical dilemma for

Mrs. Ryan and her family involved patient autonomy and self-determination (her wish to remain home and endure the risk) versus her family's wish for nursing home placement and safety (beneficence). At first, the family was reluctant to become involved, but during the family meeting at which the social worker was present, they learned the plan of care for improvement of home safety and nutritional status. Once the visiting nurse had completed the visits, the family was able to continue support of Mrs. Ryan, encouraging her to prevent deformity, increase muscle strength, and improve her range of motion. Taking a regular dose of pain medication (acetaminophen) and using a topical pain-relieving rub twice daily controlled her pain, allowing her to become more active in the home.

Critical Thinking and the Nursing Process

1. Why is the treatment of rheumatoid arthritis more complicated in the older person?

2. When teaching an older person about HIV prevention and safe sex practices, what information would you include?

(continued)

CARE PLAN **A Patient With Joint Pain From an Autoimmune Disease** *(continued)*

3. What factors place older people at risk for developing nosocomial infections in hospitals and long-term care facilities?

4. Identify behaviors you have observed during your clinical experiences that place older adults at risk for the development of nosocomial infections. What education can the nurse provide to older adults to prevent illness and strengthen the immune system?

■ Evaluate your responses in Appendix B. ⊂⊐

Chapter Highlights

■ The three major biological defense mechanisms are:
  ■ Anatomical and biochemical barrier of skin and mucous membranes
  ■ Mechanical clearance
  ■ Immune response.

■ Self-recognition, specificity, and memory are the three characteristics that are unique to the immune system.

■ Immunity can be natural or acquired. Acquired immunity can be either active or passive.

■ Lymphocytes are the white blood cells primarily concerned with immunity.

■ The humoral immune response is initiated when an antigen binds with antibody receptors on the surface of mature B cells. This results in production of plasma cells that secrete one of five types of antibodies.

■ The first exposure to foreign antigen results in production of antibodies in about 5 days. With a second exposure, there is a more rapid production of large amounts of antibodies.

■ The cell-mediated immune response is characterized by the entire T cell binding to the foreign antigen in multiple areas on the surface of the cell.

■ Immune changes with aging result in a decrease in functioning of both B cells and T cells. The primary deficit is in the proliferation of T cells in the body.

■ Stress, comorbidity, exercise, and nutrition all affect immune system function.

■ Hypersensitivity and autoimmunity are overreactions or abnormal reactions of the immune system. Rheumatoid disorders are autoimmune reactions.

■ Deficient immune responses occur when there is a functional decrease in one or more components of the immune system. Susceptibility to infections is common. HIV is a primary immunodeficiency disease.

■ Secondary immune deficiencies include physical, nutritional, environmental, psychosocial, and pharmacological factors.

■ Pneumonia, urinary tract infections, bacteremia, tuberculosis, and skin infections are common in the older person.

■ A variety of nursing interventions can improve immune status. Relieving stress, encouraging positive coping strategies, exercise, diet supplements, immunizations, and HIV teaching and screening are a few.

Pearson Nursing Student Resources
Find additional review materials at
nursing.pearsonhighered.com
Prepare for success with additional NCLEX®-style practice questions, interactive assignments and activities, web links, animations and videos, and more!

References

Buttaro, T. M., Trybulski, J., Bailey, P. P., & Sandberg-Cook, H. (2012). *Primary care: A collaborative practice* (4th ed.). St. Louis, MO: Mosby.

Centers for Disease Control and Prevention (CDC) (2011). *Pneumococcal disease in short.* Retrieved from http://www.cdc.gov/vaccines/vpd-vac/pneumo/in-short-both.htm

Centers for Disease Control and Prevention (CDC). (2012a). *Antibiotic/antimicrobial resistance.* Retrieved from http://www.cdc.gov/drugresistance

Centers for Disease Control and Prevention (CDC). (2012b). *HIV/AIDS: The elderly.* Retrieved from http://www.cdcnpin.org/scripts/population/elderly.asp

Centers for Disease Control and Prevention (CDC). (2012c). *Influenza vaccination: A summary for clinicians.* Retrieved from http://www.cdc.gov/flu/professionals/vaccination/vax-summary.htm

Centers for Disease Control and Prevention (CDC). (2012d). Recommended adult immunization schedule—United States, *MMWR, 61*(4), 1–7.

Centers for Disease Control and Prevention (CDC). (2012e). *Tuberculosis (TB).* Retrieved from http://www.cdc.gov/tb

Centers for Disease Control and Prevention (CDC). (2012f). *Urinary tract infections.* Retrieved from http://www.cdc.gov/ncidod/dbmd/diseaseinfo/urinarytractinfections_t.htm

Cronenwett, L., Sherwood, G., Barnsteiner, J., Disch, J., Johnson, J., Mitchell, P., Sullivan, D., & Warren, J. (2007). Quality and safety education for nurses. *Nursing Outlook, 55*(3), 122–131.

Friedrich, M. J. (2008). Exercise may boost aging immune system. *Journal of the American Medical Association, 299*(2), 160–161.

Huether, S. E., & McCance, K. L. (2009). *Pathophysiology: The biologic basis for disease in adults and children* (6th ed.). St. Louis, MO: Mosby.

Kemeny, M. E., & Schedlowski, M. (2007). Understanding the interaction between psychosocial stress and immune-related diseases: A stepwise progression. *Brain Behavior and Immunity, 8,* 1009–1018.

Lupus Foundation of America. (2012). *Late onset lupus fact sheet.* Retrieved from http://www.lupus.org/webmodules/webarticlesnet/templates/new_aboutindividualized.aspx?articleid=111&zoneid=18

Mocchegiani, E., Romeo, J., Malavolta, M., Costarelli, L., Giacconi, R., Diaz, L. E., & Marcos, A. (2012). Zinc: Dietary intake and impact of supplementation on immune function in elderly. *Age (Dordr)* Jan 6. [Epub ahead of print] (Retrieved from http://www.ncbi.nlm.nih.gov/pubmed/22222917)

NANDA International. (2012). *NANDA International nursing diagnoses: Definitions and classification, 2012–2014.* Philadelphia, PA: Wiley-Blackwell.

National Center for Complementary and Alternative Medicine. (2012). *Herbs at a glance: Asian ginseng.* Retrieved from http://www.nccam.nih.gov/health/asianginseng

National Institute of Allergy and Infectious Diseases (NIAID) & National Cancer Institute (NCI). (2007). *Understanding the immune system: How it works* (NIH Publication No. 07-5423). Washington, DC: U.S. Department of Health and Human Services. Retrieved from http://www.niaid.nih.gov/topics/immuneSystem/Documents/theimmunesystem.pdf

National Institutes of Health. (2012a). *Flu—Get the shot.* Retrieved from http://www.nia.nih.gov/health/publication/flu-get-shot

National Institutes of Health. (2012b). *HIV, AIDS and older people.* Retrieved from http://www.nia.nih.gov/health/publication/hiv-aids-and-older-people

National Library of Medicine [NLM]. (2012). *Aging changes and immunity.* Retrieved from http://www.nlm.nih.gov/medlineplus/ency/article/004008.htm

Reuben, D., Herr, K., Pacala, J., Pollock, B., Potter, J., & Semla, T. (2010). *Geriatrics at your fingertips* (12th ed.). Malden, MA: American Geriatrics Society, Blackwell.

Seaward, B. L. (2012). *Managing stress: Principles and strategies for health and well-being* (7th ed.). Burlington, MA: Jones & Bartlett.

Senchina, D. S., & Kohut, M. L. (2007). Immunological outcomes of exercise in older adults. *Clinical Interventions in Aging, 2*(1), 3–16.

Smeltzer, S. C., & Bare, B. B. (2010). *Brunner & Suddarth's textbook of medical-surgical nursing* (12th ed.). Philadelphia, PA: Lippincott.

Sompayrac, L. (2012). *How the immune system works* (4th ed.). West Sussex, UK: Wiley-Blackwell.

Wimalawansa, S. J. (2012). Vitamin D in the new millennium. *Current Osteoporosis Reports.* March 10(1), 4-15.

Wintergerst, E. S., Maggini, S., & Hornig, D. H. (2007). Contribution of selected vitamins and trace elements to immune function. *Annals of Nutrition & Metabolism, 51*(4), 301–323.

Yang, Y., Verkuilen, J., Rosengren, K. S., Mariani, R. A., Reed, M., Grubisich, S. A., Woods, J. A., & Schlagal, B. (2008). Effects of a traditional taiji/qigong curriculum on older adults' immune response to influenza vaccine. *Medicine and Sport Science, 52,* 64–76.

Caring for Frail Older Adults with Comorbidities

KEY TERMS

adverse drug events (ADEs) *689*
confusion *683*
failure to thrive *677*
frailty *677*
futile therapy *692*
geriatric cascade *677*
iatrogenesis *681*

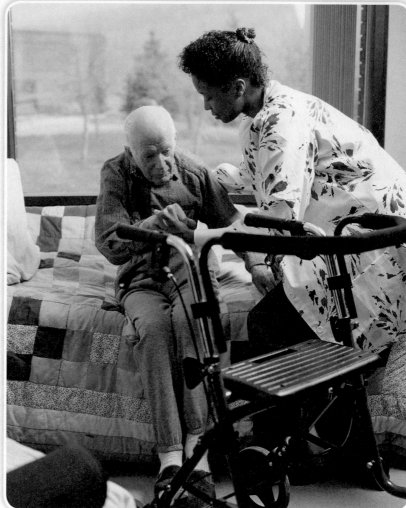

Stockbyte/Getty Images

LEARNING OUTCOMES

On completion of this chapter, the reader will be able to:

1. Describe age-related changes that affect overall health and function and that contribute to frailty.
2. State the impact of age-related changes and comorbidities on organ function.
3. Identify risk factors of health for the older person at risk for acute care hospitalization.
4. Describe the causes of and unique presentation of frailty in the older person.
5. Design appropriate nursing interventions directed toward assisting older adults with frailty to regain baseline function.
6. Formulate and implement appropriate nursing interventions to care for the older person with multisystem problems.

omprehensive nursing care of the older adult is incomplete unless the perspective of the entire person is considered. Caring for older adults with comorbidities requires skill and knowledge because the various patterns and severity of chronic conditions can combine to produce negative cumulative effects that ultimately affect the survival of the individual (Boult & Wieland, 2010). This text, like many others, focuses on the nursing interventions appropriate for each body system in isolation from other systems. However, gerontological nurses often care for older people who have multisystem problems or comorbidities. The purpose of this chapter is to describe special needs of frail older adults with multiple comorbidities, the risk factors associated with functional decline, problems encountered during hospitalization, and methods to avoid these problems and improve care.

Medical comorbidities complicate the nursing assessment and treatment of medical conditions and place the frail older person at risk for poor outcomes because of the atypical presentation of disease, delays in the initiation of treatment, lack of knowledge and skill of healthcare providers regarding care of older adults, need for multiple pharmacological interventions, and diminished organ reserve capacity that inhibits the physiological and psychological responses to stressors. The Institute of Medicine (1991) first defined **failure to thrive** as a grouping of syndromes including unintentional weight loss of more than 5% of baseline body weight, and poor appetite and nutrition often accompanied by dehydration, immobility, depression, impaired immune function, and low cholesterol levels. Often, the term *frail* is used to describe an older person experiencing this progressive physiological decline accompanied by diagnosed chronic illness, loss of organ function, recurrent acute illness, and social risk factors such as poverty, social isolation, and functional or cognitive decline.

The terms *frailty, disability, failure to thrive,* and *comorbidity* affect each other and overlap, but **frailty** is more than each of these terms alone: it is closely related to the older person's physiology and his or her inability to maintain homeostasis or optimal regulation of internal body functions. More than 50% of older adults are diagnosed with at least three comorbidities, some of which have the potential to impact function and quality of life (Anderson, 2010). Therefore, a frail older person exhibits dependence in one or more activities of daily living, is diagnosed with two or more comorbid conditions, and exhibits impairment in multiple body systems resulting in reduced ability to maintain optimal body function or homeostasis (Bartali et al., 2006). Frailty has also been defined as the presence of three or more of the following criteria:

- Unplanned weight loss (10 lb in the last year)
- Weakness and exhaustion
- Poor endurance and energy
- Decline in grip strength and gait speed
- Slowness
- Low activity

Heuberger, 2011; Young, 2003.

Frailty is an important concept for gerontological nurses and other healthcare providers caring for older people because:

- The frail older adult is the largest consumer of health care, community services, and long-term care.
- The number of older adults over the age of 85 is increasing rapidly in the United States, and the prevalence of frailty increases dramatically with age.
- Frail older adults require specialized gerontological nursing care because they have an increased burden of symptoms, are medically complex, and have increased social needs (Boult & Wieland, 2010).
- Nurses are in an ideal position to assess frailty and begin interventions to prevent adverse outcomes such as mortality, institutionalization, loss of function, and falls (Anderson, 2010).
- Nurses and other healthcare professionals are interested in identifying frail older adults to initiate specialized geriatric services to meet their needs, including geriatric assessment, multidisciplinary care, and specialized geriatric services (Golden, Martin, Silva et al., 2011).

Risks of Frailty

A frail older person is at high risk for dependency, institutionalization, falls, injuries, hospitalization, slow recovery from illness, and mortality. The frail older adult is most in need of and most likely to benefit from specialized geriatric services (Espinoza & Walston, 2005; Kietzman, Pincus, & Huynh, 2011). The very old (age 85+), those with physical frailty and cognitive impairment, and those dependent on formal and informal supports to maintain health, function, and autonomy are most at risk for decline. Often, the frail older person will suffer a rapid decline and decompensation as a result of acute illness or worsening of a chronic condition. This phenomenon of decline has been termed the **geriatric cascade** and results from the interaction of the frail older person, acute illness, and the stress of institutional care (Fretwell, 1998; Wykle & Gueldner, 2011). Frailty independently predicts poor health outcomes. Frailty becomes more common with age and, by age 95, virtually everyone exhibits signs of frailty because of accumulation of a large number of health deficits. On average, women have more deficits than men, but at any given level of deficit accumulation—including ones that would define them as frail—women tolerated deficits better, as evidenced by a lower mortality rate. The prevalence of frailty increases with age and with age made death more likely (Song, Mitnitsky, & Rockwood, 2010). Intensive, individualized nursing interventions must be instituted immediately when a frail older person is institutionalized with an acute illness or exacerbation of a chronic illness to prevent the geriatric cascade and return the older person to levels of baseline function.

The Paths to Frailty

It has been hypothesized that older adults can become frail by one or more of three pathways: *not preventable*

- Changes of aging and loss of organ reserve and function in the very old
- Diagnosis with several chronic illnesses, each of which alone and in combination with others can cause harmful effects on overall physiological function
- Chronic use of medications that can impair immunity (corticosteroids, antineoplastic agents)
- Existence in harmful social and psychological environments

Gobbens, Liujkx, Wijnen-Sponselee, et al., 2010; Robertson & Montagnini, 2004.

Figure 24-1 ▶▶▶ illustrates the interrelationship among the causes of frailty. In this model of frailty, each of the factors not only directly influences the onset and severity of frailty, but also influences all other factors in the model. For instance, the diagnosis of diabetes mellitus is known

to accelerate systemic aging. Having diabetes mellitus adds about 10 years to the age of an older person, so a 65-year-old with diabetes mellitus will physiologically resemble a 75-year-old person. Older adults with diabetes are more at risk for heart disease, stroke, poor wound healing, and micro- and macrovascular decline, thus illustrating the interrelationship between chronic illness, physiological changes of aging, and innate inability to heal and recover from illness. Age also directly affects the prognosis when an acute or chronic illness is diagnosed. For instance, older people are more at risk for death and adverse outcomes when they are diagnosed with influenza or pneumonia. These very old persons (age 85+) are more likely to die and suffer morbid events, especially during acute care hospitalization. Table 24-1 describes the age-related changes and loss of organ reserve that can contribute to the onset of frailty in the older adult.

Many of these changes are not disease specific. It may be that a critical mass of physiological changes leads to frailty rather than any one change (Gobbens et al., 2010). Individuals age at different rates and have varying degrees of compensatory abilities to overcome these age-related declines. Further, aging is affected by genetics, lifestyle, diet, physical activity, and comorbid conditions. In general, physiological aging causes a slow progressive decline in the homeostatic reserve of organ systems (Boult & Wieland, 2010). Although organ function may remain within normal limits and homeostatic mechanisms remain intact in many older adults, under periods of stress (including acute illness or exacerbation of chronic illness) the older body is less able to compensate because of declines in physiological function and reserve.

It is hypothesized that several additional factors may affect the care of the frail older person, including decline in organ function that often prohibits or complicates aggressive treatment of illness, patient and family preference, preexisting diagnosis of other diseases that already have a negative

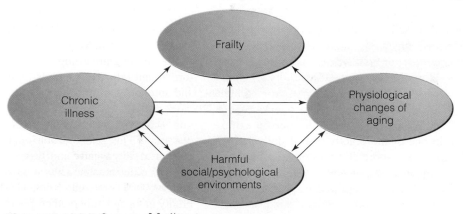

Figure 24-1 ▶▶▶ Causes of frailty.
Source: Adapted from Albert, Im, & Raveis (2002).

TABLE 24-1	**Physiological Changes of Aging and Contribution to Frailty**
Age-Related Change	**Contribution to Frailty**
Integumentary System	
• Thinning of the dermis • Decrease in eccrine and apocrine glands • Loss of subcutaneous fat • Decrease in collagen	Potential for: • Skin tears, bruising, laceration, injury, and infection • Hypo/hyperthermia • Decubitus ulcers • Decreased wound healing
Musculoskeletal System	
• Decreased bone density • Reduction in muscle mass/strength • Decreased range of motion in joints • Narrowing of intervertebral disks • Lean body mass replaced by fat • Gait instability	Potential for: • Falls and serious injury • Injury from falls and impaired balance • Gait disorders • Height loss (1 to 4 inches) with impact on chest expansion and balance • Hazards from immobility • Deconditioning • Limitation of movement and social isolation
Neurologic System	
• Increases in reaction time • Slowing of coordinated movements • Deterioration of balance mechanisms • Decreased sense of vibration, proprioception • Decreased sensation (touch, taste, hearing, vision) • Diminished deep sleep	Potential for: • Increased risk of burns/lacerations • Decreased eye–hand coordination and inability to protect self from injury • Increased risk of falls • Inability to protect self from injury • Decreased ability to interact effectively with environment • Daytime irritability and chronic fatigue
Cardiovascular System	
• Decreased arterial compliance • Deterioration of baroreceptor response • Impaired diastolic filling • Degeneration of conduction tissue • Absence of ischemic pain accompanying myocardial infarction	Potential for: • Increased risk of conduction disturbances, tachyarrhythmias • Increased risk of hypotension with dehydration • Decreased heart rate in response to stress • Increased risk of postural hypotension • Increased risk of systolic hypertension and ventricular hypertrophy • Decrease in maximum (peak exercise) heart rate
Immune System	
• Decreases in immune response	Potential for: • Atypical presentation of disease • Delayed or incomplete healing • Infections resulting from more serious pathogens • Increased susceptibility to infectious disease • Requirement for more antibiotic/antiviral treatment of infection resulting in potential for development of antibiotic-resistant organisms and systemic effects of antibiotic treatment • Increases in rate of cancer and autoimmune diseases

(continued)

TABLE 24-1	Physiological Changes of Aging and Contribution to Frailty (*continued*)
Age-Related Change	**Contribution to Frailty**
Respiratory System	
• Decreased oxygenation of tissues • Decreased lung capacity • Decreased pulmonary function • Drier mucous membranes	Potential for: • Respiratory failure under anesthesia • Respiratory depression in response to drugs • Increased risk for aspiration and infection • Decreased cough reflex • Increased sleep apnea
Renal System	
• Decreased renal function • Decrease in number of nephrons • Decreased glomerular filtration rate and creatinine production	Potential for: • Toxic drug reactions • Increased renal thresholds for glucose, electrolytes • Overhydration or dehydration
Gastrointestinal System	
• Decreased blood supply to intestines • Decreased liver function • Delayed gastric motility and emptying • Decreased gastric acid production	Potential for: • Toxic drug reactions • Digestive disorders/malabsorption syndrome • Dysphagia and aspiration pneumonia • Gastrointestinal bleeding • Gastroesophageal reflux disease, gastric and peptic ulceration • Diarrhea/constipation • Fecal incontinence
Endocrine	
• Decreased/increased secretion and action of insulin • Changes in secretion and action of thyroid hormone	Potential for: • Hypo/hyperglycemia • Hypo/hyperthyroidism
Hematopoietic	
• Decline in active bone marrow • Decreased number of red blood cells • Reduced ability to accelerate red blood cell production	Potential for: • Anemia • Decline in phagocytosis and ability to fight pathogens

Source: Adapted from Benefield & Higbee (2012); Fried et al. (2001); Gobbens et al. (2010).

impact on quality of life, and ageism in the healthcare system with older people seen as less desirable candidates for aggressive interventions (Rosenthal, Kaboli, Barnett, et al., 2002). The inevitable outcome is that older adults may not be offered or receive the same curative treatments as middle-aged or young persons, thus contributing to the higher mortality and morbidity rates based on chronological age alone rather than functional reserve. Because of the variability in aging and uniqueness of each person's compensatory ability, chronological age should never serve as a sole marker for making treatment decisions. Given the varying rates of aging among individuals and the heterogeneity of the aging process, a particular older person may have many, some, or no age-related problems or comorbidities. Fundamental mechanisms of the body decline progressively at different rates with age, giving way to a gradual incapacity to maintain homeostasis and adapt quickly to physiological and environmental insults. Older adults without adequate social support or financial resources or who have depression, cognitive impairment, or progressive apathy will progress on a path of functional decline that may be irreversible and lead to death in some cases. Optimum care is achieved by an overall understanding of the older person's current health problems, past health history, baseline levels of physical and cognitive function, financial and family support systems, and expectations and goals of care.

> **Practice Pearl ▶▶▶** Never use chronological age alone as a determinant for making treatment decisions. Be sure to include other factors such as functional ability, underlying state of health, degree of frailty, advance directives, and patient and family preference.

Social and Psychological Environments

Poverty, social isolation, depression, and cognitive impairment can undermine access to adequate health care, assistive technologies, motivation for self-care, and environmental modifications designed to encourage and maintain functional independence and overall health. Harmful social and psychological environments can directly contribute to frailty and compound the effects of chronic illness and physiological changes of aging.

Common Diagnoses Associated With Frailty

Chronic conditions and diseases such as diabetes, cardiovascular diseases, osteoporosis, and arthritis are major causes of frailty and disability in late life. Risks for disease and frailty increase with age and can be exacerbated by poor lifestyle choices and poverty (National Institute on Aging, 2011). Table 24-2 depicts common diagnoses and the mechanism by which each contributes to frailty in an older person.

Cumulative Effect of Comorbidities

Often, a frail older person will be diagnosed with several underlying chronic conditions and develop an acute condition that disrupts the stability of the chronic conditions. For instance, a person with a mild cognitive impairment might develop a urinary tract infection and might become more confused as a result of the infection. This confusion may limit the older person's ability to recognize or communicate the urinary symptoms. As a result, the urinary tract infection may go undiagnosed or untreated, leading to sepsis or pyelonephritis. Other common atypical presentations of illness in frail older adults include falls, loss of appetite, delirium, dehydration, atypical pain, dizziness, incontinence, sleep disturbances, and failures of self-care

(Amella, 2004). (See Chapter 2 ⊂▭⊃ for information on atypical presentation of disease in the older person.) Often, treatment is delayed because nurses and other healthcare providers do not recognize the importance of subtle changes in the frail older person's function. This delay in treatment can make the acute illness more difficult to treat.

> **Practice Pearl ▶▶▶** Older adults with cognitive impairment cannot adequately report symptoms of acute or chronic illness. Careful assessment of changes from baseline function, vital signs, and information from reliable caregivers is crucial.

The frail older person is more at risk for poor treatment outcomes and even death because of the interaction between normal changes of aging and common illnesses associated with age. Although evidence-based practice guidelines have been developed for many diagnoses, most have been developed based on treatment of singular diagnoses (Mutasingawa, Ge, & Upshur, 2011). Following single-disease evidence-based practice guidelines may result in overall care that is inappropriate or even harmful to frail older adults (Tinetti, Bogardus, & Agostini, 2004). Comorbidity and functional status are important factors in determining intensity of medical therapy and nursing interventions. Careful monitoring of the older person's status and effectiveness of the overall plan of care is indicated because frail older adults with poor function are at increased risk of toxicity from multiple medications, **iatrogenesis** or adverse outcomes of therapeutic interventions, and poor treatment outcomes when receiving nursing and medical treatment for acute illness. To meet the special needs of older adults during hospitalization, every effort should be made to correctly diagnose all vague symptoms and problems; treat all relevant diseases; assess the effect of current changes in the older person's health status, including the effect of the acute illness on other diagnosed chronic illnesses; and prevent complications of hospitalization (nosocomial infections, falls, delirium, polypharmacy, nutritional deficiencies) (Mitty, 2010).

Pathways to Frailty

Fried and colleagues (2001) studied frail older adults and showed linkages between disease states and the mechanisms that lead to those states, or causal pathways. One thread followed nutritional deficiencies that can reduce vision, leading to falls and serious injury. Another looked at how disease combinations such as arthritis and visual impairment, heart disease and arthritis, or stroke and high blood pressure may magnify each other's symptoms and hasten the onset of dependency. These factors combined

TABLE 24-2	Common Diagnoses and Contribution to Frailty
Diagnosis	**Contribution to Frailty**
Asthma	Toxicity of treatment, especially chronic steroid use contributing to risk of osteoporosis, elevated blood glucose levels, decreased immune response, increased risk of pulmonary infection, and decreased activity levels. Inability to engage in aerobic exercise and meet oxygen demands.
Cancer	Toxicity of treatment, anorexia, pain, systemic and metastatic nature of the disease.
Chronic obstructive pulmonary disease/emphysema	Decreased levels of blood oxygenation, chronic acute lung infections and need for antibiotic treatment, chronic fatigue and decreased activity levels.
Chronic renal failure	Potential for drug toxicity, fluid overload, dependency edema, pleural effusion, electrolyte and metabolic abnormalities.
Chronic liver disease	Potential for drug toxicity, metabolic and digestive abnormalities.
Cognitive and mood disorders	Inability to engage in self-care activities, resistiveness to care, lack of motivation for rehabilitation, toxic side effects of medications, including tardive dyskinesia and movement disorders associated with use of psychotropic medications.
Diabetes	Malabsorption, metabolic disorders, end organ damage, decreased immune response, use of multiple medications, increased risk of cardiovascular disease, potential for hyper/hypoglycemia, and exercise intolerance.
Bone fractures	Pain, toxic effects of pain medication, decreased mobility with associated risks, functional impairment, risks of surgery for open reduction, risks of hospitalization with eventual placement in long-term care facility.
Inflammatory bowel disease	Malabsorption; nutritional deficiencies; risk for dehydration; risk for fecal incontinence; potential toxic effects of medications, including antidiarrheals, steroids, and antibiotics; risk for bowel obstruction, surgery, and hospitalization.
Cardiovascular disease	Potential for treatment with many medications, including antihypertensives, cholesterol-lowering agents, diuretics, and others with risk for dehydration, metabolic and electrolyte imbalance, and other systemic adverse effects; potential for fatigue and activity intolerance.
Musculoskeletal disease	Pain and potential toxic effects of pain medications, including gastrointestinal bleeding, lethargy, liver failure, and renal impairment; functional impairment, decreased mobility, and associated risks; risks of chronic inflammation and medications associated with treatment; risk of injury, surgery, and treatment.

Source: Fried et al. (2001); Rensbergen & Nawrot (2010).

with weight loss, loss of muscle mass, and decreased strength and energy can all lead to the inactivity, decreased total energy expenditure, anorexia, and neuroendocrine dysregulation that contribute to undernutrition and negative energy balance. This vicious cycle will eventually produce frailty in the older adult (Figure 24-2 ▶▶▶).

Functional status varies considerably among older adults, with a substantial portion remaining independent in daily function throughout their lives and continuing to volunteer or work, the majority needing some assistance with instrumental activities after the age of 85, and a portion of frail older adults who are disabled. Many older people who have chronic conditions and disabilities are not frail and lead active, productive lives. However, some meet the description of frailty and are more disabled, requiring assistance with activities of daily living. Approximately 36% of older Americans with chronic conditions require assistance daily. In general, older people with lower incomes are more likely to have conditions that are more difficult or costly to treat. Native Americans and African Americans are more likely than Caucasians to have limitations in activities of daily living. Older African American men and women with arthritis are more likely to have activity limitations than other older people (U.S. Census Bureau, 2010). Nearly 60% of older African Americans report high blood pressure, and a growing number of older African Americans and Hispanics are reporting diabetes. Many of these health problems began in middle age, resulting in

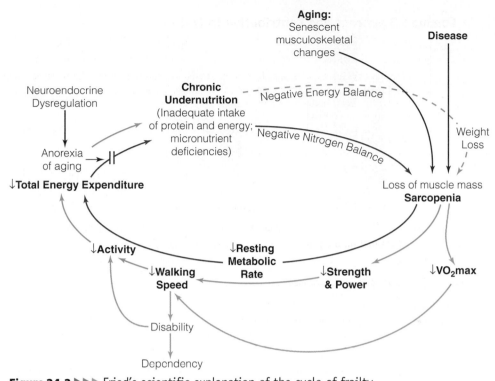

Figure 24-2 ▶▶▶ Fried's scientific explanation of the cycle of frailty.

Source: Fried et al. (2001). Frailty in Older Adults: Evidence for a Phenotype. *The Journals of Gerontology Series A 56*(3): M146–M157, Fig. 1. Reprinted with permission.

many minority older adults entering old age already carrying the burden of chronic disease and disability. Frail older adults are at risk for any number of adverse events that can be caused by a variety of stressors, some seemingly benign. For instance, an upper respiratory infection that may cause only minor inconvenience to a middle-aged or young adult may cause delirium, falls, **confusion** (impaired cognition or mental status change), dehydration, incontinence, and institutionalization in the frail older adult. Capacity to fight disease and achieve full recovery may be more difficult in frail older adults. Figure 24-3 ▶▶▶ illustrates the prevalence of hypertension, hypercholesterolemia, and diabetes in adults by race/ethnicity from 1999 to 2006.

While the number of Americans with chronic conditions is expected to increase significantly during the next several years and the prevalence of chronic conditions is also increasing, there is a simultaneous decline in the functional limitations associated with these chronic conditions. It is possible that chronic conditions are being more widely diagnosed and treated, thereby reducing their ability to cause functional limitations. Noninvasive or minimally invasive testing and screening procedures are leading to earlier diagnosis of osteoporosis, heart disease, vascular problems, cancer, and other disabling illnesses. Prescription drugs and technologies in development have the potential to contribute further to these trends (Anderson, 2010). The goal associated

with earlier diagnosis of chronic disease and more aggressive treatment is to limit accompanying disability, prevent further functional decline, and maintain or improve quality of life. If these goals are not met, early diagnosis and prolonged treatment of chronic illness results in longer periods of disability, protracted functional decline, and extension of years of life without improvement in quality of life.

Some older adults with chronic conditions remain active and independent, whereas others decline into frailty and dependence (Boult & Wieland, 2010). Several factors can affect the chronic illness trajectory:

■ Some conditions are more disabling than others. For instance, a cognitive impairment may have a greater impact on an older person's function than does osteoarthritis.
■ Many chronic conditions, such as osteoporosis and hypertension, are controllable with medications. Disabling effects and progression of symptoms may be controlled or halted with careful treatment and monitoring.
■ Many older adults have health insurance, prescription drug coverage, access to health care, social support, and adequate financial resources to manage their chronic conditions while maintaining functional ability. These older adults with these valuable resources have better outcomes than those who do not.

Anderson, 2010.

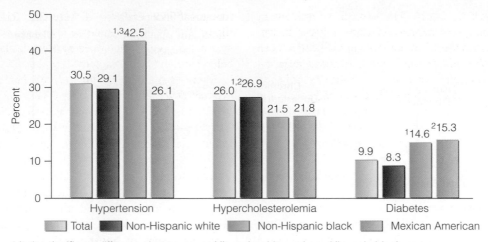

1 is the significant difference between non-Hispanic white and non-Hispanic black persons.
2 is the significant difference between non-Hispanic white and Mexican-American persons.
3 is the significant difference between non-Hispanic black and Mexican-American persons.
NOTE: Persons of other race/ethnicity included in total.

Figure 24-3 ▶▶▶ Age-adjusted prevalence of diagnosed or undiagnosed hypertension, hypercholesterolemia, and diabetes in adults, by race/ethnicity: United States, 1999–2006.

Source: Fryar, C. D., Hirsch, R., Eberhardt, M. S., Yoon, S. S., & Wright, J. D. (2010). *Hypertension, high serum total cholesterol, and diabetes: Racial and ethnic prevalence differences in U.S. adults, 1999–2006* (NCHS Data Brief No. 36). Hyattsville, MD: National Center for Health Statistics.

Trajectories of Functional Decline

Lunney and colleagues (2003) have studied older adults and document various patterns of functional decline. Frail older adults and individuals at the end of life exhibit four distinct trajectories of functional decline:

1. **Sudden death.** Physical function is optimal and a massive unpredictable event such as accident or trauma, heart attack, or stroke occurs suddenly, resulting in immediate death. Approximately 16% of study participants experienced sudden death.

2. **Diagnosis with a terminal illness.** Physical function is optimal and a terminal illness such as cancer is diagnosed with gradual, progressive, linear decline over a short and predictable period of time. Twenty-one percent of study participants experienced death from a terminal illness.

3. **Organ failure.** Physical function gradually declines with entry and reentry into the healthcare system with periods of return home between hospital stays, resulting in a downhill trajectory with periods of plateau. Twenty percent experienced death from organ failure.

4. **Frailty.** Lingering, expected deaths occur with a long, gradual downhill progression of already diminished physical function. Twenty percent experienced death with a frailty trajectory.

Glaser & Strauss, 1968; Lunney et al., 2003.

Older adults who die suddenly will not need health services, but it is likely that their survivors and loved ones will need supportive bereavement services. The majority of older Americans will experience one of the other end-of-life trajectories and will require varying clinical approaches with differing types of health services. The older adults who are diagnosed with terminal illness and who endure short-term expected death with a predictable loss of function are the only group of older adults who are likely to meet the requirements for hospice care and thus access supportive services. Those who experience entry and reentry trajectories and frailty are likely to require, but may not have access to, supportive services because of steadily diminishing reserve capacity to cope with inevitable but unpredictable acute health challenges (Lunney et al., 2003).

Frailty and Emotional Health

Chronic conditions and frailty also negatively affect emotional health. New-onset depression is frequent in older adults with significant chronic illnesses. The negative impact of these illnesses on function is increased by the presence of depression (Mezuk, Edwards, Lohman et al., 2011; Robertson & Montagnini, 2004). Women with chronic conditions are more likely to rate their health as poor, and older African American women provide the least positive assessment of their emotional well-being (National Center for Health Statistics, 2007). The careful assessment of signs and symptoms of depression using reliable instruments and judicious use of antidepressant medications can improve the quality of life and function of those suffering from depression and chronic illness. With the cost of health care rising each year, the United States already faces the challenge of providing appropriate and accessible health care to all persons. It is important to consider not only how to achieve this goal, but also how to recognize that different groups of older and chronically ill persons have different healthcare needs. The focus of health care for the frail older person will move beyond the medical model to include how to mobilize necessities for daily care, including medications, provision of nutritious meals, transportation to healthcare appointments, and home maintenance and safety (Anderson, 2010).

> **Practice Pearl** ▶▶▶ Poor health and disability are not inevitable consequences of aging; however, as we age, threats to health such as poor nutrition and an unhealthy lifestyle can become more dangerous. Normal changes of aging and diminished organ reserve result in a decreased ability to overcome these threats to health, quality of life, and function.

Americans can improve their chances for a healthy old age by simply taking advantage of recommended preventive health services and by making healthy lifestyle changes. About 70% of the physical decline that occurs with aging is related to modifiable factors such as smoking, poor nutrition, physical inactivity, and failure to use preventive and screening services (Centers for Disease Control and Prevention [CDC] & Merck Company Foundation, 2007). The challenge for healthcare professionals is to encourage people at all stages of life to reduce their chances of disability and chronic illness by undertaking healthy lifestyle changes. This strategy will increase the number of healthy years an older person is expected to live. Improvements in lifestyle choices may lead to future declines in disability rates (Anderson, 2010).

Frailty, Comorbidities, and Functional Status

Chronic diseases like diabetes, cardiovascular disease, osteoporosis, and arthritis are major causes of frailty and disability in late life (Boult & Wieland, 2010; National Institute on Aging, 2011). The established goal of the National Institute on Aging is to "add life to years" and to educate professionals and support research that establishes specific, practical ways to reduce disability and promote

functional independence in later life. Risks for chronic illness and disability increase with age, and the onset of symptoms can be accelerated by lifestyle choices and other behavioral and social factors.

Many older people who have chronic conditions and disabilities lead active, productive lives, but some are more disabled and require assistance with activities of daily living. About 44 million Americans with chronic conditions require daily assistance. Heart failure, cancer, and Alzheimer's disease represent a significant burden of care. Nurses often provide care to older adults with these diagnoses in a variety of settings. The growing number of older people with longer survival times with multiple chronic diseases illustrates the need to have expert nurses educated regarding issues of holistic geriatric care. This shifting epidemiology will dramatically alter the nature of care, because these older adults will increasingly require specialized physical and behavioral treatment across community and institutional settings. Evidence-based therapies, sophisticated levels of interprofessional care, and careful coordination characterize the health care that is necessary to provide the quality care needed by persons with heart failure, cancer, and Alzheimer's disease as well as other chronic illnesses (Boult & Wieland, 2010).

Cancer

Increasing age is directly associated with increasing rates of cancer, corresponding to an 11-fold increased incidence in persons over the age of 65. Despite these statistics, very few older adults enter into chemotherapy clinical trials. Limited information is available regarding the efficacy of various treatments such as surgery, chemotherapy, and radiation in this age group. The course of cancer treatment has shifted from relatively high mortality risks to patterns of chronic remission and recurrence in many of the most common malignancies, particularly solid tumors, with the advent of therapies that use multiple treatment modalities and collaborative care (Kumar, Katheria, & Hurria, 2010). Chronological age does not always predict the physical response of the individual to cancer treatment, but rather the presence of comorbidities. Frail older adults are particularly vulnerable to the side effects of aggressive chemotherapy and less aggressive treatment regimens may be required. The challenge is to implement evidence-based approaches to provide appropriate individualized therapies to treat cancer in the older adult without shifting the overall risk/benefit analysis of such treatments (Kumar et al., 2010).

Signs and symptoms of frailty in a person with cancer include cachexia or wasting syndrome, functional and cognitive decline, serum albumin less than 2.5 g/100 dL, recurrent diagnoses with secondary infections (pneumonia, skin infections, urinary tract infection), and unremitting pain.

Cardiovascular Disease

Cardiovascular disease is the most common cause of hospitalization and death in the older population. The underlying cause is most often coronary atherosclerosis, which occurs not only as a result of aging processes but also from the cumulative effect of poor personal health habits such as smoking, obesity, sedentary lifestyle, and poorly controlled hypertension (McCance & Huether, 2012). Separating the effects of aging from the effects of pathology is difficult and requires more ongoing study.

In the past, heart disease was thought to be a male problem. Healthcare providers are just beginning to understand that heart disease greatly affects older women, who comprise the majority of older people. One in nine women between the ages of 45 and 64 has some form of cardiovascular disease, ranging from coronary artery disease to stroke or renal vascular disease. By the time a woman reaches age 65, she has a one in three chance of developing cardiovascular disease. A number of studies show that African American women are at even greater risk than these averages.

- One in four women will die from heart disease while 1 in 30 will die from breast cancer.
- Twenty-three percent of women who have a heart attack will die within 1 year.
- Two-thirds of women who have a heart attack fail to make a full recovery.
- Within 6 years of having a heart attack, 46% of women will be diagnosed with heart failure.

Thomassian, 2012.

Men are much more likely to be stricken with heart disease in their prime middle years, whereas women tend to get it 10 to 20 years later. For most women, it is only after menopause that heart disease becomes a problem. A woman 60 years old is about as likely to get heart disease as a man of 50. By the time they are in their 70s, men and women get heart disease at equal rates. Statistics reflect an encouraging trend. Better understanding of preventive measures and increasing sophistication in diagnosis and treatment have resulted in decreasing rates of heart disease in both men and women.

A new emphasis on prevention and treatment of heart disease includes lower blood pressure goals and guidelines including lower levels for those with diabetes (see Chapter 19 ⊂⊃), new guidelines for lowering lipid levels, a greater understanding of the role of obesity on development of heart disease, use of less invasive surgical procedures to relieve arterial blockages and prevent restenosis, new drugs for the prevention and treatment of heart failure, and increasingly aggressive measures to prevent and treat

the complications and disabilities associated with stroke. Indicators of frailty in a person with cardiovascular problems might include frequent hospitalization despite optimal treatment, functional decline, elevations in blood urea nitrogen and creatinine levels, fluctuating vital signs and daily weights, persistent angina or shortness of breath even at rest, cognitive or financial problems that inhibit access to appropriate medications and treatments, and indications of drug toxicity from medications needed to sustain life and cardiovascular function.

Alzheimer's Disease

An estimated 5.4 million Americans have Alzheimer's disease, including 5.2 million people over the age of 65 and 200,000 under the age of 65 (Alzheimer's Association, 2011). By 2050, this number could double, given the population projections and growth in the numbers of older adults. A person with Alzheimer's disease will live an average of 8 years and as many as 20 years or more from the onset of symptoms (Office of Technology Assessment, 2008). More than half of all nursing home residents have Alzheimer's disease, and the average cost for nursing home care ranges from $74,000 to $82,000 per resident per year (MetLife, 2011). The cost of caring for older adults with Alzheimer's disease is expected to increase from $183 billion per year in 2011 to $1.1 trillion in 2050 (Alzheimer's Association, 2011). Currently, Medicare and Medicaid cover approximately 70% of these costs.

When cognitive capacity is impaired due to the diagnosis of Alzheimer's disease or another irreversible neurodegenerative dementia, care and treatment decisions become even more difficult. Virtually all older adults with dementia have unremitting disease courses inevitably leading to death (Alzheimer's Association, 2011). The treatment preferences of persons with dementia are often made by family members on behalf of the older person or are based on predetermined wishes such as living wills. In reality, however, treatment choices may not be so simple. There are many factors to consider, such as burden of treatment, chance of success of the intervention, relief of symptoms, reduction of a family's burden of care, the family's level of understanding and commitment, and level of acuity of the setting in which the care is provided.

Advanced age is the biggest risk factor for the development of Alzheimer's disease. One in 10 persons over the age of 65 and nearly half of those over age 85 have the disease (Alzheimer's Association, 2011). Because life expectancy in the United States is increasing and persons over age 85 represent the fastest growing segment of the population, need for care of people with Alzheimer's disease may become even more problematic during the next several decades. While more than 8 of 10 people with Alzheimer's disease live at home, the need for long-term care is nearly inevitable in the later stages of dementia to supply respite for family caregivers and to provide a comfortable and safe environment and symptomatic treatment (Alzheimer's Association, 2011).

Nearly 87% of nursing home residents with dementia exhibit one or more behavioral problems, including agitation, aggression, wandering, and sleep disorders. Delusions and hallucinations are common in all stages of dementia as the person loses contact with reality and can no longer function in his or her environment. A misplaced pair of eyeglasses may trigger a confrontation as the dementia victim accuses the caregiver of hiding the glasses or just trying to make things more difficult. The average family caregiver is usually a woman (wife, daughter, or daughter-in-law) about 60 years of age. Alzheimer's caregivers report significant physical and mental health problems, including sleep disturbances, anxiety, depression, backache, arthritis, indigestion, hypertension, and high cholesterol. Institutionalization often becomes necessary when caregivers are exhausted and can no longer provide care to their family member. This can be an especially difficult time for families, and information and support are needed by families facing these decisions.

Approximately 68% of all nursing home residents have Alzheimer's disease, and approximately one fourth of older nursing home residents will be hospitalized during a 1-year period. At any point in time, about one quarter of all hospital patients ages 65 and older are people with Alzheimer's and other dementias. The most common reasons for hospitalization of people with Alzheimer's disease include syncope, fall and trauma (26%), ischemic heart disease (17%), and gastrointestinal disease (9%) (Alzheimer's Association, 2011). Most hospitalizations will occur in the first 3 months of residence in the nursing facility.

Nursing home residents admitted to hospitals are at risk for poor outcomes based on advanced age; lack of baseline laboratory data; higher baseline levels of functional and cognitive impairment; potential for information and communication errors regarding treatments, medications, and goals of treatment during the transfer process; and diagnoses with many comorbidities. During the hospital stay, the nursing facility resident is at risk for delirium, restraints, functional decline, pressure ulcers, and medication changes that may or may not be adequately communicated to the nursing home upon discharge.

Musculoskeletal Problems

Changes in bone and muscle are associated with functional disability in later life. Osteoporosis, osteoarthritis, and age-related loss of muscle mass force many older people to become functionally dependent, suffering weakness, falls, fractures, and other problems related to immobility. Older adults diagnosed with musculoskeletal problems are at risk for frailty because weakness and immobility will compound recovery from surgery, acute illness, or chronic illness. Loss of bone and muscle mass may make position changes more difficult, complicate early ambulation attempts after surgery, necessitate the use of bedpans and catheters, and delay trips to the bathroom, thus facilitating urinary and fecal incontinence. The older person is also at risk for falls and significant injury resulting from these falls. Signs of frailty in an older person with musculoskeletal problems may include decreased stamina and physical deconditioning, shortness of breath on exertion, history of falls, dizziness, weakness, poor vision or hearing, cognitive or mood impairment inhibiting judgment and preparation for movement, and diagnoses with comorbidities such as cardiovascular or neurologic disease.

Diabetes

Older adults with diabetes are at risk for frailty because of the complicated nature of managing and treating diabetes and its association with other diseases and problems such as cardiovascular disease and declines in neural, renal, immune, and sensory function (see Chapter 19 ⊂⊃). When acute illness is diagnosed in an older person with diabetes, often eating patterns are disrupted, new medications are added, and activity levels are changed. All of these factors can greatly affect the older person's blood glucose levels and medication regimen. Because of declines in the immune system's ability to protect against infection, older adults with diabetes are more at risk for urinary tract infection, otitis media, development of peripheral ulcers, cholecystitis, and respiratory infection. When antibiotics are used in older adults with diabetes, they are usually prescribed at higher doses for longer periods of time to ensure complete eradication of the offending organism. These higher doses place the person at risk for medication side effects and drug interactions, including development of antibiotic-associated diarrhea, fungal infections, decreases in renal excretion of all prescribed medications, and development of hypo- or hyperglycemia. Older adults with diabetes may be considered frail if they exhibit any of the following characteristics: frequent need for treatment of severe hypo- or hyperglycemia indicating poor regulation and control, frequent diagnosed secondary infections, fluctuating vital signs and weight, presence of cognitive or functional impairment, financial and social problems inhibiting access to appropriate medications or treatment, and diagnosis with comorbidities complicating the assessment and treatment of the diabetes.

Long-Term Care

Factors in the acute care hospital and long-term care environment may exacerbate cognitive decline and behavioral problems. Maintaining the emotional and relational well-being of those with dementia depends on caregivers who see dignity even in those severely affected by their condition. Older patients often spend too much time in bed, often alone or attached to monitors that restrict movement. With the best intentions, an efficient nursing staff may actually reinforce the resident's dependence (Wilson et al., 2010). Many healthcare facilities are understaffed, especially at night when older adults with cognitive impairments are expected to remain in bed and asleep for 8 to 10 hours. Nurses and nursing assistants may save time by "doing for" residents rather than encouraging residents to do more for themselves. Nurses should address problem behaviors using social and environmental modifications and creative activities, thereby preserving independence and self-esteem. Drugs for behavioral control should be used cautiously and only for specific purposes such as depression, psychosis, anxiety, and sleep disturbances (Alzheimer's Association, 2011). Polypharmacy and overmedication are serious problems inherent in the care of the older person with dementia.

Behavioral approaches include training caregivers in therapeutic responses to resistiveness to care, use of calming music, therapeutic touch, and other nonpharmacological responses appropriate for each particular older person. Long-term care facilities should provide residents with safe areas to walk, access to protected outside areas, access to common rooms where activities can be enjoyed 24 hours a day, and more privacy in individual rooms. Sleep disturbances are common when two older residents share the same room and one resident requires frequent staff supervision and monitoring. Long-term care facilities should shift their focus of care delivery to become more resident centered and construct systems of care that enhance quality of life for individuals with dementia.

Post (1995) described effective quality of life for persons with dementia to include:

1. Adjustment to and coping with the experience of increasing forgetfulness prior to the point of forgetting that one forgets
2. Attainment of optimal emotional–behavioral conditions in the more advanced stages
3. Avoidance of treatment-induced agitation, fear, and pain

According to Post (1995), "Because memories and sense of self are lost to the ravages of the disease, the existential moment assumes paramount importance. When care providers can establish a system of care that enhances positive adjustment and a relatively calm emotional life, life becomes more worth living for the dementia victim" (p. 99). The nurse can greatly improve the quality of a person's life by providing a safe and consistent environment, predictable pleasures and things to look forward to, avoidance of pain and invasive interventions when possible, and abundant and generous reassurance and support in times of stress.

Long-term care facilities support daily living activities for frail older people with limited functional abilities, and this objective is conceptually different from the objectives of other healthcare facilities. However, occupancy rates in nursing homes have been falling, as have the number of private-pay residents (MetLife, 2011). Two factors may be responsible for this trend: (1) Nursing homes are reorienting themselves more toward postacute care and intensive rehabilitation and somewhat away from services provided to the traditional long-term care resident. (2) Other care settings are emerging in the marketplace for elders with disabilities who can pay for their own care. Many of these financially able elders will choose to purchase home care services or move to upscale assisted-living facilities rather than live in nursing homes. Therefore, the average nursing home resident is becoming more frail with increasing financial and physical dependency.

Making Treatment Decisions

The health care of persons with dementia or other frailty is complicated. The caring process is often prolonged and accompanied by ethical questions regarding the intensity and type of care that is delivered. In general, the provision of care for the seriously ill long-term care resident should honor the resident's preferences, reflect the needs and wishes of families, be consistent with accepted public policy, and not inflict undue burden or harm to the resident without a reasonable chance of success. Although treatment decisions must be cost indifferent, fairness demands that treatments should be provided for those older adults most likely to benefit and begin to be discouraged from those older adults with slim or no chance of benefit (Cashman, Wright, & Ring, 2010). Ineffective treatments, delivered by clinicians who are rewarded on a fee-for-service basis and requested by distraught families and older adults, strain limited resources within the healthcare system and produce suffering on the part of older adults who may already have poor quality of life. When making healthcare decisions for frail older adults, the burden of treatment should be considered along with the risks and benefits.

Palliative care can be provided to the seriously ill older person at any time during the disease process (see Chapter 11). Unlike hospice, which is a system of care that is intended for individuals close to death, palliative care can be delivered for extended periods and throughout all phases of the treatment process. Palliative care emphasizes development of a therapeutic relationship through the provision of stable healthcare providers, alleviation of pain and management of troublesome symptoms, respite for families, reduction in use of acute care hospitals for death and unnecessary hospitalization, and increases in patient and family satisfaction with healthcare delivery (City of Hope & American Association of Colleges of Nursing [AACN], 2012).

The demand for newer and more expensive services and treatments continues to grow, while the equitable delivery of high-quality health care at reasonable costs remains an unresolved challenge in the American healthcare system (Paris, Reardon, & Browne, 2003). Healthcare providers are often reticent to discuss advance directives and treatment options within the context of dementia or other forms of frailty with healthy older adults. For instance, a person may be perfectly willing to undergo a serious operation when he or she has coping abilities and mental faculties to deal with pain, spend time in a hospital away from family and friends, and participate in rehabilitation with eventual return to home. Any person who has had a serious operation knows that the experience is stressful and difficult, and most older adults cannot wait to be discharged to home. The same serious operation carries a more significant burden for an older person with dementia or physical frailty. Nurses providing care to older adults with dementia or physical frailty should be experts in pain assessment and treatment techniques, address safety issues, administer medications carefully while being alert for adverse effects, and involve the interdisciplinary healthcare team as much as possible from the moment of admission to develop and facilitate treatment goals and a discharge plan.

Physically frail older adults with cognitive impairment become even more confused with social isolation, exposure to narcotic pain medications and drugs used for anesthesia, and changes in their usual care routine. They are less able to participate in rehabilitation after surgery. Older adults with dementia and others with aphasia are much less likely to verbalize pain and request pain medications.

Often, physical and chemical restraints are needed to control agitation in older adults with dementia or delirium. An older person with dementia will often have a hand restrained to protect intravenous lines, drains, and oxygen tubing from being removed. One can only imagine how frightening this must be to an already confused and seriously ill older person. The "do everything" philosophy, nurtured in medical and nursing schools and encouraged by a litigious culture, promotes aggressive cure-oriented treatment (Post et al., 2001). Many times, significant others and families do not realize that they have the options of choosing less aggressive care that may be more appropriate for the frail older person who is at risk for adverse treatment outcomes. Nurses can play a key role in educating families, providing support, and involving the interdisciplinary team.

Acute Illness and Hospitalization

Common causes of hospitalization include pneumonia, influenza, heart failure, ischemic heart disease, urinary tract infection, hip fracture, digestive disorders, and dehydration. Heart failure and pneumonia are the most common conditions associated with rapid readmissions (Golden, Tewary, Dang et al., 2010). Stroke, hip fracture, poorly controlled diabetes, and chronic obstructive pulmonary disease are also associated with high rates of hospital readmission. Factors associated with an increased risk for rapid rehospitalization include:

- Age over 80 years
- Diagnosis of five or more comorbidities
- Functional impairment
- Current or past history of depression and/or alcohol abuse
- Inadequate social support system
- Residing in a low-income community

Golden et al., 2010.

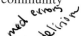
med errors
delirium

Hospital care is associated with increased use of medications, invasive procedures, diagnostic testing requiring food and fluid restriction, nosocomial infections, and occurrence of adverse events and poor outcomes to hospitalized older patients. More than 177,000 older people visit the emergency department each year and are seven times more likely to be hospitalized after an emergency department visit as a result of **adverse drug events (ADEs)** or poor outcome or toxicity resulting in real or potential harm to an individual (CDC, 2010). Older adults with comorbidities are more likely to take many medications and thus experience a higher risk of adverse drug events. Even in the absence of polypharmacy, older adults are inherently at higher risk of adverse drug events due to normal changes of aging and the resulting impact on drug metabolism and distribution. Adverse drug events can be minimized by implementing preventive strategies. Use of computerized entry systems, monitoring of prescriptions by a clinical pharmacist, and identification of the correct patient and drug using bar-code technology are methods that have been shown to decrease the frequency of medication errors. Adverse drug events can result from the following errors:

- Missed dose
- Wrong technique

- Illegible order
- Duplicate therapy
- Drug–drug interaction
- Equipment failure
- Inadequate monitoring
- Preparation error

CDC, 2010.

In 2009, Medicare began withholding payment for serious preventable adverse events, resulting in significant financial penalties to hospitals that do not provide adequate care. The responsibility of the hospital is to adequately measure and describe the occurrence of adverse events; identify and implement evidence-based practices to prevent these events; and ensure that these adverse conditions occurring during hospitalization were not present on admission. It is hoped that these efforts will provide incentives for necessary system improvements of patient safety (Wachter, Foster, & Dudley, 2008).

> **Drug Alert ▶▶▶** Medications that can cause delirium through intoxication or withdrawal include anesthetics, analgesics, antiasthmatics, anticonvulsants, antihypertensives, antimicrobials, antiparkinsonian medications, corticosteroids, gastrointestinal H_2 blockers, muscle relaxants, hypnotics, and psychotropic medications.

Some evidence suggests that sensory deprivation experienced by older adults placed in windowless hospital rooms is associated with higher rates of delirium (Tullmann, Mion, Fletcher et al., 2008). Additional factors include not wearing hearing aids or eyeglasses, separation from personal objects, and lack of clocks and calendars. Falls can occur when older people are moving about in unsafe environments and trying to ambulate with intravenous poles on slippery or wet floors without appropriate footwear. Very old persons may arrive at the hospital in later and more severe stages of illness, may have other diagnosed chronic illness, may have sensory or cognitive impairment, and may be less able to adapt to their new environment. Thus, they are more at risk from adverse events and poor outcomes during hospitalization. Entering the hospital from a nursing home is associated with many of the attributes (including cognitive impairment) predicting poor outcomes during hospitalization (Golden et al., 2010). Nursing home residents are more at risk for adverse events, and nurses are required to provide special monitoring of their progress. Delirium and functional decline should be recognized as signs of the failure or side effects of the treatment regimen and of inadequate efforts to maintain function.

Common problems experienced by nursing home residents before, during, and after hospitalization are listed in Table 24-3. To facilitate better care of hospitalized nursing home residents, the nurse should attempt to communicate with the nursing home staff and gain as much information as possible. Hospital and nursing home nurses can work together to develop a standardized transfer database to include all necessary information and keep open lines of communication to better meet the needs of nursing home residents requiring acute care.

Two general issues should be considered in caring for older adults in the hospital: (1) determining the goals of care and (2) designing and implementing strategies to achieve those goals. Failure to address these issues leads to frustration on the part of older adults, families, and caregivers. Setting realistic goals is an important opportunity for caregivers to engage in open and honest conversations with older adults and families. For instance, if a very old and

TABLE 24-3	Common Problems Relating to Hospitalization Experienced by Nursing Home Residents
Time Period	**Examples**
Upon transfer to the hospital	Incomplete data regarding medications, baseline cognitive and physical function
	New care providers
	Lack of clarity regarding predetermined wishes and code status
	Vague reports of signs and symptoms prompting the hospital transfer
	Family members in crisis with information received from a variety of unfamiliar care providers
During hospitalization	Delirium, physical and chemical restraints, urinary catheters, decubitus ulcers, malnutrition, functional decline, invasive testing, medication changes, falls
On return to the nursing home	Poor communication from the hospital regarding new diagnoses, medications, treatments, need for follow-up, and monitoring
	Loss of function from illness/hospital experience and disease progression
	Congestive heart failure from overhydration and aggressive fluid replacement
	Indwelling catheter still in place
	Nosocomial infection diagnosed on return

Source: Adapted from Reuben et al. (2012). *Geriatrics at your fingertips.* 14th edition. New York: The American Geriatrics Society.

frail person suffers a major heart attack, the family may benefit from honest information about chances for survival, opportunities for and chances of success in rehabilitation, and possibility of returning to the prior living situation. The family may have different goals, and by engaging in conversation and development of a therapeutic and trusting relationship, the plan of care will have more chance of success. The goal may be to provide aggressive intervention including invasive testing and surgery, modified interventions such as drug administration and minimally invasive procedures, or comfort care in which pain and symptom control are the predominant issues. Table 24-4 illustrates goals and levels of care. Code status and goals of care should be discussed, clarified, and clearly noted on the chart as early as possible during the hospital admission process. Disagreements between family, older adults, and caregivers are red flags that signal trouble during the caring process. The multidisciplinary team can be mobilized to help resolve conflicts.

Aggressive care is usually appropriately delivered to older adults with high functional ability, satisfactory quality of life, high rehabilitation potential, and the physical health and ability to endure and cooperate with the demands of therapy. Modified aggressive treatment is usually appropriate for older adults with higher degrees of frailty or multiple comorbidities who still have sufficient reserve capacity to respond to the treatment. Palliative care is

appropriate for all older adults and can be delivered alone or in conjunction with aggressive or modified care. Hospice care is delivered to those with a life expectancy of 6 months or less. Age alone should not dictate the appropriate level of care. The older person's predetermined wishes in conjunction with his or her underlying degree of frailty and the professional opinions of members of the healthcare team are the key factors.

Proposed screening tests for relevant comorbid conditions upon hospital admission include:

- Risk assessment and mental status testing to quantify the older person's baseline mental status and to identify cognitive deficits that may interfere with the ability to provide informed consent or to participate in the treatment and rehabilitation plan.
- Depression testing to quantify the older person's baseline level of depression, to identify older adults needing referral for counseling or treatment with antidepressants, and to identify older adults who may lack motivation, incentive, and drive to participate in the plan of care.
- Activities of daily living to identify previous level of functioning and baseline status. This is helpful information to be considered in discharge planning.
- Social support to identify family, friends, and religious and spiritual advisers who can assist and support the older person during illness and recovery.
- Presence of comorbidities, including heart disease, lung disease, chronic renal insufficiency, hypertension, diabetes, malignancy, collagen disorders, arthritis, visual impairment, and autoimmune disorders. If the older person is capable, he or she should be asked for permission to obtain and review old medical records from other hospitalizations or healthcare clinics.
- Nutrition measures, including weight, height, bone mass index, serum albumin, and cholesterol, to provide valuable information and predict responses to drug therapy and aggressive treatment.
- Polypharmacy information regarding the medications taken by the older person to prevent duplication of prescriptions during hospitalization, to avoid interactions, and to predict compliance with the discharge plan.
- Advance directives. Determine if the older person has established a living will or named a healthcare proxy. If an advance directive has not been established, determine if the older person possesses the clinical capacity to state the kind of treatment he or she would like during this hospitalization and illness. If this is not possible, identify appropriate family members who can serve as decision makers during the end-of-life period.

TABLE 24-4	Goals and Levels of Care	
Level of Intervention	**Goal**	**Examples of Intervention**
Aggressive	Extension of life is the dominant goal	Aggressive chemotherapy, invasive testing, radical surgery
Modified	Extension of life with consideration of the burden of treatment	Management of illness with medications, minimally invasive surgery, and noninvasive testing
Palliative care	Patient comfort with life extension as secondary goal	Pain management, symptom control, gentle rehabilitation, holistic care
Hospice	Comfortable death	Pain management, holistic care, symptom control

Source: Adapted from Reuben et al. (2012). *Geriatrics at your fingertips.* 14th edition. New York: The American Geriatrics Society.

Adapted from Reuben et al., 2012.

age cognitive function + IADL function prior to admission

The Best Practices feature shows the Hospital Admission Risk Profile (HARP), which can be used to quantify risk as high, medium, or low. Hospitalization also provides the opportunity for nurses to assess health promotion and disease prevention measures in older adults. For instance, older adults who smoke should be advised to discontinue smoking and be provided with information about smoking cessation programs available in the community. Influenza, pneumococcal, and tetanus vaccines can be administered if needed. Nutritional problems can be addressed. The management of comorbid conditions can be assessed and medication and treatment regimens modified if needed. For instance, an older person admitted to the hospital for a heart condition may have consistently elevated blood glucose levels and may need adjustments in antidiabetic medications and diet. Dangerous behaviors such as excessive alcohol intake, unsafe driving in the presence of cognitive or visual impairment, and history of falling can be screened for and addressed by the nurse and the interdisciplinary healthcare team. Older people without advance directives should be urged to identify healthcare proxies or complete a living will during hospitalization. The social worker and other members of the healthcare team can be consulted to collect information and coordinate the needed resources.

Many hospitals have established acute care of the elderly (ACE) units to provide specialized care to older adults and decrease the risks of adverse events during hospitalization. An ACE unit is based on four key concepts:

1. A safe environment with uncluttered halls to promote mobility, carpeted floors to decrease glare, raised toilet seats to improve continence, and a common lounge area to promote socialization and decrease isolation
2. Patient-centered interdisciplinary care guided by nurse-driven protocols to address key nursing issues such as mobility, skin care, nutrition, and continence
3. Discharge planning with the goal of returning the older person to his or her former living status
4. Careful medical and nursing interventions to prevent adverse outcomes and avoid iatrogenic problems

ACE units have been shown to prevent functional decline, decrease length of stay, and decrease nursing home placement. Additionally, ACE units have demonstrated improvement in the process of care, including increased implementation of nursing care plans to promote independent function, increased physical therapy consults, and greater satisfaction among older adults, caregivers, physicians, and nurses.

Assessing Treatment Burden

The most significant quality-of-life concern arises from the burdens that life-extending treatment can impose on people with frailty or dementia. The caregiver must examine the potential of an intervention from the very ill or disoriented person's point of view. Will the treatment be interpreted as assault or torture? Will it prolong a life with significant behavioral or physical problems? Are there indications that the older person with dementia is refusing treatment by continued attempts to remove feeding tubes, catheters, dialysis, and intravenous lines? Therapeutic interventions that impose considerable burdens on the person with dementia should not be tolerated in a humane and just healthcare system and are considered to be **futile therapy.**

Hospital care is often rushed and fragmented among many specialists, each with a limited view and perspective of the overall patient and family situation. Burdensome interventions may result in distressing conditions, including pressure ulcers, constipation, pain, and shortness of breath. However, legitimate concerns exist when advocating that dying residents receive their care in the long-term care facilities that have become their homes. Given the uneven history of care in long-term care facilities, lower nurse-to-patient ratios, and the fact that long-term care facilities exist with the objective of providing assistance to residents to compensate for functional and cognitive disabilities, the transfer to an acute care hospital may be appropriate (Post et al., 2001). Persons with end-stage dementia and physical frailty are in need of a rational approach to care at the end of life.

The cascade of illness or functional decline is the hypothesized pathway of development of complications during illness. For instance, hospitalization may trigger functional decline from falls, incontinence, not eating, and increased confusion. The medical interventions resulting from these conditions include use of physical and chemical restraints, placement of nasogastric tubes, and use of indwelling urinary catheters. Iatrogenesis and medical complications of these interventions include increased risk of thrombophlebitis, development of decubitus ulcers, aspiration pneumonia, urinary tract infection, and increased confusion or delirium. If the cascade of illness is able to progress unabated, an older person who is admitted to the hospital with mild confusion and stable chronic illness could progress to serious illness, functional decline, nursing home placement, or even death as a result of the hospitalization.

Ethical standards that guide healthcare decision making at the end of life support the self-determination of the older person (assuming the older person has made these known before becoming cognitively impaired) or best interests of the older person (in the case of the older person who did not execute advance directives before becoming impaired) (City of Hope & AACN, 2012). An ethical dilemma that may arise is whether an older person should be treated for

Best Practices Hospital Admission Risk Profile (HARP)

1. Scoring Range 0–5

A. Age

Age Category	Risk Score	
<75	0	
75–84	1	
≥85	2	SCORE =

B. Cognitive Function (abbreviated MMSE)*

MMSE Score	Risk Score	
15–21	0	
0–14	1	SCORE =

C. IADL Function Prior to Admission**

Independent IADLs	Risk Score	
6–7	0	
0–5	2	SCORE =

2. Risk Categories

Total Score	Risk of Decline in ADL Function	
4 or 5	High risk	
2 or 3	Intermediate risk	
0 or 1	Low risk	TOTAL =

*Abbreviated MMSE includes only the following 21 components of the original 30-item test: orientation (10 items: year, season, month, date, day, city, county, state, hospital, floor); registration (3 unrelated items, such as hat, ball, tree); attention (5 items, such as spelling WORLD backwards); and recall (same 3 items as in registration). Each correct answer is scored one point.

**A person is judged independent in an activity if he/she is able to perform the activity without assistance. A person is scored dependent if he/she either does not perform an activity, requires the assistance of another person or is unable to perform an activity. IADL activities include telephoning, shopping, cooking, doing housework, taking medications, using transportation, and managing finances.

a secondary problem, such as infection, if death is pending. For instance, an older person with severe dementia may develop pneumonia during the late stages of disease. The administration of antibiotics may resolve the pneumonia, but may not be justified for an older person who is suffering from dementia. In rare cases, antibiotics may improve the older person's comfort (as in treatment of bladder infections). A classic study of older adults with dementia showed there were no differences in observed discomfort before, during, or after an infectious episode regardless of whether they were treated aggressively with antibiotics or managed palliatively with antipyretics and analgesics (Hurley, Volicer, Camberg et al., 1999).

Palliative Care

The use of valuable social and financial resources on inappropriate or futile medical care depletes healthcare resources, drives up costs, and results in less money that could be spent on providing appropriate healthcare treatment and quality-of-life enhancement for older adults who may improve as a result of such treatment. Palliative care improves the quality of life of older adults and their families when facing the problems associated with life-threatening illness. This is achieved through prevention and relief from suffering; early identification, impeccable assessment, and treatment of pain; and recognition and treatment of other physical, psychosocial, and spiritual problems (City of Hope & AACN, 2012). Figure 24-4 ▶▶▶ illustrates the key concepts associated with palliative care. Although most physicians and nurses oppose active euthanasia or "mercy killing," there is no ethical or legal mandate involved with honoring the older person's or family's refusal of treatment or recommending against disproportionately burdensome treatment or treatment that will not benefit the older person (American Nurses Association, 2010). The *Code for Nurses* delineates the nursing profession's opposition to nurse participation in active euthanasia but does not negate the obligation of the nurse to provide proper and ethically justified end-of-life care, which includes the promotion of comfort and the alleviation of suffering, adequate pain control, and, at times, forgoing life-sustaining treatments.

Common reasons for withholding or withdrawing aggressive treatment include the older person's choice, excessively burdensome care, potential for further reduction in quality of life, prolongation of the dying process, and acknowledgment that the disease progression will inevitably result in death, and treatment is likely to be ineffective

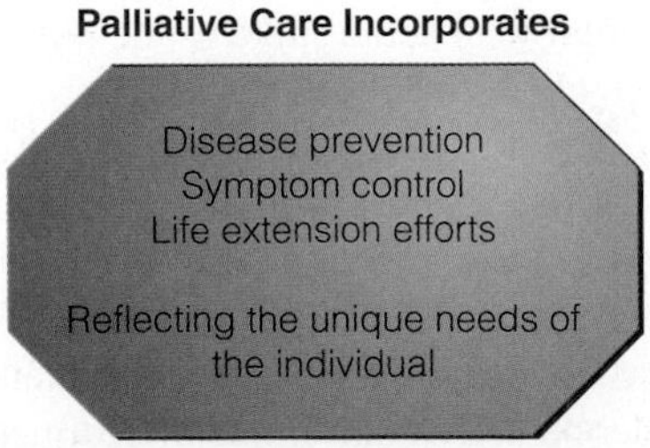

(City of Hope & AACN, 2012). Healthcare professionals may find it difficult to stop life-sustaining treatment because they have been educated to "do everything possible" to support life. Although life-sustaining treatments may be appropriate for some older adults with frailty and dementia, such treatments may only prolong suffering of other older adults. Palliative treatments such as surgery, radiation, or chemotherapy may be appropriate in that they relieve pain and suffering, but the benefit of these treatments should outweigh the burdens to ensure they are morally and ethically justified. Treatments designed to prolong life so that families have time to gather and say goodbye are most likely justifiable, but treatments designed to prolong life for family convenience (e.g., the family is going on vacation and does not want to deal with a funeral now) are most likely morally unjustifiable, especially when significant pain and suffering are involved with life extension.

> **Practice Pearl ▶▶▶** Providing comfort or palliative care is not giving up on an older person or acknowledging that nothing more can be done. Nurses providing high-quality palliative care are providing a time-intensive, individualized, and necessary service to seriously ill older adults and their family.

Healthcare providers can practice preventive ethics to promote an environment where early identification of issues and anticipation of possible dilemmas may avert potential areas of conflict. Preventive ethics involves encouraging patient choice and anticipating and preparing the person for future decision making (Nursing Ethics, 2008). The thoughtful healthcare provider will be able to anticipate where the older person and family values may be in conflict with societal and professional values. As always, conflict resolution and communication skills are the key to clarifying goals and avoiding misrepresentation.

Healthcare treatments for coexisting diseases should be modified early in the course of care for the person with dementia. Because dementia shortens the life span, some interventions designed to reduce long-term risk factors can be avoided. For instance, limiting the food choices of an older person with dementia who has high cholesterol and urging a cardiac-prudent diet may lead to weight loss, frustrate the older person, and prove to be a source of conflict with caregivers. Sometimes, aggressive treatment of disease can place the older person with dementia at risk for side effects and injury. For example, it is counterproductive to strive for low blood glucose levels in an older person with advanced dementia because of the increased danger of unrecognized hypoglycemic reactions.

Palliative Care Incorporates

Disease prevention
Symptom control
Life extension efforts

Reflecting the unique needs of the individual

Figure 24-4 ▶▶▶ Elements of palliative care.

Some interventions routinely carried out in long-term care facilities are less likely to be successful or appropriate for older adults who are physically frail or have dementia. Older adults who die in nursing homes with advanced frailty and dementia are not recognized as having a terminal condition and do not receive care that promotes palliation and comfort at the end of life. Potentially manageable symptoms (pain, shortness of breath, fever, and constipation) are not uncommon among residents dying with advanced frailty and dementia. Markers of poor quality care such as development of pressure ulcers in low-risk patients, use of physical restraints, presence of uncontrolled pain, and treatment of behavioral problems with antipsychotic medications are also common among older adults with dementia at the end of life (City of Hope & AACN, 2012). High-risk interventions that are commonly carried out and are associated with limited chance of therapeutic success include cardiopulmonary resuscitation, tube feeding, intravenous therapy, fluid restriction, and invasive laboratory testing (Mitchell, Kiely, & Hamel, 2003; Sundermann et al., 2011). Invasive medical treatments often upset the older person's emotional–behavioral adjustment, either because such treatments cannot be understood by the recipient or because the extension of life will add to mental and physical suffering (Post, 1995). Further, the failure to aggressively assess and treat pain in the older person with dementia is morally inappropriate. Older adults with dementia often cannot express pain. A skilled gerontological nurse is needed to provide high-quality palliative care.

Professional integrity is foremost in the caring relationship, and older adults and families have the right to this level of care. Palliative care can begin on the day the resident is admitted to the long-term care facility and can be applied throughout the course of illness to ensure comfort. Palliative care can enhance quality of life as older adults and families adapt to the changes brought about by the disease progression. If the older person is eligible for hospice, the older person and family should be offered that option. The caregiver is responsible for ensuring that the older person and family fully understand the options available so they can make informed decisions.

When ethical dilemmas cannot be resolved through the usual care planning and communication process, an ethics committee should be consulted. All healthcare institutions should have access to an ethics committee to provide a forum for reflection and discussion of values, to build a moral community, and to attempt to meet the needs of the older person and family through group process and consensus. Ethics committees often validate or provide options regarding ethical dilemmas and support the care team in relation to already planned options (City of Hope & AACN, 2012).

Conclusion

Older adults who are diagnosed with comorbidities, functional deficits, disadvantaged resources, and lack of organ system reserve are at risk for poor outcomes and adverse events when receiving health care. Gerontological nurses have the potential to improve the quality of life across settings by conducting effective and holistic nursing assessments, facilitating access to programs and services, educating and empowering older adults and their families, participating in and leading multidisciplinary health teams, serving as advocates and influencing the development of public policy and reform of legislation to improve long-term health care, and conducting and applying research related to aging (Young, 2003). By avoiding stereotypes, thinking holistically, using the most current and appropriate medical treatments, and trying to minimize the burden of treatment, the nurse can greatly contribute to the health and well-being of many older adults.

Nurses in all settings should practice according to the following guidelines:

- Be aware of drug interactions. Polypharmacy and drug toxicity are key problems for older adults.
- Remember that the presentation of illness is less dramatic and more vague than in other age groups. Key signs and symptoms of heart disease, infection, gastrointestinal problems, depression, and cancer may not be accompanied by the classic signs and symptoms seen in younger adults. Aggressively investigate falls, weight loss, confusion, fatigue, decline in functional ability, and incontinence.
- Conduct holistic nursing assessments when caring for frail older adults and those with comorbidities. Use valid and reliable assessment tools on admission and periodically thereafter to monitor the effect of treatments and interventions.
- Seek to access and provide the most intensive services to those considered the most frail and those diagnosed with multiple comorbidities. The comprehensive services provided by a multidisciplinary team can benefit the older adult with acute and chronic needs and deliver a full range of services across settings.
- Practice ethically according to professional standards. Try to establish advance directives and identify end-of-life preferences. Educate and empower older adults and families so that they can make more informed treatment decisions, avoid futile care, and refuse interventions that are excessively burdensome, painful, and invasive.

- Promote healthy aging in all clinical settings. Establishing a healthy lifestyle at any age will prevent or delay the onset of disability, make the pharmacological treatment of chronic illness more effective, and improve or maintain functional ability.
- Recognize and treat pain in older adults, including those with dementia or other disabilities that preclude them from adequately expressing their pain.
- Become expert at providing end-of-life care to the seriously ill and dying older person. The nurse can help provide a comfortable death that is free from pain and troubling symptoms in a supportive, caring environment.
- Seek continuing education programs and pursue advanced degrees. Keep current by reading journals. Collaborate with experts in nursing and other health professions, and advocate to improve care and services for older adults with health needs.

Amella, 2004; Benefield & Higbee, 2012; Mezey & Fulmer, 1998; Mitty, 2010; Young, 2003.

Planning for Hospitalization

The nurse will often teach older adults and their families about planning for a hospital stay for surgery or treatment of an illness. The patient–family guidelines below may help an older person at risk for adverse outcomes to have a safer and more effective hospitalization experience.

QSEN Recommendations Related to the Care of Frail Older Adults

The Quality and Safety Education for Nurses (QSEN) project addresses the challenge of preparing future nurses with the knowledge, skills, and attitudes (KSAs) to continuously improve the quality and safety of the healthcare systems in which they work (Cronenwett et al., 2007). See the QSEN table for tips on meeting QSEN standards.

Patient and Family Teaching

Gerontological nurses require skills and knowledge related to teaching patients and families about the key concepts of gerontology and gerontological nursing. The guidelines in the following feature will assist the nurse to assume the role of teacher and coach.

Meeting QSEN Standards: Frailty

	KNOWLEDGE	SKILLS	ATTITUDES
Patient-Centered Care	Involvement of patient and family in plan of care is crucial.	Family assessment and adult learning principles.	Appreciate uniqueness of each patient/family.
	Examine barriers that may keep patients from being active in formulating their plan of care.	Evaluation for depression, vision/hearing, tobacco use, and cognitive and functional status.	Provide patient-centered care to improve successful nursing outcomes.
Teamwork and Collaboration	Recognize scope of practice for interdisciplinary team members.	Use leadership skills to coordinate team and share knowledge.	Value the contribution of each member of the team to improve outcomes.
	Be aware of organizational problems that can inhibit effective team functioning.	System assessment skills. Plan for patient care at the appropriate level to maximize functioning and quality of life.	Be open to input from team members on effective means to improve communication and collaboration.
Evidence-Based Practice	Describe effective interventions to decrease iatrogenic risk factors and improve overall health and functioning.	Access current evidence-based protocols to guide interventions.	Possess confidence in necessary skills to evaluate and incorporate nursing interventions from the literature about caring for frail older adults.

Meeting QSEN Standards: Frailty *(continued)*

	KNOWLEDGE	SKILLS	ATTITUDES
Quality Improvement	Recognize the importance of measuring patient outcomes to improve patient-centered care.	Skills in data management, technology, and U.S. government and ALA sites describing current incidence and prevalence of chronic disease.	Value the use of data and outcomes as a key component of QI efforts.
Safety	Describe common medication and treatment errors and health system characteristics that increase the likelihood of such errors occurring.	Use appropriate strategies to deliver patient/family education and provide written information to compensate for memory loss (if present).	Appreciate the impact of frailty and cognitive loss on the occurrence of adverse drug reactions.
	Recognize the factors that increase the risk of nosocomial infections, falls, skin breakdown, and hazards of immobility.	Avoid the use of NG tubes, IVs, inappropriate antibiotics, and other interventions that increase the risk burden when palliative care is indicated.	Institute infection control practices to decrease the incidence of secondary nosocomial infections including removal of indwelling urinary catheters.
Informatics	Provide input into the formation and maintenance of patient databases needed for gathering QSEN data and providing patient care.	Utilize the electronic health record.	Protect patient confidentiality according to HIPAA standards.

Patient–Family Teaching Guidelines

The following are guidelines that the nurse may find useful when instructing older adults and their families about planning for hospitalization.

INSTRUCTIONS FOR HOSPITALIZATION

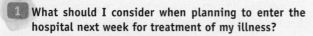

1 What should I consider when planning to enter the hospital next week for treatment of my illness?

Bring complete medical records with you to the hospital. Ask your doctor for a copy of your most recent laboratory values, your last physical examination, and an accounting of your past medical history including all hospitalizations, surgical interventions, invasive testing, and so on. Also bring a list of your current medications and dosing schedule, all of your contact information, contact information for your healthcare proxy, insurance information, and living will (if you have one).

RATIONALE:

The more information shared with the hospital providers, the less likely the chance of errors, including adverse drug events.

Carrying as much information to the hospital as possible will facilitate a smooth admission and decrease the risk of iatrogenesis.

2 What should I tell the nurses at the hospital when I am admitted?

Tell them why you are there and what goals you would like to accomplish. Also tell them if you have allergies to food or medication, problems walking, bowel or bladder problems, sleep problems, chronic pain, or other important issues relating to your care. If you wear a hearing aid or glasses, please let the nurses know. Answer all of their questions as openly and honestly as you can. Your family or significant other can help, if you wish.

(continued)

Patient–Family Teaching Guidelines *(continued)*

RATIONALE:

Sharing information about daily function and goals of treatment will assist the nurses in planning safe, effective, and appropriate nursing care. This information is crucial to development of an individualized nursing care plan.

3 **What personal items should I bring with me?**

Bring good walking slippers, a bathrobe, medical records, a book if you are a reader, a CD player for music, a small amount of money for incidental purchases, and pictures of your family. Avoid bringing valuable jewelry and large or bulky items. Ask your friends to send flowers when you go home instead of to the hospital because they can be difficult to carry out and can clutter up a small hospital room.

RATIONALE:

Good planning and bringing a few personal items can make the hospital experience more enjoyable. Large items and valuables present storage and safety problems. They should be left at home if possible.

4 **Besides my family, who should I notify regarding my hospitalization?**

You may want to let some close friends know and notify them of your visiting preferences. Some hospitalized patients like to have visitors and others prefer phone calls or cards. If you are religious, you should notify your priest, minister, or rabbi.

RATIONALE:

Sometimes, lots of visitors and phone calls can be exhausting to an older patient during the hospital experience. Helping older adults think about the number and types of visitors they would like ahead of time can head off potential problems and hurt feelings.

5 **How can I prepare myself to come back to my home after my hospitalization?**

Your nurse and social worker will work with you and your family from the moment you are admitted so that you will be able to return to your previous level of function and living arrangement. Some older people find that after treatment for an illness or an operation they are too weak to go directly home, and a short stay at a rehabilitation facility may be indicated. You should discuss these options with your nurse, physician, and social worker when you reach the hospital.

RATIONALE:

The older person and family may need warning that a direct return to home may not be possible after hospitalization for surgery or serious illness. A short-term stay in a rehabilitation unit may be needed. Some patients and families may investigate these options and other discharge options beforehand, thus easing the transition and hospital discharge.

6 **I am worried that they will hitch me up to a machine and if something goes wrong, I will be a burden to my family.**

Discuss the goals of your hospitalization and your fears with your healthcare providers and your family. Your predetermined wishes are critical to your care and will be clearly noted on your chart. If you do not have a current healthcare proxy, you will be asked to name one when you reach the hospital in the unlikely event that you will be unable to make decisions for yourself.

RATIONALE:

Having a valid and current advance directive in place is a benefit for all involved. A discussion before the hospital admission allows time to come to agreement and verbalize preferences. Even if an advance directive is in place already, repeating the discussion and reinforcing preferences is advantageous to all involved.

CARE PLAN Nursing Care of a Frail Older Person

Case Study

Mr. Krane is an 84-year-old man who has just been admitted to the acute care hospital from the emergency department. He is a nursing home resident with the following medical problems: moderate Alzheimer's disease, history of falls with injury, atrial fibrillation, and fever of unknown origin. The emergency department notes that he has a low-grade temperature, and a chest X-ray reveals a possible area of consolidation in the right lower lobe. Mr. Krane is restless, irritable, and agitated. He was held in the emergency department for 8 hours because there were several victims of a motor vehicle accident brought in for treatment of trauma shortly after he arrived. The environment was chaotic because of the trauma victims. Mr. Krane has an intravenous line in his left arm and an indwelling urinary catheter. He has not eaten a full meal since he came to the hospital. His daughter is his only living relative and she lives out of state. The social worker is attempting to contact her and has left several messages on her telephone answering machine. Code status is unknown.

Applying the Nursing Process

Assessment

The gerontological nurse should immediately assess Mr. Krane's comfort level. He is agitated and has endured a long stay in the emergency department. If his diet order has not been specified by the admitting physician, the nurse should contact the physician immediately and obtain an order for a regular or no-added-salt diet. Mr. Krane should be asked what kind of food he likes, if he has allergies or food intolerances, and what assistance he needs while eating. The nurse may wish to call the nursing home staff and request information regarding Mr. Krane's nutritional status and dietary preferences. It is hoped that food will improve his irritability and level of comfort. An additional assessment priority is patient safety. Because Mr. Krane has a history of falls, a fall prevention program should be immediately instituted. The next priority is to assess what medications he usually takes and when the last doses were administered. Because he has been diagnosed with atrial fibrillation, he is most likely on warfarin, and every effort should be made to keep his dosing schedule intact to prevent the increased risk of stroke. Additional medications to treat his dementia and pneumonia may have been ordered and should be obtained from the pharmacy as quickly as possible.

Diagnosis

The current nursing diagnoses for Mr. Krane include the following:

- *Body Temperature: Imbalanced, Risk for*
- *Confusion, Chronic*
- *Falls, Risk for*
- *Nutrition, Imbalanced: Less Than Body Requirements*
- *Tissue Perfusion: Cardiac, Risk for Decreased*
- *Social Isolation*
- *Skin Integrity, Risk for Impaired*
- *Mobility: Physical, Impaired*

NANDA-I © 2012.

Expected Outcomes

The expected outcomes for the plan of care specify that Mr. Krane will:

- Not suffer injury or adverse outcomes during his hospital stay.
- Receive appropriate medications to manage his acute and chronic illness.
- Return to the nursing home at approximately the same level of baseline function.
- Receive appropriate care consistent with his and his family's specified values and expected outcomes.

(continued)

CARE PLAN   **Nursing Care of a Frail Older Person** (continued)

Planning and Implementation

The following nursing interventions may be appropriate for Mr. Krane:

■ A fall prevention plan will be instituted with measures to include lowering the bed to the lowest position, placing the call light within easy reach, instructing Mr. Krane to call for assistance when needed, asking him not to attempt to leave the bed without assistance, and placing him in a room close to the nurses' station in order to routinely observe him.

■ If Mr. Krane is on warfarin, he is at increased risk for injury from falls due to increased clotting times as a result of anticoagulation therapy. Careful monitoring of his international normalized ratio is warranted, especially with the addition of new medications.

■ Nonpharmacological measures to improve his agitation will include approaching him calmly, calling him by name, decreasing noise and light (he is probably overstimulated from his emergency department stay),

and playing calm music. If the hospital has a volunteer program, the nurse could request a volunteer be sent to sit with Mr. Krane and read or talk to him while he is awaiting care and treatment.

■ Because Mr. Krane is at high risk for the development of delirium, careful monitoring of his cognition and level of consciousness is warranted. Appropriate parameters include mental status changes, inattention, evidence of disorganized thinking, and altered level of consciousness. The nurse should carefully note Mr. Krane's baseline level of function so changes can be detected early. Psychoactive medications should be avoided if at all possible, and behavioral and environmental interventions should be utilized to manage agitation and improve sleep.

■ Mr. Krane should wear his glasses and hearing aids during the day to improve his communication ability. Food and fluid intake should be monitored.

Evaluation

The nurse will consider the plan a success based on the following criteria:

■ Mr. Krane and his family will specify an advance directive noting the appropriate level of healthcare interventions and outcomes desired.

■ He will maintain his weight and nutritional status.

■ He will receive appropriate medications to resolve his pneumonia without toxic side effects or drug interactions.

■ He will be discharged from the hospital to the nursing home at his previous level of function.

Ethical Dilemma

During Mr. Krane's hospitalization for pneumonia, he is found to have a suspicious lesion on his lung. A CT scan reveals it is most likely the result of lung cancer. The daughter states, "I'd like to have it removed so that Dad can live out his natural life." Mr. Krane is unsure if he wants the operation, but if his daughter thinks it is necessary, he will go along with it. Mr. Krane's pulmonologist notes that there is very little chance that a lung resection will improve his prognosis or improve the quality or length of his life.

The nurse should consult with the social worker and physician regarding the need to consult the ethics committee. Disputes about appropriate care for frail older adults with

dementia can be emotional and require the input of the multidisciplinary team. Assuming that the daughter has her father's best interests at heart, she may need education and support to reconsider her decision. Additionally, Mr. Krane should be assessed for his ability to make decisions regarding his own medical care. Even with the diagnosis of dementia, Mr. Krane may have an understanding of his situation and be able to state his preferences and fears. When conflict arises regarding treatment decisions, it is often unclear who should make the final decision. The patient, the family member, the physician, and other members of the healthcare team all may have opinions regarding the best course of action. The ideal situation is

CARE PLAN Nursing Care of a Frail Older Person *(continued)*

to begin a dialogue until consensus can be reached and all parties are satisfied with the decision. Ethics committees usually have members who are experts in the mechanics of conflict resolution. It is hoped that early involvement of this committee will lead to satisfactory resolution of the conflict regarding Mr. Krane's treatment plan.

Critical Thinking and the Nursing Process

1. Imagine that you will be admitted to a hospital for a surgical procedure. If a hospital procedure allowed you to bring only five personal items, what items would you select?
2. Choose a classmate and engage in a civilized debate of the following issue: Older people with dementia should or should not receive the same medical and nursing interventions as those without dementia. Argue one point of view for 5 minutes and then switch sides to argue the opposite point of view.
3. What are the advantages and disadvantages of having special units for caring for acutely ill hospitalized older patients?
4. What suggestions can you make to improve the nursing care provided to older adults during transfer between the hospital and nursing home?

■ Evaluate your responses in Appendix B. ⊂⊃

Chapter Highlights

■ Multisystem problems and comorbidities complicate the delivery of care to older adults. People who are frail and very old are especially at risk for adverse events and poor outcomes as the result of acute illness, exacerbation of chronic illness, and hospitalization.

■ Nursing home residents are the most at risk for adverse outcomes based on their extreme frailty and high degree of cognitive impairment.

■ Hospital care can be improved for older adults. Multidisciplinary teams, patient-centered care, ACE units, and careful assessment and monitoring all increase the chances of success during hospitalization.

■ Pain management, advance care planning, treatment cessation, and resource allocation are all issues of organizational ethics.

■ To address the provision of fair and equitable long-term care, healthcare professionals and policymakers should begin public education and awareness campaigns; enhance professional education and staff development regarding delivery of palliative care; establish policies and procedures within long-term care facilities to support timely, comprehensive, and compassionate care; and advocate for funding of clinical research to evaluate the benefits and burdens of medical interventions related to caring for frail older adults with dementia in the long-term care facility.

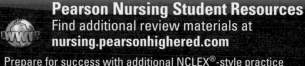

Pearson Nursing Student Resources
Find additional review materials at
nursing.pearsonhighered.com

Prepare for success with additional NCLEX®-style practice questions, interactive assignments and activities, web links, animations and videos, and more!

References

Albert, S., Im, A., & Raveis, V. (2002). Public health and the second 50 years of life. *American Journal of Public Health, 92*(8) 1–3.

Alzheimer's Association. (2011). *Alzheimer's disease facts and figures.* Retrieved from http://www.alz.org/national/documents/Facts_Figures_2011.pdf

Amella, E. (2004). Presentation of illness in older adults. *American Journal of Nursing, 104*(10), 40–51.

American Nurses Association. (2010). *Code for nurses with interpretive statements.* Retrieved from http://www.nursingworld.org/MainMenuCategories/EthicsStandards/CodeofEthicsforNurses/Code-of-Ethics.pdf

Anderson, G. (2010). *Making the case for ongoing care.* Princeton, NJ: Robert Wood Johnson Foundation.

Bartali, B., Frongillo, E., Bandinelli, S., Laurentani, F., Semba, R., Fried, L., et al. (2006). Low nutrient intake is an essential component of frailty in older persons. *Journals of Gerontology Series A–Biological Sciences & Medical Sciences, 61*(6), 589–593.

Benefield, L. E., & Higbee, R. L. (2012). *Want to know more: Frailty and its implications for care.* Hartford Institute for Geriatric Nursing. Retrieved April 6, 2012, from http://consultgerirn.org/topics/frailty_and_its_implications_for_care_new/want_to_know_more

Boult, C., & Wieland, D. (2010). Comprehensive primary care for older patients with multiple chronic conditions. *Journal of the American Medical Association, 304*(17), 1936–1943.

Cashman, J., Wright, J., & Ring. (2010). The treatment of co-morbidities in older patients with metastatic cancer. *Support Care Cancer, 18*(5), 651–655.

Centers for Disease Control and Prevention (CDC). (2010). *Adults and older adults adverse drug events.* Retrieved from http://www.cdc.gov/MedicationSafety/Adult_AdverseDrugEvents.html

Centers for Disease Control and Prevention (CDC) & Merck Company Foundation. (2007). *The state of aging and health in America 2007.* Retrieved from http://www.cdc.gov/aging/pdf/saha_2007.pdf

City of Hope & American Association of Colleges of Nursing (AACN). (2012). *End of life nursing care at the end of life (ELNEC) graduate curriculum* (Education Consortium). Bethesda, MD: National Cancer Institute.

Cronenwett, L., Sherwood, G., Barnsteiner, J., Disch, J., Johnson, J., Mitchell, P., Sullivan, D., & Warren, J. (2007). Quality and safety education for nurses, *Nursing Outlook, 55*(3) 122-131.

Espinoza, S., & Walston, J. (2005). Frailty in older adults: Insights and interventions. *Cleveland Clinic Journal of Medicine, 72*(12), 1105–1112.

Fretwell, M. (1998). Acute hospital care for frail older patients. In W. Hazzard, E. Bierman, J. Blass, W. Ettinger, & J. Halter (Eds.), *Principles of geriatric medicine and gerontology.* New York, NY: McGraw-Hill.

Fried, L., Tangen, C., Walston, J., Newman, A., Hirsch, C., Gottdiener, J., et al. (2001). Frailty of older adults: Evidence for a phenotype. *Journals of Gerontology: Biological Sciences and Medical Sciences, 56A*(3), M146–156.

Glaser, B., & Strauss, A. (1968). *A time for dying.* Chicago, IL: Aldine.

Gobbens, R., Liujkx, K., Wijnen-Sponselee, M., & Schols, J. (2010). Toward a conceptual definition of frail community dwelling older adults. *Nursing Outlook, 58*(2), 76–86.

Golden, A., Martin, S., Silva, M., & Roos, B. (2011). Care management and the transition of older adults from a skilled nursing facility back to the community. *Care Management Journals, 12,* 54–59.

Golden, A., Tewary, S., Dang, S., & Roos, B. (2010). Care management's challenges and opportunities to reduce rapid rehospitalization of frail community-dwelling older adults. *The Gerontologist, 50*(4), 451–458.

Heuberger, R. A. (2011). The frailty syndrome: A comprehensive review. *Journal of Nutrition of Gerontology and Geriatrics, 30*(4), 315–368.

Hurley, A., Volicer, L., Camberg, L., Ashley, J., & Woods, P. (1999). Measurement of observed agitation in patients with dementia of the Alzheimer type. *Journal of Mental Health and Aging, 5*(2), 117–133.

Institute of Medicine (1991). Extending life, enhancing life: A national research agenda on aging. Washington, DC: National Academy Press, 1991.

Kietzman, K., Pincus, H., & Huynh, P. (2011). Coming full circle: Planning for future pathways of transitions of care for older adults. *Annual Review of Gerontology and Geriatrics, 31,* 231–254.

Kumar, S., Katharia, V., & Hurria, A. (2010). Evaluating the older patient with cancer: Understanding frailty and the geriatric assessment. *CA: A Cancer Journal for Clinicians, 60*(2), 120–132.

Lunney, J., Lynn, J., Foley, D., Lipson, S., & Guralnik, J. (2003). Patterns of functional decline at the end of life. *Journal of the American Medical Association, 289*(18), 2387–2392.

McCance, K. L., & Huether, S. E. (2012). *The biologic basis of disease in adults and children.* St. Louis, MO: Mosby.

MetLife. (2011). *Market survey long-term care costs.* Retrieved from http://www.metlife.com/mmi/research/2011-market-survey-long-term-care-costs.html#findings

Mezey, M., & Fulmer, T. (1998). Quality care for the frail elderly. *Nursing Outlook, 46*(6), 291–292.

Mezuk, B., Edwards, L., Lohman, M., Choi, M., & Lapane, K. (2011). Depression and frailty in later life: A synthetic review. *International Journal of Geropsychiatry.* Retrieved from http://onlinelibrary.wiley.com/doi/10.1002/gps.2807/abstract;jsessionid=A7F2F0AA4610429386232D7FAE41A9DA.d02t02?userIsAuthenticated=false&deniedAccessCustomisedMessage=

Mitchell, S., Kiely, D., & Hamel, M. (2003). Dying with advanced dementia in the nursing home. *Archives of Internal Medicine, 164,* 321–326.

Mitty, E. (2010). Iatrogenesis, frailty and geriatric syndromes. *Geriatric Nursing, 31*(5), 368–374.

Mutasingawa, D., Ge, H., & Upshur, R. (2011). How applicable are clinical practice guidelines to elderly patients with comorbidities? *Canadian Family Physician, 57*(7), 253–262.

NANDA International. (2012). *NANDA International nursing diagnoses: Definitions and classification, 2012–2014.* Philadelphia, PA: Wiley-Blackwell.

National Center for Health Statistics. (2007). *Health United States 2007. With chartbook on trends in the health of Americans.* Retrieved from http://www.cdc.gov/nchs/data/hus/hus07.pdf

National Institute on Aging. (2011). *Frailty in older adults linked to Alzheimer's disease pathology.* Retrieved from http://www.nia.nih.gov/alzheimers/announcements/2009/04/frailty-older-adults-linked-alzheimers-disease-pathology

Nursing Ethics. (2008). *Preventive ethics with the elderly.* Retrieved from http://www.nursingethicsce.com/co7c3preventiveethics.asp

Office of Technology Assessment. (2008). Funding the fight against Alzheimer's disease. Retrieved from http://www.fas.org/ota/2008/03/

Paris, J., Reardon, F., & Browne, J. (2003). An economic, ethical, and legal analysis of problems in critical care medicine. In R. Irwin, F. Cerra, & J. Rippe (Eds.), *Intensive care medicine* (5th ed.). Hagerstown, MD: Lippincott.

Post, L., Mitty, E., Bottrell, M., Dubler, N., Hill, T., Mezey, M., et al. (2001). Guidelines for end-of-life care in nursing facilities: Principles and recommendations. *NAELA Quarterly, 14*(2), 24–30.

Post, S. (1995). *The moral challenge of Alzheimer disease.* Baltimore, MD: Johns Hopkins University Press.

Rensbergen, G., & Nawrot, T. (2010). Medical conditions of nursing home admissions. *British Medical Journal of Geriatrics, 10*(46). doi:10.1186/1471-2318-10-46. Retrieved from http://www.biomedcentral.com/1471-2318/10/46

Reuben, D., Herr, K., Pacala, J., Pollock, B., Potter, J., & Semla, T. (2012). *Geriatrics at your fingertips.* New York, NY: American Geriatrics Society.

Robertson, R., & Montagnini, M. (2004). Geriatric failure to thrive. *American Family Physician, 70*(2), 343–350.

Rosenthal, G., Kaboli, P., Barnett, M., & Sirio, C. (2002). Age and risk of in-hospital death: Insights from a multihospital study of intensive care patients. *Journal of the American Geriatrics Society, 50,* 1205–1212.

Sager, M.A., Rudberg, M.A. Jalaluddin, M., Franke, T., Injouye, S.K., Landefeld,C.S.,

Siebens, H., & Winograd, C.H. (1996). Hospital admission risk profile (HARP): Identifying older patients at risk for functional decline following acute medical illness and hospitalization. *Journal of the American Geriatrics Society, 44*(3), 251–257.

Song, X., Mitnitsky, A., & Rockwood, K. (2010). Prevalence and 10-year outcomes of frailty in older adults in relation to deficit accumulation. *Journal of the American Geriatrics Society, 58*(4), 681–687.

Sundermann, S., Dademasch, A., Praetorius, J., Kempfert, J., Dewey, T., Falk, V., Mohr, F.W., & Walther, T. (2011). Comprehensive assessment of frailty for elderly high-risk patients undergoing cardiac surgery. *European Journal of Cardio-thoracic Surgery, 39*(1), 33–37.

Thomassian, M. (2012). Heart disease: The number one killer in women. *HealthCentral.* Retrieved from http://www.healthcentral.com/heart-disease/c/7291/18967/heart-women

Tinetti, M., Bogardus, S., & Agostini, J. (2004). Potential pitfalls of disease-specific guidelines for patients with multiple conditions. *New England Journal of Medicine, 351,* 2870–2874.

Tullmann, D., Mion, L., Fletcher, K., & Foreman, M. (2008). Delirium. Retrieved

from http://consultgerirn.org/topics/delirium/want_to_know_more

U.S. Census Bureau. (2010). Disability characteristics. Retrieved from http://factfinder2.census.gov/faces/tableservices/jsf/pages/productview.xhtml?pid=ACS_10_1YR_S1810&prodType=table

Wachter, R., Foster, N., & Dudley, R. (2008). *Medicare's decision to withhold payment for hospital errors: The devil is in the detail.* Retrieved from http://psnet.ahrq.gov/resource.aspx?resourceID=6760

Wilson, R., Aggarwal, N., Barnes, L., Mendes de Leon, C., Herbert, L., & Evans, D. (2010). Cognitive decline in incident Alzheimer's disease in a community population. *Neurology, 74*(12), 951–955.

Wykle, M., & Gueldner, S. (2011). *Aging well.* Sudbury, MA: Jones & Bartlett.

Young, H. (2003). Challenges and solutions for care of frail older adults. *Online Journal of Issues in Nursing, 8*(2), Manuscript 4. Retrieved from http://www.nursingworld.org/MainMenuCategories/ANAMarketplace/ANAPeriodicals/OJIN/TableofContents/Volume82003/No2May2003/OlderAdultsCareSolutions.aspx

NANDA-Approved Nursing Diagnoses, 2012–2014

Activity, Deficient Diversional
Activity Intolerance
Activity Intolerance, Risk for
Activity Planning, Ineffective
Activity Planning, Risk for Ineffective
Adaptive Capacity: Intracranial, Decreased
Adverse Reaction to Iodinated Contrast Media, Risk for
Airway Clearance, Ineffective
Allergy Response, Risk for
Allergy Response, Latex
Allergy Response, Latex, Risk for
Anxiety
Anxiety, Death
Aspiration, Risk for
Attachment, Risk for Impaired
Bleeding, Risk for
Blood Glucose Level, Risk for Unstable
Body Image, Disturbed
Body Temperature: Imbalanced, Risk for
Bowel Incontinence
Breast Milk, Insufficient
Breastfeeding, Ineffective
Breastfeeding, Interrupted
Breastfeeding, Readiness for Enhanced
Breathing Pattern, Ineffective
Cardiac Output, Decreased
Caregiver Role Strain
Caregiver Role Strain, Risk for
Childbearing Process, Ineffective
Childbearing Process, Readiness for Enhanced
Childbearing Process, Risk for Ineffective
Comfort, Impaired
Comfort, Readiness for Enhanced
Communication, Readiness for Enhanced
Communication: Verbal, Impaired
Confusion, Acute
Confusion, Chronic
Confusion, Risk for Acute

Constipation
Constipation, Perceived
Constipation, Risk for
Contamination
Contamination, Risk for
Coping: Community, Ineffective
Coping: Community, Readiness for Enhanced
Coping, Defensive
Coping: Family, Compromised
Coping: Family, Disabled
Coping: Family, Readiness for Enhanced
Coping: Readiness for Enhanced
Coping, Ineffective
Decision Making, Readiness for Enhanced
Decisional Conflict (Specify)
Denial, Ineffective
Dentition, Impaired
Development: Delayed, Risk for
Diarrhea
Disuse Syndrome, Risk for
Dry Eye, Risk for
Dysreflexia, Autonomic
Dysreflexia, Autonomic, Risk for
Electrolyte Imbalance, Risk for
Energy Field, Disturbed
Environmental Interpretation Syndrome, Impaired
Failure to Thrive, Adult
Falls, Risk for
Family Processes, Dysfunctional
Family Processes, Interrupted
Family Processes, Readiness for Enhanced
Fatigue
Fear
Fluid Balance, Readiness for Enhanced
Fluid Volume: Deficient
Fluid Volume: Deficient, Risk for
Fluid Volume: Excess
Fluid Volume: Imbalanced, Risk for

Gas Exchange, Impaired
Gastrointestinal Motility, Risk for Dysfunctional
Gastrointestinal Motility, Dysfunctional
Grieving
Grieving, Complicated
Grieving, Risk for Complicated
Growth: Disproportionate, Risk for
Growth and Development, Delayed
Health: Community, Deficient
Health Behavior, Risk-Prone
Health Maintenance, Ineffective
Home Maintenance, Impaired
Hope, Readiness for Enhanced
Hopelessness
Human Dignity, Risk for Compromised
Hyperthermia
Hypothermia
Immunization Status, Readiness for Enhanced
Impulse Control, Ineffective
Infant Behavior: Disorganized
Infant Behavior: Disorganized, Risk for
Infant Behavior: Organized, Readiness for Enhanced
Infant Feeding Pattern, Ineffective
Infection, Risk for
Injury, Risk for
Insomnia
Jaundice, Neonatal
Jaundice, Neonatal, Risk for
Knowledge, Deficient
Knowledge, Readiness for Enhanced
Lifestyle, Sedentary
Liver Function, Risk for Impaired
Loneliness, Risk for
Maternal/Fetal Dyad, Risk for Disturbed
Memory, Impaired
Mobility: Bed, Impaired
Mobility: Physical, Impaired
Mobility: Wheelchair, Impaired
Moral Distress
Nausea
Neglect, Unilateral
Neurovascular Dysfunction: Peripheral, Risk for
Noncompliance
Nutrition, Imbalanced: Less than Body Requirements
Nutrition, Imbalanced: More than Body Requirements
Nutrition, Imbalanced: More than Body Requirements, Risk for
Nutrition, Readiness for Enhanced

Mucous Membrane: Oral, Impaired
Pain, Acute
Pain, Chronic
Parenting, Impaired
Parenting, Readiness for Enhanced
Parenting, Risk for Impaired
Perfusion: Gastrointestinal, Risk for Ineffective
Perfusion: Renal, Risk for Ineffective
Perioperative Positioning Injury, Risk for
Personal Identity: Disturbed
Personal Identity: Disturbed, Risk for
Poisoning, Risk for
Post-Trauma Syndrome
Post-Trauma Syndrome, Risk for
Power, Readiness for Enhanced
Powerlessness
Powerlessness, Risk for
Protection, Ineffective
Rape-Trauma Syndrome
Relationship, Ineffective
Relationship, Risk for Ineffective
Relationship, Readiness for Enhanced
Religiosity, Impaired
Religiosity, Readiness for Enhanced
Religiosity, Risk for Impaired
Relocation Stress Syndrome
Relocation Stress Syndrome, Risk for
Resilience: Individual, Impaired
Resilience, Readiness for Enhanced
Resilience, Risk for Compromised
Role Conflict, Parental
Role Performance, Ineffective
Self-Care, Readiness for Enhanced
Self-Care Deficit: Bathing
Self-Care Deficit: Dressing
Self-Care Deficit: Feeding
Self-Care Deficit: Toileting
Self-Concept, Readiness for Enhanced
Self-Esteem, Chronic Low
Self-Esteem, Chronic Low, Risk for
Self-Esteem, Situational Low
Self-Esteem, Situational Low, Risk for
Self Health Management, Ineffective
Self Health Management, Readiness for Enhanced
Self-Mutilation
Self-Mutilation, Risk for
Self Neglect
Sexual Dysfunction

Sexuality Pattern, Ineffective
Shock, Risk for
Skin Integrity, Impaired
Skin Integrity, Risk for Impaired
Sleep Deprivation
Sleep Pattern, Disturbed
Sleep, Readiness for Enhanced
Social Interaction, Impaired
Social Isolation
Sorrow, Chronic
Spiritual Distress
Spiritual Distress, Risk for
Spiritual Well-Being, Readiness for Enhanced
Sudden Infant Death Syndrome, Risk for
Stress Overload
Suffocation, Risk for
Suicide, Risk for
Surgical Recovery, Delayed
Swallowing, Impaired
Therapeutic Regimen Management: Family, Ineffective
Thermal Injury, Risk for
Thermoregulation, Ineffective
Tissue Integrity, Impaired

Tissue Perfusion: Cardiac, Risk for Decreased
Tissue Perfusion: Cerebral, Risk for Ineffective
Tissue Perfusion: Peripheral, Ineffective
Tissue Perfusion: Peripheral, Risk for Ineffective
Transfer Ability, Impaired
Trauma, Risk for
Trauma: Vascular, Risk for
Urinary Elimination, Impaired
Urinary Elimination, Readiness for Enhanced
Urinary Incontinence, Functional
Urinary Incontinence, Overflow
Urinary Incontinence, Reflex
Urinary Incontinence, Stress
Urinary Incontinence, Urge
Urinary Incontinence, Urge, Risk for
Urinary Retention
Ventilation: Spontaneous, Impaired
Ventilatory Weaning Response, Dysfunctional
Violence: Other-Directed, Risk for
Violence: Self-Directed, Risk for
Walking, Impaired
Wandering

Answers to Critical Thinking Exercises

Chapter 1

1. Thinking about your own aging is a great way to face your fears, realize your hopes, and prepare for the future. This exercise will not only help you to prepare for your own aging, but also allow you to be more effective when working with older patients.

2. Your actions in youth will form the foundations of health in old age. Your lifestyle now will be crucial to your function as you get older. If you are engaging in choices that will compromise your health in old age, make changes today. The earlier you make positive changes, the better.

3. Some common themes you might discover include strength of character, zest for life, positive outlook, avoidance of bad health habits, ability to form at least one loving and caring relationship with another, and genetic hardiness.

4. Often, gerontological nursing is not perceived as glamorous and therefore it is not promoted as a recruitment technique. Pictures showing student nurses caring for babies are more popular than pictures showing nurses with older people. Hopefully, this will change in the future and many more students will want to work with older people and make contributions to improving the health and quality of life of older people.

Chapter 2

1. You may be pleasantly surprised at what you hear from your older patients and older people in your family and community. Most often, by spending time getting to know an older person "up close and personal," younger people begin to realize and appreciate diversity and richness in aging. Try to understand the older person's circumstances today in light of past decisions and actions.

2. Because many healthcare professionals (including nurses) are educated in isolation from other healthcare professionals, the understanding and appreciation of the various professional roles is often not truly understood by others. Our professional role as gerontological nurses is evolving and we are assuming more responsibility daily in response to the complex healthcare needs of our patients. Take every opportunity you can to educate others if they have misconceptions about important and crucial roles assumed by gerontological nurses.

3. Some of your colleagues from other professions and even some nurses themselves feel trapped in the medical model. The role of nursing may be viewed too narrowly. Educate others about the use of nursing diagnosis and the ways its use complements and enriches the medical diagnosis and validates the nurse's actions specified on the nursing care plan. The nursing diagnosis is holistic and usually defines the older person's reaction to their illness, identifies immediate or possible nursing problems, and lists health promotion activities. The medical diagnosis usually is focused on an actual or potential disease process.

4/5. Many nurses choose to work with older patients because they want to help people and improve the quality of their lives. The nurse's holistic focus can enrich the interdisciplinary team perspective. The nurse can provide input whether the topic is health and wellness, spirituality, nutrition, coping and stress, or any other number of related subjects. A multidisciplinary team requires the input of nursing to function efficiently and effectively.

Chapter 3

1. This older patient should be reassured by the healthcare team that no one will go against his wishes if he becomes impaired near the time of death; however, if he changes his mind, his wishes will be honored. The social worker and other members of the interdisciplinary team should meet with the family and patient and carefully document Mr. Turner's preferences in the medical record.

2. Mrs. Lee is considered an elder at risk. A referral to the Area Council on Aging is needed. A social worker will perform an assessment. If Mrs. Lee is considered unsafe to live alone or a threat to others, a guardian will be appointed to help her make decisions to get help in her home or move to a more supportive living environment.

3. Explain the importance of protecting the patient's confidential records from unauthorized viewing by others. Ask your colleague to voluntarily discuss this issue with the supervisor. If the behavior continues to occur, you may be

required by workplace policy to report these confidentiality lapses to someone in authority.

Chapter 4

1. You may be amazed at both the culturally competent and the culturally incompetent nursing interventions you find listed now that your awareness has been raised.

2. Many nurses are unaware of their own stereotypes on aging. The nurse you interview may deny that age plays a factor in thinking about culture and care planning, but it may become apparent that the nurse is influenced by unconscious attitudes and beliefs.

3. Truth telling is a great topic to investigate, as it will incorporate many different underlying cultural values and beliefs, including legitimate role of the patient and provider, hope, reliance and trust in authority, faith in the future, and so on.

4. Many students are surprised to find that they are from a specific cultural background. Most of us have been influenced by the beliefs and attitudes of our parents and grandparents who may have immigrated from other parts of the world. Interview some older people in your family to discover your own roots. Videotape the interview if you can. This video may be viewed by future generations and become a vital record of your family's history.

5. Most older people will welcome the opportunity to talk with you about their beliefs and values. You will be the wiser.

6. Family and community support systems vary according to basic beliefs about life, death, health, suffering, role of elders, and so on. This examination will clarify some key concepts regarding various cultures. If you have traveled to other countries, this is a plus. International travel will open your eyes to differences and commonalities between that culture and the American culture.

Chapter 5

1. Risk factors for undernutrition can include depression, multiple chronic illnesses, immobility, advanced age, and other factors included in Box 5–5. Appropriate nursing interventions are presented in Box 5–8. Some risk factors are modifiable and others are not. The nurse is urged to try to come up with novel and creative solutions to maintain good nourishment in the older person.

2. Nutrition and hydration concerns for a homebound older person with arthritis include:

  - Ability to shop for or obtain groceries and prepare meals (grasping utensils, cutting, standing, carrying dishes or containers).

  - Effect of any pain or discomfort or medications taken to control pain on appetite.
  - Effect of medications on nutrition, taste perception, digestion.
  - Potential for voluntary fluid restriction to limit need to travel to bathroom.
  - Poor access to fluids due to potential immobility.

Careful monitoring by the nurse and creative approaches are needed for this older person at risk for undernutrition.

3. Nursing interventions appropriate for a cognitively impaired nursing home resident with no documentation on ability to self- or hand-feed include:

  - Provide mealtime assistance to assess ability to self-feed.
  - Provide finger foods and/or one food at a time with the appropriate utensil.
  - Cue appropriately.
  - Allow adequate unhurried time to feed.
  - Minimize environmental distractions during mealtime.
  - Assist with proper positioning for feeding.
  - Assess for any difficulties with swallowing.
  - Obtain food preferences from family or significant others.
  - Encourage family to visit at mealtime and assist with feeding.

Be sure to ask all three shifts to observe and document the resident's eating pattern as the pattern may vary according to meal, time of day, level of fatigue, staffing, and other factors.

4. Nursing interventions appropriate for an older person in long-term care at risk for dehydration include:

  - Obtain fluid preferences.
  - Prompt to drink fluids at regular intervals throughout the day.
  - Educate resident of need to drink to a schedule and not wait for thirst.
  - Offer larger volumes of fluid with snacks and medication passes.
  - Flag meal trays or room door to alert staff to leave fluids at bedside table within reach. Offer nonspillable drinking containers if needed.
  - Monitor for signs and symptoms of dehydration.

Document the fluids preferred by the resident in the nursing care plan. Offer the desired fluid frequently, but remember to vary the choice. Variety is the spice of life!

5. Appropriate nursing assessment for an older person with new dentures and weight loss might include:

  - Assess fit and comfort of dentures and check for oral pain and alterations in mucosal integrity. Refer back to dentist if indicated.

- Assess for alteration in taste perception due to dentures.
- Conduct diet history and assess for texture modifications and other diet changes or omissions, which may account for nutrition deficit of calories and other nutrients. Specifically assess protein intake since many high-protein foods, such as meats, can be difficult to chew and therefore may be avoided.
- Assess the older person's ability to care for the dentures and keep them clean. Poor oral hygiene can detract from appearance, cause bad breath, and make the older person dread placing the teeth in his or her mouth.
- Monitor the older person's weight. Even a slight weight loss (5 to 10 lbs) can cause the dentures to slip, cause pain and irritation, and inhibit ability to chew. Be proactive and urge the patient to revisit the dentist if weight changes.

Once your patient adjusts to the new dentures, you may note improvements in appearance, nutritional intake, self-confidence, and rate of smiling. Frequent modifications may be needed in the adjustment period, but it is worth it.

Chapter 6

1. Many healthcare professionals have no idea of the cost of the medications they are prescribing. Even with a drug benefit or discount card, the copayment may be extremely expensive, especially when the patient is taking many medications.

2. Often, the older patient's medication regimen is changed but the medical record is not updated. This can lead to confusion and errors. Make sure to review the medication list with your older patients on a regular basis.

3. Some older patients take their medications by size or color (e.g., "the big white one is for my joints and the little yellow one is for my heart"). This can be an unsafe and risky practice for an older person taking many medications. Colors and shapes may change when generic brands of the same medication are used. Many states now mandate that when a generic medication is dispensed, an information sheet describing the color, shape, and markings on the medication must be included.

4. Some students are surprised to discover that anyone can become confused when taking a complicated medication regimen. Even young and middle-aged persons can make errors.

Chapter 7

1. Remember to consider the physical, psychological, spiritual, and social causes in your list. Compare your list with your classmates' lists and see if there is any commonality in your perspectives.

2. Older persons with poor vision or hearing may misinterpret normal conversations and events in daily life. These mistakes can be frightening to the older person who is "seeing" things that are not there and "hearing" things that have not been said.

3. Because many older persons live alone, they can successfully conceal the amount of alcohol they consume. A person who is still working may be missed from work due to excessive alcohol intake, but the flexible schedule in retirement allows the older person to sometimes escape detection from others.

4. The older person may be unwilling to admit mental health problems. A stigma against mental health problems and fear of seeing a psychiatrist or psychologist may cause the older person to conceal feelings of depression or anxiety. Remember some older people feel that having a mental health problem is a sign of weakness.

5. Public education, continued education of health professionals, and evidence-based protocols can all enhance the mental health of older persons.

Chapter 8

1. Excessive alcohol consumption can disrupt normal sleep patterns and result in further problems such as daytime sleepiness, hangovers, dehydration, interaction with medications, and falls. Excessive alcohol consumption is a high-risk behavior in an older person.

2. Mrs. Johnson may be lonely, depressed, experiencing chronic pain, or physically ill. As she has recently had a complete physical examination and health assessment that was within normal limits, it is most likely that she is experiencing a psychological problem that may be discovered with a complete nursing assessment. A mental status examination and a depression screen would be a good place to start.

3. Proper diet, exercise, appropriate recreational activities, and alcohol avoidance may be behaviors Mrs. Johnson would carry out if she believes they will allow her to live independently and stay out of a nursing home. Sleep hygiene measures and establishment of a satisfactory nighttime ritual may be appropriate interventions.

4. While the nurse is establishing a therapeutic relationship with Mrs. Johnson, it is important to convey that she is a valuable person with a potentially serious problem and that she can regain control of her situation and achieve satisfactory sleep. A values clarification will help this patient to begin thinking about long-term goals and how she wishes

to spend the rest of her life. Asking Mrs. Johnson what is important to her and what actions she is willing to take to maintain these values is a good place to start. If she values independence and wishes to remain living in her own apartment, she may be more likely to engage in behaviors that are health promoting. Referral and counseling from a mental health worker would increase her chances of success.

5. The nurse should inform Mrs. Johnson that taking a sleep medication is indicated for short-term use only (usually less than 2 weeks) and that a long-term solution to her problem is indicated. If she is depressed or in pain, treatment of these conditions may improve her sleep patterns. Taking any medication with alcohol increases the risk of an adverse drug event and should be avoided.

Chapter 9

1. A chronic, degenerative joint problem generates pain because bone surfaces come in contact with one another and produce an inflammatory response. This inflammatory response includes increased fluid in the joint, swelling, and pain signals transmitted to the brain.

2. Mr. Adams may be lonely and depressed while experiencing chronic pain. As he recently had a complete physical examination and health assessment that was within normal limits, it is likely that he is experiencing depression as a result of social isolation and fears for his future independence. Mr. Adams requires a complete nursing assessment. A depression screen would be a good place to start.

3. Proper diet, exercise, and appropriate recreational and social activities may be behaviors Mr. Adams would carry out if he believes they will allow him to live independently. His inability to obtain needed groceries is of concern. His ability to climb stairs should be improved, or alternative living situations should be explored.

4. While the nurse is establishing a therapeutic relationship with Mr. Adams, it is important to convey to him that it is very risky to take acetaminophen on a regular basis and consume any amount of alcohol. The probability of hepatic failure is greatly increased in older persons who ingest alcohol. If he values independence and wishes to remain living in his own apartment, he may be more likely to engage in behaviors that are health promoting.

Chapter 10

1. Many caregivers experience anger directed toward the abuser. Caring for a frail older person who has been mistreated can trigger a variety of emotions. Although painful, try to identify your emotions, record them, and discuss them with an advisor or mentor. Identifying and discussing your emotional response can prevent stress and burnout.

2. Every community is different. Each has strengths and weaknesses that may indirectly contribute to elder mistreatment. Does your community have services for stressed caregivers? Are there high rates of drug and alcohol abuse? Are there respite services for elders at risk? Are there services to monitor older adults at risk for self-neglect? Make a list of strengths and weaknesses in your community and begin to advocate for services to older people by addressing weaknesses.

3. Sometimes older patients are treated harshly in the clinical setting by stressed caregivers. This cannot be excused or tolerated. Nurses and nurse's assistants may scold older patients, neglect their psychological and physical needs, or touch them harshly. This may result in emotional distress, anxiety, and skin tears and bruising. Be alert for such incidents and report them to your instructor or the charge nurse immediately.

4. Stressed family caregivers are at high risk for mistreating the older adults for whom they care. Engaging in healthy lifestyle habits and good coping mechanisms can help. Suggestions might include arranging for respite to engage in daily exercise, prayer, or meditation; listening to music; having someone to trust and confide in to receive needed support; and involving others as much as possible so as not to "go it alone." A caregiver who can maintain good emotional and physical health is an asset.

Chapter 11

1. Many nurses and nursing assistants are experts in pain assessment and will pick up on verbal and nonverbal cues when working with their patients. Others are less expert and may not be able to identify relevant factors such as grimacing, avoidance of moving about, refusal of care, and so on. Start to identify the clinical experts and learn by observing them.

2. Some students have not faced their own feelings about death and dying. Sometimes they have not faced the loss of a loved one in their own families or close friends and are relatively unfamiliar with the death and dying process. Films, stories, role-playing, and other techniques help prepare the student to face death in the clinical setting and can help prepare them for the emotions they will experience as they provide end-of-life care.

3. Journaling is a technique that helps us to sort out and record feelings and emotions as we progress through growth and developmental processes. Keeping a small journal by your bed allows you to record a few observations regarding the day's experiences and the emotional responses to those experiences. Later, when rereading the journal, you may be surprised at your responses and how you have grown

in insight and strength over time. Identify a trusted teacher or mentor to help you through this sometimes difficult process.

4. Identifying key people to help you is important because you may need to seek them out for support now or in the future. Often, the first time you see a patient who is in your care die stimulates feelings of sadness, remorse, and inadequacy. Having someone you can talk to openly and honestly about your feelings is important. Try not to repress your feelings or turn away from your emotions. You will become stronger by addressing your fears and emotions. Having a trusted mentor is a big advantage and the advice you receive can guide you through times of emotional distress.

Chapter 12

1. Intrinsic factors such as age, nutritional status, genetic predisposition, level of skin pigmentation, and degree of sun damage are all important to identify. Extrinsic factors such as medication use, degree of dryness, and temperature of the environment also have an impact. Consider both sets of factors to improve your management of dermatological problems.

2. Good nutrition forms the basis for many areas of health, including dermatological health. Poor fluid intake can cause skin dryness and flakiness. Poor protein intake can cause dull, thin skin and many other skin problems both now and in the future. Lack of certain vitamins can cause skin to crack, become prone to skin tears, and fail to heal after injury. Beauty may be skin deep but good nutrition is the foundation of healthy skin!

3. Many healthcare facilities have protocols and procedures for skin care based on habit, tradition, provider and staff preference, or trial and error. If you find discrepancies between current guidelines and clinical practices, bring in a copy of current guidelines from the Agency for Healthcare Research and Quality Website to key decision makers. Become a change agent. Once you have chosen an evidence-based protocol for treating your older patient's skin problems, make sure to stick with it for at least a week or two. Skin healing takes time and patience and frequent treatment protocol changes will only delay the overall process.

4. Often despite the best efforts of staff, older patients are overly positioned on their backs and thus can develop skin breakdown on the coccyx and other bony prominences. Pillows, rolled blankets, reclining chairs, air mattresses, wedge cushions, padding of bony prominences, and other positioning aids can assist patients to comfortably use alternative positions. Careful attention and supervision of

nursing assistants will ensure that the older patient is repositioned every 2 hours to ensure that pressure ulcers can heal and new ulcers will not develop.

Chapter 13

1. Many people are uncomfortable with others giving them oral care. This exercise will increase your sensitivity toward the feelings of your older dependent patient.

2. It is natural to feel sad when caring for someone with oral cancer and perhaps feel anger toward things the older person may have done to develop the disease. However, many older people began smoking before the risks were clearly known, and your patient may have tried many times to "kick" this addictive habit. The best bet is to assist your patients to quit smoking and urge others never to start while caring for patients with oral cancer.

3. Many nursing home patients rely on Medicaid for reimbursement and are financially indigent. Reimbursement for dental care may be absent or very low, and many patients cannot manage the cost of dental care. It is distressing to realize you are caring for a patient with unmet needs and be unable to locate a dental provider. Advocate for your patient and try to locate providers who can assist older nursing home residents with dental needs.

4. The aid should be spoken to immediately and informed that the approach was not appropriate. The nurse can role-model appropriate behavior such as using a pleasant tone, smiling, explaining the reason for the intervention, and returning at a later time if the resident refuses to cooperate at this time.

Chapter 14

1. Appropriate interventions to the nurse may be completely unacceptable to the older person. For instance, a pet who is always underfoot is a fall hazard. From the perspective of the nurse, the pet should be eliminated from the home to prevent falls and promote safety. However, the older person may rely on the friendship and companionship of the pet and feel socially isolated and lonely if the pet were to be forced from the home. Therefore, each suggestion should be discussed and a mutually agreed upon plan instituted.

2. Each nurse should report safety hazards as they occur in the clinical setting. Many hazards exist in hospitals and nursing homes, including dangling wires, wet floors, uneven surfaces, medical equipment crowding the walkways, and uneven lighting in hazardous areas. The nurse should be prepared to call upon housekeeping services to quickly clean up spills and leaks that could cause frail older persons to fall and endure injury.

3. The problem may be reframed to be more positive. For instance, the nurse might say, "Instead of seeing a cane as a sign of weakness, think of it in a new way. The cane indicates a person with a vision problem who is getting around independently. Instead of a sign of weakness, it is a sign of self-sufficiency."

4. Assess the lighting in your dining area, the degree of contrast between the food and the plate, and the help available to older persons with vision problems. You may find areas for improvement.

5. You may find that wearing gloves somewhat separates you from fully experiencing your environment. This is a reasonable emotional response to the situation and indicates the need for creativity for engaging older adults with neurological disorders and parasthesias.

6. Often, nurses only touch patients in a clinical and professional manner. Older patients may feel "touch deprived" or miss the caring and loving touch from others. Most cultures define appropriate areas for touching as the hands, face, shoulders, and upper back but if you are unsure, be sure to check first.

Chapter 15

1. The underlying process of atherosclerosis has not been changed by invasive procedures. Changing diet and exercise can help atherosclerotic changes from recurring. Lifestyle changes are needed and the postoperative period is the ideal time to help a motivated older person make these changes. Rehabilitation also provides support for smoking cessation and stress reduction.

2. When a nurse knows a patient, even subtle changes are more apparent. The older patient may be developing decreased cardiac output, which may be evident in levels of energy or mood. If a patient develops sudden confusion or change in function, this will be more obvious to a person who knows that patient. Further, the older patient and his/her family are also more likely to trust the person giving health information.

3. Rehabilitation programs provide socialization, group support, monitoring during activity progression, dietary instruction, and stress reduction techniques. There is much more to a good rehabilitation program than exercise.

4. Older persons who live alone and have heart failure need to learn self-management of their condition. This includes medication management, daily weights, healthy food choices, and knowing when to call the healthcare provider to report changes in condition. Learning all these things will require ongoing support. A meals-on-wheels program may be required to provide balanced nutrition. Adult day health programs might be appropriate to provide socialization and

assessment. Having an accessible and caring primary care provider and caring nurse can make all the difference to controlling HF and maintaining independence.

5. Rehabilitation programs that would be ideal for people of all ages include socialization, cooking classes, exercise that is like a dance class, and stress reduction through meditation. Problems such as obesity, depression, family violence, and poverty cross all age, sex, and cultures in our society. The community residents will most likely appreciate the support for all of its members.

Chapter 16

1. There are community programs (sponsored by the American Lung Association, for example) that can assist older persons to quit smoking. There are also pharmacological (nicotine patches, bupropion) and nonpharmacological techniques (relaxation, counseling) to help older people to quit. Try to identify resources in your clinical and community setting to assist your patients.

2. The best advice is not to start at all. Smoking is addictive and it is often very difficult to quit. Smoking will yellow your teeth, cause premature wrinkles, and make your breath smell stale. Further, cigarettes are very expensive and a waste of money that could be spent on education, clothing, or entertainment. Stress the immediate negative impact of smoking because sometimes teenagers cannot contemplate long-term negative health outcomes.

3. Portable oxygen use improves the quality of life and daily function of older people with chronic lung disease. Unfortunately, there is added expense and difficulty in the maintenance and use of the equipment. Newer oxygen tanks are smaller and easier to use, so encourage their use if appropriate. Help your patients anticipate their feelings as they adjust to daily oxygen use and help them rehearse answers to questions they may be asked by others.

Chapter 17

1. Human sexuality is a complex subject, and discussing it with older adults requires great sensitivity on the part of the nurse. It is important to recognize one's own practice limits and to know when a referral to another healthcare provider is needed. It is equally important to know when a referral is not needed and when a concern can be addressed with your knowledge base. By becoming comfortable with your own feelings toward sexuality, you will be better able to counsel and support your older patients.

2. Nurses have a wealth of knowledge and a powerful array of skills that should not be underestimated. Sometimes, accurate information and an empathetic listener are the most

appropriate interventions. The person who makes ageist or negative remarks about sexuality in old age is probably misinformed. There are many societal stereotypes about sexuality, especially in old age. Provide accurate information about the need for and enjoyment of sexual activity in older people.

3. Ask your colleagues in your clinical setting if they have advisors, counselors, resources, or educational materials for older persons with sexual problems. There may be more materials available for men with erectile dysfunction problems because of educational campaigns initiated by pharmaceutical manufacturers. You may have to search more widely for information for older women.

4. Many of the things that enhance sexual activity for the older adult are similar to those used by other age groups such as soft lighting, background music, and romantic food and beverages. Urge older adults to conserve energy before sexual activity so that they do not become fatigued, to take pain medications to ease arthritic aches, to use appropriate positioning techniques to enhance pleasure, and to keep lubricants and other sexual aids handy so they can be used when needed. Sexual activity between consenting adults is fun and should be enjoyed, so urge them to approach each encounter without performance anxiety and to keep an open mind.

Chapter 18

1. Nursing considerations include patient safety (they are more at risk for fracture as the result of a fall), prevention of further bone loss (daily calcium and vitamin D intake and use of an antiresorptive medication if appropriate), weight-bearing exercise, avoidance of smoking and ongoing medical assessment (bone density scans every other year). Aggressive nursing intervention is needed to prevent unnecessary injury and disability as the result of further bone loss.

2. Remove clutter, secure scatter rugs, ensure adequate lighting, mark the edge of stairs with red reflective tape, and use nonskid mats and grab bars in the bathroom. Pets who may run underfoot should wear a bell to announce their movements. Older persons may have additional ideas to prevent falls, especially if they have fallen in the past. It is important to include the patient and family in the plan.

3. Many nurses are uncomfortable recommending exercise because they fear the older person will fall, suffer injury, or not take their suggestion seriously. A regular, moderate exercise program is crucial for maintaining cardiovascular conditioning and strength. Walking, swimming, and stretching are all appropriate activities for older people. Chair exercise can be recommended for older persons with balance problems or those confined to wheelchairs. Urge your patients to see their primary healthcare provider for

assessment of exercise ability if you are in doubt. Call your local YMCA and see if they have exercise classes for older people. Sit in on one. You may be pleasantly surprised.

Chapter 19

1. Many older people are overweight, do not exercise, and have other risk factors for the development of type 2 DM. They may be unwilling to discuss lifestyle modification if they are overwhelmed and intimidated by all the changes they will need to make. When educating older persons about lifestyle modification, try to begin with one or two simple suggestions. They will be more likely to come back for a second appointment.

2. Remember that you are a role model for your older patients. Try to maintain your own health and wellness as a good example.

3. Educate your colleagues about the importance of the thyroid in the regulation and maintenance of many of the body's activities and metabolic processes. When the older person complains of vague signs and symptoms, it will become your habit to suspect the thyroid as the underlying cause.

4. Most people have difficulty reorganizing his or her life to deal with type 1 DM. It involves regularly checking blood glucose, watching diet and nutrition, calculating insulin doses, recognizing and managing signs and symptoms of hypoglycemia, and carrying syringes, insulin, lancets, and a glucose monitor at all times. Many people will be overwhelmed and frightened. By understanding these fears, you will be in a better position to support and counsel your patients.

5. Some of your colleagues may feel that genetics is more important than lifestyle; others may feel that lifestyle is the key determinant. Either way, it is crucial to consider both factors. Older persons have the power to modify their lifestyles, but genetic risks are nonmodifiable. Urge your patients to change the things that can be changed.

Chapter 20

1. Many older people feel embarrassed and defer scheduling a sigmoidoscopy or colonoscopy because of their fears. Urge them to speak with others who have had the procedure and can reassure them. Even if your patient refuses the first request for a colonoscopy, try again. Over time, your patient may come to realize the importance of this lifesaving procedure.

2. Because some lifestyle modifications that are associated with GI problems relate to food and food consumption habits, it is sometimes difficult to motivate older people to change. Referral to a dietitian or nutritionist who can make practical suggestions and encourage healthy food choices

can be beneficial. When older persons engage in lifestyle modification and enjoy improvement of GI symptoms, they may be motivated to engage in additional healthy behaviors such as increasing consumption of fluids and healthy foods and getting regular exercise.

3. The societal stereotype is that all older persons are bowel obsessed and concerned about constipation. Although this is true for some older persons, many older people do not fit this stereotype. As you work with older people who are excessively concerned with bowel function, try to identify factors in their lifestyle or background that are contributing to the problem. Many times, there are contributing factors such as preexisting illness, medications, or immobility that can be recognized by the nurse rather than attributing the problem to the aging process.

Chapter 21

1. Older persons who are in chronic atrial fibrillation are more at risk for stroke because a thrombus can form in the heart as a result of incomplete emptying of the ventricles. This thrombus can travel to any part of the body and if lodged in the brain can cause a cerebrovascular accident (CVA), brain attack, or stroke. If the use of warfarin is indicated, it is necessary to maintain an INR of about 2.5 to 3.0 to prevent stroke.

2. Mr. Thayer is at risk for bleeding from trauma or injury because of his elevated INR. If he is at risk for falling, he should be urged to walk only with assistance and to exercise extreme caution to prevent bleeding and injury. He should avoid all strenuous activities, report any blood in the stool or urine, and avoid vigorous toothbrushing until his INR returns to normal limits.

3. Mr. Thayer should be urged to eat foods high in vitamin K like green leafy vegetables for the next few days. After that, he should eat foods high in vitamin K in a consistent pattern to make titration of his dose of warfarin more stable and consistent.

4. Mr. Thayer, like other older persons with chronic health problems and complicated disease management regimens, may need additional help and support from the interdisciplinary team. Appropriate interventions may include consultation and referral to social workers, nutritionists, and recreational, physical, or occupational therapists. By addressing the older person's problem holistically, the chances of good outcomes and increased quality of life are expanded.

Chapter 22

1. Because there is no one key test or procedure that definitively diagnoses Alzheimer's disease, the diagnosis is a process of exclusion. This process involves eliminating or ruling out all other possible causes of dementia. Families will often exhibit frustration and stress during the period of diagnosis. They may experience relief when the cause of the dementia is known, but feel fear and frustration when told of the devastating diagnosis.

2. Many communities offer support groups sponsored by the Alzheimer's Association. These groups meet regularly and provide information, support, and tips on caring for persons with dementia. Contact the social worker at your clinical agency to find out more about support and resources available in your community.

3. Environmental modifications often can ease agitation and improve the quality of life for older persons with dementia. Many factors in the institutional environment (hospital or long-term care facility) may complicate the care of persons with dementia. Some of these factors include noise, light, waking patients up at night for assessment of vital signs, bathing schedules that may not conform to the best time to approach the patient, and so on. Identifying a few changes to the clinical environment is a good way to begin your professional career.

4. Many nurses would benefit from formal or informal support groups, ongoing professional education (in-service and attendance at professional conferences), training videos, and written materials. It is natural to feel frustration, anger, and other negative feelings when providing care to an older person who may be resistive, hostile, or resentful because of a cognitive impairment. Keep a journal and record the feelings (positive and negative) that you experience when caring for a resistive older person with a cognitive impairment. Share your feelings with a friend, and you may find others experience similar emotional responses. Explore some of the Websites listed in this chapter to identify sources where you can gain valuable practical information to solve clinical problems.

Chapter 23

1. Rheumatoid arthritis requires medications and interventions to relieve pain, prevent further joint destruction, and improve the quality of life. Many of these medications can be toxic to older persons and cause drug interactions when taken with other medications. Careful monitoring of drug levels and ongoing assessment of drug interactions is needed.

2. Many older people are hesitant to discuss sex and sexual behavior with a person of the opposite sex or a younger person. If you sense resistance or embarrassment on the part of older patients, question them as to why they are uncomfortable. If possible, make a referral to someone on

your team who may have the skills and experience to work with older persons and teach them safe sex practices. In general, the information you provide to the older person would be similar to the information given to younger patients. They should avoid risky sexual behaviors such as unprotected sexual intercourse and intravenous drug use. Although blood transfusion safety has increased since the 1980s, HIV antibodies in a donor may go undetected if the infected donor has been exposed but has not yet seroconverted (a process that may take up to 6 months). Therefore, many professionals urge autodonation of blood for scheduled surgery.

3. When large numbers of older, frail, and acutely ill persons are placed together in congregate living facilities, drug-resistant bacteria can thrive. Proper sanitation and hand washing are necessary to prevent transmission from person to person, with isolation of those who are at high risk for acquiring infections (patients who are immunosuppressed or have multiple comorbidities) and those who may spread infection (acutely ill with infectious disease such as tuberculosis). Cross-contamination can occur when individuals are transferred for treatment between institutions and are cared for by multiple providers.

4. The main risk factors include inappropriate use of antibiotics (including prescription for viral infections, improper administration and dosing practices, and failure to complete the entire course of treatment); poor hand washing practices of healthcare workers; use of contaminated equipment between patients, including telephones, blood pressure cuffs, stethoscopes, and eating utensils; exposure to contaminated surfaces, including taking medications dropped on the floor; placing fingers, pens, eyeglasses, hairclips, and so on in the mouth; use of indwelling urinary catheters that encourage development of urinary tract infections; failure to wear gloves or protect clothing when caring for patients who are incontinent; and failure to use aspiration precautions in patients with dysphagia. Develop good habits so that you do not place yourself or your patients at risk for developing nosocomial infections. An education program designed to educate older persons

and avoidance of the risk factors described above is a good learning activity and will benefit the older persons in your community or clinical setting.

Chapter 24

1. Entering a hospital is a stressful situation for any person, regardless of age. Some people are fearful that they will become a number instead of a person. Taking a few personal items can help strengthen the individual patient's identity and provide a stimulus for conversation with the staff. In general, advise older persons to bring items with them to the hospital that have emotional value such as family photographs and grandchildren's artwork. Avoid bringing items with financial value such as expensive jewelry or electronics as they could be misplaced or damaged during hospitalization.

2. This exercise may clarify and identify opinions that you and others have about the treatment of patients with cognitive impairment. You may find yourself engaging in this discussion with others many times during your professional career. It is a valuable exercise to learn how to argue your point of view and disagree respectfully with others.

3. Advantages may include improved care by the segregation of older patients on units with specialized resources and caregivers. Disadvantages may include the fact that older people who are not placed on these special units may not enjoy the benefits of specialized care. Segregating older patients on one unit may communicate the unfortunate message that caring for older patients is not a priority for all caregivers on the general units.

4. The most important factor is communication and sharing of crucial information, especially focusing on medications, dosing information, baseline function, food preferences, and advance directives. If there is a close relationship between a nursing home and hospital, the nurses become familiar with one another and will often just pick up the phone and call for information needed to improve the care of the older hospitalized patient.

GLOSSARY

abandonment The desertion or willful forsaking of an older adult by a caretaker, or foregoing of duties, withdrawal or neglect of duties and obligations owed to the older adult by a caretaker or other person responsible for his or her care.

abnormal sleep behaviors Behaviors such as night terrors, sleepwalking, and restless legs syndrome.

accommodation The ability of the lens to change shape in order to focus on an image.

achalasia A neurogenic esophageal disorder of unknown cause characterized by impaired esophageal peristalsis and a lack of lower esophageal sphincter relaxation.

achlorhydria Lack of hydrochloric acid in the stomach.

actinic keratosis These lesions are red-tan scaly plaques that occur on sun-exposed surfaces. The lesions increase in size and become raised with a rough surface.

acute pain Pain occurring from a time-limited illness, a recent event such as surgery, medical procedures, or trauma. Acute pain is usually limited to about 10 to 14 days.

acute-phase reactants Proteins that increase serum concentration in response to acute and chronic inflammation.

addiction Having an intense need and compulsive dependence to such an extent that not having these drugs causes severe yearning and triggers physiological withdrawal symptoms.

adjuvant drugs Medications used along with analgesics to increase the effectiveness of the analgesics and prevent and treat associated symptoms.

adrenergic receptors Receptors for the sympathetic nervous system that when stimulated cause increased heart rate, vascular tone, and contractility of the left ventricle.

adult protective services (APS) An agency that provides services to adults, including older adults, who are victims of domestic violence. Each state has APS, but available services will vary. Healthcare providers need to be familiar with the contact information for the APS that services their area.

advance directives Refers to the document signed by the patient indicating the individual's choice or wishes for medical treatment. It may also designate another to make those choices/decisions if the patient is unable.

advanced practice registered nurse (APRN) A nurse practitioner or clinical nurse specialist who holds a master's degree, has advanced clinical experience, and demonstrates depth and breadth of knowledge, competence, and skill in the practice of gerontological nursing.

adverse drug events (ADE) A poor outcome or response to a drug that results in toxicity, lack of therapeutic effect, or an interaction with another drug, resulting in actual or potential harm to the older person.

adverse drug experience Any adverse event associated with the use of a drug in humans, whether or not considered drug related, including the following: an adverse event occurring in the course of the use of a drug product in professional practice; an adverse event occurring from drug overdose whether accidental or intentional; an adverse event occurring from drug abuse; an adverse event occurring from drug withdrawal; and any failure of expected pharmacological action (FDA, 2011).

adverse drug reaction (ADR) Any response to a drug that is noxious and unintended, and that occurs at doses normally used in humans for prophylaxis, diagnosis, or therapy of disease, or for the modification of physiological function.

aerophagia Swallowing of air.

afterload The pressure against which the ventricle ejects blood.

ageism The attribution of negative stereotypes to a person based solely on that person's age.

age-related macular degeneration (ARMD) Degenerative visual disorder of the macula affecting central vision and focus.

agnosia Inability to recognize familiar objects.

alcohol abuse Use of alcoholic beverages to excess despite problems resulting from continued use.

alcohol dependence Craving or reliance on alcohol despite problems resulting from continued use.

alveoli Tiny sac-like air spaces in the lungs where the transfer of oxygen and carbon dioxide occurs.

Alzheimer's disease (AD) A type of dementia of unknown cause with symptoms that show a gradual onset and relentless progression. AD involves a sufficient loss of intellectual ability to interfere with social or occupational functioning, memory loss, possible personality change, and impairments in abstract thinking, judgment, spatial orientation, and/or language. Histopathology reveals characteristic senile plaques and neurofibrillary tangles.

anemia A condition characterized by a decrease in hemoglobin in the blood to levels below the normal range.

angular cheilosis Cracking at the corners of the mouth.

anhedonia Loss of pleasure from activities that were once enjoyable.

anomia   A severe problem with word finding and/or retrieval.

anorexia   Loss of appetite.

anorexia of aging   Diminished appetite associated with aging and related to physiological changes in digestion and metabolism.

anthropometric measurements   Measurements of the body, such as for height, weight, body fat, and muscle mass.

antibody   Antigen-specific glycoproteins that attach to the antigen and render it harmless.

antigens   A wide range of substances that are identified as "nonself" and stimulate an immune response.

anxiety   A state of apprehension, uneasiness, or distress.

apraxia   Inability to initiate purposeful motor functions and/or use objects properly in the absence of known physical problems.

asthma   A chronic inflammatory disease of the airways in which many cells and cellular elements contribute to the process, including mast cells, eosinophils, lymphocytes, macrophages, neutrophils, and epithelial cells.

atrophic gastritis   Atrophy of the gastric mucosa, which leads to achlorhydria.

atrophic vaginitis   Thinning and loss of elasticity of vaginal tissues after menopause, resulting in increased rates of infection, ulceration, and uncomfortable sexual intercourse.

autoimmunity   Response that occurs when the body loses self-recognition.

autolytic debridement   The use of enzymes to remove necrotic or dead tissue from a wound to promote healing.

balance exercises   Exercises that increase confidence in balance and help to prevent falls and fractures.

bedtime rituals   Activities undertaken by persons before going to bed that promote relaxation and sleep.

benign prostatic hyperplasia (BPH)   Non-cancerous enlargement of the prostate gland.

bereavement   Includes the feelings and outward expressions of loss, grief, and mourning of those who survive the death of someone important to them.

beta cells   Cells found in the areas of the pancreas called the islets of Langerhans that make insulin.

bladder training   Behavioral intervention in which the nurse and client establish a voiding schedule to decrease episodes of incontinence and increase bladder tone and capacity.

blood glucose   The main sugar that the body produces from ingested nutrients carried via the general circulation to all cells of the body for energy.

bone marrow   Myeloid tissue confined to the cavities in the bone. Hematopoietic bone marrow is responsible for the formation and storage of red blood cells.

breakthrough pain   Pain that manifests while a patient is receiving scheduled pain relief medication. Often described as a flare-up of pain.

bronchi   Larger air passages of the lungs.

bronchioles   Smaller air passages of the lungs.

cancellous bone   The spongy or trabecular tissue in the center of bone (vertebrae, etc.) and at the end of long bones.

cardiac output   The amount of blood the heart can pump in one minute.

caries   Cavities.

cataracts   An opacity of the lens of the eye that reduces visual acuity to 20/30 or less.

cell-mediated immune response   The reaction that occurs when mature lymphocytes contact and attack antigens.

cellulitis   An infection of the skin and subcutaneous tissue.

certification   The formal process by which clinical competence is validated in a specialty area of practice.

cerumen   A substance, commonly known as ear wax, produced by sebaceous and apocrine glands in the outer portion of the external auditory canal.

chemical debridement   The use of chemicals to remove necrotic or dead tissue from a wound to promote healing.

chemical restraints   Drugs used to quiet a person or subdue certain behaviors rather than using nonmedication measures.

chorea   Involuntary twitching of the limbs or facial muscles.

chronic obstructive pulmonary disease (COPD)   A disease state characterized by the presence of chronic airflow obstruction due to chronic bronchitis or emphysema.

circadian rhythms   A rest/activity pattern controlled by the brain using environmental cues within a 24-hour period.

CLAS standards   The collective set of CLAS mandates, guidelines, and recommendations issued by the Health and Human Services Office of Minority Health intended to inform, guide, and facilitate required and recommended practices related to culturally and linguistically appropriate health services.

Clostridium difficile   An organism, normally residing in the bowel, that can proliferate as the result of administration of antibiotics and can cause diarrhea and colonic inflammation.

cognitive function   The ability to think, reason, remember, and communicate.

cognitive impairment   A condition that causes problems with memory or other mental function.

comfort measures only (CMO)   Nursing interventions delivered not to treat disease but to improve pain, function, or quality of life.

communication   Communication differences present themselves in many ways, including language differences, verbal and nonverbal behaviors, and silence. Language differences are possibly the most important obstacle to providing CULTURALCARE because they affect all stages of the patient–caregiver–nurse relationship.

compact bone   Bone structure that is solid and strong and supports blood vessels and nerves within its core.

competence   A legal determination of the match between an individual's cognitive abilities and environmental demands.

comprehensive geriatric evaluation   An interdisciplinary approach to assessment of the older person using a biopsychosocial functional model that systematically collects data from a multidimensional, complex base and focuses the plan of care on issues of greatest concern to patients and families.

conductive hearing loss Hearing loss related to inability to conduct sound secondary to external ear problems such as impacted cerumen, infection, or tumor.

confusion Impaired cognition or orientation to time, place, or person.

continuous positive airway pressure (CPAP) A mechanical ventilation technique used to deliver continuous positive airway pressure.

contractility The strength of the cardiac contraction.

coping mechanisms Methods used by individuals to adjust to or accept a threat or challenge.

cortical bone The dense outer layer of bone.

Crohn's disease A chronic inflammatory disease affecting the terminal ileum or colon characterized by inflammation, lineal ulcerations, and granulomas.

CulturalCare A concept that describes professional nursing care that is culturally sensitive, culturally appropriate, and culturally competent. CulturalCare is critical to meet the complex nursing care needs of a given person, family, and community. It is the provision of nursing care across cultural boundaries and takes into account the context in which the patient lives as well as the situations in which the patient's health problems arise.

culturally appropriate services Healthcare services that are respectful of and responsive to cultural needs.

culturally competent care Implies that within the delivered care, the healthcare provider understands and attends to the total context of the patient's situation. Cultural competence is a complex combination of knowledge, attitudes, and skills.

culturally sensitive Implies that the healthcare providers possess some basic knowledge of and constructive attitudes toward the health traditions observed among the diverse cultural groups found in the setting in which they are practicing.

culture The nonphysical traits, such as values, beliefs, attitudes, and customs, that are shared by a group of people and passed from one generation to the next.

debridement The removal of devitalized tissue. It may appear as necrotic (black) or yellow slough.

dehydration Abnormal loss of water from the body because of a medical condition or physical exertion.

delirium Potentially reversible acute-onset confusional state.

delusions A fixed or false belief that is firmly held despite convincing evidence to the contrary.

dementia Acquired, progressive state of long duration (months to years) of decreased mental ability that impairs daily activities in a previously alert individual.

dementia with Lewy bodies (DLB) A type of dementia characterized by a fluctuating course of cognitive impairment that includes episodic confusion and lucid intervals similar to delirium and (1) visual and/or auditory hallucinations resulting in paranoid delusions, (2) mild extrapyramidal symptoms or adverse extrapyramidal response to standard doses of neuroleptics, or (3) repeated, unexplained falls; histopathology reveals presence of Lewy bodies. Also called diffuse *Lewy body disease*.

demographic disparity A variation below the percentages of the profile of the total population with a specific entity, such as poverty, or professional, such as nursing; comparison with the demographic profile of the total population.

demographic parity An equal distribution of a given entity, such as registered nurses, and the demographic profile of the total population.

dependency on others Relying on someone else for support or care.

depression Mental disorder marked by symptoms of long-lasting despondent mood often described as overwhelming sadness or emptiness, changes in appetite or weight or sleeping pattern, feeling either agitated or slowed down, loss of interest in usual activities, decreased energy, feeling worthless and guilty, difficulty thinking and concentrating, and thoughts of death or suicide.

desquamation The loss of the epidermis or top layers of skin.

detrusor muscles The muscle layer in the urinary bladder consisting of longitudinal, spiral, and circular sheets of muscle; contractions of the detrusor cause urine to flow out of the bladder through the urethra.

diabetic retinopathy Microvascular changes to the blood vessels in the eye commonly found in people with type 1 and type 2 diabetes, especially those with poor glycemic control.

diastole The period in the cardiac cycle between contractions in which the heart muscle is at rest.

diverticula A saclike mucosal projection through the muscular layer of the gastrointestinal tract.

diverticulitis Presence of diverticula with inflammation or infection.

diverticulosis Presence of diverticula without inflammation.

domestic violence Mistreatment of individuals such as spouses or intimate partners, children, and elders.

durable power of attorney for health care An agent (and an alternate if the primary proxy is not available) designated to make decisions for the older adult if he or she is unable to do so.

dysgeusia An impairment in the sense of taste.

dyspareunia Pain that is associated with sexual intercourse in a woman; may be related to atrophic vaginitis, urinary tract infection, or arthritis, among other conditions.

dyspepsia Common, usually benign upper abdominal pain or discomfort. Often called *indigestion*.

dysphagia Difficult swallowing or the perception of difficult swallowing, often resulting in delay or inability to transport ingested food from the oropharynx to the stomach.

dyspnea The subjective sensation of breathlessness, labored breathing, or feeling of being starved for air.

dysthymia Chronic feelings of sadness and lack of enjoyment in life.

dystonia Involuntary muscle contractions that force certain parts of the body into abnormal and sometimes painful movements or positions.

edentulism Lack of teeth.

edentulous Without teeth.

ejection fraction The proportion of blood that is pumped out in each heartbeat.

elder mistreatment The result of actions of abuse, neglect, abandonment, sexual abuse, and/or exploitation of the older adult.

elopement Leaving a setting of care without permission.

emphysema A condition characterized by permanent enlargement of the air spaces in the lungs with destruction of the cell walls.

epidemiology The study of the distribution and determinants of diseases and injuries in human populations.

epilepsy A chronic condition produced by temporary changes in the electrical function of the brain causing reoccurring and unprovoked seizures that affect awareness, movement, or sensation.

erectile dysfunction (ED) The inability to achieve and/or maintain an erection sufficient for satisfactory sexual intercourse.

erythrocytes Red blood cells that transport gases between the lungs and peripheral tissues.

ethnicity Cultural group's sense of identification associated with the group's common social and cultural heritage.

euthyroid A metabolic state of normal thyroid function.

executive function Ability to plan and think abstractly; loss of executive function is detected when persons with dementia interpret proverbs literally versus their abstract meaning.

exploitation The illegal or improper use of an older adult's material possessions.

extrinsic factors Environmental factors outside the person that are associated with dermatological conditions.

failure to thrive A syndrome of decline in an older person accompanied by weight loss, poor appetite, dehydration, immobility, depression, impaired immunity, and low cholesterol levels.

first-pass effect drugs Drugs significantly metabolized when they first flow through the liver (first pass into the liver).

fissures Longitudinal breaks in the epithelium of the anal canal.

flat affect Lack of facial expression or emotional response.

frailty A term used to describe a person with dependence in one or more activities of daily living, three or more comorbid conditions, and one or more geriatric syndromes (including dementia, delirium, depression, incontinence, falls, osteoporosis, gait disturbance, or pressure ulcers).

frontotemporal dementia A type of dementia characterized by symptoms of altered personality similar to changes induced by damage of frontal lobes from other causes (injury, stroke); symptoms include behavioral disinhibition, loss of social or personal awareness, or disengagement with apathy.

functional assessment A comprehensive evaluation of physical and cognitive abilities required to maintain independence; includes objective measures of physical health, activities of daily living (ADLs), instrumental activities of daily living (IADLs), and psychological and social function.

functional health patterns An interrelated group of behavioral areas that provides a view of the whole person and his/her relationship with the environment.

functional incontinence Involuntary loss of urine due to factors external to the urinary system such as immobility and/or cognitive impairment.

futile therapy Therapies that offer no realistic hope of improvement or recovery.

gastritis Inflammation of the lining of the stomach or gastric mucosa.

gastroesophageal reflux disease (GERD) The reflux of gastric contents into the esophagus.

geriatric cascade Rapid decline or decompensation as a result of acute illness or worsening of a chronic condition.

geriatrics From the Greek word *geras* meaning "old age"; the medical specialty focusing on diagnosing and treating disease of older people.

gerontological nurse A nurse who works primarily with older adults by incorporating gerontological competencies in order to assess, manage, and implement health care to meet the specialized needs of older adults and evaluate the effectiveness of such care.

gerontological nursing A nursing specialization concerned with the provision of high-quality care to older adults.

gerontologists As a result of the multidisciplinary focus of gerontology, professionals from diverse fields, including nurses, call themselves *gerontologists*.

gerontology From the Greek word *geron* meaning "old man"; the study of aging and health problems of older people with a holistic focus including biologic, sociologic, psychologic, spiritual, and economic issues.

gingivitis Inflammation of the gums.

glaucoma A disorder of the eye characterized by increased intraocular pressure that can lead to irreversible damage to the optic nerve with accompanying loss of vision.

glossitis Inflammation of the tongue.

glossitis and cheilosis Red, swollen tongue and lips; can be symptoms of vitamin deficiency.

glycosylated hemoglobin A blood test that measures an individual's average blood sugar level during the past 2 to 3 months; also called *hemoglobin A_{1C}*.

gout A disease characterized by the deposit of urate crystals in a peripheral joint, resulting in pain, inflammation, and destruction.

gradual dose reduction (GDR) Gradual dose reduction is the stepwise tapering of a dose to determine if symptoms, conditions, or risks can be managed by a lower dose or if the dose or medication can be discontinued.

granulocytes White blood cells that ingest and digest debris and foreign material throughout the body and release powerful chemicals such as histamine and heparin that assist in the inflammatory process.

Graves' disease   The most common form of hyperthyroidism. Also known as toxic diffuse goiter, Graves' is caused by an antibody that stimulates the thyroid to produce too much thyroid hormone.

grief   The personal and individualized feelings and emotional responses to a loss.

guardianship   A legally appointed individual who is responsible for an older adult unable to care for himself or herself.

hallucinations   Sensory perceptions that occur without the appropriate stimulation of the corresponding sensory organ, such as seeing people who are not present.

Hashimoto's thyroiditis   An autoimmune inflammatory disease in which antibodies attack the thyroid gland and destroy gland function eventually leading to hypothyroidism; also called *chronic autoimmune thyroiditis*.

healthcare proxy   A person designated to make healthcare decisions for another in the event that the person designating proxy is unable to make his/her own decisions because of illness or circumstance.

hematocrit   The fraction of blood that consists of red blood cells.

hematopoiesis   The production and differentiation of red blood cells occurring in the bone marrow.

hemoglobin   A protein within the red blood cell that carries gases and regulates diffusion through the cell's plasma membrane.

hemolysis   The destruction of red blood cells due to disease, toxins, or autoimmune antibodies.

hemoptysis   The coughing up of blood or production of bloody sputum.

hemorrhoids   Large blood vessels protruding into the anorectal area.

heritage consistency   The observance of the beliefs and practices of one's traditional cultural belief system.

heritage inconsistency   The observance of the beliefs and practices of one's acculturated belief system.

hiatal hernia   A diaphragmatic hernia resulting when a portion of the stomach rises into the chest.

histocompatibility antigens   Self-antigens found on body cells that will not stimulate an immune response.

homeostasis   The tendency of the body toward maintaining equilibrium.

homeostenosis   Inability of the body to restore homeostasis after even minor environmental challenges such as trauma or infection.

hospice care   A system of care that supports and cares for people in the last phase of an incurable disease so they may live as fully and comfortably as possible.

humoral immune response   Response initiated when an antigen binds with antibody receptors on the surface of the mature B cell. Antibodies are then produced.

hyperalgesia   Increased sensitivity to pain or enhanced intensity of pain sensation.

hypersensitivity   An excessive response to antigen stimulation or a normal response that is inappropriate.

hyperthyroidism   A metabolic state resulting from an excess in thyroid hormone function; also called *thyrotoxicosis*.

hypogeusia   A decreased ability to taste.

hyposmia   A decreased sense of smell.

hypothyroidism   A metabolic state resulting from a deficiency in thyroid hormone function; also called *myxedema*.

iatrogenesis   Illness or disability resulting from medical intervention.

immune deficiency   Occurs with increasing age, resulting in more difficulty defending the body from foreign invaders.

immune dysregulation   Changes in the immune system that may disrupt the regulation between the multiple components of the immune process, resulting in progressive destruction of the body cells.

immunoenhancing drugs   Drugs designed to stimulate and enhance the body's immune response to defend against foreign bodies.

immunoglobulins   Antibodies.

immunosenescence   The gradual decline in the effectiveness of the immune system that occurs as a result of changes of aging.

incompetence or insufficiency   Occurs when a valve doesn't close tightly and blood leaks back into the chamber rather than flowing forward through the heart or into an artery.

insomnia   The perception or complaint of inadequate sleep because of one or more of the following factors: difficulty falling asleep; difficulty staying asleep; frequent nighttime awakening; waking up too early in the morning; reports of unrefreshing sleep.

interdisciplinary education   An educational process that encourages the integration of different perspectives on a defined subject. The goal is to expose students to a shared knowledge base so they gain a basic understanding of core concepts, principles, and contributions of a variety of disciplines.

interdisciplinary teams   A group of people from different disciplines who assess and plan care in a collaborative manner. A common goal is established and each discipline works to achieve that goal.

intermittent positive pressure breathing (IPPB)   A device that assists intermittent positive pressure inhalation of therapeutic aerosols without the hand coordination required in the use of hand nebulizers or metered-dose inhalers.

intrinsic factors   Factors within the person, such as age, nutritional status, genetic predisposition, level of skin pigmentation, degree of sun damage, and underlying allergies that contribute to the condition of the skin.

ketones   A waste product of fat breakdown. Levels rise when the body breaks down stored fat as a secondary energy source when insufficient insulin is present to utilize blood glucose for energy.

leukocytes   White blood cells that defend the body against invading organisms and remove cellular debris.

leukoplakia   A precancerous thick white patch that develops on the inside of the mouth or other mucous membrane.

life expectancy   The average number of years from birth that an individual can expect to live.

life span   Biological limit to the length of life. Life span varies by species.

life trajectory   The historical and experiential trajectory of a given person's life—the events that occurred within the society they live in and the world, and their interpretation of them. The trajectory is predicated on countless variables, including year of birth, number of familial generations living in the United States, class, primary spoken language, and education.

ligaments   Fibrous connections between two bones that provide the joint with stability during movement.

living wills   Legal documents in which older adults describe their wishes regarding treatment at the end of life; this may include acceptance or limitation of life-sustaining treatment in the face of a life-threatening illness.

longitudinal pigmented bands   Dark, pigmented stripes or stria appearing in the nail bed that are often associated with pathological conditions.

loss   A separation from a person, thing, relationship, or situation to which one was emotionally attached.

lymphocytes   Primary white blood cells concerned with development of immunity.

lysing   Cell breakdown or disintegration.

macrocytic   When the MCV is above 100 fL and the average red cell is larger than normal.

macrophages   Monocytes that have become large phagocytic cells.

malnutrition   Poor nutrition, generally refers to protein-calorie undernutrition.

mean corpuscular volume (MCV)   A measurement of the average size of the red blood cells. Usually between 80 and 100 fL.

mechanical debridement   The use of irrigation or wet to dry dressings to remove necrotic or dead tissue from a wound in order to promote wound healing.

mediastinum   The area between the lungs containing the bronchi, heart, major blood vessels, esophagus, and trachea.

medication regimen review (MRR)   Is a process required by Medicare that involves a thorough evaluation of an individual's medication regimen by a pharmacist, in collaboration with other members of the interdisciplinary team.

melanocytes   Melanocytes produce melanin, give the skin its color, and shield the body from the harmful effects of the sun.

memory   The capacity of the immune system to develop long-lasting protection against specific invaders.

microcytic   When the MCV is below 80 fL and the average red cell is smaller than normal.

monocytes   Large phagocytic cells.

mourning   The outward, social expressions of a loss often dictated by cultural norms, customs, rituals, and traditions.

multiple sclerosis (MS)   A chronic disabling disease that affects the central nervous system causing numbness, weakness, paralysis, or loss of vision.

natural immunity   Innate resistance that is not produced by the immune response.

neglect   The refusal or failure to fulfill a person's assumed duties to an older adult.

nephropathy   A disease of the kidneys resulting in damage to the cells, small blood vessels, and parts of the kidney that filter the blood.

neuropathic pain   Pain resulting from damage to the peripheral or central nervous system.

neuropathy   A disease of the nervous system resulting in nerve damage.

nociceptive pain   Occurs as a protective, transient response to injury at the site where nociceptors (pain-sensitive nerve endings) arise and are activated by the noxious stimuli such as injury.

nocturia   Literally "night urination"; urinating two or more times per night.

nonmaleficence   The desire to do no harm.

nonprescription medicines   Drugs sold over the counter not requiring a prescription.

normocytic   When the mean corpuscular volume is between 80 and 100 fL and the average red cell is within the normal size range.

nosocomial infection   An infection acquired in a hospital or institutional setting, including those infections that develop shortly after discharge from the institutional setting.

nursing diagnosis   The naming of an individual's response to actual or potential health problems or life processes.

osteoarthritis   A disease characterized by the progressive erosion of the joint articular cartilage with the formation of new bone in the joint space.

osteoblasts   Bone-forming cells that lay down new bone.

osteomalacia   A metabolic disease in which there is inadequate mineralization of newly formed bone matrix, usually resulting from vitamin D deficiency.

osteoporosis   Characterized by low bone mass and deterioration of bone tissue leading to compromised bone strength and an increased risk of fractures.

overflow incontinence   Involuntary loss of urine due to bladder overfilling with overextended bladder muscles secondary to urethral blockage and chronic retention.

over-the-counter (OTC) medication   A nonprescription medicine.

oxyhemoglobin   The oxygen-bound form of hemoglobin (the predominant protein in red blood cells).

Paget's disease (PD)   A chronic localized bone disorder of unknown etiology in which normal bone is removed and replaced with abnormal bone, also called *osteitis deformans*.

pain An unpleasant sensory experience that evokes a complex, subjective response characterized by quantifiable measures including intensity, time, course, quality, impact, and personal meaning.

pain management Formulation and implementation of a plan to alleviate and/or reduce pain to a level of comfort that is acceptable to the patient.

palliative care Interdisciplinary team-based care for persons and family members experiencing life-threatening illness or injury that addresses their physical, emotional, social, and spiritual needs and seeks to improve quality of life along the illness/dying trajectory.

parkinsonism A neurological syndrome characterized by tremor, rigidity, and instability when walking.

Parkinson's disease (PD) A chronic, progressive neurological disorder in which a syndrome consisting of variable combinations of tremor, rigidity, and extreme slowness in movement occurs without evidence of more widespread neurological involvement.

pelvic floor exercises (Kegel exercises) Alternating contraction and relaxation of the muscles of the pelvic floor, promoting urinary continence and/or decreasing prolapse of pelvic organs.

peptic ulcer disease An erosion of the gastrointestinal mucosa either in the stomach (gastric ulcer) or the duodenum (duodenal ulcer).

periodontal disease Gum disease.

persistent pain Pain that continues for a prolonged period and may not be associated with a defined event or illness.

personality A set of personal characteristics, attitudes, and beliefs that influence how an older person interacts with the world.

phagocytes A white blood cell that ingests and destroys foreign bodies and microorganisms to help protect the body from infection.

pharmacodynamics Absorption, biotransformation, distribution, and elimination of drug (what the body does to the drug).

pharmacogenetics The investigation of genetic variations that give rise to individual and differing responses to drug therapy.

pharmacokinetics Effect of a drug on the body (what the drug does to the body).

photoaging Premature wrinkling and dryness of the skin secondary to chronic sun exposure.

physical abuse The use of physical force that may result in bodily injury.

physical dependence A state of adaptation that is manifested by withdrawal symptoms when the drug is abruptly stopped or decreased.

Pick's disease A type of dementia that is a subtype of a frontotemporal dementia and characterized by Pick bodies inside nerve cells and ballooned nerve cells.

plasma A complex aqueous liquid containing a number of organic and inorganic elements.

platelets Disc-shaped cell fragments that are essential for blood coagulation and control of bleeding.

polypharmacy The prescription, administration, or use of more medications than are clinically indicated in a given patient.

postmortem care Type of care provided to a patient after death.

prediabetes Blood glucose levels that are higher than normal but not yet high enough to be diagnosed as diabetes.

preload Amount of blood returning to the heart from the venous circulation.

presbycusis Bilateral loss of hearing due to age-related changes in the inner ear.

presbyopia A universal age-related change in the lens of the eye involving loss of accommodation. Objects held closer than 1 or 2 feet become difficult to see.

pressure ulcers Lesions caused by unrelieved pressure resulting in damage to underlying tissue.

primary immune response First exposure to foreign antigen; after 5 days, antibodies can usually be found in the blood.

pseudodementia A state of cognitive impairment caused by depression or another condition when evidence of an organic disorder is lacking.

rectal prolapse Protrusion of part of the rectum through the anus.

refractory period The brief period in which the nerves in the heart cannot respond to further stimuli.

regurgitation Occurs when a valve doesn't close tightly and blood leaks back into the chamber rather than flowing forward through the heart or into an artery.

religion Belief in a divine or superhuman power or powers to be obeyed and worshipped as the creator(s) and ruler(s) of the universe.

renal failure An acute or chronic inability of the kidneys to perform regulatory and excretory functions.

respectful care Takes into consideration the values, preferences, and expressed needs of the patient/family.

retinopathy A disease of the small blood vessels in the retina of the eye.

rheumatoid arthritis (RA) A chronic syndrome characterized by symmetric inflammation of the peripheral joints, with pain, swelling, significant morning stiffness, and general symptoms of fatigue and malaise.

risk factors Factors whose presence are associated with an increased probability that disease will develop at a later time.

sarcopenia Loss of muscle mass, occurring with aging.

scope of practice A range of nursing functions that are differentiated according to the level of practice, the role of the nurse, and the work setting. The parameters are determined by each state's nurse practice act, professional code of ethics, and nursing practice standards, as well as each individual's personal competency to perform particular activities of functions.

seasonal affective disorder A depression that occurs in the fall and spring months in older persons who have normal mental health during the rest of the year.

sebum   An oily substance that keeps hair supple and lubricates the skin.

secondary immune response   Rapid production of a large amount of antibodies due to presence of memory cells.

self-neglect   Occurs when an older adult exhibits behaviors, such as not providing self with adequate food, that threaten personal health and or safety.

self-recognition   The immune system's ability to differentiate between substances that are normal constituents of a person's body and those that are not.

senescence   Progressive deterioration of body systems that can increase the risk of mortality as an individual gets older.

senescent bone loss   Bone loss that occurs in both sexes during midlife and later.

senile purpura   Bruised and discolored areas caused by damage to the capillaries.

sensorineural hearing loss   Hearing loss related to inability of the inner ear to transmit sound waves to the brain for interpretation.

sexual abuse   Nonconsensual sexual contact of any kind with an older adult.

sexually transmitted diseases   Diseases that are transmitted via sexual intercourse.

sharp debridement   The use of a scalpel or other sharp instrument to remove necrotic tissue.

skin sensitizer   A substance that will induce an allergic response following skin contact.

sleep   A natural periodic state of rest for the mind and body.

sleep apnea   Disturbed or interrupted breathing during sleep. Usually temporary interruptions of breathing lasting 10 seconds up to 20 or 30 times per hour.

sleep architecture   The sleep cycles and phases that comprise the underlying physiological sleep mechanism. These cycles and phases can be measured by electroencephalogram (EEG) testing in a sleep center.

sleep hygiene   A rigorous program to improve sleep that mandates consistent bedtime and time of awakening with elimination of daytime napping with sleep occurring only in bed.

socialization   The process of being raised within a culture and acquiring the characteristics of the given group.

somatic pain   Pain of the muscles, joints, connective tissues, and bones that typically is well localized.

spatial disorientation   Misperception of immediate surroundings such as the inability to distinguish a two-dimensional object from a three-dimensional object or not knowing where one is in relation to the environment; leads to getting lost.

specificity   The immune response to react to only to one antigen.

standards   Authoritative statements enunciated and promulgated by a profession by which the quality of practice, service, or education of that profession's practitioners can be judged.

stenosis   Valvular thickening, stiffening, or fusing together of heart valves restricting the flow of blood.

stomatitis   Inflammatory changes of the mucous membrane in the mouth and throat including sores and ulcerations.

stress   An internal or external event that creates a nonspecific response in the older person.

stress incontinence   Involuntary loss of urine due to increased intra-abdominal pressures such as coughing or sneezing.

stroke volume   The amount of blood pumped to the aorta from the left ventricle in a typical contraction.

systole   The period in the cardiac cycle in which the heart contracts, forcing blood into the major cardiac vessels.

tinnitus   Ringing, buzzing, pulsations, or clicking when no actual sound stimulus is present.

tolerance   A state of adaptation in which exposure to a drug induces changes that result in a decrease of the drug's effects over time.

Transcultural Nursing Society Standards   Twelve standards for cultural competence in nursing practice developed by the Transcultural Nursing Society.

ulcerative colitis   A chronic inflammatory process affecting the superficial layers of the colonic wall.

undernutrition   Poor nutrition, including unintentional weight loss.

urge incontinence   Involuntary loss of urine due to forceful detrusor muscle contraction and internal sphincter weakness.

urinary catheterization   The insertion of a tube through the urethra and into the bladder to drain urine; may be removed after the urine is collected (intermittent catheterization) or left in place to continuously drain urine (indwelling catheterization). One of the most common causes of urinary tract infections in older adults. Not a treatment for urinary incontinence.

urinary frequency   More than seven voids per 24-hour period.

urinary incontinence (UI)   Involuntary release of urine; may be classified as to cause of the incontinence: functional, urge, stress, or overflow.

urinary tract infection (UTI)   The presence of bacteria in the urethra, bladder, or kidney, with or without symptoms. More common in women than in men, any UTI in a man is considered complicated. May progress to sepsis if untreated.

vascular dementia   A type of dementia caused by multiple small and/or large brain infarcts or a small strategically placed stroke and is characterized by abrupt onset, focal neurological findings, low-density areas, and/or presence of multiple strokes in CT or MRI scans.

visceral pain   Pain relating to activation of the autonomic nervous system, distention of hollow viscera, or the poorly understood mechanisms associated with hypoxia.

xerosis   Abnormal dryness of the skin.

xerostomia   Dryness in the mouth associated with decreased saliva production.

Zollinger-Ellison syndrome   A triad of symptoms including gastric hypersecretion, peptic ulceration, and hypergastrinemia as a result of a gastrin-producing tumor of the pancreas or the duodenal wall.

INDEX

The letter *f* indicates a figure appears on that page. The letter *t* indicates content appears in a table or box.